Behavior Problems of the Dog and Cat

To Susan, my perfect life partner, our fabulous children, Joanna, Mitchell, and Jordan, and my parents, who made it all possible. And, thanks to Pepper (our Havanese), for being Pepper.

Gary Landsberg

To my amazing husband and daughter for their sacrifices in order for me to complete this text. Also, to Gary Landsberg, an icon in behavioral medicine, without whose mentorship this would not have been possible.

Lisa Radosta

To my much-loved wife, Susan, and our incredible children, Nadia, Rebecca, and David. What greater inspiration could any person need or want in the pursuit of happiness and excellence.

Lowell Ackerman

Behavior Problems of the Dog and Cat

FOURTH EDITION

Gary Landsberg
DVM, MRCVS, DACVB, DECAWBM
Richmond Hill, Ontario, Canada

Lisa Radosta
DVM, DACVB
Florida Veterinary Behavior Service, Florida, USA

Lowell Ackerman
DVM, DACVD, MBA, MPA, CVA, MRCVS
Westborough, MA, USA

ELSEVIER

Elsevier
3251 Riverport Lane
St. Louis, Missouri 63043

BEHAVIOR PROBLEMS OF THE DOG AND CAT, FOURTH EDITION   ISBN: 978-0-702-08214-6

Copyright © 2024, by Elsevier Inc. All Rights Reserved.

Senior Content Strategist: Jennifer Catando
Senior Content Development Specialist: Akanksha Marwah
Senior Content Development Manager: Somodatta Choudhury
Publishing Services Manager: Deepthi Unni
Senior Project Manager: Umarani Natarajan
Design Direction: Bridget Hoette

Printed in India

Last digit is the print number: 9   8   7   6   5   4   3   2

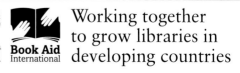

Contents

Preface

Not that long ago, animal behavior was considered an interesting diversion for veterinarians, but little emphasis was placed on this discipline in veterinary school curricula or continuing education for practitioners. Now, there is a general awakening in the veterinary profession as practitioners realize the importance of this subject to their clients, the emotional and physical well-being of their patients, the level and quality of veterinary care we provide, and the success of their practices. Attention to behavioral signs and problems is an essential part of veterinary medicine since behavioral signs and changes are often the first or only signs of underlying health problems. But behavior also plays a critical role in the relationship between the pet and its owners. The behavior, or anticipated behavior, of the pet is often the most important consideration influencing its adoption, while the pet's behavior can also lead to the dissolution of the bond between the pet and the family. Unacceptable behavior is one of the more common reasons for the abandonment and euthanasia of dogs and cats. North American statistics suggest that more pets are euthanized for behavioral reasons than for all medical reasons combined. This should be enough of an incentive for veterinary teams to incorporate behavioral evaluations and counseling into everyday practice.

Because of the importance of the human–animal bond in successful family relationships, in this edition we have chosen to refer to caretakers as "pet parents" rather than owners. Pet parent is not a legally recognized term, but it does connote a desirable status of pets within families, and recognizes the time, money, and emotionality in companion animals that mirrors the parenting of children.[1] In fact, over 75% of pet owners consider pets as members of the family, and seeing pets as part of the family and pet anthropomorphism improves human health and well-being.[2] Pet parenting often means very different things to different people in different circumstances, and yet for the purposes of this book, we believe it helps acknowledge the important role pets play within families, which is often critical in recognizing and resolving behavioral issues.

Throughout this book, you might also encounter other terms that might seem novel in our attempt to clarify concepts that have become embedded (sometimes incorrectly) in the lexicon of veterinary practice. The term "inappropriate elimination" has been commonly used for elimination in undesirable locations. However, it is clear that it is not the process of elimination that is inappropriate, but rather that the location of elimination is undesirable to the pet parent. It is actually more than just semantics, and we hope we will prove our point throughout the book as to why some terms are often a better fit for describing situations, rationalizing their causes, and contemplating management options.

The emotional state of an animal can drive or contribute to undesirable and pathologic behaviors. The most significant emotional states are fear, anxiety, stress, conflict and panic (FASCP). While each has its own definition and distinguishing characteristics, they are also difficult to distinguish entirely from each other by gross observation of the animal. In addition the specific tests needed to distinguish one emotion from another such as positron emission tomography (PET scan) are not readily available to veterinary healthcare teams. For those reasons, throughout this book, you will see FASCP used in many cases when referring to emotional drivers or contributing factors to behavior problems, rather than trying to distinguish which factor may be most appropriate in a given circumstance.

This book is designed to provide the veterinary team with the tools needed to help pet parents with concerns they might have about their pets' behavior. Most importantly, it helps veterinary teams incorporate behavior consultations into their practices in a meaningful way, and utilizes hospital paraprofessional and front-office staff to their optimum. Not only does the book introduce topics such as learning theory and behavior modification techniques, but it also covers the diagnostic and therapeutic options for the successful management of behavior problems. In this edition, we not only address neuropharmacology and psychoactive drug activity but also examine important training techniques and nutritional intervention, and explore alternative forms of therapy. Another important focus of this edition is the importance that regular veterinary care plays in maintaining not only the physical health but also the behavior and welfare of the pet. To this end, new content is devoted to making veterinary visits a positive experience and detail how best to manage pets that are fearful, anxious, or stressed. In addition, we have expanded our focus on the role that behavior plays in the health of pets and the importance of behavioral monitoring.

Throughout the text, we have included cases to illustrate real-life clinical situations. To clarify the principles best and because of veterinary–client confidentiality, our case examples are composite representatives of our caseload rather than actual clinical cases.

To be successful in managing behavior problems, veterinary teams must offer more help than just training. The proper approach to behavioral problems does not differ significantly from any other medical discipline. One needs to evaluate patient history carefully, perform a thorough physical examination, formulate differential diagnoses, conduct diagnostic testing, initiate treatment options, and monitor the patient's responses. Let this book serve as your guide.

We have also included with this book a number of the forms and handouts that we utilize in our consultations with clients. These forms and handouts, as well as our resource list and drug dosing table, have been reproduced online so that they can be printed for use in your practice. We hope that you find them valuable support aids for offering behavioral services.

To all of those who took the time to share with us their thoughts, ideas, and observations on behavior, we wholeheartedly thank you.

In this edition, we have incorporated the work of additional veterinary contributors from around the world to bring new content and new insight to our behavioral text. We thank these contributors not only for lending their expertise to the book but also for the major contributions made to offer practical and useful solutions for veterinary teams. This book is not just an academic exercise – our intention was to create a hands-on resource that can be applied by veterinary teams in everyday circumstances.

We would like to dedicate this edition to the animals whose lives will be transformed by this information and to those veterinary healthcare team members who seek to improve the welfare of animals.

We would also like to acknowledge the efforts of Dr. Wayne Hunthausen, who was our co-editor on the first three editions of this textbook. We thank him for his efforts and contributions to this project, which started before behavior was even a recognized veterinary specialty. We would also like to welcome Dr. Lisa Radosta, our newest editor and co-author, and recognize her for her invaluable contributions and expertise to this new edition. Over the last quarter century, this project has evolved from a simple behavior guide for veterinary practitioners to the current multiauthored fully referenced fourth edition for the entire veterinary team.

We would like to conclude with a very special thank you to our families who saw less of us, to our pets that received less attention and fewer walks, and to our partners and associates in practice who covered for us. You have no idea how much we appreciate your patience and value the support that you gave us while we worked on this project.

Gary Landsberg
Lowell Ackerman
Lisa Radosta

References

1. Volsche S. Pet parenting in the United States: investigating an evolutionary puzzle. *Evol Psychol.* 2021;19(3). doi: 10.117.
2. McConnell AR, Lloyd EP, Buchanan TM. Animals as friends: social psychological implications of human–pet relationships. In: Hojjat M, Moyer A, eds. *Psychology of Friendship.* Oxford, UK: Oxford University Press; 2017:157-174.

Editors

Gary Landsberg, DVM, MRCVS, DACVB, DECAWBM
Veterinary Behaviorist Consulting Services
Head, Fear Free Research, Scientific Director, CanCog Inc.

Lisa Radosta, DVM, DACVB
Medical Director, Florida Veterinary Behavior Service
www.flvetbehavior.com, www.drlisaradosta.com

Lowell Ackerman, DVM, DACVD, MBA, MPA, CVA, MRCVS
Global Consultant, Author, and Lecturer
www.lowellackerman.com

About the editors

Gary Landsberg, DVM, MRCVS, DACVB, DECAWBM
Dr. Gary Landsberg is a board-certified veterinary behaviorist, an international lecturer, and an author and editor of several veterinary books, chapters, and articles, including over 25 behavior research studies and publications. Dr. Landsberg is a graduate of the Ontario Veterinary College and a Diplomate of both the American College of Veterinary Behaviorists (ACVB) and the European College of Animal Welfare and Behavioural Medicine. He has practiced veterinary medicine at his veterinary hospital in the greater Toronto area for over 40 years and as a veterinary behaviorist for over 25 years. Throughout his career, he has appeared extensively in the media, including hosting both a call-in TV and radio show, sharing his knowledge and expertise in the field of pet health and behavior. Dr. Landsberg is currently working as a scientific advisor and consultant with Fear Free as head of research, on their advisory board and speakers, bureau, and as the veterinary scientific director for CanCog Inc. Dr. Landsberg is honored to have received awards for his contributions to the field of veterinary behavior and the veterinary profession from the American Animal Hospital Association and from the Western Veterinary Conference.

Lisa Radosta, DVM, DACVB
Dr. Radosta is a board-certified veterinary behaviorist, owner of Florida Veterinary Behavior Service, a clinical behavior specialty practice, and co-owner of Dog Nerds, an online educational resource for pet parents whose dogs have behavior disorders.

She is a sought-after speaker nationally and internationally and has contributed to over 50 media outlets, including print, radio, podcast, and national television. She is a contributing author to numerous textbooks and co-author of *From Fearful to Fear Free: A Positive Program to Free Your Dog from Anxiety, Fears, and Phobias*. During her residency, she was awarded the American College of Veterinary Behaviorist's research award for two years in a row and has authored or co-authored research papers in veterinary behavior and general veterinary journals.

Outside of behavioral medicine, Dr. Radosta can be found spending time with her eternally supportive husband, Scott, extraordinary daughter, Isabella, and her pets, Maverick and Chewie.

Lowell Ackerman, DVM, DACVD, MBA, MPA, CVA, MRCVS
Dr. Lowell Ackerman is a board-certified veterinary specialist, an award-winning author, an international lecturer, and a renowned expert in veterinary practice management. He is a graduate of the Ontario Veterinary College and a Diplomate of the American College of Veterinary Dermatology. In addition to his veterinary credentials, Dr. Ackerman holds a master's degree in public administration from Harvard University, a master's degree in business administration from the University of Phoenix, a certificate in veterinary practice administration from Purdue University, and is a certified valuation analyst (CVA) through the National Association of Certified Valuators and Analysts (NACVA). Currently, he is an independent consultant, author, and lecturer, on the Fear Free Advisory Board, and is a Fear Free certified professional. Over his career, Dr. Ackerman has been engaged in specialty practice, primary care practice, academia, consulting, industry, and teaching. He is the author or co-author of several books, including *Five-Minute Veterinary Practice Management Consult, Pet-Specific Care, for the Veterinary Team Proactive Pet Parenting, The Genetic Connection, Almost Perfect Pets, Problem Free Pets, Owner's Guide to Dog Health,* and *Cat Health Encyclopedia*.

Contributors

Lowell Ackerman, DVM, DACVD, MBA, MPA, CVA, MRCVS
Global Consultant, Author, and Lecturer
www.lowellackerman.com

Melissa Bain, DVM, DACVB (Behavior), MS, DACAW (Welfare)
Professor, Clinical Animal Behavior and Director, Professional Student Clinical Education
University of California-Davis School of Veterinary Medicine
https://www.vetmed.ucdavis.edu/faculty/melissa-bain

Kelly C. Ballantyne, DVM, DACVB
Insight Animal Behavior Services, PC
insightfulanimals.com

Leticia M. S. Dantas, MS, PhD, DVM, DACVB
Clinical Assistant Professor, UGA Behavioral Medicine Service
University of Georgia Veterinary Teaching Hospital

Ashley Elzerman, DVM, DACVB
Zoetis, Inc

Ariel Fagen, DVM, DACVB
Medical Director, Owner, Veterinary Behavior Center
www.vetbehaviorcenter.com

Alison Gerken, DVM
San Francisco SPCA

Lore I. Haug, DVM, MS, DACVB, CABC
Texas Veterinary Behavior Services
www.texasvetbehavior.com

Gary Landsberg, DVM, MRCVS, DACVB, DECAWBM
Veterinary Behaviorist Consulting Services
Head, Fear Free Research, Scientific Director, CanCog Inc.

Amy Learn, VMD, DACVB
Chief of Clinical Behavioral Medicine at the Animal Behavior Wellness Center
www.abwellnesscenter.com

Emily D. Levine, DVM, DACVB
Animal Behavior Clinic of New Jersey, Author of Doggy Dos and Don'ts
www.animalbehaviorclinicnj.com

Ellen Lindell, DVM, DACVB
Veterinary Behavior Consultations
www.lindellvetbehavior.com

Daniel S. Mills, BVSc, PhD, CBiol, FRSB, FHEA, CCAB, Dip ECAWBM (BM), FRCVS, RCVS, EBVS
European Veterinary Specialist in Behavioral Medicine
Professor, School of Life Sciences, University of Lincoln

Megan Petroff, DVM

Amy L. Pike, DVM, DACVB
Owner, Animal Behavior Wellness Center
abwellnesscenter.com

Lisa Radosta, DVM, DACVB
Owner, Florida Veterinary Behavior Service
www.flvetbehavior.com www.drlisaradosta.com

Meaghan Ropski, DVM
Friendship Hospital for Animals

Carlo Siracusa, DVM, PhD, DACVB, DECAWBM
Associate Professor of Clinical Animal Behavior and Welfare
School of Veterinary Medicine, University of Pennsylvania

Karen Sueda, DVM, DACVB
VCA West Los Angeles Animal Hospital
https://vcahospitals.com/west-los-angeles/specialty/team/karen-sueda

Wailani Sung, MS, PhD, DVM, DACVB
Director of Behavior and Welfare Programs, San Francisco SPCA
https://www.sfspca.org/behavior-training/behavior-consultations/

Andrea Y. Tu, DVM
Medical Director, Behavior Vets

Valarie V. Tynes, DVM, DACVB, DACAW
SPCA of Texas

CHAPTER 1

Behavioral medicine and the general practitioner

Amy Learn, VMD, DACVB

Behavior problems in companion animals are some of the most underdiagnosed and undertreated problems that veterinarians, pet parents, and pets struggle with. It is estimated that 13–17% of dogs have separation-related disorders and as many as 49% have noise fears or phobias.[1,2] They are a leading cause of relinquishment and degradation of the human–animal bond. Up to 20% of dogs in the United States, and over one-third of dogs in a UK study were relinquished to animal shelters for behavioral reasons.[3–6] A recent Danish study found that nearly 25% of dog and cat relinquishments were related to behavior problems.[7] While these statistics may seem discouraging, in fact, they create a significant, valuable, and critical opportunity for veterinarians because we are in the unique position of having repeated contact with most pet parents during the early, formative months of the pet's life, when pet parents are most likely to be receptive to information about preventive behavioral health. Behavioral health affects quality of life, welfare, and overall health.[8,9] Continued stress (see Chapter 7) results in chronic exposure to neurotransmitters and neurohormones which can lead to detrimental changes in heart, gastrointestinal, dermatologic, and immune functions. Veterinarians play an essential role in determining if the pet's behavior is normal or pathologic, and if diseases of other body systems (e.g., dermatologic, gastrointestinal, orthopedic, endocrine) are contributing to behavioral clinical signs. Providing behavioral care requires the education of each member of the "behavior team" in species-typical behavior, learning principles, behavioral diagnostics, and behavior case management. It is then the team's responsibility to evaluate the pet and provide education to the pet parent.

Behavioral medicine is the standard of care

The importance of companion animal behavior and welfare is recognized worldwide. Veterinary behavior is a veterinary medical specialty in North America (American College of Veterinary Behaviorists or ACVB), Europe (European College of Animal Welfare and Behavioural Medicine – Behavioral Medicine), Australia (Fellow of the Australian College of Veterinary Scientists in Animal Behaviour), and Latin American Veterinary College of Animal Welfare and Behavioural Medicine (CLEVE) as well as national veterinary specialty recognition such as AVEPA Spain (www.avepa.org). Veterinary technicians/nurses in North America can achieve specialty certification in behavioral medicine from the Academy of Veterinary Behavior Technicians (Box 1.1). Because behavior and welfare are so intimately related, behavioral medicine is, in fact, a subspecialty of the European College of Animal Welfare and Behavioural Medicine. Veterinarians often guide pet parents in the assessment of an individual pet's quality of life, yet veterinarians may not be familiar with the five freedoms of animal welfare (Figure 1.1, see also

Chapter 7). The five freedoms are regarded as the minimum elements necessary for the assessment of quality of life and the foundation on which other assessments have been built. Many commonly reported behavior problems can be attributed at least in part to a deficit in one or more of the five freedoms. By applying the five freedoms of animal welfare to companion animals, behavioral and physical well-being could be dramatically improved.

Behavioral training for the veterinary care team

While the behavioral education of new veterinarians is critical, it is still insufficient at a majority of veterinary colleges in North America and around the world. Veterinary practices must actively seek continuing education opportunities and resources for the veterinary healthcare team. Specialty training is available for those wishing to seek board certification as a veterinary behaviorist or veterinary behavioral technician (Box 1.2). However, veterinarians and technicians need not become specialists to be able to competently offer behavioral medicine services. Veterinary behavior and technician interest groups include the American Veterinary Society of Animal Behavior (AVSAB), Society of Veterinary Behavioral Technicians, the British Veterinary Behavior Association, European Society of Veterinary Clinical Ethology, the Australian Veterinary Behaviour Interest Group, and national/country behavior associations such as the STVV in Switzerland (www.stvv.ch), GTVMT in Germany (www.gtvmt.de), and Zoopsy in France (www.zoopsy.com) (see Box 1.1 and Appendix A). In addition, professional groups devoted to behavioral medicine are present on social media platforms. Continuing education can be found online and in person at most veterinary conferences. Online programs focused on behavioral education can provide an excellent behavioral foundation as well as plentiful pet parent resources. Textbooks and journals complete the resources available to the team. All members of the veterinary healthcare team should have access to online and printed resources, which can also be used for pet parent education (see Appendices A and C).

Providing behavioral services in practice

Like most disorders in veterinary medicine, treatments for behavioral disorders are most likely to result in positive outcomes when preventive, proactive, and prompt treatment is utilized as opposed to delayed or reactive treatment. A strong preventive behavioral care program and consistent monitoring of behavioral health at every veterinary visit will ensure that problems will be discovered early or ideally, prevented from occurring entirely. Behavioral screening at each visit is a critical component of complete veterinary care,

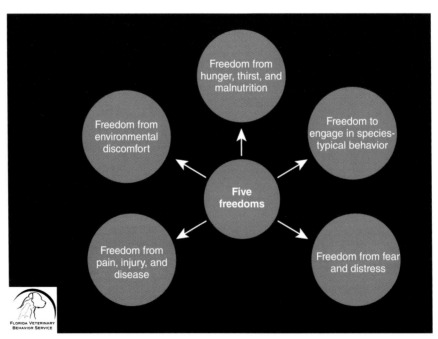

Figure 1.1 Five freedoms of animal welfare.

Box 1.2 Veterinary and technician behavior certification bodies

American College of Veterinary Behaviorists	dacvb.org
European College of Animal Welfare and Behavioural Medicine	ecawbm.org
Australian and New Zealand College of Veterinary Scientists	https://www.anzcvs.org.au/chapters/veterinary+behaviour+chapter/
Academy of Veterinary Behavioral Technicians	avbt.net
Latin American Veterinary College of Animal Welfare and Behavioural Medicine	cvlbamc.com/

not only to assess emotional wellness but also because behavioral signs are very often the first signs of systemic disease. Pet parents do not always share information about behavioral problems with their veterinarians. It is, therefore, important to regularly query pet parents specifically about behavior problems during any scheduled examination or technician/nurse visit. The most efficient way to collect information is to use a short questionnaire which can be filled out online before the appointment, or printed to be filled out at the time of the appointment (See Appendix C for list of online forms).

Veterinary care centers should offer a wide range of behavior services depending on their interest, time, availability of space, and support staff. These are highlighted in Table 1.1. Each has the effect of promoting healthy behavior in pets,

and positions the veterinary healthcare team as leaders in superior pet health care.

Services can be divided into: (1) preventive; (2) early recognition and detection of behavioral clinical signs; (3) immediate intervention for emerging behavior issues; and (4) treating behavioral disorders. Successful implementation is best achieved using a team approach, utilizing each team member's unique skills and knowledge base. Veterinarians should completely evaluate the patient for systemic disease, make a diagnosis when possible and, when necessary, create a medical treatment plan including neurochemical modulation. Veterinary technicians/nurses can educate the pet parent on management techniques to reduce stress and decrease the frequency of clinical behavioral signs, including providing resources for further learning. Behavior modification can be provided by a technician or the pet parent may be referred to a qualified positive reinforcement dog trainer (see Chapter 10).

Referral to a board-certified veterinary behaviorist can be the difference between euthanasia and relinquishment, and a positive long-term outcome. Referral to a specialist should not be considered a last resort. Puppies and kittens or any behavior case that is referred early in the progression of the problem will generally have a shorter course of treatment and more positive outcomes. The cost of an evaluation and treatment by a veterinary behaviorist is generally less than the cost of referral to other specialties for chronic diseases. For short-term treatment, the cost is comparable. Consider referral when (1) the patient has been resistant to reasonable first-line treatments; (2) the pet parent is considering euthanizing or relinquishing the pet; (3) the pet is at risk of self-injury; (4) the pet is aggressive toward people in the home and there are high-risk individuals in the home (e.g., children and elderly); (5) the pet is aggressive and the pet

Table 1.1 Behavioral services

Approach	Considerations
Preventive counseling	At each puppy and kitten visit, counsel pet parents as to normal pet behavior, socialization, and how to train desirable behaviors and prevent undesirable ones. Provide handouts, resource lists, and web links
Puppy and kitten socialization classes	Encourage pet parents to participate in puppy and kitten classes starting at 10 weeks of age to enhance early socialization and provide training advice. Consider offering these services in your practice
Behavior management products	Recommend, demonstrate, and supply control devices (head halters, body harnesses, muzzle training), enrichment toys, pet monitors and devices to manage undesirable behaviors, such as odor counteractants
Basic counseling – early intervention	As puppies and kittens mature, undesirable behaviors may develop. Early identification and timely advice can lead to successful resolution of many problems before they escalate into more difficult, serious, or refractory cases
Behavioral screening	Screening for any change in behavior at every visit is essential for early identification of signs that there might be an emerging behavior problem, or even the initial signs of a medical problem
Behavioral consultations	Every pet with a behavior problem must have a full diagnostic workup since medical problems could be a cause or contributing factor, and behavioral signs could be the first or only signs of illness
	The behavioral diagnosis primarily focuses on history taking. A movie clip, interactive discussion with the pet parent, observation of the pet and pet parent, and a written history can all be utilized
	Make sure you feel competent in performing behavior counseling for advanced problems, such as aggression or phobic behaviors. If in doubt, refer
Pharmacological management	Drug therapy (as well as natural complementary products) can be an important component or a necessity for the successful resolution of many behavior problems, such as when there is an inordinate amount of fear, anxiety, arousal, impulsivity, or behavioral pathology. A therapeutic response trial might also be warranted

parent is noncompliant and putting others at risk; (6) the veterinarian has exhausted their knowledge base or is out of their comfort zone; and (7) puppies and kittens that are moderately to severely affected. Referral can be made in person to a board-certified veterinary behaviorist or a doctor–doctor telemedicine consult can be scheduled. Just like with any other specialty, referral services are widespread. If this resource is not locally available, many veterinary behaviorists will consult by phone or virtual meeting with the primary care veterinarian.

Preventive behavioral medicine, not just for puppies and kittens

Preventive behavioral medicine does not only apply to puppies and kittens although clearly the effects of early behavioral counseling are significant. Puppies with at least one veterinary visit and cats whose pet parents were provided with behavioral educational material were at a lower rate of relinquishment.[10,11] During the socialization period, between 3 and 12 weeks (dogs) and 2 and 7 weeks (cats), puppies and kittens are the most malleable and able to develop appropriate social behavior to their own species as well as other species and to acclimate to new locations, objects, and sensory experiences (see Chapters 2 and 5). Puppies enrolled in puppy class have fewer behavior problems later in life including reduced risk of fear and aggression to unfamiliar dogs and people, fear of noises and crates, and touch sensitivity, are more obedient, and are no more likely than dogs that did not attend puppy classes to contract canine parvovirus.[2,12–17]

For these reasons, puppies should be enrolled in puppy classes after their first vaccination and deworming. (See Chapter 5 for a complete discussion of preventive behavioral medicine.)

New puppy and kitten pet parents usually have a plethora of questions. In order to cover all topics, educate the pet parent, and care for the pet physically, the veterinary care team needs to be organized. Puppy and kitten packs should include: (1) a checklist of behavior topics; (2) initial training recommendations; (3) puppy and kitten class recommendations; and (4) resources including web sites, videos, handouts, book recommendations, and brochures (see Appendix A).

However, preventive behavioral medicine can provide substantial benefits at all stages of a pet's life. This is especially true considering that at least in one study, the mean age of presentation for evaluation at a behavior specialty practice was approximately 3.5 years.[18,19] Noise aversion may present later (median 6.5 years) especially if there is concurrent musculoskeletal pain, and dogs may show changes in cognitive function as early as 7 years of age, but are more commonly seen at 11 years and older (see Chapters 8 and 15).[19–21] For cats median age of presentation was 4.5 years, with a median of 1.5 years for ingestive behaviors (e.g., pica), and >9 years for excessive vocalization[22,23] (see Tables 1.2 and 1.3). For these reasons, every visit for every pet should begin with history taking including screening for behavioral clinical signs and concerns (see Forms online listed in Appendix C), as these signs may only be evident at home and not during veterinary evaluation. Visual evaluation of the pet at every visit is essential. This should include their comfort level in the unfamiliar setting of the veterinary office, with handling, interacting with unfamiliar people, and with close proximity to unfamiliar animals. It is beneficial to educate the

Table 1.2 Behavior problems in dogs

Most common problems according to pet parents[1]	Most common problems at referral practices in the United States and Australia[2,3]	Problems leading to increased risk for relinquishment[4]	Problems leading to shelter surrender[5]
Fear/anxiety (includes all fear, anxiety, and phobia)	Aggression to people or other dogs	Aggression to pets or people	Destruction
Aggression	Fear, anxiety, nervous (including noise, situational and separation-related disorders)	Barking	Aggression to people
Jumping	Vocalization	Destructive behavior	Aggression to other pets
Vocalization	Elimination	Elimination	Hyperactive
Noise phobia	Destructive	Excitability/unruliness	Barking
Fear of veterinary visits	Repetitive		Soiling
Coprophagia			
Compulsive			
Elimination			
Separation-related disorders			

[1]Dinwoodie I, Dwyer B, Zottola V, et al. Demographics and comorbidity of behavior problems in dogs, *J Vet Behav.* 2019;32:62-71.
[2]Col R, Day C, Phillips CJC. An epidemiological analysis of dog behavior problems presented to an Australian behavior clinic, with associated risk factors, *J Vet Behav.* 2016;15:1-11.
[3]Siracusa C, Provoost L, Reisner IR. Dog- and owner-related risk factors for consideration of euthanasia or rehoming before a referral behavioral consultation and for euthanizing or rehoming the dog after the consultation. *J Vet Behav.* 2017;22:46-569.
[4]Patronek GJ, Glickman LT, McCabe GP. Risk factors for relinquishment of dogs to an animal shelter. *J Am Vet Med Assoc.* 1996;209:572.
[5]Diesel G, David Brodbelt D, Pfeiffer DU. Characteristics of relinquished dogs and their owners at 14 rehoming centers in the United Kingdom. *J Appl Anim Welf Sci.* 2010;13(1):15-30.

TABLE 1.3 Behavior problems in cats

Most common problems seen by pet parents[1,2]	Most common problems at referral practices (Australia[3])	Problems leading to increased risk for relinquishment[4]	Problems leading to shelter surrender[5]
House soiling	House soiling	Elimination	Aggression between cats
Aggression to animals	Aggression	Scratching	House soiling
Aggression to people	Anxious/fearful	Aggression	Aggression to people
Destructiveness	Vocalization		Fearful
Unruly behavior	Pica – oral compulsive		Problems with dogs
Fear	Self-grooming		Other behaviors
	Attention seeking		Scratching

[1]Bamberger M, Houpt KA. Signalment factors, comorbidity, and trends in behavior diagnoses in cats: 736 cases (1991–2001). *J Am Vet Med Assoc.* 2006;229(10):1602-1606.
[2]Kass PH, Scarlett JM. Behavioral reasons for relinquishment of dogs and cats to 12 shelters. *J Appl Anim Welf Sci.* 2000;3:93-106.
[3]Wassink-van der Schot AA, Day C, Morton JM, et al. Risk factors for behavior problems in cats presented to an Australian companion animal behavior clinic. *J Vet Behav.* 2016;14:34-40.
[4]Patronek GJ, Glickman LT, Beck AM, et al. Risk factors for relinquishment of cats to an animal shelter. *J Am Vet Med Assoc.* 1996;209:582.
[5]Casey RA, Vandenbussche S, Bradshaw JWS, et al. Reasons for relinquishment and return of domestic cats (*Felis Silvestris Catus*) to rescue shelters in the UK. *Anthrozoös.* 2009;22(4):347-358.

pet parent about reinforcement-based learning and the behavior and body language of their pet, and create a plan to improve future reactions; in fact, puppy behaviors including signs of anxiety observed during veterinary visits tend to persist into adulthood.[24]

The focus of preventive counseling should be on those behaviors that most commonly lead to relinquishment in dogs and cats including (1) aggression; (2) disobedience; (3) destruction, hyperactivity, and noisiness; (4) house soiling; (5) fearfulness and escape; and (6) unfriendliness[25] (see Tables 1.2 and 1.3). Because undesirable elimination is a risk factor for relinquishment in both dogs and cats, veterinarians should be proactive in providing advice on house training and litterbox training at all stages of life. In one study, 31% of people surrendering dogs believed that it was helpful to shove the dog's nose in the excrement and another 11.4% were uncertain, demonstrating that almost half of pet parents surveyed in the study did not understand proper house training techniques.[26] There are many opinions available to pet parents whether they are talking to their neighbors, reading a blog, or scrolling through social media. As veterinarians, it is important to be aware of the most current science-based techniques so that we can inform pet parents of the most appropriate ways to teach and interact with their pets.

Pharmacy and over-the-counter products

In decades past, veterinary care centers were one-stop shops for everything that the pet parent needed for a lifetime of pet care. Now, pet parents may purchase their dog's food from one web site and their cat's medications from an online pharmacy across the country. Even in these conditions, the veterinary care center can still be the source of good, accurate information and immediate purchase of certain products. A list of enrichment tools and over-the-counter therapies which may help to alleviate clinical signs should be available, either as a handout or as a resource or directed

link on the clinic's web site (see Appendix A for resources). In addition, pets benefit most when they can receive immediate treatment. For that reason, it is helpful for certain products to be carried at the in-house pharmacy. These might include toys, training devices, pheromone analog diffusers, puzzle or food toys, supplements, essential oil diffusers/sprays, and frequently used medications.

Gonadectomy

Gonadectomy of dogs and cats, before sexual maturity, has been the standard of care in veterinary medicine for generations. Within the last decade, evidence has mounted indicating that for some individuals, gonadectomy at a young age may have deleterious effects on physical and behavioral wellness. However, there is evidence that gonadectomy reduces relinquishment, some unruly behaviors, and sexual behaviors.[18,27–30] To further complicate matters, it may be challenging to separate undesirable, sexual, and pathologic behavior patterns, all which may respond differently to gonadectomy. While the evidence suggests that there may be an ideal age at which to gonadectomize dogs, that age has yet to be elucidated. In cats, there has been even less research conducted on the effects of gonadectomy on behavior.

Behaviors which appear similar (e.g., urination in the house) can have varying etiologies and responses to gonadectomy. In a survey of 122 pet parents of male dogs, gonadectomy reduced excessive sexual behavior toward people and other dogs by over 40%, roaming induced by bitches in heat, aggression to male dogs outside the house, and urination in the home by approximately 60%, and testosterone-related diseases by over 90%; however, mounting of inanimate objects, nonsexual roaming, and urination outside of the house were reduced by 26% or less.[28] Similarly, Hart and Eckstein found that urine marking, mounting, and fighting with other dogs were all reduced significantly or eliminated by neutering in 50–60% of the dogs and roaming reduced in 90% of the dogs.[29] Neilson and Eckstein found that neutering caused a 90% reduction in 40% of dogs with marking and roaming, and 25% with mounting.[30] In contrast, female dogs that underwent early age gonadectomy had a higher likelihood of urinary incontinence and cystitis.[27] In summary, some behaviors which are affected by sex hormones may be decreased significantly by neuter and spay procedures; however, if the behavior is not affected by sex hormones or has other inputs (e.g., environment, learning and wellness), the effect can be minimal and spaying may lead to incontinence requiring medical treatment.

Historically, gonadectomy has been recommended for aggressive behavior; however, there is substantial evidence that it is an ineffective treatment for aggression outside of intact male aggression (see above) and may, in some cases be associated with increased aggression toward certain targets. Hart and Eckstein found that aggressive behavior was eliminated in only 30% of dogs after neutering.[29] Using the C-BARQ (canine behavioral assessment and research questionnaire), out of almost 14,000 pet parents, no association was found between aggression and gonadectomy at any age toward familiar people or dogs; however, dogs gonadectomized between 7 and 12 months were 26% more likely to demonstrate aggression toward strangers compared to intact dogs.[31] In a study of 14 German Shepherds, dogs spayed between 5 and 10 months of age displayed more reactivity than intact females when approached by an unfamiliar person and dog.[32] Similarly, in dogs spayed at less than a year of age, there was a risk of increased aggression toward familiar people, with the greatest risk in puppies that had previously showed some aggression.[33]

Neutering of male cats has been shown to eliminate roaming (95%), spraying (85%), and fighting with other cats (85%).[34] In another study, the likelihood of urine spraying, sexual behaviors, and aggression toward the veterinarian were decreased in cats that were neutered prior to 5.5 months of age compared with cats that were neutered at an older age, while shyness increased in both male and female cats that underwent gonadectomy before 5.5 months of age.[35]

Regarding nonaggressive behavior disorders, the evidence is conflicting. Early age gonadectomy has been reported to increase noise phobia and decrease separation-related disorders, escape behaviors, and elimination when frightened[27] while another study of over 2500 Vizsla dogs found an increased risk of behavioral disorders in dogs neutered before six months of age, and an increased risk of storm phobias regardless of age of gonadectomy.[36] In a study of over 7800 dogs presented to a veterinary behavior clinic, neutered dogs were found to have greater problems with integration into the household, obsessive behavior, attention seeking and grieving, and a slightly lower risk for developing aggression.[18]

Development of behavioral phenotype depends on hereditary, hormonal, environmental, and health inputs. The literature investigating the effects of gonadectomy reflects the diversity in etiology. Based on so many varying findings, veterinarians cannot make blanket statements about what is right for all patients. Spaying and neutering can have behavioral benefits, eliminating some unwanted behaviors that increase the likelihood of relinquishment. On the other hand, it is clear that spaying and neutering, as a treatment, does not eliminate the behavior problems for which pet parents are most likely to seek help (e.g., aggression, noise

phobia, separation-related disorders) and may in some cases increase the likelihood or progression of negative behaviors. A risk-benefit analysis should be done for each patient when considering when to recommend spaying or neutering. This is important because in addition to behavioral consequences, there are often different recommendations made about neutering based on a pet's species, breed, gender, and risks for other medical conditions (developmental orthopedic conditions, certain cancers, female incontinence, etc.).[36,37]

Treatment of behavior disorders

Evaluation, diagnosis, and treatment of behavioral disorders can be very rewarding for the entire veterinary healthcare team. For those who lack training, like any other unknown skill, it can feel challenging. Start slow within the team's comfort level and expand the types of cases that are handled in the clinic as their competency increases. Until the team is fluent in the diagnosis and treatment of behavior disorders, referral is suggested.

The options for referral when diagnosis and treatment of a behavior disorder is beyond the scope of the veterinary care team include board-certified veterinary behaviorists, applied animal behaviorists, and certified dog training professionals. Each one has their own focus and level of training.

Board-certified veterinary behaviorists are veterinarians, certified by ACVB and/or ECAWBM, who have completed a residency in clinical behavioral medicine (three to seven years), have completed all requirements for credentialing, and have passed a board examination. Details on specialty training and the locations of board-certified veterinary behaviorists can be found on the behaviorist college web sites (see Box 1.2). Board-certified veterinary behaviorists are the only specialists in veterinary behavior with the knowledge and ability to evaluate, diagnose, and treat all body systems including prescribing medications and creating behavior modification plans.

Certified applied animal behaviorists must have a postgraduate degree in behavior, as well as sufficient clinical experience to achieve certification from the Animal Behavior Society. When referring to an applied animal behaviorist, coordinated case supervision with the referring veterinarian is essential to rule out systemic and/or physical illness. In addition, unless the applied animal behaviorist is also a veterinarian, they are not trained in psychopharmacology or licensed to diagnose, prescribe, or dispense medications meaning that the attending veterinarian is responsible for medication choices and prescribing.

A skilled, certified positive reinforcement dog training professional can be the difference between a positive and negative outcome in the treatment of behavior cases. Curating a quality list of dog training professionals in your area is essential, but not necessarily easy to do. At the time of this writing, there are no requirements in education or experience associated with the terms "dog trainer" or "behaviorist." Even the term "specialist" can be used as long as the person is not a veterinarian. Therefore, caution and close scrutiny of credentials should be exercised before referral. Also be certain not to confuse trainers, who can be an invaluable resource in helping to implement a training and behavior modification program, with a behaviorist who will fully evaluate the problem and help to determine the prognosis and the best possible management and treatment options for the pet, home, and family.

The team approach to behavioral medicine

The team approach utilizes the strengths, education, and experience of the veterinary healthcare team to provide a full range of behavior services from education to evaluation, diagnostic workups, and treatment. As with any team, a strong team leader or advocate can make the difference between success and failure. A lead technician or nurse is best suited to be the behavior team leader. Team leaders should be given time and financial resources to educate themselves and others. Implementation strategies for behavioral medicine appointments are similar to implementing any new profit center. All members of the team must be educated on the services offered, how to schedule and how to be empathetic to pet parents whose pet has a behavior disorder. For whatever reason, the veterinary healthcare team may feel more comfortable giving out advice for patients with behavior disorders than physical disorders. Just as we want each team member to fully represent their skill-set to help pet parents and their pets, we also want to coach them to stay in their own lane and not make recommendations that are outside of their scope or knowledge.

Client care representatives (client service representatives, client experience representatives, receptionists)

Client care representatives (CCR) are the first and last persons that the client hears and sees. Their influence on how the practice is perceived by the client is immeasurable. Just as the CCR team is trained to direct the wide range of client needs with which they are presented, they should also be trained to do so for those clients who call with questions about their pet that has a behavior problem. CCRs should document the pet parent's concerns, but should avoid giving quick-fix suggestions, advice, or referrals until the veterinarian has assessed the problem. CCRs can schedule an appointment with the veterinarian and direct the call to a technician/nurse for triage and early recommendations (see Appendix A).

Veterinary technicians and nurses

A highly skilled veterinary technician/nurse is essential for the efficient and effective delivery of high-quality veterinary medicine. Practicing behavioral medicine gives veterinary technicians a unique opportunity to have autonomy and play a greater role in the education of pet parents. Technicians/nurses should be trained to recognize fearful, anxious, and stressed body language in cats and dogs (as well as other companion animals that visit the clinic). They should log those observations as a behavioral or emotional record within the medical record. In addition, they can choreograph physical examinations and blood draws to keep the restraint low stress (see Chapter 16).

The technician can take primary responsibility for preselection advice, preventive counseling, puppy and kitten socialization classes, behavior products, management issues for emerging problems, and behavioral screening. If the veterinary care center has sufficient space and a technician or team member has the necessary skills, obedience training and behavior modification could be offered as clinic services. Otherwise, the clinic should identify one or more reputable trainers to whom families can be referred. For behavior problems, the behavioral technician can also play an important role in recommending behavior consultations, by discussing the protocol and scheduling the visit. During the consultation, the technician/nurse can work with the veterinarian in history taking, developing the treatment plan, and helping the pet parent implement techniques, products, and the treatment program. The technician might also provide continued training and support between visits either at home or in the clinic, and should have primary responsibility for case followup to liaise with the veterinarian until the next visit is required (see Table 1.4).

Table 1.4 Roles of trainers, technicians, applied animal behaviorists, and veterinarians in behavior counseling

Trainers, veterinary technicians, and veterinary nurses	Teaching appropriate behavior Puppy classes Dog sport classes Introduction of a new pet to the family Correcting normal but undesirable behavior Techniques and product implementation, for example, clicker training, head halter Work with pet parent to implement program after veterinary diagnosis and consultation Problem screening Management advice until time of assessment by veterinarian **Note** Trainers and veterinary should not recommend medications or make a diagnosis. ***Note*** Veterinary technicians also act as a liaison between the veterinarian and the pet parent.
Certified applied animal behaviorist (CAAB)	Diagnose behavior problems and create behavior modification treatment plans **Note** The CAAB should not be prescribing or recommending medications.
Veterinarian	Diagnosis of physical and primary behavioral problems in animals Prescribing medications for treatment of physical and primary behavioral problems Create behavior modification plans Refer to CAAB Refer to board-certified veterinary behaviorist

Veterinarians

When presented with any change in behavior, the first step is to assess overall wellness. This may include, but is not limited to a physical examination and a baseline workup [CBC, serum chemistry, fT4 (ED), urinalysis, fecal]. The question is not whether it is behavioral or medical. The question to be answered is what influence does systemic or physical disease have on the clinical behavioral signs which are being exhibited. Treatment of behavioral disorders is not secondary to resolution of physical disorders, unless it is clear that the clinical signs are definitely caused by the physical disorder. Stress and anxiety can be alleviated while waiting for the results of diagnostic tests. As discussed previously in this text, if any of the seven criteria above are met, referral to a veterinary behaviorist should be made earlier rather than later. Referral to a dog trainer is appropriate when the pet presents with unruly or obedience-related behaviors, or when the veterinarian has made a diagnosis and formulated a treatment plan. See Chapter 9 for more information on the diagnosis and treatment of behavior disorders.

Dog training professionals

While some practices may have team members who can offer training services in the clinic, most practices will have some need for referral of cases to trainers both for preventive management and training as well as for the implementation of behavioral treatments. Since dog training is an unlicensed and unregulated profession, it can be difficult to determine where to send pet parents. Only refer to science-based, certified positive reinforcement dog training professionals (see Appendix A for more information on dog training certifications). Trainers should have a basic education in psychology and learning principles, utilize humane reinforcement-based methods, and avoid the use of force or confrontation. In fact, the use of confrontational techniques, from yelling "no" to "alpha roll-overs" or "grounding techniques" on aggressive dogs, has been shown to increase aggression in dogs.[38] Devices like prong or shock collars have no place in training.[39] Dogs trained with positive reinforcement alone are likely to show less avoidance, stress, and aggression than dogs trained with positive reinforcement combined with punishment or punishment alone.[15,16] This is true even in the hands of skilled professionals who understand how to use these tools. Training techniques such as shock, choke, and pinch collars present an animal welfare concern and the risk of injury. For all of these reasons, avoid trainers who employ shock, pinch, and choke collars, use alpha rolls, physically handle or advocate dominance or confrontational techniques. On some level, you may be held accountable whether by the pet parent, through an online review or legally for recommendations which are known to depart from the standard of care and endanger the pet. Make referrals wisely. See Chapter 10 for more information about behavioral treatment techniques. See Appendix A for resources to help pet parents find a qualified dog trainer.

Before you make a referral to a dog training professional, interview them regarding their techniques, education, certifications, commitment to ongoing continuing education, and philosophy on the treatment of pets. If there is a board-certified veterinary behaviorist in the area, they may also have recommendations for appropriate trainers. In addition, watch the trainer's classes to ensure that you are comfortable with their approach.

The economics of providing behavioral services

As part of a comprehensive examination appointment, all veterinarians should be performing some behavioral services or they are not truly providing complete patient care, and are economically disadvantaging themselves. Behavior disorders in companion animals tear apart the human–animal bond and contribute to relinquishment. Addressing these problems is the responsibility of the veterinary care team. In addition, it adds flavor to the day of appointments, giving the veterinary team the opportunity to feel the reward of helping patients live more joyful lives, and restoring and strengthening the bond between patient and pet parent.

The addition of any "profit center" to a veterinary practice depends on the service being able to deliver a "profit." The best driver of pet parent expenditures is the strength of the human–animal bond, and those with the strongest bond take their pets to veterinarians more often, are more likely to follow veterinary recommendations (regardless of cost), and are more likely to seek preventive care for their pets.[40,41] When pets are in their homes, they go to the veterinarian's office many times throughout the course of their lives. As is well known, acquiring a new client is much more costly to the practice than nurturing the committed clients who we have. Clients whose pets have behavior problems are some of the most committed clients to the practice. Committed clients leave positive reviews and spread the word about their beloved veterinarian. Maintaining a pet within your veterinary practice, with regular care, for its entire life, is the most economically positive thing you can do for your bottom line.

Historically, the diagnosis and treatment of veterinary behavior problems in companion animals was viewed as taking longer when compared to problems of other body systems. Times have changed. It is now recognized that strategies such as questionnaire forms, modified history taking, evaluation of physical health, pet parent resources, and utilization of support staff together with a sound education and understanding of normal behavior, behavior management, and behavior modification principles can allow the primary care veterinarian to treat moderately complex cases effectively in primary care.

As noted above, the first step is to evaluate the overall physical wellness of the pet. Systemic disease and pain may contribute to as high as 80% of behavior problems referred to board-certified veterinary behaviorists.[42] In order to treat more complex behavioral disorders efficiently, history can be collected in a stepwise fashion with longer appointments being broken up into half-hour appointments. Because physical health is intertwined inseparably with emotional health and the development of behavior disorders, the use of diagnostic tests is just as important as with any other disease process. Technicians/nurses can be used as they would for any other appointment; as an educator for the pet parent and the primary contact person for followup. More severe cases and those within the guidelines mentioned above should be referred to a board-certified veterinary behaviorist.

Even if you never offer in-depth behavioral consultations, it is critical to hospital profits for you to counsel pet parents effectively about preventable problems. Once again, profit in a veterinary hospital is not dependent on a one-time sale of services: lifelong quality care and the ability to deliver services over the long term are always the best business decisions.[40] Potential behavioral profit centers are discussed above and in Table 1.1.

Conclusion

The idea that behavioral medicine cannot be addressed profitably in primary care practice is a misconception. Behavioral medicine is no more complex or time consuming than internal medicine. They are actually very similar. Each visit starts with a wellness check and collection of history. While diagnostic test results are pending, short-term fixes are put in place to eliminate or abate clinical signs. This may include environmental or medical interventions. Some behavior patients might be kept in the hospital until they are well (e.g., separation-related disorders) or until they are stable just as with a diabetic patient. Recheck appointments include further history and repeat wellness checks. They may also include further diagnostics. These appointments can easily be split up and spread out as with any other type of medicine.

The sad truth about pet behavior problems is that too frequently, many end with a terminal solution. Millions of pets are euthanized at shelters alone, with most due to non-medical reasons.[6,43] Behavior problems are a common reason for shelter surrender in dogs and cats, as well as being a common reason for pet parents to seek euthanasia for pets at veterinary clinics. Undesirable behavior, most commonly aggression, was the primary reason for the death of dogs under three years of age at primary care veterinarians in

Table 1.5 The top five reasons for shelter surrender

Dogs	Cats
Housing	Too many animals
Nonaggressive behavior/personality	Housing
Cannot care for animal	Family health/death
Too many animals	Litter/breeder
Caretaker or family health/death	Financial

24PetWatch Owner Surrender and Acquisition Source Analysis. https://network.bestfriends.org/tools-and-information/research/owner-surrender-acquisition-source-analysis. Accessed July 2022.

33.7% of cases in the United Kingdom and 29.7% in Australia (29.7%).[44,45] Since the pet's behavior is one of the principal factors in forging a strong pet–pet parent bond, it is not surprising that undesirable behavior can weaken the bond, leading to a decreased commitment to pet care and an increase in relinquishment. A close veterinary–pet parent relationship can be helpful to reverse this trend. It is clear that with timely and accurate behavioral advice, and setting realistic expectations beginning from the very first puppy and kitten visit, fewer pets will meet premature and untimely deaths, and a significant cause of pet parent loss can be eliminated[46,47] (see Table 1.5).

There are many reasons why veterinarians should be enthusiastic about behavior counseling. In addition to the altruistic reason of improving the lives of pets and pet parents, there are also solid economic reasons for embracing these concepts. Fewer pets will be rejected, abandoned, or destroyed. The benefits are obvious to all: by saving the pet's life and improving the bond between pet parent and pet, the pet parent's commitment to, and level of, pet care should be greatly enhanced.

References

1. Blackwell EJ, Bradshaw JWS, Casey RA. Fear responses to noises in domestic dogs: prevalence, risk factors and co-occurrence with other fear-related behaviour. *Appl Anim Behav Sci.* 2013;145:15–25

2. Dinwoodie IR, Dwyer B, Zottola V, et al. Demographics and comorbidity of behavior problems in dogs. *J Vet Behav.* 2019;32:62–71.

3. Miller DD, Staats SR, Partlo C, et al. Factors associated with the decision to surrender a pet to an animal shelter. *J Am Vet Med Assoc.* 1996;209:738–742.

4. DiGiacomo N, Arluke A, Patronek G. Surrendering pets to shelters: the relinquisher's perspective. *Anthrozoos.* 1998;11;41–51.

5. Kass PH, New Jr JC, Scarlett JM, et al. Understanding animal companion surplus in the United States: relinquishment of non-adoptables to animal shelters for euthanasia. *J Appl Anim Welf Sci.* 2001;4:4:237–248.

6. Protopopova A, Gunter LM. Adoption and relinquishment interventions at the animal shelter: a review. *Anim Welf.* 2017;26:35–48.

7. Jensen JBH, Sandøe P, Nielsen SS. Owner-related reasons matter more than behavioural problems a study of why owners relinquished dogs and cats to a Danish animal shelter from 1996 to 2017. *Animals.* 2020;10(6):1064. https://doi.org/10.3390/ani10061.

8. Berteselli G, Servida F, Dall'Ara P, et al. Evaluation of immunological, stress and behavioural parameters in dogs (*Canis familiaris*) with anxiety-related disorders. In: Mills D, Levine E, Landsberg G, et al., eds. *Current Issues and Research in Veterinary Behavioral Medicine.* West Lafayette, Indiana: Purdue University Press; 2005:18–22.

9. Hart B. Beyond fever: comparative perspectives on sickness behavior In: Breed MD, Moore J, eds. *Encyclopedia of Animal Behavior.* Oxford: Academic Press, 2010:205–221.

10. Gazzano A, Bianchi L, Campa S. The prevention of undesirable behaviors in cats: effectiveness of veterinary behaviorists' advice given to kitten owners. *J Vet Behav.* 2015;10:535–542.

11. Gazzano A, Mariti C, Alvarez S. The prevention of undesirable behaviors in dogs; the effectiveness of veterinary behaviorists; advice given to puppy owners. *J Vet Behav.* 2008;3:125–133.

12. Duxbury MM, Jackson JA, Line SW, et al. Evaluation of association between retention in the home and attendance at puppy socialization classes. *J Am Vet Med Assoc.* 2003;223(1):61–66.

13. Stepita ME, Bain MJ, Kass PH. Frequency of CPV infection in vaccinated puppies that attended puppy socialization classes. *J Am Anim Hosp Assoc.* 2013;49(2):95–100.

14. González-Martínez Á, Martínez MF, Rosado B, et al. Association between

puppy classes and adulthood behavior of the dog. *J Vet Behav.* 2019;32:36–41.

15. Blackwell EJ, Twells C, Seawright A, et al. The relationship between training methods and the occurrence of behavior problems as reported by owners, in a population of domestic dogs. *J Vet Behav.* 2008;3:207–217.

16. Cutler JH, Coe JB, Niel L. Puppy socialization practices of a sample of dog owners from across Canada and the United States. *J Am Vet Med Assoc.* 2017; 251:1415–1423.

17. Casey R, Loftus Be, Bolster C, et al. Human directed aggression in domestic dogs (*Canis familiaris*): occurrence in different contexts and risk factors. *Appl Anim Behav Sci.* 2014;152:52–63.

18. Col R, Day C, Phillips CJC. An epidemiological analysis of dog behavior problems presented to an Australian behavior clinic, with associated risk factors. *J Vet Behav.* 2016;15:1–11.

19. Bamberger M, Houpt KA. Signalment factors, comorbidity, and trends in behavior diagnoses in dogs: 1,644 cases (1991–2001). *J Am Vet Med Assoc.* 2006;229(10):1591–1601.

20. Lopes Fagundes AL, Hewison L, McPeake KJ, et al. Noise sensitivities in dogs: an exploration of signs in dogs with and without musculoskeletal pain using qualitative content analysis. *Front Vet Sci.* 2018;5:17.

21. Landsberg G. Therapeutic agents for the treatment of cognitive dysfunction syndrome in senior dogs. *Prog Neuro-Psycho Biol Psych.* 2005;29(3):471–479.

22. Bamberger M, Houpt KA. Signalment factors, comorbidity, and trends in behavior diagnoses in dogs: 736 cases (1991–2001). *J Am Vet Med Assoc.* 2006;229(10):1602–1606.

23. Wassink-van der Schot AA, Day C, Morton JM, et al. Risk factors for behavior problems in cats presented to an Australian companion animal behavior clinic. *J Vet Behav.* 2016;14:34–40.

24. Godbout M, Frank D. Persistence of puppy behaviors and signs of anxiety during adulthood. *J Vet Behav.* 2011;1(6):92.

25. Coe JB, Young I, Lambert K, et al. A scoping review of published research on the relinquishment of companion animals. *J Appl Anim Welf Sci.* 2014;17(3): 253–273.

26. New JC, Salman MD, King M. Characteristics of shelter-relinquished animals and their owners compared with animals and their owners in U.S. pet-owning households. *J Appl Anim Welf Sci.* 2000;3:179–201.

27. Spain CV, Scarlet JM, Houpt KA. Long-term risks and benefits of early-age gonadectomy in dogs. *J Am Vet Med Assoc.* 2004;224(3):380–387.

28. Maarschalkerweerd RJ, Endenburg N, Kirpensteijn J, et al. Influence of orchiectomy on canine behaviour. *Vet Rec.* 1997;140(24):617–619.

29. Hart BL, Eckstein RA. The role of gonadal hormones in the occurrence of objectionable behaviours in dogs and cats. *Appl Anim Behav Sci.* 1997;52(3–4):331–344.

30. Neilson JA, Eckstein RA, Hart BL. Effects of castration on problem behaivors in male dogs with reference to age and duration of behavior. *J Am Vet Med Assoc.* 1997;211:180–182.

31. Farhoody P, Mallawaarachchi I, Tarwater PM, et al. Aggression toward familiar people, strangers, and conspecifics in gonadectomized and intact dogs. *Front Vet Sci.* 2018;5:18.

32. Kim HH, Yeon SC, Houpt KA, et al. Effects of ovariohysterectomy on reactivity in German Shepherd dogs. *Vet J.* 2006;172(1):154–159.

33. O'Farrell V, Peachey E. Behavioural effects of ovariohysterectomy on bitches. *J Small Anim Pract.* 1990;31:595–598.

34. Hart BL, Barrett RE. Effects of castration on fighting, roaming and urine spraying in adult male cats. *J Am Vet Med Assoc.* 1973;163:290–292.

35. Spain VC, Scarlett JM, Houpt KA. Long-term risks and benefits of early age gonadectomy in cats. *J Am Vet Med Assoc.* 2004;224:372–379.

36. Zink MC, Farhoody P, Elser SE, et al. Evaluation of the risk and age of onset of cancer and behavioral disorders in gonadectomized Vizslas. *J Am Vet Med Assoc.* 2014;244(3):309–319.

37. Oberbauer AM, Belanger JM, Famula TR. A review of the impact of neuter status on expression of inherited conditions in dogs. *Front Vet Sci.* 2019;6:397.

38. Herron ME, Shofer FS, Reisner IR. Survey of the use and outcome of confrontational and non-confrontational training methods in client-owned dogs showing undesired behaviors. *Appl Anim Behav Sci.* 2009; 117(1–2):47–54.

39. China L, Mills DS, Cooper JJ. Efficacy of dog training with and without remote electronic collars vs. a focus on positive reinforcement. *Front Vet Sci.* 2020;7:508.

40. Radosta L. Incorporating behavioral medicine into general practice. *Compend Contin Educ Vet.* 2009;31:258–263.

41. Lue TW, Pantenburg DP, Crawford PM. Impact of the owner-pet and client-veterinary bond on the care that pets receive. *J Am Vet Med Assoc.* 2008;232: 531–536.

42. Mills DS, Demontigny-Bedard I, Gruen M, et al. Pain and problem behavior in cats and dogs. *Animals.* 2020;10(2):318.

43. Diesel G, Brodbelt D, Pfeiffer DU. Characteristics of relinquished dogs and their pet parents at 14 rehoming centers in the United Kingdom. *J Appl Anim Welf Sci.* 2010;13:15–30.

44. Boyd C, Jarvis S, McGreevy PD, et al. Mortality resulting from undesirable behaviours in dogs aged under three years attending primary-care veterinary practices in England. *Anim Welf.* 2018:27:251–262.

45. Yu Y, Wilson B, Masters S, et al. Mortality resulting from undesirable behaviours in dogs aged three years and under attending primary-care veterinary practices in Australia. *Animals.* 2021;11(2):493.

46. Patronek GJ, Glickman LT, Beck AM, et al. Risk factors for relinquishment of dogs to an animal shelter. *J Am Vet Med Assoc.* 1996;209:572–581.

47. Patronek GJ, McCabe GP, Ecker C. Risk factors for relinquishment of cats to an animal shelter. *J Am Vet Med Assoc.* 1996;209:582–588.

Recommended reading

Koch CS. Veterinary behaviorists should be the first, not the last, resort for optimal patient care. *J Am Vet Med Assoc.* 2018;253:1110-1112.

CHAPTER 2

Developmental, social, and, communicative behavior

Ashley Elzerman, DVM, DACVB and Lisa Radosta, DVM, DACVB

Introduction

Adult behaviors are shaped by hereditary predisposition, environmental influences, and learning (most importantly during the socialization period for each species). These factors are interrelated and severe deficits in one area cannot be completely overcome by strengths in other areas. Domestic dogs have shared a close relationship and coevolution with their human companions[1] and there has been intense selection for the development of breeds with certain physical and behavioral characteristics. Meanwhile, domestic cats have relatively recent evolutionary origins. Since cats have persisted in human cultures due to either their hunting abilities or, more recently, because of their value as pets, selective breeding for behavioral or morphological characteristics has not occurred in cats to the extent it has in dogs.

There are many similarities between cats and dogs when it comes to behavioral tendencies. In both dogs and cats, early development that starts in utero affects adult behavior; body language signals are the primary mode of communication with humans increasing or decreasing with familiarity, reinforcement, or punishment; most behavior problems stem from fear, anxiety, stress, conflict panic, or frustration; group living is common, but the social structure is fluid, not linear, and depends on the living conditions; and both species have ancestors to which we can look for guidance on natural behaviors, yet both are distant enough to be distinct species with their own genetic predispositions.

Canine development

Development of behavior begins with the genetic makeup of the individual and environmental effects in utero. After parturition, the effects of the environment and learning continue to affect the development of canine behavior. The periods of development described in dogs include the prenatal period and six postnatal developmental stages: (1) the neonatal stage (birth to 13 days); (2) the transitional stage (13–19 days); (3) the socialization period (19 days until approximately 12 weeks); (4) the juvenile period (12 weeks to sexual maturity); (5) adolescent stage; and the (6) adult stage (from sexual maturity onward).[2] The precise beginning and end of each phase of development vary somewhat from individual to individual, but the progression from one stage to the next is consistent. Within the adult stage is the social maturity stage.

Prenatal development and in utero influences

The influence of the environment on canine behavior comes into play even before birth. While studies in dogs are limited, there are many studies in other species such as humans, rodents, and production animal species to suggest that the in utero environment affects behavioral development. The importance of neurodevelopmental influences on the mental and emotional well-being of humans is a subject of intensive study and studies have shown a link between prenatal stress of the mother and cognitive, behavioral, and emotional problems in infants and children.[3–7] Animal studies have been conducted to further determine the influence of experiential, biological, and genetic factors on the developmental variation in fearfulness and anxiety. In rodents, prenatal stress can cause increased emotionality,[8] upregulation of the hypothalamic–pituitary axis, increased anxiety, and abnormal social behavior in the offspring through adulthood.[9–11] High levels of stress during pregnancy might also lead to changes in reproductive behavior of offspring when they become adults.[12] Similar results have been reported for guinea pigs.[13] Since excessive maternal stress has been shown in other mammalian species to have detrimental effects on offspring, it is likely that this phenomenon occurs in dogs and cats as well. For this reason, excessive stress should be avoided in pregnant bitches and queens. Alternatively, providing for her biological and emotional needs could potentially protect somewhat against emotionality. In addition to the effects of cortisol and other stress neurotransmitters on development, exposure of the fetus to prenatal testosterone primes the central nervous system (organizational effect), so that the male behaviors such as leg lifting begin to emerge with maturation, independent of testosterone levels at the time of onset of the behavior.[14]

Neonatal stage

During the neonatal period, the puppy spends most of its time nursing or sleeping. Puppies have limited motor ability and, up until about 5 days of age, movement is on the belly by paddling and stroking with the limbs. By 6–10 days, the forelimbs are capable of supporting weight and by 11–15 days, the hind limbs can support weight and walking begins.[15] The rooting reflex is present from birth and begins to wane after about 14 days.[16] A slow and sustained pain response to toe pinch is present from birth, but withdrawal and escape from pain do not develop until early in the transition period.[17] Eyes and ear canals are closed at birth and open by 10–14 days, by which time the palpebral reflex to touch and light and the pupillary responses have already developed.[16] Being unable to hear or see, neonatal puppies are effectively shielded from most psychological effects of the environment. Defecation and urination are reflexes that are elicited by the mother's licking and cleaning of the perineal region.[16] Temperature regulation is poor at birth and puppies huddle together. They exhibit intense distress and vocalize if they become cold.[18]

Some degree of stress (e.g., handling, cold temperature, and very brief separation) in the neonatal period may accelerate hair growth, weight gain, and maturation of the nervous system, reduce emotionality later in life, increase problem solving ability and social confidence, decrease reactivity and promote resistance to some diseases.[2] One study showed that puppies that have been exposed to daily handling and sensory stimulation from birth to 5 weeks of age had increased adrenal activity, a more mature electroencephalogram (EEG), performed better and were less aroused in a problem-solving situation, were more attracted to people and had slightly better coordination compared to controls.[19] Similar results were found in a study comparing handled and nonhandled, kennel-raised and home-raised dogs, with the handled puppies calmer, more exploratory, and with a longer latency to vocalize. Environment was a factor in emotional stability as the handled, kennel-raised puppies were better able to cope with the stress of isolation.[20]

Handling sessions from the first days of a puppy's life are, therefore, recommended. They will not only expose the puppy to a mild stress, which likely affects the pituitary–adrenocortical system in a way that helps the puppy cope later on but also facilitate socialization when the puppy gets older. In addition to handling sessions, puppies may be removed from the nest (best while someone else walks the mother) and placed singly on a cool vinyl floor for a brief time (30 seconds) before being put back into the warm nest. Flashing light, noises, and motion have also been used as mild stressors. In a study in which puppies were exposed to a program of extra socialization and sensory stimulus exposure (tactile, auditory, visual, environmental, and social) for the first 6 weeks, 5 days a week for 5–15 minutes per session, at 8 months, puppies receiving the program had significantly better scores than controls for separation-related behavior, generalized anxiety, body sensitivity, and distraction.[21]

Transitional period

Toward the end of the second week, the pup enters the transitional period of its neurological and behavioral development. During this period, the puppy changes from a condition of complete dependence upon its mother to one of increasing independence. The transitional period begins with the opening of the eyes and ears. The auditory evoked startle response usually emerges by 18 days and the puppy may begin to localize sound.[2] The brainstem auditory evoked response also attains the characteristics of the adult at this time.[22] The electroretinogram has the basic features of the adult pattern by 15 days and is fully developed by 28 days.[23] Visual and auditory orientation develops around 25 days.[17]

During the transitional period, the puppy begins to walk rather than crawl, both forward and backward. Puppies begin to exhibit voluntary control of elimination, but the mother continues to clean the puppies' excreta until the puppies are at least 3 weeks of age.[24,25] By the end of the transition period, the puppy begins to interact with other individuals and many of the patterns of adult social behavior appear. Play mouthing by puppies begins to develop and by 4 weeks of age; nipping can be quite painful[24] (see Figure 2.1).

Gently exposing the pups to all types of stimuli for short periods each day during this period is likely to enhance

physical and mental development. A simple exercise involves allowing pups to crawl or walk on surfaces with differing textures and temperatures. Objects of varying shapes can be moved in front of them to promote visual acuity and motor skills. Providing a variety of noise stimuli at low decibels and varied frequencies may facilitate auditory development. Whistles, rattles, music, recordings of environmental noises, and the human voice can be used to provide a variety of auditory stimulation. The individual puppy may have varying degrees of tolerance for any given stimulation level, so the puppy's reaction to the stimulation should be monitored and the intensity decreased if the puppy startles to the noise.

Socialization period

The onset and early stages of the socialization period are closely associated with the maturation and myelination of the spinal cord.[26] All sensory systems are functional during this period and learning capacity increases. Although the puppy can support itself and becomes more mobile during the transitional period, normal sitting and standing develop by about 28 days.[24] Teeth erupt and the pups begin taking semisolid food for the first time at about 3 weeks of age, and all of the deciduous teeth have erupted by about 6 weeks of age. A puppy's performance in classical and operant conditioning exercises reaches adult levels at about 4–5 weeks, but vision and brainwave function do not reach adult levels until about 8 weeks.[17] By 4 weeks of age, puppies tend to sleep in groups and at 6 weeks, they start to sleep alone. Weaning begins around 4–6 weeks of age. At first, the puppy begins to show an interest in food, and the mother will begin to decrease nursing contact and may regurgitate food for her young.[24,25] This is a good time to begin offering appropriate food to puppies. Most puppies are weaned and eating solid foods by about 60 days of age (approximately 8.5 weeks old). By 8–9 weeks of age, puppies are attracted by the odors of urine and feces to specific areas for elimination and begin to avoid soiling their den (sleeping quarters)[27] (see Figure 2.2).

The socialization period is one of rapid development of social behavior patterns.[25] At the beginning of this period, the puppy begins to respond to the sight or sound of persons or other animals at a distance. The behavior of puppies during the early socialization period is characterized by a willingness to approach novel objects and, in particular, moving stimuli. Investigative behavior becomes apparent, and puppies begin exploring away from the nest area. Social following and early signs of affiliative behavior emerge. During this time, there is a marked increase in interaction with littermates, the mother, and the environment. Distance decreasing and increasing social signaling begin to appear. Gradually, as the mother spends less time with the puppies, the interaction and relationship between littermates strengthens. The socialization period is an important time for puppy development and its importance cannot be overemphasized. The puppy's experiences and social familiarity during this period establish the general pattern that will affect almost every social or situational response in later life. In fact, dogs that are not well socialized as puppies are more likely to show fearful behavior, aggression to unfamiliar people, and aggression to dogs. By the end of this period, the puppy has formed patterns of response to the situations to which it has

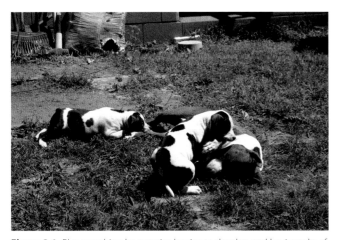

Figure 2.1 Play mouthing by puppies begins to develop and by 4 weeks of age. *(Attribution: Lisa Radosta.)*

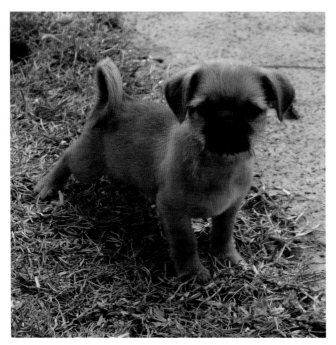

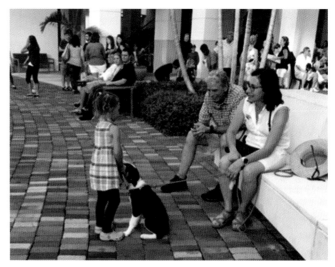

Figure 2.3 Socialization should include most things they are likely to encounter later in life including interactions with children. *(Attribution: Lisa Radosta.)*

Figure 2.2 By 8–9 weeks of age, puppies are attracted by the odors of urine and feces to specific areas for elimination and begin to avoid soiling their den. *(Attribution: Lisa Radosta.)*

been exposed and to those with which it has had a lack of exposure. If the puppy does not encounter a situation, place, person, object, or thing during this period, they are more likely to be fearful when encountering those stimuli again in the future. For well-socialized pups, this should include most things they are likely to encounter later in life[25] (see Figure 2.3). While the exact termination of the socialization period most likely varies within individuals or within breeds, there is a finite end that for most is likely between 12 and 16 weeks of age. Beyond that time, socialization does not occur. It is this finite end which makes it imperative that puppies be exposed to every possible situation in a positive way during this time. If a puppy older than 14–16 weeks presents with fear, aggression, or anxiety, the veterinarian should consider this patient to have a behavior problem, which will continue or get worse with time if not treated.

During the socialization period, the puppy develops attachments to its own and to other species that it encounters socially. It is also a time when the puppy begins to become familiar with and make attachments to places (localization or site attachment) and adapts to many of the stimuli to which it has been exposed (habituation). Since this is the time when social relationships are established, it is essential that puppies have contact with a wide variety of future social partners (people and animals), with positive consequences. Since the socialization period is also a time of increased sensitivity to psychological stress, the type of exposure is critical. Excessive stimuli, whether positive or negative, before 7 weeks of age can increase neurochemical arousal, which may lead to increased or abnormal attachments.[28] For this reason, exposures before 7 weeks of age should be varied and positive, but not overwhelming for the pup. In other words, exposure if positive is necessary for normal development. Negative, chaotic, or overexposure, where the puppy is overwhelmed or develops a conditioned arousal (see Chapter 10) to a certain

stimulus, can be negative. This underlines the importance of proper socialization as opposed to general exposure.

The sensitivity necessary to facilitate the formation of social relationships also seems to make the puppy vulnerable to psychological trauma. Fear postures begin to emerge at about 8 weeks of age,[25] and by 12 weeks, sociability begins to decrease, and the undersocialized puppy may become increasingly fearful of novel situations and people.[2] Startle reactions to sound and sudden movement become much more pronounced. With time, the puppies learn to discriminate between stimuli associated with dangerous situations and those that are insignificant. Frequent gentle handling has been found to be important for kittens in order to decrease the fear response shown to humans, and the same is probably true for puppies.[29] Compared to puppies raised indoors in the breeder's home, puppies raised in outdoor kennels showed greater submissive behavior, greater risk of fear aggression, and were less able to cope with novel situations.[30,31]

During the socialization period, social play and exploration become increasingly important[17] (see Figure 2.4). Play between puppies not only aids in physical development but also provides practice in the development of appropriate adult behaviors, including communication, predation, and sexual relationships. Pups that have the opportunity to interact with other dogs also learn from them by observation. Although solitary play does occur, most play is social, with biting, barking, chasing, pouncing, and mounting being the most frequent components.

It appears that extreme behavior can develop in pups during this period. In a pilot study, puppies were observed during their routine veterinary visit. Each puppy was observed while free in the room, during the physical examination and after the examination, and the preliminary findings suggest that there was a set of extreme behaviors displayed by 10% of the puppies in this study. These "extreme" puppies displayed active avoidance, flattened ear position, excessive motor activity, less exploration, lip licking, panting, and extremes of locomotion (increased activity or prolonged inactivity).[32] When reevaluated 12 months later, the signs of anxiety noted

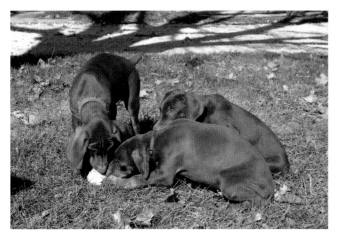

Figure 2.4 During the socialization period, social play and exploration become increasingly important. *(Attribution: Lisa Radosta.)*

in these dogs were highly correlated with the data collected during puppyhood, indicating persistence of these "extreme" behaviors into adulthood.[33] This study underscores the concept that behaviors present in puppyhood can and often do get worse with time.

Juvenile period

The juvenile period extends from the end of the socialization period to sexual maturity. By 12 weeks of age, basic learning capacities appear to be fully developed. While object and environmental exploration increase during this period, it is also a time of increasing. The speed of learning begins to slow by about 4 months, perhaps because previous learning begins to interfere with new learning.[16] By 4–6 months, males begin to show greater attraction to females showing signs of estrus.[24] While not documented in the literature, it is suspected that between 4 and 11 months of age one or more periods in which fear has a greater likelihood of developing and altering adult behavior than at other times in the puppy's development. Structured exposure to environmental stimuli during this period can have behavioral benefits later in life.[28] Therefore even though the socialization period has ended, continued meaningful, positive interactions with environmental stimuli should be recommended.

Adolescent period

The adolescent period starts with puberty and ends with attainment of social maturity, which is around 2–3 years of age.[24a] Different breeds and individuals within those breeds may come into social maturity at different times. Dogs become increasingly more independent at this stage, and cute puppy behaviors might be less tolerated by pet parents of the adolescent dog. Prevention and management of behaviors that are not under the pet parent's control will keep the dog from learning unwanted behaviors. Physical and mental exercise for the dog is essential to making this stage more enjoyable. Training problems and behavior disorders are likely to become more pronounced during this stage of development. For example, dogs might start barking at strangers entering the home or become territorial during adolescence (see Tables 2.1 and 2.2).

Table 2.1 Dog developmental periods

Developmental period	Age
Neonatal stage	Birth to 13 days
Transitional	13–19 days
Socialization	19 days–12 weeks
Juvenile	12 weeks to sexual maturity
Adolescent	9 months–3 years
Adult	3 years onward

*Stages will vary slightly depending on the individual.

Table 2.2 Dog developmental characteristics as they relate to age

Age	Developmental characteristics	Developmental period
6–10 days	Forelimbs can support weight	Neonatal
11–15 days	Walking begins	Neonatal Transitional
14 days	Rooting reflex wanes	Transitional
10–14 days	Eyes and ear canals open Palpebral reflex and pupillary response developed	Neonatal Transitional
18 days	Auditory evoked startle response Brainstem auditory evoked response = adult	Transitional
15–28 days	ERG fully develops	Transitional Socialization
19 days	Voluntary control of elimination Adult social behavior begins to develop	Transitional
21 days	Teeth erupt Begins to eat solid food	Socialization
25 days	Visual and auditory orientation	Socialization
28 days	Play mouthing develops Normal sitting and standing Teeth erupt Sleep in groups Weaning begins	Socialization
28–35 days	Performance in classical and operant conditioning exercises reaches adult levels	Socialization
42 days	All teeth erupted Begin to sleep alone	Socialization
54 days	Fear postures emerge	Socialization
56–60 days	Weaning usually complete	Socialization
56–63 days	Elimination areas emerge Avoid soiling in den	Socialization
8 weeks	First fear period	Socialization
12 weeks	Sociability decreases	Socialization
16 weeks	Speed of learning decreases	Juvenile
6–8 months	Second "fear period(s)"	Juvenile

Canine social behavior and communication

Social behavior comprises all interactions among members of the same species. To understand the biology of a domestic species, one should be familiar with both the behavior of the wild ancestor and the modifications that occurred during the domestication process.

Dogs are not wolves

Domestic dogs are a product of human domestication of wild gray wolves (*Canis lupus*) 15,000 years ago.[34] Wolves that possessed the characteristics necessary to live and work with humans were selected for domestication, most likely because they were good scavengers, protectors, and companions (see Box 2.1).

Domesticated dogs differ from wolves substantially in many ways. Through domestication, dogs have altered preferences for social interactions often preferring humans to dogs and petting from humans to food. Another difference between dogs and wolves exists in the repertoire of vocal signals, which is more extensive in dogs and may have evolved as a means of intraspecific communication among dogs, and between dogs and humans.[35] Also, dogs seem to be able to react to human visual cues in a different manner than wolves.[35,36] Dogs and wolves also vary in their affiliative behavior with people. From a very young age, dogs seek human eye contact – something not seen in wolves, even hand-raised ones.[35]

Neoteny, also called juvenilization, is the delaying or slowing of physiological development. This tends to result in pedomorphosis, which is the retention of juvenile features in adult dogs, which is a result of domestication, further underscoring the differences between wolves and dogs. Traits present in wolf pups but not in adult wolves, such as engagement in play, seeking physical contact, desire to be social and interact, barking, pawing, and nuzzling, have been retained in adult dogs but not in adult wolves. While the DNA sequence in dogs and wolves is similar, it is not identical. The forces of domestication have affected the expression of the domestic dog's genes (i.e., epigenetics) to cause changes including the size and shape of the head, frequency of heat cycles, social structure, visual and auditory communication, response of the hypothalamic–pituitary axis to stressors, levels of oxytocin and oxytocin signaling,[37,38] digestive enzymes (e.g., carbohydrate digestion),[39] frequency and context of vocalizations, and behavior patterns (i.e., domestication syndrome).

In contrast to wild wolves, studies of both urban and suburban feral dogs have also demonstrated that they do not live in packs nor do they breed cooperatively.[40] Instead, they live in small, loosely coherent groups of two to six unrelated dogs.[40] Upon the loss of members of the group, the number regenerates through the addition of abandoned or escaped pets. The range occupied by a group of dogs is less than 0.1 sq. mile (0.25 sq. km) in urban areas where there are many food sources, but no high concentration of food in one specific place. In these urban areas, dogs tend to be territorial; that is, they defend their territory against other dogs that might try to intrude and attempt to raise the puppies alone. As a result, pups born to stray dogs seldom survive to adulthood and rarely account for growth or regeneration of a pack. Predatory behavior is poorly developed in dogs compared to wolves and depends on the degree of neotenization of a breed. Dogs are predominantly scavengers, and when they hunt, they do not hunt in a cooperative way.

Scientific findings overwhelmingly show that dogs are not wolves in a different type of fur coat. Therefore, any comparison between wolves and dogs should be made with great care.

Dominance

A discussion of canine communication and social behavior would not be complete without the mention of "dominance." Studies evaluating this concept have concluded that the theory that canine social groups are organized by a dominance hierarchy "is a human projection that needs replacing."[41] The term "dominant" as it is defined in ethology describes the comparison of two individuals within a social group or dyad, not a character trait which is universally displayed in all situations. That is to say that a dog that is dominant and shows that by growling when another dog approaches her bone, may then in the same day or even a couple of minutes later be on the receiving end of the growling as another dog holds a toy that she wants. Dogs modify their behavior to avoid conflict and retain resources no matter where they are and with whom they are interacting.

It is undeniable that dominance hierarchies exist in animal societies. Depending on the species being studied, the most dominant animal may be the most or least aggressive.[42,43] It is a misconception to assume that the top of the hierarchy is achieved by the most aggressive animal. In dogs, the most aggressive individual is most likely to be the most uncertain dog in the interaction.[44] In addition, the concept that a dog is constantly driven to strive for a higher rank is unsubstantiated in the literature. The strongest evidence for aggression between dogs in the same household comes from two areas: fear, anxiety, stress, conflict, and panic (FASCP) and resource holding potential (RHP). RHP can be understood as the traits possessed by an individual which affect ability to win a competitive contest over a limited resource.[45] RHP may be a factor in aggression between dogs in the same household, as some resources such as the attention from the pet parent are considered by the dogs as scarce or limited.

Box 2.1 Characteristics in dogs which differ from wolves

- *C. familiaris*
- More extensive vocal repertoire
- More innate reaction to human visual cues
- Seek out eye contact with humans
- Retain juvenile features such as play, barking, and nuzzling
- Diverse genetically driven features
- More frequent heat cycles
- Unstructured social structure more dependent on RHP than dominance hierarchy
- More diverse visual and auditory communication
- Different levels of oxytocin and genetically driven oxytocin signaling
- Enzymes for carbohydrate digestion
- Do not form family "packs" or groups

Canine social groups

As stated above, dogs form social groups with rules for interaction based on RHP, self-defense, and maintenance of homeostasis by avoidance of fear, anxiety, stress, conflict, and panic (FASCP), with individuals giving way to each other based on their history of interaction (previous experience) and individual motivations. The dog world is not fair and equitable, as a general rule. Therefore, it is not uncommon to find social asymmetries between dogs living together in a household, where one dog is more competent in controlling resources and social interactions. Pet parents who try to equalize these asymmetries can, therefore, alter what otherwise might be a healthy social relationship between dogs. Further complicating matters is the wide diversity in physical and behavioral traits between breeds, which may compromise an individual dog's ability to communicate.

Canine communication

Dogs communicate with each other using body postures, facial expressions, physical interactions, and vocalization as appeasement to avoid confrontations. These are ritualized much like a waltz or the movements of a highly trained dressage horse. They are clear from one dog to another as long as both dogs have all their senses intact and process social interactions normally. Most ritualized behaviors are intended to avoid aggression and injury to either party.

Therefore, when humans use physical techniques (e.g., pinning, alpha rolls, and grabbing the collar) or verbal corrections, this is not the visual, olfactory, pheromonal, and vocal "language" with which dogs communicate. Instead, the dog reacts to the person's actions and emotional state.[46,47] As you might feel if your family member suddenly tossed you to the ground and held you down, dogs show signs of fear, anxiety, stress, conflict, panic and aggression during these interactions. They are not natural and, in any language, human or dog, are rude and combative. It should not be surprising, therefore, that studies have demonstrated that positive training, consistency, and rule structure led to significantly higher levels of obedience, fewer behavior problems, and lower levels of aggression and avoidance behaviors, while punishment led to significantly higher training problems, lower obedience scores, and an increase in avoidance behaviors and aggression toward unfamiliar people and dogs.[48-50] An in-depth review of the effects of using aversive training techniques found that aversive training methods have undesirable, unintended outcomes and there was no evidence to suggest that aversive training methods are more effective than reward-based methods.[50] Confrontational techniques, such as hitting, growling, alpha rolls, or even yelling "no," do nothing to encourage desirable behavior and, in fact, can lead to aggression, especially in dogs that are already aggressive to people.[51] Relationships with dogs should not be based on an ill-conceived concept of trying to achieve a dominant status. Instead, the pet parent should focus on effectively communicating what they want the dog to learn by consistently and predictably rewarding those behaviors that are desirable while ignoring or preventing those that are undesirable. See Chapter 10 for a more detailed discussion of training techniques and learning theory.

Canine senses and their role in communication

Vision

Dogs have several unique visual characteristics. The unique characteristics of the dog's eye make dogs better able to hunt small, fast-moving animals that are active in dim light.[52]

Because of the diversity of the species, sporting huge differences in skull shape and length, there are also differences in the neurons in the area centralis of the retina (involved in visual acuity) that contribute to the differences in vision between breeds.[53] Visual acuity, a measure of the sharpness of vision, is eight times worse in dogs when compared to humans, leaving dogs less likely than humans to be able to distinguish fine details at a distance. Dogs can see colors in the blue–violet and the yellow–green ranges, (i.e., dichromatic vision)[54] with cones comprising 20% of the central portion of the retina[55] and colors outside of this spectrum likely are seen as shades of gray. Dogs can distinguish colors under natural lighting conditions well enough to be successful in discrimination tests.[56] Brightness discrimination (ability to distinguish between shades of gray) is partially dependent on visual acuity and is about two times worse in dogs than in humans, varying between breeds.[57]

Dogs have good vision in dim light because of the wealth of rods in the central area of the retina when compared to humans, who have predominantly cones,[52] and the unique tapetum lucidum in the back of the eye, which reflects light back onto the retina a second time. In dogs, after exposure to bright light (e.g., flash), rhodopsin (a photopigment) takes over an hour to completely regenerate, which could explain why some dogs do not respond well to bright lights.[59-61] This could be a factor in the way that dogs respond to lightning, flash photography, and the bright light necessary for an ocular examination. This apparent loss of some of the elements of vision may be frightening to dogs. As explained in more detail in Chapter 10, any antecedent can be paired with any event. This may cause dogs to avoid situations where they have previously experienced a flash of light. A dog's total binocular field of vision varies with the different skull and facial features of the dog, but is generally about 240 degrees, which is about 60 to 70 degrees greater than a human's, enabling dogs to visualize the horizon more completely.[52]

Hearing

Dogs can hear higher pitched sounds (up to 45,000 Hz)[62a] compared to humans (20,000 Hz). They can hear sounds between −5 and −15 dB (0 dB is the softest sound that can be heard by a human). The sensitivity to sounds and ability to hear higher frequencies may contribute to storm and noise phobia. Dogs can localize the source of a noise by moving their pinnae. They are able to maximize sound capture and localize sounds by moving their pinnae and tilting their heads.[62b]

Olfaction

Dogs are 10,000 to 100,000 times better than humans at recognizing a scent in the environment, having between 220 million and 2 billion neurons in the olfactory epithelium (humans have 2 to 5 million).[63,64] It is no wonder then that dogs are used daily for search and rescue, bomb detection, cancer detection, and hypoglycemia alerts. The olfactory system is intimately linked to the limbic system (emotional system in the brain). The processing of the information from this part of the environment is like no other, triggering cascades of neurotransmitters involved in the physiologic actions related to emotions. This partially explains the strong emotional reactions that dogs have to the scents such as those of the pet parent, those associated with the veterinary clinic, and those of conspecifics.

There is controversy in the literature regarding whether this extraordinary talent in dogs is an indicator of their use of scent to a greater degree in their daily life or if through domestication while the ability to detect scent in small amounts remains, the usefulness to the domestic dog has diminished. Dogs have been shown to use this over their visual senses when light is adequate as well as when it is poor.[65] However, it is accepted that dogs use their sense of smell in food selection.[66]

Taste

Dogs have taste buds similar to human's taste buds, but there are fewer of them, and there are differences in types and distribution. Dogs have about 1700 taste buds compared to humans who have approximately 9000. Dogs can perceive six types of tastes: sweet, sour, salty, bitter, umami (savoriness), and water.[67–69] Interestingly, the taste buds which detect bitter tasting foods are mainly distributed at the back of the tongue, so a quick lick or gulping could entirely bypass those taste receptors. Dogs like any other animal can develop a taste preference or taste aversion to almost any substance. Their sense of taste is already functional at birth. Aside from taste, palatability is largely based on smell, temperature, and texture. Dogs prefer sweet-tasting foods to bitter and salty foods. Preferences develop in puppyhood and may be congenital.[70]

Touch

Dogs have sensory nerves across their body surface, just as people do, and touch is as important to dogs as it is to humans. In fact, touch may be one of the first senses developed in dogs, and dams start nuzzling and licking puppies soon after birth. The skin has receptors to sense touch, pressure, pain, body movement and position, temperature, vibration, and chemical stimulation. Touch receptors are located at the base of every hair, and especially the vibrissae which can also sense air flow. Touch can be calming, arousing, or aversive, depending on the type and circumstance. The presumption that all dogs or even most dogs appreciate petting is false. Just as we have preferences for physical interaction such as hugging, especially from strangers, dogs have preferences regarding petting. Dogs may not enjoy petting because they have a hereditary predisposition toward this behavior, they are painful, uncomfortable or pruritic and/or they are fearful because of previous interactions, or they simply do not enjoy it. Pet parents should understand that it may not be their fault at all, nor must any trauma have occurred for their dog to dislike petting. Pet parents very commonly are not aware of subtle signs of FASCP such as averting the gaze, lip licking,

or stress yawning. Unfortunately, the lack of knowledge of canine body language can lead to miscommunications and even aggression. Dogs can be conditioned to appreciate and enjoy touch. Any time that a patient presents with an intolerance of touch, pain, pruritus, and/or discomfort should always be considered a factor until proven otherwise.

Communication concepts and body language signals

Dogs use auditory, visual, olfactory, and tactile signals to communicate with members of their social group and others. In order for pet parents to understand their dogs, which in turn allows them to better assess their health and well-being, they must understand the meaning of individual canine body language signals. Social communication involves the effective and efficient exchange of clear information between individuals. The information is transferred from one individual to another when an individual (emitter) sends a signal that may modify another individual's behavior (receptor). Signals carry information that the individual wants to convey as well as information about the internal state of the signaler.

As discussed above, the communication system utilized by dogs is efficient and effective if both the sender and the recipient have normal behavior patterns because many signals are highly ritualized and preserved genetically, becoming part of the normal behavior repertoire of dogs with a specific meaning in dog–dog communication. Body language signals when understood by the recipient (e.g., other dogs) will then influence the recipient's behavior. They are used as a means of communication primarily to avoid conflict and resolve challenges over resources without injury to either party and first and foremost are an expression of FASCP and frustration. Individual postures can indicate a wide range of emotions and needs including fear, anxiety, conflict, aggression, play, happiness, or appeasement among other things. Compound messages exist being made up of more than one body language signal originating from several body parts including the ears, musculature, eyes tail, and mouth (see Figure 2.5). Some body language displays can be interpreted differently depending on the accompanying individual body language signals and the context. As discussed above, *Canis familiaris* is the most diverse species on earth. While the specific characteristics for which they were bred endear them to us and pet parents, they do not always facilitate peaceful communication. The conformation, coat color, and coat length of the dog may limit or enhance that individual's ability to display a certain body language signal and for the intended recipient to receive an accurate message. This can contribute to FASCP and aggression in the sender and recipient dog.

As with petting noted above, body language signals while innate, can be learned, punished (decreased), or reinforced (increased). For example, consider the dog that enters the veterinary clinic for a routine physical examination. When the technician/nurse approaches the dog, the dog averts his gaze and licks his lips, indicating that he is fearful, anxious, stressed, or conflicted and that he wants space from the technician. The technician approaches, talking sweetly, unaware that the dog's the signals (see Figure 2.6). The discrete body language signals

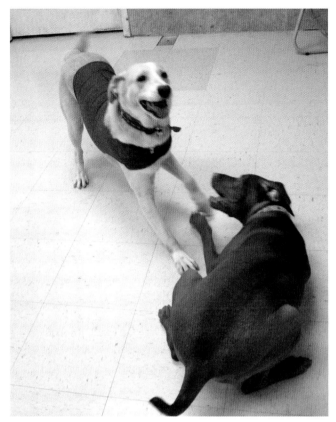

Figure 2.5 Compound messages are made up of more than one body language signal originating from several body parts including the ears, musculature, eyes, tail, and mouth. Play postures are a common example of compound messages. *(Attribution: Lisa Radosta.)*

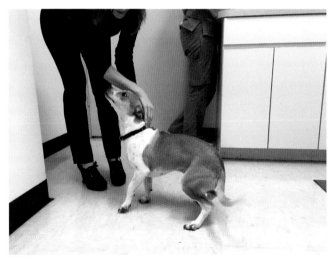

Figure 2.6 This dog is showing several signs of conflict. He willingly approached the person petting him; however, when petted, he displayed distance increasing signals including lip lick, ears back, tail down, and lowered body posture. *(Attribution: Lisa Radosta.)*

of avert gaze and lip lick have been punished, reducing the likelihood that they will be displayed in the future in that situation (see Chapter 10). With enough repetition, lip licking and averting the gaze in this situation will likely be abandoned as a tool for communication. However, the dog's motivation (FASCP) has not been appropriately addressed. In other

words, the dog still needs to communicate, however, the most benign signal exhibited was not effective in producing the desired outcome—more distance from the veterinary technician. The need for communication on the dog's part will often in this situation lead to more prominent signals such as growling, barking, or biting to repel the stimulus of which it is afraid. This is a common example of the evolution of aggression in the veterinary clinic inadvertently contributed to by the veterinary healthcare team. Think of canine body language signals as requests. Your job is to figure out the dog's "ask." Does the dog want you to approach? Move away? Play? Learning another species' language is complicated, but with study and practice, it is possible to better understand the intentions and emotions of our canine patients.

As with the assessment of any aspect of a patient's health and welfare, the assessment of body language requires the consideration of several factors: (1) the signal being emitted; (2) the context in which it occurs; and (3) the relationship between the emitter and the recipient. For body posture and facial expression resources, see Appendix A.

Vocalizations (Vocal communication)

Dogs bark, groan, growl, grunt, howl, moan, scream, whine, whimper to communicate indicating distress, alarm, care seeking, territorial threat, defense, contentment, solicitation of play, group communication, greeting, or pain, among other things.[71,72] The production of vocal signals depends on the size and anatomy specific to that individual dog and is influenced by breed. In addition, domestication by humans as in every other aspect of the life of dogs has influenced the tone and purpose of certain dog vocalizations. Vocalization of any kind can also be used in situations of conflict or frustration.

Whining/whimpering

Whimpers and whines are high pitched and often indicate a need for attention, greeting, or distress.[73] At birth, puppies are capable of whining to attract attention from the dam. As already discussed here and further in Chapter 10, vocalizations can be reinforced or punished. Pet parents may respond immediately to pets that whine, reinforcing that behavior.

Growling

The structure of growls in dogs and wolves are identical and both use growls during conflict and displays of aggression although that is where the similarities end. Adult wolves do not growl in play as dogs do, further demonstrating the effect of domestication and neoteny on dogs.[74] In general, a growl should be regarded as a response to something that the dog sees as a threat. When a dog growls, it is best to step away and reassess the situation before proceeding. When growls are ignored by the pet parent, veterinarian, or any recipient, the vocalization is effectively punished. This, as noted above, can cause the dog to escalate to more obvious (severe) aggressive displays.

Barking

Barking is a puppylike behavior in wolves, which is rare in adult wolves except perhaps in situations of conflict and as a warning. In dogs, barking is a well-developed vocalization present in a wide range of contexts, including excitement, play, attention seeking, or whenever the dog wants to raise awareness of a change in the environment. Barks can have different tones which may have originated to indicate characteristics of the sender and which might indicate size or intention.[75] Barks can classified by acoustic features (frequency, roughness/noisiness, and rhythmicity)[76] and function.[74] Variation in the aspects of the bark are most likely at least in part a function of that dog's specific anatomy, which is affected of course by their breed.

Body postures (Visual communication)

Body language postures can be classified in many ways depending on the discipline. Ethologists may characterize them as offensive or defensive and distance increasing or distance decreasing (see Table 2.3). Most often in veterinary medicine, they will be classified as relaxed, fearful, anxious, stressed, conflicted, and aggressive. Familiarity with the different terms, while not essential, is interesting and allows for a deeper understanding of the dog's intention. In this text, we will most often characterize body language as relaxed or FASCP; however, distance increasing or decreasing may be used.

A tense or stiff body posture (e.g., muscles tense and body still) indicates neurochemical arousal (activation of the sympathetic nervous system [SNS] – see Figure 2.7). Activation of the SNS is fairly nonspecific, becoming activated when the dog is excited, fearful, stressed, anxious, conflicted, or frustrated. That is to say that arousal can occur with almost any emotional state. The resultant body posture may be intended to signal a positive (play) or negative (aggression) interaction. A tense body posture should cause the recipient (pet parent, dog, or veterinary team member) to stop and assess the situation, considering context, additional body language and conformation.

A dog can shift its weight forward, down, or back, whether the dog is standing, sitting, or lying down. Weight shifted away from the stimulus or toward the ground generally

Table 2.3 Common dog body language postures, their meaning, and appropriate recipient action

Body Posture	Meaning	Recipient action
Tense or stiff musculature	Activation of the SNS system	Stop, assess the situation, other body language postures, and context before proceeding. Decrease social pressure by moving away.
Piloerection	Activation of the SNS system	Stop, assess the situation, other body language postures, and context before proceeding. Decrease social pressure by moving away.
Mounting	Sexual (less likely in gonadectomized dogs) Displacement (FASCP)	Redirect the dog to a more appropriate or calming behavior.
Paw lift	Anticipation associated with positive or negative consequences	Stop, assess the situation, other body language postures, and context before proceeding.
Play bow	Play solicitation	If appropriate for context, initiate, or continue with play.
Step back/step away	Distance increasing, FASCP	Decrease social pressure by moving away.
Shake off	An arousing (positive or negative) interaction has ended	Wait for the dog to recover. Observe for the next body language signal before proceeding.
Tail wagging	Willingness to interact associated with positive or negative emotional states	Stop, assess the situation, other body language postures, and context before proceeding.
Tail down	FASCP If tucked, severe FASCP	Stop, assess the situation, other body language postures, and context before proceeding.
Tail curled tightly over back or well above back	SNS arousal	Stop, assess the situation, other body language postures, and context before proceeding.
Head down	FASCP	Stop, assess the situation, other body language postures, and context before proceeding.
Avert gaze	Distance increasing signal	Decrease social pressure by moving away.
Ears back	Distance increasing signal Solicitation	Stop, assess the situation, other body language postures, and context before proceeding.
Dilated pupils	SNS arousal	Stop, assess the situation, other body language postures, and context before proceeding.
Lip lick	Distance increasing signal	Stop, assess the situation, other body language postures, and context before proceeding. Decrease social pressure by moving away.

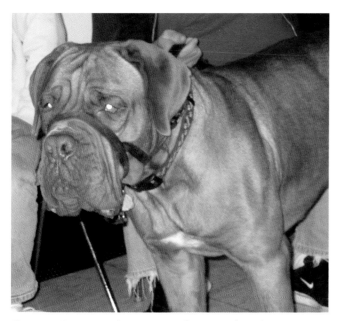

Figure 2.7 Tense musculature is a sign of SNS arousal. *(Attribution: Lisa Radosta.)*

indicates a decreased interest in interacting with the stimulus (e.g., fear, anxiety, conflict, and stress), while weight shifted forward indicates an interest in interaction (e.g., play, excitement, predation, and aggression) although not necessarily a positive one. Dogs with weight shifted away or down should cause the recipient to decrease stress by backing away or removing the stimulus. Dogs with body weight shifted forward should cause the recipient to assess the situation based on context, conformation, and additional body language.

Piloerection, indicating SNS activation, can be associated with many emotional states and could result in friendly or unfriendly interactions. As with other body language signals, piloerection should cause the recipient to pause and assess the situation (see Figure 2.8).

Mounting can be sexual; however, in gonadectomized dogs, it is most often a displacement or conflict behavior indicating a level of excitement and uncertainty, not a desire to dominate the mountee. The observer should try to redirect the dog calmly to another behavior which is inconsistent with mounting (see Figure 2.9).

Lifting of one of the front paws is an indication of anticipation of either an action on the dog's part or an action on the part of something in the environment. It may indicate excitement that a treat will be tossed, or an intention to lunge and bite. As with many other signals, a paw lift should cause the recipient to stop and assess the situation considering context, additional body language, and conformation (see Figure 2.10).

The play bow (rump in the air, front legs lowered to ground) is a play solicitation. The play bow can also be seen in other situations such as aggression in which the dog's movement is restricted. It is a combination of moving forward and an intention to jump backward. While the play bow is almost always associated with play, it can be associated with other emotional states. Action on the observer's

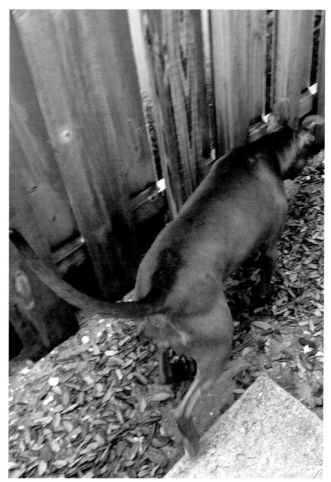

Figure 2.8 Piloerection indicates SNS activation and can be associated with many emotional states and could result in friendly or unfriendly interactions. *(Attribution: Lisa Radosta.)*

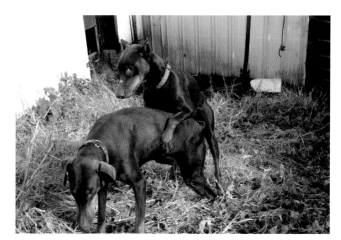

Figure 2.9 In gonadectomized dogs, mounting is most often a displacement or conflict behavior indicating a level of excitement and uncertainty, not a desire to dominate the mountee. *(Attribution: Lisa Radosta.)*

part should be based on other body language signals and context (see Figure 2.11).

A step back or step away is an indication that the dog is requesting more space from the stimulus. It may be preceded by an avert gaze (see below). As with any body posture

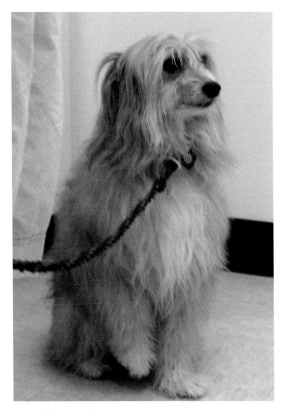

Figure 2.10 This dog is lifting one paw in anticipation of the technician's approach for a physical examination. Lifting of one of the front paws may indicate almost any emotional state associated with anticipation. *(Attribution: Lisa Radosta.)*

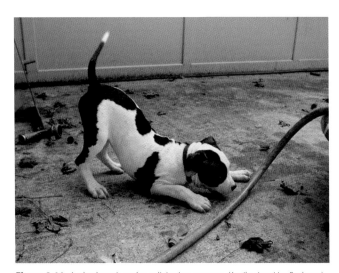

Figure 2.11 A play bow is a play solicitation posture. *(Attribution: Lisa Radosta.)*

in which weight shifted back or down, with the exception of the play bow, the dog should be given space.

The shake-off, where the dog rotates the body side to side (similar to what is displayed after a bath), indicates that the preceding incident was exciting or arousing. This is often displayed during play when a particular dog needs a break or after a physical examination has been completed. The observer should wait for the dog to recover and approach when he is ready.

Tail

The tail may be the most misunderstood part of the dog's body. As a matter of fact, a wagging tail is inaccurately interpreted by most pet parents as a sign of friendly interaction when it actually signals neurochemical arousal and a willingness to interact. As above, neurochemical arousal can be associated with FASCP, happiness, or aggression. Another consideration is the amplitude and intensity of the tail wag. A slow wagging tail generally indicates uncertainty while a very fast wagging tail or a stiff tail with just the tip wagging indicates high arousal. A large amplitude wag where the caudal part of the body moves with the tail indicates excited and friendly interaction. A wagging tail should be interpreted in the context of the situation along with other body signals exhibited.

When the tail is held below the natural carriage for an individual dog, it indicates FASCP. When it is held very far under the body, the FASCP is severe. When it is held at least 45 degrees above normal carriage for that individual, it indicates SNS activation which may indicate that aggression is to follow. The interpretation of the tail carriage should be made with consideration of the breed's normal tail carriage[77] (see Figure 2.12).

Head

Dogs that move their head away (e.g., avert gaze and look away) are indicating that they want distance from the stimulus and do not want to interact. An avert gaze is characterized by a movement of the head away from the stimulus, but the body stays still. Often the eyes will continue to engage the stimulus. In this case, the observer should move away.

Ears

Ear carriage is dependent on the conformation of the dog; however, some generalizations can be made. Pricked-up ears (or raised at their base in lop-eared dogs) indicate attentiveness. Ears that are folded back and flattened indicate FASCP or play. The farther back the ears fold, the more intense the motivation, whether that be fear or play. Since the same ear

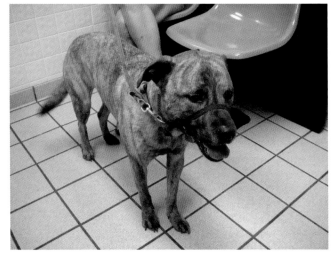

Figure 2.12 Holding the tail below the normal body posture indicates, fear, anxiety, stress, or conflict. *(Attribution: Lisa Radosta.)*

carriages can be associated with different emotional states, the observer should analyze them in context, considering other body language signals displayed concurrently.

Eyes

A direct eye stare indicates an alert and potentially highly aroused (SNS activation) dog and may precede aggression. Most dogs will not maintain direct eye contact for long if they are not neurochemically aroused, have not been taught to do so (e.g., watch me) or were not reinforced for this behavior (e.g., ball toss and treat). Completely avoiding eye contact usually indicates some degree of FASCP, although if a dog has been punished for looking at a person, that can cause him to avoid eye contact. Dilated pupils in a well-lit environment in a normal-sighted dog are a sign of SNS arousal. When a dog orients the nose toward a stimulus and moves the eyes laterally, exposing more of the sclera (i.e., whale eye), he is indicating FACS and SNS activation. The dog does not want to look away from the stimulus as it is too dangerous (by his assessment) to do so, but he is indicating that he needs space or distance (averting the gaze; see above). This is often accompanied by a tense body posture and is displayed just before an aggressive display. Dilated pupils, direct stare, and whale eye all indicate SNS activation except in the situations mentioned above. The observer or recipient should analyze them in context with the situation and concurrent body language signals.

Mouth

A lip curl that exposes the teeth indicates aggression or play. It does not indicate a motivation of FASCP or confidence. It indicates that the dog is requesting in a species-typical way for distance from the stimulus and is threatening to do harm if the interactions are not terminated (aggressive lip curl) or that he is soliciting play. Licking or nuzzling the mouth of a dog or a person is an appeasement behavior, or a way to initiate social contact in a friendly, nonthreatening way. It has also been reinforced by many pet parents as "kisses." Yawning can be displayed when the dog first wakes up from sleep or because of FASCP. Lip licking when not eating or anticipating food is a request for distance (distance increasing signal) indicating a level of FASCP. These behaviors should cause the observer to increase distance from the dog.

Olfactory communication

Olfactory signals contain information about many aspects of the dog's physical, physiological, and behavioral characteristics, including individual identity, sex, breeding condition, age, social status, and even emotional state. Consequently, chemical communication plays a fundamental role in virtually all aspects of canine social, maternal, and reproductive behavior. Dogs show specific behavior patterns related to odor communication, including tonguing and the raised-leg urination posture. Olfactory cues are found in all body secretions, from sebaceous and apocrine skin glands to saliva, urine, and vaginal discharge. Each dog seems to have an individual odor, which results from a variety of internal and environmental influences, from genetics to the effects of diet and microflora. Beyond individual recognition, dogs release

to the environment certain chemicals that possess a specific regulatory effect on the physiology and behavior of their conspecifics. Chemical signals in mammals need to be understood as modulators that exert their effect in conjunction with other elements of control, including social context and learning processes.

Olfactory communication can take place through direct contact (e.g., sniffing an individual) and investigation of scent left behind (e.g., urine marking). Dogs deposit scent via feces, urine, and glandular secretions. Dogs can recognize individuals and distinguish that scent from their own.[72] It is unclear what information the dog can glean from this type of communication, but the interest of dogs in the scents in their environment implies that the information at minimum is enriching if not essential. Raised-leg urination (posture of urine marking) serves to leave a scent communication, is a social display and a sign of anxiety. Ground scratching is a form of scent (sweat glands on feet) and visual marking.[72,79] Dogs also roll in odiferous items such as feces of other species or carrion. The function of this behavior is not understood.

Behavior patterns

Conflict behavior

Conflict is a state of stress and is defined as a psychological struggle, often unconscious, resulting from the opposition or simultaneous functioning of mutually exclusive impulses, desires, or tendencies. Conflict behaviors may be shown in situations of frustration, fear, anxiety, stress, uncertainty, and/or motivational conflict. In pet dogs, conflict often arises from an unpredictable environment where the dog lacks control over pleasant or unpleasant outcomes (see Chapter 10) including social interactions, schedule, and time of feeding. Conflict behaviors are displayed when the dog experiences two opposing motivations, such as the motivation to approach and the motivation to withdraw. Conflict behaviors can be recognized because the dog will display opposing body language signals. As with most other signals, the observer or recipient should pause and reassess.

Play

Play likely developed from predatory behavior. Not all dogs know how to play appropriately. Puppies that were are not socialized with other dogs before 12–14 weeks show deficits in social behavior and group play with their peers.[80] Play is neurochemically arousing and can include pawing with a front foot, twisting jumps, open-mouth panting, tail wagging, tail over, lower or at the back, chase, inguinal presentation, wrestling, biting, and growling. During play, there is SNS activation which can lead to aggressive and injurious interactions fairly quickly if signals are misunderstood. Dogs that are playing appropriately will display self-handicapping (one dog assuming inguinal presentation), role reversals (chaser versus being chased), loose tail carriage, relaxed body postures, quick changes from lying to standing to chasing, and inhibited bites and growls.

Aggression

The scientific literature supports the tenet that normal dogs avoid conflict and use aggression as a last resort. Aggressive outbursts are common in mammals (including humans) in reaction to the stress of having lost control of or the ability to predict the outcome of a situation. Dogs are no different. Those that are frustrated or feeling FASCP may become aggressive. Aggression at its core is a distance increasing signal with an intent to do harm if the social pressure is not reduced. Recipients and observers should step away, give the dog distance, and reassess the situation before proceeding.

Pet parents often report that their dog became aggressive "without warning." This is rarely the case. Aggression is almost always directly or historically preceded by body language signals which indicate FASCP and/or frustration. Consider the following example. As discussed above, body language signals can be punished or reinforced, decreasing or increasing their likelihood of those signals being exhibited in the future. Once a body language signal has been successful in achieving a return to homeostasis or a more relaxed state free of FASCP and frustration, that body language signal or group of signals has been reinforced and will be exhibited more frequently. This is one of the ways that dogs whose motivation is FASCP come to display aggression when the motivation is FASCP. They have been taught inadvertently through poor dog training techniques (shock, choke, and pinch collars) and misunderstanding of pet parents and veterinary healthcare team members that aggressive displays are effective and fearful body language is not. Once this has been "learned," it cannot be completely "unlearned." The stress ladder is a visual guide to the different body language signals offered by dogs (see Figure 2.13). If the lower rungs of the ladder have been punished, consider them to have disappeared. Rebuilding those rungs in the dog's behavioral repertoire in that situation can be nearly impossible.

Fear, Anxiety, Stress, Conflict, and Panic

Over the past decade, it has become clear that FASCP are the cause of almost all behavior disorders in dogs. A relaxed dog that is in homeostasis physically, physiologically, and emotionally generally does not get involved in or cause conflict. The individual behaviors associated with FASCP have been described above. Generally, a fearful or anxious dog has a low body posture, weight shifted back, ears back, tail down or tucked, and may attempt to escape. A stressed dog has an increased heart rate, respiratory rate, body temperature, and dilated pupils, and may display any or all of the body language signals listed in this text associated with fear, anxiety, stress, conflict, or panic. Fear, anxiety, and stress are closely related and cannot generally be separated by gross observation. If you observe body language associated with fear, anxiety, conflict, or panic, assume that stress is also present and vice versa.

Touch

Touch is important for the development of attachment within groups of social animals. Physical contact while resting has been observed in dogs even in hot weather, so it is believed that it has a social function and is not just used to get or conserve warmth. Physical contact can also be solicited or accepted in canine interaction with humans and proximity, including physical contact, has been identified as a bonding behavior.

Metacommunication

Metacommunication refers to a signal or a combination of signals which affect the way the subsequent behavior is understood. The best example of metacommunication in dogs is the play-soliciting posture or play bow. Whenever this posture is presented, it indicates not only the desire to play but also that all subsequent signals should be interpreted in the context of play.

Human–dog communication

The dog learns in its coexistence with humans to consider them as members of its social group. In fact, dogs may have

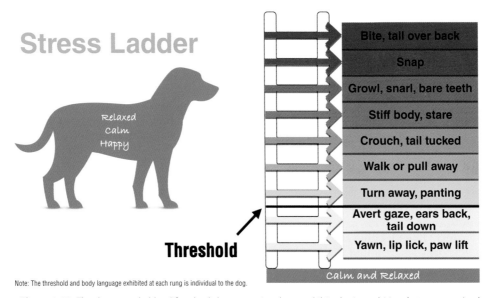

Note: The threshold and body language exhibited at each rung is individual to the dog.

Figure 2.13 The dog stress ladder. Often body language signals are exhibited prior to biting, but go unnoticed by pet parents. *(Attribution: Lisa Radosta. Modified from Shepherd, K 2009. BSAVA Manual of Canine and Feline Behaviour, 2nd edition.)*

developed the ability to use human social cues to predict human behaviors and fit into the human social system more successfully.[79] Thus, they readily learn the signals that mean humans are interested in them.[46] As long as humans are able to interpret canine body language, they will be able to understand the dog's intentions, their moods, and influence the dog's behavior in a way that makes sense to the dog. It is important to remember that while humans are basically a visual species, dogs live in a world of smells and sounds. Thus, their behavior may be in response to signals undetectable by humans.

Dogs are remarkably adaptable. When dogs are adopted by a human family, they learn to interpret the body postures, actions, words, and wishes of their pet parents and seem to have evolved to be able to better do so.[46] Unfortunately, pet parents do not spend nearly as much time learning about their dog's body language. This can be a particular problem with children, who may be less able to read the dog's body language and signals and may be less consistent in their responses. The veterinary healthcare team has an obligation to educate pet parents on proper interpretation of body language signals to strengthen the human–animal bond, prevent behavior problems and animal suffering.

Feline development

Kittens have loosely defined stages of development, although it can vary between individuals based not only on genetic factors but also on maternal factors, environmental factors such as handling and housing, and sexual differences. In this text, we use similar time periods as have been defined in dogs; however, it should be noted that these stages have not been fully investigated. In addition, while the visual and embryonic development of cats is well studied as a result of their wide use in laboratory research, as pets the research on their development is lagging behind that of dogs (see Table 2.4).

Prenatal development and in utero influences

Kittens are generally born after a 63-day gestation.[81] As with most mammals, the condition of the mother during pregnancy plays an important role in the development of the offspring. Kittens from undernourished mothers can have growth deficits in some brain regions (cerebrum, cerebellum, and brainstem), as well as delays in the development of crawling, suckling, eye opening, walking, play, exploration, climbing, and predation. These kittens may also show decreased learning ability, antisocial behavior toward other cats, and increased fear and aggression. Many of these changes do not arise until much later in the cat's development. Maternal malnutrition from a low-protein diet, can also lead to abnormalities in behavior and motor development.[82,83]

Tactile sensitivity is present in the embryo by day 24 of prenatal life and the vestibular righting reflex has developed by about day 54 of gestation.[84]

Neonatal and transitional period

The neonatal period is a time primarily of nursing and sleep, in which the kitten is fully dependent on its mother. The transitional period, where locomotion and sensory development emerge, begins in the second week. During the neonatal period, the kitten is predominantly guided by tactile, thermal, and olfactory stimuli. Kittens are born with their eyes closed and unable to hear.[29,85] Olfaction is present at birth. The external ear canal begins to open between 6 and 14 days of age and is fully open by day 17. Kittens first begin to respond to sound around day 5 and can orient to the source of sound by about 2 weeks.[29,85,86] Adultlike orienting is present by a month of age. Although the eyes open at around 7–10 days, visual orienting and following do not develop until the third week, and visual orienting and obstacle avoidance are not developed until 4–5 weeks of age.[29,85] Full visual acuity may not be achieved until 3–4 months of age. Self-grooming in the form of oral grooming and paw grooming begin to emerge in the second to third week of life.

At birth, kittens move toward warmth but cannot regulate their body temperature until around 3 weeks of age; full adult temperature regulation may not be achieved until 7 weeks of age. During the first 2 weeks of life, the kittens are fairly immobile, and walking does not begin until around 3 weeks of age.[85] Body righting, although present at birth, is not well developed until 1 month of age (see Table 2.5).

Good maternal behavior is essential for healthy kitten development. Kittens that are separated from their mother and hand raised from 2 weeks of age are more fearful of kittens and people, more sensitive to novel stimuli, and slower to learn.[87,88] Hand-raised kittens may still develop social attachments to other kittens, but this occurs much more slowly.[89] Contrary to popular thought, recent studies have found that bottle-reared kittens were not more likely to exhibit aggressive behavior compared to queen-reared kittens[89,90].

The effects of early handling on kittens

Early handling of kittens by humans is not only beneficial for improving social relationships between kittens and humans but also leads to accelerated physical and central nervous system development. Kittens that are held and lightly stroked daily for the first few weeks of life open their eyes earlier, begin to explore earlier, and are less fearful of humans.[91] Kittens that are handled for 5 minutes daily from birth to 45 days are less fearful than kittens that are not handled. They approach strange toys and people more frequently and are slower to learn avoidance.[94] In a study in which 5½–9½-week-old kittens were handled by 0, 1, and 5 people, the 5-person kittens exhibited the least fear of strangers.[93] In another study, kittens that were handled between 3 and 14 weeks of age would accept holding for longer and had less delay before approaching humans than

Table 2.4 Cat developmental periods

Developmental period	Age
Neonatal stage	Birth to 14 days
Transitional	14–21 days
Socialization	21 days to 7–9 weeks
Juvenile/adult	9 weeks to 9 months

*Stages will vary slightly depending on the individual.

Table 2.5 Cat developmental characteristics as they relate to age

Age	Developmental characteristics
0–14 days	Thermal, tactile, olfactory dominant Body righting present
5 days	Responses to sound present
6–17 days	Ear canals open
7–10 days	Eyes open
14 days	Can orient to sound Teeth begin to erupt
21 days	Olfaction matures Body temperature regulation begins Visual orientation develops Grooming begins Walking begins
28 days	Hearing well developed Mature orientation to sound developed Body righting well developed Walking improves Weaning begins Social play begins
28–35 days	Visual orientation and obstacle avoidance fully developed Mother begins to bring prey to the kittens
35 days	Running begins Teeth fully erupted Prey killing begins
35–42 days	Complete voluntary control of elimination Digging as a part of elimination begins
42 days	Body temperature regulation mature Use all gaits in adult locomotion Weaning complete Defensive reactions to large prey and fearful reactions begin
49–56 days	Play, exploration of inanimate objects, and locomotor play escalate
9–14 weeks	Social play peaks
10–11 weeks	Complex motor abilities developed
12 weeks	Predatory behaviors emerge as part of social play
18 weeks	Object play peaks

kittens that had received no handling and those that were handled between 7 and 14 weeks of age.[94] These studies indicate that the most receptive time for socializing kittens to people is up to 7 weeks of age, and that the more opportunities the kitten has for pleasant human handling, the friendlier the kitten is likely to be toward people.[95]

There may be a limit to the duration and intensity of handling which is optimal for development of bonds with people. Several studies have assessed the duration of handling required to adequately socialize kittens. Lengths of time as short as 2-5 minutes a day throughout the socialization period can be effective at altering behavior up to a year later.[95,96] Kittens may be more outgoing and confident when socialized with their littermates.[97] Establishment of a relationship with a cat may be enhanced by the act of the

provision of food.[98] The kittens may be influenced by the presence and activities of the queen when socialization is attempted, and if the queen is reserved, shy, or fearful, this behavior may be learned by the kittens. Cats may learn to expect pleasant or unpleasant interactions from either familiar or unfamiliar people.

Though further study is indicated, based on a review of the available studies, the optimally socialized cat is one sired by an outgoing, confident father and raised by a mother that is at the very least not overly fearful of humans. Ideally, the kittens should have pleasant, positive interactions with a few familiar people for 30–60 minutes a day. The people to whom a kitten is introduced should be consistently pleasant and predictable in their interactions and avoid traumatic experiences.

Socialization period

The socialization period begins in the third week and extends to 7–9 weeks of age. Maturity is not reached up to 48 months of age.[24] By 4 weeks of age, hearing, vision, temperature regulation, and mobility are sufficient for the kitten to begin moving away from the nest and developing social relationships with people and other animals in its environment. At this age, learning can be accomplished solely by visual cues. Body-righting ability is fully mature by about 6 weeks of age. Running begins in the fifth week and most adult locomotion is developed by 7 weeks of age.[29] Complex motor abilities may not be fully developed until 10 weeks or older.

During the first 3 weeks, the mother initiates nursing, and teeth begin to erupt at about 2 weeks of age. At 4 weeks, the kittens begin to eat some solid foods and weaning begins. From this point onward, the kitten initiates most bouts of nursing. At 4–5 weeks of age, in a free-living environment, the mother may begin to bring prey to the kitten.[101] Deciduous dentition is fully developed by 5 weeks of age, and kittens may start to kill mice at this time if exposed to them. Kittens generally share their mother's food choices, and this is most marked by 7–8 weeks of age. Similarly, the choice of prey is usually similar to that of the mother.[101] By 5–6 weeks of age, the kitten has full voluntary control of elimination, and digging and covering in loose soil may begin. By 7 weeks of age, most kittens are weaned, although suckling may continue intermittently for several more weeks. Defensive reactions to large prey and fearful reactions to threatening stimuli may begin to be displayed by 6 weeks of age.[103] Kittens removed from the litter before 6 weeks of age are more likely to be fearful and reactive compared with kittens weaned between 6 and 12 weeks of age,[88,102] and those weaned before 8 weeks of age are more likely to show aggression directed at unfamiliar people than those weaned after 14 weeks.[104]

Within the socialization period, social attachments are formed most easily and rapidly. Social play begins at this time, before the interest in object play. Attachments can be formed at other times, but the process is much slower and involves extensive exposure. Socializing kittens to other species, including humans, may begin as early as 2 weeks of age and may only extend to 7 weeks of age. Because of genetic differences between individuals and other factors such as early handling, maternal effects, and the cat's environment and experiences, kittens and adult cats can show a great variability in their friendliness toward people and other cats, regardless of the amount of early socialization.[105] Studies of cat personalities have explored dimensions of emotional stability (timidness and fearfulness), energy level, exploration, sociability, and goal-directed behavior. These dimensions have been utilized to propose a five-factor model of personality and create surveys to assess feline personality.[105a,106] Factors that might influence these personality types include parental genetics, early socialization, and social or observational effects of mother and littermates.[107] Kittens lacking early socialization are more likely to be fearful of people and thus more likely to display fear-induced and defensive aggression when approached or handled.[107,108,108a] Paternal temperament appears to have a large effect on the temperament of the offspring, with friendly toms more likely to sire friendly kittens even if the kittens are not exposed to the tom after birth.[107,109] The presence or absence of the queen and her behavior toward stimuli during early development of the kittens can affect the development of behavior disorders, presumably due to the effect observational learning and mimicry of behavior and exposure leading to FASCP.[88,102] Early trauma has also been linked to an increased likelihood of aggression.[110] When a kitten grows up without appropriate social interaction that discourages hard biting, such as a kitten that has been hand reared with no contact with other cats, it may bite without inhibition into adulthood and be quite dangerous.[111,112]

As with dogs, the amount of handling or socialization most likely varies depending on the genetic makeup and early life experiences of the individual. Since it is impossible to predict an animal's behavioral future, socialization should take place in every individual.

Play and predatory behavior

Playful social interactions with siblings and the queen begin at around 4 weeks and are generally well developed by 7 weeks of age. Social play includes wrestling, rolling, and biting of conspecifics and may be directed at the human hand (or other moving body part). Predatory-type behaviors may become a part of social play in the third month and agonistic social behavior also begins to emerge. Play between older kittens may become more serious and intense over time. Play, exploration of inanimate objects, and locomotor play begin to escalate at around 7–8 weeks of age and peak at around 18 weeks of age before beginning to decline. Social play, on the other hand, peaks from 9 to 14 weeks, with object play more common than social play by about week 16.[85] Object play may be social or solitary and may consist of pawing, stalking, and biting of objects. This type of play also simulates a variety of aspects of the predatory sequence. Pet parents should provide an opportunity for their kittens to engage in object play by offering a variety of preylike toys for their cats to attack and catch. Kittens that are weaned at an earlier age show earlier development of object play.[113]

Predatory behavior may be affected by social or observational learning, age of weaning, early socialization, maternal behavior, observation of other cats, genetics, and possibly by competition with littermates. A kitten's mother will gradually introduce it to prey, so maternal effects can be an important factor in prey preferences and hunting ability.[114] At first, dead prey is brought to the kitten, progressing to live prey, which the mother releases for it. If the kitten loses control or pauses too long, the mother may intervene so the kitten's skills become more finely tuned through observation and interaction.[115] Lack of familiarity with a species or socialization to that species may inhibit predation on that species. Despite a lack of familiarity with prey and even in the absence of maternal experience and learning, many cats still develop into competent hunters. Early weaned kittens develop predatory behavior earlier and show an earlier increase in object play, while normally weaned kittens are less likely to become predators and have a later onset of object play.[115] Hunger has been shown to increase the incidence of killing prey, while increasing prey size reduces the probability of killing. Similarly, studies of object play found that hunger increases the motivation to play and reduces fear of larger toys.[116]

Juvenile period/adulthood

The juvenile phase continues until sexual maturity, at which time the cat may become increasingly independent. Age of sexual maturity depends in females on genetics, breed, and the environment. Sexual maturity is usually observed at 5–9 months of age, although the first heat cycle may occur as early as 4 months in some cats. Although male kittens may be mature enough for spermatogenesis by about 5 months of age, mating and sexual maturity are usually not observed until around 9–12 months of age.

Social behavior and communication in cats

The domestic cat (*Felis catus*) is a small, crepuscular (most active during dawn and dusk), solitary hunter of the felid family. Molecular, archeological, and behavioral evidence suggests that the domestic cat was derived from near Eastern and Egyptian populations of *Felis silvestris libyca*, the African wildcat.[117,118] There are genetic and morphological similarities to *Felis silvestris* (the European wildcat), but behavioral evidence suggests *F. silvestris* is not likely to accept human contact, as displayed by severe fierceness and extreme shyness even under ideal handling and rearing of first-generation hybrid offspring.[118]

The cat evolved in arid areas and hunted small animals such as rodents, frogs, birds, and reptiles. Among felines, domestic cats are small, tending to weigh between 2 and 8 kg, and have large, forward-facing eyes, large, mobile ears, and sensitive vibrissae on their face that aid in detecting prey in dim light. They have large, laterally flattened canine teeth and sharp retractable claws on front toes to catch, hold, and kill prey. The cat is an ambush hunter. It locates prey using its sensitive hearing, vision, and sense of smell. It then stalks silently until it is close enough for a sudden rush and grab. Domestic cats do not possess the stamina to chase prey for long periods. They are able to climb and to jump up to five times their own height. Being small, they are potentially prey for other larger animals, so being agile gives the cat an advantage not only when hunting but also in escaping when being hunted.

Social organization and density

Of all the domestic species, cats are unique in western countries, as there is a flow of individuals between three distinct populations: owned cats, semiowned cats, and feral cats. The normal social organization of cats is variable, depending on the presence of resources, and as such cannot be described by one social system paradigm.[119] Cats are solitary hunters, as their prey consists of small animals that are best caught by a single animal, but it is generally accepted that cats are a social species that form complex social groups.[120] Cats can live in a variety of social group structures from solitary life to living in large, stable colonies. The composition of the groups varies with the distribution and abundance of food, gender, and the social nature of the individual. Where food is abundant, cats will gather together and form structured groups.

A population of cats within an area can be considered a colony.[85,120] Within a colony, the cats will form affiliative and antagonistic relationships. Affiliated cats are identified by their greeting each other, rubbing heads and bodies, and sometimes entwining their tails. They may also groom each other.[120] It is thought that this helps create a group odor that identifies all members. Long-term associates and related individuals will be generally found together, may share sleeping spaces, and share food.[122,123] Antagonistic encounters are rare in a stable colony, meaning, as with dogs and most other mammalian species, aggression is avoided if at all possible. Cats that do not get along tend to avoid each other and use time-sharing to access common areas. With the group, dominant–subordinate relationships (social asymmetry) may be established as a means of resolving conflicts without aggression, just as in the dog.[120]

Queens will generally form groups with their kittens. Queens may raise their kittens with other queens. Natural colonies are matrilineal, comprising females and successive generations of young.[120,124] Neutered males behave more like females, while relationships with males may vary from solitary to affiliative.

For intact male cats, spending time with queens is important to their developing familiarity with them so there is a chance the queen will mate with the male when next in estrus. However, spending too much time with one group of queens reduces the time available to spend with other queens.

Territory boundaries are maintained with visual and olfactory signals in the form of scratching on vertical surfaces, facial rubbing, and deposition of urine and/or feces. Aggression is displayed by colony members to unfamiliar cats. Noncolony members may be gradually accepted to the colony after many interactions between the noncolony members and the colony members.[120]

When presented with conflict, rather than fighting, it is more common for cats to defer to or avoid a cat that already has a resource, whether a resting area, litter box, or access to a passageway (first come, first served).[125] On the other hand, a social asymmetry helps to maintain healthy social relationships without the need for conflict. Much has been said about dominance in dogs, but what do we know about dominance in cats? Cats appear to some extent to have a hierarchy based on RHP (how likely the cat is able to keep the resource if there is aggression) and relative resource value (how important the resource is to the cat), similar to dogs. In this type of dominance hierarchy, the dominance is not static, but instead fluid based on the value of the resources and the interactions between the cats at that resource. For example, in one study of feral cats, the male cats were higher ranking away from food (they had preferential access to resources), while the female cats were higher ranking near food

(they ate first).[126] Also in this study, kittens between 4 and 6 months of age were more likely to feed first compared to either sex of adult cat, indicating that dominance is not absolute.[126] In some cases, the female cat is higher ranking, even though she is of smaller body size than the male cat.[128] Similarly to dogs, the highest-ranking cat is not necessarily the most aggressive cat.[120] The overwhelming majority of the aggression that is seen in domestic cats presented to veterinarians is a result of fear, anxiety, stress, conflict, panic, discomfort, or pain, not dominance.

Feline senses

Vision

Cats' eyes have many characteristics to maximize the visual field and the collection of light entering the eye to stimulate the retinal cells. The cornea is larger and more curved and, therefore, collects more light than the human eye. The cat retina has approximately 25 light-sensitive rods for every color-sensitive cone, compared to about 20:1 in humans.[125] The tapetum lucidum under the retina reflects light back to maximize the chance of rods being stimulated. This layer is what makes cat eyes glow yellowish green when light is shone into them. These retinal differences allow cats to see in about one-sixth the light or three to eight times the threshold of detection sensitivity than humans.[85,125] Cats have little need for color vision, as they hunt mainly at night and most prey species do not have a wide range of coat colors. It appears that cats can see in the green–yellow spectrum and blue wavelengths of light and can be taught to distinguish between red and other colors.

The lens of the eye has a limited capacity for accommodation. Because of this, cats can see best about 75 cm (30 in) from the viewed object and have a loss of ability to focus on objects closer than 25 cm.[85,125] To maximize visual acuity, they have multifocal lenses, which focus light at particular wavelengths. The slit pupil prevents the loss of visual fields that can focus at set wavelengths and maximizes the cat's vision.[129] Binocular vision aids the cat in judging distances for catching prey, climbing, and jumping. The binocular overlap is about 98 degrees, allowing cats to judge distances very accurately.[125]

Hearing

The cat's large, mobile pinnae act to collect and funnel sounds into the ear canal. Each ear can move independently of the other and can swivel almost 180 degrees, effectively giving them surround sound. When tracking a sound such as that of a prey animal, cats use a combination of the interaural time differences for sounds to reach both pinnae, level differences between the pinnae, and directional amplification effects of the pinnae to localize the sound and orient their head.[130] They are able to do this as the prey animal and the cat are both moving. Cats can hear one of the largest ranges of frequencies of any mammal.

Olfaction

Cats have a well-developed sense of smell at birth. These nerves are myelinated at birth, in contrast to most other neurons in the nervous system, and the sense of smell is fully developed by the time that the kitten is 3 weeks of age.[131] This allows signals to pass rapidly to the brain. Kittens use their sense of smell and touch to find the queen's teats.[132] If they are unable to smell, either experimentally or due to illness such as an upper respiratory infection, kittens cannot find the queen's nipples to feed.[133]

Cats use their sense of smell for locating prey and for evaluating communication signals left by other cats. Odors play an important role in social organization of cats and in reproduction. The cat has two olfactory structures. Scent molecules are detected by receptors of olfactory sensory neurons in the olfactory mucosa (smell), and by the vomeronasal organ (VNO), which is connected to the nasal and oral cavity by the nasopalatine duct.[134] The VNO sits between the oral cavity and the nasal cavity, has connections to both, has unique receptors outside of those associated with the nasal epithelium, and is associated with the processing of social signals.[125,134]

The gape or flehmen response may be performed after the cat has sniffed or even licked at a scent source. By wrinkling the upper lip and opening the mouth, the cat opens the ducts of the VNO and pumps saliva and the semiochemical molecules including pheromones into the VNO.[24] Cats cannot fully evert their upper lip like horses and cattle because of the frenulum between the upper lip and the upper jaw. The gape reaction is seen when tom cats find urine from another cat. However, queens will also show the behavior (see Figure 2.14).

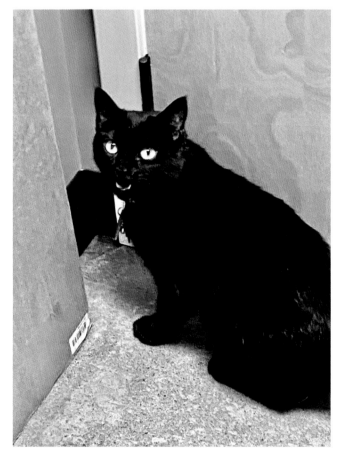

Figure 2.14 Gape or flehmen response. *(Attribution: Deborah Bryant, DVM, DACVB.)*

Taste

Cats have two types of taste buds on their tongues: mushroom-shaped papillae at the front and sides of the tongue and cup-shaped papillae at the back of the tongue. Cats can taste salty, bitter, and acid. Like dogs, they also have water receptors. Cats have little reaction to sucrose and will tend to drink sweet water only if the sugar is masked by salt.

Touch

Cats have sensory nerves across their body surface, just as dogs and people do, and touch is important to cats. Touch may be one of the first senses developed, and queens start nuzzling and licking kittens soon after birth. Like dogs, cats have many specialized touch receptors, including vibrissae on the face that can sense air flow. Just as noted above in the case of dogs, cats do not inherently appreciate petting or touch of any sort. In fact, petting is a common cause of aggression in cats. Cats may not like petting because it does not feel good, they are pruritic or painful, they learned through negative physical interactions that petting was uncomfortable, or the petting is in an unnatural location. Cats groom each other typically no farther caudal than the shoulders. Yet, pet parents stroke their cats down the back and to the tip of the tail. Even this seemingly small change in the way that the cat is touched can cause fear, anxiety, stress, and conflict, leading to aggression. Cat body language is subtle or unknown to pet parents and as such, it is easily missed or misinterpreted. Like any other behavior, petting can be conditioned to be a positive interaction. This is one of the treatments for cats with petting-induced aggression.

Communication concepts and body language signals

Cats communicate via specific body language signals, body postures, and vocalizations similar to dogs. As with dogs, each body language signal by itself has a specific meaning. Compound body language signals exist whose meaning is the sum of the body language signals within it. For this reason, all body language should be viewed in the context of the situation, the sender, and the recipient. Most cat behavior problems stem from FASCP, just as in dogs and most other animals. Since cats are social animals, body language signals also facilitate affiliative behavior and help them avoid conflict (for body posture and facial expression resources, see Appendix A).

Visual communication

The perceived size and shape of the body, ear position, pupil size, movement and position of the tail, and visibility of teeth all convey important messages to others. Cats can increase their perceived size via piloerection and by standing at their full height. Cats arch their backs when extremely fearful (Halloween cat), which is often accompanied by piloerection (see Figure 2.15).

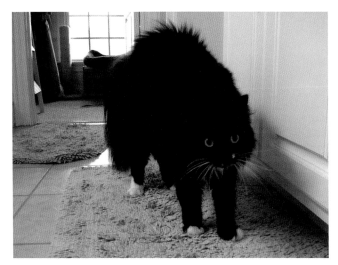

Figure 2.15 Fearful cat: arched back, dilated pupils, and piloerection. *(Attribution: Courtesy Katy Cohen.)*

Ears

An interested cat will have its ears forward. A frightened cat will have its ears flat and backward facing. Between forward and flat back, there are many positions which can indicate anything from relaxation to agitation. When the ears are turned to the side slightly so that the internal part of the pinna cannot be visualized, but they are not flat back, this indicates agitation (SNS arousal). This may be the first noticeable signal that a cat does not desire interaction and is often accompanied by mildly dilated pupils (see Figures 2.16–2.18).

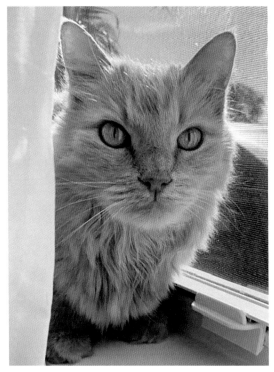

Figure 2.16 Ears forward indicates an alert cat. This cat has a small pupil size and a relaxed body posture, indicating that he is alert and not stressed. *(Attribution: Alison Gerken, DVM.)*

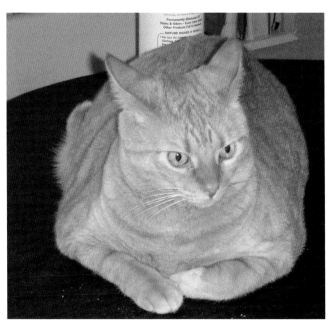

Figure 2.17 Ears midway back indicates fear, anxiety, stress, or agitation. This cat is also lying in a defensive body position and averting his gaze from the camera indicating that he is stressed by this interaction. *(Attribution: Lisa Radosta.)*

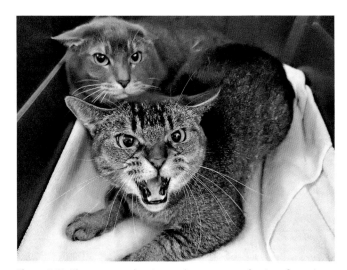

Figure 2.18 These cats are showing moderate to severe fear (ears flat and back, hissing, dilated pupils). *(Attribution: Gary Landsberg, DVM, DACVB.)*

Eyes

The unique pupil shape of domestic cats and often light iris color when compared to dogs makes the eyes an especially obvious way to read what the cat is thinking. While it is true that a direct stare between two cats can be regarded as a threat and that averting the eyes is a distance increasing signal, it is also true that cats can be taught to make direct eye contact with people through reinforcement (see Chapter 12). Cats then might use this body language signal to communicate to the pet parent a need such as hunger. When cats approach, they often do not approach head on with a direct stare but instead slightly avert the gaze. Dilated pupils in a well-lit room indicate SNS arousal (see Figure 2.19).

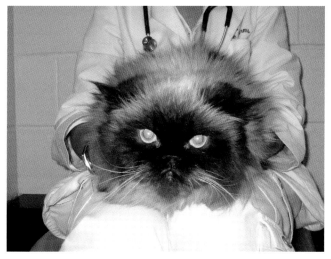

Figure 2.19 Dilated pupils in a bright room indicate severe fear, anxiety, and stress. This cat also has his ears held midway back indicating fear, anxiety, stress, and/or agitation. *(Attribution: Lisa Radosta.)*

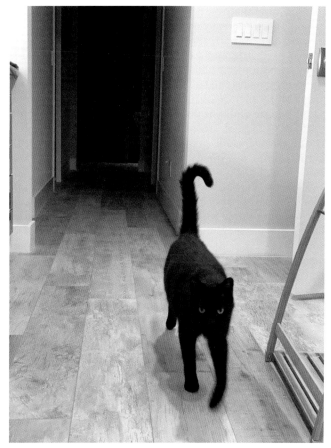

Figure 2.20 Question mark tail indicates affiliative interaction. *(Attribution: Lisa Radosta.)*

Tail

Cat tails are extremely expressive and very rarely still. In contrast with dogs, positioning of the feline tail is often clearer in its meaning. The natural tail carriage of most cats is slightly below the back with a gentle curve. Vertical raised tails (especially those with an inverted U or question mark shape) indicate amicable approach and familiar recognition[135] (see Figure 2.20). This particular posture is only observed in two species of felines: the domestic cat and the African lion. Interestingly, these are two of the only three species of felines showing a gregarious social structure.

A thrashing, thumping, or piloerect tail indicates SNS activation and FASCP. A tail which is upright but not curled at the end indicates interest and potentially a calm state of arousal, but this body language signal can also be considered transitional. The cat could be initiating an affiliative interaction after approach or could simply be moving through the space. When the tail is held close to the body, the cat is showing FASCP. This can be displayed as wrapped around the body or curled between the legs (see Figure 2.21).

Body postures

Similar to dogs, cats that shift their weight back and down are fearful, anxious, or stressed. Cats that stand with their weight evenly distributed or onto their front feet are alert and engaged. Cats in any posture can show aggression. As noted above, the classic Halloween cat with an arched back is consistent with extreme fear.

An appeasing posture is defined as one that induces relaxation or reduces the aggressive motivation of the other individual. Young cats will sometimes approach adult males and roll onto their side or back. Many believe this is an appeasement posture. Kittens will also approach another cat and roll over as an invitation to play. Purring is often observed together with this body posture. However, in adult cats, rolling over onto the back should be considered with other body language signals and the context of the situation. Cats rarely

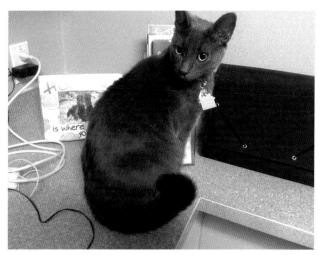

Figure 2.21 This cat's tail is curled around his body and his pupils are dilated, indicating a state of FASCP. *(Attribution: Lisa Radosta.)*

solicit attention in this way and it is often misinterpreted by pet parents, causing bites.

Auditory communication

Vocalizations convey general information regarding the underlying emotional or motivational state of the cat within four main contexts: (1) social interactions with other cats (conflict or affiliative); (2) sexual behavior; (3) parental behavior; and (4) interactions with people.

Some texts purport that the many distinct vocalizations uttered by the domestic cat at least in part developed as a way to communicate with humans oblivious to the olfactory and body language signals which would be used to communicate with other cats. This appears to be true as cats rarely communicate with vocalizations with each other. Most are confined to sexual, agonisic, and caregiving situations.[134] Vocalizations include purr, trill/chirrup, miaow, female call, mowl (male call), howl, growl, yowl, snarl, hiss, spit, and pain shriek.[134]

Like any behavior, vocalizations can be reinforced or punished, increasing or decreasing the likelihood of occurrence in the future. In addition, selective breeding has produced breeds that are more likely to be vocal, such as the Siamese. Since these types of vocalizations do not occur very frequently between cats, it is challenging to decipher what each type of sound means. Meowing, for example, can be a sign of happiness, fear, defensiveness, stress, anxiety, conflict, frustration, and illness.

Growling is a vocalization of high intensity, long duration, and low frequency, which is typically observed in aggressive interactions. Hissing is an involuntary (autonomic) defensive response emitted with the mouth opened and the teeth exposed. Cats in the veterinary hospital are most likely to acting defensively, meaning that the underlying motive is fear and self-preservation.

Purring is caused by contraction of the laryngeal muscles closing the glottis and a subsequent buildup of pressure forcing the glottis open and separating the vocal folds. Adult cats purr when they are interacting with people, objects, or animals, or doing something pleasurable such as rolling or rubbing. Purring can be solicitous, meaning the cat may be asking for attention, food, or another need.

Cats are born with this ability, being able to purr within 3 days of birth, first observed in young kittens during the queen's lactation. Purring while nursing could be a way for the kitten to communicate that everything is right and may contribute to reinforce the mother–infant bond. Cats sometimes purr when they are afraid, such as during a veterinary visit. One potential reason for this might be the initial cause of purring in kittens, which is to solicit help or care from the queen. Cats purr at frequencies between 25 and 150 Hz and exhibit strong purring 25 and 50 Hz. These frequencies correspond with the frequencies used in the treatment of fractures and pain. These frequencies may also assist in muscle growth, flexibility, and wound healing.[136]

Humans listening to recordings of solicitation and non-solicitation purrs could identify the solicitation purrs as the more urgent and less pleasant of the nonsolicitation purrs. Individuals who owned a cat did significantly better at identifying the purrs, indicating that learning may play a role in identifying feline communications[137] (see Table 2.6).

Table 2.6 Common cat body language postures, their meaning, and appropriate recipient action

Body posture	Meaning	Recipient action
Dilated pupils	SNS arousal	Stop, assess the situation, other body language postures, and context before proceeding.
Ears forward	Alert Activation of SNS	Stop, assess the situation, other body language postures, and context before proceeding.
Ears slightly back	Fear, anxiety, stress, conflict, or panic	Stop, assess the situation, other body language postures, and context before proceeding.
Ears flat back	Extreme fear	Increase distance.
Piloerection	SNS arousal	Increase distance
Rolling over onto the back	Appeasement (kittens)	Decrease social pressure by moving away.
Arched back	SNS arousal, extreme fear	Increase distance.
Tail thumping	SNS arousal, agitation	Stop, assess the situation, other body language postures, and context before proceeding. Increase distance.
Tail tucked under abdomen	Severe fear, anxiety, stress, conflict, or panic	Stop, assess the situation, other body language postures, and context before proceeding. Increase distance.
Tail above back in question mark posture	Solicitation of positive interactions	Proceed with interaction.
Avert gaze	Distance increasing signal	Decrease social pressure by moving away.
Lip lick	Distance increasing signal	Stop, assess the situation, other body language postures, and context before proceeding. Decrease social pressure by moving away.
Slow eye blink	Distance increasing signal	Stop, assess the situation, other body language postures, and context before proceeding. Decrease social pressure by moving away.

Tactile communication

From a practical perspective, tactile communication can be divided into two main patterns: allorubbing and allogrooming. Allorubbing occurs when a cat rubs (head, body, and tail) its body against another individual and is an affiliative behavior. It also provides olfactory and tactile enrichment and may be used to spread colony scent. In a friendly interaction, a cat may rub its head, body, and tail toward a person or another cat. Between cats, allorubbing is more frequently observed between females and between males and females. Allorubbing helps to reinforce social bonds through the release of different neurotransmitters and neurohormones, including dopamine, endorphins, and oxytocin. Allogrooming occurs when one cat licks or otherwise grooms another individual and is an affiliative behavior most likely to occur between conspecifics in a social relationship.[24]

Besides allorubbing and allogrooming, cats often seek physical contact with other cats during periods of rest. This behavior is understood as a sign of social tolerance and would indicate a good social relationship between the individuals that expressed it.

Olfactory communication

For cats, much like their solitary ancestors (and most carnivores), olfactory communication (chemical signals) in the way of urine, saliva, scratching, feces, allorubbing, and allogrooming is essential for effective communication and avoidance of conflict.[134] Solitary animals utilize chemical signals to establish territory and communicate characteristics to others without actually having to come in contact with other individuals. Although not fully investigated in cats to date, is it presumed that cats that live in social groups combine their individual scents through allorubbing and allogrooming to create a colony scent. Cats have sebaceous scent glands on each side of the forehead, corners of the lips, under the chin, feet, and perianal area. Cats also utilize facial pheromones, of which five have been identified, to communicate.[138]

Human–cat communication

Within the framework of social relationships between people and cats, communication should be understood as a bidirectional phenomenon. Therefore, it is important for pet parents not only to understand feline communication but also to respond properly to the different signals emitted by a cat. This will strengthen the bond between the pet parent and the pet, help the pet parent to detect illness and discomfort, and decrease the likelihood of miscommunications leading to behavior problems.

References

1. Markwell PJ, Thorne CJ. Early behavioural development of dogs. *J Small Anim Pract.* 1987;28:984–991.
2. Serpell J, Jagoe JA. Becoming a dog: early experience and the development of behavior. In: Serpell J, ed. *The Domestic Dog.* Cambridge, UK: Cambridge University Press; 2017:93–117.
3. Bergman K, Sarkar P, O'Connor TG, et al. Maternal stress during pregnancy predicts cognitive ability and fearfulness in infancy. *J Am Acad Child Adolesc Psychiatry.* 2007;46:1454–1463.
4. Davis EP, Glynn LM, Schetter CD, et al. Prenatal exposure to maternal depression and cortisol influences infant temperament *J Am Acad Child Adolesc Psychiatry.* 2007;46:737–746.
5. Van den Bergh BRH, Mulder EJH, Mennes M, et al. Antenatal maternal anxiety and stress and the neurobehavioural development of the fetus and child: links and possible mechanisms. A review. *Neurosci Biobehav Rev.* 2005;29:237–258.
6. Nazzari S, Fearon P, Rice F, et al. Neuroendocrine and immune markers of maternal stress during pregnancy and infant cognitive development. *Dev Psychobiol.* 2020;62:1100–1110.
7. Davis EP, Sandman CA. Prenatal psychobiological predictors of anxiety risk in preadolescent children. *Psychoneuroendocrinology* 2012;37:1224–1233.
8. Vallee M, May W, Dullu F, et al. Prenatal stress induces high anxiety and postnatal handling induces low anxiety in adult offspring: correlation with stress-induced corticosterone secretion. *J Neurosci.* 1997;17:2626–2636.
9. Braastad BO. Effects of prenatal stress on behavior of offspring of laboratory and farmed mammals. *Appl Anim Behav Sci.* 1998;61:159–180.
10. Fride E, Weinstock M. Prenatal stress increase anxiety related behavior and alters cerebral lateralization of dopamine activity. *Life Sci.* 1988;42:1059–1065.
11. Weinstock M. Prenatal stressors in rodents: effects on behavior. *Neurobiol Stress.* 2017;6:3–13.
12. Dahlöf L-G, Hård E, Larsson K. Influence of maternal stress on offspring sexual behaviour. *Anim Behav.* 1977;25:958–963.
13. Kapoor A, Matthews SG. Short periods of prenatal stress affect growth, behaviour and hypothalamo-pituitary-adrenal axis activity in male guinea pig offspring. *J Physiol.* 2005;566:967–977.
14. Ranson E, Beach FA. Effects of testosterone on ontogeny of urinary behavior in male and female dogs. *Horm Behav.* 1985;19:36–51.
15. Fox MW, Scott, JP. *Canine Behavior.* Springfield, IL: Charles C. Thomas; 1965.
16. Thorne C. *The Waltham Book of Dog and Cat Behaviour.* Oxford: Pergamon Press; 1992.
17. Fox MW. Socialization, environmental factors, and abnormal behavioral development in animals. In: Fox MW, ed. *Abnormal Behavior in Animals.* Philadelphia: WB Saunders; 1968.
18. Fredericson E, Gurney N, Dubois E. The relationship between environmental temperature and behavior in neonatal puppies. *J Comp Physiol Psychol.* 1956;49:278–280.
19. Fox MW, Stelzner D. Behavioural effects of differential early experience in the dog. *Anim Behav.* 1966;14:273–281.
20. Gazzano A, Mariti C, Notaro L, et al. Effects of early gentling and early environment on emotional development of puppies. *Appl Anim Behav Sci.* 2008;110:294–304.
21. Vaterlaws-Whiteside H, Hartmann A. Improving puppy behavior using a new standardized socialization program. *Appl Anim Behav.* 2017;197:55–61.
22. Strain G, Tedford B, Jackson R. Postnatal development of the brain stem auditory-evoked potential in dogs. *Am J Vet Res.* 1991;52:410–415.
23. Parry HB, Tansley K, Thomson L. Electroretinogram during development of hereditary retinal degeneration in the dog. *Br J Ophthalmol.* 1955;39:349.
24. Houpt KA. *Domestic Animal Behavior for Veterinarians and Animal Scientists.* 6th ed. Hoboken, NJ: John Wiley & Sons; 2018.
24a. Hammerle M, Horst C, Levine E et al. 2015 AAHA Canine and Feline Behavior Management Guidelines; https://www.aaha.org/aaha-guidelines/behavior-management/behavior-management-home

25. Scott JP, Fuller JL. *Genetics and Social Behavior of the Dog.* Chicago: University of Chicago Press; 1965.

26. Fox MW. *Integrative Development of Brain and Behavior in the Dog.* Chicago: University of Chicago Press; 1971.

27. Ross S. Some observations on the lair dwelling behavior of dogs. *Behaviour* 1950;2:144–162.

28. Scott JP. Critical periods in behavioral development. *Science* 1962;138:949–958.

29. Bateson P. Behavioural development in the cat. In: Turner DC, Bateson P, eds. *The Domestic Cat: The Biology of its Behaviour.* 3rd ed. Cambridge: Cambridge University Press; 2014;11–26.

30. Appleby DL, Bradshaw JWS, Casey RA. Relationship between aggressive and avoidance behavior by dogs and their experience in the first six months of life. *Vet Rec.* 2002;150:434–438.

31. Majecka K, Pąsiek M, Pietraszewski D, et al. Behavioural outcomes of housing for domestic dog puppies (*Canis lupus familiaris*). *Appl Anim Behav Sci.* 2020;222:104899.

32. Godbout M, Palestrini C, Beauchamp G, et al. Puppy behavior at the veterinary clinic: a pilot study. *J Vet Behav.* 2007;2:126–135.

33. Godbout M, Frank D. Persistence of puppy behaviors and signs of anxiety during adulthood. *J Vet Behav.* 2011;6:92.

34. Sablin MV, Khlopachev GA. The earliest ice age dogs; Evidence from Eliseevichi 11. *Curr Anthropol.* 2002;43(5):795–799.

35. Miklósi Adm. *Dog Behaviour, Evolution, and Cognition.* 2nd ed. Oxford: Oxford University Press; 2015.

36. Hare B, Tomasello M. Human-like social skills in dogs? *Trends Cogn Sci.* 2005;9: 439–444.

37. Wirobski G, Range F, Schaebs F, et al. Endocrine changes related to dog domestication: comparing urinary cortisol and oxytocin in hand-raised pack-living dogs and wolves. *Horm Behav.* 2021;128:104901.

38. Nagasawa M, Mitsui S, En S, et al. Social evolution. Oxytocin-gaze positive loop and the coevolution of human–dog bonds. *Science.* 2015;348:333–336.

39. Axelsson E, Ratnakumar A, Arendt ML, et al. The genomic signature of dog domestication reveals adaptation to a starch-rich diet. *Nature.* 2013;495: 360–364.

40. Boitani L, Ciucci P, Ortlani A. Behaviour and social ecology of free-ranging dogs. In: Jensen P, ed. *The Behavioural Biology of Dogs.* Wallingord: CAB International; 2007.

41. Semyonova A. The social organization of the domestic dog; a longitudinal study of domestic canine behavior and the ontogeny of domestic canine social systems. The Carriage House Foundation, The Hague; 2003.

42. Premnath S, Sinha A, Gadagkar R. Dominance relationship in the establishment of reproductive division of labour in a primitively eusocial wasp (*Ropalidia marginata*). *Behav Ecol Sociobiol.* 1996;39:125–132.

43. Furuichi T. Agonistic interactions and matrifocal dominance rank of wild bonobos (*Pan paniscus*) at Wamba. *Int J Primatol.* 1997;18:855–875.

44. Silk MJ, Cant MA, Cafazzo S, et al. Elevated aggression is associated with uncertainty in a network of dog dominance interactions. *Proc Royal Soc B.* 2019;286:20190536. doi:10.1098/rspb.2019.0536.

45. Allen AL, Krofel M. Resource holding potential. In: AG Vonk J, Shackelford TJ, eds. *Encyclopedia of Animal Cognition and Behavior*, Cham, Springer; 2017:63.

46. Gácsi M, Miklósi Á, Varga O, et al. Are readers of our face readers of our minds? Dogs (*Canis familiaris*) show situation-dependent recognition of human's attention. *Anim Cogn.* 2004;7:144–153.

47. Huber A, Barber ALA, Faragó T, et al. Investigating emotional contagion in dogs (*Canis familiaris*) to emotional sounds of humans and conspecifics. *Anim Cogn.* 2017;20:703–715.

48. Blackwell EJ, Twells C, Seawright A, et al. The relationship between training methods and the occurrence of behavior problems, as reported by owners, in a population of domestic dogs. *J Vet Behav.* 2008;3:207–217.

49. Hsu Y, Sun L. Factors associated with aggressive responses in pet dogs. *Appl Anim Behav Sci.* 2010;123:108–123.

50. Ziv G. The effects of using aversive training methods in dogs—a review. *J Vet Behav.* 2017;19:50–60.

51. Herron ME, Shofer FS, Reisner IR. Survey of the use and outcome of confrontational and non-confrontational training methods in client-owned dogs showing undesired behaviors. *Appl Anim Behav Sci.* 2009;117:47–54.

52. Miller PE, Murphy CJ. Vision in dogs. *J Am Vet Med Assoc.* 1995;207:1623–1634.

53. McGreevy P, Grassi TD, Harman AM. A strong correlation exists between the distribution of retinal ganglion cells and nose length in the dog. *Brain Behav Evol.* 2004;63:13–22.

54. Neitz J, Geist T, Jacobs G. Color vision in the dog. *Visual Neurosci.* 1989;3:119–125.

55. Parry HB. Degenerations of the dog retina, I: structure and development of the retina of the normal dog. *Br J Ophthalmol.* 1953;37(8):385–444.

56. Kasparson AA. Badridze J, Maximov VV. 2013 Colour cues proved to be more informative for dogs than brightness. Proc. R. Soc. B. 28020131356

57. Pretterer G, Bubna-Littitz H, Windischbauer G, et al. Brightness discrimination in the dog. *J Vis.* 2004;4:241–249.

59. Kemp CM, Jacobson SG. Rhodopsin levels in the central retinas of normal miniature poodles and those with progressive rod-cone degeneration. *Exp Eye Res.* 1992;54:947–956.

60. Jacobs GH, Deegan JF, Crognale MA, et al. Photopigments of dogs and foxes and their implications for canid vision. *Vis Neurosci.* 1991;10:173–180.

61. Parkes, JH, Aquirre G, Rockey JH, et al. Progressive rod-cone degeneration in the dog: characterization of the visual pigment. *Invest Ophthalmol Vis Sci.* 1982;23:674–678.

62a. Cox C. Investigation of hearing loss in dogs. *In Pract.* 2002;24:494–501. doi:10.1136/inpract.24.9.494.

62b. Thompson RF. The Brain: a Neuroscience Primer. New York: WH Freeman; 1993.

63. Moulton DG. Minimum odorant concentrations detectable by the dog and their implications for olfactory receptor sensitivity. In: Muller-Schwarz D, Mozell MM, eds. *Chemical Signals in Vertebrates.* New York: Plenum Press; 1977:455–464.

64. Siniscalchi M, d'Ingeo S, Minunno M, et al. Communication in dogs. *Animals.* 2018;8:131. doi:10.3390/ani8080131.

65. Gazit I, Terkel J. Domination of olfaction over vision in explosives detection by dogs. *Appl Anim Behav Sci.* 2003;82:65–73.

66. Houpt KA, Hintz HF, Shepherd P. The role of olfaction in canine food preferences. *Chem Senses.* 1978;3:281–290.

67. Lindemann B. Taste reception. *Physiol Rev.* 1996;76(3):719–766.

68. Kumazawa T, Kurihara K. Large synergism between monosodium glutamate and 5′-nucleotides in canine taste nerve responses. *Am J Physiol.* 1990;259(3):R420-R426.

69. Kurihara K, Kashiwayanagi M. Physiological studies on umami taste. *J Nutr.* 2000;130(4):931S-934S.

70. Stokke T. *The Effect of Reward Type and Reward Preference on the Performance of Detection Dogs* (Master's thesis). Norwegian University of Life Sciences; 2014.

71. Beaver B. *Canine Behavior. Insights and Answers.* 2nd ed. St. Lous: Saunders Elsevier; 2011.

72. Bradshaw JW, Rooney N. Dog social behavior and communication. In: Serpell J, ed. The Domestic Dog. Cambridge, UK: Cambridge University Press; 2016: 133–159. ISBN 978-0521425377.

73. Fox, MW. *Behaviour of Wolves, Dogs, and Related Canids.* London: Jonathan Cape Ltd; 1971.

74. Cohen JA, Fox MA. Vocalizations in wild canids and possible effects of domestication. *Behav Processes.* 1976;1(1):77–92.

75. Pongracz P, Molnar C, Miklosi A. Barking in family dogs: an ethological approach. *Vet J.* 2009;183:141–187.

76. Tembrock G. Canid vocalisations. *Behav Processes.* 1976;1:57–75.

77. Lindsay S. *Handbook of Applied Dog Training. Vol. 1:* Adaption and Learning. Ames, IA: Iowa State University Press; 2000.

78. Bekoff JM. Scent marking by free ranging domestic dogs. Olfactory and visual components. *Biol Behav.* 1979;4:123–139.

79. Topál J, Gácsi M, Miklósi Á, et al. Attachment to humans: a comparative study on hand-reared wolves and differently socialized dog puppies. *Anim Behav.* 2005;70:1367–1375.

80. Fox MW, Stelzner D. The effects of early experience on the development of inter and intraspecies social relationships in the dog. *Anim Behav.* 1967; 15:377–386

81. Hemmer H. Gestation period and postnatal development in felids. *Carnivore*. 1979;2:90–100.

82. Smith BA, Jansen GR. Brain development in the feline. *Nutr Rep Int*. 1977;16:487–495.

83. Gallo PV, Werboff J, Knox K. Protein restriction during gestation and lactation: development of attachment behavior in cats. *Behav Neural Biol*. 1980;29(2):216–23.

84. Windle WF, Fish MW. The development of the vestibular righting reflex in the cat. *J Compar Neurol*. 1932;54:85–96.

85. Bradshaw JWS, Casey RA, Brown SL. The Behaviour of the Domestic Cat. 2nd ed. Oxfordshire: UK, CABI, 2012

86. Olmstead CE, Villablanca JR. Development of behavioral audition in the kitten. *Physiol Behav*. 1980;74:705–712.

87. Mellen JD. Effects of early rearing experience on subsequent adult sexual behavior using domestic cats (*Felis catus*) as a model for exotic small felids. *Zoo Biol*. 1992;11:17–32.

88. Seitz PF. Infantile experience and adult behavior in animal subjects: II. Age of separation from the mother and adult behavior in the cat. *Psychosom Med*. 1959;21:353–378.

89. Chon E. The effects of queen (*Felis sylvestris*)-rearing versus hand-rearing on feline aggression and other problematic behaviors. *5th International Veterinary Behavior Meeting*. Minneapolis (MN): Purdue University Press; 2005:201–202.

90. O'Hanley KA, Pearl DL, Niel L. Risk factors for aggression in adult cats that were fostered through a shelter program as kittens. *Appl Anim Behav Sci*. 2021;236:105251.

91. Meier GW. Infantile handling and development in Siamese kittens. *J Compar Physiol Psychol*. 1961;54:284.

92. Collard RR. Fear of strangers and play behavior in kittens with varied social experience *Child Dev*. 1967:877–891.

93. Wilson M, Warren J, Abbott L. Infantile stimulation, activity, and learning by cats. *Child Dev*. 1965:843–853.

94. Karsh EB. Factors influencing the socialization of cats to people. In: Anderson RK, Hart BL, Hart LA, eds. *The Pet Connection: Its Influence on Our Health and Quality of Life*. Minneapolis: University of Minnesota Press; 1984.

95. Karsh E. The effects of early handling on the development of social bonds between cats and people. In: Katcher A, Beck A, eds. *New Perspectives on Our Lives with Companion Animals*. Philadelphia: University of Pennsylvania Press; 1983.

96. Casey RA, Bradshaw JWS. The effects of additional socialization for kittens in a rescue centre on their behavior and suitability as a pet. *Appl Anim Behav Sci*. 2008. 114:196–205.

97. Mendl M. The effects of litter-size variation on the development of play behaviour in the domestic cat: litters of one and two. *Anim Behav*. 1988;36:20–34.

98. Stammbach-Geering K. *Der Einfluss der Fütterung auf die Katze-Mensch-Beziehung (The Influence of Feeding on the Cat-Human Relationship)*. Verlag nicht ermittelbar; 1986.

101. Caro TM. Effects of the mother, object play, and adult experience on predation in cats. *Behav Neural Biol*. 1980;29:29–51.

103. Kolb B, Nonneman AJ. The development of social responsiveness in kittens. *Anim Behav*. 1975;23:368–374.

104. Ahola MK, Vapalahti K, Lohi H. Early weaning increases aggression and stereotypic behaviour in cats. *Sci Rep*. 2017;7:1–9. doi:10.1038/s41598-017- 11173-5.

105. Baerends-van Roon JM, Baerends GP. *The Morphogenesis of the Behaviour of the Domestic Cat*. Amsterdam: Elsevier Science; 1978.

105a. Ley JM. Feline Social Behavior and Personality. *August's Consultations in Feline Internal Medicine*. Elsevier, Inc.; 2015: 941–950.

106. Litchfield CA, Quinton G, Tindle H, et al. The 'Feline Five': an exploration of personality in pet cats (*Felis catus*). *PLoS One* 2017;12:e0183455.

107. McCune S. The impact of paternity and early socialisation on the development of cats' behaviour to people and novel objects. *Appl Anim Behav Sci*. 1995;45:109–124.

108. Turner DC. The human-cat relationship. In: Turner DC, Bateson P, eds. *The Domestic Cat: The Biology of Its Behaviour*. Cambridge: Cambridge University Press; 2000:4e6.

108a. Lowe SE, Bradshaw JWS. Ontogeny of individuality in the domestic cat in the home environment. *Anim Behav*. 2001;61:231e7.

109. Reisner IR, Houpt KA, Erb HN, Quimby FW. Friendly to humans and defensive aggression in cats: the influence of handling and paternity. *Physiol Behav*. 1994;55:1119e24.

110. Ramos D, Mills DS. Human directed aggression in Brazilian domestic cats: owner reported prevalence, contexts and risk factors. *J Fel Med Surg*. 2009;1:835e841. doi:10.1016/j.jfms.2009.04.006.

111. Mellen J. Effects of early rearing experience on subsequent adult sexual behavior using domestic cats (*Felis catus*) as a model for exotic small felids. *Zoo Biol*. 1992;11:17.

112. Seitz PFD. Infantile experience and adult behavior in animal subjects: II. Age of separation from the mother and adult behavior in the cat. *Psychosom Med*. 1959;21:353.

113. Bateson P, Barrett P. The development of play in cats. *Behaviour*. 1978;66.

114. Caro TM. The effects of experience on the predatory patterns of cats. *Behav Neural Biol*. 1980;29:1–28.

115. Tan PL, Counsilman JJ. The influence of weaning on prey-catching behaviour in kittens. *Z Tierpsychol*. 1985;70:148–164.

116. Hall SL, Bradshaw JWS. The influence of hunger on object play by adult domestic cats. *Appl Anim Behav Sci*. 1998;58:143–150.

117. Ottoni C, Van Neer W, De Cupere B, et al. The palaeogenetics of cat dispersal in the ancient world. *Nat Ecol Evol*. 2017;1:1–7.

118. Serpell JA. Domestication and history of the cat. In: Turner D, Bateson P, eds. *The Domestic Cat: The Biology of its Behaviour*. 3rd ed. Cambridge: Cambridge University Press; 2014:83–100.

119. Iwaza M, Doi T. Flexibility of the social system of the feral cat, *Felis catus*. *Anim Soc*. 1994;29:237–246.

120. Crowell-Davis SL, Curtis TM, Knowles RJ. Social organization in the cat: a modern understanding. *J Fel Med Surg*. 2004;6:19–28.

122. Alger JM, Alger SF. *Cat Culture*: The Social World of a Cat Shelter. Philadelphia: Temple University Press; 2005.

123. Curtis TM, Knowles RJ, Crowell-Davis SL. Influence of familiarity and relatedness on proximity and allogrooming in domestic cats (*Felis catus*). *Am J Vet Res*. 2003;64:1151–1154.

124. Macdonald DW, Yamaguchi N, Kerby G. Group-living in the domestic cat: its sociobiology and epidemiology. In: Turner DC, Bateson P, eds. *The Domestic Cat: The Biology of Its Behaviour*. 3rd ed. Cambridge: Cambridge University Press; 2014.

125. Beaver BV. *Feline Behavior*: a Guide for Veterinarians. 2nd ed. St. Louis: Saunders; 2003:142–143.

126. Bonanni R, Cafazzo S, Fantini C, et al. Feeding-order in an urban feral domestic cat colony: relationship to dominance, rank, sex and age. *Anim Behav*. 2007;74:1369e1379. doi:10.1016/j.anbehav.2007.02.029.

128. Natoli E, Baggio A, Pontier D. Male and female agonistic and affiliative relationships in a social group of farm cats (*Felis catus* L.). *Behav Processes*. 2001;53:137e143.

129. Malmstrom T, Kroger RH. Pupil shapes and lens optics in the eyes of terrestrial vertebrates. *J Exp Biol*. 2006;209:18–25.

130. Beitel RE. Acoustic pursuit of invisible moving targets by cats. *J Acoust Soc Am*. 1999;105:3449–3453.

131. Villablanca JR, Olmstead CE. Neurological development in kittens. *Dev Psychobiol*. 1979;12:101–127.

132. Raihani G, Gonzalez D, Arteaga L, et al. Olfactory guidance of nipple attachment and suckling in kittens of the domestic cat: inborn and learned responses. *Dev Psychobiol*. 2009;51:662–671.

133. Kovach JK, Kling A. Mechanisms of neonate sucking behaviour in the kitten. *Anim Behav*. 1967;15:91–101.

134. Brown SL, Bradshaw JWS. Communication in the domestic cat species. In: Turner DC, Bateson P, eds. *The Domestic Cat: The Biology of Its Behaviour*. 3rd ed. Cambridge: Cambridge University Press; 2014, 37-59.

135. Cafazzo S, Natoli E. The social function of tail up in the domestic cat (*Felis silvestris catus*). *Behav Processes*. 2009;80:60–66.

136. Von Muggenthaler E. The felid purr: a healing mechanism? *J Acoust Soc Am.* 2001;110:2666. doi:10.1121/1.4777098.

137. McComb K, Taylor AM, Wilson C, et al. The cry embedded within the purr. *Curr Biol.* 2009;19:R507-R508.

138. Pageat P, Gaultier E. Current research in canine and feline pheromones. *Vet Clin North Am Small Anim Pract.* 2003;33:187–211.

Resources and recommended reading

2015 AAHA Behavior Management Guidelines - https://www.aaha.org/aaha-guidelines/behavior-management/behavior-management-home.

Beaver BV. Feline behavior: a guide for veterinarians. 2nd ed. St. Louis: Saunders; 2003

Bradshaw JWS, Casey RA, Brown SL. The Domestic Cat, 2nd ed. Oxfordshire: CABI, 2012

Fear Free – fearfreepets.com.

Fear free Happy homes – fearfreehappyhomes.com - https://www.fearfreehappyhomes.com/kit/dogs-101/.

https://www.fearfreehappyhomes.com/kit/cats-101/.

Miklosi A. *Dog Behaviour, Evolution and Cognition.* 2nd ed. Oxford: Oxford University Press; 2015.

Scott JP, Fuller JL. *Genetics and the Social Behavior of the Dog.* Chicago, IL: The University of Chicago Press; 1965.

Serpell J, ed. *The Domestic Dog: Its Evolution, Behavior, and Interaction with People.* 2nd ed. Cambridge: Cambridge University Press; 2017.

Turner D, Bateson P, eds. *The Domestic Cat: The Biology of Its Behavior.* 3rd ed. Cambridge: Cambridge University Press; 2014.

Martin, D, Martin K. Puppy Start Right.

Puppy Socialization. What it is and how to do it. Marge Rogers and Eileen Anderson. Bright Friends Productions; 2021.

Kitten Kindergarten. How to educate your kitten successfully from the very first day. Sabine Schroll, DVM. Books on Demand; 1st ed. (April 13, 2017).

CHAPTER 3

Pet selection and the genetics of behavior

Lowell Ackerman, DVM, DACVD, MBA, MPA, CVA, MRCVS

Pet selection

One of the most valuable services a veterinarian can perform for pet parents is to assist them in picking the pet that best suits their home and lifestyle. This is an extremely useful, but underutilized facet of veterinary practice. Insufficient effort and forethought about the selection of a pet and the preparation for its arrival are significant factors associated with later relinquishment and euthanasia. Some pet parents spend more time picking a houseplant than they do a pet that will live with them for over a decade. For additional information on this important topic, please also see Chapter 4.

A prepurchase selection consultation is the best way to determine the needs of the prospective pet parent. There are several ways of determining whether the family is suited to pet parentship and, if so, which type of pet would be most compatible. Most veterinary associations, kennel groups, breed clubs, and humane societies have produced handouts and/or have websites on the subject (www.akc.org, www.ckc.ca, www.thekennelclub.org.uk, www.avma.org, www.aaha.org). Everyone has a stake in making sure the right pet ends up in the right household (see Table 3.1).

Some veterinarians feel uncomfortable discussing pet selection because they do not know much about the process other than consequences associated with physical disease. Acquiring a pet is an emotional experience, and veterinarians would do well to put themselves in the place of pet parents when considering what recommendations to make. You may need to consider what kind of pet would be best for a young family that has never owned a dog or cat

before. How about a family without children whose home is lavishly and expensively decorated? Consider an elderly pet parent on a pension who loves animals but cannot afford to spend much on the purchase and upkeep of a pet (see Box 3.1).

Since the pet selection consultation is so important, a questionnaire that provides all the necessary information for making an informed recommendation can be very helpful. It should be made clear to the pet parent, however, that it is not the role of the consultant to choose a particular breed, age, or sex for the family. Rather, the consultant should discuss the advantages as well as any concerns about each breed, and give suggestions on sex, age, and how to choose an individual dog or cat

Be certain also to take the opportunity at the selection consultation to provide the family with the health, feeding, and housing information and in particular, behavior and training that they will need to get started on the right track. Setting realistic expectations and providing behavioral advice at each puppy or kitten visit can lower the risk for future relinquishment.[1,2]

Breed considerations

The primary focus of selective breeding was to develop dogs that were best able to perform specific working functions such as herding, hunting, retrieving, or protection as well as more specific tasks such as search and rescue. Many dogs continue to be bred for working ability or for more specialized tasks such as therapy and assistance, while others are

Table 3.1 Some of the breed selector tools on the internet

Organization	Website
Iams (dog)	https://www.iams.com/breedselector/
Pedigree (dog)	https://www.pedigree.com/getting-a-new-dog/breed-match
Purina (dog)	https://www.purina.com/dogs/dog-breed-selector
Purina (cat)	https://www.purina.com/cat-breed-selector
Vetstreet (dog & cat)	http://www.vetstreet.com/breed-finder
Whiskas (cat)	https://www.whiskas.co.uk/cat-breed-selector

Modified from: Ackerman, L. Problem Free Pets. The Ultimate Guide to Pet Parenting. Dermvet; 2020.

Box 3.1 Factors for consideration in pet selection

- Species (dog, cat)
- Breed (purebred versus hybrid versus mixed)
  - Heritable medical and behavioral problems
  - Hybrid vigor
  - Breeding versus pet quality
- Age (puppy, kitten versus adult)
- Physical characteristics
  - General appearance
  - Size
  - Hair coat
- Breed behavioral characteristics
  - Breed function/work
  - Activity requirements
  - Temperament
  - Protective behavior/tendency to bark
- Sex (male versus female; neutered versus intact)
- Source (breeder, shelter, private home, retail) – assess care and upbringing
- Parent assessment (behavior, physical appearance, health)
- Pet parent considerations
  - Purpose of pet parentship – pet's function
  - Expense
  - Limitations of family members (e.g., allergy and disabilities)
  - Schedules and activities of family
  - Family's experience with pets
  - Environment – type of home, location, fencing

---

bred specifically for show. Therefore, there can be dramatic differences between the behavioral needs and the temperament of working lines and show lines.

By selecting a mixed-breed animal from a shelter, an abandoned animal can be saved from death, and the initial cost is very reasonable. One can even argue that there may be genetic advantages to obtaining mixed-breed animals ("hybrid vigor"). Selective breeding has produced dogs with a range of extreme proportions from giant breed to toy and from brachycephalic to chondrodysplastic, which in turn contributes to health problems. Furthermore, inbreeding can increase the likelihood of heritable diseases of both

health and behavior.[3,4] Eliminating genetic defects requires the identification and removal of affected individuals from the breeding pool, yet ironically, removal of these individuals further narrows the breeding pool. Therefore, outbreeding or even crossbreeding may be the most practical solution. With genetic testing available, the process can be facilitated when genotype can be conclusively demonstrated. Although kennel clubs and breed associations may be resistant to crossbreeding, this is the very way that today's breeds were originally developed.[5]

Therefore, the issues with respect to breed selection are (1) whether the prospective pet parent wants a purebred pet; (2) understanding the function for which the breed was originally developed; (3) whether the dogs are bred for work or show; (4) the potential health and behavior issues of the breed; and (5) whether the dog is likely to be suitable to the pet parent's home, lifestyle, and goals of pet parentship. Despite the downsides to inbreeding, predictability is likely to be highest for size, coat, function, health, and behavior from selecting a purebred dog with known parentage (see Box 3.1). Of course, while physical and behavioral attributes tend to be most noticeable in dogs, it is important to appreciate that the same concepts are applicable to cats. It is just that physical and behavioral variabilities tend to be less evident in cats, although each breed definitely has distinctive attributes.

With hundreds of breeds of dogs and dozens of breeds of cats to choose from, it is advisable that the pet parents first narrow the selection process down to a few breeds that appeal to them before attending a selection consult at the veterinary hospital. This can be accomplished by providing suggested reading and websites (see Appendix A) as well as having the pet parent attend dog or cat shows to see a variety of breeds and meet breeders and/or handlers. The pet parents might also be encouraged to contact groomers, trainers, or kennel clubs for additional input. The websites of national breed clubs and veterinary organizations can provide useful information on pet selection for pet parents although the wording used on the websites can be misleading. For example, words such as "aloof" and phrases such as "one-owner dog" might seem benign to a pet parent. However, dogs described as aloof are very often prone to fearful and anxious behavior and dogs that are one-owner dogs can very well be dogs that show aggression or fear to those outside of the family. Helping pet parents decipher the language of dog breed standards can help them to better understand the breed's predispositions. Another option is to visit one of the computerized selection services on the internet (see Table 3.1).

Two of the most important aspects of pet selection include determining the family's reason for desiring a pet as well as any limitations the family may envision for the pet. This may not only help them to choose the right type of pet but also eliminate certain breeds from consideration (see Table 3.2). For example, a family that includes a member allergic to cats may want to favor a dog as a better pet in that circumstance. A family that is interested in obtaining a pet primarily for activities might be interested in engaging in agility training, flyball, or herding trials, or might be a sedentary couple or incapable of providing intensive exercise or training. Similarly, potential pet parents may want to consider breeds for a particular type of work (herding, hunting, or

Table 3.2 Breed tendencies that might be important in the selection process

Condition	Breed(s)
Tendency to drool and slobber	Basset Hound, Black and Tan Coonhound, Bloodhound, Bluetick Coonhound, Boxer, Bullmastiff, Chinese Shar-Pei, Clumber Spaniel, Dogue De Bordeaux, English Bulldog, English Setter, French Bulldog, Great Dane, Great Pyrenees, Irish Water Spaniel, Kuvasz, Mastiff, Neapolitan Mastiff, Newfoundland, Plott Hound, Pyrenean Mastiff, Redbone Coonhound, Saint Bernard, Spanish Mastiff
Tendency to snore	Boston Terrier, Boxer, Chinese Shar-Pei, English Bulldog, English Toy Spaniel, French Bulldog, Pekingese, Pug, Shih Tzu
Tendency to shed	Akita, Alaskan Malamute, American Eskimo Dog, Beagle, Belgian Sheepdog, Belgian Tervuren, Bernese Mountain Dog, Boston Terrier, Chow Chow, Dalmatian, German Shepherd Dog, Great Pyrenees, Keeshond, Lakeland Terrier, Maltese, Newfoundland, Pekingese, Pomeranian, Pug, Samoyed, Shetland Sheepdog, Shiba Inu, Shih Tzu, Siberian Husky, Sussex Spaniel
Considered less troublesome for those with pet allergies*	Affenpinscher, American Hairless Terrier, Bedlington Terrier, Bichon Frise, Bolognese, Bouvier des Flandres, Chinese Crested, Coton de Tulear, Dandie Dinmont Terrier, Giant Schnauzer, Havanese, Irish Water Spaniel, Lagotto Romagnolo, Lhasa Apso, Maltese, Miniature Poodle, Peruvian Inca Orchid, Poodle, Polish Lowland Sheepdog, Portuguese Water Dog, Puli, Silky Terrier, Skye Terrier, Soft-Coated Wheaten Terrier, Standard Schnauzer, Welsh Terrier, Xoloitzcuintli, Yorkshire Terrier

*Not necessarily nonallergenic or hypoallergenic, but tends to shed less and/or produce less dander. However, studies have demonstrated that there does not appear to be any significant difference in the levels of the major dog allergen (Can f 1), regardless of breed. (Nicholas CE, Wegienka GR, Havstad, SL, et al. Dog allergen levels in homes with hypoallergenic compared with nonhypoallergenic dogs. *Am J Rhinol Allergy.* 2011;25:252–256.)

household protection), a particular size range, or behavioral characteristics.

If a pet parent then has a query about a breed with which you are less familiar, the veterinarian should be prepared to do the research before making recommendations. If time is taken to document pros and cons for each breed as you experience or read about them, eventually an impressive array of facts could be collected for the would-be pet parent. In addition, resources in the way of books, journals, videos, blogs, and websites can be valuable.

Pet parents will need information on:

- breed standards (physical attributes)
- breed function (i.e., the selection pressures on this breed when it was developed)
- potential genetic and health problems
- breed behavioral characteristics
- behavior disorders or clusters of clinical signs that have been reported or documented in the breed

Although there are a number of books that provide breed behavioral profiles (see recommended reading, on page 46.) there can be a great deal of variability between lines, across different geographical areas, and even between individuals within the same litter. Veterinarians should have some idea of the characteristics that are most predictable and which traits are more affected by environment and training. Veterinarians should also be cognizant of potential problems such as tendencies toward aggression, high activity level, fear, sensitivity to pain and noise, and specific conditions such as flank sucking in Doberman Pinschers, wool sucking in Siamese cats, spinning in Bull Terriers, and tail chasing in German Shepherd Dogs. With that said, veterinarians should stick to the facts and their clinical experience, avoid broad generalizations that rely solely on opinion. For example, there is a factual difference between the following statements:

"German Shepherd Dogs are genetically predisposed to tail chasing and lumbosacral disease." "Chihuahuas are land sharks. They are all aggressive." Stick with factual representations and clinical impressions, not opinion.

Pet age

Puppies less than 3 months and kittens less than 7 weeks are most receptive to socialization, adapting to new environments, and habituating to new stimuli. Young pets may also be a better mix for families with existing pets. Conversely, puppies and kittens require a committed family to provide the appropriate time and energy to socialize properly and train the puppy or kitten at this highly impressionable age. Adult dogs and cats may already be insufficiently socialized or improperly trained so that problems may be difficult or impossible to correct. Adult pets may have difficulty adapting to an environment or social group that is dissimilar from their previous household. In fact, one study found that adult cats are more likely than kittens to be returned to shelters due to behavior problems and incompatibility with other pets. By comparison, adult pets may be able to handle longer pet parent departures; may present fewer problems with overexuberant play, nipping, and chewing; and may already have some basic training.[6] In addition, while behavior assessment tests in young puppies and kittens may be poorly predictive of adult behavior, predictability may be greater when assessing older puppies and kittens and adult pets (see below).

Pet gender

Male dogs and cats are slightly larger in stature than females. Male dogs may mark, mount, masturbate, and display aggression toward other male dogs. Some studies suggest that male dogs may be more trainable for certain tasks, such as scent work.[7] A study of pet dogs suggested that male dogs are more likely to score above the median on aggression directed at social group members.[8]

Source

The best source for a purebred pet is a breeder who carefully considers the behavioral and medical aspects of the animals they are breeding, although rescue groups and shelters may also be good options. With that said, obtaining a puppy from a breeder does not guarantee that the puppy will be without serious physical or behavioral genetic predispositions. Breeders may not breed for the traits most important to pet parents, such as temperament; cannot completely control the genetic makeup of any individual; often lack education on the behavioral characteristics which would indicate a potential problem later on; and finding an excellent breeder may be challenging. If puppies and kittens are obtained directly from the breeder, the prospective parent can better assess and ensure that they have been properly cared for and have been socialized prior to adoption (see Chapter 2).[9] Quality breeders should have at least one parent on site. If the puppies are less than 8 weeks old, they should ideally be with the dam and the litter. One of the best predictors of the behavior of the puppy or kitten in the future is the behavior of the parents. For example, if the breeder will not allow interaction with the sire or dam if onsite; if the sire and/or the dam barks, growls, or lunges at the prospective pet parent; or if the sire or dam will not permit petting or seems fearful/standoffish, the potential for a hereditary predisposition to those behaviors is likely to be present in the puppies. Similarly, if the queen or tom are friendly and seek social interaction, they very likely have passed the genes for those tendencies to their offspring. Studies in cats have clearly demonstrated that paternal genes are more likely to influence boldness, resistance to handling or restraint, and perhaps even friendliness.[9,10] Therefore, whenever possible, especially in cats, observe and assess the tom. Reputable breeders should be happy to provide references (veterinarians and previous buyers) and should be proud to show you their kennel/cattery and other dogs/cats that may be related. Veterinarians or educated members of the veterinary healthcare team can offer to watch videos or view images of the litter or parents prior to adoption and give an educated opinion of any red flags.

Purebred dogs and cats that are obtained from pet stores, breeding farms, puppy mills, and animal shelters usually have unknown medical and genetic histories, although each source should be judged on its own merits. Such pets may be stressed by weaning, transport, handling, and housing, and have high levels of exposure to other animals at a time when their resistance is low or suspect. They are also at higher risk for respiratory and intestinal diseases than those from private pet parents.[11] Dogs obtained from pet stores or commercial breeders are up to two times more likely to display aggression toward familiar and unfamiliar people and dogs, fear on walks, fear of people and other pets, fear of objects, increased separation-related behaviors, and increased reactivity when compared to puppies obtained from other sources.[12-17] In addition, they are reported to be less trainable and more excitable than those acquired from other sources.[15] For the reasons stated above, advise caution when pet parents plan to acquire a dog or cat from a retail store or a commercial breeder that they cannot personally visit.

Saving the life of a pet from a breed rescue organization or shelter is often preferred by well-meaning pet parents. Like any source, there are risks and benefits associated with adoption of a pet that has been rehomed, whether through a rescue, shelter, or from a friend. Sometimes the background and reason for relinquishment are known but often, the quality of the previous environment and the extent of socialization are unknown. In fact, health or behavior issues may have

been and often are a factor in relinquishment. The same guidelines which are used to assess dogs and cats at a breeder's home can be used in the shelter. With that said, there are no validated, easy to implement, publicly available temperament tests which can be used to assess current behavior with the goal of predicting future behavior. Shelters are stressful places. Dogs and cats behave differently there. Even a change in environment from the breeder's home or a foster parent's home to the adoptive parent's home can cause behaviors to appear or to terminate. The best thing to advise pet parents to do is to look for objective signs of fear, anxiety, and stress in the new pet prior to adoption. If the pet parent is told that the pet is not aggressive or is not fearful, that should be considered carefully based on the current information of the lack of predictive value of shelter temperament testing.

For mixed-breed dogs, DNA testing is commercially available to help determine the relative proportion of possible breeds in the mix. These tests are based on the presence of genetic markers which are not completely predictive but may prove to be useful in determining the behavioral characteristics of the pet, behavioral expectations, and potential health concerns that might arise. In one study of 20 mixed-breed dogs, in only four of the dogs did the DNA testing match with the breed type that had been selected on the basis of visual identification.[18] It is important to realize that these tests rely on matching an individual's genetic markers with known purebreds in its database, so the determination is a reflection of its database rather than a measure of genes attributable to specific breeds.

Many pet parents decide on a particular breed because of a pet that they have met through a relative, friend, or acquaintance, or pets they have shared their lives with previously. If that pet was healthy and had a desirable personality, it may be possible to contact the breeder to see if related individuals from more recent litters might be available. In those cases, the pet parent should be informed that even though a dog or cat comes from the same breeder or is of the same breed as their previous pet or a beloved neighbor's pet, they will have their own genetic predispositions which will be affected by the environment in which they live. Veterinarians might also consider collecting listings of breeders who have proven to produce problem-free pets. In addition, the kennel clubs of most countries publish directories of breed and rescue associations either in print or online. (See resources and recommended reading).

Temperament testing

While numerous puppy temperament tests have been developed, there is no evidence that they accurately predict adult behavior, other than fear and reactivity.[19-27] One study found no correlation between puppy biting and the development of aggression at 1 and 3 years.[23] Testing of 8–16-week-old puppies was not predictive for separation related disorders.[24] On the other hand, in a study in which puppies were assessed during veterinary visits between 8 and 16 weeks of age, about 10% displayed extreme behaviors, including vocalization, panting, ears flattened, and avoidance, that correlated with data collected 1 year later.[20] By 3-4 months, following the primary sensitive period, assessment testing may have increased predictive value as problems such as fears, possessive and territorial aggression, barking, and resistance to handling begin to emerge.[19,21,26,27] In addition, there is variability as to when traits might be identifiable for specific functions. For example, when testing potential police dogs, retrieval was predictable at 8 weeks of age, while aggression was not predictable until 9 months.[19] Therefore, when selecting a puppy, prospective pet parents should combine breed information and observation of the parents with evaluation of the puppy to identify extremes of behavior, including fear, avoidance, or excessive reactivity, that might be warning signs for future problems.

A number of assessment tests have also been developed for shelter dogs to assist in matching and adoption success.[28-36] These tests assess factors such as response to cage approach, handling, food bowl, toys, unfamiliar people, toddlers, dolls, stuffed dogs, and an artificial hand.[28,30-31,35,37-38] However, behaviors observed during these evaluations do not reliably predict future behavior in the home, and are impacted by stress, personnel, familiarity, and human-memory bias, and subject to false-positives, false-negatives, and lack of test-retest and interrater reliability.[30,33-40]

In a 2019 study, Patronek et al. found that none of the canine shelter assessment protocols had sufficient evidence of reliability and validity.[39] Using a hypothetical statistical analysis, Patronek and Bradley determined the prediction that a dog would exhibit threat or bite problems after adoption was "no better than flipping a coin."[40] Similarly in several studies evaluating aggression assessment protocols, there was insufficient validity for use as a method of decision making about adopting or keeping dogs as pets.[29,33-39] In fact, most recently, it was shown that even though owners report problem behaviors, most had a high level of satisfaction with their dogs. For example, despite failing food guarding tests, many owners reported that adopted dogs did not exhibit food aggression in the home, or did not consider food guarding to be a challenge to keeping the dog.[35,42] Instead of provocative tests shelter staff should collect behavior histories at relinquishment, verify serious reported incidents, screen out dogs that are too threatening to handle, and spend resources on engaging dogs in enjoyable activities including walks, socialization with people, training, and dog play groups.[40]

For cats, the sensitive period for socialization begins to wane by 7-9 weeks of age. Therefore, for the assessment of kitten temperament, 2-3 months may be more accurate than for puppies. Based on observer ratings, Feaver et al. proposed three cat personality dimensions a) bold, confident, and easy going b) shy/nervous, and c) active and aggressive.[43] (Also see chapter 2). Initial estimates were that 15% of cats seem to be resistant to socialization with humans.[44] While temperament assessment may be an aid in predicting behavior in the home, cat personality and adoption compatibility are based not only on the cat's behavior at the time but by owner personality, owner expectations, and the quality and level of initial counseling and resources they receive on introducing the cat to the home, behavioral needs, and learning.[45,46] The modified Feline-ality program, which evaluates cats based on posture, greeting when cage opened, cage condition, and novel room and social interactions, may aid adopters in matching the appropriate cat to their needs and household.[46]

Behavioral genetics

We are now at a stage where major advances are being made in the association of traits (both physical and behavioral) with genetic variants. In addition to a variety of genetic tests indicating disease susceptibility in a variety of breeds, there are also a number of traits and characteristics for which genetic associations have been determined. In the dog, this includes shedding tendency (MC5R), skull diversity (BMP3), hair length (FGF5), altitude adaptation (ESPA1), double versus single coat (CFA28), and multiple colors (various genes). In the cat, in addition to coat color genes, there are gene associations with long versus short hair (FGF5), curly coat (LPAR6 and KRT71), and several others.

While we are currently not in a position to identify tail chasing in Bull Terriers or aggression in English Springer Spaniels with a direct DNA test, the time may not be far off. There are tests for behavior propensity in the Belgian Malinois, associated with polymorphisms of the dopamine transporter gene (SLC6A3), which can be associated with seizures, episodic biting behaviors, "glazing over," and general loss of clarity. There are also numerous genetic tests for a variety of neurological disorders that can be associated with aberrant behaviors such as cerebellar ataxia, cerebellar cortical degeneration, psychomotor epilepsy, glycogen storage diseases, juvenile epilepsy, episodic falling, exercise-induced collapse, myasthenic syndrome, and several other presentations.[3] While dogs and cats (and humans) are clearly a lot more than their collective DNA, the field of behavioral genetics is coming into its own as gene mutations are being recognized that have a direct effect on behavior.

It is suspected that approximately 30% of the estimated 20,000 or so genes in the human genome are expressed primarily in the brain, and of course it is the brain that governs everything humans do, think, or perceive. Should we suspect otherwise in animals? Genetics plays a key role in predicting behaviors, and yet we are very early in the evolution of characterizing the process. Behaviors such as herding and retrieving are firmly entrenched in some breeds, and we are getting closer to understanding the genetic basis for these traits. The same can be said for trainability and boldness in dogs.[47] In addition, it appears that dogs have evolved a social-cognitive specialization that allows them unusual skill in cooperating and communicating with humans.[48] In fact, dogs and humans accept each other into a mutual social structure, which appears to have been the result of genetic selection.[49] Genetics may even play a central role in why pets are so willing to consider us as their loving family members, and genetic alterations similar to those seen in human Williams syndrome may be a clue to how pets became so sociable. Behavioral traits do have a genetic basis, and there is often a high degree of genetic correlation between traits.[50]

There have been some developments in identifying quantitative trait loci (QTLs) important in some behavioral conditions, but there is much more to be learned in years to come. Since behaviors are often conserved within breed groups, individual qualities (e.g., retrieving ability) can often be achieved by the appropriate selection of specific breeds, especially if representative family members can be observed. For mixed-breed dogs, a rough approximation might be accomplished by discerning which breeds primarily contributed to an individual animal through commercially available heritage profiles see Box 3.2.

Box 3.2 Disorders that have a behavioral component for which DNA testing is currently available

Alaskan Husky encephalopathy	Late-onset ataxia
Alexander disease	Lysosomal storage disease
Border Collie collapse	L2-hydroxyglutaric aciduria
Centronuclear myopathy	Malignant hyperthermia
Cerebellar abiotrophy	Mannosidosis
Cerebellar ataxia	Mucopolysaccharidosis IIIb
Cobalamin malabsorption	Multidrug resistance I (MDRI) mutation
Charcot–Marie–Tooth disease	Muscular dystrophy
Dandy–Walker malformation	Musladin–Leuke syndrome
Deafness	Myasthenic syndrome
Degenerative myelopathy	Myoclonic epilepsy
Episodic falling	Narcolepsy
Exercise-induced collapse	Necrotizing meningoencephalitis
Fucosidosis	Neonatal encephalopathy
Globoid cell leukodystrophy	Neuronal ceroid lipofuscinosis
Glycogen storage diseases	Paroxysmal dyskinesia
GM-1 gangliosidosis	Periodic aggression (behavior propensity)
GM-2 gangliosidosis	Polyneuropathy
Greyhound polyneuropathy	Pyruvate dehydrogenase phosphatase I deficiency
Hypothyroidism with goiter	Sensory neuropathy
Juvenile epilepsy	Startle disease (hyperekplexia)
Lafora body disease	Van Den Ende–Gupta syndrome

Abstracted from: Ackerman L. *Proactive Pet Parenting: Anticipating Pet Health Problems Before They Happen*. Problem Free Publishing; 2020.

Grounds to suspect a genetic basis for behavioral problems

We clearly appreciate several inherited behavior traits in animals, including the sophisticated herding ability of the Border Collie, the signaling antics of the Nova Scotia Duck Tolling Retriever, the tracking ability of many hounds, and the fetching ability of many retrievers. In fact, most of the breeds created today have unique physical and behavioral traits which have been accentuated with each passing generation. There is no reason to suspect that many other behavioral traits, desirable and undesirable, are not heritable to at least some extent. For example, shyness or fearfulness appears to demonstrate high heritability.[51] For traits such as aggression toward strangers, trainability, and chasing, genes may contribute 60–70% of behavioral variation among breeds.[52] Other studies suggest that the heritability of many behavioral traits in dogs is low.[53]

In dogs, there is interesting evidence to suggest that the species was domesticated intentionally, with selection to retain juvenile traits, a process known as pedomorphosis. Thus, both physical and behavioral traits of the young, such as skulls that are unusually broad for their length, whining, barking, and submissiveness, are retained in dogs throughout their lifespan, but are typically outgrown by wolves as they mature. Domestication of many species has led to interesting traits not seen in the wild, such as the appearance of dwarf and giant varieties, piebald coat color, curly tails, rolled tails, shortened tails, floppy ears, and changes in reproductive cycles. It is reasonable to predict that selection for tameness may alter regulatory mechanisms for neurochemistry, and the developmental pathways they govern. Animals may have participated more directly in the process, as tamer animals tended to succeed with close proximity to humans and access to their food and care. It is not unreasonable to

conclude that anomalies in these behaviors could have both heritable and environmental components.

One of the most studied aspect of this process is often referred to as the farm-fox experiments (Balyaev's foxes) in which a population of foxes was subjected to selection on the basis of tameness alone.[54] Over successive generations, the foxes had both morphologic changes and behavioral changes that made them tamer to handle, suggesting that there are genetic loci that influence tame behavior. However, domestication likely requires a more comprehensive approach focused on essential adaptations to human-modified environments.[55]

When it comes to traits like aggression, heritability appears to play a role in addition to environmental influence which also affect the expression of genes. Nature versus nurture need not be a zero-sum game. For several years, investigators have examined how two neurotransmitters, serotonin and vasopressin, interact to control aggression. In many species, aggressive behavior is inversely correlated with the level of serotonin in the brain. Vasopressin seems to have the opposite effect. In fact, serotonin may decrease aggressive behavior in part by inhibiting the activity of the vasopressin neurons. Potentially, an inefficient serotonin system may let vasopressin build up in the central nervous system, priming the body for aggressive behavior. The important point to be made here is that there is unlikely to be an aggression gene that codes for the expression of growling or barking. It is more likely that a gene exists that codes for some protein that codes for variable functionality of serotonin and which, in turn, alters other neurotransmitters, including vasopressin and many others.

There have been many studies to suggest that a variety of behaviors have a heritable basis, and may even purport to have associations with certain genetic variants. This could prove to be very useful when attempting to select pets for a specific purpose. However, at present, even though some genetic variants have been identified to be "associated" with a variety of behaviors, such a selection process is not imminent in the near future, and most of these variants are not available for veterinary teams to select for testing.

This goal of detecting genetic variants associated with behavioral risk is shared with human medicine, and many candidate genes have been assessed in pets. For example, some genomic regions associated with fearfulness in dogs appear to overlap human neuropsychiatric loci associated with anxiety.[56,57] It is possible that reduced fear and aggression variants at such loci may have been involved in the domestication process.[58]

There are many studies that suggest that behaviors are strongly influenced by genetic variants, including hunting performance,[59,60] capacity to defend,[61] and impulsivity.[62] In more recent studies, there may be associations suggested between allelic variants or polymorphisms and genetic traits; however, such associations may have low specificity. For example, the DRD4 gene, associated with polymorphisms of the dopamine D4 receptor, have been implicated in both human and canine behavior studies, and this makes intuitive sense because dopamine D4 receptors are abundant in the limbic system, which is responsible for emotions and cognitive functions. While there may be some association of such polymorphisms with behaviors such as excitability, reactivity, or even aggression, such work requires a lot more validation before it has clinical utility. Similarly, serotonin transport (5HTT) and tyrosine hydroxylase genes may eventually prove useful in assessing pets for certain behaviors, but are not yet suitable to be clinical tools. Artificial selection has likely resulted in the relatively rapid evolution of brain-expressed genes during the domestication process.[63]

Such studies are not limited to dogs. It is interesting to note that individuals may even attribute personality traits on the basis of coat color of cats. For example, orange cats may be considered friendlier, tricolored cats as intolerant, and white cats as aloof.[64] Coat color is definitely genetic in origin, and yet perceptions of personality on the basis of coat color may possibly reflect personal bias rather than science. It has also been suggested the oxytocin receptor gene (OXTR) polymorphisms may be involved in feline social behaviors, especially friendliness and roughness.[65] It actually appears that signatures of selection in the cat genome are linked to genes associated with memory, fear-conditioning behavior, and stimulus-reward learning, potentially all attributes associated with domestication.[66]

The other likelihood is that genetics alone is probably not sufficient for clinical manifestations of disorders like aggression. We know of the critical socialization period for dogs and cats, and that tractability is directly related to whether or not animals were properly socialized during that period. This could serve as one of the many potential triggers for clinical forms of aggression. So, theoretically, a dog (for example) could have a genetic predisposition toward aggression, but it only becomes clinically manifested if the dog was improperly socialized during the sensitive period for socialization, or affected by some other trigger, such as diet, hormonal levels, or any number of other potential moderators of behavior. Does this likely occur in dogs? Probably. One small study demonstrated that supplementing the diet of a dog with aggression toward people with tryptophan and changing to a low-protein diet with a high relative tryptophan to large neutral amino acids ratio may reduce aggression. The rationale here is that tryptophan is a precursor of serotonin and that supplementation with tryptophan (or relatively increasing the ratio of tryptophan to competing amino acids) will increase brain serotonin levels and reduce aggression. The presumption is thus that aggression is somehow associated with defective neurotransmitter metabolism, which is likely (at least partially) a heritable event that can be moderated, at least in part, by diet (see Chapter 13). Similarly, it has been proposed that oral tyrosine may induce increased levels of catecholamine (norepinephrine and epinephrine) in the brain, at least in certain breeds, perhaps affecting the ability to focus attention.[67] These are certainly interesting concepts, but not sufficiently supported to be relied upon for reliable behavioral management.

Genes causing behavioral problems

Hoping that genetics will explain all behavioral problems is simplistic, and does not reflect the way that genes actually work. Genes do not cause disorders—they code for proteins that interact with other proteins and the environment to cause variable effects. Even in single-gene defects such as von Willebrand disease in Doberman Pinschers, the resultant level of von Willebrand factor is a continuous trait that does not match well with our clinical impression of a classic recessive disorder. Thus, while an individual animal with this monogenic disorder is clear, affected, or a carrier, there is a huge overlap in von Willebrand factor levels between carrier and affected individuals. It is this variability in penetrance and expressivity that keenly complicates our understanding of even simple genetic disorders and confounds our ability to appreciate complex relationships between genes, proteins, and environmental impact. So, while we have successfully navigated the genomic revolution, a much more complicated fate awaits us as we start to investigate the new field of proteomics, an arena in which we must contend not with 20,000 or so genes written in a four-letter alphabet, but the mind-boggling world of a million proteins written in combinations of 20 amino acids. The structure of these proteins is important, but it is the patterns in which they fold three-dimensionally and their interaction with other proteins and the universe around them that produce almost infinite variability in presentation. Thus, in human medicine, detecting a hypothetical genetic variant for schizophrenia may indicate some heightened risk of developing the condition, but it is not a foregone conclusion that having the gene mutation makes schizophrenia inevitable. The same is true for traits in both dogs and cats.

Another likelihood as we explore the genetics of behavioral conditions is that different mutations in different genes may cause the same apparent end result, at least in some breeds. For most behavioral problems seen in animals, we are not expecting to find a single genetic mutation responsible for a major behavioral problem, such as aggression, and certainly not in all breeds. Even if aggression was controlled by a single genetic mutation in one breed, we would not expect it necessarily to be the same in other breeds. For example, the gene that causes progressive retinal atrophy (PRA) in the Irish Setter is significantly different from the gene that causes PRA in the Siberian Husky, or the Cardigan Welsh Corgi, or the Abyssinian, for that matter. Accordingly, while are DNA tests for PRA in each of these breeds (and in several others), the mutation seen in one breed is rarely shared with other than closely related breeds. Thus, while Siberian Huskies share the same gene mutation for PRA with Samoyeds and the DNA test can therefore be used in both breeds, this is fortuitous (given the potential relatedness of those breeds) rather than commonplace. So, even if we ever developed a DNA test of a risk factor for aggression (or a compulsive disorder, for example) in a particular breed, we should not presume that the behavior results from that same variant in other breeds as well.

Unfortunately, for the majority of behavioral clinical signs and disorders seen in animals (and humans), we are not expecting to find a single genetic mutation to explain the problem. For these types of continuous traits that exist along a spectrum of behaviors, attempts have been made to map contributing genes with QTLs. Polygenic traits are usually caused by a relative handful of genes rather than many genes. This bolsters our hopes that genetic tests will eventually be available for most complex problems, including aggression and compulsive disorders (as well as hip dysplasia and many other heritable problems). It remains possible, for these and other complex disorders, that there may be a small number of genes that have fairly major effects and a larger number of genes that play a more minor role. If this is true, it should make the task of finding at least the first few QTLs that much easier. That being said, most of these traits are also likely to be multifactorial and influenced by factors other than just genetics.

Quantitative traits vary on a continuous scale and are determined by the action of genes at many loci (QTLs) as well as by many nongenetic environmental factors.[68] These QTLs are regions of DNA that have been associated with phenotypic traits; they may be located on different chromosomes, they may have a major or minor influence on expression of the trait, and they may raise or lower the risk of that trait manifestation. While still in its infancy, this approach will likely become extremely important as we look to determine risk for the development of traits controlled by more than one gene, such as diabetes mellitus, cancer, hip dysplasia, and many behavioral disorders. While it is unlikely that we will ever find a single gene responsible for many of these conditions, it is quite possible that we will find several genes (or markers) that are associated with increased or decreased risk for a specific condition that can be considered in aggregate to help predict risk. For example, we might find that the presence of some QTLs are associated with an increased risk of flank sucking in Doberman Pinschers, while others are associated with decreasing the risk, and the aggregate risk can then be characterized for a specific animal. There are already some preliminary findings to support such associations for canine traits such as compulsive disorder (stereotypies and repetitive behaviors)[69] and certain phenotypes (including size, trainability, herding ability, and even longevity).[70]

There are hopes that genetic screening might eventually help detect risk for problematic behaviors, such as aggression. While there are clearly genetic factors underlying fear and aggression, the genetic predisposition for aggression to a pet parent or family dog has been demonstrated to be distinct from aggression toward unfamiliar humans and dogs.[71] Prevalence studies also provide an indication of breed propensities and trends, and certain breeds often appear to be overrepresented in such studies. Studies have also demonstrated breed-specific differences in sociability, fearfulness, aggression, and behavior consistency between breeds.[72] While both nature and nurture determine behavior, there is also evidence that environmental effects (e.g., nutrition and stress) can be conserved in genes and even passed to the next generation (epigenetics).[3]

Conclusion

It is likely that many of the behavioral problems noted in this book have at least some heritable component. However, even with a genetic predisposition, environmental triggers are likely necessary for full manifestation of the trait. Research is actively under way to find genetic links for behavior disorders, beginning with those that are common or exclusive to specific breeds.[3]

Finding a genetic mutation or marker-based tests for behavior problems such as impulsive aggression in English Springer Spaniels or English Cocker Spaniels, spinning in Bull Terriers, tail chasing in German Shepherd Dogs, or fearfulness in German Shorthaired Pointers would provide a means of identifying and removing affected individuals from the breeding population. In addition, knowledge of the precise genetic anomaly presents intriguing possibilities for new and more effective forms of treatment. It is, however, important to temper enthusiasm with practicality. While the prospects for genetic testing are tantalizing, it is important to realize that most behavioral traits will not be the result of single-gene interactions, but complex multifactorial representations of a collection of genetic variants, many breed specific, and combined with certain environmental aspects. Screening pets for such variants is unlikely to be diagnostic but is rather meant to detect risk factors that might possibly contribute to phenotypic outcomes.

We should anticipate that optimal behavior outcomes are shaped by genetic selection, the presence of certain genotypes, prenatal health, maternal behavior, neonatal experience, appropriate environment and enrichment, socialization, and the ongoing experiences, behavioral management, and training after adoption into the new home. When it comes to genetic screening in such a selection process, while studies of various genomic regions have provided some tantalizing prospects for associating behaviors in certain breeds, most such tests are not commercially available, so are not yet practical screening tests to be used by today's veterinary team. Stay tuned!

References

1. Patronek GJ, Glickman LT, Beck AM, et al. Risk factors for relinquishment of cats to an animal shelter. *J Am Vet Med Assoc.* 1996;209(3):582–588.

2. Patronek GJ, Glickman LT, Beck AM, et al. Risk factors for relinquishment of dogs to an animal shelter. *J Am Vet Med Assoc.* 1996;209(3):572–581.

3. Ackerman L. *Proactive Pet Parenting*: Anticipating Pet Health Problems Before They Happen. Westborough, MA: Problem Free Publishing; 2020.

4. Gough A, Thomas A, O'Neill D. *Breed Predisposition to Disease in Dogs and Cats.* 3rd ed. Ames, Iowa: Wiley Blackwell; 2018.

5. Bradshaw J. *Dog Sense*: How the New Science of Dog Behavior Can Make You a Better Friend to Your Pet. New York: Basic Books; 2011.

6. Powell, L, Reinhard C, Satriale D. et al. Characterizing unsuccessful animal adoptions: age and breed predict the likelihood of return, reasons for return and post-return outcomes. *Sci Rep.* 2021;11:8018. https://doi.org/10.1038/s41598-021-87649-2

7. Fattah AFA, Abdel-Hamid SE. Influence of gender, neuter status, and training method on police dog narcotics, olfaction performance, behavior and welfare. *J Adv Vet Anim Res.* 2020;7:655–662.

8. Hsu Y, Sun L. Factors associated with aggressive responses in pet dogs. *Appl Anim Behav Sci.* 2010;123:108–123.

9. McCune S. The impact of paternity and early socialisation on the development of cats' behaviour to people and novel objects. *Appl Anim Behav Sci.* 1995;45:109–124.

10. Reisner IR, Houpt KA, Erb HN, et al. Friendliness to humans and defensive aggression in cats: the influence of handling and paternity. *Physiol Behav.* 1994;55:1119–1124.

11. Scarlett JM, Saidla JE, Pollock RVH. Source of acquisition as a risk factor for disease and death in pups. *J Am Vet Med Assoc.* 1994;204:1906–1913.

12. McMillan FD. Behavioral and psychological outcomes for dogs sold as puppies through pet stores and/or born in commercial breeding establishments: current knowledge and putative causes. *J Vet Behav.* 2017;19:14–26.

13. Jagoe JA. *Behaviour Problems in the Domestic Dog*: A Retrospective and Prospective Study to Identify Factors Influencing Their Development. Unpublished Ph.D. thesis. Cambridge, UK: University of Cambridge; 1994.

14. Bennett PC, Rohlf VI. Owner-companion dog interactions: relationships between demographic variables, potentially problematic behaviours, training engagement and shared activities. *Appl Anim Behav Sci.* 2007;102:65–84.

15. McMillan FD, Serpell JA, Duffy DL, et al. Differences in behavioral characteristics between dogs obtained as puppies from pet stores and those obtained from noncommercial breeders. *J Am Vet Med Assoc.* 2013;242:1359–1363.

16. Casey RA, Loftus B, Bolster C, et al. Human directed aggression in domestic dogs (*Canis familiaris*): occurrence in different contexts and risk factors. *Appl Anim Behav Sci.* 2014;152:52–63.

17. Pirrone F, Pierantoni L, Pastorino GQ, et al. Owner-reported aggressive behavior towards familiar people may be a more prominent occurrence in pet shop-traded dogs. *J Vet Behav: Clin Appl Res.* 2016;11:13–17.

18. Voith V, Ingram E, Mitsouris K, et al. Comparison of the adoption agency breed identification and DNA breed identification in dogs. *J Appl Anim Welf Sci.* 2009;12:253–262.

19. Wilsson E, Sundgren PE. Behaviour test for eight-week old puppies-heritabilities of tested behaviour traits and its correspondence to later behaviour. *Appl Anim Behav Sci.* 1997;58:151–62.

20. Godbout M, Frank D. Persistence of puppy behaviors and signs of anxiety during adulthood. *J Vet Behav.* 2011;6:92.

21. Goddard ME, Belharz RG. Early prediction of adult behavior in potential guide dogs. *Appl Anim Behav Sci.* 1986;15:247–60.

22. Jones AC, Gosling SD. Temperament and personality in dogs (*Canis familiaris*): A review and evaluation of past research. *Appl Anim Behav Sci.* 2005;95:1–53.

23. Godbout M, Frank D. Excessive mouthing in puppies as a predictor of aggressive behavior in adult dogs. *J Vet Behav.* 2011;6:93.

24. Cannas S, Frank D, Minero M, et al. Puppy behavior when left home alone: changes during the first few months after adoption. *J Vet Behav.* 2010;5:94–100.

25. Dollion N, Paulus A, Champagne N et al. Fear/reactivity in working dogs; an analysis of 37 years of behavioural data from the Mira Foundation's future service dogs. *Appl Anim Behav Sci.* 2019;221:104864.

26. Beaudet R, Chalifoux A, Daillaire A. Predictive value of activity level and behavioral evaluation on future dominance in puppies. *Appl Anim Behav Sci.* 1994;40:273–84.

27. Weiss E, Greenberg G. Service dog selection tests: Effectiveness for dogs from animal shelters. *Appl Anim Behav Sci.* 1997;53:297–308.

28. Netto WJ, Planta DJU. Behavioural testing for aggression in the domestic dog. *Appl Anim Behav Sci.* 1997;52:243–63. (doll)

29. Diesel G, Brodbelt D, Pfeiffer DU. Reliability of assessment of dogs' behavioural responses by staff working at a welfare charity in the UK. *Appl Anim Behav Sci.* 2008;115:171–181.

30. van der Borg JAM, Beerda B, Ooms M et al. Evaluation of behaviour testing for human directed aggression in dogs. *Appl Anim Behav Sci.* 2010;128:78–90.

31. Kroll T, Houpt KA, Erb HN. The use of novel stimuli as an indicator of aggression in dogs. *J Am Anim Hosp Assoc.* 2004;40:13–9.

32. De Meester RH, Bacquer DD, Peremans K. Aerament of dogs. *J Vet Behav.* 2008;3:161–170.

33. Bräm M, Doherr MG, Lehmann D, et al. Evaluating aggressive behavior in dogs: a comparison of 3 tests. *J Vet Behav.* 2008;3:152–160.

34. Svartberg K. A comparison of behaviour in test and in everyday life: evidence of three consistent boldness-related personality traits in dogs. *Appl Anim Behav Sci.* 2005;91:103–108.

35. Marder AM, Shabelansky A, Patronek GJ et al. Food-related aggression in shelter dogs: A comparison of behavior identified by a behavior evaluation in the shelter and owner reports after adoption, *Appl Anim Behav Sci.* 2013;148:150–156.

36. Bennett SL, Weng H, Walker SL et al. Comparison of SAFER behavior assessment results in shelter dogs at intake and after a 3-day acclimation period. *J Appl Anim Welf Sci.* 2015;18:153–168.

37. Shabelansky A, Dowling-Guyer S, Quist H et al. Consistency of shelter dogs' behavior toward a fake versus real stimulus dog during a behavior evaluation, *Appl Anim Behav Sci.* 2015;163:158–166.

38. Christensen E, Scarlett J, Campagna M, et al. Aggressive behavior in adopted dogs that passed a temperament test. *Appl Anim Behav Sci.* 2007;106:85–95

39. Patronek GJ, Bradley J, Arps E. What is the evidence for reliability and validity of behavior evaluations for shelter dogs? A prequel to "No better than flipping a coin". *J Vet Behav.* 2019;31:43–58.

40. Patronek GJ, Bradley J. No better than flipping a coin: Reconsidering canine behavior evaluations in animal shelters. *J Vet Behav.* 2016;15:66–77.

41. Patronek GJ, Bradley J, Arps E. Saving Normal: A new look at behavioral incompatibilities and dog relinquishment to shelters. *J Vet Behav.* 2022;49:36–45.

42. Mohan-Gibbons H, Dolan ED, Reid P et al. The impact of excluding food guarding from a standardized behavioral canine assessment in animal shelters. *Animals (Basel)*;2018;8:27.

43. Feaver, J, Mendl M, Bateson PJ. A method for rating the individual distinctiveness of domestic cats. *Anim. Behav.* 1986;34:1016–1025.

44. Mertens C, Shar R. Practical aspects of research in cats. In: Turner DC, Bateson P, editors. The domestic cat; the biology of its behavior. 2nd ed. Cambridge: Cambridge University Press; 1988. p. 179–90.

45. Travnik IdC, Machado DdS, Gonçalves LdS et al. Temperament in Domestic Cats: A Review of Proximate Mechanisms, Methods of Assessment, Its Effects on

Human—Cat Relationships, and One Welfare. *Animals.* 2020;10:1516.

46. Weiss E, Gramann S, Drain N et al. Modification of the Feline-Ality. Assessment and the ability to predict adopted cats' behaviors in their new homes. *Animals.* 2015;5:71–88.

47. Turcsan B, Kubinyi E, Miklosi A. Trainability and boldness traits differ between dog breed clusters based on conventional breed categories and genetic relatedness. *Appl Anim Behav Sci.* 2011;132:61–70.

48. Hare B, Tomasello M. Behavioral genetics of dog cognition: human-like social skills in dogs are heritable and derived. In: Ostrander EA, Giger U, Lindblad-Toh K, eds. *The Dog and Its Genome.* Woodbury, New York: Cold Spring Harbor Laboratory Press; 2006:497–514.

49. Kukekova AV, Acland GM, Oskina IN, et al. The genetics of domesticated behavior in canids: what can dogs and silver foxes tell us about each other? In: Ostrander EA, Giger U, Lindblad-Toh K, eds. *The Dog and Its Genome.* Woodbury, New York: Cold Spring Harbor Laboratory Press; 2006:515–537.

50. Wayne RK, Ostrander EA. Lessons learned from the dog genome. *Trends Genet.* 2007;23:557–567.

51. Goddard ME, Beilharz RG. A multivariate analysis of the genetics of fearfulness in potential guide dogs. *Behav Genet.* 1985;15:69–80.

52. MacLean EL, Snyder-Mackler N, vonHoldt BM et al. Highly heritable and functionally relevant breed differences in dog behaviour. *Proc R Soc B.* 2019;286:20190716.

53. Hradecka L, Bartos L, Svobodova I, Sales J. Heritability of behavioural traits in domestic dogs: a meta-analysis. *Appl Anim Behav Sci.* 2015;170:1–13.

54. Belyaev DK, Plyusnina IZ, Trut LN. Domestication in the silver fox (*Vulpes fulvus* Desm): changes in physiological boundaries of the sensitive period of primary socialization. *Appl Anim Behav Sci.* 1985;13:359–370.

55. Lord KA, Larson G, Coppinger RP, Karlsson EK. The history of farm foxes undermines the animal domestication syndrome. *Trends Ecol Evol.* 2020;35:125–136.

56. Sarviaho R, Hakosalo O, Tiira K, Sulkama S. Two novel genomic regions associated with fearfulness in dogs overlap human neuropsychiatric loci. *Transl Psychiatry.* 2019;9(1):18.

57. Sarviaho R, Hakosalo O, Tiira K, et al. A novel genomic region on chromosome 11 associated with fearfulness in dogs. *Transl Psychiatry.* 2020;10:169.

58. Zapata I, Serpell JA, Alvarez CE. Genetic mapping of canine fear and aggression. *BMC Genomics.* 2016;17:572. doi:10.1186/s12864-016-2936-3.

59. Brenoe UT, Larsgard AG, Johannessen K-R, Uldal SH. Estimates of genetic parameters for hunting performance traits in three breeds of gun hunting dogs in Norway. *Appl Anim Behav Sci.* 2002;77:209–215.

60. Lindberg S, Strandberg E, Swenson L. Genetic analysis of hunting behaviour in Swedish Flatcoated Retrievers. *Appl Anim Behav Sci.* 2004;88:289–298.

61. Courreau J-F, Langlois B. Genetic parameters and environmental effects which characterize the defence ability of the Belgian shepherd dog. *Appl Anim Behav Sci.* 2005;91:233–245.

62. Fadel FR, Driscoll P, Pilot M, et al. Differences in trait impulsivity indicate diversification of dog breeds into working and show lines. *Sci Rep.* 2016;6:22162

63. Li Y, Vonholdt BM, Reynolds A, et al. Artificial selection on brain-expressed genes during the domestication of dog. *Mol Biol Evol.* 2013;30(8):1867–1876.

64. Delgado MM, Munera JD, Reevy GM. Human perception of coat color as an indicator of domestic cat personality. *Anthrozoos.* 2012;25(4):427–440.

65. Arahori M, Hori Y, Saito A, et al. The oxytocin receptor gene (OXTR) polymorphism in cats (*Felis catus*) is associated with "roughness" assessed by owners. *J Vet Behav.* 2016;11:109–112.

66. Montague MJ, Li G, Gandolfi B, et al. Comparative analysis of the domestic cat genome reveals genetic signatures underlying feline biology and domestication. *Proc Nat Acad Sci.* 2014;111(48):17230–17235.

67. Kano M, Uchiyama H, Ohta M, Ohtani N. Oral tyrosine changed the responses to commands in German shepherds and Labrador retrievers but not in toy poodles. *J Vet Behav.* 2015;10(3):194–198.

68. Nicholas FW. *Introduction to Veterinary Genetics.* 3rd ed. Ames, Iowa: Wiley-Blackwell; 2010.

69. Dodman NH, Karlsson EK, Moon-Fanelli A, et al. A canine chromosome 7 locus confers compulsive disorder susceptibility. *Mol Psychiatry.* 2010;15:8–10.

70. Jones P, Chase K, Martin A, et al. Single-nucleotide-polymorphism-based association mapping of dog stereotypes. *Genetics.* 2008;179:1033–1044.

71. Zapata I, Serpell JA, Alvarez CE. Genetic mapping of fear and aggression. *Genomics.* 2016;17:572. doi:10.1186/s12864-016-2936-3.

72. Svartberg K, Tapper I, Temrin H. Consistency of personality traits in dogs. *Anim Behav.* 2005;69:283–291.

Resources and recommended reading

Ackerman L. *Proactive Pet Parenting: Anticipating Pet Health Problems Before They Happen.* Problem Free Publishing; 2020.

Ackerman L. *Problem Free Pets. The Ultimate Guide to Pet Parenting.* Dermvet; 2020.

Ackerman L. *The Genetic Connection: A Guide to Health Problems in Purebred Dogs.* 2nd ed. Lakewood, Colorado: AAHA Press; 2011.

Alderton D. *The right dog for you: how to choose the perfect breed for you and your family.* London: Ivy Press 2021.

Alderton D. *The cat selector; how to choose the right cat for you.* B.E.S. Publishing 2011.

Bell JS, Cavanagh, KE, Tilley, LP, Smith, FWK. *Veterinary Medical Guide to Dog and Cat Breeds.* Teton NewMedia; 2012.

Bradley J. *The relevance of breed in selecting a companion animal dog.* National Canine Research Council. 2011.

Crispin S. The advisory council on the welfare Issues of dog Breeding. *Vet J.* 2011; 189: 129–131.

DVM 360. https://www.dvm360.com/view/helping-make-perfect-match-pet-selection-counseling.

Hart B, Hart L. *The Perfect Puppy: Breed selection and care by veterinary science for behavior, neutering, age and longevity.* Academic Press, 2022.

Marder A, Duxbury MM. Obtaining a pet: realistic expectations. *Vet Clin North Am Small Anim Pract.* 2008;38(5):1145–62.

Morrill K, Hekman J, Li X et al. Ancestry-inclusive dog genomics challenges popular breed stereotypes. *Science,* 2022;376(6592), p.eabk0639.

Morris D. *Dogs: The Ultimate Dictionary of 1000 Breeds.* London: Trafalgar Square; 2008.

National Canine Research Council. Evidence-based canine genome and behavior research library. https://nationalcanineresearchcouncil.com/research-library-home/

Overall KL, Tiira K, Broach D, Bryant D. Genetics and behavior: a guide for practitioners. *Vet Clin Small Anim.* 2014;44:483–505.

Rigterink A, Houpt K. Genetics of canine behavior: a review. *World J Med Genet.* 2014;4(3):46–57.

Scott JP, Fuller JL. *Genetics and the Social Behaviour of the Dog.* The University of Chicago Press; 1998.

The complete cat breed book. 2nd ed. Dorling Kindersley 2020

The complete dog Breed Book, New edition. Dorling Kindersley 2020.

Vet Girl - https://vetgirlontherun.com/how-to-counsel-your-pet-owners-on-how-to-pick-a-pet-vetgirl-veterinary-continuing-education-blog/

Internet (web) resources

American Association of Feline Practitioners: https://catfriendly.com/be-a-cat-friendly-caregiver/making-the-commitment/

American Kennel Club: akc.org,

American Veterinary Medical Association: https://www.avma.org/resources/pet-owners/petcare/selecting-pet-dog

Best Friends: https://resources.bestfriends.org/article/choosing-pet

Blue Cross: https://www.bluecross.org.uk/advice/pets/finding-the-right-pet

Canadian Kennel Club: https://www.ckc.ca/en/Choosing-a-Dog

Canadian Veterinary Medical Association: https://www.canadianveterinarians.net/

public-resources/animal-owners/selecting-and-owning-a-pet/

The Kennel Club (UK) https://www.thekennelclub.org.uk/getting-a-dog/;

Petfinder https://www.petfinder.com/pet-adoption/

CHAPTER 4

Pets and the family dynamic

Emily D. Levine, DVM, DACVB

Chapter contents

Introduction

Having children and pets in the same household can result in mutually beneficial relationships; however, it can also lead to relationship breakdowns which can result in relinquishment of the pet. There are social, emotional, cognitive, health, and educational benefits for children who have pets in the home.[1] One recent study found that children aged 9–11 years who lived with dogs reported more positive qualities and less conflict with friends than those without dogs in the home.[2] From the dog's point of view, living in a home with children may be beneficial or it may be stressful. Chronic stress negatively affects the dog's quality of life (QOL) and increases the risk of certain diseases (see Chapter 7).[3,4] The effect on the QOL of companion animals living with children has been grossly understudied. Ensuring the pet's QOL should always be a top consideration for the family. However, in reality, that is not always the case. The veterinarian can help ensure the safety of children and the QOL of pets by 1) asking about interactions between the pets and children and 2) monitoring the pet's health at each visit for physical disease (e.g., musculoskeletal, neurologic, endocrine, dental, gastrointestinal, decline in hearing or visual abilities) that may be causing or exacerbating bite risk to the children in the home or those who visit (see Chapter 6). The purpose of this chapter is to highlight how the family should prepare pets and the children to live together and understand the contexts and causes of injury to children in order to ultimately reduce the risk to children and maintain a good QOL for the pet.

The number of bites to children by family dogs is astounding. According to the Centers for Disease Control and Prevention (CDC), in the 10 years from 2011 and 2020, for children between 0 and 4, there was an estimated 335,000 emergency department visits in the United Statues for nonfatal dog bites, and approximately 720,000 for children 0–9.[5] As high as those numbers are, the actual number of bites to children is likely significantly higher, as these data only accounted for children whose family sought medical treatment. Parents may not bring their child to the emergency room after a bite so as to not implicate the dog. In addition, often children will not tell their parents when they have been bitten if the parent did not see the bite happen.[6,7] Eighty-six percent of these bites result from the child initiating interactions that they and many parents view as benign but the dog does not (e.g., petting, hugging, kissing, etc.).[8–11] Most bites to the child are to the face, neck, and head area.[12–16] While the causes of bites to children need further examination, one potential reason is a result of innate "leaning in" behavior exhibited by children when examining something of interest to them.[17,18]

It is important to note that the vast majority of these bites are from the family dog in the home, not an unfamiliar or stray dog.[14–18] When these bites occur, it is common that the parents are in the room with the child and dog.[11,13] This happens when the type of supervision is passive versus active (see Figure 4.1). Many of these bites are preventable with implementation of basic dog–child safety rules. See Figure 4.2 for a list of rules in a pet parent-friendly format. This is also available online as a printable handout. While the statistics on cat bites are not as readily available, cats can certainly harm children by biting or scratching.

Most cats and dogs bite children out of fear, anxiety, stress, conflict, panic, and/or frustration. The pet is not biting to exert dominance or establish itself as a pack leader but instead is merely trying to communicate that the interaction makes him uncomfortable. One of the best and most powerful ways to prevent bites is to be able to recognize and understand pet body language. This enables supervising adults to teach children how to recognize when the pet is uncomfortable, thereby preventing bites before happen. Pet parents may be aware of their pet's stress level but may not recognize early signs of stress as they apply to aggression.[19,20] When earlier signs of stress such as lip licking, head turns, growling, and attempts to escape are ignored or punished (e.g., yelling, hitting, shock, leash corrections), dogs often escalate to biting. In cats, body language may include tail thumping/thrashing, ears back, pupils dilated, hunched body, attempts

to escape, hissing, or swatting. Once a dog or cat learns that biting is the most effective way to communicate fear, anxiety, and stress, and to remove the threat, it is challenging to teach them to display a more benign behavior when they are stressed. All recommendations here apply to dogs and cats unless otherwise noted.

Considerations when selecting a dog for a family with children

For families who are ready to bring a dog into the home, the first consideration should be *why* they want a dog. Do they want a family dog that can participate in family activities; a dog to engage in competitive dog sports; a dog that will work on the farm; or a protection dog? The second consideration should be the *age* of the dog. Some families want to get a puppy, whereas others are more open to any age as long as it is a good fit for the family. See Chapter 3 for more information on pet selection.

For families who desire a typical family dog but would like to adopt a puppy from a breeder, the family should make sure the puppy is from nonworking lines and is being raised

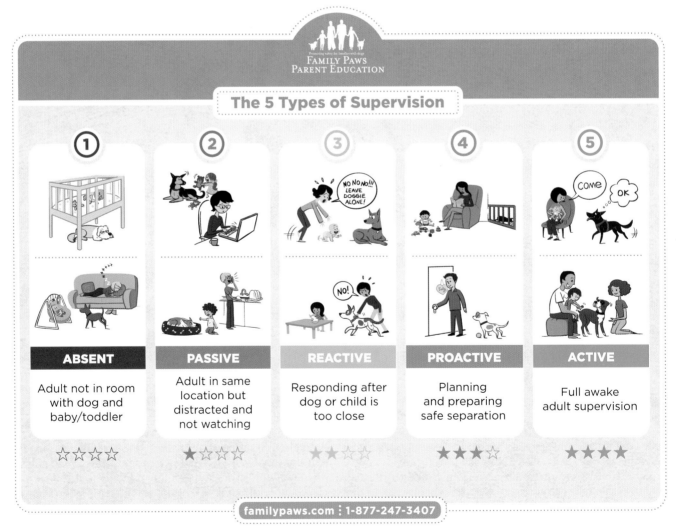

Figure 4.1 Proactive supervision may not be fully understood by parents.

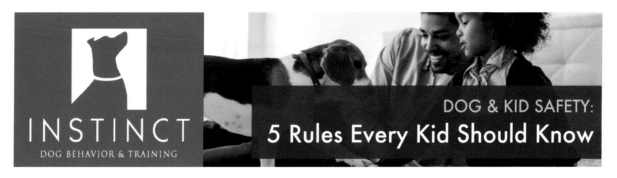

Are You Managing a Dog-and-Kid Household?

Here are 5 dog safety rules EVERY kid should know:

Learning when to
IGNORE
dogs

#1. Dog Sleeping or Eating? No Time for a Greeting!

Every kid should understand that it is not safe to approach a dog when they are sleeping, resting, or eating.

#2. Dog with a Toy or Bone? Leave 'Em Alone!

All kids should learn it is dangerous to approach a dog who has something in or near their mouth, such as a toy, bone, or "stolen" item.

Learning how to
INVITE
dogs to interact

#3. Be an Inviter, Not an Invader

We can teach our kids to invite dogs to come to *them* to interact, rather than the kid invading the dog's space. Dogs always have the right to say "No thanks" to an invitation.

#4. The Face is NOT the Place!

We must teach our kids that face-to-face contact with a dog is NEVER a safe thing to do. When kids lean in close, even an innocent warning snap can result in a devastating face bite.

Learning how to
ENGAGE
dogs safely

#5. Be a Gentle Friend

We can teach our kids that hitting, poking, grabbing, and climbing on dogs is both dangerous and unkind. Instead, they should pet with one hand in soft, slow strokes along a dog's shoulder or back.

Instinct Online School | *the* DOGS & KIDS *course* | by Dr. Emily Levine, DACVB
onlineschool.instinctdogtraining.com

Figure 4.2 Handouts like this one make parent education more effective.

in a home setting, ideally with children. At minimum, the breeder should be taking steps to actively expose the puppies in a positive manner to children starting as early as 3 weeks of age. Within an individual breed, there are genetic differences between dogs from working and nonworking lines. Those differences within the same breed are larger than between different breeds.[21] It is not possible to generalize for a particular breed whether it is best to advise pet parents to adopt a puppy from conformation, working or pet lines. Studies in English Springer Spaniels suggest that dogs that were bred for conformation were more likely to have owner, dog and stranger aggression,[22,23] while another study found that conformation dogs were less playful, curious, and aggressive.[23] Conversely, in Labrador Retrievers, field stock has been shown to have more aggression than conformation lines.[24] Ideally, the puppy would be from a repeat breeding. While there are no guarantees for any puppy's behavior and temperament, knowing that the first litter of puppies did well in homes with families would be an indicator that the next breeding of the same dogs would be similar. In addition, the adoptive pet parents should have an opportunity to visit with the breeding pair or their offspring prior to purchasing a puppy. Pet parents should be advised to resist adopting puppies from anxious, timid, or aggressive bitches or sires.

For those choosing to adopt a puppy from a rescue or shelter, the family should look for any behaviors or body language that are associated with fear, anxiety, and stress, as these temperamental traits indicate that the puppy may not be suitable for a home with children (see Chapter 2). These behaviors and body postures may manifest as hiding, shaking, tail down, ears back, avoidance, cowering, growling, barking, biting, and being easily startled when exposed to sounds, touch, handling, or the sight of various stimuli. Hiring a qualified positive reinforcement trainer would be a smart approach to help the family pick out a puppy.

For families that do not wish to adopt a puppy and/or would like to have a better sense of the temperament of the dog they are bringing into their home, an adult dog that has completed both adolescence and social maturation is an option. While more research is needed on the developmental stages of dogs, there is evidence that dogs go through an adolescent phase between 8 and 11 months of age, which can result in behavior changes that families may find difficult to live with.[25,26] This phase is generally thought to end by 36 months of age, but there is a lack of data pertaining to the age when this is complete.[27] It is likely no coincidence that 8–36 months of age are common times for dogs to be relinquished.[28,29] Given the ambiguity of when this process ends for each individual dog, the family may want to select a dog that is at least 3 years old in order to have a sense of the dog's personality and temperament.

Older dogs are more likely to be available for adoption from shelters or rescues. The environment of rescues and shelters can be stressful and the behavior of the dog in these environments may not reflect what the dog's behavior will be in the home.[8,30–32] Ideally, families would adopt dogs that were fostered in a family home with children so a more accurate picture of the dog's behavior would be known. Because this may not be possible in most situations, the family should consider hiring a qualified positive reinforcement dog training professional to help them identify any red flags and facilitate the assimilation of the dog into the family and home.

Preparing pets and children to live together

With proper preparation, harmonious and loving relationships can be built between children and the pets in the home. Preparation should include: 1) exposure of the pet to the sights and sounds of children in a positive way; 2) prevention of negative interactions after the child or dog arrives

in the home; 3) introduction of the child to the pet; 4) keeping both the child and the pet safe; 5) ensuring that the pet copes well with a child in the home; and 6) building a long-term positive relationship between the pet and the child.

Many families take for granted a positive relationship between children and pets. However, pets do not innately know how to behave around children and children do not innately know how to behave around pets. Learning how to read dog and cat body language, how to approach them, and safely interact with them are skills that must be learned. See resources in Appendix A. While it is typically expected that the parent will teach these skills to the children, studies illustrate that many adults, including dog-owning adults, have limited knowledge of dog behavior and are unaware of the factors that might lead to dog bites to children.[33] Cats, too, typically signal their level of comfort with child–pet interactions before biting or scratching. Fortunately, most problems can be avoided with some forethought and training, leading to positive interactions between children and pets. Even with proper training and socialization, the reality is that most pets will have some limits on when, how frequently, with whom, and the quality and type of contact that they will tolerate or enjoy. These boundaries, which will be different for every pet, need to be respected to ensure a good QOL for the pet and the child's safety.

For families who have a pet in the home, the focus should be on preparation of the cat or dog for the environmental, social, and routine changes that inevitably occur with arrival of a child into the home. While some of the approaches will be the same regardless of the species or age of the pet, there are certain exercises that can and should be done with a puppy that may not be suitable for an adult dog or a cat, depending on its temperament. For all pets, regardless of species or age, a sanctuary space where they can escape the sounds and sights of the family is essential.

Parents often assume that jealousy is the cause of problem behaviors associated with the arrival of a new child into the home, but this is not the case. Most problems result from fear, anxiety, stress, conflict, panic, and/or frustration. caused by alterations in the pet's environment and family interactions. Changes in feeding, exercise, and play schedules; what the pet is allowed to do; how the pet gets attention; inconsistencies in the way family members interact with the pet; and the pet's level of familiarity and socialization with children may all be factors which lead to conflict between pets and children. Preparing the family pet for the arrival of a new baby or any child (e.g., adoption, remarriage) includes gradual environmental change, review of household rules for interactions, and positive reinforcement training of desired behaviors with an ultimate goal of giving the pet environmental and social predictability.[34]

Preparing a puppy for a child in the home

Preparation for a good relationship between the dog and children begins in puppyhood. To accomplish this, there should be frequent opportunities for the pup to meet children before 16 weeks of age. The puppy should be introduced to children when the children are calm, and food rewards should be used to facilitate introductions. Puppy classes that encourage family attendance can be a way of meeting children in a controlled environment. Early positive interactions regarding handling and petting help prevent the development of fear, avoidance behavior, and aggression toward children when the pet is older.

The exercises below are intended for behaviorally healthy puppies. Any puppies exhibiting fear, apprehension, or aggressive behaviors need a behavior management and modification treatment plan developed by a qualified positive reinforcement trainer, veterinarian, or board-certified veterinary behaviorist, and may need the help of medications and/or supplements (see Chapter 11). If the puppy shows any signs of fear, anxiety, stress, conflict, panic, and/or aggression during these exercises, the pet parents should stop practicing them and seek veterinary guidance immediately.

All family members should make a point of gently and positively handling the puppy in all of the ways that a child might touch it. Making positive associations using food rewards or play while touching the tail, ears, and body; grasping the collar; brushing teeth; grooming; and nail trimming should help the dog adapt to contact with all parts of the body, which might be similar to what might be encountered with a child. Any type of physical punishment, threats with a hand, or forceful interactions (e.g., pinning, rolling over, or hugging aggressively) should simply not be done. All pets must learn that the human hand is friendly and not to be feared (i.e., associated with food, receiving toys, and gentle affection). If the pet associates hand movement with discomfort, it might bite when the child moves a hand toward it.

The puppy should be exposed to the sights and sounds of children being loud and playing from a safe distance while being given food rewards or playing. Because many dogs are sound sensitive in adulthood, the puppy should be exposed to the sounds associated with having children in the home. Another common situation in which dogs show aggression is being approached while eating. This behavior pattern can often be avoided by using counterconditioning to create a positive emotional response to the approach of a person to the food bowl. During mealtime, a person should stand a distance away that does not upset the puppy. The person can call the puppy's name and then toss a treat more exciting than the kibble that the puppy is eating into the food bowl. Then, over many sessions, the person can move closer to the food bowl when performing this exercise. By doing these exercises, the pup will learn to look forward to having people nearby at meal times, understanding that humans will not steal their food but instead will drop delicious food into the bowl. Once the puppy understands basic cues, training can be instituted to teach him to walk away from his bowl calmly so that the bowl can be picked up if needed (see Chapter 10).

These conditioning techniques should be thought of as a "behavioral vaccine" in that they will not 100% prevent an incident but would lessen the likelihood of an incident in that specific situation. Children should taught or encouraged to not pet or touch a dog while it is eating and to keep their hands away from the bowl. The real purpose of these exercises is to condition the puppy to be comfortable with these actions should the child do this in the event there is a failure of management or proactive supervision. Taking the food bowl away while the pet is eating serves to teach the puppy that people who approach while he is eating will take his food, which often leads to fear, anxiety, stress, and aggression around the food bowl. As for adult dogs, puppies should learn cues such as sit, down, go to place, and leave it. Young puppies learn quickly; however, they may have short attention spans and are easily distracted. Training expectations should be commensurate with the age of the puppy.

Preparing a kitten for a child in the home

Kittens, like puppies, need direction, structure, and enrichment in order to successfully live with children. Kittens should be exposed to children in a positive way with food rewards or play. Kittens benefit from enrichment in the way of vertical resting space, hiding spaces, sanctuary spaces, food toys, and predatory toys. Rotating toys so that there are 3 different toys per day kept out of rotation for 5 days can keep kittens focused on their own toys instead of the child's items. The use of food puzzle toys for meals, catnip, or silver vine can encourage independent play, giving the family time to be with the baby.

Kittens should never be taught to chase fingers, pounce on feet, or grab body parts. These types of behaviors can lead bites later in life, which could be injurious to the child. Most certainly, kittens can be trained. Kittens that will be living with children should understand how to come when called, go to the top of a cat tree, and stay in place on a bed. Kittens may get bursts of energy, leaping into the air and onto furniture. This behavior, while normal, can be dangerous. A sanctuary space to which the kitten is accustomed can be a viable solution. The room can be set up with toys, food and water, and a litterbox so that the kitten is comfortable there. Conditioning the kitten to stay in that space happily and calmly will be beneficial not only when the child is young but throughout the cat's life. See Appendix A for cat training resources.

Preparing an adult dog for a child in the home

Pet parents may feel that because the dog historically got along well with visiting children or children in the neighborhood that the dog will inherently refrain from exhibiting aggression toward their child. Alternatively, they may feel that even though their dog has shown fear or aggression toward other children that the dog will inherently love their own children. Even if the dog gets along well with children historically, a child living in the same home with a dog full-time is a very different experience for the dog than occasionally seeing kids for brief periods of time. Unfortunately, there are no validated, 100% accurate predictors of aggression by dogs to children. In the authors' experience, dogs that are fearful may be safe with the new children and dogs that are friendly may be frightened of the children. For this reason, preparation of all dogs regardless of temperament is essential. In addition, all dogs should be regarded as a potential danger to the child, with privileges and freedom being added as the dog's and the child's behavior patterns become more apparent.

Before preparations begin, an assessment of the dog's temperament should be made by the veterinarian. There is not a validated temperament test for the evaluation of dog behavior at the time of this writing. This leaves the veterinarian with a thorough history and their personal experience with the dog as the foundation of the assessment. All types of aggression should be considered potentially dangerous, regardless of how minor the aggression is deemed. Aggression includes growling, lunging, biting, snapping, baring teeth, muzzle punching, barking, and grumbling. It is not uncommon for pet parents to regard growling as safe, putting only biting in the "dangerous" category. Furthermore, overt signs of fear such as averting the gaze, lowering the head, lowering the tail, attempting to escape, quickly turning the head toward the child or person, and avoidance should be regarded as predisposing factors for the development of aggression (see Figure 4.3). Some dogs will not be safe with children, no matter what training is completed. For those dogs, creation of a sanctuary space as part of a "crate, gate, and separate" plan is necessary for the safety of the child and the QOL of the dog.

Aggression toward the child is not the only concern. If the dog has any behavior issues that are not related to aggression but could endanger the welfare of a child (e.g., jumping on people, jumping on windows, pulling on leash, stealing items), those behavioral issues should be addressed as soon as possible. One example would be a dog that charges to the window or door, plowing through anything in its way. Pet parents should have a realistic and practical understanding of their dog's limitations, even if he is only overly friendly, and structure the interactions with children accordingly. Preparation should start when the family knows that they will be bringing a child into the home, whether through pregnancy or adoption. Expect baby preparation to take about 3 months of training. For pregnant mothers, preparation should start no later than the first trimester. A dog is likely to become anxious or frustrated if the routine, environment, or the way

the pet parent interacts with it changes or lacks predictability. Therefore, gradual adjustments should be made before the baby arrives. Feeding, exercise, and play schedules; sleeping and resting areas; and any new rules (e.g., rooms the dog is permitted to enter, furniture on which the dog is allowed to sleep, jumping up during greeting, barking at the window), will need to be put into place ahead of time to fit the family's situation once the baby is home. If the family plans to walk the dog with the baby in a stroller, training walks on leash while a parent pushes a stroller should begin.

If the pet parents are consistent and predictable in their responses, the dog should quickly learn which behaviors get rewards and which do not. This is particularly important when giving attention. If the pet gets attention by nudging, head pressing, pawing, or licking, the pet parents must stop rewarding these behaviors, as they are not acceptable ways to get attention and could be problematic once the child comes. By consistently ignoring these behaviors, they should eventually cease via extinction (see Chapter 10). However, the pet should also be provided with a new way to earn attention, such as to sit. The pet may initially be confused and frustrated which results in an increase in the negative behavior, (extinction burst, see Chapter 10). If the pet parents even occasionally give attention when these behaviors are exhibited, they will inadvertently reinforce them, causing them to continue to occur but more intensely than before. It takes time to complete this process and is best done before the stress of the last trimester. The pet parent should begin a program of structured interactions and predictable consequences so that the pet learns that calm and settled behaviors are the way to get rewards prior to the baby's arrival. This effectively puts the rewards (e.g., affection, eating, treats) under the dog's control by consistently and predictably training that only calm responses (sit–watch, down–stay, lying on a bed/mat) will be

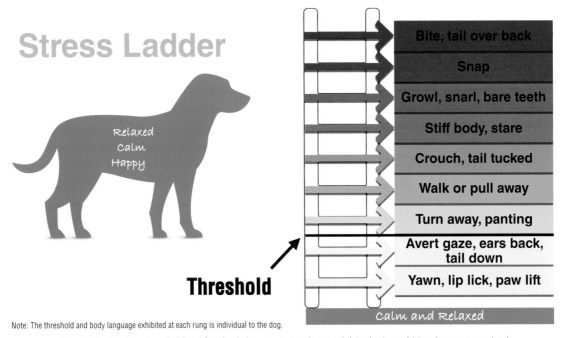

Note: The threshold and body language exhibited at each rung is individual to the dog.

Figure 4.3 The dog stress ladder. Often body language signals are exhibited prior to biting, but go unnoticed by pet parents. *(Attribution: Lisa Radosta. Modified from Shepherd, K 2009. BSAVA Manual of Canine and Feline Behaviour, 2nd edition.)*

rewarded. If the pet parents are consistent and predictable, the pet should soon learn that these calm behaviors are the way to get attention. The pet parent should reach out to a positive reinforcement trainer to help implement these steps in a manner that will teach the dog the cues using a humane, science-based approach.

Cue words should precede any reward (e.g., sit, focus, down and settle, or go to a mat or crate) to ensure the dog learns to respond to these cues immediately and consistently in a variety of locations and situations. Giving rewards inconsistently will delay training, add to the dog's confusion and anxiety about how to get what it wants, and may ultimately reward undesirable behaviors. If the soon-to-be parents have not been using cue words on a regular basis, it is critical they start teaching the dog what these cues mean and the positive consequences to performing desired behaviors. Using cues will not only provide the necessary structure and predictability for the dog, but the basic cue words will be important and practical tools for use in a variety of situations. While it may seem unnecessary to recommend training for the dog early in pregnancy, it is not uncommon in the author's experience for parents to wait to address training until after the baby arrives.

Other behaviors that are permitted now but will not be permitted after the baby has arrived must also be addressed. Such behaviors may include: jumping up, barking at windows, lying on furniture, climbing into the lap. Dogs can be trained to exhibit desired behaviors such as sit for all greetings and rest on a mat by rewarding these behaviors instead of the undesirable behaviors. Most pet parents are not dog trainers, so encouraging them to get a qualified positive reinforcement trainer is advisable if the dog needs training.

Another critical step to prepare the dog for the child is to ensure that the dog can cope with being separated from the child and family. There will be times when the safest thing to do is simply to separate the dog from the child or guests. Prior to the arrival of the child, the family should practice separating the dog using a barrier like a baby gate. The family should start with short, positive sessions such as feeding the dog a meal out of a food or puzzle toy while separated from the family behind a baby gate with the adults in sight on the other side of the gate. The time of separation can be slowly expanded over several sessions. If the dog experiences moderate to significant distress (e.g., anxiety, fear, frustration, aggression) when separated by a barrier, the family veterinarian or a board-certified veterinary behaviorist should be consulted to determine if medications or supplements will be needed (see Chapters 11 and 12) in addition to a behavioral treatment plan.

The dog should also be prepared for the baby's homecoming by exposing it to the sounds and smells of the new baby. If the dog gets upset when it hears certain sounds, a recording of baby noises (e.g., cooing, crying, screaming) can be used in a desensitization and counterconditioning program (see Appendix A for product sources). The recording should first be played at a sufficiently low volume that the dog shows no anxiety, while the dog is engaged in something positive such as positive reinforcement training, play, or eating a meal. Very gradually the volume can be increased as the weeks go by until the pet seems comfortable with the sounds at high volumes.

Once the baby arrives, a towel or blanket with the baby's scent can be taken home from the hospital to prepare the pet for the new smells that will arrive with the baby. The object with the scent should be presented while the dog is relaxed and taking treats or playing with a favored toy. Some dogs will be anxious when the parent is carrying or nursing the new baby. Testing the dog by carrying around and fussing with a doll (especially one that moves and makes crying sounds) can be useful. If there is any anxiety, a positive association should be made with this doll using favored food rewards, affection, or a favored play toy.

While it is prudent that parents start preparing the dog for a child if they are even thinking of having children in the future or when they first find out they are pregnant, many veterinarians will experience the pet parent asking for advice when they are due in a few weeks. The authors suggest advising the pet parent as follows:

- Get baby gates so they can separate the dog and baby when needed. When they first put up the baby gates, use food-filled toys to keep the dog happily occupied.
- Brush up the dog's cue words: sit, down, stay, go to place, and come. Even if they have never learned these words, most dogs can learn this very quickly when taught by a qualified positive reinforcement trainer (no punishment-based techniques!).
- Get a baby doll that cries which can be readily found on the internet, and carry it around while playing baby sounds, all the while using food and toys to make positive associations.

Preparing an adult cat for a child in the home

The guidelines written here apply to dogs as well as cats. Cats, however, may be less understood than dogs despite the fact that their body language is just as obvious. How the cat responds to a new baby or children will depend upon previous experiences as well as the cat's temperament. Some cats will adapt quickly to children and new babies by either ignoring them or eventually seeking them out for investigation or social contact (e.g., bunting or cheek rubbing), while others may immediately be inquisitive, playful, and affectionate. While investigation, seeking affection, and social contact may be desirable, these behaviors must be well supervised, since they can still lead to injury to the child or inappropriate responses from the child to the pet. Just as with dogs, cats need a space to retreat from the chaos of children in the household. Creation of a sanctuary area outside of the living space is essential.

Pet parents should consider how the daily schedule, social interactions, and household will need to be changed when the new child arrives and begin to adapt the cat slowly in advance of the new arrival. Many cats can become stressed and anxious when there are changes to their daily routine, social interactions, or environment. The cat's response may be a change in behavior or attitude with respect to humans or other cats (e.g., fear, avoidance, irritability, aggression), elimination outside of the litterbox, and/or overgrooming. There may also be an impact on the cat's physical health, such as an increase or decrease in appetite, activity, and/or sleep. Conditions with a stress-induced component (e.g., feline interstitial cystitis) may also be more likely to occur.[35] Whenever possible, changes should be made slowly and should be associated with positive events and interactions such as food, treats, affection, and play. For example, if the cat initiates play by chasing and attacking moving objects, the pet parents should initiate and provide play sessions and toys to meet the cat's needs. If there are rooms, counters, and areas of the house that will be out of bounds for the cat when the child arrives, pet parents should begin in advance to keep the cat out of these areas, and teach the cat where it is allowed to sleep, play, and explore. New furniture should be set up in advance of the child's arrival, as some cats can be particularly sensitive or reactive to new structures and new odors.

Some cats are anxious when they hear strange sounds. For these cats, a recording can be obtained of baby noises (e.g., cooing, crying, screaming; see resources in Appendix A). The recording should be played at a level that is low enough to cause no anxiety while offering tasty food treats, play, or catnip toys. The volume should be gradually increased over several weeks until the cat seems comfortable with these noises at high volumes. To prepare the pet for the new smells that will arrive with the baby, a towel or blanket with the baby's scent can be brought home from the hospital. The cat should then be taught to associate the object with favored rewards. On occasion, some cats may become anxious or overly investigative when the pet parent carries, changes, or nurses the new baby. Testing the cat by carrying around and fussing with a doll (especially one that moves and makes crying sounds) can be useful. A positive association should be made with this doll, using favored toys, treats, or food rewards before the baby arrives. Pheromone analog diffusers may be helpful in reducing anxiety in cats.[36] Cats that show moderate to severe fear, anxiety, stress, conflict, panic, and/or aggression, in general or when the baby arrives will likely need medication or supplements to help (see Chapter 11 and Chapter 12). Just like dogs, cats can be taught how to respond to cue words such as sit, go to place, and stay. Similar to dogs, cats may need to be separated from the family at times. If the cat has difficulty coping with this, the parents should reach out to their veterinarian or a board-certified veterinary behaviorist for help. Understanding cat body language is also essential to identify when a cat may be feeling stressed (see Chapter 2 and resources in Appendix A).

Introducing the baby to the pets

When the baby first comes home, it is important to set up the pet for success by anticipating problems and taking steps to prevent them. If the pet has not seen both parents for several days, there will probably be a great deal of excited greeting behavior when they arrive with the baby. In situations such as this, one parent should go inside without the baby and greet the pet to avoid overexcitement and potential injury to the baby. That parent should then go back outside and hold the baby while the other parent goes in to meet the pet. If only one of the parents has been gone during the childbirthing process, that parent should enter the home to greet the pet without holding the baby. With this approach, the pet is being set up for success when meeting the baby, since he will have an opportunity to excitedly greet the pet parents. The pet parents should wait until the excitement has died down and the pet is calm before introducing him to the baby. That may be later in the same day or a few days afterward. Some dogs and cats will never be introduced to the baby if, for example, they have shown aggression previously. The baby will be in the house for 18 years at least. There is no rush to introduce the pet to the baby. The parents should

not put the baby on the floor with the pet, on the pet, or in the pet's face. Dogs and cats have an acute sense of smell; they can smell the baby without being close enough to touch it. The family should *never*, no matter how sweet, trustworthy, or friendly the pet appears, allow an unsupervised pet around the baby. Any pet can hurt a child, whether showing aggression, innocent investigation, or play. Children and pets should never be left in the same room unsupervised for any length of time. When a pet parent leaves the room, the baby or the pet should come with them.

Careful judgment must be exercised in deciding if and when to allow the pet close enough to sniff. If there is *any* likelihood that the pet might bite or if the dog has any history of aggression (see above), do not allow the pet to meet the baby at all but instead focus on helping the pet get comfortable with separation. For dogs, any introductions should be made when the dog is calm and under good control, on a loose leash held by an adult with another adult in charge of the baby. If the dog becomes overly excited when on leash or when wearing the gear used for walking, introductions can be made with the dog behind a baby gate. During these times, it is wise to train a desirable response such as a "down–stay" away from the baby and give favored rewards, or have the dog go to its room, mat, or yard with a special chew toy.

It is especially important to be vigilant when the baby is crying, kicking, or waving its arms. This could cause a curious dog to jump up and injure the infant. Cats can become scared and redirect with aggression to the pet parent, the baby, or another pet. The pet parents should immediately separate the pet from the baby and seek guidance from their veterinarian if the pet exhibits any predatory signs such as stalking, strong focus, and unusual interest around the baby. Whenever the pet is in the room with the baby, there should be one family member in charge of the baby and one in charge of the pet, rewarding acceptable behaviors (e.g., lying on a bed away from the baby, orienting to the baby in a calm manner) with treats, food, play, or affection. The idea is to promote relaxed behaviors and to condition a positive emotional response to the baby by pairing the baby's presence with calm behaviors and pleasurable rewards. This association can be made more dramatic by reducing the amount of attention or treats the pet gets when the baby is not around. In this way, the dog learns that the presence of the baby is associated with positive events and the absence of the baby is not. The biggest mistake pet parents make when they try to shape their pet's behavior is to concentrate on telling the dog what is wrong instead of rewarding what is right.

Some families may benefit from boarding the pet for the first few days after the baby comes home if they simply feels it will be too much for them to have the dog in the home while they themselves are adjusting. For dogs, a dog walker may be hired to come and play with the dog and walk the dog since for the first several weeks, the parents are likely going to be sleep deprived, exhausted, and overwhelmed with the new responsibilities of parenting.

Interactions change as the child grows

As the baby continues to grow and mature, the risk of a dog bite to the child increases. The QOL of the dog may concurrently decrease as the child is more mobile. Therefore, even if the dog has adapted nicely to a particular stage in the child's life, parents must always be prepared for a change in the relationship between the child and dog as the child goes through various developmental stages (e.g., crawling, walking).

Kids also go through phases where they mimic their parents and test boundaries that likely further increase the risk of a bite. Many parents have experienced this phenomenon after watching their child apparently purposefully do something that they were told not do, such as approach the dog while eating. Parents may also notice that the child engages with the dog in the way that they see their parents engaging with the dog (e.g., hugging, petting, kissing, picking up, scolding, removing something directly from the dog's mouth). Parents should demonstrate safe ways of interacting with the dog whenever the child is in the same room. If the dog is not comfortable with the interaction, signs of fear or aggression (see above) will most likely be displayed. All too often, pet parents are not actively supervising the dog and the child resulting in a lack of knowledge of the dog's body language signals. Pet parents may report that the dog displayed aggression "out of the blue" or "unpredictably" when in fact, the dog had been exhibiting signs of fear, anxiety, stress, panic, and/or conflict. Dogs might then be punished for behaviors which are indicative of an attempt to communicate in the only way that they can that they are uncomfortable with certain interactions. It is the adults' responsibility to ensure bites do not happen by proactively supervising dogs and children.

Reading a dog's body language is not intuitive. It is a skill that needs to be learned. Studies have shown that children often confuse a fearful or angry dog with a friendly dog.[37,38] While children are able to read humans faces with greater than 90% correct responses with respect to that person being happy or angry, 69% of 4-year-old kids misread aggressive dog faces as happy faces.[37] Adults do not necessarily understand dog body language signaling, and dog pet parentship does not predict correct interpretations of dog body language particularly fear, anxiety, and stress.[19,20,39,40] Aldridge and Rose presented 15 videos and images of happy, frightened, and aggressive dogs to 117 children ranging from ages 4 to 7. Approximately 45% of 4- to 5-year-olds incorrectly identified the frightened dog. Regardless of interpreting this emotion correctly or incorrectly, the kids were equally inclined to approach both happy and fearful dogs.[41] Guiding pet parents and their children on how to read dog body language and/or providing resources for them to do this, (e.g. Blue Dog), is important (see Chapter 2, and Appendix A our online handouts for a pet parent handout).[34,41]

In addition to being able to read dog body language, it is essential to teach kids appropriate ways to approach, handle, interact, and play with their dog and to know what environmental accommodation can be made to help the dog cope when stressed and or wanting to avoid a situation. Many interactions which end in bites are initiated by the child. Dogs should not be expected to tolerate any and all interactions. The child must be taught appropriate ways of interacting with the dog. See recommended reading, Appendix A. This will not only reduce the incidents of bites but also increase the chances the family dog has a good QOL.

The stress the dog experiences when living with children does not always stem from direct physical interactions. Several nondirect physical interactions have been identified as being stressful for dogs (see Table 4.1) and while bites were

Table 4.1 Nondirect physical interactions that increase risk for a lower QOL for the dog

The child having a meltdown and/or a tantrum
Having child visitors in the home
Having the child and dog in the car together
The child playing with loud and wheeled toys
Change in routine due to child's needs/schedule
The dog not having a safe space to retreat away from the child

Reference: Hall et al., 2017, 2019.

not a common finding for the nondirect physical interactions, anything causing stress can lower thresholds for biting in the more "typical high-risk dog-child interactions."[3,4] Recent evidence highlights interactions and environmental adjustments that may benefit the dog.[3,4] The environmental adjustments should ensure the dog has a safe place to retreat to get away from the child and reduce noise in the household.[3,4] Children are too inconsistent in their actions to result in a reliably trained dog. All training should be positive reinforcement and completed by an adult before the child is permitted to interact with the dog. Child participation in positive reinforcement training can begin once the child is talking and has reasonable motor control. All interactions should be supervised by an adult whose attention is solely focused on the child and dog. The adult can hold the child on their lap then ask the dog for a behavior that the dog knows well. The child can then toss the food as a reward. Over time, the child can give the verbal cue for the behavior at the same time as the adult, as well as following up with a reward. Finally, the child can give the cue word and then reward the dog. This can be done with as many behaviors as are known by the dog. When the child is old enough, he or she can be taught the same rule structure as the adults so that the dog consistently learns to lie down or sit calmly before it gets things that it wants (e.g., toys, treats, play). Since babies, toddlers, and young children cannot be expected to understand dog body language, management strategies (see Table 4.2) must be used as a cornerstone for bite prevention.

Nonfamily dogs

The information in this chapter applies to interactions between children and dogs, regardless of how well they know the dog. Children should be reminded of the rules before going over to friends' or relatives' homes where there are have dogs or when seeing dogs out in public. It is especially important to remind them of these rules if they happen to live with a dog that is tolerant of children and does not show aggressive behavior. See Table 4.3 and Appendix A. Any interaction with someone else's dog should only happen if express permission is given by the adult responsible for that pet. If the child is approached by a dog that is acting aggressively, he or she should stand very still like a tree, say nothing, hold their arms against their body, and avoid eye contact. If the child is on the ground or knocked down, they should curl into a tight ball, cover their ears with their fists, and remain still and quiet until the animal moves far away.

Table 4.2 Management techniques intended to reduce the risk of injury to children

Management tool	Description
Baby/pet gates	There are a great variety of options for indoor gates for all types of home layouts. These are great to use for most dogs and are especially helpful for dogs that do not cope well in smaller, confined spaces.
Exercise pen (X-pen)	These allow the dog to have more room than a crate and to be in the same room with the family. This is also a good option for younger dogs that may not be able to be trusted not to get into things they should not.
Crates	These are only acceptable tools to use if the dog appears calm and comfortable in crates. There are many dogs that exhibit clinical signs of fear, anxiety, stress, conflict, panic, and/or aggression when crated. For dogs that do not cope well in crates, these are not safe or ethical to use. For those that can be in a crate, it needs to be large enough for the dog to comfortably stand up, lie down, stretch out completely, and turn around.
Separate room	This can be a great way to give the dog space to play, rest, walk around, and stretch as long as the dog does not display signs of fear, anxiety, stress, conflict, panic, and/or aggression when the door to that room is closed or a tall baby gate is used to prevent the dog and child from being in the same room at certain times.
Basket muzzle	This tool will prevent a bite but parents should be discouraged from putting it on and subsequently leaving the kids and dog alone or letting the child do whatever they please to the dog. It is essential to use a basket-style muzzle so the dog can pant comfortably and drink water. It is also essential to use positive training techniques to acclimate the dog to the muzzle.

Management techniques are the cornerstone of bite prevention.

Table 4.3 Rules to teach kids

Do not bother a dog if the dog is resting.
Do not hug/kiss a dog.
Do not pet a dog without asking for permission.
Do not take anything out of a dog's mouth.
Do not bother a dog while they are eating a meal, snack, bone, treat.
Do not bother a dog if they are actively working on a toy.
Do not put your face next to a dog's face.
Do not physically be rough with the dog or tease a dog.

A family-friendly handout of these rules can be found online in a printable format. See Appendix A

Final thoughts

The physical and emotional benefits of living with pets are clear. What is also clear is that children are particularly vulnerable to bites and that life with a child can be stressful for pets. One of our many responsibilities as veterinarians is to maintain a positive QOL for pets and a strong human–animal bond while also considering the public health aspects of pet ownership, including the risk of dog bites. Pet parents can be resistant to preparation of their pet for the baby. Veterinarians must be vigilant, honest, and empathetic to keep pets in their homes and keep children safe.

References

1. Purewal R, Chirstley R, Kordas K, Johnson C, Meinte K, Gee N, et al. Companion animal and child/adolescent development: a systemic review of the evidence. *Int J Env Res Public Health.* 2017;14:234.
2. Kerns KA, Koehn AJ, van Dulmen MHN, Stuart-Parrigon KL, Coifman KG. Preadolescents' relationships with pet dogs: relationship continuity, and associations with adjustment. *Appl Develop Sci.* 2017;21:67–80.
3. Hall SS, Wright HF, Mills DS. Parent perceptions of the quality of life of pet dogs living with neuro-typically developing and neuro-atypically developing children: an exploratory study. *PLoS One.* 2017;12:e0185300.
4. Hall SS, Brown BJ, Mils DS. Developing and assessing the validity of a scale to assess pet dog quality of life: Lincoln P-QoL. *Front Vet Sci.* 2019;6:326.
5. Centers for Disease Control and Prevention. Wisqars non-fatal injury data.

https://www.cdc.gov/injury/wisqars/index.html
6. Wilson F, Dwyer F, Bennet P. Prevention of dog bites: evaluation of brief educational intervention program for preschool children. *J Commun Psychol.* 2003;31:75–86.
7. Lakenstani NN, Donaldson Ml, Verga M, Waran N. Keeping children safe: how reliable are children at interpreting dog behavior? In: M. Mendl, OHP. Burman, A. Butterworth, MJ et al (eds). ISAE 2006: *Proceeding of the 40th International Congress of the International Society for Applies Ethology.* University of Bristol; 2006:233.
8. Valsecchi P, Barnard S, Stefanini C. Temperament test for re-homed dogs validated through direct behavioral observation in shelter and home environment. *J Vet Behav.* 2011;6(3):161–177.
9. Chun YT. Dog bites in children less than 4 years old. *Pediatrics.* 1982;69:119–120.

10. Avner R, Baker MS. Dog bites in urban children. *Pediatrics.* 1991;88:55–57.
11. Reisner I, Shofer F, Nance M. Behavioral assessment of child-directed canine aggression. *Inj Prev.* 2007;13:348–351.
12. Mannion C, Graham A, Shepherd K, Greenberg D. Dog bites and maxillofacial surgery: what can we do? *Br J Oral Maxillofac Surg.* 2015;56:479–484.
13. Kahn A, Bauche P, Amoureux J, Dog Bites research Team. Child victims of dog bites treated in emergency departments. *Eur J Pediatr.* 2003;162:254–258.
14. Schalamon J, Ainoedhofer HM, Singer G, et al. Analysis of dog bites in children who are younger than 17 years. *Pediatrics.* 2006;117:e374-e379.
15. Dwyer JP, Douglas TS, van As AB. Dog bite injury in children- a review of data from a South Africa pediatric unit. *S Afr Med J.* 2007;97:597–600.

16. Reisner IR, Nance ML, Zeller JS, Houseknech EM, Kassam-Adams N, Weibe DJ. Behavioral characteristics associated with dog bites to children presenting to an urban trauma center. *Inj Prev.* 2011;17:348–353.

17. Meints K, Syrnyk C, De Keuster T. Why do children get bitten in the face? *Inj Prev.* 2010;16(supply 1):A172.

18. Meints K. Children and dogs - risks and prevention. In: Mills D, Westgarth C, eds. *Dog Bites A Multidisciplinary Perspective.* Sheffield: 5M Publishing Ltd; 2017:393.

19. Mariti C, Gazzano A, Moore JL, Baragli P, Chelli L, Sigheri C. Perception of dogs' stress by their owners. *J Vet Behav.* 2012;7:213–219.

20. Bloom T, Friedman H. Classifying dogs' (Canis familiaris) facial expressions from photographs. *Behav Processes.* 2013;96: 1–10.

21. Fadel FR, Driscoll P, Pilot M, Wright H, Zulch H, Mills D. Differences in trait impulsivity indicate diversification of dog breeds into working and show lines. *Sci Rep.* 2016;6:22162.

22. Reisner IR, Houpt KA, Shofer FS. National survey of owner-directed aggression in English Springer Spaniels. *J Am Vet Med Assoc.* 2005;227:1594–1603.

23. Svartberg K. Breed typical behavior in dogs – historical remnants or recent constructs? *Appl Anim Behav Sci.* 2005;96:293–313.

24. Duffy DL, Hsu Y, Serpell JA. Breed differences in canine aggression. *Appl Anim Behav Sci.* 2008;114:441–460.

25. Overall KL, Love M. Dog bites to humans -demography, epidemiology, injury, and risk. *J Am Vet Med Assoc.* 2001; 1923–1934.

26. Asher L, England GC, Sommerville R, Harvey ND. Teenage dogs? Evidence for adolescent-phase conflict behavior and an association between attachment to humans and pubertal timing in the domestic dog. *Biol Lett.* 2020;16(5): 10.1098/rsbl.2020.0097.

27. Overall KL. Normal canine behavior and ontogeny. In: Overall KA, ed. *Manual of Clinical Behavioral Medicine for Dogs and Cats.* St. Louis: Elsevier; 2013:122–161.

28. Weiss E, Slater M, Garrison L, Drain N, Dolan E, Scarlett JM, et al. Large dog relinquishment to two municipal facilities in New York City and Washington, D.C.: identifying targets for intervention. *Animals.* 2014;4(3):409–433.

29. New JC, Salman MD, King M, Scarlett JM, Kass PH, Hutchison JM. Characteristics of shelter relinquished animals and their owners compared with animals and their owners in U.S pet-owning house-holds. *J Appl Anim Sci.* 2000;3:179–201.

30. Walker JK, Dale AR, D'Eath RB. Qualitative Behavior Assessment of dogs in the shelter and home environmental and relationship with quantitative behaviour assessment and physiological responses. *Appl Anim Behav.* 2016;184:97–108.

31. Marder AR, Shabelansky A, Patronek GJ, Dowling-Guyer S, D'Arpino S. Food-related aggression in the shelter dogs: a comparison of behavior identified by a behavior evaluation in the shelter and owner reports after adoptions. *Anim Behav.* 2013;148:150–156.

32. Hennessy M, Voith V, Mazzei S, Buttram J, Miller D, Linden F. Behavior and cortisol levels of dogs in a public animal shelter, and an exploration of the ability of these measures to predict problem behavior after adoption. *Appl Anim Behav Sci.* 2001;73(3):217–233.

33. Reisner IR, Shofer S. Effects of gender and parental status on knowledge and attitudes of dog owners regarding dog aggression toward children. *J Am Vet Med Assoc.* 2008;233:1412–1419.

34. Bergman L, Haskins L. Expanding families: preparing for and introducing dogs and cats to infants, children, and new pets. *Vet Clin Small Animal Pract.* 2008;38:1023–1043.

35. Buffington TCA, Pacak K. Increased plasma norepinephrine concentration in cats with interstitial cystitis. *J Urol.* 2001;165:2051–2054.

36. Feliway (CEVA). www.feliway.com (worldwide); us.feliway.com (USA)

37. Meints K, Racca A, Hickey N. How to prevent dog bite injuries? Children misinterpret dog facial expressions. *Inj Prev.* 2010;16(supplement 1)A68.

38. Amici F, Waterman J, Kellermann CM et al. The ability to recognize dog emotions depends on the cultural milieu in which we grow up. *Sci Rep.* 9(1):16414.

39. Kerswell KJ, Bennett PJ, Butler KL, Hemsworth, PH. Self reported comprehension ratings of dog behavior by puppy owners. *Anthrozoos.* 2007; 22:183–193.

40. Demirbas YS, Ozturk BE, Kockaya M, et al. Adults ability to interpret canine body language during a dog-child interaction. *Anthrozoos.* 2016;29:581–596.

41. Aldridge GL, Rose SE. Young children's interpretation of dogs' emotions and their intentions to approach happy, angry, and frightened dogs. *Antrozoos.* 2019;32:361–374.

Resources and recommended reading

(For comprehensive references for child safety, bite prevention, and communication and body language, see appendix A.)

The Blue Dog — http://thebluedog.org/en/.

Cat Body Language — https://www.maddiesfund.org/feline-communication-how-to-speak-cat.htm.

Family dog – Stop the 77 — https://www.thefamilydog.com/stop-the-77/.

Jakeman M, Oxley JA, Owczarczak-Garstecka SC, et al. Pet dog bites in children: management and prevention. *BMJ Paediatr Open.* 2020;4:e00726. doi:10.1136/bmjpo-2020-000726.

Levine ED, *Doggie Dos and Don'ts.* Instinct Dog Behavior & Training; 2020.

Pelar C. *Living with Kids and Dogs...without Losing Your Mind.* 2nd ed. Dream Dog Productions; 2012.

Tudge N. A Kids' *Comprehensive Guide to Speaking Dog.* Joanne Tudge; 2017.

CHAPTER 5

Prevention: the best medicine

Andrea Y. Tu, DVM and Lisa Radosta, DVM, DACVB

Introduction

The old adage "An ounce of prevention is worth a pound of cure," still holds true. Early intervention generally shortens treatment times and improves outcomes. Pet parents often think that their dog or cat will grow out of negative behavior patterns. While dogs and cats may calm down and play less as they get older, especially if gonadectomized, they do not grow out of serious behavior problems. Instead, behavioral clinical signs get worse with age.[1] The best approach is to prevent behavior problems in puppies, kittens, or any pet of any age. When a problem does arise, treat early and immediately (see Chapter 1). When thinking of preventive behavioral medicine, puppies and kittens immediately come to mind; however, pets adopted at any age and seen by the veterinary team at any stage of life can be helped with preventive measures.

Setting the pet up for success

Pet parents should understand that it is far more productive and effective to train and guide the puppy, kitten, or new pet into acceptable responses (e.g., what to chew, where to scratch, where to eliminate, what to do to gain attention), rather than trying to punish the pet for every behavior that might be undesirable. The pillars of prevention of behavior problems include consistent interactions; reward-based training; environmental enrichment, reading and recognizing communication; meeting the behavioral needs of the species and breed; individual, proactive supervision; and independence training (see Box 5.1).

A major driver of fear, anxiety, stress, and conflict (FASC) is inconsistency in interactions between the pet parent and the pet. Dogs and cats are able to adapt to different styles of interaction within and outside of the family. However, when there are inconsistencies with interactions with a single person or broad inconsistencies in the way family members interact with the pet, the risk of an increase in FASC is high. Pet parents should be consistent and fair in their interactions with their pets. This may require that individual family members attend training classes, read or view resources, or meet with the veterinary healthcare team for education (see Chapters 2 and 10).

Puppies, kittens, and new pets to the household are much like toddlers in that they need proactive supervision. Proactive supervision entails watching the pet carefully and never leaving the pet unattended until it is completely capable of

1. Consistent interactions and predictability
2. Reward-based training
3. Proactive supervision
4. Environmental enrichment
5. Independence training and confinement
6. Reading and recognizing communication
7. Meeting the behavioral needs of the species, breed, and individual

being alone without causing harm to him- or herself or damage to the pet parent's property. This very simple concept eludes most pet parents. Very often, they leave new pets of any age unattended before they are ready. This can lead to disappointment by the pet parent, resulting in punishment to the pet. This causes confusion on the part of the pet that does not know why it is being punished. Appropriate supervision may entail using a leash and collar or harness as an umbilical cord to keep the pet with the pet parent.

Reward-based training is essential for a strong relationship between pet and pet parent. No person or animal enjoys being hurt. Pain and discomfort do not make for strong relationships, no matter to which species you are referring. Shock, choke, and pinch collars are painful. Hitting or yelling can cause fear, anxiety, and stress. Even the squirt from a water bottle can traumatize a dog or cat, depending on their individual sensitivities. There will be times where pet parents will be frustrated and will use punishment inappropriately. If given the proper tools at the outset by the veterinary healthcare team and a positive reinforcement training professional, the pet parent will be much less likely to fall into the trap of punishment. See Chapter 10 for more information on training.

We control everything about our pets, lives from what they eat to where they go to where they are permitted to sleep to when they are permitted to eliminate. In addition, our pets do not leave the house nearly as often as we do, often leading underenriched lives. This can lead to many behavior problems and an overemphasis on the relationship with the pet parent, potentially leading to separation-related disorders. Environmental enrichment is as important as anything else that we do to maintain the health and wellness of our patients. Environmental enrichment provides outlets for normal behavior and enhances physical and emotional well-being with positive, enjoyable activities away from locations, targets, and stimuli that might be a problem for the pet parent or the pet. Many indoor cats receive only minimal environmental enrichment, particularly with interactive social play and exploration. Additionally, the pet parents often do not understand normal behavior, enrichment (particularly for indoor cats), the risk of behavior problems if the cat's needs are not met, and how to provide sufficient resources to minimize social conflict.[2]

Overall success can only be achieved if all of the pet's innate needs are considered and met, including, for example, chewing, scratching, climbing, perching, bedding, food, water, elimination, and security. Other needs include play, mental stimulation, physical exercise, and social interaction. Once the pet learns undesirable behaviors because appropriate outlets are not provided and is reinforcing for them (e.g., chewing on baseboards), even when the environment is brought up to par, the undesirable (but normal) behaviors persist. Once a behavior is learned, it is very difficult and, in many cases, impossible for the pet to "unlearn" that behavior. It is much easier, more effective, and efficient to prevent undesirable behaviors by providing a properly enriched environment from the start.

Independence is a skill to be learned by the pet regardless of the age at which they are adopted. Independence is a gift that supports the pet parent's and pet's happiness. Access to areas and objects that might be targets of undesirable behavior should be prevented. Family possessions and dangerous or toxic items should be put out of reach. The pet should be confined when it cannot be supervised. Pets that must eliminate during the time that the family is away for long periods will need to be provided with access to an elimination area that is acceptable to the family. Pets should be provided with a sanctuary space in which they can get away from it all, whether a scary visitor, another pet, a child, or a storm. Every being needs a safe place to go!

Working with new puppies and kittens – the team approach

Providing timely behavioral advice to new puppy and kitten pet parents can help prevent undesirable behaviors as well as help correct existing problems before they become resistant to change. The first veterinary visit is the time to introduce the family to important concepts about behavior, learning, and training. Do not assume that the family knows how to raise a pet in the healthiest way for that individual pet. Preventive advice should be offered to all new pet parents so that they know what is needed and what to expect when raising their pet. Unrealistic pet parent expectations, insufficient or incorrect counseling and instructive material, lack of training, allowing the pet to roam outdoors, improper gonadectomy (or at the wrong time), destructive behavior, and house soiling have been shown to increase the risk of pet parent relinquishment.[3–6] These are issues that need to be discussed with all pet parents. In fact, a single behavior counseling session at the first puppy or kitten visit can affect a lasting change. In dogs, one session of behavioral advice reduced the risk of house soiling, mounting, mouthing, excessive play, demanding food at the table, and fear of unfamiliar people in dogs, and in cats, undesirable climbing of furniture and curtains, vocalization, disturbing pet parents while resting, and fewer issues with body handling.[7,8] A list of topics that should be discussed can be found in Box 5.2.

A new pet checklist for all puppy and kitten appointments will ensure that all veterinary healthcare team members address all points in an orderly manner and important topics do not get missed (See Appendix C, online resources). Advice to pet parents can be spread out over the course of puppy and kitten visits. As long as the information is properly prioritized and given at an appropriate time in the pet's development, not all information needs to be provided at once. Preadoption consultations and puppy or kitten classes provide additional opportunities to educate and counsel the new pet parent.

Technicians and nurses have come to be the educators in veterinary practices; puppy and kitten appointments are no different. Properly trained team members can be very effective in this role, providing another important facet to the practice's team approach to health care, giving the veterinarian more

Box 5.2 Behavioral topics that should be discussed with each new pet parent and that can be a major focus of staff training and involvement in preventive behavior counseling

- Socialization with people, situations, and animals of all types
- List of appropriate reading material, web sites, videos
- Providing a safe environment by pet proofing the home and yard
- Supervision, confinement, crate training, carrier training
- Housetraining, litterbox training
- Handling and husbandry
- Enrichment, play, and exercise
- Chewing, scratching, and destructive behaviors
- Reward-based training and shaping desirable behaviors
- Giving pets control to make choices that are acceptable to pet parents
- Basic grooming needs, nail trimming
- Outdoor safety and pet ID (e.g., microchip)
- Pet health insurance and other risk management strategies
- Training tools (e.g., head collars, leashes, harnesses, toys)

time to concentrate on the more intricate aspects of the diagnosis and treatment of behavioral disorders. A designated team member (behavioral medicine advocate) can be responsible for ensuring that the information is correct, up to date, and in line with the current science and literature. This information can be gleaned through veterinary continuing education, journals, and textbooks, as well as online resources. Dog training seminars may be used to further expand a team member's knowledge; however, veterinary behavior resources should be used as the foundation of all recommendations.

Because there are many types of learners and pet parents may be distracted during their appointment, lists of resources (e.g., handouts, videos, web sites reading lists) in a handout or on the practice's web site should be made available. See Appendix A for a comprehensive list of resources. Review the contents of all premade packets prior to sharing with your pet parent to ensure that the information and recommendations contained in the packet are appropriate and up to date with the most current behavioral recommendations. Behavioral medicine advocates or supervising team members should be adequately compensated, and time scheduled for continuing education. Opportunities are plentiful and webinars are common, so team members never even have to leave the office to get a great education. The hospital can also enroll team members in certification programs such as Fear Free certification (www.fearfreepets.com). For a more complete discussion of the role of veterinary healthcare team members in the implementation of preventative behavioral medicine, see Chapter 1.

Pet parents find information about their new puppy or kitten in lots of places, but mostly online. Unfortunately, veterinarians report that only about 20% of pet parents talk to them about what they find online.[9] Not only are pet parents unlikely to offer information to their veterinarian, but many may also be unaware themselves of what constitutes a reportable problem in a kitten or puppy. Pet parents should be asked about their puppy's or kitten's behavior at each visit. A one-page behavior intake questionnaire (e.g., see Chapter 1) for each puppy's and kitten visit can assist with history taking without sacrificing efficiency. Unless veterinary team members take a proactive approach, pet

parents may not realize that members of the team are important resources for behavioral advice or that early intervention may prevent the development of more serious problems. During each physical exam, observe the pet for any undesirable behaviors (e.g., fear, aggression, impulsivity) and advise on how these might best be handled. If the pet shows evidence that it may become dangerous to family members, it is incumbent upon the veterinarian to inform the pet parents fully and give them appropriate options. When behavioral advice is given, it is important for the veterinarian or team members to record the findings and recommendations in the pet's medical or behavioral records, and to follow up by telephone, e-mail, or in person to ensure that the pet is being managed and improvement is being made. As outlined in Chapter 2, clinical signs in puppies and kittens should be addressed immediately.

Socialization

Socialization has been discussed in Chapter 2. It is such an important topic for puppies and kittens that it is mentioned again here.[10] Socialization is a special learning process by which puppies and kittens develop a positive association with people, animals, locations, and all other stimuli in their environment.[11–13] Puppies and kittens need to be handled frequently and have positive contact with a variety of people and other animals, objects, and environments early in their lives in order to become normal, friendly, confident adults. Puppies and kittens that develop social relationships during these periods are often capable of maintaining these relationships for life and are likely to be friendly and form stable attachments.[10,14]

The most critical period for socialization (sensitive period) in puppies starts at 2–1/2–3 weeks and declines at 12 weeks of age, while the most receptive period for kittens is from two to seven weeks of age.[10,14] Often, pet parents believe that socialization entails just bringing their new pet out to various environments to meet people and other animals of the same species. However, socialization is a much more active process than exposure alone. Proper socialization involves helping the pet form *positive* associations with the people, animals, situations, and stimuli, including the veterinary environment, that it will encounter throughout life. Fear of veterinary visits has been associated with negative or indifferent experiences during veterinary visits as a puppy.[15] It is essential that the exposures are positive. Negative exposures during this time have an equally amplified effect on later behavior. Advise pet parents to stop the interaction if the pet shows signs of moderate or severe fear, anxiety, or stress, preventing negative associations resulting in lifelong consequences for the pet. During this period, strong fear-eliciting situations and stimuli must be avoided. Pheromone analogues may also be helpful during the socialization period. In one study, puppies wearing dog-appeasing pheromone (Adaptil) collars were less fearful and anxious, had more positive interactions, and in followup surveys for one year were consistently more social and faster to adapt to new situations than puppies wearing placebo collars.[16] See Chapter 2 for more information on puppy socialization.

While much has been written about puppy socialization, it is equally important for kittens to develop and maintain proper social relationships with other cats, people, other species, and the stimuli within their environment. However, since the sensitive period for socialization in cats begins to wane as early as seven weeks of age, before most pet parents adopt their kittens, socialization must begin immediately after adoption.

Pet parents may not feel that socialization of their new kitten is important or may not know how to implement proper socialization. While cats do not generally go as many places outside of the home as dogs, lack of exposure to stimuli can significantly contribute to fear aggression, fear at the veterinarian's office, noise aversion or phobia, fear of adults or children, and separation-related disorders. Positive exposure of kittens to sounds, animals, and people can primarily, with the exception of the veterinarian's office, occur at home (see Figure 5.1). Pet parents should attempt to maintain their kitten's social skills with other cats by having more than one cat in the home, visiting friends with healthy, vaccinated, sociable cats, or by attending kitten kindergarten.

While proper socialization of puppies and kittens during the periods outlined above are extremely important to prevent the development of behavior disorders, positive exposure prior to and after the socialization period is ideal for long-term behavioral stability and wellness. See Chapter 2 for more information on how the prenatal and early environment affects behavioral development. There are many factors involved in proper prevention of fear-based behavior disorders in dogs and cats (Box 5.3). Pet parents should understand that socialization is one of the most important ways to ensure the health and wellness of their pet, as important as heartworm prevention or vaccination. Puppies and kittens with a nondomestic (kennel-reared with minimal human interaction) maternal environment and insufficient socialization are at increased risk for developing avoidance behavior near unfamiliar people, conspecifics, noises, and places, and fear-induced aggression.[17]

Unfortunately, the practice of recommending that puppies stay home or avoid contact with much of the outside

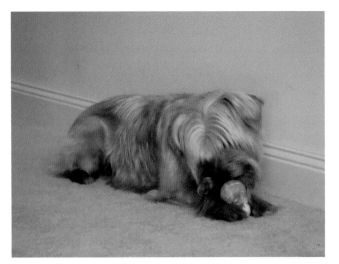

Figure 5.1 Food toys can keep dogs occupied during stressful situations in the home. *(Attribution: Lisa Radosta.)*

world still exists in veterinary medicine. Yet poor socialization as a puppy, infrequent participation in training, living in an urban environment, and receiving less than adequate daily exercise have all been associated with social fearfulness.[18] Social deprivation (e.g., isolation until 16 weeks) prevents the establishment of normal socialization and can affect learning, fear responses, sexual behavior, and social behavior.[19–21] This means that if puppies are not socialized during the socialization period (3–12 weeks) due to the recommendation of the veterinary healthcare team, the puppy is more likely to be afflicted with behavior disorders which often lead to relinquishment or death. In short, the recommendation to keep an otherwise healthy pet at home or isolated from a range of people, animals, environments, and stimuli until 16 weeks when the last vaccination has been administered is harmful to the pet.

Puppy class and kitty kindergarten

One way to achieve successful socialization is to take puppies to puppy classes and kittens to kitty kindergarten (Figures 5.2–5.4). Puppies that attend properly conducted puppy classes had reduced risk of fear and aggression to unfamiliar people; familiar and unfamiliar dogs; reduced nonsocial fears, including thunder, vacuum cleaners, crates; less touch sensitivity; improved trainability; and pet parents who were less likely to use punishment.[22–25] In addition, puppies had more effective behavior problem intervention, fewer behavior problems later in life, and higher retention rates in the home as adults. Puppies were no more likely to contract canine parvovirus compared to puppies that do not attend puppy class.[26–28] Puppy classes have also been demonstrated to have a positive effect on puppies that were separated from their litter prematurely (30–45 days) in reducing fearfulness on walks, intraspecific aggression, barking, and possessiveness.[29] In summary, there is overwhelming scientific evidence that puppies that are socialized via a puppy class have long-lasting benefits, including avoidance of relinquishment and euthanasia and were no more likely to get infectious diseases.

One major concern of some veterinarians and pet parents is the risk of disease to puppies and kittens that have not yet finished their vaccination series. However, in order for socialization classes to be optimally effective, they

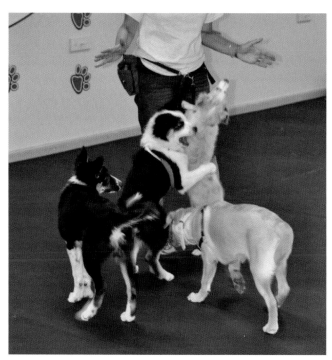

Figure 5.2 Puppy classes can aid in successful socialization. *(Cheryl VanVoorhies, M.ed.)*

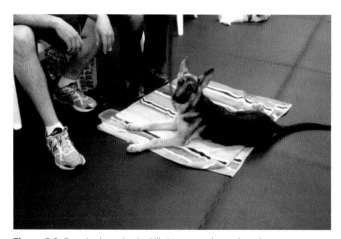

Figure 5.3 Puppies learn basic skills in puppy class, when they are most amenable to acquiring behaviors. *(Cheryl VanVoorhies, M.ed.)*

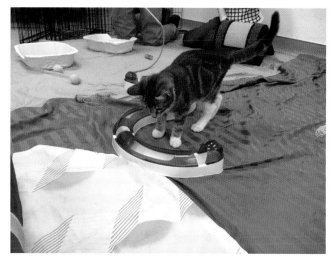

Figure 5.4 Kitten kindergarten gives kittens exposure to stimuli that they will encounter later in life. *(Attribution: San Francisco SPCA.)*

should begin well within the primary socialization period (i.e., before 12 weeks of age). Therefore, the risk of disease must be weighed against the potential benefits of early socialization and training. If puppies and kittens have been examined and found to be in good health and free of parasites, have been vaccinated with their first puppy or kitten vaccine at least seven days earlier, and continue to receive their vaccinations in a timely manner, then bringing them into an indoor training environment with other pets their own age should be a minimum risk compared with the benefits that might be achieved. In fact, this type of well-screened and supervised environment may be less

risky than a walk along the street or a trip to other areas frequented by pets. Indeed, the risk of disease to puppies and kittens when proper precautions are taken are minimal for the lifelong welfare of the pet when one further considers that behavioral concerns is the top and second most frequent reason for canine and feline relinquishment to a shelter (respectively), and behavior problems are one of the most significant barriers to adoption.[30,31] For these reasons, puppies and kittens should start socialization, ideally in puppy classes after their first vaccination and deworming.

Classes can be taught by a veterinary healthcare team member or a positive reinforcement dog trainer. The goals of these classes are to provide socialization to a variety of stimuli, educate pet parents in the training and management of pets, and prevent behavior problems. Offering puppy and kitten classes in the veterinary hospital also provide the optimal agenda, counseling, and guidance, and to positively condition the pet to the hospital, handling, and healthcare equipment and procedures. In one study in a veterinary hospital that introduced a 5-week-long puppy socialization and reinforcement training class, there was a 94% retention rate in the home after two years, compared to five years earlier when up to two-thirds of the dogs were no longer in their home after two years.[32]

Structured and supervised play with conspecifics (especially in dogs that have no other dogs in their home environment) provides an opportunity to develop socially acceptable behaviors and refine communication skills between members of the species. Social interaction with people and other pets as well as some demonstration and guidance on reward-based training techniques should also be covered. Any emerging problems should be identified and appropriate management and solutions discussed. See Box 5.4 for a list of topics covered in puppy and kitten classes.

Veterinary hospitals that are not able to offer full classes and do not have a dog training professional to which to refer may consider having a monthly 1-hour to 2-hour puppy

1. Routine health care
2. Training for good manners (at home and when out)
3. Socialization
4. Positive handling and cooperative care (including grooming and veterinary procedures)
5. Normal behavior and providing for the pet's behavioral needs
6. How animals learn and shaping desirable behavior
7. Setting the household up for success
8. House/litter training
9. Destructive behavior
10. Play biting
11. Unruly behavior
12. Giving animals choices as a part of building a trusting relationship

or kitten socialization "party" at the hospital. During this get-together (open house), families can bring their new pets, meet the team, take a tour of the hospital, and get additional information on behavior, nutrition, grooming, and dental care, while the pets have social time with other people and pets under the watchful eye of a trained team member. A few refreshments and samples for pet parents and pets might also be a good way to encourage attendance.

Foundational concepts for pet parent education

Whether a puppy, kitten, or an older dog or cat, there are challenges for the pet and for the pet parents when transitioning to a new home. Most pet parents, even those who are experienced, do not understand species-typical behavior or communication in dogs and cats. These are foundational parts of the education of the pet parent, which are the responsibility of the veterinary healthcare team. See Chapter 2 for a discussion of communication and body language.

The new home should provide a predictable routine: appropriate outlets for each of the pet's needs at each stage of development; secure and comfortable housing; and predictable consequences that focus on rewarding what is desirable and preventing what is undesirable. Reinforcement-based training can quickly enhance the bond between pet and pet parent while improving communication and shaping those behaviors that are desirable. In addition, pet parents often forget that cats can and do need the same type of structured interactions and training from which dogs benefit.

Punishment-based training (see Chapter 10) often causes FASC, which is the cause of most behavior disorders requiring treatment by veterinarians. In addition, this type of training degrades the bond between pet and pet parent at best and only teaches the pet who, what, and when to avoid, rather than training the pet to do what is desirable. Focusing on the prevention of problems and setting up an environment in which the pet can succeed improves the welfare of the pet and the pet–family bond, and reduces those behavioral problems that can damage or break the bond.[33–35]

It is important for the family to understand that they must provide for all of the pet's needs. Besides nutrition, health, and shelter, dogs and cats have very important social, physical, and mental stimulation requirements. If these are not met, a variety of undesirable behaviors may develop, including unruliness, hyperactivity, undesirable play behavior, unwanted exploratory behavior, destructiveness, conflict-induced behaviors such as self-trauma, nocturnal activity, and attention-seeking behaviors. In cats, the consequences might include periuria and perichezia, scratching, aggression, anxiety, vocalization, and excessive activity.[36] For these reasons, lack of understanding of the pet's needs or ability to meet those needs will produce a less than satisfactory family–pet relationship.[37] It is never too early to introduce the Five Freedoms of Animal Welfare to pet parents, as this can be a guide not only for newly adopted pets but end-of-life decisions (see Figure 5.5).

Providing opportunities for species-typical behavior which may be considered undesirable by pet parents through environmental enrichment and management can make the difference between a positive and negative relationship between the pet and the family. Environmental enrichment increases positive utilization of the environment, can reduce the frequency of unacceptable behaviors, and increases the pet's ability to cope with challenges in a more productive and healthy manner.[38]

All animals require an environment that allows them to be physically stimulated (exercised) as well as mentally stimulated (cognitively and/or emotionally motivated/exercised). Pets need to be provided with complex, stimulating environments that allow them to carry out activities that give them choices, both physically and psychologically, to the extent with which they can cope. Pets with FASC need the enrichment to be appropriate to their needs, as too much can exacerbate their issues, as can too little. Confined animals are often understimulated because choices are not available or choices are made for them that do not meet their needs. Indoor-only cats can be considered for all intents and purposes confined animals. While some cultures and home environments offer cats the opportunity to safely spend time outdoors to engage in some of these daily activities, the challenge is much greater for pet parents who live in urban areas and high-rise apartments and house their cats entirely indoors.[39]

Dogs and cats are social species that often benefit from regular interaction with others, be it with their own or other species. It is not behaviorally healthy for dogs or cats to live alone for extended periods of time without social interaction or alternative forms of stimulation.

As with human beings, one size does not fit all. Many dogs and cats do not desire or benefit from interactions with certain stimuli, which may include people, dogs, cats, or other species. In addition, social exposure does not equal a constant stream of interaction. Sleep is as important for cats and dogs as it is for us. Constant interaction can be stressful. Exercise can be a positive aspect of enrichment. However, if walks or play are stressful, the activity is counterproductive and can lead to chronic stress, which has serious detrimental effects on the pet's overall wellness. See Chapter 7 for more detail on chronic stress.

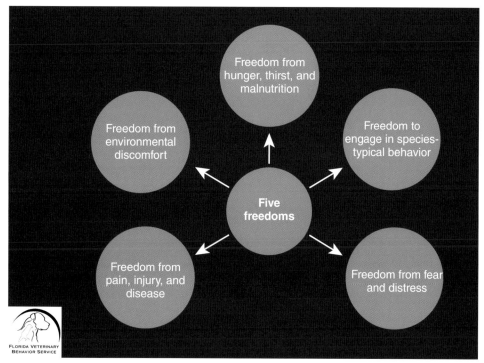

FLORIDA VETERINARY
BEHAVIOR SERVICE

Figure 5.5 Five freedoms of animal welfare. *(Attribution: Lisa Radosta.)*

Environmental Enrichment

Much of this chapter is devoted to environmental enrichment, emphasizing the importance of this topic on dog and cat well-being, behavior, and health. It is important for dogs and cats to live in an environment that is interesting, complex, and stimulating, so it is not surprising that they may engage in behaviors that help to fill the void or develop displacement behaviors when frustrated, underenriched, or prevented from exhibiting their normal repertoire of behaviors. The family should consider the pet's normal behavioral repertoire and include outlets for predation and chase, social interactions, eating multiple small meals, object play and exploration, scratching, climbing, comfortable places for perching and resting, and providing sufficient resources to prevent social conflict (see Boxes 5.5–5.7).

Food and puzzle toys

One opportunity for quick and easy enrichment is to utilize the time that would normally be spent eating a meal to mentally challenge the dog or cat. Feeding from food toys should start as soon as the new pet enters the home, regardless of age. Older pets, those that have been isolated or feral, or those suffering from FASC may be frightened or confused by the food toy. In those cases, slow introduction is best while giving some of the meal or a more desirable type of food in the food toy and less desirable food in the food bowl (see Figures 5.1 and 5.6).

Cats are especially suspicious, requiring patience and fortitude in some cases. Encourage pet parents to stick with it. This is all the more reason to introduce food toys immediately to puppies or kittens. Remember socialization? Food toys are a stimulus in the environment, as is the texture and taste of food. Exposure to these things (e.g., different foods and ways to acquire food) is beneficial, as the pet's life inevitably changes over time, which may cause changes to food, administration of medications in food, and how the pet is fed. Feeding from food and puzzle toys is one of the easiest things to do and it reaps big rewards in behavior (Figures 5.7 and 5.8).

Organization of the environment

Dogs and cats alike need environments in which they can live comfortably, find places to get away and hide, and have places to rest. Sanctuary spaces are places where dogs and cats can get away from it all. In addition, they allow the pet to be confined when needed. Training this behavior (being able to stay alone in a space) can be useful for visitors, when moving, when introducing another pet to the home, for a new baby, and natural disasters (e.g., hurricanes). A sanctuary space can be a bathroom, bedroom, crate, or closet, for example. Sometimes pets are trained to stay in a space with a closed door (e.g., when visitors will be present) and sometimes an open door is more appropriate (e.g., storms) (see Figures 5.9 and 5.10).

The simplest form of prevention of undesirable behaviors involves separating the pet from the site of the problem or confining it so that the undesirable behavior cannot be performed.[40,41] A common misconception is that confinement is cruel or unfair. On the contrary, leaving a pet unsupervised to investigate, destroy, and perhaps get injured is far more inhumane. For kittens, crating may be useful, but most

Box 5.5 Suggestions for environmental enrichment for dogs

Auditory
- Radio
- Television
- Pet-specific music
- Calming music
- Classical music
- Toys that squeak, grunt, or squeal
- Access to outdoors

Oral/gustatory
- Food hidden around the home
- Frozen or fresh fruit or vegetables (small chunks)
- Rotation of foods for meals or treats
- Ice cubes of meat or broth
- Treats or kibble in plastic water bottles
- Nosework
- Timed feeder
- Food toys such as Kong or other puzzle toys
- Pieces of food tossed down the hall, up the stairs, in the kennel, or around the yard
- Natural products – bones, antlers, etc.
- Manufactured chews – Nylabones, rubber chews
- Soft toys
- Rubber toys
- Fabric toys

Olfactory
- Lavender
- Mint
- Chamomile
- Pheromone analogues
- Prey scent placed on toys
- Rotation of foods or treats
- Outdoors/new environments

Exercise
- Retrieving
- Tug of war
- Flying disc
- Soccer
- Swimming
- Walking
- Jogging
- Agility
- Barn Hunt
- Tracking
- Herding
- Flyball
- Lure coursing

Social
- Dog walker
- Another pet of the same species or different species
- Day care if it is enjoyed by the dog
- Dog beach if safe to take to the beach
- Private play sessions
- Grooming
- Dog training classes

Arrangement of home
- Several resting areas designated for the dog
- Hiding area
- Crate or area where the dog can move away from others, away from the front door or stressors

Tactile
- Toys of varying textures
- Areas to explore and dig in the yard

Box 5.6 Suggestions for environmental enrichment for cats

Auditory
- Radio
- Television
- Pet-specific music
- Calming music
- Classical music
- Toys that squeak, jingle, or make high-pitched sounds
- Access to outdoors through a catio, harness, and leash or patio
- Hammock near a window

Oral/gustatory
- Food hidden around the home
- Rotation of foods for meals or treats
- Timed feeder
- Food toys such as Catit toys
- Pieces of food tossed down the hall, up the stairs, in the kennel, or around the yard
- Cat grass
- Silver vine
- Catnip
- Drinking fountains
- Rawhide
- Freeze-dried meat strips

Olfactory
- Lavender
- Mint
- Chamomile
- Pheromone analogues
- Prey scent placed on toys
- Rotation of foods or treats
- Outdoors/new environments

Exercise
- Stuffed toys that can be chased
- Motorized toys
- Ping pong balls, walnuts, and hair ties
- Feather or rubber toys on flexible wires
- Toys that hang from a door

Social
- Another pet of the same species or different species
- Private play sessions
- Training sessions

Arrangement of home
- Multilevel resting area
- Cat shelves
- Kitty condos
- Hammock next to window
- Perch on windowsill
- Aquarium

Tactile
- Different scratching surfaces
- Different resting surfaces
- Toys of varying textures

- Destructive chewing, digging, and scratching
- Investigative behavior, garbage raiding
- Hyperactivity, excitability, nocturnal activity
- Unruliness, knocking over furniture, jumping up
- Excessive play
- Rough play
- Attention-soliciting behaviors such as barking and whining
- Aggression
- Nocturnal wakening
- Biting
- Barking or meowing for attention
- Barking at the door and windows

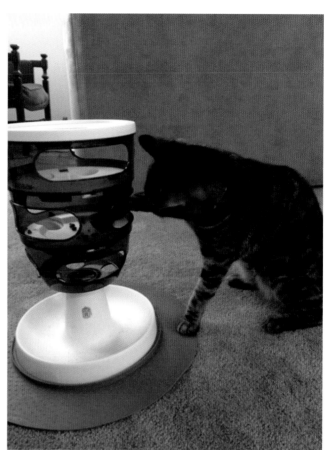

Figure 5.8 Food toys are widely available for cats. *(Attribution: Elizabeth MacHaffee.)*

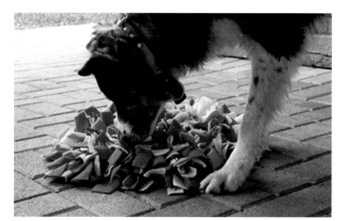

Figure 5.6 Food toys (dog). A snuffle mat is an easy toy to make at home to keep dogs busy. *(Attribution: Mindy Cox, CPDT-KSA.)*

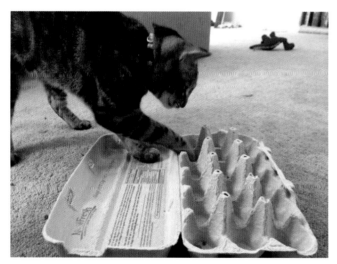

Figure 5.7 A food toy can be made out of almost any item. *(Attribution: Elizabeth MacHaffee.)*

kittens can be housed in a sanctuary room with toys, food, water, a scratching post, and litterbox, provided there are no objects that can be damaged by climbing or chewing.

Crate training, while not a necessity for all families and all pets, can be helpful in many circumstances. As mentioned above, it can be used as a sanctuary space. Feeling comfortable in a crate can ease FASC when in the veterinary clinic, when moving, during times of family transition (e.g., children, marriage, divorce, elderly parents) and in case of emergencies (e.g., hurricane, flood, fire). Pet parents who seldom leave their pets alone and those who house their pets outdoors when they cannot be supervised may require little or no indoor confinement. However, because a pet is not confined now does not predict that it will not need this skill in the future. Preventive behavior medicine entails to some extent the prediction of what the pet will experience over its lifetime. It is very likely that the pet will need to be confined and left alone at some point. For these reasons, independence and confinement training should be taught early on to all pets. Regardless of future intentions, when pet parents must leave a new pet unsupervised inside the home, it is essential that it be confined to an area where it will not injure itself, cause household damage, escape, or eliminate in unacceptable locations. When crate training is used, the crate should be big enough for the pet to stand up and turn around comfortably with space for water, food, a bed, and a litterbox (cats). Pets should not be left alone in the crate for extended periods of time.

Regardless of whether a crate or a room is being used as the confinement or sanctuary space, it should be associated with positive things such as feeding and resting. Pet parents can feed their pets in the sanctuary space, toss treats there for their pet to find, and put new chewies or enrichment items in that space. It should never be used as punishment. Unless the pet

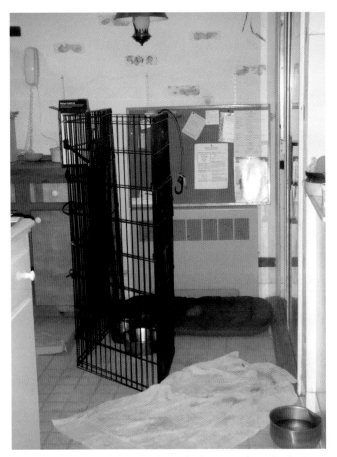

Figure 5.9 A sanctuary space can be made almost anywhere. *(Attribution: Lisa Radosta.)*

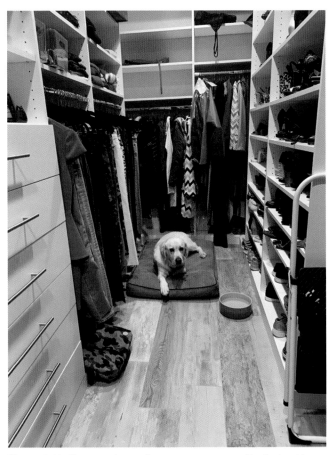

Figure 5.10 Closets make excellent sanctuary spaces. *(Attribution: Lisa Radosta.)*

needs to be confined immediately for safety or house training, the sanctuary space or crate should be introduced slowly with longer periods of confinement occurring as the pet can tolerate it. Some dogs suffer from confinement distress and cannot be confined in a crate. They may, however, be able to be confined in an exercise pen, closet, or bathroom.

Cats are unique in that they utilize high spaces as well as moderate- and low-level spaces. Inside the home, shelves on which to climb, cubbies, cardboard boxes, tunnels, and paper bags that provide hiding and resting places enhance and increase the size of the cat's environment, as well as improve the chances that multiple cats can successfully share the home. The cat carrier can be especially stressful for cats. Confinement training should include the cat carrier which will be used for transport to the veterinary office (see Appendix A and Resources and Recommended Reading). Carrier training should be completed slowly over many sessions, using food or play to help condition a positive emotional response.

Exercise and exposure to outdoors

Exercise can be beneficial for the pet's overall health and can provide a wealth of environmental enrichment. Young dogs should be given sufficient exercise to dissipate an ample amount of energy. A 15-minute exercise period once or twice daily may be suitable for many dogs, but this may not meet the behavioral needs of some working dogs. On the other hand, it may be too much for a more sedentary dog. The recommended amount of exercise is dependent on the pet's overall health, tolerance for exercise, and tolerance for the stimuli in the environment. Puppies and dogs with health issues (including most brachycephalic breeds) may be at risk for medical problems when exercised at too high of an intensity or for a prolonged length of time. Active families may prefer to jog, run, or take long walks to satisfy their dog's needs. More sedentary families can accomplish the same goals by throwing a ball, toy, or flying disc for the dog to retrieve. Meeting the physical and mental needs of some breeds (e.g., Border Collies, German Shorthaired Pointers, Bengal cats) may be more challenging to achieve for the average pet parent. Pet parents should make plans to spend time each day with their pet and then honor that commitment – both will benefit. Exercise periods are not only healthy for pet parent and pet, but are wonderful interactive sessions that help in the bonding process and can also prevent unwanted attention-soliciting behaviors.

The pet parent may believe that they can exercise the anxiety, fear, or stress out of their pet. This is untrue. While exercise has its benefits, significant reductions in FASC in pets that are moderately to severely affected is not one of them, provided that the pet's needs are being met for enrichment, exploration, and play. If the pet shows FASC when outside, it is counterproductive to go outside with risks outweighing the benefits. The pet parent should seek help from the veterinary team or find alternate ways to exercise and enrich the pet. For pets that benefit from going outside but have limitations physically or emotionally, using a stroller, carry bag (smaller pets), or wagon may be helpful (Figure 5.11). For cats, outdoor enclosures or catios (also known as cat patios) can be utilized. Often, cats can be trained to walk on a harness, similarly to a dog. In addition, interactive play with family members and tossing toys or treats up and down stairways can help increase the energy output for cats that will participate (Figure 5.12).

When pet parents provide a routine program of interactive, regularly scheduled daily exercise or training, this provides a more predictable daily routine. When the dog or cat knows what to expect, they are more likely to be relaxed between outings or training sessions. Sufficiently enriched pets are likely to exhibit fewer attention-getting behavior problems.

Destructive behaviors

Dogs need to chew and cats need to scratch. These are innate behaviors which are necessary for a good quality of life. Dogs should be provided from puppyhood with safe and varied objects on which to chew. This will reduce the likelihood of destruction in the house. Cats need access to suitable surfaces to scratch for claw maintenance and to express normal marking behavior. An indoor garden box with grass, catnip, silver vine, or catmint for cats to nibble

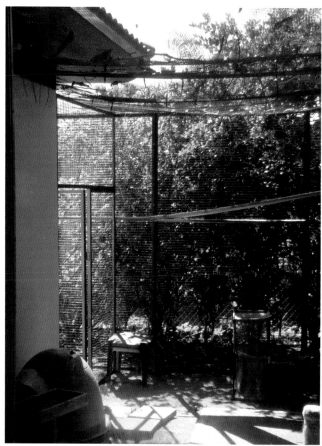

Figure 5.12 Catios can offer the enrichment of outside with the safety of inside. *(Attribution: Lisa Radosta.)*

and roll in can provide enjoyment for many cats. Destructive behaviors are discussed in more detail in Chapters 19 and 20.

Play

Play should be part of the daily routine or problems might result. Play is important for maintaining physical exercise, mental stimulation, and physical health, and building the relationship between family members and the pet.[42,43]

Pet parents should be encouraged to provide a supply of safe and interesting toys the pet can manipulate when alone. While interactions with the family are important, so is independence and independent play. Both types of play, social and object, should be readily available to cats and dogs.

Selection of an appropriate type and amount of play should be based on the individual pet, breed (especially important for dogs), the pet parents, the household, and the dog's age and activity level. In cats, pet parents who played for 5 minutes or more per session reported significantly fewer problems than those with play bouts of 1 minute.[44]

When selecting chew and feeding toys, whether for a dog or a cat of any age, begin with a variety of toys to determine which type the pet prefers. Most pets will make it clear by playing with their favorite toys. Then, the pet parent can purchase more of what their pet likes and donate the rest to a

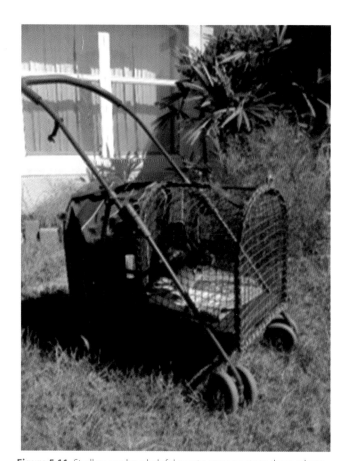

Figure 5.11 Strollers can be a helpful way to expose cats to the outdoors safely. *(Attribution: Lisa Radosta.)*

local shelter or rescue. Rotating toys (three new toys per day) will keep the pet motivated. Toys should stay out of rotation for five days. A toy box with more toys less desirable than the three which are on daily rotation can be kept out so that the pet has adequate options. Throughout this book, we have and will continue to discuss reinforcing and capturing desirable behaviors. This also applies to enrichment strategies. When a dog or cat is performing an appropriate behavior, such as gnawing on a chew toy (dog) or scratching on a scratching post (cat), the behavior should be reinforced with calm verbal acknowledgment or small pieces of food tossed to or near the pet. See Appendix A for enrichment resources.

Object play/independent play

Dogs

Most pet parents seem to regard play as something that their dog engages in with them or another animal. However, dogs can and should play independently. Encouraging independence in this and other ways (e.g., sanctuary space training), allows healthy separation from the pet parent. This may help the dog to adjust in the future to times of separation. Using interactive toys that the dog turns on, food toys, and automated ball machines are just some of the ways that dogs can learn independent play. Pet parents may need to reinforce this play at first to get the dog interested.

Dogs may be less particular than cats about the toys with which they play; however, they too have preferences. Pet parents should be encouraged to pay attention to what their pet likes and purchase more toys of that style. Sometimes pet parents stop giving their dog toys because they destroy them. This is normal behavior and demonstrates that individual dog's need to tear something up. Pet parents can seek out more durable toys, or restuff and sew back together toys which have been destroyed. Always focus on providing suitable and appealing alternatives and outlets for undesirable behavior. Eliminating toys altogether is not an acceptable solution to the problem.

Cats

Object play in the form of games of pounce and chase appears to resemble predatory patterns closely in cats. Hungry cats show increased biting attacks and hunting behavior, and play may become more intense with increasing hunger.[45–47] Therefore, as mealtimes approach, the cat might be most in need of play. On the other hand, since feeding may decrease the frequency or intensity of hunting, feeding multiple small meals a day might reduce the intensity of play.[48]

Toys that are most similar to normal prey in size, movement, and texture are most likely to motivate the cat to stalk, chase, and pounce.[45,49,50] In addition, interest and play with toys have been shown to increase with scent and with novelty.[51–53] Safety must also be considered when choosing a suitable toy. Toys (e.g., cardboard, plastic, leather, feathers) attached to ropes, strings, or wands can be kept away from the body and moved in such a way as to encourage stalking, chasing, pouncing, and biting. If the cat contacts human body parts, play should immediately cease. In one study, a used hair band was the most interesting of a group of toys,

followed by a small plastic toy stuffed with food. Each was attached to a length of string to initiate the chase sequence.[54] In another study comparing three different toy preferences, significantly more cats preferred interacting with a movement toy over a feather or mouse toy.[55] Stuffing food, silver vine, or catnip in a toy may encourage chase and a reward offered when captured. Toys should be sufficiently small and light so that the cats can carry them with their mouths and easily remove any food stuffed inside.

Studies have found that cats will rapidly habituate to a toy, but this does not mean that they have lost their interest in playing.[50] In fact, in one study, even after a cat is interested in a toy, for the next 5 minutes play interest is heightened (disinhibition) and may not wane for 25–40 minutes. Therefore, even as interest in one toy wanes, extending the play session by immediately providing alternative toys is advisable, after which the cat might be fed a small meal.[50]

Feral cats have been reported spending up to 12 hours per day searching for food and eating 8–10 small meals a day. With this in mind, multiple small meals and multiple chase and play sessions may be beneficial.[56,57] While there are many commercial cat enrichment products available, common household items such as ping pong balls or empty boxes provide opportunities for play and exploration. Dry food can be hidden around the house for the cat to "hunt" for its meal. Dry and canned food can be placed in food manipulation toys, but an empty soda bottle, empty plastic food container, or the inner cardboard tubes of a used roll of paper towels with a few strategically placed holes can be used for dry food. Ice cube trays or egg cartons can be used to dispense canned food in small portions. Freezing canned food in an ice cube tray further slows feeding.

Some cats also seem to engage in their own "moments" of active play, such as tearing around the house for several minutes each evening. Although it might be preferable to engage the cat in alternative acceptable activities such as chase and feeding toys, this can be an "acceptable" outlet if damage and injury can be prevented. Recently, however, new outlets for feline exercise have become available, including activities such as agility course training and competitions as well as at-home exercise wheels, which may provide cat pet parents with more options to ensure their cat receives the exercise they require. Motorized or motion-activated toys are a fantastic way to encourage independent object play in cats.

Social play

Dogs

The family should initiate play sessions to avoid reinforcing excessively demanding, excitable, and attention-soliciting behavior. The appropriate amount and type of play should be based on the needs of the individual (breed, age, energy level), as well as the lifestyle, health, and ages of the pet parents. While there is individual and breed variability, fetch, hide and seek, toss and find the treat, chase, round-robin recalls, and tug of war are all games most dogs enjoy. Although there has been some controversy about whether games that involve pulling, tugging, and rough play might be problematic, these types of play have not been shown to lead to the development of other behavior problems, except perhaps in dogs that become too aroused and excitable and use their mouths inappropriately to grab and bite arms, legs, hands, or clothing, and those that cannot be sufficiently calmed down at the end of the play session.

Some dogs may not know how to play, while others simply may not desire social play. This often stresses pet parents; however, there is no reason that any one dog must play with other dogs to have a great quality of life. The type of enrichment provided should match what the dog needs, not what the pet parent wants. Play is discussed extensively in Chapter 2.

Cats

Play and exercise sessions provide the cat with social interaction with the family and an outlet for exploration and play. In a study comparing human social interaction, food, toy, and scent, human social play (with a feathered toy attached to a rod) in both shelter and pet cats was the most preferred stimulus by a majority of cats.[55]

If a kitten's or cat's needs for play, exercise, and social contact are satisfied, undesirable behaviors such as excessive nocturnal activity, destructive exploration, scratching, overly exuberant activity sessions, play aggression toward people and other cats, and annoying attention-soliciting behaviors are less likely to develop. Feline predatory and play behaviors tend to occur as short periods of high activity. If the goal is to wear the cat out to curb undesirably exuberant play behavior, the play session should continue until the cat calms down and loses interest in the activity. However, even though a cat loses interest in one toy when the novelty wears off, it may still be raring to go if another toy is offered. If the pet loses interest after two or three play attempts with different toys, it might be time for a break, or time to give the cat a small food-filled toy to change its focus to another activity. Play sessions should be designed to provide active chase-and-pounce targets. The family is most likely to engage cats in play by using moving objects that can be stalked, chased, swatted, or pounced upon. Cats may also engage in play

with other housemates, which can be encouraged if there are no untoward consequences.

Interactive cat toys include long wands with dangling toys that resemble prey, wiggling ropes, and objects that are thrown or rolled for the cat to chase. Hands should never be used for play. This type of interaction promotes the biting and swatting of hands. Why would we ever do that?

Handling and restraint

It is essential that any new pet to the household, regardless of age, learn at minimum to accept and potentially enjoy forms of handling from responsible family members, which will be necessary for the maintenance of their health and well-being. For puppies and kittens, this can occur via puppy class or kitten kindergarten. For pets adopted after the socialization period and for whom associations with handling have most likely been made, exposure must be slow and is often best done with the help of a qualified positive reinforcement trainer. All handling should be gentle, slowly increasing to the level at which it will be necessary for health and wellness. Handling exercises should include gentle handling of the face, ears, feet, tail, collar, and haircoat. All handling should be followed by a food reward at each step. See Chapter 10 for more information on desensitization and counterconditioning. Provided there are no signs of fear, anxiety, or resistance, the pet parent should gradually proceed to tooth brushing, grooming, lifting (if appropriate), nail trimming, and handling the face and neck. A pet that is not accustomed to being handled may resist or become fearful or aggressive when handled by a groomer, veterinarian, trainer, or child.[58]

Conclusion

Prevention is always preferred over treatment of a behavior problem. As with most situations in veterinary medicine, education of pet parents is the most important step in the prevention of behavior problems in dogs and cats.

References

1. Handegard KW, Storengen LM, Lingaas F. Noise reactivity in standard poodles and Irish soft-coated wheaten terriers. *J Vet Behav.* 2019; doi:10.1016/j.jveb.2020.01.002.

2. Grigg EK, Kogan LR. Owners' attitudes, knowledge, and care practices: exploring the implications for domestic cat behavior and welfare in the home. *Animals.* 2019;9:978. doi:10.3390/ani9110978.

3. Hart BL, Hart LA, Thigpen AP, et al. Assisting decision-making on age of neutering for 35 breeds of dogs: associated joint disorders, cancers, and urinary incontinence. *Front Vet Sci.* 2020;7:388.

4. Hart BL, Hart LA, Thigpen AP, et al. Assisting decision-making on age of neutering for mixed breed dogs of five weight categories: associated joint

disorders and cancers. *Front Vet Sci.* 2020;7:472. doi:10.3389/fvets.2020.00472.

5. Patronek GJ, Glickman LT, Beck AM. Risk factors for relinquishment of dogs to an animal shelter. *J Am Vet Med Assoc.* 1996; 209:572–581.

6. Patronek GJ, Glickman LT, Beck AM, et al. Risk factors for relinquishment of cats to an animal shelter. *J Am Vet Med Assoc.* 1996;209:582–588.

7. Gazzano A, Mariti C, Alvares S, et al. The prevention of undesirable behaviors in dogs: effectiveness of veterinary behaviorists' advice given to puppy owners. *J Vet Behav.* 2008;3:125–133.

8. Gazzano A, Bianchi L, Campa S, et al. The prevention of undesirable behavior in cats: effectiveness of a veterinary

behaviorists' advice given to kitten owners. *J Vet Behav.* 2015;10:535–542.

9. Kogan L, Schoenfeld-Tacher R, Simon A, et al. The internet and pet health information: perceptions and behaviors of pet owners and veterinarians. *Int J Vet Med.* 2009;8:1.

10. Horwitz DF. Feline socialization: how environment and early learning influence behavior. *Vet Med-US.* 1993;August:14–16.

11. Freedman DG, King JA, Elliott O. Critical periods in the social development of dogs. *Science.* 1961;133(3547):1016–1017.

12. Scott JP. Critical periods in social development. *Science.* 1962;949–958.

13. Scott JP, Fuller JL. *Genetics and the Social Behavior of the Dog.* Chicago: University of Chicago Press; 1965.

14. Karsh EB, Turner DC. The human-cat relationship. In: Turner DC, Bateson P, eds. *The Domestic Cat: The Biology of its Behaviour*. Cambridge: Cambridge University Press; 1988:159–177.

15. Stellato AC, Flint HE, Dewey CE, et al. Risk-factors associated with veterinary-related fear and aggression in owned domestic dogs. *Appl Anim Behav Sci*. 2021;241:105374. doi:10.1016/j.applanim.2021.105374.

16. Denenberg S, Landsberg GM. Effect of dog-appeasing pheromones on anxiety and fear in puppies during training its effects on long term socialization. *J Am Vet Med Assoc*. 2008;233:1874–1882.

17. Appleby DL, Bradshaw JWS, Casey RA. Relationship between aggressive and avoidance behaviour by dogs and their experience in the first six months of life. *Vet Rec*. 2002;150:434–438.

18. Puurunen J, Hakanen E, Salonen MK, et al. Inadequate socialisation, inactivity, and urban living environment are associated with social fearfulness in pet dogs. *Sci Rep*. 2020;10:3527. doi:10.1038/s41598-020-60546-w.

19. Collard RR. Fear of strangers and play behavior in kittens varied with social experience. *Child Dev*. 1967;38:877.

20. Fox MW, Stelzner D. Behavioral effects of differential early experience in the dog. *Anim Behav*. 1966;14:273–281.

21. Angameier E, James WT. The influence of early sensory-social deprivation on the social operant in dogs. *J Genet Psychol*. 1961;99:153–158.

22. González-Martínez Á, Martínez MF, Rosado B, et al. Association between puppy classes and adulthood behavior of the dog. *J Vet Behav*. 2019;32:36–41.

23. Blackwell EJ, Twells C, Seawright A, et al. The relationship between training methods and the occurrence of behaviour problems as reported by owners in a population of domestic dogs. *J Vet Behav*. 2008;3:207–217.

24. Casey R, Loftus BE, Bolster C, et al. Human directed aggression in domestic dogs (*Canis familiaris*): occurrence in different contexts and risk factors. *Appl Anim Behav Sci*. 2014;152:52–63.

25. Cutler JH, Coe JB, Niel L. Puppy socialization practices of a sample of dog owners from across Canada and the United States. *J Am Vet Med Assoc*. 2017; 251:1415–1423.

26. Duxbury MM, Jackson JA, Line SW, et al. Evaluation of association between retention in the home and attendance at puppy socialization classes. *J Am Vet Med Assoc*. 2003;223(1):61–66.

27. Stepita ME, Bain MJ, Kass PH. Frequency of CPV infection in vaccinated puppies that attended puppy socialization classes. *J Am Anim Hosp Assoc*. 2013;49(2):95–100.

28. Seksel K, Mazurski EJ, Taylor A. Puppy socialisation programs: short and long term behavioural effects. *Appl Anim Behav Sci*. 1999;62:335–349.

29. Pierantoni L, Albertini M, Sammartano V, et al. Puppy classes may positively affect the behaviour of adult dogs separated from their litters too early. *Proc European Veterinary Animal Behaviour and Welfare Congress*. Berlin; 2018:146–147.

30. Salman MD, New Jr JG, Scarlett JM, et al. Human and animal factors related to the relinquishment of dogs and cats in 12 selected animal shelters in the United States. *J Appl Anim Welf Sci*. 1998;1(3):207–226.

31. Salman MD, Hutchison J, Ruch-Gallie R, et al. Behavioral reasons for relinquishment of dogs and cats to 12 shelters. *J Appl Anim Welf Sci*. 2000;3(2):93–106.

32. DePorter T, Schulkey R. Evaluation of the association between attendance at veterinary hospital based puppy socialization classes and long term retention in the home. *Proc VBS*. Indianapolis; 2017:14–15.

33. Horwitz D, Landsberg G, Luescher A, et al. Enriching the environment of our pets: roundtable on the psychology of play and behavior modification. *Vet Forum*. 2003;20:46.

34. Hunthausen W, Seksel K. Preventative behavioral medicine. In: Horwitz D, Mills DS, Heath S, eds. *BSAVA Manual of Canine and Feline Behavioural Medicine*. Gloucester, UK: BSAVA; 2009:49–60.

35. Leuscher A. Enriching the environment of our pets: the psychology of play and behavior modification. Vet Forum December 2002.

36. Jongman EC. Adaptation of domestic cats to confinement. *J Vet Behav*. 2007;2:193–196.

37. Neville PF. An ethical viewpoint: the role of veterinarians and behaviourists in ensuring good husbandry for cats. *J Feline Med Surg*. 2004;6:43–48.

38. Ellis S. Environmental enrichment. Practical strategies for improving feline welfare. *J Feline Med Surg*. 2009;11:901–912.

39. Rochlitz I. A review of the housing requirements of domestic cats (*Felis silvestris catus*) kept in the home. *Appl Anim Behav Sci*. 2005;93:97–109.

40. Landsberg GM. Confinement training. *Vet Pract Staff*. 1993;5:19–22.

41. Milani MM. Crate training as a feline stress reliever. *Feline Pract*. 2000;28:8–9.

42. Rooney NJ, Bradshaw JWS. An experimental study of the effects of play upon the dog–human relationship. *Appl Anim Behav Sci*. 2002;75:161–176.

43. Mertens C, Shar R. Practical aspects of research in cats. In: Turner DC, Bateson P, eds. *The Domestic Cat; the Biology of its Behavior*. Cambridge: Cambridge University Press; 1988:179–190.

44. Strickler BL, Shull EA. An owner survey of toys, activity problems and behavior problems in indoor cats. *J Vet Behav*. 2014;9:207–214.

45. Hall SL, Bradshaw JWS. The influence of hunger on object play by adult domestic cats. *Appl Anim Behav Sci*. 1998;58:143.

46. Adamec R, Stark-Adamec C, Livingston KE. The development of predatory aggression and defense in the domestic cat (*Felis catus*): III. Effects on development of hunger between 180 and 365 days of age. *Behav Neural Biol*. 1980; 30:435–447.

47. Biben M. Predation and predatory play behavior of domestic cats. *Anim Behav*. 1979;27:81–94.

48. Fitzgerald BM, Turner DC. Hunting behavior of domestic cats and their impact on prey populations. In: Turner DC, Bateson P, eds. *The Domestic Cat; the Biology of its Behaviour*. 3rd ed. Cambridge: Cambridge University Press; 2014.

49. Bradshaw JWS, Casey RA, Brown SL. *The Behaviour of the Domestic Cat*. 2nd ed. Oxfordshire: CABI Press; 2012:128–141.

50. Hall SL, Bradshaw JWS, Robinson IH. Object play in adult domestic cats: the roles of habituation and disinhibition. *Appl Anim Behav Sci*. 2002;79:263–271.

51. Machado JC, Genaro G. Influence of olfactory enrichment on the exploratory behavior of captive-housed cats. *Aust Vet J*. 2014;92:492–498.

52. Myatt, AE. *An Olfactory Enrichment Study at the Ashland Cat Shelter*. Diss. Ashland University; 2014. <https://etd.ohiolink.edu/apexprod/rws_etd/send_file/send?accession=auhonors1399629978&disposition=inline/> Accessed August 7, 2021.

53. Ellis SLH, Wells DL. The influence of olfactory stimulation on the behaviour of cats housed in a rescue shelter. *Appl Anim Behav Sci*. 2010;123:56–62.

54. Denenberg S. Cat toy play trial: a comparison of different toys. In: *Proceedings of the Annual Scientific Symposium of Animal Behavior*. Denver, CO; 2003:25–33.

55. Vitale Shreve KR, Mehrkam LR, Udell MAR. Social interaction, food, scent or toys? A formal assessment of domestic pet and shelter cat (*Felis silvestris catus*) preferences. *Behav Proc*. 2017;141:322–328.

56. Overall KL, Rodan I, Beaver BV, et al. Feline behavior guidelines from the American Association of Feline Practitioners. *J Am Vet Med Assoc*. 2005; 227:50–84.

57. Turner DC, Meister O. Hunting behaviour of the domestic cat. In Turner D, Bateson P, eds. *The Domestic Cat; the Biology of its Behavior*. Cambridge: Cambridge University Press; 1988: 111–121.

58. Yin S. *Low Stress Handling, Restraint and Behavior Modification of Dogs and Cats: Techniques for Developing Patients Who Love Their Visits*. Davis: Cattledog Publishing; 2009.

Resources and recommended reading

Ackerman L. *Proactive Pet Parenting: Anticipating Pet Health Problems Before They Happen.* Problem Free Publishing; 2020.

American Association of Feline Practitioners (AAFP). Client resources: catvets.com.

American Association of Feline Practitioners (AAFP). Environmental Needs Guidelines. <https://catvets.com/guidelines/practice-guidelines/environmental-needs-guidelines/>.

American Association of Feline Practitioners (AAFP). What your cat needs to feel secure. <https://catfriendly.com/cat-friendly-homes/what-your-cat-needs-to-feel-secure/>.

American College of Veterinary Behaviorists, Herron M, Horwitz DF. *Decoding Your Cat.* Houghton Mifflin Harcourt Publishing Company; 2020.

American College of Veterinary Behaviorists, Ciribassi J, Horwitz DF. *Decoding Your Dog.* Houghton Mifflin Harcourt Publishing Company; 2015.

American Veterinary Society of Animal Behavior (AVSAB) position statement on puppy socialization: <https://avsab.org/wp-content/uploads/2018/03/Puppy_Socialization_Position_Statement_Download_-_10-3-14.pdf/>.

Bradshaw J, Ellis S. *The Trainable Cat – a Practical Guide to Making Life Happier for You and Your Cat.* New York, NY: Basic Books; 2016.

Catalyst council. https://www.youtube.com/user/catalystcouncil.

Cat Friendly Homes - catfriendly.com.

Fear free happy homes. fearfreehappyhomes.com.

Ohio State University – Indoor pet initiative. <https://indoorpet.osu.edu/cats/>.

Serpell J, Barrett P, eds. *The Domestic Dog: its Evolution, Behavior and Interactions with People.* 2nd ed. Cambridge: Cambridge University Press; 2017.

Turner DC, Bateson P, eds. *The Domestic Cat; the Biology of its Behavior.* 3rd ed. Cambridge: Cambridge University Press; 2014.

CHAPTER 6

All body systems affect behavior

Alison Gerken, DVM

Introduction

Physical health can have direct or indirect effects on behavior, contributing to how a pet might behave in certain situations or respond to specific stimuli. Alternatively, emotional health can affect the development of systemic diseases. The effects of the interplay of health and behavior may be influenced by genetics, neonatal development, early experience (including maternal deprivation, environmental isolation, and socialization), age, type of health problems, nutrition, and environmental variables.

Lethargy, altered social interactions, irritability, anxiety, aggression, anorexia, depression, decreased response to stimuli, reduction in grooming, house soiling, and night waking are just some of the behavior changes that may present due to an underlying physical health issue. For some conditions, such as sensory decline, cognitive dysfunction syndrome, and pain, behavioral changes may be the only presenting signs.

For each behavioral clinical sign, a list of differentials should be made for all contributing body systems, whether they be physical or mental? emotional? Behavioral is not a body system. Medications and supplements currently being administered should be determined to evaluate their role in the pet's behavior. To ensure early diagnosis and intervention and to evaluate improvement and response to therapy, pet parents should be asked about behavior changes at each visit and encouraged to seek guidance as soon as signs arise (see Chapter 1).

Veterinarians, when presented with a patient who has behavior changes, have been trained to ask themselves, "Is it medical or behavioral?" and then to proceed to rule out the medical diseases. What is left must surely be behavioral, right? As veterinary medicine has evolved, so has the understanding that behavioral disorders and medical diseases are not separate entities. The word "medical" often refers to practices related to the treatment of illness and injuries. Behavior disorders are illnesses with clinical signs caused at least in part, and oftentimes in total, by neurochemical and hormonal changes in the brain and in the body. As with illnesses of other body systems, behavior disorders can result from epigenetic factors such as diet, medications, systemic illness, experience, trauma, and environment. For these reasons, behavioral medicine should be regarded as medical, not a separate process from medical disease.

Many patients referred for behavioral evaluation and treatment have an underlying physical disease contributing or causing the behavioral clinical signs. In one study, 15% of dogs brought to veterinarians for behavior problems had a physical problem,[1] while a multicentered study of cases at referral practices reported a prevalence of 28–82% of behavior problems to be related to pain.[25] Because of the potential for concurrent, interacting disorders, differentials for all body systems must be considered and fully investigated for any behavioral clinical sign in order to arrive at a correct diagnosis and to institute appropriate and efficacious treatment (see Tables 6.1 and 6.2). Simple therapeutic trials can be completed after diagnostics have been run if a final diagnosis has not been elucidated. For example, if a repetitive behavior responds to treatment with glucocorticoids, analgesics, gabapentin or opioids, an immunotherapeutic medication, or

anticonvulsants, then the primary cause is most likely not behavioral. In addition, if clinical signs such as licking, biting, and chewing improve even to some extent with glucocorticoid, antiemetic/nausea, or immunotherapy treatment, there is likely a dermatologic or gastrointestinal disease contributing to those clinical signs.

Physical health decreases the threshold for fear, anxiety, and stress. Although physical issues can directly affect behavior, such as when diabetes or cystitis incites house soiling or pain leads to aggression, the threshold theory (as in dermatology when multiple subclinical pruritic stimuli combine to cause clinical pruritus) also applies to behavioral problems, since multiple stimuli (e.g., pain, discomfort, pruritus, anxiety, fear, stress) can combine to push the pet beyond a threshold at which a behavioral clinical sign will be exhibited. This is especially important in senior pets where concurrent compromise of organ function, sensory decline, painful conditions, age-related nervous system pathology, or other health issues can all affect behavior. For example, a dog may maintain a healthy relationship with other dogs in

Table 6.1 The effects of health on behavior[42,72,80]

Organ system pathology	Possible behavioral consequences/clinical signs
Neurologic	
Central (intracranial/extracranial), particularly if affecting forebrain, limbic/temporal, and hypothalamic regions	Altered awareness, altered response to stimuli, loss of learned behaviors, reduced trainability, house soiling, disorientation, altered activity levels, altered sleep-wake patterns, vocalization, change in temperament (fear, anxiety), altered appetite, aggression, docility
Focal seizures – temporal lobe epilepsy	Repetitive behaviors, self-traumatic disorders, chomping/chewing, staring, alterations in temperament (e.g., episodic or intermittent states of fear or aggression), aimless wandering
Sensory dysfunction – auditory, visual	Altered response to stimuli, decreased greeting, altered social interactions, disorientation, irritability, aggression, vocalization, house soiling, fear, anxiety, altered-wake cycles, reduced appetite, decreased grooming, decreased response to commands
Peripheral neuropathy	Self-mutilation, irritability, aggression, circling, hyperesthesia
Endocrine	
Hyperthyroidism or hypothyroidism, hyperadrenocorticism or hypoadrenocorticism, diabetes mellitus, insulinoma, functional gonadal tumors	Altered emotional state, irritability/aggression, lethargy, decreased response to stimuli, anxiety, polyuria, polydipsia, house soiling/marking, altered sleep-wake cycles, altered activity levels, altered appetite, pica, sexual behaviors (e.g., mounting, marking)
Hepatic encephalopathy	Disorientation, fear, anxiety, irritability, personality changes, dullness/lethargy, pacing, agitation, aggression
Urogenital	
Lower urinary tract disease, renal disease	Polyuria, polydipsia, dysuria, house soiling, stranguria, reduced appetite, waking at night
Musculoskeletal	
Pain (degenerative joint disease)	See Table 6.2
Gastrointestinal	
Gastrointestinal – esophageal/gastric/bowel disease, pancreatitis	Licking, polyphagia, air snapping, chewing/chomping, pica, coprophagia, fecal house soiling, aggression
Dermatologic	
Otitis, chronic dermatitis, pyoderma, claw disorders	Overgrooming, acral lick dermatitis (dogs), nail biting, hyperesthesia, other self-trauma (chewing/biting/sucking/scratching), aggression, irritability, avoidance
Oral	Pawing/rubbing at face, ptyalism, fear, withdrawal, inactivity, irritability, aggression, decreased interest in food, decreased grooming, vocalization
Cardiovascular	Lethargy, decreased activity, exercise intolerance, withdrawal, hiding, irritability, reduced appetite

Table 6.2 Signs of pain in dogs and cats[72,80,98,147]

Loss of normal behavior	Decreased activity including play, exercise, exploration, climbing, jumping, scratching, greeting, response to stimuli grooming, appetite, social interaction altered sleep, litterbox use
Development of new or abnormal behaviors	Elimination, aggression/irritability, fear/anxiety/phobia, vocalization, disrupted sleep, hyperesthesia, altered interactions with people/other pets, licking, pica, repetitive behaviors, self-trauma, house soiling
Response to palpation of affected area	Tension, avoidance, withdrawal, threat, distress vocalization, aggression
Physiologic measures	Tachycardia, tachypnea, increased blood pressure, pupil dilation, increased cortisol levels, increased endorphins Poor correlation with subjective measures may be due to pain, fear/anxiety/stress, surgical procedures, or other medical pathology (i.e., acidosis, hypovolemia)
Locomotion, gait, mobility	Lameness, altered ability to climb, jump, stretch, rise, scratch

the house by avoiding agonistic interactions and communicating when to stay away using visual signals and body postures. However, should the pet then develop osteoarthritis or sensory decline (auditory or visual), he may resort to aggression to keep the other dogs away if his opportunities to avoid, signal, and perceive are lost. As another example, Hyperthyroid cats might be more irritable and hence more likely to spray if exposed to the sights, sounds, or odors of new cats on the property.

Stress may also affect both physical and behavioral health and well-being. Stress alters immune health and may be a contributing or exacerbating factor in dermatologic, gastrointestinal, respiratory, cardiac, and neurologic diseases, as well as behavioral pathology. To complete the cycle, pain, discomfort, illness, or irritability will exacerbate stress and anxiety. (See Chapter 7 for further discussion on the effects of stress on behavior.)

Is it physical or behavioral? Often, it is both!

Very often, behavior disorders result from the interplay between systemic disease and mental disease, physical changes and emotional changes. Behavioral changes may be subtle and therefore go unrecognized by the pet parents until they have progressed in severity. Some pets, especially cats, may seclude themselves from family members, making detection of a problem and monitoring by the pet parent difficult.

Determining the etiology of a behavioral sign requires a thorough history, evaluation of all concurrent signs, and direct observation of the patient. Suspicion of a non-behavioral etiology should increase when behavior changes develop acutely, occur in the very young or old, or when there is a sudden change in the nature of a preexisting behavior condition.

A comprehensive diagnostic assessment, including physical examination and diagnostic tests that are appropriate based on the presenting signs, are essential components of each behavior case. For example, bloodwork, urinalysis, and urinary tract imaging should be completed in patients that present for urinary house soiling. Pets with self-traumatic disorders require a comprehensive dermatologic evaluation which might include skin scrapings, cytology, bacterial and fungal culture, elimination diet trials, and anthelmintics. Blood and urine tests should also be part of the behavior screening for any pet that might be placed on behavioral medication(s) to determine if there are any potential contraindications and to obtain baseline data for future comparisons.

Assuming the absence or resolution of any abnormalities on diagnostic tests and physical examination, it may seem clear that the problem is primarily behavioral. However, even if it appears that there is no underlying systemic disease and a behavioral inciting factor can be identified, physical problems cannot always be entirely ruled out by physical examination and diagnostic tests alone. The diagnostic dilemma is further complicated by the fact that some issues may persist despite diagnosis and treatment of a causative or contributive physical disease because of learned habits, inadvertent reinforcement or punishment by pet parents, or alterations in receptors and neurotransmitters in the brain. For example, if the pet becomes aggressive when approached due to pain or discomfort, the aggression may continue after the pain is treated if the pet has learned that aggression successfully leads to retreat of a perceived threat or improved control of social situations, or he may continue to be guarded about any hand movement toward him if he anticipates that touch might still trigger pain. House soiling caused by diabetes mellitus or feline idiopathic cystitis might persist even after the inciting systemic disease is resolved due to newly learned substrate preferences and aversion.

Reaching a diagnosis for a behavioral problem may not be a simple matter since physical problems can affect behavior as well as exacerbate stress, stress can affect health and behavior, and consequences (learning) will have a far-reaching impact on how a problem progresses. In all cases, the practitioner should work to identify and address any underlying stress, since, even if stress does not play a role in the problem that is being evaluated, it is essential for the pet's and pet parent's health and welfare.

Specific body systems and their contribution to behavioral clinical signs

Neurological system

The central nervous system is directly involved in the control of behavior; therefore, neurological diseases can cause a multitude of changes in behavior. Neurological diseases that affect behavior may be intracranial or extracranial (see Box 6.1). Alterations in awareness, responsiveness to stimuli, and consciousness might arise from any disease that involves the forebrain or brainstem. Altered responsiveness to stimuli can also arise from sensory or motor dysfunction.

Box 6.1 Physical causes of behavioral signs

Degenerative/**D**evelopmental: cognitive dysfunction syndrome, sensory decline, degenerative arthritis, acquired portosystemic shunt, hypoplasia of organ, compromised cerebrovascular circulation

Anomaly/**A**utoimmune: storage diseases, idiopathic epilepsy, autoimmune hemolytic anemia, granulomatous meningoencephalitis, congenital portosystemic shunt, congenital blindness or deafness

Metabolic diseases: hypothyroidism and hyperthyroidism, hypoadrenocorticism and hyperadrenocorticism, diabetes mellitus, diabetes insipidus, hepatic, renal, sex hormone imbalances, enzyme deficiencies

Nutritional/**N**eoplasia: imbalances, excesses or deficiencies (may be primary or secondary to disease), brain tumor, any tumor causing pain or illness, interstitial cell tumor

Inflammatory/**I**nfectious/**I**schemic/**I**mmune/**I**diopathic/**I**nherited/**I**atrogenic: vasculitis, meningoencephalitis, feline infectious peritonitis, feline leukemia virus, feline immunodeficiency virus, toxoplasmosis, rabies, distemper, rickettsial diseases

Trauma/**T**oxin: head injury, any painful injury, lead, pesticides, illicit drugs

Behavioral/psychological disorders, abnormal behavior: compulsive disorders, stereotypies, sleep disorders, phobias, separation-related disorders, fear/anxiety disorders, posttraumatic stress disorder, hypersensitivity, hyperactivity, attention deficit hyperactivity disorder, impulsivity, hyperreactivity

Pet parents may complain of circling, which may be caused by many neurological disorders including forebrain and brainstem lesions. Circling has also been associated with hydrocephalus in Bull Terriers and Yorkshire Terriers;[3,4] however, other studies have found no abnormalities on MRI or histologic exam.[5] The limbic system is associated with emotion so diseases affecting it, including areas such as the hypothalamus, can also affect behavior.[6]

Neurologic disease may or may not be appreciated on the neurological exam. There are areas in the central nervous system that are considered silent zones (e.g., frontal lobe) in that disease in these areas may not lead to changes on the neurological examination or laboratory tests.[7,8] The forebrain is responsible for cognition, so forebrain lesions are often associated with behavior changes like change in personality or mood, inability to recognize or respond appropriately to stimuli, and loss of previously learned behaviors.

Seizures are the most common neurological problem reported in dogs, with idiopathic epilepsy being the most common diagnosis of canine seizures.[7,9] Generalized and focal or partial seizures have been associated with behavior changes, cognitive impairment, and reduced trainability, as have the medications used for treatment,[10–16] which can make differentiating seizure disorders from behavior disorders challenging.

Air snapping, tail chasing, pouncing, fixed staring, star gazing, head shaking, chewing, spinning, tremors, aimless wandering, or episodic aggression have all been associated with focal seizures[10–20] as well as postictal signs in dogs.[10,13] Fly biting may be a manifestation of a focal seizure, peripheral neuropathy, compulsive disorder, or underlying medical disorder including gastrointestinal disease.[3,21–24,25] Differential diagnoses for tail chasing or spinning include central neurologic disease, myelopathy, anal sac disease, gastrointestinal disease, and urogenital tract disease. Bull Terriers that presented for a range of abnormal behavior including tail chasing, fly catching, unprovoked aggression, and extreme fear had abnormal electroencephalograms with five of the seven affected dogs improving with phenobarbital treatment.[26] More recently, an association has been demonstrated between compulsive tail chasing, trance like behavior, and episodic aggression in Bull Terriers, with similarities in phenotype and serum neuropeptides to autism spectrum disorders.[3,27,28]

Focal seizures in cats may manifest as abnormal motor activity, including twitching and tremors, as well as altered mental status where affected cats do not respond to stimuli normally.[29] Aberrant behavior including hissing in the absence of an overt cause, growling, running blindly into objects, self-chewing, biting, and circling have been observed in cats experiencing focal seizures.[10,29,30] Focal seizures are a differential for any repetitive behavior including fly biting, tail chasing, fixed staring, star gazing, light or shadow chasing, head shaking, chewing, licking, checking, or aimless wandering.

There appears to be an association between psychiatric disorders and seizure disorders. Dogs with epilepsy have a higher risk of displaying fear and anxiety behaviors (i.e., approached by an unfamiliar dog, groomed, left alone), defensive aggression, barking without apparent cause, chasing shadows and lights, aimless pacing, increased agitation when their caretakers showed affection to other people or dogs, staring into space, chasing cats and other small animals, excitability, and cognitive decline.[11–16]

A therapeutic response to phenobarbital, potassium bromide, levetiracetam, gabapentin, carbamazepine, zonisamide, or perhaps clonazepam (cats) may help to rule in or out a seizure focus as a cause. However, because many of these drugs might also reduce anxiety or neuropathic pain, an improvement in clinical signs does not necessarily confirm a seizure disorder as a diagnosis. While a therapeutic response to serotonin reuptake inhibitors such as fluoxetine would be suggestive of a compulsive or behavioral disorder,[22] these drugs may decrease the epileptic threshold.[32]

Primary or metastatic tumors affecting the central nervous system may cause various behavior changes. Clinical signs vary with the size, rate of growth, location of the tumor, and biochemical changes. Forebrain tumors may result in behavioral changes with or without the presence of neurological deficits including depression, loss of learned behaviors such as house soiling, disorientation, changes in appetite and thirst, pacing or circling, altered social interactions, vocalization, aggression, diminished vision or blindness, head pressing, and seizures.[33–35] Seizures and altered mentation were the primary presenting signs of 173 dogs with primary cranial neoplasia, while in 6 dogs, the tumors were an incidental finding.[33] In a study of 43 dogs with tumors affecting the rostral brain, 5 presented only with behavior changes and 31 had normal neurological examinations at the time of presentation.[8] Of 160 cats with intracranial neoplasia, the most common signs were altered mental status, circling, and seizures with 15.6% presenting with behavior changes, of which 60% were aggressive. No specific neurological signs were seen in 21% of the cats and in 18%, the tumors were an incidental finding.[35] Onset of behavioral signs in a middle-aged or senior pet would be a strong indicator for a medical cause.[7]

Cognitive dysfunction syndrome is a progressive neurodegenerative disease of senior dogs and cats which can lead to a multitude of behavioral changes such as disorientation, altered interaction with the family, changes in sleep-wake cycles, house soiling, changes in activity, increased anxiety, and/or vocalization.[36-38] (see Chapter 8). Cognitive dysfunction may affect up to 60% of older dogs[36] and 50% of cats aged 15 or older.[38]

Sleep disorders can also cause behavior changes. Narcolepsy is a chronic sleep disorder in dogs and cats that is characterized by acute recurring attacks of sleep.[39] It may be confused with seizures given its abrupt onset.[39] Clinical signs include excessive daytime sleepiness, sleep paralysis, and cataplexy, which is a sudden loss of muscle tone in response to stimulation, for which eating is the most common precipitating factor.[39] Narcolepsy may be inherited or sporadic in dogs,[39] so it can present in young or older dogs. Genetic testing is available for several variants of narcolepsy in dogs in which it is inherited as an autosomal recessive trait with full penetrance in the Dachshund, Doberman Pinscher, and Labrador Retriever. Most inherited forms of narcolepsy will be evident in the first six months of life, while the clinical onset in sporadic cases is much more variable. Rapid eye movement sleep disorders, which might include signs of panic, howling, barking, growling, chewing, aggression, or violent limb movements during sleep, have been diagnosed in dogs.[40,41]

Peripheral neuropathies or spinal cord disease (i.e., intervertebral disc disease, trauma, inflammatory central nervous system disease, tumors, ischemia) may lead to pain-related changes, self-mutilation, scratching, repeatedly looking at the same bodily area, yelping, lethargy, decreased appetite, and aggression.[42,43] Dogs with spinal meningiomas may develop behavior changes including restlessness and irritability before they develop gait changes.[44]

Feline hyperesthesia is a presenting complaint in which the hallmark sign is rippling and twitching of the skin over the lumbar spine that may arise from any number of medical or behavioral causes, including dermatologic diseases, spinal disease, feline leukemia virus (FeLV) myelitis, myositis, myopathy, neurological disease, including focal seizures, orthopedic and neuropathic pain, compulsive disorders, and any condition leading to behavioral arousal. Clinical signs may also include dilated pupils, biting and chasing of the tail, licking, biting and pulling out hair, excessive grooming, and behaviors associated with high arousal, including anxiety, aggression, restlessness, running, defecation, and vocalization.[45] The rippling of skin in response to gentle touch in some likely occurs due to abnormal sensory states where relatively innocuous touch sensations elicit unpleasant sensations such as pain or pruritus.[45,46]

Hyperactivity in dogs is a common complaint of pet parents, and may not be a result of a physiological disorder. However, in some cases, dogs that demonstrate frenetic energy or overactivity (including pacing, barking, chewing), distractibility, short attention spans, impulsiveness, repetitive behavior, aggression, lack of trainability, sleep perturbation, and failure to settle in calm, quiet environments, along with somatic signs including tachycardia, tachypnea, and salivation, may have canine hyperactivity or hyperkinesis syndrome.[47-49] This syndrome has been reported in the literature since the 1970s and has been likened to attention deficit hyperactivity disorder (ADHD) in people. While the pathophysiology of ADHD is unknown, it is a highly inheritable neurodevelopmental disorder.[50,51] Similar to ADHD in people, canine hyperactivity or hyperkinesis syndrome is hypothesized to result from dysregulation of dopamine and/or noradrenergic and serotonergic neurotransmission.[49,52]

Canine hyperactivity or hyperkinesis syndrome is presently considered rare, but pet parents often insist that their dogs demonstrating "hyperactivity," "overactivity," or unruly behaviors have ADHD. More often, this is not true hyperactivity or ADHD, but instead increased energy which is not pathologic but is instead due to breed disposition, conditioned responses, inadvertent reinforcement, underexercise, and/or insufficient mental stimulation. In addition, numerous physiological and behavioral disorders may account for ADHD-like behaviors, such as metabolic derangements,[53] thyroid gland dysfunction,[54] neurological conditions,[55] hepatoencephalopathy,[56] pain,[49] cognitive decline,[57] and fear or anxiety-based disorders. Additionally, dogs that did not undergo training may be more likely to demonstrate undesirable or unruly behaviors, causing pet parents to assume the problem lies within their pet. Further, the use of punishment-based techniques,[58-61] such as scolding, yelling, hitting, and the use of aversive tools such as electronic (shock) and prong collars, may increase fear, stress, anxiety, and attention-seeking behaviors.

Several terms have been used to describe ADHD-like behavior in dogs, including hyperkinesis, hyperactivity, impulsivity, and inattention.[49] While impulsivity, which is characterized by impaired motor inhibitory control and an inability to tolerate a delay in gratification,[62] is a component of hyperkinesis and human ADHD, it may be a normal variation of behavioral styles or traits.[51] Studies suggest that 12–15%[63] and 20%[64] of dogs naturally manifest high levels of hyperactivity, impulsivity, and inattention. However, high levels of impulsivity, hyperactivity, and inattention may be abnormal and associated with other behavioral comorbidities,[47,51] such as aggression,[51] compulsive disorders,[51,63] and fear disorders.[51,63]

Studies have found that hyperactivity, impulsivity, and inattention are more common in certain breeds,[51] smaller dogs,[65] and younger dogs.[51,66-68] One study did not find a correlation between impulsivity and a dog's age,[69] and other studies have found no significant difference between the sexes[65,67] or have found females to be more hyperactive and impulsive.[66] Furthermore, studies have found higher hyperactivity and impulsivity in dogs that spend more time alone,[51] receive less exercise, and rarely participate in training.[51,67] In these cases, high levels of hyperactivity, impulsivity, and inattention may be due to limited opportunities to release energy and frustration.[51]

Canine hyperactivity or hyperkinesis syndrome cannot be diagnosed based on clinical signs alone, and no clear consensus for the diagnosis of canine hyperactivity or hyperkinesis syndrome or ADHD exists in either human or veterinary medicine.[49] Therefore, a behavioral history is critical in distinguishing abnormal behaviors from normal but undesirable behaviors. The behavior history should include a detailed description of the dog's behavior over a 24-hour period, including his activities, social interactions, exercise, and other opportunities for enrichment, whether the dog settles (if so, how often and under what circumstances), the dog's response to activities, and the family's response to unwanted behavior, including the use of punishment.

Some researchers purport that true canine hyperactivity or hyperkinetic syndrome can be diagnosed from a stimulant-response test. This was historically performed by administering dextroamphetamine orally in the veterinary clinic and then monitoring the dog's activity levels, pulses, respiratory rates, and salivation for 1–2 hours.[47] An alternative method is to perform testing in the home environment. The pet parent should keep a journal of their dog's motor activity, using a Likert scale to rank the intensity of his activity levels, daily activities, and physiological parameters including respiratory rate and heart rate, for at least several days. As dogs with true hyperkinesis demonstrate a paradoxical calming response to amphetamines,[47,51] methylphenidate administration is initiated and the pet parent continues the activity log as described above. Higher doses of fluoxetine of 2–4 mg/kg PO q24h have also been used to treat hyperkinesis syndrome.[49] (See Chapter 11 for more information on methylphenidate administration for canine hyperactivity or hyperkinesis syndrome.)

A positive response to methylphenidate or dextroamphetamine has been utilized to make a presumptive diagnosis of hyperkinesis, though this technique is not reliable.[47,48] As there is individual variability in response to treatment,[68,69] some nonhyperkinetic dogs respond physiologically to amphetamines in a similar way as dogs with true hyperkinesis.[69] Response depends on the treatment protocol;[69] the dog's behavior may be influenced by his environment and pet parent bias may influence the results. For these reasons, this protocol is not validated as a means of diagnosing hyperkinesis in dogs. Validated questionnaires evaluating a pet dog's impulsivity, motor skills, and inattention have been established,[67,69] but these questionnaires alone are not sufficient to make a diagnosis of hyperkinesis. One study showed that an accelerometer is a reliable tool in assessing motor activity but is not sufficient alone to diagnose hyperkinetic syndrome.

The use of stimulant medication is inappropriate and not justified in the absence of a strong suspicion for a diagnosis of canine hyperactivity or hyperkinesis syndrome, as these medications are not without risk, especially in dogs without true hyperkinesis. Initial treatment should consist of increasing mental and physical stimulation by increasing exercise, providing structured interactions with the family, using food puzzles and other food-dispensing devices, eliminating all forms of punishment, ignoring attention-seeking behaviors, and pursuing positive reinforcement-based training with a skilled dog training professional to reduce impulsivity. (See Chapter 10 for more information on behavior modification for impulsivity) If these treatments are instituted and clinical signs persist for more than 3–6 months, then institution of methylphenidate may be considered as an adjunct to behavior modification. Pet parents must be informed that their dog's behavior may worsen and physiological parameters including heart rate, respiratory rate, and motor activity may increase as a result of stimulant administration. While medication for canine hyperactivity or hyperkinesis syndrome can sometimes be discontinued once behavior modification is effective, in some cases, treatment must be prolonged, possibly for the remainder of the dog's life.[47]

For any case presenting with behavioral clinical signs, a full neurological examination should be performed. If the history and clinical signs support the presence of a possible neurological disease, a complete blood count, biochemical panel, urinalysis, thyroid panel, bile acids, and referral to a neurologist for advanced diagnostics like neuroimaging, cerebrospinal fluid analysis, electroencephalogram, brainstem auditory evoked response testing, and electromyography may be indicated.

Endocrine system

Endocrine diseases can contribute to a multitude of behavior changes including anxiety, irritability, changes in activity level, and aggression (see Table 6.1).

Deficiencies in thyroxine affect several body systems, making the presentation of hypothyroidism extremely varied. Classic signs of hypothyroidism include lethargy, weight gain, hair loss, seborrhea, pyoderma, exercise intolerance, bradycardia, and cold intolerance.[42,70–72] Behavioral changes associated with hypothyroidism in dogs may also include lethargy, mental dullness, sluggishness, decreased mentation, disorientation, and altered social interactions, as well as anxiety, fears, phobias, and aggression.[7,34,70,72,73–75] In some cases, aggression has been reported to be the only presenting complaint, and improvement in aggression has been reported with thyroid replacement therapy.[7,70,73,75] In contrast, a study comparing eight thyroid analytes (TT3, fT3, TgAA, T3AA, T4AA, TT4, fT4, TSH) in aggressive and nonaggressive dogs found a significant difference in only one value, T4AA, which was within normal limits and considered nondiagnostic for hypothyroidism in dogs.[76] In a study of dogs with aggression and with low or low normal total T4 or total or free T3, or the presence of thyroid autoantibodies, there were no significant group differences in aggression after six weeks of thyroid treatment.[74] In dogs treated with levothyroxine for hypothyroidism, an increase in activity was reported after six weeks, but no other behavior changes were observed over six months.[77] As there is evidence that hypothyroidism may be a primary cause of behavior disorders, but its role is unclear, thyroid assessment should be part of the diagnostic workup for any dog that presents for anxiety, fear, or aggression.[7] However, caution must be exercised when diagnosing and treating hypothyroidism. Though it is the most commonly diagnosed endocrinopathy in dogs, its true prevalence is estimated to be about 0.4%.[71] It is likely overdiagnosed due to the many nonthyroidal factors that may decrease total thyroxine (T4) concentrations including normal serum thyroxine fluctuations, breed variations, age, medications, nonthyroidal illness, and stress.[71,74] Total T4 is a sensitive but nonspecific screening test, so additional testing including free T4 by equilibrium dialysis, thyroid stimulation hormone (TSH), antithyroglobulin antibodies (TgAA), and ultrasonography (though rarely necessary) should be pursued when hypothyroidism is suspected.[71,72] While there are reports of dogs with aggression improving with thyroid replacement therapy,[36,74,75] thyroxine supplementation for the treatment of behavioral disorders in dogs is not recommended in the absence of aberrant thyroid function revealed through testing.[7,25]

Hyperthyroidism has a major effect on the nervous system and has been associated with hyperactivity,[78] increased vocalization, irritability, aggression, panting, reactivity to stimuli, increased appetite, increased thirst and urination, house soiling, muscle wasting, and weight loss [34,42,79,80] (see Table 6.1). In one study, iatrogenic hyperthyroidism in rats changed the levels of serotonin, dopamine, and norepinephrine, which are neurotransmitters important in behavioral control.[78] Hyperthyroidism is the most common endocrine disorder in cats, affecting about 13.9% of cats 11 years of age and older.[79] Therefore, a routine thyroid screen should be instituted for any type of feline behavioral disorder in middle-aged and senior cats with onset of or increase in anxiety, irritability, or aggression.[79]

Hyperadrenocorticism (Cushing's disease) occurs in dogs and cats and may be the result of a pituitary adenoma or a functional cortisol-secreting adrenal tumor. Cushing's disease, in addition to polyuria, polydipsia, polyphagia, and dermatologic changes, may also cause behavior changes including depression, weakness, restlessness, panting, disrupted sleep, increased irritability, and house soiling[34,42,72] (see Table 6.1). Pituitary adenomas may create neurologic changes by growth and expansion into the hypothalamus, causing blindness, depression, confusion, pacing, circling, aggression, seizures, and signs of endocrine disease including polyuria and polydipsia.[30,35] Hyperadrenocorticism in cats may cause lethargy, polyphagia, polyuria, polydipsia, and house soiling. In two case reports of cats with hyperadrenocorticism, both developed urine spraying and aggression.[81,82]

Diabetes mellitus can result in a variety of behavioral and neurological signs. As insulin deficiency results in failure of glucose transport into the muscle and adipose tissue, early signs of diabetes mellitus may include lethargy, weakness, exercise intolerance, gait change, or impaired jumping.[34,42] The classic clinical signs of polydipsia, polyuria, and polyphagia do not develop until the blood glucose concentration exceeds the renal tubular threshold for glucose.[83]

Several endocrine diseases, including hyperthyroidism, Cushing's disease, and diabetes mellitus, frequently cause polyphagia, which can lead to begging for food, counter-surfing (stealing food off of kitchen counters), trash raiding, coprophagia, aggression around food or other items, and predatory aggression. Diseases that cause polydipsia and polyuria can lead to sleep disruption and to house soiling in otherwise house- or litter-trained pets.

For all behavior cases, diagnostics should include a complete blood count (CBC), biochemistry panel, urinalysis, and serum total T4 and free T4 (ED) thyroid function testing. Based on these results, performing a more comprehensive thyroid panel including TSH and TgAA, a fructosamine test, urine cortisol:creatinine ratio test, adrenocorticotropic stimulation test, low-dose dexamethasone suppression test, imaging including abdominal ultrasound, and blood pressure measurements may be indicated.

Gastrointestinal system

There is an increasing amount of evidence in humans and animals showing a link between the gut microbiome and behavior.[84,85] The term "gut-brain axis" refers to the bidirectional communication between the gastrointestinal tract and the brain. In dogs, intestinal inflammation, whether chronic or acute, is associated with significant differences in the composition of the intestinal microbiota.[86] There is evidence that alterations in the microbiota of the gut may lead to a variety of behavior changes including aggression.[87]

Gastrointestinal diseases and behavioral diseases may share the same presenting signs including withdrawal, inactivity, restlessness, pacing, lip licking, polyphagia, hyperphagia, irritability, house soiling, disrupted sleep, fly snapping, coprophagia, pica, and grass and plant eating.[34,72,80,88–91] (see Table 6.1). Polyphagia may lead to begging, stealing, garbage raiding, and counter surfing, as well as to coprophagia, aggression around food or other items, and predatory aggression. Inflammatory bowel disease[34,42] and pancreatitis may cause decreased appetite, inactivity, restlessness, irritability, aggression, nighttime waking, lip licking, and pica (see Table 6.1). Medications that might increase appetite include corticosteroids and benzodiazepines, while appetite might be suppressed by some medications such as antidepressants, cyclosporine, ketoconazole, or any medication that causes gastrointestinal upset. Similarly, pets on calorie restriction may have increased appetite, irritability, aggression, and restlessness. For pets presenting with coprophagia and grass eating, gastrointestinal, nutritional, and metabolic disorders should be ruled out; however, both pica and coprophagia are considered normal behaviors. See Chapter 13 for more information on these disorders.

For fecal house soiling or perichezia (the inappropriate deposition of feces outside of acceptable locations), medical conditions including inflammatory or infiltrative bowel disease, dietary intolerance, infectious diseases, parasitism, constipation, colorectal disease, megacolon, metabolic and endocrine diseases, malabsorptive disease, orthopedic disease, neurologic disease, cognitive dysfunction, and pancreatic disease should be considered as the cause or contributing factors. Keep in mind that the pet may also have litterbox aversion or substrate preference, for example, while still having an underlying systemic cause.[7,34,80] See Chapters 21 and 22 for more information on canine and feline house soiling.

Unusual oral behaviors, including fly snapping, star gazing, excessive licking, sucking, pica, smacking lips, or gulping have been associated with a variety of gastrointestinal disorders even when other gastrointestinal signs are not present. In a study of 19 dogs with excessive licking of surfaces, 14 were diagnosed with gastrointestinal disorders, including eosinophilic and lymphoplasmacytic infiltration, delayed gastric emptying, irritable bowel syndrome, giardiasis, pancreatitis, and gastric foreign bodies. Clinical signs in 9 of 17 dogs resolved after 90 days of medical treatment. Four additional dogs showed a decrease in licking after 180 days of treatment.[88] In another study, all 7 dogs with fly-biting behavior were diagnosed with a gastrointestinal abnormality, with 6 of the 7 responding to medical treatment alone.[89]

Pica occurs in dogs and cats. It may be a compulsive disorder that might have a genetic basis in some individuals; however, very often, pets with pica have underlying gastrointestinal disease. Cats with pica vomit more frequently than cats without pica.[90] Additionally, in a study of eight cats with pica, six were diagnosed with gastric or intestinal eosinophilic infiltrates, four with suspected delayed gastric emptying, one with suspected gastric influx, and one with *Giardia* spp.[91] For diagnosis and treatment of picas, see Chapter 13.

Gastrointestinal disease should remain on the differential list for many behavior problems. The presence of gastrointestinal signs might suggest the presence of an underlying or contributing gastrointestinal cause of the behavioral signs. Underlying gastrointestinal disease must be diagnosed and treated in order to improve or resolve the behavioral clinical signs. The veterinarian should question pet parents about gastrointestinal signs in every appointment when pets are presented for behavioral clinical signs. In animals with possible gastrointestinal disease, diagnostics may be extensive and may include a complete blood count, biochemical panel, urinalysis, serum thyroxine levels, gastrointestinal panel including cobalamin, folate, and serum trypsin-like immunoreactivity, canine or feline pancreatic lipase, fecal parasite detection, gastrointestinal infectious disease testing using polymerase chain reaction, imaging including abdominal radiographs, ultrasound and endoscopy, and biopsies. In addition to appropriate gastrointestinal diagnostics, a positive response to a therapeutic diet trial and/or medications to alleviate gastrointestinal signs such as antinausea medications or gastrointestinal protectants, might elevate suspicion for potential medical causes.

Musculoskeletal

Joint and skeletal disorders are the most common musculoskeletal diseases in animals. Twenty percent of dogs older than one year in North America reportedly have osteoarthritis.[92,93] Studies in cats show that up to 92% had radiographic evidence of osteoarthritis; however, one-third or less of cats with radiographic osteoarthritis had signs of mobility impairment and only 16.7% were lame.[94–96] Musculoskeletal diseases cause pain, with a change in behavior sometimes being the only clinical sign. Behavioral changes associated with pain are extremely varied and may include reluctance to walk, run, jump, climb, exercise or play, aggression, irritability, fear, anxiety, altered sleep, changes in interactions with pet parents or other pets, altered facial expressions, altered posture, restlessness, hiding, lethargy, reactivity or sensitivity when touched, decreased social interaction, vocalization, attention seeking, and house soiling[25,34,42,72,79,80,98–101] (see Table 6.2). Pain has also been associated with repetitive behaviors.[7,25,102]

In one study of 137 declawed cats, 63% showed radiographic evidence of residual P3 fragments.[103] These cats were almost three times more likely to be diagnosed with back pain than non-declawed cats and were also more likely to manifest undesirable behaviors such as house soiling and aggression, including biting. These adverse behaviors were not eliminated when onychectomy was performed using optimal surgical techniques.[103]

Obesity is on the rise in pets and has a number of behavioral and physiological ramifications. In 2018 the Association for Pet Obesity Prevention (petobesityprevention.org) classified 55.8% of dogs and 59.5% of cats as overweight or obese. Obesity often causes reduced activity and lethargy. In dogs, obesity increases the risk of osteoarthritis,[97] intervertebral disc disease,[104] and cardiovascular effects,[105] while in cats, obesity and overweight status increase the risk of diabetes,[80] osteoarthritis,[95,106] and oral and lower urinary tract diseases,[107] all of which can cause behavioral changes and compromise quality of life.

Dermatological

Any dermatologic issue, whether the result of allergies, bacterial or fungal infections, neoplasia, trauma, or endocrine disease, that causes pruritus or pain can present as behavior changes like increased reactivity, anxiety, and aggression. It is well documented in humans that pruritus can lead to secondary behavioral disorders.[108] Self-traumatic disorders including biting, chewing, scratching, licking, or excessive barbering should always suggest pain or pruritus. Overgrooming is most commonly due to underlying pain (e.g., orthopedic, abdominal, urinary, pancreatic, gastrointestinal) or systemic disease. Rarely is overgrooming a primary behavioral disorder. Some cats with histologically normal skin still can have a dermatologic cause of overgrooming.[109]

For acral lick dermatitis (ALD), atopic dermatitis, adverse food reactions, deep pyoderma (which is often multidrug resistant), and a variety of medical causes, including osteoarthritis, tumors (soft tissue or osseous), trauma, and protozoal and fungal infections may all be factors in its pathogenesis.[3,110] For claw (nail) biting in dogs, immune-mediated, inflammatory, or infectious causes including *Malassezia* must first be ruled out.

Psychological stress can exacerbate pruritus by activating the release of neuropeptides that act along afferent and efferent central nervous system pathways that may be responsible for sensations such as pruritus and pain and that may stimulate behaviors including scratching, licking, and biting.[3,111] Just as stress may exacerbate pruritus, pruritus increases stress. Therefore, stress associated with a physical lesion can increase the likelihood of the development of undesirable behaviors.[111] A recent study found that the severity of pruritus in dogs with atopic dermatitis was directly associated with behaviors including mounting, chewing, coprophagia, hyperactivity, begging for and stealing food, attention seeking, and excessive grooming.[111]

Severe pruritus may result in an itch-scratch or itch-lick cycle in which the scratching or licking persists even after the underlying dermatologic issue has been resolved. In some cases, a dog may start to lick a lesion such as a dermal or subcutaneous mass, wound, or sutures, which may lead to persistent licking of that site or of other parts of the body. This may cause lick granulomas (ALD) to form, which can lead to increased irritability and increased sensitivity at the site, further exacerbating the licking and leading to self-mutilation. In addition, pet parents may inadvertently reinforce licking, biting, and scratching with attention perpetuating the pattern after the inciting cause has been resolved.

When it comes to pruritus, it is not unusual that pets have multiple inciting factors in what is often referred to as a pruritic threshold. There may be multiple causes of subclinical inflammation that cumulatively result in the pet being pruritic. So there may be subthreshold inflammation associated with atopic dermatitis or adverse food reactions for which the pet can compensate and not need to scratch excessively, but eventually some other condition (such as flea bite dermatitis) will cause inflammation to rise above the threshold, at which point the pet is clinically pruritic.

Similarly, pets may experience what might be referred to as the allergic (or atopic) march, which is the natural progression or evolution of allergies over time. While it is unusual in dogs or cats for this "march" to evolve from dermatologic to respiratory signs, as often occurs in humans, it is not a rare occurrence that it could progress from seasonal to nonseasonal or from localized to more generalized involvement.

Clinical signs including, licking, biting, chewing, scratching, overgrooming, spinning, chasing, biting, and chewing on the tail may have a dermatologic etiology or contributing cause and should trigger a full dermatologic workup.[3,110] Behavioral diagnoses can be made prior to workup and treatment can be initiated to improve quality of life, but rarely do disorders with the clinical signs listed above have a primary behavioral etiology. Dogs with ALD may have allergic disease or pyoderma.[110] Up to 76% of cats referred to a veterinary behaviorist for excessive grooming and presumed psychogenic alopecia have an underlying dermatologic issue such as allergies, food intolerance, or parasites causing or contributing to the problem.[109] Therefore, dermatologic diseases must be ruled out with skin scrapings, cytology, fungal and bacterial cultures, and biopsies if indicated, as well as elimination diet trials, antibiotics, corticosteroids, and parasite control trials when a dog or cat presents with any of these behaviors before a final behavioral diagnosis is made.

Urogenital

The onset of urinary house soiling in a house-trained or litter-trained pet can be due to any medical problem that causes an increased volume of urine, increased discomfort during elimination, or decreased control of urination, or that affects cortical homeostasis. Lower urinary tract diseases including urinary tract infection, cystolithiasis, urethrolithiasis, and neoplasia may lead to urinary house soiling. In a retrospective study of cats with problem elimination behavior, 60% of the cats had a history of feline lower urinary tract disease.[112] On the other hand, urinary tract disease may be less likely to be a factor in urine marking in cats.[113] However, a recent case-controlled study found a similar frequency (39%) of medical problems in both toileting and spraying cats.[114] Systemic illnesses could also contribute to marking in dogs or cats by altering hormonal states or increasing anxiety. Assessment of every elimination disorder should therefore begin with a physical examination, complete blood count, biochemical profile, urinalysis, urine culture and sensitivity serum thyroxine concentration, and abdominal radiographs and any other imaging such as abdominal ultrasound or urethrocystography if indicated. In marking cats, evidence of masculinization such as penile barbs or odorous urine might indicate that hormonal assessment is warranted. In one study, a number of castrated dogs and cats that presented with intact male sexual characteristics were diagnosed with extratesticular tumors, while in a case report of a 9-year-old neutered male, signs of aggression toward other cats, urine marking, and excessive vocalization were associated with an adrenal cortical adenoma.[115] Therefore, when marking or other sexual behaviors arise in dogs or cats, examination for a scrotal mass and testosterone levels in response to gonadotropin-releasing hormone response test should be considered. See Chapters 21 and 22 for more details on the role of medical problems in canine and feline house soiling.

Oral

The World Small Animal Veterinary Association's most recently published Global Dental Guidelines state that dental disease is the most common medical issue in small animals and that it is underdiagnosed and undertreated in small animal practice, as many pets rarely show overt signs of dental pain.[116] In studies, periodontal disease was found in about 85–90% of dogs[117,118] and in about 60–70% of cats.[119,120] In a study evaluating the periodontal health status of 109 colony cats, only 4% of the cats were free of gingival inflammation.[120]

Oral disease may present with signs of pain-related behaviors such as aggression, irritability, decreased activity and playfulness, withdrawal, decreased interest in food, head shyness, repetitive behaviors such as aimless pacing, licking, digging, and vocalization[34,72,117,119,122,123] (see Table 6.1). In one study comparing cats with minimal oral disease to cats with severe dental disease, cats with severe dental disease were less active and playful and had more difficulty grasping food.[124] Treatment of the periodontal disease may lead to improved or resolved behavior, but some behaviors such as avoidance or aggression around handling may persist due to the pet learning new behaviors.

Feline orofacial pain syndrome is a neuropathic condition that presents with behavioral signs indicative of severe oral discomfort. Affected cats most commonly present with pawing and mutilation of the mouth, especially the tongue, exaggerated licking and unusual chewing, and these signs may be elicited by movements like eating, drinking, or grooming. The condition can be exacerbated by stress and social tension between household cats.[125]

Sensory

Sensory decline, namely reduction in vision and hearing, is increasingly prevalent in older pets.[126] One study found that 54% of dogs in a sample of veterinary practices had an eye anomaly affecting vision over the course of the dog's lifespan.[127] Another study found that 5–10% of dogs in the United States are deaf or have reduced hearing.[128] Sensory-impaired pets may demonstrate increased anxiety, confusion and frustration, disrupted sleep, vocalization, altered social interactions, and house soiling, and may withdraw as navigating their familiar environment and routine becomes more difficult[72,79,80] (see Table 6.1). Pets with vision or hearing reduction may also startle more easily and show aggression toward people or other animals in the house when approached. Pet parents may complain that their pet no longer responds when called or spoken to or no longer greets them after an arrival home. One study found that auditory or visually impaired dogs were more prone to chewing, licking, and barking.[126] There are a number of genetic anomalies that can produce deafness and blindness across many purebred and mixed-breed animals[127,128] that may lead to behavior abnormalities in young pets. Changes in taste and smell may also occur in older pets, potentially leading to altered food preferences and a decline in appetite. Reduction or loss of olfaction in cats is especially important as their willingness to eat is closely dependent on their ability to smell their food. Hyporexia or anorexia in cats can lead to serious medical problems including nutritional deficiencies and hepatic lipidosis.

Immunological

There are a number of viral, bacterial, or parasitic infections that can lead to a wide range of behavior changes. The most commonly seen ones in small animals are discussed here.

Rabies virus is a well-known cause of profound behavior changes. Rabies virus is often characterized by three phases: the prodromal phase presents as mentation changes from more docile to more agitated; the furious phase consists of hyperactivity, aggression, and ataxia; and a paralytic form with progressive paralysis which may follow the furious form, especially in cats.[129]

Feline infectious peritonitis (FIP), in the earliest stages, may present with nonspecific signs of malaise, inappetence, weight loss, and fever.[130] The noneffusive (dry) form of FIP commonly involves central nervous system involvement, with over 50% of cats with inflammatory disease of the central nervous system having FIP.[130] Central nervous system involvement in cats with dry FIP is varied in clinical presentation but may include personality changes such as aggression, rage, withdrawal, hyperesthesia, and pica.[130,131]

FeLV and feline immunodeficiency virus (FIV) can also cause behavioral changes in cats.[38] In a report on FeLV-associated myelopathy in 16 cats, clinical signs in affected cats included fly biting, abnormal behavior, abnormal vocalization, pica, hyperesthesia, and urinary incontinence.[132] Cats with FIV may develop deficiencies in learning new tasks, loss of socialization, decreased grooming, house soiling, aggressive behaviors, dementia, disorientation, polyphagia, stereotypies, decreased sleep, and overall more abnormal behaviors with more severe signs than in a control group of cats.[133,134,136]

Canine distemper virus may result in respiratory and gastrointestinal signs, but the neurological changes that occur later in the course of the illness can cause the most notable behavior changes. Up to 30% of infected dogs develop central nervous system signs which may include obtundation, compulsive pacing, vocalization, and circling.[137]

Rickettsial diseases, including Rocky Mountain spotted fever and canine ehrlichiosis, may present with behavioral changes including lethargy, depression, and decreased appetite.[138] Mentation changes due to the development of meningoencephalitis may also occur.[30]

Though most cats infected with *Toxoplasma gondii* show no clinical signs, the development of toxoplasmosis can cause behavior changes in affected cats.[139] The most common signs of toxoplasmosis are lethargy and decreased appetite. When toxoplasmosis affects the central nervous system, it can cause behavior changes, circling, and head pressing.[38] Dogs are rarely affected.[139]

Cardiorespiratory

Cardiac diseases, including chronic valvular disease, myocardial fibrosis, cardiomyopathy, rhythm disturbances, and pericardial disease as well as respiratory diseases, including chronic rhinitis, chronic lower airway disease, tracheal collapse, and laryngeal paralysis, may cause reduced perfusion and oxygenation to the central nervous system, leading to

decreased activity, exercise intolerance, unwillingness to participate in normal activities, hiding or withdrawal from the family, and reduced appetite.

Vascular

Hypertension affects both cats and dogs. It may be situational (due to excitement or anxiety), secondary to an endocrinopathy (e.g., hyperadrenocorticism, hyperthyroidism, diabetes mellitus), renal insufficiency, cardiomyopathy, a side effect of medications (e.g., glucocorticoids, phenylpropanolamine), or idiopathic. Hypertensive encephalopathy has been reported in dogs and cats.[140,141] Neurologic signs were reported in 29%[142] and 46%[143] of hypertensive cats in two studies. Hypertensive encephalopathy is more likely to occur in cats with a sudden increase in blood pressure, a systolic blood pressure that exceeds 180 mmHg, or both.[144] Hypertension may cause nonspecific signs including confusion, vocalization, sleep disruption, pacing, lethargy, decreased activity, altered appetite (increased or decreased), restlessness, and agitation.[34,80]

Medications that can cause behavioral side effects

Since drugs are utilized for improving physiological or psychological health and well-being, often an improvement or resolution in behavioral signs will be achieved. However, therapeutic effects, side effects, and adverse effects of medications can also contribute to changes in behavior that may or may not be the intended, desired, or expected effect. Antihistamines such as diphenhydramine might cause sedation or could have a paradoxical effect of increasing restlessness or agitation. Drugs that have an anxiolytic effect such as benzodiazepines or buspirone may disinhibit some behaviors, leading to an increase in aggression in cases where fear might have been inhibiting the aggressive response. In addition, benzodiazepines might sedate, increase appetite, or cause paradoxical agitation and restlessness. Mirtazapine, a tetracyclic antidepressant, is most commonly used in pets as an appetite stimulant and antiemetic; it may calm or sedate, or it may lead to increased agitation and vocalization, especially in cats. While tricyclic antidepressants and selective serotonin reuptake inhibitors are less likely to lead to disinhibition, they can have variable effects on behavior, including anorexia, the potential for urine retention, or sedation in the more anticholinergic or antihistaminic antidepressants, or a more activating effect with fluoxetine. Corticosteroids can cause behavior changes, including polydipsia and polyphagia contributing to begging, food stealing, pica, house soiling, night waking, and panting. In addition, dogs treated with corticosteroids may be more nervous, fearful, aggressive around food, aggressive when disturbed, likely to bark, and easily startled, while being less playful and confident.[145] Excess thyroid supplementation can contribute to increased anxiety, restlessness, reactivity, weight loss, and possible aggression. Phenylpropanolamine and theophylline can cause increased irritability, agitation, excitability, restlessness, and panting. Phenobarbital, though often sedating, may cause anxiety and agitation. Oclacitinib (Apoquel) has been associated with aggression.[146] Whenever a pet presents with behavior changes, the history should always include a list of current and previous medications.

Pain and its effects on behavior

Pain is defined as "an aversive sensory and emotional experience which elicits protective motor actions and results in learned avoidance and modification of behavior traits including social behavior" (iasp-pain.org). Pain is generally classified as acute or chronic. Acute pain (adaptive) describes pain that lasts a short time and subsides once healing is completed, while chronic pain (maladaptive or long term) describes pain that extends beyond the expected period of tissue healing, creating numerous physiological changes in the central and peripheral nervous systems that allow pain to persist in the absence of an inciting stimulus.[98,147]

Clinical presentation will vary depending on the cause of pain, source of pain (e.g., surgery, trauma, medical), body system (e.g., gastrointestinal, dental, ophthalmic, otic, musculoskeletal), species and individual differences, type of pain (nociceptive, inflammatory, neuropathic), and whether the pain is acute or chronic.[25,98,147]

Pain should be considered a differential diagnosis for any behavior problem, including aggression, fear, anxiety, phobia, avoidance, pica, decreased activity, inappetence, irritability, restlessness, house soiling, vocalization, changes in sleep patterns, hyperesthesia, and repetitive behaviors[7,25,42,72,80,98,99,100,147,148] (see Table 6.2). Any change from normal behavior and the development of new behaviors can be due to underlying pain. Based on a multicenter study of veterinary behaviorists, 28–82% of cases were reported to involve painful conditions. The association between behavior problems and pain might be a direct manifestation of pain, pain associated with secondary concerns within the behavior problem, exacerbation of signs, or adjunctive behavioral signs.[25] Therefore, even if a physical cause cannot be identified, if there is a change from normal behavior, development of new behaviors or behavioral signs, these might be associated with pain for which an analgesic response trial would be indicated.[25,98,147]

New onset or worsening of aggression is a common sign of pain in pets. Pain may be a cause or contributing factor to aggression in dogs perhaps by lowering the threshold for aggression or as a defensive/protective mechanism.[7,25,99,100] Pain may also manifest as aggression as the pet learns that aggressive behaviors like growling, snapping, or biting are effective ways to avoid physical contact that may lead to an exacerbation of pain.

Pain can also induce fear and anxiety in animals, which may lead to new or persistent behavior problems, while fear and anxiety may trigger or exacerbate pain.[7,25,34,98,102,147] Animals that begin licking a specific bodily region due to underlying pain, such as a cat licking his ventrum due to cystitis or a dog licking his flank due to osteoarthritis, may be further perpetuated by the increased stress of pain. Licking is also reinforced because it may temporarily alleviate the pain and because pet parents may interact more with their pets when they are excessively licking, even if their intention is to interrupt or cease the licking. The combination of increased stress and reinforcement of the licking may lead to the development of a repetitive behavior or compulsive disorder where the pet continues to lick despite resolution of the underlying pain. In human medicine, it is well documented that fear, anxiety, and stress can increase pain.[7,25,102] Children with higher preoperative anxiety had greater postoperative pain and patients with higher anxiety states had higher pain scores.[149,150] In pets, fear and anxiety may also exacerbate pain and negatively affect emotional health and affective state, which can be improved with pain management.[7,25,98,147,152] In turn, pain will contribute to heightened fear and anxiety. In one study, dogs with chronic musculoskeletal pain were more likely to experience fear-related noise sensitivity and to generalize fear to other contexts.[148] Therefore, for patients with anxiety and pain, both conditions should be treated to effectively address patient health, welfare, and quality of life.

Additionally, if the pet has experienced pain in a specific location or context, this can lead to a conditioned fear or avoidance of the situation or associated stimuli. For example, cats with lower urinary tract disease may experience pain when eliminating in the litterbox and develop a subsequent aversion to using the litterbox, leading to house soiling that may persist despite resolution of the urinary tract disease. Pain-related changes such as aggression due to otitis externa may persist following treatment if a pet has associated pain with handling by the pet parents, especially if the pet parents cleaned or instilled otic medications into the pet's ears. Similarly, pain or discomfort associated with veterinary care may lead to fear of the environment, equipment, or the sights, sounds, or scents of the hospital.

The need for pain assessment

Pain assessment is central to veterinary practice and patient welfare and should be a component of every physical examination as a "4th vital sign" after temperature, pulse, and respiration.[98,147,153] Acute pain may result in chronic pain[154] and chronic pain, such as that caused by osteoarthritis, may lead to central sensitization, an increased sensitivity of the nociceptive system,[155] so early recognition and treatment of acute and chronic pain are essential in the prevention of chronic pain syndromes. While several pain assessment tools have been validated for the evaluation of acute and chronic pain in dogs and cats, they are not regularly and consistently used in veterinary practices. In a survey, over 80% of veterinary nursing staff felt that pain-scoring tools would be useful but only 8.1% of practices utilized a scoring system.[156] Another study found that the lack of pain assessment was one of the main reasons that analgesic administration had been neglected in cats.[157] This is unacceptable and it must be a goal of all clinicians to identify pain and provide effective analgesia to all painful patients. Veterinary practices should select pain assessment measures for in-hospital use, patient discharge, and ongoing evaluation based on the latest available data for validity and reliability and what might be most practical for staff and pet parents. Veterinarians must take a proactive approach in educating staff and pet parents on procedures and methods for pain monitoring and assessment.

For veterinary practitioners, there are three areas of pain management on which to focus: (1) assessment of pain in ill or postoperative patients in the hospital; (2) informing and educating pet parents about monitoring, assessment, and management of pain after hospital discharge; and (3) advising pet parents about the significance of any change in behavior or emergence of abnormal behavior to be able to identify the onset and progress of pain, especially chronic disease states such as degenerative joint disease.

In-clinic assessment and evaluation of acute pain

A method of evaluating pain in hospitalized surgical and medical patients should be implemented in each veterinary clinic so that ongoing pain management can be performed and modified to suit the needs of each pet on a case-by-case basis.[98,147] Pets that might be experiencing pain should be monitored regularly every 2–4 hours for improvement or deterioration when determining response to pain medication or the need for additional medication.

While pain assessment should combine physical examination, diagnostic tests, and behavioral signs, there appears to be a poor correlation between subjective signs and more objective physiologic measures including heart rate, respiratory rate, blood pressure, pupil dilation, body temperature, or a rise in beta-endorphins or cortisol.[1,2,98,106,147,158–160] Numerous studies have found that behavioral measures, including the absence of normal behaviors or the expression of abnormal behaviors, may be of greater importance in diagnosing and monitoring some forms of pain, as changes in physical and physiological parameters could be related to nonpainful conditions including fear, stress, concurrent disease, and medications.[98,106,147,158,161,162] Behavioral responses to pain can range from hiding, avoidance, and escape to agonistic body postures and expressions. Expressive behaviors and postures such as attention soliciting, whining or purring, and head rubbing might also be indicative of attempts to relieve pain (Table 6.2). However, since animals have adaptive mechanisms which may mask signs of pain, the absence of overt signs does not mean an absence of pain. For example, some species, especially cats, may tend to mask signs of illness and discomfort. Some dogs may continue to wag their tails and cats may continue to purr even though they may be experiencing severe pain. To address pain in pets adequately, veterinarians and pet parents should begin with the assumption that procedures and medical conditions that are painful in humans would cause similar pain in pets, and any change from normal behavior may be an indicator of pain.

Differentiating signs of pain from the depression or dysphoria associated with some narcotics can be difficult. To assist in distinguishing pain from dysphoria, an analgesic challenge can be performed by administering analgesia; a decrease in the dysphoric behaviors suggests the presence of pain, whereas no change or no worsening of behaviors suggests dysphoria.[106]

Monitoring scales

Behavioral measures are necessary for prompt and accurate diagnosis and treatment of pain. In-clinic monitoring should focus on attitude and demeanor behavior including grooming, elimination, vocalization, and sleep patterns; as well as body postures, facial expressions, appetite; activity, mobility, and gait, and attention to painful sites.[161–168] Mobility and gait

may be difficult to assess in pets that require confinement or are immobile, and changes in these behaviors can be due to anxiety rather than discomfort. Vocalization and aggression may be associated with many other stimuli (e.g., noises) as well as reactions to drugs used for anesthesia and premedication. Therefore, pain-scoring systems that rely solely on agitation, movement, and vocalization are unreliable.

For dogs, together with physical examination and vital signs, primary measures of evaluation include posture, activity, vocalization, mental status, attention to affected area, demeanor, mobility, and response to palpation.[98] A validated assessment tool for measuring acute pain in dogs is the Glasgow Short Form Composite Measure Pain Scale, which can be applied quickly and reliably in a clinical setting.[98,147,154,161,164,165] It includes 30 descriptors in 6 behavioral pain categories, including mobility, vocalization, attention to wound, response to touch, posture/activity, and demeanor.

Another approach is a simple, although not well validated, picture-guided, four-point numeric acute pain scale developed at Colorado State University (CSU).[98,147,161] The scale is intended primarily as a teaching tool and to guide observations of clinical patients. The CSU scale includes behavioral signs of pain, response to palpation as well as body tension, which is a parameter not addressed in other scales. To the authors' knowledge, this is the only scale that emphasizes the importance of delaying assessment in a sleeping patient while prompting the observer to recognize patients that may be inappropriately obtunded by medication or more serious health concerns.

Cats do not always demonstrate pain overtly, making recognition difficult. Evaluation involves physical examination, pet parent questionnaires, observation of behavioral changes, and interactive or evoked measures.[98,106,147,151,162,166] Physiologic changes are important aspects of patient and health evaluation but are poorly correlated with pain.[98,106]

Licking or biting at the surgical site or a decrease in eating might be indicative of pain.[151,162,166] Body postures and facial expressions may include orbital tightening, ear position changes, head down, abdomen tucked up, crouching, or stiffened or tense.[101,106,166,167] Cats may sit quietly, avoid attention, appear depressed, hide, and attempt to avoid petting or handling.[106,151,162,166] Some cats growl, hiss, vocalize, and become aggressive with attempts to handle.[106,162,166] While gauging the cat's reaction to gentle handling and palpation is useful, some cats may be too fearful or painful to allow social interaction.[106,147]

For hospitalized cats, several validated pain scales exist.[106,162,166] The UNESP-Botucatu Multidimensional Composite Pain Scale (MCPS) consists of three subscales with ten variables including pain expression, psychomotor, and physiologic measures.[106,162] A recent study has demonstrated validity of a four-item UNESP-Botacatu short-scale assessing posture, activity, attitude, and reaction to touch.[151] The Feline Grimace Scale, a facial expression scoring system evaluating ears, eyes, muzzle, whiskers, and head position, and the Glasgow Composite Measure Scale-Feline, which also incorporates facial expressions, have both been validated for acute feline pain assessment.[161,166,167,169] The Colorado State University Acute Feline Pain Scale may be a reliable tool for interrater postoperative pain assessment but is not validated.[106,161,171] For the UNESP-Botacatu, Glasgow, and CSU scales, patients are first evaluated without interaction, followed by observation with

Table 6.3 Various pain scales used in small animal practice

ACVS Canine Orthopedic Index (COI)	https://www.vet.upenn.edu/research/clinical-trials-vcic/our-services/pennchart/canine-orthopedic-index
Canine Brief Pain Inventory (CBPI)	https://www.vet.upenn.edu/research/clinical-trials-vcic/our-services/pennchart/cbpi-tool
Cincinnati Orthopedic Disability Index (CODI)	https://www.fourleg.com/media/Cincinnati%20Orthopedic%20Disability%20Index.pdf
Colorado State University Acute Canine Pain Scale	http://csu-cvmbs.colostate.edu/Documents/anesthesia-pain-management-pain-score-canine.pdf
Colorado State University Acute Feline Pain Scale	http://csu-cvmbs.colostate.edu/Documents/anesthesia-pain-management-pain-score-feline.pdf
Feline Grimace Scale	https://www.felinegrimacescale.com
Feline Musculoskeletal Pain Index	Painfreecats.org
Glasgow Composite Measure Pain Scale, short form (CMPS-SF)	https://www.newmetrica.com/acute-pain-measurement
Glasgow Composite Measure Scale-Feline	https://www.newmetrica.com/acute-pain-measurement
Helsinki Chronic Pain Index (HCPI)	https://www.fourleg.com/media/Helsinki%20Chronic%20Pain%20Index.pdf
Liverpool Osteoarthritis in Dogs (LOAD) Canine Osteoarthritis Staging Tool	https://www.galliprantvet.com/us/en/coast-tools
UNESP-Botucatu Multidimensional Composite Pain Scale (MCPS)	http://www.animalpain.com.br/en-us

cage open, and then with gentle handling.[106,151,172,160,166] The Feline Grimace Scale is a solely observational scoring assessment that can be done quickly, which is a benefit in a practice with a large number of postsurgical patients or in an intensive care unit.[167,169] See recommended reading at the end of this chapter for more resources on pain scales.

Each pain assessment tool for dogs and cats has its limitations that may lead to false decreases or increases on the pain scale, and each continues to be refined (Table 6.3). The effects of the pet's disease and sedation on pain assessment are unknown.

Pet parent monitoring after discharge from the hospital

Upon their pet's discharge from hospitalization following surgery, illness, or injury, pet parents should be advised that the pet is likely to feel pain in much the same way a person would in the same situation. Cat parents should be advised to monitor closely and report any changes in both mobility and behavior, including overall activity, time spent sleeping, playfulness, and any change from what was previously normal in behavior or temperament (e.g., increase or decrease in avoidance or aggression).[106,173] Appetite, drinking, and elimination habits should also be closely monitored. For dogs, similar measures to what are used in the veterinary clinic can also be used in the home. Dogs should be monitored for posture, activity, vocalization, attention to wound area, appetite, a change in demeanor, mobility, and response to touch. The Glasgow Pain Scale or a picture guide like the Colorado Pain Scales or Feline Grimace Scale might improve pet parent monitoring. For pet parent resources, see https://catfriendly.com/feline-diseases/signs-symptoms/know-cat-pain/ and https://ivapm.org/animal-owners/animal-pain-awareness/.

When pain medications have been dispensed, the goal should be a return to normal behavior and mobility, with specific attention to any change in behavior when pain medications are withdrawn. Pet parents should be advised

that any change in mobility or behavior may not only be an indication of pain but could also be an indication of stress, surgical complications, drug side effects, or a progression of the underlying illness.

Assessing chronic pain

Dogs

In dogs with pain due to degenerative joint disease, pet parents may report signs of lameness or alterations in gait or mobility which might then be confirmed by veterinary orthopedic exam and gait analysis and supported by radiographic findings.[163,174,175] However, radiographic variables do not correlate well with either pet parent or veterinary pain scores.[155,174] Alterations in behavior and demeanor are also commonly reported signs of pain and may be the initial, primary, or only sign of pain in some dogs. Therefore, any change from normal behavior, including activity, social interactions, and play, the appearance of new behavioral signs (e.g., house soiling, vocalization) or a change in temperament or mood (e.g., aggression, avoidance) might be due to pain and can be used to identify arthritis in dogs and monitor response to therapy.[7,25,98,99,147,174–176]

Standardized multifactorial canine monitoring scales for chronic pain are the Canine Brief Pain Inventory (CBPI), Helsinki Chronic Pain Index (HCPI), Cincinnati Orthopedic Disability Index (CODI), ACVS Canine Orthopedic Index (COI), and Liverpool Osteoarthritis in Dogs (LOAD).[98,147,161,175,176,177]

Cats

While lameness and gait alterations may be the primary presenting sign of degenerative joint disease in dogs, this is seldom the case in cats, with less than half of these cats showing lameness or gait alterations.[106,163,178,179] Even when there is

Box 6.2 Behavioral/observation signs of degenerative joint disease in cats[80,98]

Mobility	Decreased, hesitancy, or difficulty with walking, running, jumping, stretching, climbing, and litterbox access and use; stiffness, weakness; change in sleeping or resting areas or position
Activity	Sleeping more, decreased sleep/night waking, playing less, reluctance to engage in normal daily activities
Grooming	Increased scratching and licking, decreased coat maintenance
Temperament	Decreased or increased interaction with people; increased irritability; aggression; less interest in or tolerance of other pets
Behavior	House soiling, vocalization, decreased greeting; withdrawal/hiding; increased "clinginess"; hissing if touched

radiographic evidence of arthritis, lameness was present in only 4–17.5% of these cats.[94–96,106] In addition, cats can be painful despite normal imaging.[83] Common causes of chronic pain include osteoarthritis, neoplasia, dental, gastrointestinal, persistent postsurgical, and neuropathic.[106,161] In cats, studies consistently show that changes in lifestyle (including activity and mobility) and behavior (including grooming and temperament) are the most sensitive signs of arthritic pain.[106,178–180] (Table 6.2). One study showed that pet parent measures of alterations in activity were consistent with objective measures of activity using an accelerometer.[180] Pet parents commonly report that their cats experienced alterations in their ability to jump or in the height of their jump secondary to pain[178] (see Box 6.2).

Veterinary professionals should keep in that mind that while osteoarthritis is common in cats, radiographic evidence does not correlate with clinical signs of pain that clinical examination may lead to an overestimation of pain as cats may resent joint palpation; and that fear, anxiety, and stress may affect (inhibit or exacerbate) the response.[7,98,106,147,153,155] Pet parent education in observation and reporting of changes in mobility, activity, grooming, temperament, and behavior is necessary for identifying pain and assessing response to therapy. Chronic pain scales that have been validated for some application in cats are the Feline Musculoskeletal Pain Index and the Montreal Instrument for Cat Arthritis Testing (for the pet parent and for the veterinarian).[106,171,177,170,181] There is also evidence that health-related quality of life questionnaires can be used to assess the effects of chronic disease including pain and osteoarthritis on quality of life.[106,161,182]

Managing pain

Current pain management guidelines emphasize the proactive and preemptive prevention of pain and early multimodal intervention, since both peripheral and central sensitization or "windup" (increased responsiveness to stimuli and reduced threshold to stimulation) pose one of the greatest challenges to managing chronic pain.[98,106,147,183] In fact, there is a strong correlation between postoperative pain and the development of chronic pain.[183] Therefore, preoperative and perioperative analgesia are the most effective means of minimizing postoperative pain and improving outcome (Table 6.4). The simplified assumption that a pet under sufficient depth of anesthesia will not perceive pain is no longer valid. Although anesthetics inhibit the perception of pain, anesthetic recovery can be improved, and postoperative pain and the need for pain medications reduced by blocking transduction at the site of injury, blocking the transmission of pain, and enhancing spinal modulation to prevent noxious stimuli from sensitizing the nervous system. An understanding of the potential for pain with each procedure and the drug regimen that might best prevent this pain is therefore an important aspect of humane care.

For other conditions causing acute pain, balanced analgesia that involves the combination of two or more classes of analgesic drugs is generally most effective since it likely addresses different mechanisms for pain sensation. For example, the use of nonsteroidal antiinflammatory drugs (NSAIDs) or local anesthetic can inhibit transduction at the site of injury, and a local nerve block can be used to prevent transmission of the nerve impulse and pain modulation pathways in the spinal cord.

Chronic pain, such as from osteoarthritis, is one of the most common indications for long-term pain management and yet misconceptions on proper use of medications for this purpose are commonplace. The medications most commonly used for this purpose are the NSAIDs and related coxibs, which have both analgesic and antiinflammatory effects by inhibiting the synthesis of prostaglandins through cyclooxygenase inhibition. Since NSAIDs are the most common drugs used to manage chronic pain in veterinary practices, it is important for them to be selected and used appropriately.[98,147] For pets that are not candidates for or that do not tolerate a NSAID or require adjunctive medication for pain management, gabapentin is widely used to treat pain clinically, with 69.0% of veterinarian respondents in a survey study indicating that they prescribed gabapentin as an analgesic on a daily or weekly basis, but current evidence of its efficacy as an analgesic medication in dogs is low. There is a paucity of studies evaluating the efficacy of gabapentin

Table 6.4 Pain and analgesia resources

2022 AAHA Canine and Feline Behavior Management Guidelines	https://www.aaha.org/globalassets/02-guidelines/2022-pain-management/resources/2022-aaha-pain-management-guidelines-for-dog-and-cats.pdf
International Veterinary Academy of Pain Management	www.ivapm.org
NewMetrica	https://www.newmetrica.com/publications/
Veterinary Anesthesia and Analgesia Support Group	www.vasg.org
WSAVA Guidelines for Recognition, Assessment and Treatment of Pain (2022)	https://onlinelibrary.wiley.com/doi/10.1111/jsap.13566

in chronic pain in dogs. One retrospective study suggested that gabapentin offered some analgesic benefit in dogs whose chronic pain was not fully controlled with NSAIDs or nutraceuticals alone.[187] There is also limited data that suggests some efficacy in cats with pain due to osteoarthritis.[98] Gabapentin has not been shown to be effective for acute pain in dogs.[98,185] Some Studies in dogs have suggested the need for higher doses (e.g., 10–20 mg/kg) or more frequent dosing (every 8 hours), with patient-specific adjustments until side effects are noted or analgesia is achieved.[184–188] One study evaluating long-term use of gabapentin for musculoskeletal or head trauma in 3 cats at an average dose of 6.5 mg/kg every 12 hours found that satisfactory pain management was achieved in all of the cats.[189] Other neuromodulatory agents such as pregabalin, tricyclic antidepressants, serotonin norepinephrine reuptake inhibitors, amantadine, acetaminophen (in dogs) (with hydrocodone or codeine), lidocaine, and tramadol (in cats), as well as opioids, may be beneficial in patients with maladaptive chronic pain.[98] Synthetic dog-appeasing pheromone also appears to affect behavioral and neuroendocrine perioperative stress responses by modification of lactotropic axis activity and may improve the recovery and welfare of dogs undergoing surgery.[190]

While improvement in behavioral signs, gait, or mobility might be an indication of the efficacy of pain medication, some behavior problems may persist even after the pain is successfully controlled due to the pet having learned new behavioral strategies or conditioned responses to stimuli. In these cases, concurrent pain medication in combination with behavioral therapy or environmental management may be needed to achieve successful outcomes.

Neuropathic pain

Neuropathic pain is defined as pain arising as a lesion or disease affecting the somatosensory system (pain arising from nerve injury). It can be extremely difficult to diagnose, may have a greater impact on quality of life than other forms of pain, and is poorly or partially responsive to NSAIDs. In humans, the pain is described as burning, pulsing, shooting, or stabbing. As with other forms of pain, changes in behavior and demeanor, reactivity to palpation, and gait or locomotor changes may be seen depending on the cause and location of the lesions. Neuropathic pain in pets may be associated with trauma (accidental or surgical), neck and back pain, nervous system disease including Chiari-like malformation, diabetic neuropathy, and hyperesthesia, oro-facial pain syndrome, and interstitial cystitis in cats.[153,177,184] Signs of self-trauma such as tail mutilation, paw chewing, or face scratching might also arise as a result of neuropathic pain.[191]

References

1. Conzemius MG, Sammarco JL, Perkowski SZ, et al. Correlation between subjective and objective measures used to determine severity of postoperative pain in dogs. *J Am Vet Med Assoc*. 1997; 210:1619–1622.
2. Cambridge AJ, Tobias KM, Newberry RC. Subjective and objective measurements of postoperative pain in cats. *J Am Vet Med Assoc*. 2000;217:685–690.
3. Tynes V, Sinn L. Abnormal repetitive behavior in dogs and cats: a guide for practitioners. *Vet Clin Small Anim*. 2014; 44:543–564.
4. Woo DC, Choi CB, Nam JW, et al. Quantitative analysis of hydrocephalic ventricular alterations in Yorkshire terriers using magnetic resonance imaging. *Vet Med*. 2010;55:125–132.
5. Escriou C, Renier S, Tiira K, et al. Phenotypic and genetic characterization of "spinning" or "tail-chasing" in Bull Terriers. *J Vet Behav*. 2012;7:e4–e5.
6. Mori Y, Ma J, Tanaka S, et al. Hypothalamically induced emotional behavior and immunological changes in the cat. *Psychiatry Clin Neurosci*. 2001; 55:325–332.
7. Camps T, Amat M, Manteca X. A review of medical conditions and behavioral problems in dogs and cats. *Animals*. 2019;9:1–17.
8. Foster ES, Carrillo JM, Patnaik AK. Clinical signs of tumors affecting the rostral cerebrum in 43 dogs. *J Vet Intern Med*. 1988;2:71–74.
9. Kearsley-Fleet L, O'Neill DG, Volk HA, et al. Prevalence and risk factors for canine epilepsy of unknown origin in the UK. *Vet Rec*. 2013;172:338.
10. Berendt M, Farquhar RG, Mandigers PJJ, et al. International veterinary epilepsy task force consensus report on epilepsy definition, classification and terminology in companion animals. *BMC Vet Res*. 2015;11:182.
11. Levitin H, Wallis Hague D, Ballantyne KC, et al. Behavioral changes in dogs with idiopathic epilepsy compared to other medical populations. *Front Vet Sci*. 2019;6:396.
12. Shihab N, Bowen J, Volk HA. Behavioral changes in dogs associated with the development of idiopathic epilepsy. *Epilepsy Behav*. 2011;21(2):160–167.
13. Packer RMA, Volk HA. Epilepsy beyond seizures: a review of the impact of epilepsy and its comorbidities on health-related quality of life in dogs. *Vet Rec*. 2015;177:306–315.
14. Packer RMA, McGreevy PD, Pergande A, et al. Negative effects of epilepsy and antiepileptic drugs on the trainability of dogs with naturally occurring idiopathic epilepsy. *Appl Anim Behav Sci*. 2018;200: 106–113.
15. Packer RMA, Law TH, Davies E, et al. Effects of a ketogenic diet on ADHD like behavior in dogs with idiopathic epilepsy. *Epilepsy Behav*. 2016;55:62–68.
16. Packer RMA, McGreevy PD, Salvin HE, et al. Cognitive dysfunction in dogs with naturally occurring epilepsy. *PLoS One*. 2018;13(2):e0192182.
17. Berendt M, Farquhar RG, Mandigers PJJ, et al. International veterinary epilepsy task force consensus report on epilepsy definition, classification and terminology in companion animals. *BMC Vet Res*. 2015;11:182.
18. Dodman NH, Miczek KA, Knowles K, et al. Phenobarbital-responsive episodic dyscontrol (rage) in dogs. *J Am Vet Med Assoc*. 1992;201:1580–1583.
19. Dodman NH, Branson R, Gliatto J. Tail chasing in a Bull Terrier. *J Am Vet Med Assoc*. 1993;202:758–760.
20. Breitschwerdt EB, Breazilc JW, Broadhurst JJ. Clinical and electroencephalographic findings associated with ten cases of suspected limbic epilepsy in the dog. *J Am Anim Hosp Assoc*. 1979;15:37–50.
21. Rusbridge C. New considerations about Chiari-like malformation, syringomyelia and their management. *In Pract*. 2020;42:252–267.
22. Wrzosek M, Plonek M, Nicpon J, et al. Retrospective multicenter evaluation of the "fly-catching syndrome" in 24 dogs: EEG, BAER, MRI, CSF findings and response to antiepileptic and antidepressant treatment. *Epilepsy Behav*. 2015;53:184–189.
23. Brewer DM, Cerda-Goncalez S, Dewey CW, et al. Diagnosis and surgical resection of a choroid plexus cyst in a dog. *J Small Anim Pract*. 2010;51:169–172. doi: 10.1111/j.1748-5827.2009.00855.x.

24. Tynes V, Sinn L. Abnormal repetitive behaviors in dogs and cats. *Vet Clin North Am Small Anim Pract.* 2014;44: 543–564. doi:10.1016/J.CVSM.2014. 01.011.

25. Mills DS, Demontigny-Bedard I, Gruen M, et al. Pain and problem behavior in cats and dogs. *Animals.* 2020;10:318. doi:10.3390/ani10020318.

26. Dodman NH, Knowles KE, Shuster L, et al. Behavioral changes associated with suspected complex partial seizures in Bull Terriers. *J Am Vet Med Assoc.* 1996;208(5): 688–691.

27. Tsilioni I, Dodman N, Petra AI, et al. Elevated serum neurotensin and CRH levels in children with autistic spectrum disorders and tail-chasing Bull Terriers with a phenotype similar to autism. *Transl Psychiatry.* 2014;4(10):e466.

28. Moon-Fanelli AA, Dodman NH, Famula TR, et al. Characteristics of compulsive tail chasing and associated risk factors in Bull Terriers. *J Am Vet Med Assoc.* 2011; 238(7):883–889.

29. Barone G. Neurology. In: Little SE, ed. *The Cat.* St. Louis: Elsevier Saunders; 2012:734–767.

30. Lorenz MD, Coates JR, Kent M. Systemic or multifocal signs. In: *Handbook of Veterinary Neurology.* 5th ed. London: Saunders; 2011:432–487 [chapter 15].

31. Levitin H, Wallis Hague D, Ballantyne KC, et al. Behavioral changes in dogs with idiopathic epilepsy compared to other medical populations. *Front Vet Sci.* 2019;6:396.

32. Simpson BS, Landsberg GM, Reisner IR, et al. Effects of Reconcile (fluoxetine) chewable tablets plus behavior management for canine separation anxiety. *Vet Ther.* 2007;8(1):18–31.

33. Snyder JM, Shofer FS, Van Winkel T, et al. Canine intracranial neoplasia: 176 cases (1986–2003). *J Vet Intern Med.* 2006;20: 669–675.

34. Denenberg S, Leibel FX, Rose J. Behavioral and medical differentials of cognitive decline and dementia in dogs and cats. In: Landsberg G, et al. eds. *Canine and Feline Dementia. Molecular Basis, Diagnosis and Therapy.* Cham, Switzerland: Springer International Publishing; 2019:13–58.

35. Troxel MT, Vite CH, Van Winkle TJ, et al. Feline intracranial neoplasia: retrospective review of 160 cases (1985–2001). *J Vet Intern Med.* 2003;17(6):850–859.

36. Neilson JC, Hart BL, Cliff KD, et al. Prevalence of behavioral changes associated with age-related cognitive impairment in dogs. *J Am Vet Med Assoc.* 2001;18:1787–1791.

37. Fast R, Schütt T, Toft N, et al. An observational study with long-term follow-up of canine cognitive dysfunction: clinical characteristics, survival, and risk factors. *J Vet Intern Med.* 2013;27:822–829.

38. Gunn-Moore DA, Moffat K, Christie LA, et al. Cognitive dysfunction and the neurobiology of aging in cats. *J Small Anim Pract.* 2007;48:546–553.

39. LeClerc M-K. Narcolepsy and cataplexy. In: Tilley LP, et al. eds. *Blackwell's Five- Minute Veterinary Consult: Canine and Feline.* 7th ed. Hoboken: John Wiley and Sons; 2021:954.

40. Hendricks JC, Lager A, O'Brien D, et al. Movement disorders during sleep in cats and dogs. *J Am Vet Med Assoc.* 1989;194:686–689.

41. Schubert TA, Chidester M, Chrisman CL. Clinical characteristics, management and long-term outcome of suspected rapid eye movement sleep behaviour disorder in 14 dogs. *J Small Anim Pract.* 2011; 52:93–100.

42. Rajapaksha E. Special considerations for diagnosing behavior problems in older pets. *Vet Clin North Am Small Anim Pract.* 2018;48(3):443–456.

43. Affenzeller N, McPeake KJ, McClement J, et al. Human-directed aggressive behaviour as the main presenting sign in dogs subsequently diagnosed with diskospondylitis. *Vet Rec Case Rep.* 2017;5(4):e000501.

44. Fingeroth JM, Prata RG, Patnaik AK. Spinal meningiomas in dogs: 13 cases (1972–1987). *J Am Vet Med Assoc.* 1987; 191:720–726.

45. Batle PA, Rusbridge C, Nuttall, et al. Feline hyperaesthesia syndrome with self-trauma to the tail; restrospective study of seven cases and proposal for an integrated multidisciplinary diagnostic approach. *J Feline Med Surg.* 2019;21: 178–185.

46. Drew LJ, MacDermott AB. Neuroscience: unbearable lightness of touch. *Nature.* 2009;462:580–581.

47. Luescher UA. Hyperkinesis in dogs: six case reports. *Can Vet J.* 1993;34:368–370.

48. Stiles EK, Palestrini C, Beauchamp G, et al. Physiological and behavioral effects of dextroamphetamine on Beagle dogs. *J Vet Behav.* 2011;6(6):328–336.

49. Bleuer-Elsner S, Muller G, Beata C, et al. Effect of fluoxetine at a dose of 2-4 mg/kg daily in dogs exhibiting hypersensitivity-hyperactivity syndrome, a retrospective study. *J Vet Behav.* 2021; 44:25–31.

50. Olsen D, Wellner N, Kaas M, et al. Altered dopaminergic firing pattern and novelty response underlie ADHD-like behavior of SorCS2-deficient mice. *Transl Psychiatry.* 2021;11(1):74. doi:10.1038/s41398-021-01199-9.

51. Sulkama S, Puurunen J, Salonen M, et al. Canine hyperactivity, impulsivity and inattention share similar demographic risk factors and behavioural comorbidities with human ADHD. *Transl Psychiatry.* 2021;11(501). doi:10.1038/s41398-021-01626-x.

52. Bacanli A, Unsel-Bolat G, Suren S, et al. Effects of the dopamine transporter gene on neuroimaging findings in different attention deficit hyperactivity disorder presentations. *Brain Imag Behav.* 2021;15(2):1103–1114.

53. Puurunen J, Sulkama S, Tiira K, et al. A non-targeted metabolite profiling pilot study suggests that tryptophan and lipid metabolisms are linked with ADHD-like behaviours in dogs. *Behav Brain Funct.* 2016;12(27). doi:10.1186/s12993-016-0112-1.

54. Scharf VF, Oblak ML, Hoffman K, et al. Clinical features and outcome of functional thyroid tumours in 70 dogs. *J Small Anim Pract.* 2020;61:504–511.

55. Prikryl M, Cherubini GB, Palus V. Neurogenic hyperkinetic movement disorders in dogs. *Comp Anim.* 2018; 23(4):230–235.

56. Lidbury JA, Cook AK, Steiner, JM. Hepatic encephalopathy in dogs and cats. *J Vet Emerg Crit Care.* 2016;26(4): 471–487.

57. Dewey CW, Davies ES, Xie H, et al. Canine cognitive dysfunction: pathophysiology, diagnosis and treatment. *Vet Clin North Am Small Anim Pract.* 2019;49(3):477–499.

58. Schalke E, Stichnoth J, Ott S, et al. Clinical signs caused by the use of electric training collars on dogs in everyday life situations. *Appl Anim Behav Sci.* 2007; 105(4):369–380.

59. Blackwell EJ, Twells C, Seawright A, et al. The relationship between training methods and the occurrence of behavior problems, as reported by owners, in a population of domestic dogs. *J Vet Behav.* 2008;3:207–217.

60. Ziv G. The effects of using aversive training methods in dogs - a review. *J Vet Behav.* 2017;19:50–60.

61. Fernandes JG, Olsson IAS, Vieira de Castro AC. Do aversive-based training methods actually compromise dog welfare?: a literature review. *Appl Anim Behav Sci.* 2017;196:1–12.

62. Riemer S, Mills D, Wright H. Impulsive for life? The nature of long-term impulsivity in domestic dogs. *Anim Cogn.* 2014;17(3):815–819.

63. Dinwoodie IR, Dwyer B, Zottola V, et al. Demographics and comorbidity of behavior problems in dogs. *J Vet Behav.* 2019;32:62–71.

64. Salonen M, Sulkama S, Mikkola S, et al. Prevalence, comorbidity and breed differences in canine anxiety in 13,700 Finnish pet dogs. *Sci Rep.* 2020;10:2962.

65. Tonoike A, Nagasawa M, Mogi K, et al. Comparison of owner-reported behavioral characteristics among genetically clustered breeds of dog (*Canis familiaris*). *Sci Rep.* 2015;5:17710. doi:10.1038/srep17710.

66. Lit L, Schweitzer JB, Iosif AM, et al. Owner reports of attention, activity and impulsivity in dogs: a replication study. *Behav Brain Funct.* 2010;6:1. doi:10/1186/1744-9081-6-1.

67. Wright HF, Mills DS, Pollux PMJ. Development and validation of a psychometric tool for assessing impulsivity in the domestic dog (*Canis familiaris*). *Int J Comp Psychol.* 2011;24:210–225.

68. Ley JM, Bennett PC, Coleman GJ. A refinement and validation of the Monash Canine Personality Questionnaire

(MCPQ). *Appl Anim Behav Sci.* 2009;116:220–227.

69. Vas J, Topál J, Péch É, et al. Measuring attention deficit and activity in dogs: a new application and validation of a human ADHD questionnaire. *Appl Anim Behav Sci.* 2007;103:105–117.

70. Beaver B, Haug L. Canine behaviors associated with hypothyroidism. *J Am Anim Hosp Assoc.* 2005;39:431–434.

71. Lathan PA. Hypothyroidism. In: Tilley LP et al., eds. *Blackwell's Five-Minute Veterinary Consult: Canine and Feline.* 7th ed. John Wiley and Sons; 2021:747–749.

72. Bellows J, Colitz CM, Daristotle L, et al. Defining healthy aging in older dogs and differentiating healthy aging from disease. *J Am Vet Med Assoc.* 2015;246:77–89.

73. Aronson LP, Dodds WJ. The effect of hypothyroid function on canine behavior. In: Mills D, Leviine E, Landsberg G, et al., eds. *Current Research in Veterinary Behavioral Medicine.* West Lafayette: Purdue University Press; 2005:131–138.

74. Dodman N, Aronson L, Cottam N, et al. The effect of thyroid replacement in dogs with suboptimal thyroid function on owner-directed aggression: a randomized, double-blind, placebo-controlled clinical trial. *J Vet Behav.* 2013;8(4):225–230.

75. Fatjo J, Stub C, Manteca X. Aggression and hypothyroidism. *Vet Rec.* 2002;151:547–548.

76. Radosta LA, Shofer FS, Reisner RI. Comparison of thyroid analytes in dogs aggressive to familiar people and in non-aggressive dogs. *Vet J.* 2012;2:472–475.

77. Hrovat A, De Keuster T, Kooistra HS, et al. Behavior in dogs with spontaneous hypothyroidism during treatment with levothyroxine. *J Vet Intern Med.* 2019;33:64–71.

78. Hassan WA, Rahman TA, Aly MS, et al. Alterations in monoamines level in discrete brain regions and other peripheral tissues in young and adult male rats during experimental hyperthyroidism. *Int J Dev Neurosci.* 2013;31:311–318.

79. Sordo L, Breheny C, Halls V. Prevalence of disease and age-related behavior changes in cats: past and present. *Vet Sci.* 2020;7:85.

80. Bellows J, Center S, Daristotle L, et al. Evaluating aging in cats: how to determine what is healthy and what is disease. *J Feline Med Surg.* 2016;8:551–570.

81. Boag AK, Neiger R, Church DB. Trilostane treatment of bilateral adrenal enlargement and excessive sex steroid hormone production in a cat. *J Small Anim Pract.* 2004;45:263–266.

82. Millard RP, Pickens EH, Wells KL. Excessive production of sex hormones with an adrenocortical tumor. *J Am Vet Med Assoc.* 2009;234:505–508.

83. Behrend E, Holford A, Lathan P, et al. AAHA diabetes management guidelines for dogs and cats. *J Am Anim Hosp Assoc.* 2018;54:1–21.

84. Shen, HH. Microbes on the mind. *Proc Natl Acad Sci U S A.* 2015;112:9143–9145.

85. Dinan TG, Cryan JF. Gut-brain axis in 2016: brain-gut-microbiota axis - mood, metabolism and behaviour. *Nat Rev Gastroenterol Hepatol.* 2017;14:69–70.

86. Pilla R, Suchodolski JS. The role of the canine gut microbiome and metabolome in health and gastrointestinal disease. *Front Vet Sci.* 2020;6:498.

87. Kirchoff NS, Udell MAR, Sharpton TJ. The gut microbiome correlates with conspecific aggression in a small population of rescued dogs (Canis familiaris). *Peer J.* 2019;7:e6103.

88. Bécuwe-Bonnet V, Bélanger MC, Diane Frank D, et al. Gastrointestinal disorders in dogs with excessive licking of surfaces. *J Vet Behav.* 2012;7:194–204.

89. Frank D, Belanger MC, Becuwe-Bonnet V, et al. Prospective medical evaluation of 7 dogs presented with fly biting. *Can Vet J.* 2012;53:1279–1284.

90. Demontigny-Bedard I, Beauchamp G, Belanger MC, et al. Characterization of pica and chewing behaviors in privately owned cats: a case-control study. *J Feline Med Surg.* 2016;18:652–657.

91. Demontigny-Bedard I, Belanger MC, Helie P, et al. Medical and behavioral evaluation of 8 cats presenting with fabric ingestion: an exploratory pilot study. *Can Vet J.* 2019;60:1081–1088.

92. Johnston SA. Osteoarthritis. Joint anatomy, physiology, and pathobiology. *Vet Clin North Am Small Anim Pract.* 1997;27:699–723.

93. Anderson KL, Zulch H, O'Neill DG, et al. Risk factors for canine osteoarthritis and its predisposing arthropathies: a systemic review. *Front Vet Sci.* 2020;7:220. doi:10.3389/fvets.2020.00220.

94. Clarke SP, Mellor D, Clements DN, et al. Prevalence of radiographic signs of degenerative joint disease in a hospital population of cats. *Vet Rec.* 2005;157:793–799.

95. Lascelles BDX, Henry III JB, Brown J, et al. Cross-sectional study of the prevalence of radiographic degenerative joint disease in domesticated cats. *Vet Surg.* 2010;39:535–544.

96. Godfrey DR. Osteoarthritis in cats: a retrospective radiological study. *J Small Anim Pract.* 2005;46:425–429.

97. Mirza U, Bin Farooq U, Makhdoomi DM, et al. Osteoarthritis in dogs - effect on diet. *Int J Food Sci Agri.* 2021;5(4):670–673.

98. Gruen ME, Lascelles DBX, Colleran E, et al. AAHA pain management guidelines for dogs and cats. *J Am Anim Hosp Assoc.* 2022;58:55–76.

99. Barcelos A-M, Zulch H, Mills DS. Clinical indicators of occult musculoskeletal pain in aggressive dogs. *Vet Rec.* 2015;176:465.

100. Camps T, Amat M, Mariotti VM, et al. Pain-related aggression in dogs: 12 clinical cases. *J Vet Behav.* 2012;7:99–102.

101. Holden E, Calvo G, Collins M, et al. Evaluation of facial expression in acute pain in cats. *J Small Anim Pract.* 2014;55(12):615–621.

102. Asmundson GJG, Katz J. Understanding the co-occurrence of anxiety disorders and chronic pain: state-of-the-art. *Depress Anxiety.* 2009;26:888–901.

103. Martell-Moran NK, Townsend HG. Pain and adverse behavior in declawed cats. *J Feline Med Surg.* 2018;20:208–287.

104. Packer RM, Hendricks A, Volk HA, et al. How long and low can you go? Effect of conformation on the risk of thoracolumbar intervertebral disc extrusion in domestic dogs. *PLoS One.* 2013;8:e69650.

105. Pelosi A, Rosenstein D, Abood SK, et al. Cardiac effect of short-term experimental weight gain and loss in dogs. *Vet Rec.* 2013;172:153.

106. Steagall PV, Monteiro B. Chronic pain in cats. Recent advances in clinical assessment. *J Feline Med Surg.* 2019;21:601–614.

107. Lund EM, Armstrong PJ, Kirk CA, Klausner JS. Prevalence and risk factors for obesity in adult cats from private US veterinary practices. *Int J Appl Res Vet Med.* 2005;3:88–96.

108. Tey HL, Wallengren J, Yosipovitch G. Psychosomatic factors in pruritus. *Clin Dermatol.* 2013;31(1):31–40.

109. Waisglass SE, Landsberg GM, Yager JA, et al. Underlying medical conditions in cats with presumptive psychogenic alopecia. *J Am Vet Med Assoc.* 2006;228(11):1705–1709.

110. Grace SF. Acral lick dermatitis. In: Tilley LP, et al. eds. *Blackwell's Five-Minute Veterinary Consult: Canine and Feline.* 7th ed. Hoboken: John Wiley and Sons; 2021:16–17.

111. Harvey ND, Craigon PJ, Shaw SC, et al. Behavior differences in dogs with atopic dermatitis suggest stress could be a significant problem associated with chronic pruritus. *Animals.* 2019;9(10):813.

112. Horwitz D. Behavioral and environmental factors associated with elimination behavior problems in cats: a retrospective study. *Appl Anim Behav Sci.* 1997;52:129–137.

113. Tynes VV, Hart BL, Pryor PA, et al. Evaluation of the role of lower urinary tract disease in cats with urine marking behavior. *J Am Vet Med Assoc.* 2003;223:457–461.

114. Ramos D, Reche-Junior A, Mills DS, et al. A closer look at the health of cats showing urinary house soiling (periuria): a case-control study 2018. *J Feline Med Surg.* 2019;21:772–779.

115. Reche Junior A, Ramos D, Ferreira M, et al. A case of behavioral changes in a castrated male cat due to a functional adrenocortical adenoma producing testosterone and androstenedione. *J Feline Med Surg Open Rep.* 2021;7(1):2055116920981247.

116. Niemiec B, Gawor J, Nemec A, et al. World Small Animal Veterinary Association global dental guidelines. *J Sm Anim Prac.* 2020;61:E36–E161.

117. Kyllar M, Witter K. Prevalence of dental disorders in pet dogs. *Vet Med.* 2005;50: 496–505.

118. Fernandes NA, Batista Borges AP, Carlo Reis EC, et al. Prevalence of periodontal disease in dogs and owners' level of awareness – a prospective clinical trial. *Rev Ceres.* 2012;59(4):446–451.

119. Wiggs RB, Lobprise HB. Periodontology. In: *Veterinary Dentistry, Principals and Practice.* Philadelphia: Lippincott-Raven; 1997:186–231.

120. Lommer MJ, Verstraete FJM. Prevalence of odontoclastic resorption lesions and periapical radiographic lucencies in cats: 265 cases (1995–1998). *J Am Vet Med Assoc.* 2000;217:1866–1869.

121. Sordo L, Breheny C, Halls V, et al. Prevalence of disease and age-related behavioural changes in cats: past and present. *Vet Sci.* 2020;7(3):1–19.

122. Landsberg G, Arajuo JA. Behavior problems in geriatric pets. *Vet Clin Small Anim.* 2005;35(3):675–698.

123. Wallis C, Holcombe LJ. A review of the frequency and impact of periodontal disease in dogs. *J Small Anim Pract.* 2020;61:529–540. doi:10.1111/jsap.13218.

124. Watanabe R, Frank D, Steagall PV. Pain behaviors before and after treatment of oral disease in cats using video assessment: a prospective, blinded, randomized clinical trial. *BMC Vet Res.* 2020:16:100.

125. Rusbridge S, Heath S. Feline orofacial pain syndrome. In: Rodan I, Heath S, eds. *Feline Behavioral Health and Welfare.* St. Louis: Elsevier; 2016:213–226 [chapter 16].

126. Farmer-Dougan V, Quick A, Harper K, et al. Behavior of hearing or vision impaired and normal hearing and vision dogs (*Canis lupus familiaris*): not the same but not that different. *J Vet Behav* 2013;9:316–323.

127. Tamilmahan P, Zama MMS, Pathak R, et al. A retrospective study of ocular occurrences in domestic animals: 799 cases. *Vet World.* 2014;6:274–276.

128. Strain G. *Deafness in Dogs and Cats.* Wallingford, UK: CAB International; 2013.

129. Barber R. Rabies. In: Tilley LP, et al. eds. *Blackwell's Five-Minute Veterinary Consult: Canine and Feline.* 7th ed., Hoboken: John Wiley and Sons; 2021: 1178–1179.

130. Pedersen NC. A review of feline infectious peritonitis virus infection: 1963–2008. *J Feline Med Surg.* 2009;11:225–258.

131. Diaz JV, Poma R. Diagnosis and clinical signs of feline infectious peritonitis in the central nervous system. *Can Vet J.* 2009;50:1091–1093.

132. Carmichael KP, Bienzle D, McDonnell JJ. Feline leukemia virus-associated myelopathy in cats. *Vet Pathol.* 2002;39: 536–545.

133. Dow SW, Dreitz MJ, Hoover EA. Exploring the link between FIV infection and neurologic disease in cats. *Vet Med.* 1992;87:1181–1184.

134. Power C. Neurological disease in feline immunodeficiency virus infection: disease mechanisms and therapeutic interventions for NeuroAIDS. *J Neurovirol.* 2017;24(2):220–228.

135. Power C. Neurological disease in feline immunodeficiency virus infection: disease mechanisms and therapeutic interventions for NeuroAIDS. *J Neurovirol.* 2017;24(2): 220–228.

136. Steigerwald ES, Sarter M, March P, et al. Effects of FIV on cognition and behavioral function in cats. *J Acquir Immune Defic Syndr Hum Retrovirol.* 1999;20:411–419.

137. Sykes J. Canine distemper virus infection. In: *Canine and Feline Infectious Diseases.* St. Louis: Elsevier Health Sciences; 2013:152–165. [chapter 15].

138. Levin ML, Killmaster LF, Zemtsova GE, et al. Clinical presentation, convalescence and relapse of Rocky Mountain Spotted Fever in dogs experimentally infected via tick bite. *PLoS One.* 2014;9(12):e115105.

139. Calero-Bernal R, Gennari SM. Clinical toxoplasmosis in dogs and cats: an update. *Front Vet Sci.* 2019(6):54. doi:10.3389/fvets.2019.00054.

140. Church ME, Turek BJ, Durham AC. Neuropathology of spontaneous hypertensive encephalopathy in cats. *Vet Pathol.* 2019;56(5):778–782.

141. O'Neill J, Kent M, Glass EN, et al. Clinicopathalogic and MRI characteristics of presumptive hypertensive encephalopathy in two cats and two dogs. *J Am Anim Hosp Assoc.* 2013;49(6):412–420.

142. Maggio F, DeFrancesco TC, Atkins CE, et al. Ocular lesions associated with systemic hypertension in cats: 69 cases (1985–1998). *J Am Vet Med Assoc.* 2000;217:695–702.

143. Littman MP. Spontaneous systemic hypertension in 24 cats. *J Vet Intern Med.* 1994;8:79–86.

144. Acierno MJ, Brown S, Coleman AE, et al. ACVIM consensus statement: guidelines for the identification, evaluation, and management of systemic hypertension in dogs and cats. *J Vet Intern Med.* 2018; 32:1803–1822.

145. Notari L, Burman O, Mills D. Behavioral changes in dogs treated with corticosteroids. *Physiol Behav.* 2015;151: 609–616.

146. Cosgrove SB, Wren JA, Cleaver DM, et al. Efficacy and safety of oclacitinib for the control of pruritus and associated skin lesions in dogs with canine allergic dermatitis. *Vet Dermatol.* 2013;24(5): 479–e114.

147. Mathews K, Kronen PW, Lascelles D, et al. WSAVA Guidelines for recognition, assessment and treatment of pain. *J Small Anim Pract.* 2014;55:E10–E68.

148. Fagundes ALL, Hewison L, McPeake KJ, et al. Noise sensitivities in dogs: an exploration of signs in dogs with and without musculoskeletal pain using qualitative content analysis. *Front Vet Sci.* 2018;5:17.

149. Chieng YJ, Chan WC, Klainin-Yobus P, et al. Perioperative anxiety and post-operative pain in children and adolescents undergoing elective surgical procedures: a quantitative systematic review. *J Adv Nurs.* 2014;70: 243–255.

150. Storm H, Günther A, Sackey PV, et al. Measuring pain—physiological and self-rated measurements in relation to pain stimulation and anxiety. *Acta Anaesthesiol Scand.* 2019;63:668–675.

151. Belli M, de Oliveira AR, de Lima MT, et al. Clinical validation of the short and long UNESP-Botucatu scales for feline pain assessment. *Peer J.* 2021;9:e11225. doi:10.7717/peerj.11225.

152. Blake JE, Adran D, Grady K, et al. Evidence of increased positive affective state in dogs after treatment with firocoxib for osteoarthritis pain. In: *Proc ACVB Vet Behav Symp.* 2020:3–4.

153. Steagall PV, Monteiro B. Acute pain in cats. Recent advances in clinical assessment. *J Feline Med Surg.* 2019;21:25–34.

154. Rousseau-Blass F, O'Toole E, Macroux J, et al. Prevalence and management of pain in dogs in the emergency service of a veterinary teaching hospital. *Can Vet J.* 2020;61(3):294–300.

155. Klinck MP, Mogil JS, Moreau M, et al. Translational pain assessment. *Pain.* 2017;158(9):1633–1646.

156. Robertson S. Managing pain in feline patients. *Vet Clin North Am Sm Anim Pract.* 2008;38:1267–1290.

157. Simon BT, Scallan EM, Carroll G. The lack of analgesic use (oligoanalgesia) in small animal practice. *J Small Anim Pract.* 2017;58:543–554.

158. Hernandez-Avalos I, Mota-Rojas D, Mora-Medina P, et al. Review of different methods used for clinical recognition and assessment of pain in dogs and cats. *Int J Vet Sci Med.* 2019;7(1):43–54.

159. De Jonckheere J, Bonhomme V, Jeanne M, et al. Physiological signal processing for individualized anti-nociception management during general anesthesia: a review. *Yearb Med Inform.* 2015;10(1): 95–101.

160. Brondani JT, Luna SPL, Padovani C. Refinement and initial validation of a multidimensional composite scale for use in assessing acute postoperative pain in cats. *Am J Vet Res.* 2011;72(2):174–183.

161. Reid J, Nolan AM, Scott EM. Measuring pain in dogs and cats using structured behavioural observation. *Vet J.* 2018;236: 72–79.

162. Brondani JT, Mama KR, Luna SPL, et al. Validation of the English version of the UNESP-Botucatu multidimensional composite pain scale for assessing postoperative pain in cats. *BMC Vet Res.* 2013;9:143.

163. Muir W, Wiese AJ, Wittum TE. Prevalence and characteristics of pain in

dogs and cats examined as outpatients at a veterinary teaching hospital. *J Am Vet Med Assoc*. 2004;224:1459–1463.

164. Murrell JC, Psatha EP, Scott EM, et al. Application of a modified form of the Glasgow pain scale in a veterinary teaching hospital in the Netherlands. *Vet Rec*. 2008;162:403–408.

165. Reid J, Nolan AM, Hughes JML, et al. Development of the short-form Glasgow Composite Measure Pain Scale (CMPS-SF) and derivation of an analgesic intervention score. *Anim Welf*. 2007;16:97–104.

166. Reid J, Scott EM, Calvo G. Definitive Glasgow acute pain scale for cats: validation and intervention level. *Vet Rec*. 2017;180:449.

167. Evangelista MC, Watanabe R, Leung VSY, et al. Facial expressions of pain in cats: the development and validation of a Feline Grimace Scale. *Sci Rep*. 2019;9(1):9128.

168. Merola I, Mills DS. Systematic review of the behavioural assessment of pain in cats. *J Feline Med Surg*. 2015;18(2):60–76.

169. Evangelista MC, Benito J, Monteiro BP, et al. Clinical applicability of the Feline Grimace Scale: real-time versus image scoring and the influence of sedation and surgery. *Peer J*. 2020;8:e8967. doi:10.7717/peerj.8967.

170. Gruen ME, Griffith EH, Thomson AE, et al. Criterion validation testing of clinical metrology instruments for measuring degenerative joint disease associated mobility impairment in cats. *PLoS One*. 2015;10:e0131839.

171. Gruen ME, Griffith E, Thomson A, et al. Detection of clinically relevant pain relief in cats with degenerative joint disease associated pain. *J Vet Intern Med*. 2014;28:346–350.

172. Merola I, Mills DS. Systematic review of the behavioural assessment of pain in cats. *J Feline Med Surg*. 2015;18(2):60–76.

173. Vaisanen M, Tuomikoski SK, Vainio OM. Behavioral alterations and severity of pain in cats recovering at home following elective ovariohysterectomy or castration. *J Am Vet Med Assoc*. 2007; 231:236–242.

174. Hielm Bjorkman AK, Kuusela E, Liman A, et al. Evaluation of methods for assessment of pain associated with chronic osteoarthritis in dogs. *J Am Vet Med Assoc*. 2003;222:1552–1558.

175. Brown DC, Boston RC, Coyne JC, et al. Ability of the canine brief pain inventory to detect response to treatment in dogs with osteoarthritis. *J Am Vet Med Assoc*. 2008;15:1278–1283.

176. Walton MB, Cowderoy E, Lascelles D, et al. Evaluation of construct and criterion validity for the 'Liverpool Osteoarthritis in Dogs' (LOAD) clinical metrology instrument and comparison to two other instruments. *PLoS One*. 2013;8(3):e58125.

177. Lascelles BDX, Brown DC, Conzemius MG, et al. Measurement of chronic pain in companion animals: discussion from the Pain in Animals Workshop (PAW 2017). *Vet J*. 2019;250:71–78.

178. Clarke SP, Bennett D. Feline osteoarthritis: a prospective study of 28 cases. *J Small Anim Pract*. 2006;47:439–445.

179. Bennett D, Morton C. A study of owner observed behavioural and lifestyle changes in cats with musculoskeletal disease before and after analgesic therapy. *J Feline Med Surg*. 2009;11: 997–1004.

180. Lascelles BD, Hansen BD, Roe S, et al. Evaluation of client-specific outcome measures and activity monitoring to measure pain relief in cats with osteoarthritis. *J Vet Intern Med*. 2007;21: 410–416.

181. Klinck MP, Gruen ME, del Castillo JRE, et al. Development and preliminary validity and reliability of the Montreal instrument for cat arthritis testing, for use by caretaker/owner, MI-CAT(C) via a randomised clinical trial. *Appl Anim Behav Sci*. 2018;200:96–105.

182. Noble CE, Wiseman-Orr LM, Scott ME, et al. Development, initial validation and reliability testing of a web-based, generic feline health-related quality-of-life instrument. *J Feline Med Surg*. 2019; 21:84–94.

183. Gurney MA. Pharmacological options for intra-operative and early postoperative analgesia: an update. *J Small Anim Pract*. 2012;53(7):377–386.

184. Mathews A. Physiologic and pharmacologic applications to manage neuropathic pain. In: Mathews KA, Sinclair M, Steele AS, et al. *Analgesia and Anesthesia for the Ill or Injured Dog and Cat*. Hoboken: John Wiley and Sons; 2018:17–50.

185. Wagner AE, Mich PM, Uhrig SR, et al. Clinical evaluation of perioperative administration of gabapentin as an adjunct for postoperative analgesia in dogs undergoing amputation of a forelimb. *J Am Vet Med Assoc*. 2010;236:751–756.

186. Aghighi SA, Tipold A, Piechotta M, et al. Assessment of the effects of adjunctive gabapentin on postoperative pain after intervertebral disc surgery in dogs. *Vet Anaesth Analg*. 2012;39:636–646.

187. Davis LV, Hellyer PW, Downing RA, et al. Retrospective study of 240 dogs receiving gabapentin for chronic pain relief. *J Vet Med Res*. 2020;7(4):1194.

188. Kukanich B, Cohen RL. Pharmacokinetics of oral gabapentin in greyhound dogs. *Vet J*. 2011;187:133–135.

189. Lorenz ND, Comerford EJ, Iff I. Long-term use of gabapentin for musculoskeletal disease and trauma in three cats. *J Feline Med Surg*. 2013;15(6): 507–512.

190. Siracusa C, Manteca X, Cuenca R, et al. Effect of a synthetic appeasing pheromone on behavioral, neuroendocrine, immune, and acute-phase perioperative stress responses in dogs. *J Am Vet Med Assoc*. 2010;237: 673–681.

191. Cashmore RG, Harcourt-Brown TR, Freeman PM. Clinical diagnosis and treatment of suspected neuropathic pain in three dogs. *Aust Vet J*. 2009;87:45–50.

Resources and recommended reading

Amadei L, Cantile C, Gazzano A, et al. The link between neurology and behavior in veterinary medicine: a review. *J Vet Behav*. 2021;46:40–53.

Czopowicz M, Szalu-Jordanow O, Frymus T. Cerebral toxoplasmosis in a cat. *Medycyna Wet*. 2010;66(11):784–786.

Gruen ME, Lascelles BDX, Colleran E, et al. AAHA Pain management guidelines for dogs and cats. *J Am Anim Hosp Assoc*. 2022; 58(2):55–76.

McAuliffe LR, Koch CS, Serpell J et al. Associations between atopic dermatitis and anxiety aggression, and fear-based behaviors in dogs. *J Am Anim Hosp Assoc*, 2022;58(4):161–167.

Schering Corporation. Leventa (levothyroxine sodium) [product information]. Summit, NJ, USA; 2010. Available at: https://dailymed.nlm.nih.gov/dailymed/drugInfo.cfm?setid=8fe4aef5-086a-4747-a60b-c2d0c0513285. Accessed August 18, 2022.

Siracusa C. Treatments affecting dog behaviour: something to be aware of. *Vet Rec*. 2016;179(18):460–461.

WSAVA guidelines for the assessment, recognition and treatment of pain. 2022. https://onlinelibrary.wiley.com/doi/10.1111/jsap.13566

CHAPTER 7

Physiologic stress and its effect on health and welfare

Melissa Bain, DVM, DACVB (Behavior), MS, DACAW (Welfare)

Introduction

Veterinarians strive to improve the health of their patients. Recently there has been a more concentrated effort to understand the relationship between stress, physical health, and emotional health. We have progressed beyond "is it medical OR behavioral," but instead are turning our focus to identifying all of the factors that can affect the way in which an animal acts and treat the animal as a whole.

What is stress?

Mental and physical health

One must first define health to address the relationship between mental and physical health. In the wake of World War II, the World Health Organization (WHO) stated as the first principle of its constitution that, "Health is a state of complete physical, mental and social well-being and not merely the absence of disease or infirmity."[1] Although the definition applies to humans, it seems to be a reasonable starting place for a definition of mental and physical heath for animals in general.

More recently, Broom observed that views on the concept of health differ among food animal producers, ethologists, and some veterinarians.[2] He observed that, "…for most people, health refers to the state of the body and brain in relation to the effects of pathogens, parasites, tissue damage or physiological disorder," that is, physical pathology. Studies of confined animals, however, in zoos, production facilities, and people's homes have found that the quality of the environment also can affect animal's mental and physical health.

Defining the concept of "mental health" is particularly tricky, since mental processes appear to be an emergent property of brains that cannot (yet) be measured directly but might be inferred from the behavior of animals. Just as organ functions are emergent properties of their cell biology, we perceive mental processes to be generated from and dependent upon neural activity but nonetheless separate from it.[3,4] From this perspective, mental health implies brain health, which largely results from variable contributions of genetic, epigenetic, and environmental interactions.

Animal welfare, well-being, and stress

There are many definitions used to describe welfare. A working definition is that animal welfare refers to the "state of the animal." A broader definition is the provision of animal care that encompasses all aspects of an animal's well-being, including husbandry, medical care, and opportunities to perform species-typical behaviors. Welfare can be considered poor, adequate, or good.

An identifiable framework of animal welfare is that of the "Five Freedoms," developed from the Brambell Report in response to the book *Animal Machines* by Ruth Harrison. These Five Freedoms are as follows:

- Freedom from hunger or thirst;
- Freedom from discomfort;
- Freedom from pain, injury, or disease;
- Freedom to express normal behavior; and
- Freedom from fear and distress.[5]

However, this definition can be limiting. Another approach by McMillan focuses on a balance of quality of life, recognizing that there are pleasant and unpleasant feelings in many areas, while understanding that there are individual differences.[6]

Well-being is equally difficult to define, as it stems from an individual's perspective. The National Institute of Food and Agriculture states that "animal well-being is a complex topic."[7] It is a balance between an animal's negative and positive affect, and its ability to cope and obtain its needs. It is a combination of positive and negative aspects of its welfare, quality of life, and happiness, including environmental conditions in which an animal lives.

The word "stress" means different things to different people.[8] In the context of health and welfare, we define stress to mean "effects of the (internal and external) environment on the organism." The eminent neuroendocrinologist and "stress scientist" Bruce McEwen describes three categories of stress responses: "good stress," where an individual can perceive opportunities, take risks, rise to challenges, and feel rewarded by (often) positive outcomes; "tolerable stress," where an individual can perceive threats but still has enough of a perception of control to cope with the challenges presented; and "toxic stress," which occurs when threats exceed the individual's perception of control of their environment.[9,10] When sustained, it is this level of perception of threat that is most damaging to mental and physical health.[11]

How stress and behavior affect physical and mental health

Causes of stress

Causes of mild stress responses, defined as brief in duration and mild to moderate in magnitude, can help develop stress coping skills. Mild stress responses are part of normal development when they occur in the safe, predictable environments of stable and supportive relationships. Examples of events resulting in positive stress responses in young animals include nonthreatening veterinary visits and exposure to novel environments and foods.

Moderate stress responses result from exposure to experiences that present greater threats, such as lack of stimulation/boredom or household instability, illness or injury, or exposure to a natural disaster. As with mild stress responses, when the event occurs in an otherwise safe environment, recovery to normal is likely. Thus, the essential feature that makes moderate stress response tolerable is the extent to which one's protective surroundings permit retention of

sufficient perception of control to permit adaptive coping to occur.

In the most threatening circumstances, severe stress responses can result. Toxic stress responses, strong, frequent, or prolonged, are the most dangerous to long-term health and welfare. Examples of events that can result in severe stress responses include chronic abuse, severe or chronic disease, and adverse early life events like nutritional deprivation, maternal separation, or significant maternal threat during pregnancy.[12,13]

Stress can have both physical and psychological causes. Physical stress can be caused by disease or illness, pain, exposure to temperature extremes, sleep deprivation, thirst, or hunger. Psychological stressors might include exposure to fear-evoking stimuli, social conflict, disturbing the pet when sleeping or eating, frustration, unpredictable consequences (rewards or punishment), environmental deprivation, scheduling changes, or situations leading to conflict (competing motivations).

The effects of adverse events, particularly during the vulnerable period of early life, on the long-term mental and physical health of animals demonstrate the importance of identification of risk factors and provision of effective education by the veterinary team and animal owners about appropriate environments for confined animals across the lifespan.[14-17] From this perspective, initial vaccination appointments become anything but "routine," and may in fact be the most important appointments of the animal's life, as they present opportunities to teach husbandry appropriate for the animal based on the environment in which it will be living at a time when pet parents are likely to be motivated and responsive to recommendations.

The stress response

Understanding the relationships between mental and physical health also requires consideration across levels of analysis. For animals, these include the interactions of the macroenvironment and microenvironment with the individual's genetics, epigenetics (how behavior and environment affect genetic expression), molecules, cells, circuits, physiology, and behavior.

The term stress can be defined in various ways. From the perspectives of health and disease, stress is often defined in terms of stressors, which are events in the internal and external environment that result in a stress response. We think of stressors as events that are perceived as threats to one's perception of control. From this perspective, a stressor is anything that activates the central threat response system (CTRS).[18] Stressors vary along a continuum: positive to negative; short term to long term; acute to chronic; and mild to toxic intensity. All events that activate the CTRS are not equally threatening, and a conceptual taxonomy comprises three distinct types of CTRS responses: mild (positive), moderate (tolerable), and severe (toxic). The taxonomy is based on the differences in their potential to cause enduring physiologic disruptions because of the intensity and duration of the response.

The first component of the stress response is the hypothalamic-pituitary-adrenal (HPA) axis, in which the hypothalamus releases corticotropin-releasing hormone, which stimulates the release of adrenocorticotropic hormone. The second component is the sympathetic–adrenal–medullary system, which releases norepinephrine (noradrenaline) and epinephrine (adrenaline). Norepinephrine is associated with sensitization and fear conditioning (see Figure 7.1).

In cats, transient hyperglycemia may occur with stress. If stress is persistent or chronic, there is continued stimulation of the HPA axis and an increase in cortisol with depression of the catecholamine system, leading to alterations in the immune system and possible development of stress-related diseases.[19] There are many papers documenting physiological responses to stress in dogs.[20] Oxytocin and vasopressin have also been implicated in stress responses, and correlate to behavioral responses in dogs.[21–25] In one study, levels of salivary arginine vasopressin, a mediator of the HPA axis, were decreased in dogs after noise and environmental stimulation in the more stressed group but not in the less stressed group.[26]

A recent study found higher plasma levels of dopamine and serotonin in pets with stress compared to controls.[27] Increases in dopamine may enhance aggressive behavior and lead to an increase in stereotypic and grooming behaviors. Elevated prolactin levels were found in dogs with chronic stress, stereotypic behaviors, fear aggression, and autonomic signs, while lower levels of prolactin were associated with acute fearful and phobic events.[28,29] Therefore, there can be marked differences in the way that acute and chronic stress affects health and behavior.[28,30]

While it is common to consider the effects of disease on behavior, acute and chronic stress can also have an impact on both health and behavior.[31] Stress is an altered state of homeostasis which can be caused by physical or emotional factors. This results in psychological, behavioral, endocrine, and immune effects that are designed to help cope with stress.[27] Response to stress will vary between individuals and may be affected by breed, early experience, sex, age, health, and the pet's behavioral profile. In dogs and cats, exposure to mild stressors and handling early in life stimulates hormonal, adrenal, and pituitary systems that result in animals that perform better in problem-solving tasks, have greater resistance to disease, and can better withstand stress later in life.[32] Thus, not only can health affect behavior, but behavior can affect health. Improving or resolving any underlying stress and anxiety can be essential to the health and welfare of the pet and the strength of the pet–pet parent bond.

A summary of signs displayed by animals in stress-inducing situations can be found in Table 7.1.

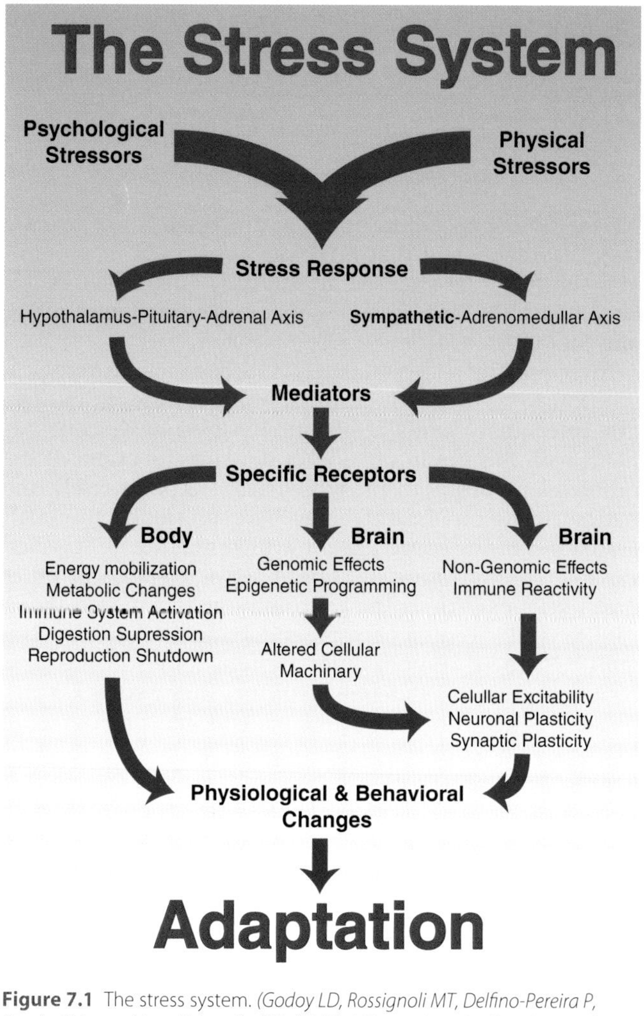

Stress and physical health

In humans, there are correlations between stress and poor health, poor immune function, cardiovascular disease, skin disease, asthma, gastrointestinal disorders, and cellular aging. Similarly, in pets, stress may alter immune function and has been shown to be a contributing or aggravating factor in gastrointestinal diseases, dermatologic conditions, respiratory and cardiac conditions, behavioral disorders, and a shortened lifespan.[33] In one study, behaviors associated with illness, including disorders of the gastrointestinal and urinary tract, skin, other sickness behaviors, and problem behaviors including avoidance, periuria, and perichezia, were associated with environmental stressors in a colony of cats.[34] Lymphopenia and changes in neutrophil:lymphocyte ratios were seen in cats diagnosed with feline interstitial cystitis (FIC).[35] See Chapter 6 for a discussion of how diseases of each body system can cause behavioral signs.

Urinary tract and stress

Abnormal signs referable to the lower urinary tracts (LUTs) of domestic cats include variable combinations of increased voiding urgency and frequency, decreased volume, blood in the urine, and urination outside the litterbox. Although there are many possible causes of these signs, the most common causes include: "idiopathic cystitis," a stone, or a urinary tract infection (usually in older cats with upper tract disease). In addition to infection and inflammation, stress responses also can activate the lower urinary tract, although some of the fundamental neural mechanisms and pathways linking psychosocial stress to altered behaviors and physiological disorders are still unclear. Holstege has pointed out that micturition plays a much more important role in the context of the survival of individuals and species in most mammals than it does in humans.[36] For most mammals, urine also signals important

Figure 7.1 The stress system. (*Godoy LD, Rossignoli MT, Delfino-Pereira P, Garcia-Cairasco N, and Umeoka EHL (2018) A Comprehensive Overview on Stress Neurobiology: Basic Concepts and Clinical Implications. Front. Behav. Neurosci. 12:127. doi: 10.3389/fnbeh.2018.00127*)

Table 7.1 Physiological and behavioral signs displayed by animals in stress-inducing situations

Category	Nonthreatened	Threatened
Physiological	Normal temperature	Elevated temperature
	Normal heart rate	Elevated heart rate
	Normal blood pressure	Elevated blood pressure
	Normal respiratory rate	Elevated respiratory rate
	Normal pupil diameter	Dilated pupils
		Flushing
		"Sweaty" paws
		Excessive shedding
Behavioral	Affiliative behaviors – purring, rubbing, etc.	Attempts to flee
	Appetitive lip licking	Apprehensive lip licking
	Interest in eating and drinking	Decreased or absent eating or drinking
	Normal eliminations	Decreased or absent eliminations for longer than 48 hours
	Approach behaviors	Defensive aggression (hissing, growling, spitting, tail twitching, ear flicking, scratching, biting)
	Relaxed postures	Trembling, vigilance
	Slow eye blinks	Freezing, hiding, or other fearful postures
		Averting gaze or other displacement behaviors increased vocalization or marking, altered grooming, or sleep
Sickness behaviors	Absent	Present

messages such as the demarcation of territory of a specific individual[37] and estrus.[38] These urine functions demonstrate that voiding can occur for reasons other than to empty a full bladder, including the contexts of perception of threat and reproduction. Micturition responses in these situations require and imply supraspinal control of micturition.[36]

Part of the interest in feline stress biology arose from studies of cats with severe recurrent chronic LUTs. Lower urinary tract signs have long been recognized in domestic cats, being described as "very common" in Kirk's 1925 veterinary textbook.[39] Clinicians historically interpreted signs referable to the LUT to suggest an external (e.g., infectious agent, urinary stone) or structural disorder of the LUT (e.g., stricture or incontinence), although environmental conditions were recognized as a risk factor by Kirk in 1925 and subsequently confirmed to be relevant by other investigators.[40,41]

In 1996, Osborne et al. summarized the literature on feline LUTs, identifying some 30 distinct causes of LUTs.[42] That so many potential causes result in similar LUTs demonstrates that the signs in themselves only represent the limited repertoire available to the LUT to respond to any insult. During this time, a syndrome described as "FIC" also was being studied.[43] These studies found that additional problems outside the lower urinary tract were commonly present in these cats and could be mitigated by multimodal environmental modification (MEMO).[44] Subsequent research has revealed the complex nature of this condition. For example, some cats with severe chronic LUTs seem to

have a functional, rather than a structural, lower urinary tract disorder,[45] and that LUTs can occur even in presumably healthy cats exposed to stressful circumstances.[34,46] See Chapter 24 for further discussion of feline housesoiling and MEMO.

These findings suggest that terms such as "feline urological syndrome,"[47] "feline lower urinary tract disease,"[48] and "feline interstitial cystitis"[43] historically used to describe patients with this syndrome do not describe the extent of the problems occurring in many afflicted cats. Conversely, the narrow focus on the LUT may have precluded thorough evaluation of the entire patient, which might have revealed variable combinations of clinical signs referable to other organ systems such as the gastrointestinal tract, skin, lung, cardiovascular, central nervous, endocrine, and immune systems.[44,49] These comorbidities include some of the most common problems in feline medicine. They also lack a predictable pattern of onset across patients and often precede the appearance of LUTs. This situation is similar in human beings with "central sensitivity syndromes," suggesting that individual patterns of comorbidities may represent an amplification of underlying familial sensitivities.[50,51] One must also consider other comorbidities for cats that are inappropriately eliminating, including renal insufficiency.[52]

Gastrointestinal and ingestive disorders and stress

Stress and anxiety in humans can alter bacterial flora, inhibit gastric emptying, increase colonic activity, and increase intestinal permeability, leading to irritable bowel syndrome, inflammatory bowel disease, gastrointestinal reflux, stress-induced hypersensitivity, and heartburn.[53] More investigation is being done into how the gut–brain connection relates to behavior and using this connection for therapeutic intervention.[54-56]

In pets, acute fear and anxiety can lead to a decrease in appetite or anorexia, diarrhea, vomiting, or colitis. With chronic anxiety, such as during a move, when a new pet is introduced into the home, or with the loss of a human or pet in the family, there may be more profound effects on behavior and health. In a pilot study, dogs with inflammatory bowel disease appeared to be more anxious when exposed to novel stimuli, indicating a possible relationship between gastrointestinal disorders and the dogs' response to stressors.[57] However, studies of racing sled dogs have shown limited correlation between the stress of racing and gastritis.[58,59]

Stress also appears to be a risk factor for coprophagia in some dogs.[60] In addition, stress associated with unexpected environmental events in colony cats had increased risks for decreased food intake and no elimination for 24 hours, as well as elimination outside of the litterbox.[34] In cats, prolonged anorexia can have serious hepatic consequences. Pica, polyphagia, and polydipsia may also be stress induced. As with all interactions between physiological and psychological symptoms, one should not forget to investigate underlying medical conditions. In one study of dogs presenting for excessive licking, the majority of them had an underlying physiological reason for this behavior.[61]

Dermatologic signs and stress

Although stress leads to an immune response intended to enhance defense mechanisms, in some individuals, rather than helping to achieve homeostasis, these stressors may contribute to inflammatory dermatoses.[62,63] This brain–skin connection is comprised of psycho-neuro-endocrino-immunological factors which, under situations of stress, may play a role in the pathogenesis of dermatoses such as atopic dermatitis, psoriasis, and urticaria.[64,65] In humans with atopic disease, stress has been shown to increase levels of immunoglobulin E and eosinophils, causing an overreactive sympathetic adrenomedullary system and a decrease in HPA responsiveness.[66-69] Stress may also lead to increased release of vasoactive neuropeptides from dermal nerve endings that may contribute to atopic disease, psoriasis, and other chronic skin diseases.[70-73] In addition, an association between asthma and atopy has been demonstrated in humans.[74] A link has also been established between stress and increased epidermal permeability.[75] Skin barrier permeability may be further altered by cortisol release.[64,76,77] A similar alteration in skin barrier function and an increase of epidermal permeability in pets might exacerbate atopic disease in a genetically predisposed individual. Finally, skin disease itself can affect quality of life and lead to further stress. Stress intervention in humans can improve both well-being as well as cutaneous manifestations.[77,78] Self-traumatic disorders in humans may fall into the obsessive-compulsive spectrum such as the impulse control disorders trichotillomania, skin picking and nail biting; compulsive washing and grooming; or psychiatric disorders leading to psychogenic excoriation.

In dogs and cats, there is a similar interplay between the brain and skin.[79] Although self-traumatic disorders may not be caused by psychiatric disease but instead underlying pain or pruritus, they may have a psycho-neuro-immuno-endocrinological component, may be a primary behavior disorder, or may be a cutaneous sensory disorder.[80] An increased severity and frequency of skin disorders in dogs with nonsocial fear and separation-related disorders have been identified.[33] In one study of dogs with recurrent pyoderma, psychogenic factors were identified and successfully treated.[81] While there may not be a confirmed association between pruritus and aggressive, anxious, or fearful behavior in dogs, concurrent behavioral abnormalities cannot be assumed to result from dermatoses and be expected to resolve with treatment of the skin disease alone; treatment of both conditions is needed.[82]

Psychodermatoses have also been reported in dogs and cats, where the onset of pruritic behavior was associated with emotionally unstable events. In those studies, all skin and behavior problems were improved with behavioral therapy.[83,84] Primary behavior disorders of the skin might include compulsive disorders, displacement behaviors, reinforced behaviors, and possibly psychotic disorders. However, since medical problems can incite self-traumatic behavior, can be a component of psychodermatoses, or can develop secondary to a behavioral cause (e.g., deep pyoderma), they must first be diagnosed and treated.[85,86] Drug therapy with fluoxetine or clomipramine can dramatically improve compulsive disorders, with a 50% or greater improvement expected.[86-88] See Chapter 18 for a more detailed description of compulsive disorders and their treatment. One must not ignore primary medical conditions that could present as a problem behavior, such for cats with so-called "psychogenic alopecia" and dogs with acral lick dermatitis.[89,90]

Stress and aging

Aging is the sum of the deleterious effects of time upon the cellular function, microanatomy, and physiology of each body system. With age, there is a general deterioration in physical condition, tissue hypoxia, alterations in cell membranes, increased production and decreased clearance of reactive oxygen species, a decline in organ function, sensory function, and mental function, and a gradual deterioration of the immune system. Studies in multiple species have found that adverse early life experiences and other stressors can also result in accelerated telomere shortening.[16,91-95] With increasing age, along with additive effects of diet and environment, there is an increase in reactive oxygen species, leading to oxidative damage to organ tissues, including the brain.[96,97] These changes reduce the pet's ability to respond to stress and maintain homeostatic balance, thus resulting in increased susceptibility to tumors, disease, and behavior problems. Senior pets may be less able to cope with environmental, schedule, and social changes. See Chapter 8 for details.

Direct effects of behavior on health

Another important consideration with respect to the effects of behaviors on health is that of pets that engage in potentially dangerous or self-injurious activities. With extreme fear, anxiety, and phobic behaviors, pets' attempts to avoid the stimulus or situation or escape from confinement may result in property damage as well as the pets being seriously injured during these attempts. Foreign body ingestion, poisoning, or accidental electrocution can be a result of exploration and scavenging (e.g., stealing, garbage raiding) or picas (see Chapter 13). In addition, self-traumatic disorders ranging from hair loss to tail mutilation may also be a result of primary behavior problems (see Chapter 18). And, of course, without adequate confinement or supervision, pets roaming the streets could be seriously injured or killed by cars, predators, and fights with other animals, or from the gunshots of property owners who might have been protecting their homes or livestock.

Stress and behavioral health

Behaviors often associated with poor mental health include aggression, withdrawal, hiding, and sickness behaviors, whereas those often associated with good mental health include play, exploration, and the like, the specifics of which may depend on the animal's species and environmental context. Although behaviors may appear maladaptive when they develop secondary to a physical condition, one must be careful to avoid thinking of all behaviors associated with poor health or welfare as inappropriate, maladaptive, or malfunctional. Responses to conflict and frustration might include aggression or avoidance (to distance the pet from the source of conflict), urine marking, redirected aggression, depression or apathy, or displacement behaviors, such as self-trauma, spinning, tail chasing, or hyperesthesia, might be exhibited. Displacement behaviors might be more likely to arise in pets that are overly anxious or reactive and those that are genetically predisposed. In addition, genetics will likely contribute to the specific signs that the pet is most likely to display. For example, sucking disorders have been shown to have an inherited susceptibility in Doberman Pinschers, tail chasing and spinning are more commonly associated with German Shepherd Dogs and Bull Terriers, and Siamese and Birman cats have a greater susceptibility to wool sucking.[98-102] Recurrent or ongoing stress along with genetic susceptibility likely contributes to the development of compulsive disorders (Chapter 18).

Adaptive sickness behaviors that contribute to greater well-being by increasing insulating ability and water conservation, and decreasing heat loss and energy expenditure, include piloerection and lack of grooming. The increase in metabolic energy expenditure during a febrile episode can be made up later, after the inappetence due to lack of desire to hunt or forage for food that occurs during this episode has subsided, which may have served to protect the animal from predation.[103,104]

Chronic anxiety and stress can contribute to behavioral disorders in humans, including panic disorders, separation-related disorders, social and other phobias, obsessive-compulsive disorders, generalized anxiety disorders, post-traumatic stress disorders, impulse control disorders, and sleep disorders, all of which may have animal correlates.[105,106] In one study, unexpected stressful environmental events led to an increase in avoidance behaviors and elimination of both urine and stools outside the litterbox in a group of colony cats.[34]

In situations of conflict (competing motivations) and frustration (where the pet is unable to achieve its goals), or when the behavioral needs of the pet are not addressed, the pet may be unable to find appropriate mechanisms to cope. Displacement behaviors, those behavioral responses to an external stimulus, such as a sound, confinement, or aggression that are performed out of context in response to the trigger, that arise in response to a specific stimulus (e.g., visual, auditory, odor, tactile) or event (e.g., car ride, veterinary visit, pet parent departure or homecoming) might be resolved if inciting factors are avoided and pet parent responses are consistent and predictable.[107-110] However, secondary problems (e.g., pain, pruritus, infection) may be perpetuating factors.

When displacement behaviors begin to be exhibited outside the original context and begin to interfere with normal daily activities and function, they may fall under the obsessive-compulsive spectrum,[87,111] but not all repetitive behaviors can be considered "compulsive."[112] Compulsive disorders generally have some degree of dyscontrol in their initiation or termination of the behavior. Signs are often repetitive, exaggerated, sustained, or so intense that they are difficult to interrupt. A behavior might be considered compulsive when it does not provide a mechanism for the pet to settle (achieve behavioral homeostasis) and the signs persist even after the anxiety-evoking situation is resolved. Compulsive disorders in pets might include: (1) neurological and locomotory signs such as air snapping and spinning; (2) ingestive signs such as picas, licking, and wool sucking in cats; or (3) self-directed behaviors such as acral lick dermatitis and flank sucking in dogs, psychogenic alopecia, and tail chasing in cats. Since self-traumatic disorders often develop secondary medical complications, concurrent medical and behavioral therapy is often required.[84,113] Abnormal serotonin transmission may be the primary mechanism by which stereotypies are induced.[86] Opioid involvement, dopaminergic stimulation, and altered glutaminergic neurotransmission may also play a role. For details on the diagnosis and treatment of compulsive disorders, see Chapter 18.

Stress management

Animals need environments that are compatible with their physical and behavioral needs to enjoy mental and physical health. Provision of effective environmental enrichment is built on the foundation of the Five Freedoms of Animal Welfare, mentioned earlier in this text. These have now been extended and updated.[114,115] Not only must we think about the effects of the physical environment on an animal's behavior, but there is evidence of the effects of human behavior and even chemosignals on animal behavior.[116-121]

A program to reduce stress and maintain quality of life should optimize pleasant feelings and minimize unpleasant ones.[122] Since stress can play an important role in the development of both medical and behavior problems, and both medical and behavior problems may further add to the pet's stress, close attention to identifying and resolving stress should be one of the first considerations in the treatment (and prevention) of behavior problems.

A behavioral program to ensure maximal quality of life should include social companionship, mental and physical enrichment, identifying and reducing stressors, and providing the pet with control. Pets can best handle stress if they have a sense of control, including appropriate opportunities to avoid unpleasant situations. Pets should also have control over their environment by being offered opportunities to engage in their normal repertoire of behaviors and by allowing them to make choices (e.g., climbing, perching, bedding, play) that are acceptable to the pet and to the pet parent. The focus should be on encouraging and reinforcing what is desirable and preventing or avoiding what is unacceptable. If consequences are consistent and predictable, desirable behaviors can be increased with reinforcers and undesirable behaviors can be reduced. Since positive punishment is likely to increase fear and anxiety, it should not be utilized. See Chapter 10 for details.

Prevention and treatment should focus on consistency, gradual change, and enrichment in the form of: (1) safe social interactions; (2) physical activity; (3) object and exploratory play that is motivating to each of the senses (sight, smell, texture, taste); and (4) activities that are designed to meet the needs of the species and individual (e.g., climbing, predatory play toys, and perches for cats, and chewing, retrieving, or herding activities for dogs).[123] Often this is termed "environmental enrichment." We define environmental enrichment as provision of resources that effectively improve the animal's mental and physical health. Environmental enrichment is a relatively new concept but is based on the ancient art of animal husbandry. There are many research studies that have evaluated the effects of enrichment programs on the behavior and welfare of animals.[124–126] As shown in Figure 7.2, a total of 1930 papers on EE were published from 1967 through 2018, the majority after 2000.

Effective enrichment that addresses the needs of an animal has been found to decrease sickness behaviors in confined domestic cats, to improve mental and physical health in a variety of species, and to normalize behavioral and physiological parameters associated with markers of stress.[127–132]

Pet parents should focus on minimizing or avoiding environmental events that might incite stress, such as loud or unfamiliar noises, sudden or unexpected movements, novel or unfamiliar places and objects, interactions with unfamiliar

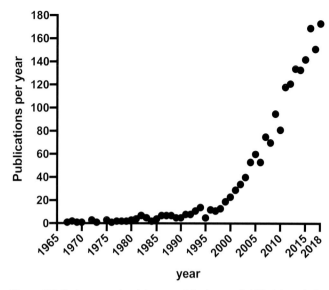

Figure 7.2 Environmental enrichment publications on PubMed. A total of 2298 papers on the topic were published from 1967 through 2020.

animals or pets, and sudden or dramatic changes in routine. The response of an individual to stress may vary with genetics, early handling, socialization, and previous experience. When changes are likely to be stressful for individual pets, they should be made gradually whenever possible. While some degree of novelty is generally appealing, maintaining familiarity and making changes slowly are particularly important for pets that might be more sensitive to change. Positive outcomes can help the animal to adapt more quickly to a new situation.

Conclusion

Over the past number of years, more interest has been paid to identifying and alleviating stress in animals. Problem behaviors are often linked to or exacerbated by stressful situations, and the focus is morphing from purely treating the animal to working on ways to manage their environments so that external stressors are less likely to affect animals and treatment plans are more effective.

References

1. *World Health Organization Constitution.* <https://www.who.int/about/who-we-are/constitution/>; Accessed November 9, 2020.
2. Broom DM. Behaviour and welfare in relation to pathology. *Appl Anim Behav Sci.* 2006;97:73–83.
3. Anderson NB. Levels of analysis in health science. A framework for integrating sociobehavioral and biomedical research. *Ann N Y Acad Sci.* 1998;840:563–576.
4. Voneida TJ. Sperry's concept of mind as an emergent property of brain function and its implications for the future of humankind. *Neuropsychologia.* 1998;36:1077–1082.
5. *Council FAW.* Five Freedoms. <https://webarchive.nationalarchives.gov.uk/20121010012427/http://www.fawc.org.uk/freedoms.htm/>; 2012; Accessed November 11, 2020.
6. McMillan FD. Development of a mental wellness program for animals. *J Am Vet Med Assoc.* 2002;220:965–972.
7. *United States Department of Agriculture NIoFaA.* Animal Well-Being. <https://nifa.usda.gov/program/animal-well-being/>; Accessed November 9, 2020.
8. Del Giudice M, Buck CL, Chaby LE, et al. What is stress? A systems perspective. *Integr Comp Biol.* 2018;58:1019–1032.
9. McEwen B. *When is Stress Good for You?* <https://aeon.co/essays/how-stress-works-in-the-human-body-to-make-or-break-us/>; Accessed November 9, 2020.
10. McEwen BS. Neurobiological and systemic effects of chronic stress. *Chronic Stress.* 2017;1:2470547017692328.
11. Shonkoff JP, Boyce W, Cameron J, et al. Excessive stress disrupts the architecture of the developing brain. National Scientific Council on the Developing Child, Working Paper 2005;3:2014.
12. Guzman DB, Howell B, Sanchez M. Early life stress and development: preclinical science. In: Bremner JD, ed. *Posttraumatic*

Stress Disorder. Hoboken, NJ: John Wiley & Sons, Inc; 2016;61–80.

13. Bouret S, Levin BE, Ozanne SE. Gene-environment interactions controlling energy and glucose homeostasis and the developmental origins of obesity. *Physiol Rev*. 2015;95:47–82.

14. Dietz L, Arnold A-MK, Goerlich-Jansson VC, et al. The importance of early life experiences for the development of behavioural disorders in domestic dogs. *Behaviour* 2018;155:83–114.

15. Nishi M, Horii-Hayashi N, Sasagawa T. Effects of early life adverse experiences on the brain: implications from maternal separation models in rodents. *Front Neurosci*. 2014;8:166.

16. Price LH, Kao H-T, Burgers DE, et al. Telomeres and early-life stress: an overview. *Biol Psychiatry*. 2013;73:15–23.

17. Wilsson E. Nature and nurture-how different conditions affect the behavior of dogs. *J Vet Behav*. 2016;16:45–52.

18. Elman I, Borsook D. Threat response system: parallel brain processes in pain vis-a-vis fear and anxiety. *Front Psychiatry*. 2018;9:29.

19. Dhabhar FS. Effects of stress on immune function: the good, the bad, and the beautiful. *Immunol Res*. 2014;58:193–210.

20. Hydbring-Sandberg E, von Walter LW, Hoglund K, et al. Physiological reactions to fear provocation in dogs. *J Endocrinol*. 2004;180:439–448.

21. MacLean EL, Gesquiere LR, Gee N, et al. Validation of salivary oxytocin and vasopressin as biomarkers in domestic dogs. *J Neurosci Methods*. 2018;293:67–76.

22. MacLean EL, Gesquiere LR, Gruen ME, et al. Endogenous oxytocin, vasopressin, and aggression in domestic dogs. *Front Psychol*. 2017;8:1613.

23. Petersson M, Uvnäs-Moberg K, Nilsson A, et al. Oxytocin and cortisol levels in dog owners and their dogs are associated with behavioral patterns: an exploratory study. *Front Psychol*. 2017;8:1796.

24. Pirrone F, Pierantoni L, Bossetti A, et al. Salivary vasopressin as a potential non-invasive biomarker of anxiety in dogs diagnosed with separation-related problems. *Animals*. 2019;9:1033.

25. Srithunyarat T, Hagman R, Höglund O, et al. Catestatin, vasostatin, cortisol, and visual analog scale scoring for stress assessment in healthy dogs. *Res Vet Sci*. 2018;117:74–80.

26. Jeong Y-K, Oh Y-I, Song K-H, et al. Evaluation of salivary vasopressin as an acute stress biomarker in healthy dogs with stress due to noise and environmental challenges. *BMC Vet Res*. 2020;16:331.

27. Riva J, Bondiolotti G, Michelazzi M, et al. Anxiety related behavioural disorders and neurotransmitters in dogs. *Appl Anim Behav Sci*. 2008;114:168–181.

28. Pageat P, Lafont C, Falewee C, et al. An evaluation of serum prolactin in anxious dogs and response to treatment with selegiline or fluoxetine. *Appl Anim Behav Sci*. 2007;105:342–350.

29. Siracusa C, Manteca X, Cuenca R, et al. Effect of a synthetic appeasing pheromone on behavioral, neuroendocrine, immune, and acute-phase perioperative stress responses in dogs. *J Am Vet Med Assoc*. 2010;237:673–681.

30. Beerda B, Schilder MB, van Hooff JA, et al. Manifestations of chronic and acute stress in dogs. *Appl Anim Behav Sci*. 1997;52:307–319.

31. Berteselli G, Servida F, Dall'Ara P, et al. Evaluation of immunological, stress and behavioural parameters in dogs (*Canis familiaris*) with anxiety-related disorders. *Curr Issues Res Vet Behav Med*. 2005:18–22.

32. Battaglia CL. Periods of early development and the effects of stimulation and social experiences in the canine. *J Vet Behav*. 2009;4:203–210.

33. Dreschel N. Anxiety, fear, disease, and lifespan in domestic dogs. *J Vet Behav: Clin Appl Res*. 2009;6:249–250.

34. Stella JL, Lord LK, Buffington CT. Sickness behaviors in response to unusual external events in healthy cats and cats with feline interstitial cystitis. *J Am Vet Med Assoc*. 2011;238:67–73.

35. Stella J, Croney C, Buffington T. Effects of stressors on the behavior and physiology of domestic cats. *Appl Anim Behav Sci*. 2013;143:157–163.

36. Holstege E. Micturition and the soul. *J Comp Neurol*. 2005;493:15–20.

37. Pryor PA, Hart BL, Bain MJ, et al. Causes of urine marking in cats and effects of environmental management on frequency of marking. *J Am Vet Med Assoc*. 2001;219:1709–1713.

38. Hart BL. Facilitation by estrogen of sexual reflexes in female cats. *Physiol Behav*. 1971;7:675–678.

39. Kirk H. Retention of urine and urine deposits. In: Kirk H, ed. *The Diseases of the Cat and its General Management*. London: Bailliere, Tindall and Cox; 1925;261–267.

40. Caston HT. Stress and the feline urological syndrome. *Feline Pract*. 1973;3:14–22.

41. Stella JL, Lord LK, Buffington CA. Sickness behaviors in response to unusual external events in healthy cats and cats with feline interstitial cystitis. *J Am Vet Med Assoc*. 2011;238:67–73.

42. Osborne CA, Kruger JM, Lulich JP. Feline lower urinary tract disorders. Definition of terms and concepts. *Vet Clin N Am - Small Anim Pract*. 1996;26:169–179.

43. Buffington CAT, Chew DJ, Woodworth BE. Feline interstitial cystitis. *J Am Vet Med Assoc*. 1999;215:682–687.

44. Buffington CT, Westropp JL, Chew DJ, et al. Clinical evaluation of multimodal environmental modification (MEMO) in the management of cats with idiopathic cystitis. *J Feline Med Surg*. 2006;8:261–268.

45. Buffington CA. Idiopathic cystitis in domestic cats-beyond the lower urinary tract. *J Vet Intern Med*. 2011;25:784–796.

46. Westropp JL, Kass PH, Buffington C. Evaluation of the effects of stress in cats with idiopathic cystitis. *Am J Vet Res*. 2006;67:731–736.

47. Osbaldiston G, Taussig R. Clinical report on 46 cases of feline urological syndrome. *Vet Med Small Anim Clin*. 1970;65:461.

48. Osborne CA, Johnston GR, Polzin DJ, et al. Redefinition of the feline urologic syndrome: feline lower urinary tract disease with heterogeneous causes. *Vet Clin N Am: Small Anim Pract*. 1984;14(3):409–438.

49. Buffington CT, Westropp JL, Chew DJ, et al. Risk factors associated with clinical signs of lower urinary tract disease in indoor-housed cats. *J Am Vet Med Assoc*. 2006;228:722–725.

50. Buffington CA. Developmental influences on medically unexplained symptoms. *Psychother Psychosom*. 2009;78:139–144.

51. Yunus MB. Editorial review (thematic issue: an update on central sensitivity syndromes and the issues of nosology and psychobiology). *Curr Rheumatol Rev*. 2015;11:70–85.

52. Ramos D, Reche-Junior A, Mills DS, et al. A closer look at the health of cats showing urinary house-soiling (periuria): a case-control study. *J Feline Med Surg*. 2019;21:772–779.

53. Bhatia V, Tandon RK. Stress and the gastrointestinal tract. *J Gastroenterol Hepatol*. 2005;20:332–339.

54. Gambaro E, Gramaglia C, Baldon G, et al. "Gut–brain axis": review of the role of the probiotics in anxiety and depressive disorders. *Brain Behav*. 2020;10:e01803.

55. Konturek PC, Brzozowski T, Konturek S. Stress and the gut: pathophysiology, clinical consequences, diagnostic approach and treatment options. *J Physiol Pharmacol*. 2011;62:591–599.

56. O'Mahony SM, Clarke G, Borre Y, et al. Serotonin, tryptophan metabolism and the brain-gut-microbiome axis. *Behav Brain Res*. 2015;277:32–48.

57. Monte F, Basse C, Lynch A. Stress as a factor in inflammatory bowel disease; pilot study to investigate whether affected dogs differ from unaffected controls in their response to novel stimuli. In: *Proceedings of the European Veterinary Behavioral Meeting*. 2010:46–49.

58. Fergestad ME, Jahr TH, Krontveit RI, et al. Serum concentration of gastrin, cortisol and C-reactive protein in a group of Norwegian sled dogs during training and after endurance racing: a prospective cohort study. *Acta Vet Scand*. 2016;58:24.

59. Royer CM, Willard M, Williamson K, et al. Exercise stress, intestinal permeability and gastric ulceration in racing Alaskan sled dogs. *Comp Exerc Physiol*. 2005;2:53.

60. Hart BL, Hart LA, Thigpen AP, et al. The paradox of canine conspecific coprophagy. *Vet Med Sci*. 2018;4:106–114.

61. Bécuwe-Bonnet V, Bélanger M-C, Frank D, et al. Gastrointestinal disorders in dogs with excessive licking of surfaces. *J Vet Behav*. 2012;7:194–204.

62. Joachim RA, Handjiski B, Blois SM, et al. Stress-induced neurogenic inflammation in murine skin skews dendritic cells towards maturation and migration: key role of intercellular adhesion molecule-1/leukocyte function-associated antigen interactions. *Am J Pathol.* 2008;173:1379–1388.

63. Liezmann C, Klapp B, Peters E. Stress, atopy and allergy: a re-evaluation from a psychoneuroimmunologic persepective. *Dermatoendocrinol.* 2011;3:37–40.

64. Arndt J, Smith N, Tausk F. Stress and atopic dermatitis. *Curr Allergy Asthma Rep.* 2008;8:312–317.

65. Panconesi E, Hautmann G. Psychophysiology of stress in dermatology: the psychobiologic pattern of psychosomatics. *Dermatol Clin.* 1996;14:399–422.

66. Buske-Kirschbaum A, Geiben A, Höllig H, et al. Altered responsiveness of the hypothalamus-pituitary-adrenal axis and the sympathetic adrenomedullary system to stress in patients with atopic dermatitis. *J Clin Endocrinol Metab.* 2002;87:4245–4251.

67. Buske-Kirschbaum A, Gierens A, Höllig H, et al. Stress-induced immunomodulation is altered in patients with atopic dermatitis. *J Neuroimmunol.* 2002;129:161–167.

68. Buske-Kirschbaum A, Hellhammer DH. Endocrine and immune responses to stress in chronic inflammatory skin disorders. *Ann N Y Acad Sci.* 2003;992:231–240.

69. Dickerson SS, Kemeny ME. Acute stressors and cortisol responses: a theoretical integration and synthesis of laboratory research. *Psychol Bull.* 2004;130:355.

70. Hall JMF, Cruser d, Podawiltz A, et al. Psychological stress and the cutaneous immune response: roles of the HPA axis and the sympathetic nervous system in atopic dermatitis and psoriasis. *Dermatol Res Pract.* 2012;2012:403908.

71. Pasaoglu G, Bavbek S, Tugcu H, et al. Psychological status of patients with chronic urticaria. *J Dermatol.* 2006;33:765–771.

72. Saraceno R, Kleyn CE, Terenghi G, et al. The role of neuropeptides in psoriasis. *Br J Dermatol.* 2006;155:876–882.

73. Schmid-Ott G, Jaeger B, Boehm T, et al. Immunological effects of stress in psoriasis. *Br J Dermatol.* 2009;160:782–785.

74. Barone S, Bacon SL, Campbell TS, et al. The association between anxiety sensitivity and atopy in adult asthmatics. *J Behav Med.* 2008;31:331–339.

75. Garg A, Chren M-M, Sands LP, et al. Psychological stress perturbs epidermal permeability barrier homeostasis: Implications for the pathogenesis of stress-associated skin disorders. *Arch Dermatol.* 2001;137:53–59.

76. Mitschenko A, Lwow A, Kupfer J, et al. Atopic dermatitis and stress? How do emotions come into skin? *Hautarzt.* 2008;59:314–318.

77. Denda M, Tsuchiya T, Elias PM, et al. Stress alters cutaneous permeability barrier homeostasis. *Am J Physiol-Regul Integr Comp Physiol.* 2000;278:R367–R372.

78. Ersser SJ, Cowdell F, Latter S, et al. Psychological and educational interventions for atopic eczema in children. *Cochrane Database Syst Rev.* 2014:1–51.

79. Harvey ND, Craigon PJ, Shaw SC, et al. Behavioural differences in dogs with atopic dermatitis suggest stress could be a significant problem associated with chronic pruritus. *Animals.* 2019;9:813.

80. Virga V. Behavioral dermatology. *Vet Clin N Am - Small Anim Pract.* 2003;33:231.

81. Nagata M, Shibata K. Importance of psychogenic factors in canine recurrent pyoderma. *Vet Dermatol.* 2004;15(s1):42.

82. Klinck MP, Shofer FS, Reisner IR. Association of pruritus with anxiety or aggression in dogs. *J Am Vet Med Assoc.* 2008;233:1105–1111.

83. Nagata M, Shibata K, Irimajiri M, et al. Importance of psychogenic dermatoses in dogs with pruritic behavior. *Vet Dermatol.* 2002;13:211–229.

84. Titeux E, Gilbert C, Amaury B et al. From Feline Idiopathic Ulcerative Dermatitis to Feline Behavioral Ulcerative Dermatitis: Grooming Repetitive Behaviors Indicators of Poor Welfare in Cats. *Front Vet Sci.* 2018;5:81

85. Shumaker A, Angus J, Coyner K, et al. Microbiological and histopathological features of canine acral lick dermatitis. *Vet Dermatol.* 2008;19:288–298.

86. Irimajiri M, Luescher AU, Douglass G, et al. Randomized, controlled clinical trial of the efficacy of fluoxetine for treatment of compulsive disorders in dogs. *J Am Vet Med Assoc.* 2009;235:705–709.

87. Overall KL, Dunham AE. Clinical features and outcome in dogs and cats with obsessive-compulsive disorder: 126 cases (1989–2000). *J Am Vet Med Assoc.* 2002;221:1445–1452.

88. Yalcin E. Comparison of clomipramine and fluoxetine treatment of dogs with tail chasing. *Tierärztl Prax Kleintiere.* 2010;2010:295–299.

89. Waisglass SE, Landsberg GM, Yager JA, et al. Underlying medical conditions in cats with presumptive psychogenic alopecia. *J Am Vet Med Assoc.* 2006;228:1705–1709.

90. Denerolle P, White SD, Taylor TS, et al. Organic diseases mimicking acral lick dermatitis in six dogs. *J Am Anim Hosp Assoc.* 2007;43:215–220.

91. Chatelain M, Drobniak SM, Szulkin M. The association between stressors and telomeres in non-human vertebrates: a meta-analysis. *Ecol Lett.* 2020;23:381–398.

92. Cram DL, Monaghan P, Gillespie R, et al. Effects of early-life competition and maternal nutrition on telomere lengths in wild meerkats. *Proc R Soc B: Biol Sci.* 2017;284:20171383.

93. Gil D, Alfonso-Iñiguez S, Pérez-Rodríguez L, et al. Harsh conditions during early development influence telomere length in an altricial passerine: links with oxidative stress and corticosteroids. *J Evol Biol.* 2019;32:111–125.

94. Nettle D, Andrews C, Reichert S, et al. Early-life adversity accelerates cellular ageing and affects adult inflammation: experimental evidence from the European starling. *Sci Rep.* 2017;7:1–10.

95. Xavier G, Spindola LM, Ota VK, et al. Effect of male-specific childhood trauma on telomere length. *J Psychiatr Res.* 2018;107:104–109.

96. Cotman CW, Head E. The canine (dog) model of human aging and disease: dietary, environmental and immunotherapy approaches. *J Alzheimer's Dis.* 2008;15:685–707.

97. Head E, Liu J, Hagen T, et al. Oxidative damage increases with age in a canine model of human brain aging. *J Neurochem.* 2002;82:375–381.

98. Bradshaw JW, Neville PF, Sawyer D. Factors affecting pica in the domestic cat. *Appl Anim Behav Sci.* 1997;52:373–379.

99. Demontigny-Bédard I, Beauchamp G, Bélanger M-C, et al. Characterization of pica and chewing behaviors in privately owned cats: a case-control study. *J Feline Med Surg.* 2016;18:652–657.

100. Dodman NH, Karlsson EK, Moon-Fanelli A, et al. A canine chromosome 7 locus confers compulsive disorder susceptibility. *Mol Psychiatry.* 2010;15:8–10.

101. Moon-Fanelli AA, Dodman NH, Cottam N. Blanket and flank sucking in Doberman Pinschers. *J Am Vet Med Assoc.* 2007;231:907–912.

102. Moon-Fanelli AA, Dodman NH, Famula TR, et al. Characteristics of compulsive tail chasing and associated risk factors in Bull Terriers. *J Am Vet Med Assoc.* 2011;238:883–889.

103. Hart B. Beyond fever: comparative perspectives on sickness behavior. In: Breed MD, Moore J, eds. *Encyclopedia of Animal Behavior.* Oxford: Academic Press; 2010:205–210.

104. Hart BL. Behavioural defences in animals against pathogens and parasites: parallels with the pillars of medicine in humans. *Philos Trans R Soc B: Biol Sci.* 2011;366:3406–3417.

105. Overall KL. Natural animal models of human psychiatric conditions: assessment of mechanism and validity. *Progress Neuro-Psychopharmacol Biol Psychiatry.* 2000;24:727–776.

106. van der Staay FJ, Arndt SS, Nordquist RE. Evaluation of animal models of neurobehavioral disorders. *Behav Brain Funct.* 2009;5:11.

107. Bain MJ, Fan CM. Animal behavior case of the month. *J Am Vet Med Assoc*. 2012;240:673–675.

108. McPeake KJ, Collins LM, Zulch H, et al. The Canine Frustration Questionnaire—development of a new psychometric tool for measuring frustration in domestic dogs (*Canis familiaris*). *Front Vet Sci*. 2019;6:152.

109. Bain MJ, Good KL. Animal behavior case of the month. *J Am Vet Med Assoc*. 2015; 247:352–355.

110. Beaver B. *The Veterinarian's Encyclopedia of Animal Behavior*. Ames, IA: Iowa State University Press: 1994.

111. Hewson CJ, Luescher UA, Ball RO. The use of chance-corrected agreement to diagnose canine compulsive disorder: an approach to behavioral diagnosis in the absence of a 'Gold Standard'. *Can J Vet Res*. 1999;63:201–206.

112. Frank D. Repetitive behaviors in cats and dogs: are they really a sign of obsessive-compulsive disorders (OCD)? *Can Vet J*. 2013;54:129.

113. Shumaker AK. Diagnosis and treatment of canine acral lick dermatitis. *Vet Clin N Am - Small Anim Pract*. 2019;49: 105–123.

114. Mellor DJ. Updating animal welfare thinking: moving beyond the "Five Freedoms" towards "a Life Worth Living". *Animals*. 2016;6:21.

115. Mellor DJ, Beausoleil N. Extending the 'Five Domains' model for animal welfare assessment to incorporate positive welfare states. *Anim Welf*. 2015;24:241.

116. D'Aniello B, Semin GR, Alterisio A, et al. Interspecies transmission of emotional information via chemosignals: from humans to dogs (*Canis lupus familiaris*). *Anim. Cogn*. 2018;21:67–78.

117. Diverio S, Menchetti L, Riggio G, et al. Dogs' coping styles and dog-handler relationships influence avalanche search team performance. *Appl Anim Behav Sci*. 2017;191:67–77.

118. Hoummady S, Péron F, Grandjean D, et al. Relationships between personality of human–dog dyads and performances in working tasks. *Appl Anim Behav Sci*. 2016;177:42–51.

119. Jamieson LTJ, Baxter GS, Murray PJ. You are not my handler! Impact of changing handlers on dogs' behaviours and detection performance. *Animals*. 2018;8:176.

120. Jezierski T, Adamkiewicz E, Walczak M, et al. Efficacy of drug detection by fully-trained police dogs varies by breed, training level, type of drug and search environment. *Forensic Sci Int*. 2014; 237:112–118.

121. Sorge RE, Martin LJ, Isbester KA, et al. Olfactory exposure to males, including men, causes stress and related analgesia in rodents. *Nat Methods*. 2014;11:629–632.

122. McMillan FD. Maximizing quality of life in ill animals. *J Am Anim Hosp Assoc*. 2003;39:227–235.

123. Veasey JS. In pursuit of peak animal welfare; the need to prioritize the meaningful over the measurable. *Zoo Biol*. 2017:1–13.

124. Wells DL. A review of environmental enrichment for kennelled dogs, *Canis familiaris*. *Appl Anim Behav Sci*. 2004;85: 307–317.

125. Wells DL. Sensory stimulation as environmental enrichment for captive animals: a review. *Appl Anim Behav Sci*. 2009;118:1–11.

126. Foreman-Worsley R, Farnworth MJ. A systematic review of social and environmental factors and their implications for indoor cat welfare. *Appl Anim Behav Sci*. 2019;220:104841.

127. Eisinger BE, Zhao X. Identifying molecular mediators of environmentally enhanced neurogenesis. *Cell Tissue Res*. 2018;371:7–21.

128. Mármol F, Rodríguez CA, Sánchez J, et al. Anti-oxidative effects produced by environmental enrichment in the hippocampus and cerebral cortex of male and female rats. *Brain Res*. 2015;1613:120–129.

129. Mármol F, Sanchez J, Torres M, et al. Environmental enrichment in the absence of wheel running produces beneficial behavioural and anti-oxidative effects in rats. *Behav Process*. 2017;144: 66–71.

130. Montes S, Yee-Rios Y, Páez-Martínez N. Environmental enrichment restores oxidative balance in animals chronically exposed to toluene: comparison with melatonin. *Brain Res Bull*. 2019;144:58–67.

131. Sadek T, Hamper B, Horwitz D, et al. Feline feeding programs: addressing behavioural needs to improve feline health and wellbeing. *J Feline Med Surg*. 2018;20:1049–1055.

132. Sale A, Berardi N, Maffei L. Environment and brain plasticity: towards an endogenous pharmacotherapy. *Physiol Rev*. 2014;94:189–234.

Reading and Resources

Environmental Needs Guidelines: https://catvets.com/guidelines/practice-guidelines/environmental-needs-guidelines

Kartashova IA, Ganina KK, Karelina EA et al. How to evaluate and manage stress in dogs – A guide for veterinary specialist, *Appl Anim Behav Sci*. 2021;243:105458

Lefman SH, Prittle JE. Psychogenic stress in hospitalized patients; causation, implications and therapies. *J Vet Emerg Crit Care*. 2019;29:2017-120

McMillan FD (editor). Mental Health and Well-Being in Animals, 2nd edition. Boston, MA, USA: CABI, 2019.

Mills D, Karagiannis C, Zulch H. Stress - Its effects on health and behavior: A guide for practitioners. *Vet Clin North Am Small Anim Pract*. 2014;44:525-541

Tynes VV, Sinn L. Abnormal repetitive behaviors in dogs and cats: A guide for practitioners. *Vet Clin North Am Small Anim Pract*. 2014;44:543-564.

Zhang L, Bian Z, Liu Q et al. Dealing with stress in cats: What is new about the olfactory strategy? *Front Vet Sci*. 2022;9:928943.

CHAPTER 8

The effects of aging on behavior in senior pets

Gary Landsberg, DVM, MRCVS, DACVB, DECAWBM

Chapter contents

Introduction

As pets age, there are likely to be an increasing number of health concerns where a change in behavior is noticed as the first sign of illness. In fact, for some of the more common physical problems associated with age, including pain, sensory decline, and neurologic disease, the only presenting signs might be behavioral. Senior pets are also at increased risk for behavior problems because of cognitive decline or cognitive dysfunction syndrome (CDS), or they may have had a behavior disorder earlier in life that has progressed with age. In many cases, family members do not even report these signs to the veterinary healthcare team if they are subtle or mild, especially with cats that may not overtly display early signs of pain or illness, or where the behavior is desirable for pet parents, such as pets that are more sociable and affectionate or less active and "appear" to be calmer. Even when pet parents do recognize the signs, they may view them as a normal part of aging and be unaware of what they might signify for the pet's health and welfare. Early identification and reporting is an essential element in the prompt diagnosis of medical and behavioral conditions that might be treatable, manageable, or where the progression might be slowed, and to maximize mental, physical, and social well-being and longevity.[1-3] Additionally, the veterinary healthcare team may not be trained to recognize these changes and their relevance and the importance of asking about them. This bilateral lack of understanding is detrimental to patient welfare.

Age-related changes in cognition and behavior

Age-related changes in cognition and behavior may include changes in activity levels, altered responses to stimuli, altered social interactions, altered sleep–wake cycles, house soiling, confusion, deficits in learning and memory, altered response to previously recognized stimuli, increases in fear, anxiety, stress, conflict or panic, altered cognition and altered response to pet parent cues, and altered appetite, self-hygiene, and control of feeding or drinking behaviors.[1–9] Geriatric behavioral changes can be a result of CDS (described below), systemic diseases including endocrinopathies, organ dysfunction, hypertension, sensory decline, pain, brain disease, behavioral disorders, and the interplay of these factors. Indeed, senior pets can have multiple concurrent problems, making diagnosis much more challenging[1,2,9,10] (see Chapter 6). In addition, prevalence, number, and severity of clinical signs increase with age.[8,11–13] The age at which signs are recognized (not necessarily reported) and at which signs are most likely to be reported by pet parents varies.

Epidemiology of behavior problems in senior pets

In several studies looking at the epidemiology of behavior problem distribution in senior pets, an increasing number of problems are reported with advancing age, with significant progression observed over the course of as little as six months.

Of 270 dogs over seven years of age presented for behavior problems at a Spanish veterinary behavior clinic, 32% were aggressive to family members, 16% aggressive to family dogs, 9% barking, 8% separation-related disorders, 6.4% disorientation, 6% aggression toward unfamiliar people, 5% house soiling, 4.2% destructive, 4% compulsive disorders, and 3% noise fears.[14] Sixteen percent of these cases were diagnosed as CDS.[14] Seventy-four percent were reported to have at least one problem, 19.8% with two problems, 4.6% with three problems, and 1.3% with four problems. In a US veterinary behavior practice 30% were separation-related disorders, 27% pet parent aggression, 17% aggression to other dogs, 8% compulsive disorders, 5% phobias, 4% anxiety, 3% house soiling, and 1% vocalization. Seven percent of these cases were diagnosed as CDS.[15] By comparison, when examining the presentation across all age groups at behavioral practices, aggression represented between 37% and 75% of cases with anxiety disorders representing 12–19%.[16,17] In an internet-based survey of dogs over eight years of age, 826 out of 957 dogs (86.3%) were diagnosed as "successful agers" in which canine cognitive dysfunction had been ruled out using a validated Canine Cognitive Dysfunction Rating Scale or CCDR (described below).[11] Over the course of six months, significant age effects on the percentage of dogs deteriorating were seen in nine items related to ingestion, locomotion, and arousal, nine items related to learning and memory, and three behavior problems, house soiling, fears and phobias, and vocalization.[11] Over half of the items declined by greater than 10%, particularly activity, play, response to commands, and fears and phobias. In cats over 10 years of age referred to three behavioral practices, 73% were marking or soiling, 16% aggressive, 6% vocalizing, and 6% restlessness.[3]

Most recently, in an online survey of pet parents evaluating age-related behavioral changes in 883 cats 11 years and older in the United Kingdom, the most noticeable and consistent change in social behavior was the cats becoming more sociable and affectionate to their pet parents and demanding more attention. Behavior changes included 59% vocalizing during the day, 56% house soiling, 44% vocalizing at night, 74% intermittent agitation, 59% decreased willingness to go outside, alterations in sociability with people (36% more and 7% less), sociability with other animals (19% less and 13% more), sleeping (26% more and 3% less), and grooming (36% less and 10% more).[9] There was a significant association with increasing age with increased daytime and nighttime vocalization, decreased sociability with other cats in the home, increased sleeping, less time spent outside, and increased house soiling.[9] Medical conditions associated with these signs are discussed under Cognitive Dysfunction Diagnosis below.

The onset and prevalence of these behavioral findings serve to demonstrate the importance of biannual proactive screening of senior pets for changes in behavioral and physical health (see approach to the senior pet appointment below).

Cognitive dysfunction syndrome

CDS is a neurodegenerative disorder of senior dogs and cats characterized by increasing brain pathology and gradual and progressive cognitive decline.[1-4,6,10,18-25] Advancing brain pathology is expressed by signs related to deficits and/or alterations in learning, memory, perception, awareness, social interactions, sleep, and activity.[2,3,6-8,10,13,19-22] Clinical signs have been described by the acronym **DISH**, including **D**isorientation, altered social **I**nteractions and **S**leep–wake cycles, and loss of **H**ouse training, and deficits or alternations in learning, memory, and previously learned behaviors.[7,8,12,26,27] Alterations in activity are also associated with CDS in both dogs and cats.[2,5,6,9,11,28-30] While activity levels may initially decrease with age, an increase in spontaneous and aimless activity has been identified with greater severity and advancing CDS in dogs.[5,31-34] Increasing anxiety, irritability, and agitation (including increased attention seeking and vocalization) may also be associated with CDS in dogs and cats.[2,3,6,9,28,35] In dogs, increased anxiety and agitation was seen in 46% of CDS-affected dogs compared to 4% of unaffected dogs, while another study identified 61% of dogs with CDS to have signs of anxiety.[28,36] These signs may be analogous to the anxiety, troubled sleep, and agitation often associated with diseases causing cognitive decline and frontal lobe dysfunction in humans.[37,38] Furthermore, senior dogs may express more passive responses of stress and anxiety (e.g., withdrawn, depressed activity, avoidant), which may be subtle and more difficult to recognize but equally as intense mentally and physiologically.[39,40] Therefore in dogs and likely also cats, the acronym **DISHAA**, including the four categories of DISH as well as both **A**nxiety and altered **A**ctivity would encompass all of the categories for assessing CDS[1,41-45] (see Form 8.1).

Prevalence and signs of cognitive dysfunction syndrome

CDS is a highly prevalent yet grossly underreported condition of senior dogs and cats in which the prevalence, severity, number, and progression of signs is significantly associated

Form 8.1 Cognitive dysfunction (DISHAA) screening checklist

Senior pet cognitive dysfunction syndrome (DISHAA) behavior screening questionnaire	Score
Instructions: Indicate your assessment by entering a score for each question. The purpose of this questionnaire is to identify behavior changes that have arisen or changed in your patient's senior years. Therefore, please ask the pet parents to consider their dogs' current behaviors and any behavioral changes that have developed since their pet was seven years of age, or compared to previous assessments (6–12 months ago). **Scoring Key (severity):** **0** = *None (no change)* **1** = *1 to 2 times per month or mild* **2** = *1 to 2 times per week or moderate* **3** = *Every day or severe*	
A: Disorientation	
Gets stuck, shows difficulty getting around objects or goes to the hinged side of door	
Stares blankly at walls, floor, or into space	
Does not appear to recognize familiar people/familiar pets	
Gets lost in the home or yard	
Less reactive to visual (sights) or auditory (sounds) stimuli	
Has difficulty finding food dropped on the floor	
B: Altered social interactions	
More irritable/fearful/aggressive with visitors, family members, or other pets	
Decreased interest in approaching people or greeting or receiving affection/petting	
C: Sleep–wake cycles	
Pacing, restless, sleeping less, or waking at night	
Vocalization at night	
D: House training, learning and memory	
Less able to learn new tasks or response to previously learned commands/name/work	
Indoor soiling of urine ___ stools ___ or decreased signaling to go out *(check if relevant)*	
Difficulty getting dog's attention/increased distraction/decreased focus	
E: Anxiety/response to stimuli	
Increased anxiety when separated from pet parents	
More reactive/fearful to visual (sights) or auditory (sounds) stimuli	
Increased fear of places/locations (e.g., new environments/going outdoors)	
F: Activity	
Decrease in exploration or play with toys, family members, or other pets	
Increased activity including aimless pacing or wandering	
Repetitive behaviors, for example, circling ___ chewing ___ licking ___ star gazing ___ *(check if relevant)*	

A score of 4–15 is consistent with mild CDS.
A score of 16–33 is consistent with moderate CDS.
A score >33 is consistent with severe CDS.
Copyright Gary Landsberg and CanCog Inc. Used with permission.

with increasing age.[6–8,11–13,28,29,46,47] Prevalence, distribution, and severity of signs vary greatly with the population surveyed and the questions posed. It is clear from numerous prevalence studies that pet parents do not voluntarily report many of these behavioral changes, especially those that are mild, unless they are actively questioned by the veterinary care team.[7,8,46,48] For example, pet parents are more likely to report the most troublesome concerns or severe signs about their senior pet's behavior, while those that are subtle and of minimal concern to the pet parent are seldom reported or go unnoticed even if they might be more common. In addition, the prevalence of CDS in dogs and cats is likely greatly underestimated since deficits in learning and memory likely arise several years before the first clinical signs of cognitive decline appear (discussed below). While there is no cure for CDS, early detection and intervention may slow progression, prevent complications, and increase quality of life and lifespan.

Overall, across all published studies, prevalence in dogs over eight years of age has been reported to range from 14% to over 70%,[7,8,12,30,46] while a study of cats 11 and older reported a prevalence of approximately 35%.[29]

In a University of California Davis study of 180 owners of dogs aged 11–16 whose medical records had been screened to rule out any health abnormalities that would have caused behavioral signs, pet parents were called to inquire if their pet had any noticeable behavioral changes in four DISH categories of cognitive dysfunction: Disorientation, Social Interactions, Sleep–wake cycles, or House soiling. Twenty-eight percent of dogs aged 11 to 12 years and 68% of dogs 15 to 16 years of age were positive for one category, while and 10% of 11- to 12-year-old and 35% of 15- to 16-year-old dogs were positive for two or more categories.[7] Altered sleep–wake cycles were the most commonly affected category in the 11- to 12- and 13- to 14-year-old age groups, while social interactions followed by disorientation and sleep–wake cycles were most affected in 15- to 16-year-old dogs. Twenty-two percent of the dogs that did not have any signs developed signs 12–18 months later, while 48% of dogs with impairment in one category developed impairment in two or more categories.[13]

In a 2009 Spanish study of 325 dogs over the age of 9 using a similar DISH questionnaire, prevalence of CDS was 22.5%, with social interactions and house soiling most commonly reported (37%), followed by sleep–wake cycle (20%) and disorientation (16%).[12]

In a 2007 Italian study of 124 dogs over seven years of age, using a questionnaire with an added category for anxiety (DISHA), 22 of the dogs (18%) were excluded due to clinical health concerns and/or severe sensory impairment. Prevalence of dogs with at least one sign of CDS was 73%, with 41% having alterations in one category and 32% having signs in two or more categories.[30] And in a Danish study of 94 dogs over eight years of age, 57% of dogs with CDS had decreased daytime activity, 51% altered social interactions, and 41% anxiety.[28] Of the dogs diagnosed with borderline CDS, 70% had increased daytime sleep and 11% anxiety, while only 4% of dogs with no CDS were reported to have anxiety. Over the course of three years, 58% with no CDS developed borderline CDS, and 11% converted from borderline to CDS status.[28]

Using a CCDR in a large web-based cross-sectional study of 497 dogs eight years of age or over, the prevalence in 10- to 12-year-old dogs was 5%, 23.3% in dogs 12–14, and 41% in dogs over 14, with an overall prevalence of 14.2%.[46] Yet over 85% of CDS cases had not yet been identified.

Most recently in a "prospective" study of 300 dogs over eight years of age visiting a veterinary hospital in Slovakia, for either preventive care or health complaints, 215 dogs were enrolled for cognitive dysfunction diagnostic screening, using a validated Canine Dementia Scale (CADES) with the four DISHA categories. The remaining 85 dogs (28%) were excluded because of medical causes (although this does not preclude these dogs from also having CDS). Of the 215 dogs, 159 (74%) were diagnosed as cognitively impaired. Of these, 80 dogs had mild cognitive impairment, most of which had not been noticed or reported by the pet parents, primarily altered social interactions, less daytime and greater night time activity. Dogs with moderate impairment (49) had signs such as house soiling and hyperactivity at night, while dogs with severe impairment (49) were affected in all

four DISH domains. Over the course of six months, 42% of dogs with no impairment converted to mild impairment and 24% of dogs from mild to moderate, while over a year, this almost doubled to over 71% from no impairment to mild and 50% from mild to moderate.[8]

In one study of 154 apparently healthy cats aged 11 and older presented for routine preventive care, 28% of 95 cats aged 11–14, and 50% of 46 cats aged 15 and older had at least one behavioral change related to cognitive dysfunction, representing an overall prevalence of 35%. Nineteen of the 154 cats were excluded based on abnormal findings on examination and/or laboratory screening, although these cats may have also had concurrent CDS. The most predominant signs in cats aged 11–14 were altered social interactions, while cats 15 had predominantly increased vocalization and altered activity, including increased aimless activity.[29]

The onset and progression of CDS and its behavioral signs further demonstrate the importance of biannual proactive screening of senior pets for changes in behavioral and physical health (discussed below). In addition, if veterinarians do not educate pet parents that these signs might be indicative of emerging health and welfare concerns, many of which can be resolved, improved, or progression slowed if diagnosed early, then pet parents will not know the importance of reporting these signs.

Cognitive dysfunction screening and assessment scales

Proactive and standardized behavioral and cognitive screening should be part of every senior care visit for dogs from 6–8 years of age and cats over 10.[1,2,6,9–11,41,43,49,50] The assessment questionnaire, together with pet parent educational resources on aging, senior pet health, and behavior, can be posted on or linked to the clinic web site, or sent by email to the pet parent in advance of the scheduled visit. The forms should also be kept in the medical record to track changes at each subsequent visit.

A broad range of screening and diagnostic criteria for behavioral signs have been developed to identify pets with signs consistent with cognitive dysfunction. These include a screening questionnaire with the DISHAA categories (Form 8.1); the CCDR,[51] a validated scale with high negative predictive value based on the onset, progression, and change in frequency of 13 signs including activity, house soiling, awareness, recognition, and social interactions; CADES, a validated scale based on the frequency of 17 signs in the four categories of DISH which may have greater sensitivity in differentiating mild, moderate, and severe cognitive impairment[8]; and an age-related cognitive and affective disorder (ARCAD) scale, as described in the French veterinary psychiatric literature by Dr. Patrick Pageat,[4] which assesses both affective (emotional) and cognitive signs. A significant correlation has been shown between the ARCAD score and beta-amyloid deposits in the temporal cortex and the hypothalamus.[4] Recently, another screening checklist has been proposed for senior cats with the acronym VISHDAAL, which represents Vocalization, altered social Interactions, altered Sleep–wake cycles, House soiling, Disorientation, altered Activity, Anxiety, and Learning and Memory deficits.[2,9,35] Although clinical signs related to vocalization, learning, and memory are included in the DISHAA acronym, the VISHDAAL scale places a more specific emphasis on assessment of senior cats and signs of vocalization. Studies have shown that 60% of cats 11 and older may vocalize excessively during the day and/or night and that vocalization is one of the most common signs of CDS and its differential diagnosis.[2,3,9,29,35]

While the CCDR and CADES (DISH) scales may be most specific for the diagnosis of CDS, the DISHAA and the VISHDAAL evaluation questionnaires may provide more sensitive screening tools for identifying all clinical signs that might be caused by CDS; however, to date, the VISHDAAL scale has not been validated or used in any studies. The DISHAA questionnaire encompasses all six categories of signs attributed to cognitive dysfunction and has been used in several scientific studies for the diagnosis assessment, and treatment of CDS.[36,42,43,45,48] The current version of the questionnaire (see Form 8.1) includes all pertinent behavioral signs from CADES and CCDR assessment tools, and has been initially validated for prevalence, internal consistency, factor analysis, and test–retest reliability based on an initial sample size of 100 dogs with signs of CDS.[42] A version of this questionnaire can be viewed at https://www.purinainstitute.com/sites/g/files/auxxlc381/files/2018-08/DISHAA.pdf. Signs that are components of other assessment scales include altered self-hygiene and control of feeding and drinking behaviors.[4,5,28,47] For cat specific questionnaires see References 35 (VISHDAAL) and AAFP Senior Care Guidelines 41.

Learning and memory assessment

While the initial and hallmark signs of cognitive decline and dysfunction relate to a decline in learning and memory, the onset and progression of these signs may be difficult for pet parents to recognize, as the average pet may appear minimally challenged until the dysfunction becomes severe. In fact, while pet parents most commonly begin to recognize and report signs associated with CDS beginning around 9–11 years or older,[2,7–9,12,28,29,46] using a standardized test apparatus, to assess different cognitive domains, cognitive decline has been identified in dogs and cats as early as 6 to 7 years of age in dogs and cats.[20,21,52–58] This also correlates with functional changes beginning at six to seven years of age in the neurons of the caudate nucleus in cats (See Figure 8.1), leading to impaired information processing[59,60] as well as a decline in cerebral glucose metabolism in dogs at six years of age compared to one year.[61]

Much of the primary research into brain aging and cognitive decline in dogs began with collaborative studies between several researchers in laboratory Beagles as models for human brain aging. Initially, the neuropsychological assessment was developed at the University of Toronto, which led to the founding of CanCog Incorporated. The studies initially focused on developing a test apparatus, methodology, and validated protocols for assessing cognitive function in dogs and more recently, for use in cats[2,20–22,52–57,62–68] (see Figure 8.1). These measures provide an objective means of assessing executive function, attention, and memory impairment in dogs and cats.[1–3,10,19–22,53–56,62] These functions are highly dependent on the frontal lobe, which shows atrophy and beta-amyloid accumulation prior to other brain areas.[4,25] The tests provide both a standardized measure of cognitive function as well as a mechanism by which the effects of therapeutic

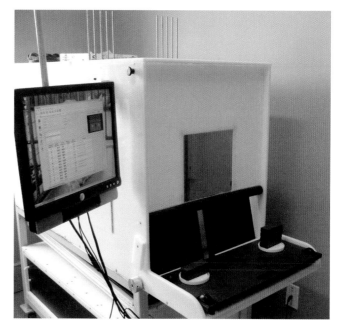

Figure 8.1 Toronto general test apparatus. In discrimination learning, the dog or cat learns to find food under one of the objects (e.g., the large object), the position of which is randomly presented. When discrimination learning reaches criterion (over 70% success), the dog or cat can then be tested on reversal learning, where the food is presented under the opposite (small) object, until the pet reaches criterion. This task is significantly more difficult for senior dogs and cats to learn compared to young adults. (*Courtesy CanCog Inc.*)

agents can be assessed on several different cognitive domains.[52,53,64–68]

In these tests, dogs and cats are trained to use visual and/or spatial information to solve different problems. The object discrimination task provides an initial measure of learning ability. In this task, the subject is presented with two different distinct objects, only one of which covers a food reward. Subjects must learn to displace the correct object (regardless of position) to recover the food. The rate of learning, of simple discrimination tasks in older dogs and cats does not differ from younger counterparts[19,22,55,56,69]; however, if the task is made more complex or demanding such as when objects are more similar or of two different sizes, aged animals have more difficulty in learning the task compared to younger animals[20–22,54–56,62,70] (see Figures 8.1 and 8.2).

Tasks requiring the inhibition of a previously learned behavior, as in reversal learning, are also sensitive to age. In the reversal task, reward contingencies are reversed such that food is now hidden under the object that was not previously rewarded.[19,22,53,56,62] In contrast to simple learning tasks, older dogs and cats require significantly more trials to learn to alter their response in this task compared to young dogs and are not readily able to modify learned behaviors, indicating dysfunction of the prefrontal cortex.[19,20,22,56,62,69] This is a brain region in dogs in which the earliest and most consistent neuropathology tends to arise. Other behaviors that might be associated with prefrontal cortex dysfunction might include changes in personality, including fearfulness and aggression, stereotypic pacing or circling, and a loss of previously learned behaviors, for example, house soiling.

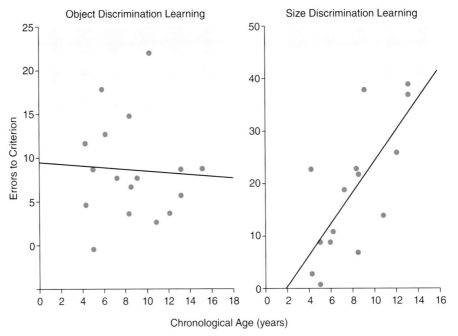

Figure 8.2 Object discrimination learning is not sensitive to age in dogs (correlation between age and error scores on object discrimination is $r = 0.05$). In contrast, size discrimination error scores increase significantly with age (correlation between age and error scores on size discrimination is $r = 0.728$) *(Reproduced from Head E, Callahan H, Muggenburg BA, et al. Discrimination learning ability and beta amyloid accumulation in the dog. Neurobiol Aging. 1998;19:415-425, with permission from Elsevier Science.)*

The aging process has also been demonstrated to affect spatial memory, which is measured by the ability of dogs to remember where they had last obtained a food reward with increasing delays (Figures 8.3 and 8.4). Memory testing has identified three groups of aged dogs: (1) unimpaired, (normal aging); (2) mild cognitive impairment (MCI) and

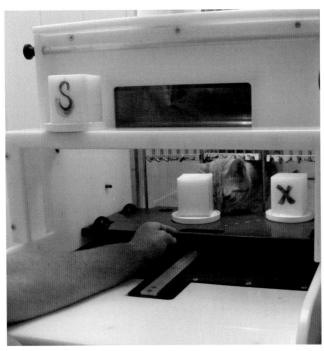

Figure 8.3 Feline testing. Cat being tested on two-choice memory task (delayed nonmatching to position DNMP). *(Courtesy CanCog Inc.)*

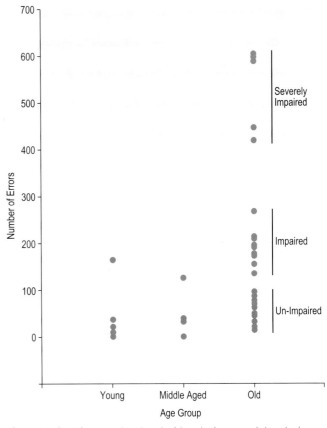

Figure 8.4 Spatial memory is unimpaired, impaired, or severely impaired in three different subsets of aged dogs. *(Reproduced from Head E, Milgram NW, Cotman CW. Neurobiological models of aging in the dog and other vertebrate species. In: Hof AP, Mobbs C, eds. Functional Neurobiology of Aging. San Diego, CA: Academic Press; 2001:457-468, with permission from Academic Press.)*

(3) severely impaired (Figure 8.4). This is consistent with the findings in the geriatric human population.[71] In fact, the level at which performance declines on memory tasks might correspond to the stages of Alzheimer's disease (AD).[15,20,21,53,54, 55,56,62,69,71,72] Clinically dementia these may present as wandering, getting lost, and disorientation, disrupted sleep wake–cycles, and a decline in recognition of familiar people and animals.

The CanCog neuropsychological test apparatus has also been modified for assessment of cognitive function in cats. Three groups of cats, an adult group (3–3.8 years of age), old group (7.7–9 years), and senior group (10.5–15) were assessed on a battery of cognitive tasks (see Figure 8.2). The findings parallel those in dogs, with minimal age differences on the simple discrimination tasks, but with adult cats performing more accurately than old and senior cats on more complex tasks, including reversal and spatial memory (two-position DNMP). However, in contrast to dogs, cats were unable to learn a three-position DNMP task.[56]

Other laboratory models have also been utilized to evaluate age-related deficits in cats. In one study, deficits in eye blink conditioning, found in Alzheimer's patients, were also demonstrated in a subset of aged cats.[73] In a second study, evaluating performance on a hole board task, aging did not appear to affect spatial learning compared to younger cats (<3 years old); however, memory errors were more abundant.[74]

Clinical signs tend to parallel a decline in performance in these tasks.[53] Deficits in cognition tasks have been shown to correlate with alterations in activity, social interactions and exploration, disorientation, house soiling and other learned behaviors, decreased exploratory and play with toys (see Figure 8.5), and sleep disturbances.[20,22,31–34]

Adapting and validating these tasks for clinical use in pet dogs and cats is challenging, as these tests are lengthy, complex, and require trained personnel to administer.[75–77] However, one task, a food search test, may provide a methodology for pet parents to assess and track their pets in the home environment as it has been demonstrated to decline with age (>9 years) and with increasing cognitive dysfunction.[76]

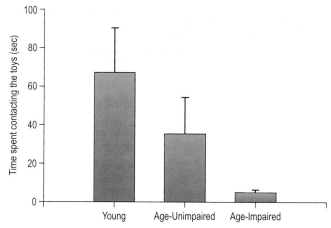

Figure 8.5 The amount of time spent playing or contacting the various toys in the room is plotted against cognitive group. Young dogs play with the toys more than age-impaired ($P < 0.027$) dogs, which rarely touched the toys. Aged, unimpaired dogs explored the toys a little. *(Courtesy Dr. Bill Milgram, CanCog Inc.)*

Risk factors for cognitive dysfunction syndrome

Increasing age is the primary risk factor for the onset and progression of CDS in dogs and cats.[7,8,28–30,43,46,78,79] Across all studies, there were no other consistent or significant risk factors for CDS for sex, neuter status, size, housing, and environment, although there have been some conflicting findings that might warrant further evaluation of the effects of sex, neuter status, and environment.[7,8,12,28,30,43,46,78,80] This may be a functional of substantially different recruitment methods and populations, screening scales, and diagnostic criteria between studies. In addition, one study has identified quality of nutrition as a risk factor. This is consistent with evidence that dietary therapeutics and supplements particularly when combined with environmental enrichment may improve or slow the progression of cognitive decline and dysfunction[42,43,52,57,63,64,66, 68,79,81,82] (see CDS treatment below).

The evidence surrounding the effect of gonadectomy and gender is not definitive. Females and neutered males were significantly more affected than intact males in one study,[2] while another study identified a trend toward a higher prevalence in neutered males.[12,83] In the majority of studies, there was no difference found between the sexes or between gonadectomized and intact dogs.[7,28,46,80]

The impact of body size does not appear to be large if present at all, although in one study, smaller dogs appeared to be more likely to develop CDS when compared to larger dogs,[12] which is consistent with their longer lifespan. Five other studies have found no impact of body size, or longevity on the age of onset, signs, or progression of memory or cognitive impairment.[7,20,28,46,80] However in another study in the 11–13 year age group, dogs >15 kg had significantly higher prevalence (65%) than dogs < 15 kg (43%).[80] Prevalence did not differ between breeds even though large-breed dogs have a shorter lifespan than small-breed dogs.[78,84]

Dogs fed low-quality commercial diets or table scraps were significantly 2.8 times more likely to develop CDS than dogs fed commercial diets formulated for age, size, or health.[80]

Environment may also play a role in the development of neurodegenerative disease. Dogs from areas with high air pollution exhibited early occurrence of beta-amyloid plaques and elevation of proinflammatory markers which preceded by several years similar changes in the brains of dogs living in environments with low air pollution.[85] Humans and pets living together also share the same environmental risk factors. Therefore, since brain aging and AD in humans share many similarities with brain aging and CDS in dogs and cats, the same risk factors would also apply. Poor environmental stimulation and prolonged or chronic stress may also contribute to the development of cognitive decline and CDS.[35,79]

Approach to the senior pet appointment

In 2005, the American Animal Hospital Association senior care task force published guidelines for dogs and cats for twice yearly health care visits for senior pets, to include: a thorough medical and behavioral history, physical examination: laboratory evaluation, focused client education and proactive screening for changes in behavior and cognition.[86] This has been further reiterated as the standard of care in the

2019 AAHA Canine Life Stage Guidelines, the 2021 AAFP Feline Senior Care Guidelines and the 2021 AAHA/AAFP Canine and Feline Life Stage Guidelines.[41,49] (See Resources and Recommended Reading).

These biannual wellness visits should include three essential components: (1) pet parent history including behavioral and cognitive assessment (2) physical examination including blood pressure, neurological, sensory and pain assessment and (3) laboratory screening. Together the assessment should identify and proactively evaluate for any onset, change or decline in the pet's physical, behavioral, and cognitive health and well-being. The veterinarian and health-care team should also counsel the pet parents on pet-specific recommendations for the prevention and management of nutritional and environment risk factors for cognitive decline and for maximizing physical and behavioral well-being.

Pet parent history and cognitive dysfunction syndrome screening

The behavioral and medical history, together with the cognitive dysfunction screening questionnaire (i.e., pet parent history), is the first of three steps in the senior pet health evaluation. Together with the veterinary examination and laboratory screening tests, early identification and reporting of any changes in health or behavior allows for the prompt diagnosis and treatment of any medical, behavioral, and cognitive health issues that might have begun to arise.

As detailed previously, many pet parents do not notice or report changes that are mild or subtle or that they perceive as a normal part of aging if they are not informed and educated about what these signs might signify for the pet's health and welfare, and the value and benefits to the pet of early identification, diagnosis, and treatment.[2,5] In fact, 85% or more of cases go undiagnosed, with new signs arising or signs progressing over the following 6–12 months, unless pet parents are actively informed and questioned on the identification and reporting of changes in behavior.[8,46,51]

Handouts and web links can be used to educate pet parents further about geriatric care, and questionnaires can be used to screen for problems quickly and extensively at each visit (Form 8.1). In fact, use of a history screening questionnaire, which can be attached or linked to the clinic web site or sent to the pet parent in advance of the visit, can serve as an educational tool on senior care, inform the pet parent of what to look for and report, as well as help to expedite and facilitate history taking and data collection so that more time can be allotted to assessing and diagnosing any behavior or health concerns and counseling the pet parent. A recent innovative approach to preventive senior canine care offered 4-week group classes for pet parents with dogs >8 years of age to provide education on senior care, cognitive dysfunction identification and screening, reinforcement-based training, and managing undesirable behavior, as well as an interactional portion with training and enrichment. Based on assessment with a DISHAA scale, signs of CDS were found to develop and worsen with age, with dogs attending the class showing no significant difference over 12 months, while dogs that did not attend the class had significantly increased CDS scores, further supporting the value of pet parent **education**, behavior **counseling,** behavior

screening, reward training, and enrichment in mitigating progression of CDS and improving quality of life.[43] While both the CCDR[51] and CADES (DISH)[8] questionnaire have been validated for diagnosis of CDS, the DISHAA questionnaire may provide a more sensitive tool to identify all clinical signs that might be caused by CDS[42,43,45,48] (see Form 8.1).

Veterinary examination and laboratory screening tests

Biannual physical exams and laboratory screening tests of senior pets can effectively identify emerging and subclinical problems that would otherwise go unrecognized or diagnosed until sufficiently clinically advanced or problematic to the pet and/or pet parent. In two recent trials, 100 apparently healthy senior and geriatric dogs and 100 middle-aged (6–10) and geriatric (>10) cats were assessed by routine physical examination and laboratory blood and urine screening. In the dog trial, 53 were identified as having elevated systolic blood pressure, 22 had heart murmurs, over 20% had hypophosphatemia, leukopenia, increased serum creatinine, ALT, and alkaline phosphatase, and 4 had bacterial cystitis. Platelets were significantly higher and temperature, hematocrit (HCT), albumin, and TT4 were lower in geriatric compared to senior dogs.[87] In the cat trial, systolic blood pressure was increased in 8 cats (>160 mm), 72 had gingivitis, 32 had submandibular lymphadenopathy, 20 had an enlarged thyroid, 11 had heart murmurs, 41 crystalluria, at least 25% had increased creatinine, proteinuria, and/or hyperglycemia, 14 were FIV positive, and 3 had increased thyroxine. Compared to middle-aged cats, old cats had significantly higher systolic blood pressure, heart rate, platelet count, urine protein-creatinine ratios, bilirubin, and frequency of murmurs, and significantly lower HCT, calcium, and albumen.[88]

Taken together, pet parent screening for health and behavioral history, including the use of a cognitive dysfunction scale, veterinary examination, and laboratory screening underscore the importance of biannual health screening to identify changes in behavior health and welfare, for early identification and treatment, often before they are clinically evident or become problematic to the pet or pet parent.

Historically, behavioral changes in animals have been regarded as separate from physical (medical) problems, with veterinarians encouraged to rule out physical differential diagnoses before considering behavioral differential diagnoses or to delay treatment for behavior problems while physical disease was ruled out. However, both behavior disorders and physical disorders have a physiologic component and both cause stress, which further impacts and compounds both health and behavior problems. A one-medicine approach to behavior changes supports the concept that both emotional and physical processes influence behavioral clinical signs. See Chapter 7 for more information on the stress response associated with behavioral clinical signs and Chapter 9 for more information on how to apply the one-medicine approach to behavioral cases.

Neuropathology of brain aging

In dogs, advancing age is associated with frontal lobe and hippocampal atrophy, an increase in ventricular size, widening of sulci, and evidence of meningeal calcification, demyelination, increased lipofuscin and apoptotic bodies, neuroaxonal degeneration, decreased neurogenesis a loss of neurons, and decline in markers of neuronal health[4,5,8,19,23 25,44,71,79,89-92] (see Figures 8.6 and 8.7). There is also brain pathology in cats progresses with age, including atrophy of the cerebral cortex and basal ganglia, region-specific neuronal loss, increased ventricular size, lipofuscin accumulation, and widening of the sulci, although not as marked as seen in dogs or people.[1,2,6,10,18,59,91,93,94] Compared to young cats (less than three years), loss of neuronal function in the caudate nucleus may be seen in cats as young as six to seven years, which may impact motor function and habituation to stimuli.[2,59,60] Neuronal loss has also been observed in the molecular layer of the cerebellum in 12- to 13-year-old cats and in the hippocampus, associated with Aβ plaques and hyperphosphorylated tau deposits, particularly after the age of 14.[93,94]

Compromised circulation in both dogs and cats, including microhemorrhage, infarcts, arteriosclerosis of the nonlipid variety, and cerebral amyloid angiopathy (CAA), an accumulation of beta-amyloid in the walls of the cerebral vessels, may also be responsible for signs of CDS.[1,2,6,10,18,23,24,91,95,96] With increasing age, hypertension, heart disease, anemia, neuropathology of blood vessels, and altered blood viscosity may also compromise cerebral circulation and perfusion in dogs and cats, which may contribute to neuronal hypoxia and loss and cognitive decline.[1,2,6,11,18,19,23,24,68,95,96]

Functional changes that may occur in the aging brain include a possible depletion of catecholamines and an increase in monoamine oxidase B (MAOB) activity in dogs.[97] As in humans with AD, impairment in cholinergic function has also been identified in dogs and cats, which may contribute to declining cognitive and motor function and a disruption in sleep–wake cycles.[1-5,10,44,72,91,98,99] Cognitively impaired dogs also show a significant reduction in the noradrenergic neurons in the local coeruleus, which is also implicated in AD.[18,100]

In dogs, cats, and humans, there is an accumulation of diffuse beta-amyloid plaques and perivascular infiltrates which increases with age.[2,4,18,19,24,44,70,71,93,96,101-115] Beta-amyloid can be detected as early as 7–8 years of age in dogs and cats, and both the quantity and frequency of distribution increase with age.[2,5,18,21,24,70,91,93,105,114] In both dogs and cats, the deposits appear in the cerebral cortex with later progression into the hippocampus,[2,10,18,91,102,107] Vasculopathies including CAA, similar to that in human brain aging and AD, are frequently found in aged dogs and in some but not all studies or less commonly in aged cats.[5,18,79,93,101-105,109-111] (see Figure 8.8).

Dogs display highly similar age related Aβ pathology to humans both in the sequence and the pattern and progression of distribution.[24,25,44,71,104] Furthermore, in dogs, the

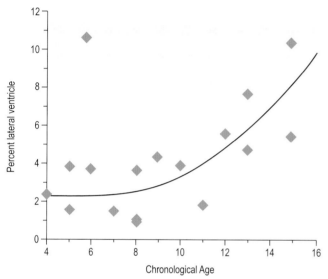

Figure 8.6 The plot of percentage lateral ventricle volume (normalized by the total cerebral volume) with age. The relationship with age was not linear; rather, it was stable before age 10 and progressed very rapidly thereafter. A 6-year-old dog was obviously falling out of the age dependence trend and was marked as an outlier. Excluding the outlier, the age correlation was significant. The solid curve is for visual guidance. (Reproduced from Su M-Y, Head F, Brooks W, et al. Imaging of anatomic and vascular characteristics in a canine model of human aging. Neurobiol Aging. 1998;19:479-485, with permission from Elsevier Science.)

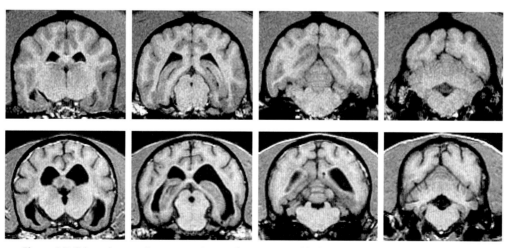

Figure 8.7 Selected magnetic resonance images from a 2-year-old (above) and a 15-year-old (below) dog. The old dog showed marked ventricular enlargement and cortical atrophy (deep gyri and widened sulci). (Courtesy L. M.-Y. Su.)

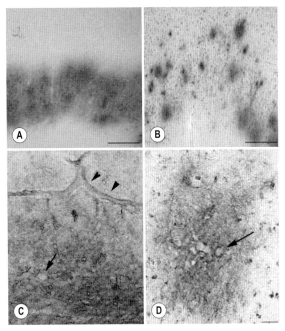

Figure 8.8 Diffuse Aβ deposition in the parietal cortex of (A) an aged cat with symptoms of cognitive dysfunction syndrome (tissue provided by Dr. Kelly Moffat) versus (B) in the aged canine brain. Note that Aβ in the cat is present as a large diffuse cloud whereas, in the dog, more discrete deposits form. Higher magnification of Aβ in (C) cats and (D) dogs. Note the Aβ deposition associated with blood vessels (arrowheads) in the cat and that, in both animals, intact neurons (arrows) are present within diffuse clouds of Aβ. Bars in (A) and (B): 500 μm; (C) and (D): 50 μm. *(Courtesy Dr. E. Head.)*

amount and location of Aβ plaque deposition has been linked to the severity of cognitive deficits, although not all studies have found this association.[4,5,10,18,19,24,25,70,91,104,105,112–114] Aβ Plaques in dogs are diffuse with no dense core, that may progress into more compact deposits.[4,10,18,24,25,70,71] Reversal learning deficits indicative of executive dysfunction tend to show more extensive Aβ deposition in the prefrontal cortex, while size discrimination learning ability is associated with amount of Aβ in the entorhinal cortex.[10,19,24,70] Genetics may be a contributing factor in the extent of amyloid distribution, as some breeds develop beta-amyloid at an earlier age and there is high concordance within litters in the extent of beta-amyloid.[106]

Soluble Aβ can also be measured in the cerebrospinal fluid (CSF) of dogs, making it a potentially useful marker for aging and cognition studies for predicting levels of Aβ in brain as well as the extent of plaque formation.[45,108] In the brain increases in Aβ42 are detected at a younger age, before increases in Aβ40, and correlate with increased amyloid load. In the CSF, there is an inverse relationship, with brain amyloid deposition increasing while CSF Aβ42 decreases, since soluble CSF pools decrease as Aβ is deposited in the brain.[108] A recent study found CSF Aβ42 to be lower in aged dogs with MCI compared to cognitively unimpaired.[45] Taken together, levels of CSF Aβ42 and the ratio CSF Aβ42/40, combined with clinical cognitive assessment, may predict Aβ levels in the brain, and provide a methodology for identifying MCI in aged dogs.[45,108] In addition plasma levels of Aβ42 and Aβ42/40 may also hold promise as blood biomarkers.[26,49,113]

Aged cats spontaneously develop Aβ plaques, most typically after 10 years of age but have been reported by 7.5 years of age years.[2,18,93,96,101,103,104,107,110] Compared to dogs Aβ plaques in cats are even more diffuse, which may progress into denser patches.[2,6,10,18,93,96,101–104,107,110,111] Although plaques have been found in cats with behavioral dysfunction and increasing cognitive decline, a correlation has not been established between the behavioral signs and the extent of Aβ.[2,6,18,91,93,96,101,103,104,110] In fact, the pattern and distribution of Aβ in aged cats, may be more similar to the non-demented brain of elderly humans, rather than AD.[2,10,91,93,96,101,103,104,110]

Aging dogs and cats develop tauopathies which share many features of human AD. Although these rarely if ever progress to mature neurofibrillary tangles (NFT), where NFT have been reported in dogs and cats, they are considered to be pre-tangles, an early form of NFT seen in AD.[2,9,10,18,91,93,101,103,107,109,111–115] While no definitive correlation has been established between tau and CDS in dogs and cats[2,6,18,93,101] elevated synapse related phosphorylated tau in the cortex and intracellular phosphorylated tau together with Aβ deposition in the cerebral cortex and hippocampus, have been identified in dogs with CDS.[79,91,109,112,114] In cats, several studies have shown that elderly cats with tau pathology display behavior changes associated with CDS, and that tau pathology is associated with significant cortical atrophy and neuron loss.[2,91,93,111] While the greatest neuron loss was found in cats with concurrent tau and Aβ deposits, tau pathology has been identified independent of Aβ deposits in several aged cats.[93,101,111]

Recent evidence points to beta-amyloid oligomers, a soluble form of Aβ that is particularly toxic to synapses and associated with cognitive dysfunction in humans, in being responsible for the neurotoxic and cognitive deficits of CDS in dogs and cats; however a clear role has not been established.[2,18,44,45,91,93,108,109,112,115] In one study in dogs with CDS the hyperphosphorylated tau did not co-localize with Aβ plaques but did co-localize with intraneuronal Aβ oligomers in the frontal cortex and hippocampus.[111]

Several studies demonstrate the role of oxidative damage and mitochondrial dysfunction on brain aging in dogs, which is also speculated to be a factor in aging cats.[2,6,18,52,62,81,116,117] Normally, the body's antioxidant defenses, including enzymes such as superoxide dismutase, catalase, and glutathione peroxidase, and free radical scavengers such as vitamins A, C, and E, eliminate free radicals as they are produced. With age, an increased production and decreased clearance of free radicals can lead to a net increase that may react with DNA, lipids, and proteins, leading to cellular damage, dysfunction, and even cell death. The brain is particularly susceptible to the effects of free radicals because it has high lipid content, a high demand for oxygen, and limited ability for antioxidant defense and repair. It therefore follows that diets rich in antioxidants and mitochondrial cofactors have been shown to improve learning and memory in senior dogs.[52,81]

Brain glucose metabolism may also be compromised with increasing age with a significant decline at around six years of age in Beagle dogs that further declines with age.[61,79] Recent studies have shown that dietary supplementation with medium-chain triglycerides (MCTs) which are converted in the liver to a ketone body, beta-hydroxybutyrate, can provide the brain with an alternative source of energy that improves executive function, learning, and memory in senior dogs.[64]

Together these studies demonstrate that dogs and cats with CDS display age related neuropathologic features including Aβ deposition, tauopathy with neuronal loss, intracellular beta-amyloid oligomers, neuronal loss and brain atrophy, together with learning and memory deficits and clinical signs of CDS, which strongly supports that the aging dog and cat are a naturally occurring model of brain aging and AD in humans.AD.[2,5,18,26,44,90–94,100,101,109,114,115]

Therefore studies into the risk factors, prevention, and treatment in one species may translate into breakthroughs and advances for all! However, in contrast to humans dogs and cats Aβ plaques are diffuse and lack a central dense core, and full blown NFT's, and seldom progresses to mortality.[10,18] In fact, in one study of 74 dogs with CDS, in only six of the cases was CDS the cause of death or euthanasia.[28]

Threshold theory of behavior change

Factors contributing to the development of behavioral clinical signs at any age include genetics, epigenetics (effect of environment and external factors on the expression of genes), the pet's coping style, maternal care, neonatal handling and socialization, environmental experience, physical health, and learning. Physical conditions can act in concert with other factors to lower thresholds of inhibition and result in exhibition of behavioral clinical signs such as fear, anxiety, stress, conflict, panic, phobia, frustration, and aggression. For example, pain (e.g., osteoarthritis, dental disease) can lead to fear of being handled, which can result in avoidance of the family and other pets, and aggression. If mobility is affected, the pet may become increasingly fearful, reclusive, or aggressive, or may have more difficulty accessing its elimination area. These problems may appear to be acute when in fact the pet has finally reached a threshold at which an overt, grossly observable sign is present. This can be especially noticeable in cases of interpet aggression. While pet parents may present two household pets for aggression to each other and state that the younger dog clearly knows that the older dog is impaired, causing the younger dog to be aggressive to elevate his status in the pack, what is likely is that the older dog is suffering from physical disease and sensory decline that does not permit recognition or acknowledgement of the body language through which the younger dog communicates, combined with the inability to the situation due to cognitive, sensory or physical decline. In these cases, controlling the younger dog's behavior and separating the dogs when proactive supervision is not possible is essential.

Causes of senior pet behavior problems

When presented with a senior patient with a change from normal behavior, the onset of a new problem, or progression of an existing problem, the veterinary team must evaluate each case to determine if there is a contributing physical cause for the problem. Any disease that affects the central or peripheral nervous system (e.g., CDS, hepatic encephalopathy, tumors, intervertebral disk disease), the cardiovascular system (e.g., cardiac disease, anemia, hypertension), bones and joints (e.g., osteoarthritis, neoplasia), the dermatologic system (e.g., atopic dermatitis, adverse food reaction), gastrointestinal (GI) system

(e.g., inflammatory bowel disease, food intolerance, neoplasia), renal/urinary system (e.g., renal disease, feline interstitial cystitis [FIC] or the endocrine system (e.g., hyper-or hypothyroidism, hyper- or hypoadrenocorticism) can affect behavior.[10] In fact, medical health conditions have been identified in up to 80% of dogs with behavioral problems, with arthritic pain and sensory decline in particular causing, contributing to, or exacerbating signs associated with CDS.[118–120] Therefore, both pet parent and veterinary recognition and assessment of pain, vision, hearing and neurologic signs are a particularly important part of the senior pet diagnostic assessment.[10,121]

As senior pets are prone to the development of an increasing number of health conditions including CDS, it can be extremely challenging to determine the cause of the behavioral signs. In addition, a diagnosis of a medical or a primary behavior problem does not rule out a concurrent diagnosis of CDS. In fact, visual decline, olfactory decline, swaying and falling, tremors, and a tendency toward hearing decline, were all found to be associated with CDS[118,122] (see Box 8.1).

Medical differentials for behavioral clinical signs are discussed in detail in Chapter 6.

Illness results in behavioral signs both as a consequence of the illness itself (fever, discomfort, pain) and as a mechanism for healing and staying safe from harm. Any change in behavior, temperament, appetite, or activity may be a result of illness. For example, cats may have alterations in vocalization, appetite, grooming, sociability (increased, decreased), play, sleep, elimination, going outside, and irritability.[9,35,123]

When pets are presented with behavior changes that might be due to CDS, a neurological cause might be diagnosed if there were neurological deficits or other concurrent signs such as cranial nerve involvement, seizures, sensory or motor deficits, tremors, emesis, altered eating or drinking, appearing blind or lost, pacing, circling to one side, or head pressing. However, the changes in behavior may precede any of these neurological signs.

Behavior and memory circuits are mainly located in the forebrain, including the limbic system, which typically includes the amygdala, hippocampus, thalamus, hypothalamus, basal ganglia, and cingulate gyrus. Therefore, a change in personality or mood, inability to recognize or respond appropriately to stimuli, and loss of previously learned behavior might be indicative of forebrain involvement. Alterations in awareness and responsiveness to stimuli and consciousness might arise from disease of the brainstem or

---

Box 8.1 Physical problems affecting behavior in senior pets (for a more comprehensive list of health issues and their effects on behavior, see Table 6.1)

- Neurological (central, cognitive dysfunction syndrome, peripheral)
- Cardiovascular/respiratory
- Neuromuscular/musculoskeletal
- Sensory dysfunction (e.g., hearing, sight)
- Metabolic/degenerative disorders (e.g., hepatic, renal)
- Urogenital/gastrointestinal
- Endocrine disorders (e.g., thyroid, adrenal, pancreas, gonadal)
- Dermatologic (e.g., pruritus, otitis, anal sacculitis, intertrigo)
- Infection/inflammation (e.g., prostatitis, cystitis)
- Pain and discomfort (e.g., dental, degenerative arthritis, neuropathy)
- Neoplasia

forebrain, as well as from deficits in the sensory system. Diseases affecting the limbic system and hypothalamus can affect emotional state.

Sensory dysfunction or motor dysfunction may contribute to altered responsiveness to stimuli, increased fear, anxiety, aggression, reduced ability to cope with change, altered appetite, as well as decreased desire (or ability) to go outside or use a litterbox, reluctance to climb or jump, and hiding.

Endocrine diseases including hyperthyroidism, hyperadrenocorticism, and hypothyroidism can also contribute to anxiety. Since cortisol inhibits thyroid stimulating hormone (TSH) release, stress can also diminish thyroid levels. Classical signs of hypothyroidism include thin coat, seborrhea, lethargy, bradycardia, and heat seeking. However, in the early stages of hypothyroidism, it has been suggested that dogs may present with fear-based behaviors, hyperactivity, poor learning, anxiety, and aggression, especially toward family members, perhaps due to lower 5HT turnover or lowered threshold for aggression.[124,125] In a placebo-controlled study of dogs presented with aggression with low to low normal thyroid levels, there was a significant decrease in aggression in both thyroxine and placebo-treated groups but no differences between groups.[126] In two other studies comparing thyroid levels in dogs with and without problem behaviors, thyroid levels were normal.[127] Therefore, a therapeutic trial might be considered if clinical signs and laboratory diagnostics are suspicious of hypothyroidism. However, thyroid supplementation that is not indicated could lead to hyperthyroid levels. In cats, hyperthyroidism is the most common endocrine condition affecting behavior. Behavioral signs might include increased activity, hyperphagia, polydipsia, increased irritability, house soiling, and intercat or pet parent-directed aggression. Signs of hypertension associated with thyroid disease might include night waking, vocalization, confusion, irritability, aggression, and altered activity levels.

Diabetes mellitus is associated with altered appetite, polyuria, and polydipsia, and may lead to house soiling. There may also be signs of lethargy, fatigue, and altered social interactions and sleep–wake cycles. Diabetes insipidus can lead to house soiling, altered sleep, night waking, lethargy, irritability, and resource guarding of water.

Hyperadrenocorticism (hypercortisolism) may be associated with behavioral signs primarily related to elevated cortisol. Signs might include anxiety, exercise intolerance, altered social interactions including increased irritability, aggression, reduced interest in play, night waking, panting, and polydipsia and polyphagia. In fact, a recent study has demonstrated that hypercortisolism may accelerate neurodegeneration, resulting in more intense behavioral and cognitive changes.[128]

Hepatic disease may lead to behavioral signs related to altered absorption, digestion and breakdown of nutrients, pain, discomfort, and hepatoencephalopathy. Dogs and cats may show avoidance, irritability, aggression, altered sleep, listlessness, confusion, ataxia, and repetitive behaviors (e.g., staring, pacing).

Compromised circulation, hypotension, and hypertension may alter blood flow to the brain, leading to hypoxia in the brain. Cardiovascular disease can cause exercise intolerance, reduced activity, anxiety, lethargy, altered social interactions, reduced awareness, altered sleep, and confusion.

Any disease associated with increased intestinal motility, diarrhea, constipation, or decreased control may cause house soiling. Diseases of the GI tract causing pain, discomfort, and nausea may lead to altered appetite, anxiety, irritability, night waking, repetitive pacing, vocalization, and avoidance, as well as lip licking, environmental licking, stretching, sucking, and pica. Oral behaviors including licking, sucking, pica, smacking lips, gulping, and fly snapping may be due to GI disorders.[129,130] In cats with pica, seven out of eight had mild to moderate gastritis or enteritis and three improved by 50% or greater with treatment.[131]

Pain can have both behavioral and physical signs that vary between dogs and cats and with the source of pain. Behavioral signs might include altered response to stimuli, a decline in activity, a change in behavior or alterations in normal daily activities (climbing, scratching, going outdoors, going for walks, play), altered social interactions, night waking, reduced sleep, restlessness, increased irritability or aggression, hiding and avoidance, altered appetite, vocalization, or house soiling. While dogs are more likely to show overt signs of pain (e.g., lameness, attending to painful location), cats show more behavioral signs including avoidance-related behavior and a decline in activity including climbing, jumping, scratching, and hunting (See chapter 6).

Medications can also affect behavior. Therefore, if there are behavioral signs, the effects of any medications the pet is taking should be considered. In one study, dogs on glucocorticoids were significantly less playful, more nervous, more fearful, less confident, food aggressive, more prone to bark, startle, and react aggressively when disturbed, and avoided people or unusual situations.[132]

The role of stress in health and behavior

While it is common to consider the effects of disease on behavior, stress (an altered state of homeostasis which can be caused by physical or emotional factors) can adversely impact both physical and behavioral health and welfare. As discussed in Chapters 7, 9, and 14, stress is an adaptive measure that affects the hypothalamic-pituitary axis (HPA) and noradrenergic system and triggers psychological, behavioral, endocrine, and immune effects that are designed to handle stress and a return to homeostasis. However, chronic, prolonged, or recurrent stress can lead to reduced immune function, increased susceptibility to infection, delayed healing, diseases of the urinary tract (e.g., FIC), cardiovascular and respiratory disease, cellular aging, GI disease, dermatologic conditions, and behavioral disorders. These health conditions will further aggravate stress for the pet and often for the pet parent, while the behavioral consequences (e.g., self-trauma, ingestive, destructive) might further impact physical health and welfare.

In the aging pet, there is a general deterioration in physical and behavioral health; tissue hypoxia; alterations in cell membranes; increased production and decreased clearance of reactive oxygen species; a decline in organ, sensory, and mental function; a gradual deterioration of the immune system; and decreased ability to cope with change. Thus, the senior pet is less able to respond to stress and maintain homeostatic balance. Pet parents should be encouraged to maintain a stable and predictable environment and schedule; to plan and make any necessary changes gradually; and to monitor pet enrichment programs, especially for cats (see below) to ensure that they have a positive and desired effect.

Diagnosis of behavior problems in senior pets

As with pets of any age, the diagnosis of a behavior problem requires: (1) the recognition and reporting of behavioral and medical signs by the pet parent; (2) a behavioral history to determine the role of the pet, the pet parents, and the social and physical environment in the onset, progress, and consequences of the problem itself (see Chapters 1 and 9 for more information about the approach to behavior cases in clinical practice); and (3) a physical examination and diagnostic tests with a focus on the health issues that are most likely to be associated with the clinical signs and signalment. See causes of behavior problems above and in Chapter 6.

The behavioral history should focus on what might have changed in the pet's health or environment that could have caused or contributed to the problem. Any change from previous behavior should immediately prompt further questions to determine if there are any other concurrent signs that might be consistent with an underlying physical problem and a more thorough behavioral history to rule out any changes in the pet's schedule or household that may have caused or contributed to the signs. Video recordings of the behaviors can also be particularly helpful to visualize what the pet parent is describing and to observe and evaluate the pet's behavioral signs and body language.

In some cases, the pet parents are seeking help for a problem that has been longstanding but has recently become less tolerable. This may be due to changes in the home such as the vocal dog that is now a greater concern because of pet parent health issues, new neighbors, or new family members (e.g., spouse, new baby). For some pet parents, a preexisting problem may have significantly increased in intensity or frequency to become a serious concern for the pet and/or pet parent, such as a fear of noises that progresses to a severe storm aversion or phobia. Underlying health issues such as sensory decline and pain are common causes and contributing factors.[120,121,133] Since senior pets may also be less adaptable and more sensitive to change, modifications to the pet's schedule or routine, social environment (e.g., baby, spouse, new pet) or physical environment (e.g., moving, renovations) can have a greater impact on the behavior of an older pet compared to a younger one.

Another important diagnostic consideration is that even if physical problems can be effectively resolved, some or all of the behavior problems might persist through inadvertent intrinsic and extrinsic reinforcement and/or punishment (see Chapter 9) of the behavior, requiring concurrent behavior guidance to manage, modify, and improve the behavior. The history will therefore also need to evaluate if there are any environmental factors, relationship issues, or learned factors that might have played a role in the cause or persistence of a behavioral problem. Pet parents should be informed of this possibility.

Because dogs and cats cannot directly report symptoms, the behavioral workup is comprised of the behavioral history including the onset, progression, and description of all presenting medical and behavioral clinical signs, a complete physical examination including neurological, sensory, mobility and pain evaluation, and laboratory screening as determined by the pet's signalment, health, behavior, and medical signs, and the findings of the physical examination with a minimum database that should include a complete blood profile, serum chemistry, thyroid evaluation, urinalysis, fecal antigen + giardia. If physical problems are diagnosed, it can be a challenge to determine whether the problem is actually causing the behavioral signs. Response to therapy may therefore be an important step in the workup; however, treatment which will not interfere with diagnosis and treatment of another disorder should not be delayed while results for tests are awaited. Thus, a patient suffering emotionally or physically from pain, fear, anxiety, stress, conflict, and panic should be treated immediately. Waiting to rule out physical disease before providing behavioral guidance and treatments that immediately address the pet's physical and emotional welfare may cause needless patient suffering.

Unfortunately, with age, not all physical problems can be resolved or improved, and some may continue to progress. Therefore, the pet parent should be provided with realistic expectations and modifications to the pet's environment or schedule to help the family and pet best manage the situation.

Diagnosis of cognitive dysfunction syndrome

To diagnose CDS, veterinarians must rely on the pet parent to recognize and reporting any changes in behavior or the onset of new behavior problems, represented by the acronym DISHAA (disorientation, alterations in social interactions or sleep–wake cycles, loss of house soiling or other learned behaviors, signs of anxiety or altered activity), ideally with the aid of one of the cognitive screening questionnaires described above (see Cognitive Dysfunction Screening and Assessment Scales and Form 8.1). Only with careful questioning and history taking is it likely that signs would be detectable in the earliest stages of development. Requesting the pet parent to complete the assessment tool prior to the appointment and return it or bring it to the visit can inform and educate the pet parent on the reason and importance of identification and reporting of changes in behavior and expedite data collection so that time can be spent assessing the pet and addressing the pertinent issues during the veterinary visit. In addition, the questionnaire aids in tracking the onset and progression of any signs from the previous visit.

As CDS is a diagnosis of exclusion, all possible medical as well as behavioral causes of the signs must be considered and ruled out. Any change from normal behavior may be the first or only sign of a physical health condition and is a critical component in the monitoring of patients for progression and for response to therapeutic interventions.

In addition, both behavioral and medical health problems and their consequences can cause or contribute to emotional and physiological stress, impaired welfare, and further health and behavioral conditions associated with chronic stress. The components of the diagnostic workup for cognitive dysfunction include: (1) pet parent history; (2) veterinary examination including neurological, sensory, pain, mobility, and blood pressure; and (3) diagnostic tests as determined by the presenting signs, medical history, and physical examination findings.[1,2,9–11,18,35,41,49–51,86] Therapeutic trials (e.g., analgesic response) and ongoing follow-up and monitoring may also be essential to assess outcome and progress, confirm the diagnosis, and make necessary modifications to the therapeutic plan for optimum health and welfare (see Box 8.2).

In one senior dog cognitive therapeutic trial, 100 apparently healthy dogs were initially screened for signs of CDS with a DISHAA questionnaire. Fifteen of the dogs identified as having signs of CDS were subsequently excluded due to underlying medical problems identified on laboratory screening, including liver, kidney, or Cushing's disease or bacterial cystitis.[42] In the study by Madari et al. of dogs with signs consistent with a diagnosis of CDS, of 300 dogs visiting the veterinary clinic for preventive care or health complaints, 85 were found to have underlying medical problems.[8] In the Sordo et al. cat study evaluating the prevalence of disease in cats with age-related behavior signs that might be attributed to cognitive dysfunction (see Epidemiology of Behavior Problems above), of 883 cats ranging from 11 to over 20 years of age, cats showed significant associations between increased sleeping and blindness, deafness, arthritis, and kidney disease; increased daytime vocalizing with deafness, arthritis, hyperthyroid, and kidney disease; increased night vocalizing with blindness, deafness, arthritis, and hyperthyroid; increased soiling with kidney disease, blindness, and urinary tract disease; increased agitation and irritability with blindness, arthritis, and kidney disease; decreased sociability with other animals with blindness, deafness, arthritis, kidney, and dental disease; and increased sociability with people with blindness, arthritis, and kidney disease.[9]

Behavior problems of senior pets

Anxiety, fears, and phobias

Increasing anxiety is a relatively common complaint of pet parents of older pets. Increasing sensitivity to stimuli, increasing fear of unfamiliar pets and unfamiliar people, increased irritability, decreased tolerance of handling and restraint, increased following and desire for contact, and increasing anxiety during pet parent departures are some of the more common family concerns. Discomfort related to orthopedic and neurologic disease is a common cause of fear of walking on certain surfaces in older dogs. The presenting complaint may appear to be totally unrelated, such as house soiling (fear of walking on a surface leading to the door out of which the dog goes for elimination) or aggression (resulting from pet parent attempts to move the dog), and the reluctance to walk on certain surfaces may be incidentally found after taking the history. By the same token, pain (e.g., osteoarthritis) can cause cats to show aggression when lifted or when pet parents attempt to move them, something that they may have tolerated for years. The initiating event may have been a particularly fearful or uncomfortable experience that may have gone unnoticed by the pet parents.

Physical problems that affect the CNS, including cognitive dysfunction and other age-related brain pathology, decreased sensory acuity, endocrinopathies, and painful conditions such as arthritis and dental disease, must be ruled out. The locus ceruleus and its neurotransmitter norepinephrine are vital in the genesis of fear and panic, so that age-related changes that affect the limbic system, the locus ceruleus, and norepinephrine transmission can either aggravate or reduce fearful and phobic responses. The history may indicate that these pets have previously had less intense fears but that with repetition over the years (and perhaps contributing physical factors), the problem may have intensified (e.g., storm phobias). The pet parent's response to the pet may further compound the problem, either by inadvertently reinforcing the behavior or aggravating the anxiety (e.g., responding with anger, frustration, or punishment). Thus, many of these problems are likely to be multifactorial, with physical, environmental, and pet parent influences.

Separation-related disorders may be comorbid with other fears and phobias, or may be related to a recent change to the household, schedule, or social partners (family members, other pets).[134] Senior pets may have greater difficulty adapting to change, and health issues can further contribute to the problem. Crating or confining the pet to prevent further damage or soiling may further add to the pet's anxiety if the pet has not been sufficiently accustomed to confinement. Pet parents may confine an older dog to a crate assuming that because the dog could be confined without stress earlier in life that this type of confinement can be reintroduced without retraining the pet. In these cases, the confinement and the pet parent's departure both contribute to the pet's anxiety. The history, physical assessment, and findings of diagnostic testing as well as video recording or web monitoring of the pet's behavior during departures are useful in making a diagnosis and developing a treatment plan. See Chapter 17 for more information on separation-related disorders.

Increased fear and anxiety in cats can lead to avoidance behaviors, vocalization, house soiling, or redirected aggression. Novel noises or odors can increase fear and anxiety. In many cases, a physical cause such as pain, sensory decline, cognitive dysfunction, or other age-related brain pathology are likely contributing factors, since behavioral signs are often the first or only indication that a cat has a health problem. The history should evaluate all physical and behavioral signs, combined with physical, orthopedic, and neurologic examinations and diagnostic tests (complete blood count, serum chemistry, proBNP, urinalysis, thyroid assessment, and fecal antigen + giardia), as well as any changes or alterations to the pet's lifestyle or household. Cats, especially senior cats and those with physical problems, can be particularly sensitive to the effects of change. Pet parent responses can further aggravate the situation, since alterations in the pet parent's response to the cat or adjustments to the environment to deal with the problem can further add to the cat's stress. Improvement can best be achieved by providing a predictable environment, predictable consequences, enriching the environment, and using reinforcement-based techniques to increase desirable behaviors while ignoring or preventing undesirable behaviors (see Chapters 20, 22, and 24).

Excessive vocalization

In cats and dogs, vocalization can become a problem if it becomes excessive and uncontrollable, or occurs at undesirable times (e.g., when the family is sleeping). Sensory dysfunction (particularly auditory dysfunction), age-related cognitive dysfunction, CNS pathology, and pain- and age-related physical conditions may contribute to increased anxiety, noise sensitivity, and vocalization. Hearing loss may lead to an inability of the pet to audit its own vocalization level or volume. Distress vocalization (dogs) and house soiling (dogs and cats) when the family is absent may be due to separation-related disorders. If excessive vocalization occurs when the family is at home, then the history will need to be evaluated to determine when and under what circumstances the dog or cat vocalizes. Cats and dogs with polyphagia may vocalize in an attempt to acquire food, which is reinforced if the pet parents acquiesce. Dogs might vocalize to signal pet parents if they have an increased need to eliminate or in response to specific stimuli (noises, visitors) and is particularly problematic if it wakes the pet parents at night. Attempts to quiet the pet may reinforce the behavior (if the pet parent gives attention or uses treats or toys to quiet the dog or cat) or increase the anxiety (by responding with anger, frustration, or punishment). Treatment and control of vocalization in dogs is covered in Chapter 17 and 19 and excessive vocalization in cats in Chapter 20.

House soiling

House soiling in dogs and cats may be indicative of a wide range of physical problems that can affect the older pet. Sensory decline, painful neurological or neuromuscular conditions that affect mobility, age-related cognitive dysfunction, other forms of CNS pathology, any physical condition that might affect behavior (e.g., endocrinopathies, hepatic encephalopathy), and physical conditions that increase the volume or frequency of elimination, discomfort during elimination, or a decrease in control may all be contributing factors. In cats, litter avoidance may arise from physical problems that make accessing the litterbox difficult, uncomfortable, or more frightening (e.g., sensory decline, arthritis, obesity). It is worth noting that cats are particularly difficult to assess regarding pain and illness and pet parents often are unaware of the early clinical signs of disease. Pets with disease conditions that affect the CNS (e.g., brain tumors, cognitive dysfunction) may begin to eliminate in the home, often in more random locations. This may be a sign of advanced cognitive dysfunction in dogs than in cats, since there are numerous learned components to the behavioral sequence, including: (1) voluntary control of elimination when the pet feels the urge; (2) signaling the family to be taken outdoors to eliminate; (3) seeking out the appropriate location; (4) responding to an elimination cue (if trained in this manner); and (5) voluntarily voiding at the appropriate site.

House soiling that occurs only during a perceived or actual separation from the pet parent may be a result of a separation-related disorder. However, separation-related disorders are not the only reason that a pet would soil only when the pet parent is away from home. Some dogs will not soil as long as the pet parents are available to take the dog outdoors to eliminate. Cats may not soil if the litterbox is cleaned appropriately. Because senior pets are more resistant and less able to adapt to change, any alteration in the pet's schedule or environment may contribute to soiling. Anxiety and conflict could contribute to urine marking behavior, feline periuria, and feline perichezia.

Whether the cause is physical or behavioral, once the pet begins to use new indoor locations regularly, even with sufficient cleaning, the pet is likely to return to the site, as elimination itself is intrinsically reinforced (pressure on the bladder, colon, and associated sphincters is reduced immediately) and that reinforcement is associated with a location in the house. Therefore, in addition to the physical assessment and diagnostics as outlined above, the history is an essential component in making a diagnosis as well as formulating a treatment plan. This would include determining the distribution (random or specific locations), frequency, and location of elimination (hidden locations or near exit doors), whether the pet eliminates when the pet parent is home or absent, any changes in the schedule or household at the time of onset, other concurrent changes in health or behavior including mobility, sensory loss, or incontinence, what the family has done to date to try and improve the behavior and the pet's response to each. While the treatment program is essentially the same for any house soiling problem (see Chapters 21 and 22), there may be limitations on what can be achieved in the senior pet if its health problems or cognitive dysfunction cannot be entirely resolved. For example, dogs with polyuria may need more frequent access to elimination areas or an indoor litter location might be required, while cats may require more frequently cleaned litterboxes, boxes with lower sides, change in location of boxes (to avoid other cats), bigger boxes or more boxes (to account for social interactions, physical limitations, or increased urgency/frequency). Pets with mobility and sensory issues may need help accessing their elimination area, better lighting, or environmental modifications to improve accessibility, including an easier access to the outdoors or ramps for dogs, lower sides or a ramp for entry to litterboxes for cats, a much larger litterbox, or a new site for the litterbox. Incontinence issues may require the use of diapers or confinement on surfaces with absorbable material (provided it is not ingested by the pet) if medication cannot be found to improve the problem.

Repetitive (compulsive) and stereotypic behaviors

Repetitive (compulsive) and stereotypic behaviors encompass a wide spectrum of behaviors with numerous causative factors. Conflict, stress, frustration, or anxiety-producing stimuli or situations may lead to displacement and redirected behavior, which over time might become repetitive or compulsive. Pet parent responses may further reinforce or aggravate the problem. Physical conditions, cognitive dysfunction, sensory decline, and other related brain pathology and alterations in neurotransmitters may cause or contribute to the problem in the aging pet. Repetitive pacing and aimless wandering are commonly reported in pets with cognitive dysfunction. Many oral behaviors seen in senior pets, including picas, licking, sucking, or chewing of household objects, may be due to physical conditions that cause polyphagia or GI upset (see Chapters 6, 13, and 18).

Aggression

Aggression may also arise in the older pet, although it is more commonly reported earlier in life. Physical conditions affecting appetite, mobility, cognition, sensory function, or hormonal status, and conditions leading to increased pain or discomfort, lower the threshold for exhibition of aggression. Aggression to family members may arise from physical problems contributing to pain and discomfort, changes in family makeup such as the birth of a new baby or marriage, or other changes in the schedule or household that lead to anxiety or conflict. Aggression to other family pets might arise from the introduction or maturation of a younger pet, or age-related changes in the older pet that alter the way in which the pet responds to or interacts with the other family pets. Increased aggression toward unfamiliar animals and people may result from increasing anxiety and altered sensitivity to stimuli with age. In addition, health and cognitive status may cause or influence aggression (see Chapters 23 and 24).

Restlessness/waking at night

Pets that disrupt the pet parent's sleep will impact on the pet parent's health and well-being as well as the bond with the pet. In some cases, the pet parent's frustration and concern are just as much for their pet's well-being as their own. The pet should first be closely evaluated for any physical problems that might lead to an increased frequency of elimination, restlessness, or discomfort. Sensory changes can affect the pet's depth of sleep. With age, there may also be altered sleep–wake cycles and decreased rapid eye movement (REM) sleep, which may be a component of cognitive dysfunction or other forms of CNS pathology. Pets that sleep more during the day and evening hours may be more awake through the night. In dogs, an altered response to environmental stimuli, such as paper delivery or a garage door opening, may trigger nocturnal activity and vocalization. Keeping a diary may be helpful for identifying that type of problem. Very often, pet parents report that no matter what they do or how they interact with the pet, the restlessness does not abate until morning. This can help the veterinarian distinguish between cognitive decline, physical causes, and attention-seeking behavior (should decrease when the pet parent gives attention and worsen when they withdraw attention).

Treatment of common behavior problems in senior pets

The diagnosis and treatment of behavior problems in senior pets is identical to treatment of those problems in younger pets taking into account the pet's physical, sensory, health, and cognitive limitations. Treatment plans must address the five freedoms of animal welfare: freedom to engage in species-typical behavior, freedom from fear and distress, freedom from environmental stress, freedom from pain and discomfort, and freedom from hunger and thirst (see Chapter 7).

For diagnosis and treatment for specific problems see ingestive behaviors (Chapter 13), fears, phobias, and anxiety (Chapter 14), noise aversion (Chapter 15), separation-related disorders (Chapter 17) repetitive behaviors (Chapter 18), unruly behaviors such as barking and feline vocalization (Chapters 19 and 20), house soiling (Chapters 21 and 22), and aggression (Chapters 23 and 24). However since physical health and CDS may limit the improvement that can be realistically achieved, and modifications may have to be made to the environment or schedule to cope with the problems satisfactorily such as warming canned food to promote food consumption in cats with reduced interest in eating.[123] In addition medical problems, sensory decline, and CDS may alter the pet's ability to communicate with people and other pets, and impede learning. Honest and frank discussion with the family is essential to ensure that they have realistic expectations about what might be achieved both in the short term and over time. At some point, the conversation will need to turn to quality of life, palliative and hospice care, and end-of-life issues. While these topics are not discussed directly in this text, emotional suffering is as significant as physical suffering and should be considered as a part of welfare.[41,86] For more information on welfare see Chapter 7 and the reading and resource references below.

Behavioral treatment plans for older pets should include the following recommendation categories:
1. Avoidance of triggers.
2. Modulation of fear, anxiety, stress, conflict, panic, and pain through environmental management, medications, diet, and supplements as needed.
3. Management of the environment to provide adequate outlets necessary to address breed-typical needs, increase enrichment, allow the declining pet to engage in species-typical behaviors safely and without pain and discomfort; keep the pet and the family safe and remove reinforcement for undesirable behaviors.
4. Pathways to teach desirable behaviors with positive reinforcement.
5. Education on proper interactions with the pet, species-specific body language, and proper training.
6. Discontinuation of all positive punishment techniques.
7. Discussion of quality of life and welfare.

There are times when all of these recommendations cannot be made due to time constraints or individual deficits in the veterinarian's abilities and pet parent overwhelm. When that is the case, focus on alleviation of distress and pain and avoidance of triggers. Recheck appointments can be made to address issues which could not be addressed in the initial appointment. Resources which can be found online or handouts given to pet parents can help fill in the gaps. Referral to a board-certified veterinary behaviorist is necessary when the veterinarian feels that they have exhausted their resources for creating a treatment plan.

When used in combination with medical and nutritional therapies, physical and mental exercise and enrichment have been shown to slow the progression of cognitive impairment.[66,81,135] Aged dogs trained to run on a treadmill for 10 minutes daily showed acutely improved performance on both a concurrent discrimination task and a novel object task.[136] When this exercise regimen was continued, dogs showed improved performance on an object location memory task. In humans, exercise is known to benefit brain function and has been shown to delay the onset of cognitive decline associated with AD. Finally, behavioral enrichment in aged dogs protected against neuronal loss in the hippocampus.[137]

Once established and especially when there is an impact of other body systems in combination with cognitive decline (e.g., renal, pain, and discomfort such as from degenerative joint disease or neoplasia, sensory loss, cognitive dysfunction, degenerative myelopathy, or the side effects of medications such as steroids) while significant improvement can be made in the behavioral clinical signs, relapses and adjustments to the treatment plan are inevitable as diseases of the body and cognitive decline progress. In addition, even if the health issues can be controlled or resolved, once the pet's sleep cycles are altered or the pet has learned that aggression can successfully achieve its goal, it may require a concerted effort to resolve the problems. This might involve using a combination of environmental management, behavior modification, medications, or supplements, as well as physical treatment of health problems and cognitive dysfunction. Senior pets may be more sensitive to medications with anticholinergic or sedating effects.[2,6,10,86] Combinations of supplements, medications, or higher dosages (which may have been tolerated in a younger pet) may cause side effects in older pets. Liver and renal disease (or normal aging of these organs) may cause decreased or slowed metabolism and excretion of some medications. In older pets, it is prudent to start medications and supplements at a low dose and work up the dosing range, be thoughtful and cautious regarding medication and supplement combinations, consider interactions with other medications, and be aware of P450 CYP enzyme inhibition and activation before prescribing.

Aggression

The contribution of physical problems (including pain) and cognitive dysfunction to the development and perpetuation of aggression may be difficult to assess until treatment has been implemented and any improvement can be evaluated. Management and prevention by identifying and avoiding situations that trigger aggression may be the best option. This is often in the best interest of the pet that clearly does not want to engage in the interactions.

Treatment requires a combination of identifying and avoiding triggers for aggression (e.g., keeping the pet away from potential problems, avoiding situations that incite aggression), associating positive outcomes with aggression-eliciting stimuli (counterconditioning), teaching new behavioral responses (differential reinforcement of other or incompatible behaviors), often, together with medications or supplements to treat the underlying physical issues or treat the behavior.

If the older pet is fearful, anxious, or aggressive around other pets with which it has been living previously, investigate the interactions between the pets prior to presentation. Did the pets get along well historically? Were there occasional fights? Along with the cognitive changes, sensory decline, pain, mobility, and other health issues that arise in geriatric pets, visual, olfactory, and auditory communication (the principal methods by which the dogs communicate) may be altered by changes in the way that the aged dog receives and responds to signals. This can change the nature of even a long standing relationship, causing aggression to develop. Pain or altered cognition may also contribute to failing social relationships and an increase in aggression. Once threats or aggression are displayed, learning and consequences can lead to a further deterioration in the relationship. Pet parent responses (e.g., to protect one dog or punish the offender) may also increase the pet's anxiety or interfere with the ability of the pets to learn new strategies to avoid aggression. Identifying the circumstances and locations in which problems arise and recommending avoidance will help pet parents to develop preventive strategies. If the senior pet is physically and mentally capable, it should be possible to use differential reinforcement of an alternate or other behavior and counterconditioning to help reduce anxiety and teach new behaviors that are acceptable to both pets. Pet parents may come in focused on the older dog's aggression; however, the behavior of the younger pet will be easier to modify in many cases. If both pets are not treated, poor outcomes are more likely. Even if some degree of separation is required, continuing to engage in enjoyable shared activities in which the pets show no fear, anxiety, or aggression (e.g., walks, play sessions, reward training) can help to maintain positive social relationships. With that said, past behavior does not accurately predict future behavior. Because of the level to which pet parents cannot assess accurately their pet's behavior, it is better to recommend that the pets be separated at all times unless there is an adult to engage in proactive supervision. The primary goal should be the safety of the pets and the family.

Many pet parents get a younger dog or cat as their older one ages in order to prevent having a petless household when the older pet dies or potentially as a friend to the older pet. Even friendly older dogs and cats often receive a puppy or kitten coolly. The introduction of a new pet may lead to increased anxiety because of the alterations in the attention, play, or exercise the pet receives, painful interactions which are intended as play by the puppy or kitten, and inability to have reasonable access to resources. If the older pet is sufficiently healthy and has had adequate socialization, problems can usually be prevented with controlled introductions and training for the newcomer. Hopefully, the new pet might add valuable social companionship and enrichment for the senior dog, while a young dog can benefit from the social interactions and observational learning of the senior pet. However, if the elderly dog has physical problems, has been inadequately socialized to other pets, or is fearful or anxious about meeting unfamiliar dogs, introduction of a new pet should be avoided, or the introductions will need to be done very gradually and positively while avoiding as much disruption as possible to the senior pet's home or lifestyle. If an older dog becomes fearful or aggressive when a new puppy is introduced, the dogs should be separated whenever they cannot be proactively supervised. Not only does this affect the quality of life of the older dog that deserves peaceful golden years, but also the development of the younger dog that may develop its own behavior disorder as a result of the negative interactions. The family may at first have to provide play, exercise, and training with each dog independently. In some cases, the dogs may engage successfully in positive activities such as reward training, walks, and play but become aggressive over pet parent attention and resources in the home. Pet parents are often distressed that the older dog is showing aggression to the new dog or puppy. It is not uncommon for older pets to be presented for euthanasia or relinquished for this very problem. Pet parents should be counseled that the older dog, much like some older people, finds comfort in the structure routines and predictability of the household, may have underlying deficits in physical health or cognition, and the added unfamiliarity with the dog that just entered the home. In this case, there is a disparity in the needs of the two dogs. The needs of each must be met separately at first. The younger or new dog must have appropriate training before it is allowed to interact with the older dog. It is often easier to control the younger dog rather than alter the behavior of the senior dog. It is possible to countercondition the older dog to accept the younger dog's presence; however, without proper training the younger dog will continue to interact in undesirable ways with the senior dog. If the family can achieve and reinforce successful outcomes when the dogs interact, it should be possible to shape a healthy social relationship successfully in most cases.

Cats that are not well socialized may react with aggression (often due to fear, but territorial aggression is also possible) toward new cats and kittens. Introductions to new cats and kittens should always be done slowly. Separating the new cat into a room of its own and slow and gradual introduction with counterconditioning may be successful (see Chapter 24), but the prognosis can be guarded for achieving success since the genetics, sociability, previous experience, environment, or health of the senior cat may preclude the development of a healthy social relationship with other cats. If the new cat is an adult that is social and calm around other cats, or perhaps a social young kitten (7–9 weeks), there may be a more successful long-term outcome, but introductions will still need to be gradual. Another issue is that physical problems and cognitive decline could contribute to a breakdown in the social relationships between existing cats. Treatment of underlying physical problems, desensitization, counterconditioning, medications, supplements, and pheromones (e.g., Feliway) may be effective, but it can be difficult to reestablish a healthy social relationship between an aging cat and other cats in the home once it has been altered. As is the case with dogs, pet parents may need reminding that the quality of life of the older pet is paramount. Helping them understand that the cat or dog did not get a vote in whether there would be another pet in the household and most likely would have voted against the adoption if permitted can go a long way in helping pet parents understand the plight of the older animal. Another way to help the pet parents understand would be to draw analogies to their own lives. Would they desire to live with a roommate not of their choosing? What if it was a toddler? Most people will answer no to these questions, opening the door for an honest conversation of what the pet is experiencing. For full treatment of aggression, see Chapters 23 and 24.

Restlessness/waking at night

Some of the common contributing factors for night waking in dogs and cats include CDS and other neurological diseases, pain, an increased need to eliminate, sensory decline, hypertension, and the side effects of medications prescribed to treat diseases of other body systems (see Chapter 6). Further compounding the problem is that even if the underlying cause can be identified and controlled or resolved, once the pet's sleep cycle is altered, it will often require a combination of physical and behavioral approaches to reestablish an acceptable sleep/wake cycle or to manage the problem successfully.

Some pets may have difficulty settling and falling asleep; others may fall asleep normally but wake multiple times a night, while some pets may be unable to settle through the entire night. It is also important to review the entire behavioral history, including the pet's activity level during the daytime, since some pets may have no appreciable decline in daytime activity, while others can display unsettled and repetitive daytime activity or excessive sleep, low activity levels, a decreased desire for play and social interactions, and what might be described as "apathy." Some dogs and most cats wake up at a set time each night. This is an essential part of the history which should be obtained to properly dose medications or modify the environment to help the patient sleep.

Since cats tend to be more active at night or especially around dawn, it is important to determine if the nighttime waking is a change from previous sleep patterns. If the night waking is accompanied by increased activity with aimless wandering and repetitive behaviors, decreased response to stimuli, altered social interactions with pet parents, or an overall decline in play and activity, these signs are consistent with cognitive dysfunction, provided other physical causes are ruled out.

Cats and dogs may wake more frequently at night if there is an increase in nighttime activities (e.g., noise, other animals) outside the home. Noise sensitivities may be more pronounced at night, presumably due to reduced ambient noise, which may lead to nighttime waking even if the stimulus is not audible to the family. In addition to ruling out all possible health issues, the history should focus on the pet's daily routine, the pattern of nighttime waking, and any other changes in health or behavior.

Treatment of nighttime waking without formally diagnosed CDS generally involves treatment of any disorders which cause pain or discomfort, medications to help induce sleep, changes to the schedule to assist with sleep, and enrichment during the day. Basic recommendations begin with an attempt to increase predictability and enrichment during the daytime hours. Exposure to fresh air and ambient light may help to reduce anxiety and improve cognition and nighttime sleep. When health problems or cognitive decline limit the pet's daytime activity, the pet parents should find alternate forms of play and enrichment (see Treatment of Cognitive Dysfunction, below). At bedtime, helping the dog to settle with reward training, massage, gentle petting, or quiet time can help calm dogs that cannot fall asleep because of agitation or arousal. Reducing ambient noises using white noise devices (assuming they do not interfere with sleep) and keeping a night light turned on might help some pets. Finding and reinforcing the use of a bedding location or surface where the pet is most comfortable can be helpful. Most pets benefit from having a specific resting area where they would prefer to sleep; this may be in a crate or dog bed, and/or in a family member's bedroom. A heated bed or memory foam padding may be attractive to some pets and ease pain or discomfort. A baby gate at the doorway, closing the bedroom door, or using a crate at night (if the pet is conditioned and appreciates being in a crate) may prevent the pet from wandering at night. The preferred location for some pets may be in another room, away from family members. The key is to find what comforts the pet, does not contribute to its distress, and helps the pet parent sleep.

Throughout the day, the pet parents should consistently and predictably reinforce only desirable behaviors (e.g. relaxed, social, play) and not vocal or attention seeking behaviors. Increased play, exercise (within the pet's ability), and reward-based training can be helpful. Relaxation can be taught to both dogs and cats (see Chapters 17 and 24). Clicker training or training with a remote treat dispenser which can remotely deliver treats at the pet's resting site can help to more immediately reward and shape desired behaviors. Another option for some cats that wake early is to utilize a timed feeder so that the pet can occupy itself without gaining pet parent attention.

Advise families that punishment or scolding can contribute to the pet's fear, anxiety, stress, conflict, panic, or frustration and while it may make them feel better, it most certainly will make the pet's problem worse. In addition, their pet is giving them trouble because it is having trouble and suffering. Punishment is contraindicated. Attending to the vocalization of the pet (especially during the night) by feeding, affection, allowing the pet outdoors or onto the bed may temporarily quiet the pet but can perpetuate these behaviors by reinforcing the behavior and schedule. Nonetheless, the pet parents are often suffering too from sleep deprivation and worry about their pet. Many times, they do whatever they can to get some sleep. While academically, the veterinarian understands that this is the wrong course and should advise the pet parent of such, this is also a time for empathy for the pet parent. It is best to try to make reasonable treatment plans which take into account the welfare of the pet and the pet parent.

When nighttime waking is related to cognitive dysfunction, treatment with medications and products for CDS and increased environmental enrichment in conjunction with the behavioral techniques discussed above may markedly improve the problem. Natural therapeutics such as melatonin, pheromones, l-theanine or alpha-casozepine supplements, aromatherapy or essential oils (See chapter 12) or drugs such as gabapentin, pregabalin, trazodone or some benzodiazepines may aid in calming, and alleviating signs associated with FASCP and for inducing or maintaining sleep if dosed prior to bedtime. For the dog or cat that has difficulty settling at night but then sleeps well, situational use of anxiolytics which may promote sleep may be beneficial as adjunctive therapy to behavior modification. Benzodiazepines may be useful due to their rapid onset and short-acting anxiolytic and sedative effects, but cognitive impairment, increased activity and paradoxical excitement may be seen in some pets. In senior pets, especially where liver function might be compromised, clonazepam, lorazepam, or oxazepam might be preferable to diazepam or clorazepate since they have no active intermediate metabolites. Since pain may contribute to unsettled sleep or night waking, consider pain management products. Gabapentin might be a consideration both as an adjunctive therapy for pain management as well as for its behavioral calming effects. Dose nighttime medications intended to relieve anxiety and or help pet's sleep 1 to 2 hours prior to the time when the patient usually wakes up. If the pet wakes up at 4 am, and the pet parent goes to sleep at 11 pm, the medication should be administered at bedtime. If the pet wakes up at 12 am and the pet parent goes to sleep at 11 pm, the medications should be administered at 10–10:30 pm. If the pet does not settle at all at bedtime and the pet parent goes to sleep at 11 pm, the medications should be administered at 9 to 9:30 pm.

For senior pets with generalized anxiety, noise phobias, or separation-related disorders that are not restricted to nighttime anxiety, ongoing continuing use medications may be required alone, or in combination with situational medications. Consider medications with fewer side effects such as sertraline or buspirone (which are not effective for situational problems and typically require 2–4 weeks to full effect). Before prescribing check for any potential drug interactions, and their potential impact on organ health and cognition.

Treatment of cognitive dysfunction

When cognition is impaired, diet, medications, or supplements can be useful in improving signs, slowing the progress of CDS, and making pets more amenable to environmental changes and behavior modification. Canine studies have also shown that mental stimulation is an essential component in maintaining quality of life and that continued enrichment in the form of training, play, exercise, and novel toys can help to maintain cognitive function (i.e., use it or lose it).[43,66,81,135,136] Maintaining a regular, predictable enriched daily routine and providing the pet with control to engage in pleasant interactions and avoid unpleasant ones can help to reduce stress and anxiety, improve cognitive function and quality of life, and maintain temporal orientation.[41,86] This is analogous to human studies in which education, Mental (brain) activities, and physical exercise have been found to delay the onset of dementia. However, excessive change can be stressful, especially to the senior pet, so any change in the household or routine should be gradual. Inconsistency and lack of control can cause stress and negatively impact health and behavioral well-being.

Since physical problems may reduce the pet's ability or interest in engaging in some forms of enrichment, pet parents should find alternative activities (e.g., short walks, tug toys, find-and-seek, reward training) and new forms of object play (e.g., food manipulation toys, chew toys, hanging feeding toys for cats) that are within the pet's physical and mental capabilities. See Chapters 5 and 13 for more information on food toys (see Figures 8.9 and 8.10). As sensory acuity, sensory processing, and cognitive function decline, adding new olfactory, tactile, and sound cues might help the pet better navigate its environment and maintain some degree of environmental familiarity and comfort.

Additional modifications may be required if mobility is affected or urinary frequency or control becomes an issue. Dogs

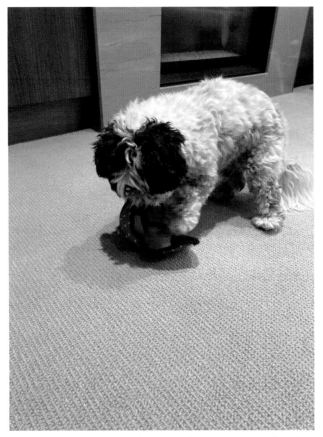

Figure 8.9 Canine enrichment food manipulation toy – Kong Hide and Treat. *(Courtesy Gary Landsberg.)*

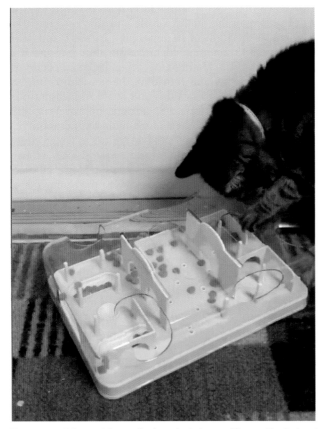

Figure 8.10 Feline enrichment food manipulation toy. *(Courtesy Lisa Radosta.)*

may require more frequent trips outdoors, a dog walker, or an indoor elimination area if they have physical conditions leading to polyuria or incontinence. Ramps and physical support may be required for pets with mobility issues. More litterboxes, larger boxes, or more frequent cleaning may be required for cats with polyuria. Ramps, litterboxes with lower sides, larger boxes, boxes on every floor of the home, or relocation of litterboxes may be required for cats with mobility problems. Provision of nonslip surfaces or rugs are a must for pets that tend to fall or slip, especially on stairs. Helping the pet feel secure in its environment will lower stress.

Medications

A comprehensive evaluation of the pet's physical health, including any concurrent medications (or natural supplements) should precede the use of any medication in senior pets. Selegiline Anipryl, Zoetis, https://www2.zoetisus.com/content/_assets/docs/Petcare/anipryl-pi.pdf) is licensed and labeled for dogs in North America for the treatment of CDS and is classified as MAOB inhibitor (although the extent to which it affects MAOB in dogs has not been well documented).[97,138] It may enhance dopamine and other catecholamines in the cortex and hippocampus and has been shown both in the laboratory and clinical setting to enhance cognitive function.[139,140] Selegiline has been shown to increase 2-phenylethylamine (PEA) in the dog brain. PEA is a neuromodulator that enhances dopamine and catecholamine function and may itself enhance cognitive function.[141] Selegiline may also alleviate CDS by increased release and decreased reuptake of norepinephrine. Catecholamine enhancement may lead to improved neuronal impulse transmission. Selegiline metabolites l-amphetamine, and l-methamphetamine may also enhance cognitive function. Selegiline may contribute to a decrease in free radical load in the brain. By inhibition of MAOB, fewer toxic free radicals may be produced. In addition, in dogs, selegiline increases enzymes that scavenge free radicals such as superoxide dismutase.[142] Selegiline may also have neuroprotective effects on dopaminergic, noradrenergic, and cholinergic neurons. Some dogs improve within the first two weeks, while a few do not show improvement until the second month.[140] Selegiline should not be used concurrently with other MAO inhibitors such as amitraz and medications that might increase serotonin transmission such as SSRIs, serotonin reuptake inhibitors/antagonists, and tricyclic antidepressants.

Since the elderly are particularly susceptible to the effects of anticholinergic drugs, it is prudent to consider therapies with less anticholinergic effects in both dogs and cats.[10,98,99] While drugs that enhance cholinergic transmission might be beneficial, acetylcholine inhibitors currently in use for humans, such as donepezil and phenserine, do not have established pharmacokinetic profiles for use in pets, although there have been case reports of donepezil use.[143] Laboratory studies with donepezil at 1.5 mg/kg demonstrated improvement in DNMP memory on a longer delay while phenserine at 0.5 mg/kg also significantly improved memory performance on a longer delay as well as an oddity discrimination task.[144]

Propentofylline is licensed in some countries (outside of North America) for the treatment of dullness, lethargy, and depressed demeanor in old dogs. Propentofylline may increase blood flow to muscles and brain. It inhibits platelet aggregation and thrombus formation. Drugs that may enhance the noradrenergic system such as adrafanil and modafinil might be useful in older dogs to improve alertness and help maintain normal sleep–wake cycles by increasing daytime exploration and activity.[145] These medications might therefore be a consideration to increase mental alertness and daytime activity.

Other treatment strategies may include the N-methyl-D-aspartate receptor antagonist memantine and some newer therapeutics under investigation including crisdesalazine (GedaCure) an inhibitor of microsomal prostaglandin E synthase-1 (https://www.businesswire.com/news/home/20210210005036/en) and a novel butyrylcholinesterase inhibitor.[146–148]

No medications are presently approved for use in cats; therefore, the possibility of improving signs must be weighed against the potential risks. Selegiline has been anecdotally reported to be useful in clinical cases of CDS in senior cats.[23,6,10,41,149] Improvement in disorientation, vocalization, and affection have been reported in cats at a dose of 0.5–1 mg/kg in the morning and a small study found no evidence of toxicity at a dose up to 10 mg/kg.[2,3,6,10,149,150] Except for occasional vomiting and excess salivation at the highest dose, adverse effects were not reported.[148] Propentofylline has been anecdotally reported to be useful in cats at one-quarter of a 50-mg tablet (12.5 mg/CAT) daily.[2,3,6,35] In addition, telmisartan (an angiotensin receptor blocker, is also currently being studied.[2,35]

Nutritional and dietary therapy

Another strategy in the treatment of CDS is the use of diets and supplements to improve antioxidant defenses and reduce the toxic effects of free radicals. The use of combined ingredients may have a synergistic effect to reduce cognitive decline. Risk factors that have been associated with accelerated brain aging and the risk of AD in humans include DHA deficiency; high homocysteine; low vitamin B6, vitamin B12, and folic acid; chronic oxidative stress; and chronic low-grade inflammation.[78,116] Therefore, nutritional supplements and diets that target these risk factors might improve brain function and slow decline. In humans, a number of studies have found that dietary management together with physical activity dietary management with fruits, vegetables, whole grains, legumes, nuts, fish and polyunsaturated fatty acids (PUFA's) in the form of fish oils might reduce the risk or delay the onset of cognitive impairment.[79,149]

In dogs, a senior diet (Canine b/d, Hill's Pet Nutrition) has been shown to improve the signs and slow the progress of cognitive decline.[52,63,66,81,82,118,135] It is supplemented with a combination of omega-3 fatty acids, antioxidants (vitamins C and E, beta carotene, selenium, ascorbic acid, flavonoids, and carotenoids), DL-alpha-lipoic acid, and L-carnitine, which are intended to enhance mitochondrial function.

The diet improved performance on a number of cognitive tasks when compared to a nonsupplemented diet, beginning as early as 2–8 weeks after the onset of therapy.[63] After two years, a control group (no enrichment, control diet) showed a dramatic decline in cognitive function, while those in either the enriched diet or the environmental enrichment group alone continued to do better than controls. The combined effect of the enriched diet plus the enriched environment provided the greatest improvement.[52,66,81,82,118,135]

Supplementing diets with MCT can provide an alternative source of energy for aging neurons, in the form of ketone bodies, as brain glucose metabolism declines with age.[61,79] Adding MCT oils to the diet increases levels of the ketone body beta-hydroxybutyrate, which has been shown to improve cognition in memory-impaired humans and to improve cognitive dysfunction significantly in canine patients.[42,64,79,152] Diets supplemented with MCTs have also been shown to improve mitochondrial function, increase PUFA's and decrease amyloid precursor protein in the parietal cortex of aged dogs.[153,154] Compared with controls, dogs fed a diet supplemented with 5.5% MCT over eight months showed significantly better performance on complex learning tasks compared to controls. Treated dogs demonstrated elevated levels of the ketone body beta-hydroxybutyrate.[64] In another 6-month study in Beagles aged 9–11.5 years, dogs fed the Brain Protection Blend- (BPB) supplemented diet showed significantly better performance on complex discrimination tasks.[68] The blend contains B vitamins, antioxidants including selenium and vitamins E and C, fish oil containing DHA and EPA and arginine, which were selected to address risk factors for cognitive decline.[42,68,79] Purina Bright Minds Senior Dog Foods are supplemented with both BPB plus 5.5% MCT. A double-blind, placebo-controlled clinical trial of ProPlan Veterinary Diets Neurocare with both 6.5% MCT and the BPB blend, in dogs with CDS resulted in significant improvement in all six categories of DISHAA signs over a 3-month period and five of the categories after the first month.[42]

In middle aged and older cats, cognitive performance was improved with a BPB supplemented diet.[57] In other studies in aged cats, diets containing tocophorols, vitamin C, beta-carotene, l-carnitine, DHA, cysteine, and methionine or a combination of essential fatty acids, chondroprotectants, l-carnitine and lysine improved activity and signs of CDS.[2,3,35,155] Although diets targeting brain aging in senior cats, are not commercially available, these studies provide some insight as to the potential effect of these ingredient blends. PUFAs are considered fundamental to brain function. They play an important role in maintaining cell membrane structure, fluidity, and cell-to-cell communication.[149] Studies in humans with fish oil supplements containing DHA and EPA have demonstrated an ability to improve cognition and may slow cognitive decline in alone or in combination with B vitamins those with mild impairment.[149,157] For aging dogs and cats, PUFAs are frequently combined with other supplements or in diets for brain health.

A number of clinical trials have shown improvements in clinical signs associated with CDS in dogs using dietary supplements containing phosphatidylserine, a membrane phospholipid, that may facilitate neuronal activities such as signal transduction and stimulate acetylcholine release.[30] One product, Senilife (Ceva Animal Health) was tested on dogs using a memory task after administration of 60 days of either a placebo or the product. Performance accuracy was significantly improved in the treated group compared to baseline, and dogs receiving the supplement in the first portion of the study maintained their improved performance.[67] The product also contains vitamin B6 (pyridoxine), vitamin E, resveratrol, which may protect against oxidative damage, and reduce beta-amyloid secretion and gingko biloba, which may have neuroprotective and antioxidant effects, improve cerebral blood flow, and enhance dopaminergic transmission. Although also labeled for use in cats, efficacy studies have not been published. Another product containing phosphatidylserine, in combination with omega-3 fatty acids, vitamins E and C, L-carnitine, alpha-lipoic acid, coenzyme Q, and selenium (Aktivait, Vet Plus), demonstrated significant improvement over placebo in signs of disorientation, social interactions, and house soiling in dogs.[27] A feline version of Aktivait, with no alpha-lipoic acid due to its potential toxicity in cats, is also available, but has not been tested in clinical trials.[158] Choline and phosphatidylcholine are precursors of acetylcholine and, as such, may enhance acetylcholine transmission, although there is no evidence to support their efficacy.

Another nutraceutical supplement, DiSenior, containing a mixture of krill oil, gingko biloba, vitamin E, glucosamine, and several botanical ingredients, has shown a positive effect on learning in aged dogs and on neuronal function in vitro.[51,159]

S-AdenosylMethionine (SAMe) is formed from methionine and adenosine triphosphate. SAMe may help to maintain cell membrane fluidity and receptor function and regulate neurotransmitter levels as well as increase the production of glutathione. Improvement has recently been demonstrated in executive function in laboratory studies in both dogs and cats.[65] In addition, in a placebo-controlled trial, greater improvement in activity and awareness was reported in dogs in the SAMe group after eight weeks.[36] Since SAMe may enhance central serotonin levels, caution should be used when combining with other drugs that might increase serotonin.

Several other therapeutic options that may have applications for the treatment of CDS in dogs include Huperzine A, curcurmin, an ultramicronized palmitoethynolamide supplement,

---

Box 8.3 Management of behavior problems in senior pets

1. Treat underlying physical problems (resolution or improvement will not be possible for some physical conditions). Therefore, the pet parent's expectations will need to be modified and accommodations may need to be made to the pet's schedule or environment to meet the needs or limitations of some senior pets.
2. Treat cognitive dysfunction if present or suspected. This may lead to an improvement in clinical signs. Retraining may not be possible if cognitive function is impaired.
3. Assess response to therapy:
   (a) If behavioral signs have been resolved following physical treatment, then the physical problem or cognitive dysfunction has likely been the cause of the behavioral problem.
   (b) If there has been some but incomplete, improvement, then review the diagnosis to determine if additional contributing problems may be improved with treatment.
   (c) Consider the impact of any drug, dietary, or alternative therapy on behavior, and if this is a factor, consider whether an alternative drug or dose might be appropriate and whether the benefits outweigh potential side effects.
   (d) Review the progress of the problem, as there may be learned and conditioned factors that will also need to be addressed with behavior therapy and environmental modification.
4. Treat primary or secondary behavior problems.
5. Continue or increase enrichment through increased social interactions, ongoing training, and novel ways to engage in exploration and object play, for example, food manipulation toys.
6. Make changes slowly to reduce potential stress. Identify sources of stress or anxiety, prevent or avoid in the short term, and work to resolve with response substitution and counterconditioning in the long term.

---

and a novel lipid extract containing brain-derived phopsholipids and DHA in aged pets.[10,123,160]

For a summary of management options for senior pet behavior problems, see Box 8.3.

CASE EXAMPLES

Case 1

Presentation

Tony, an 11-year-old, 5 kg, orange male, neutered tabby cat, was presented for spraying on the patio doors.

History

Tony had been seen spraying on the patio doors intermittently for a month. Neighborhood cats frequented the patio, but until recently, Tony had exhibited no indoor spraying. A complete behavioral assessment revealed no obvious changes to Tony's household or environment. He had two litterboxes, both of adequate size and scooped daily.

Workup

The physical examination was within normal limits. A complete blood count, serum chemistry, T4, ProBnp, urinalysis, fecal antigen + giardia were performed.

Differential diagnoses

Differential diagnoses included endocrine, renal, metabolic diseases, CDS and urine marking due to social or environmental causes. Tony's thyroxine level was markedly elevated, and hyperthyroidism was diagnosed. His score on the CDS screening tool was consistent with mild signs of CDS. After diagnostics were received, he was diagnosed with urine marking due to underlying hyperthyroidism.

Treatment

Tony was referred to a specialist for radioiodine treatment. The pet parent was educated about the risks of encouraging stray cats to come into the back yard. In addition, she received information on environmental enrichment.

Followup

The veterinary technician called Tony's pet parent two weeks after discharge from the specialty hospital and she reported that Tony had not been seen spraying since returning from the specialty hospital. Approximately six months later, Tony was again presented for spraying near the patio door. After careful questioning, the pet parent shared that her mother and her cat were living in the house with them indefinitely. The other cat was kept in a separate room in the house and she was not planning to introduce the cats. Differential diagnoses included endocrine, renal, and metabolic diseases, and urine marking due to social or environmental causes. A physical examination and repeat laboratory testing were completed. All findings were within normal limits. In light of this, he was diagnosed with urine marking due to social stress. The pet parent was given several resources for trapping feral cats humanely and several rescue and shelter resources. The veterinarian also recommended using window film so that he could not see the stray cats, continue cleaning the boxes as she had been, clean the areas where he had sprayed with one of the recommended cleaners, and plug in pheromone diffusers. Finally, the recommendation was made to keep the cats separated. The pet parent was educated about how stress can accumulate in the environment to lower inhibitions for stress-related behaviors. These changes were successful in stopping the recurrence of the urine spraying.

Case 2

Presentation

Jody was a 13-year-old, 6 kg spayed female Beagle cross that had begun to wake the pet parents every night at about 12 am by pacing and vocalizing.

History

Jody traditionally slept in her dog bed on the bedroom floor. When the problem first began, the pet parents attempted to leave Jody outside the bedroom with the door closed. This only led to louder vocalization as well as digging and scratching at the door. The pet parents would attempt to put Jody outdoors to eliminate when she woke, but she merely waited outside the door to be allowed back in. They had tried feeding her, petting her, and playing with her. She did not eat when food was offered and although she tolerated petting, it did not comfort her. During the daytime, there was no apparent increased frequency of elimination, and the pet parents noted no other apparent changes except a decreased responsiveness to previously trained cues and occasional restless pacing. The pet parents also felt there was a decrease in hearing ability, although she could successfully be woken by calling her name loudly when she was sleeping. Her score on the CDS screening tool was consistent with moderate CDS.

Workup

Physical evaluation, CBC, serum chemistry, urinalysis and fecal antigen + giardia were performed. The only abnormality was a moderate increase in serum alkaline phosphatase. Further studies were conducted in consideration of a possible diagnosis of hyperadrenocorticism. Results of a low-dose dexamethasone suppression test were equivocal, but there was no measurable increase in water intake and specific gravity of the urine of first morning sample showed a concentration of >1.025. A diagnosis of hyperadrenocorticism could not be confirmed at this time. The pet parents declined further diagnostics.

Differential diagnoses

Differential diagnoses included cognitive dysfunction, discomfort due to endocrine, metabolic or orthopedic disease, attention-seeking behavior, cognitive dysfunction, loss of hearing, panic attacks, and aversion to sounds during the night. There were no obvious sounds at night, and she did not have a history of noise aversion. Laboratory testing did not yield any definitive diagnoses and she was not placated when being petted. Her CDS screening tool score was moderate and CDS was considered as a potential final diagnosis.

Treatment

The pet parents were instructed to provide an additional play, exercise, and training session in the afternoon and prior to bedtime, and to try and keep Jody awake and stimulated with feeding and chew toys during the evenings. They were also instructed to teach her to go to her bed on cue with the help of the handouts on the veterinary practice web site. The Hills B/D diet was sent home with them, along with a SAMe supplement and Senilife. Gabapentin was dispensed at a dose of 10 mg/kg PO at 9 pm. The pet parents were instructed that they could give up to 20 mg/kg if they did not see up to a 50% difference in Jody's behavior after 2 nights. If Jody woke the pet parents up, they were to direct her back to her bed in the room. They were further instructed to keep a log of the medication doses that they were using, the time that it

was dosed, and the effect. If she did not sleep well for 2 consecutive nights, they were to call the veterinary hospital.

Followup

The veterinary technician followed up in three days to see how Jody was doing. The pet parents reported that she loved the food toys, and they were shocked that she was able to learn anything at her age, but she was learning how to go to her bed on cue. They had been giving the supplements as directed and had started to wean her onto the new food. The veterinary technician reminded them that these treatments would take about 6–12 weeks to achieve their full efficacy. They had been giving 10 mg/kg of gabapentin at 9 pm and she was sleeping through the night.

Jody presented to the veterinarian two weeks after the initial appointment. Her parents reported that she was up again and that nothing was working. The gabapentin was not working at all. A physical examination was completed and a history taken. The veterinarian reminded them that the supplements and diets can take some time to work, that they needed to keep a log of her behavior and the dose of medication that they had given, and contact the hospital immediately when she did not sleep for 2 consecutive nights. They were instructed to increase the gabapentin to 20 mg/kg PO at 9 pm each night. They were further instructed to increase the dose by 5–10 mg/kg up to 50 mg/kg if needed if they did not see at least a 50% improvement in her clinical signs within two days and they were not seeing any side effects. A recheck was scheduled for two weeks with the doctor.

Three months later, Jody was presented for pacing and whining at night. The pet parents had canceled their 2-week recheck appointment because she was doing very well. At this time, she was waking up at 11 pm, as soon as the pet parents went to sleep. The pet parents were giving her the B/D diet Senilife, SAMe, and gabapentin at 30 mg/kg PO at 9 pm. They reported that she seemed to have more spunk during the day, was more responsive to their cues, and she was enjoying training. When asked why they had not increased the dosage of gabapentin as directed, the pet parents stated that they did not want to drug their dog. They had taught her to go to her bed and they were able to direct her earlier on in treatment to go there, but now she was too distressed. The veterinarian completed a physical examination (within normal limits), CBC, serum chemistry, and urinalysis. In the meantime, the pet parents were reminded of the previous gabapentin dosing range, and the recommendation to call the clinic if she did not sleep for 2 nights. It was recommended that they continue training, enroll her in a trick training class at the local training center, and continue the diet and the supplements. It was explained that the supplements and diet slowed the progression of brain disease and were most likely responsible for the changes in her personality for the better. The pet parents were counseled that gabapentin was a safe medication and without increasing the dosage, adding in another medication, or changing medications, it was unlikely that she would sleep.

A week later, the veterinary technician called the pet parents to give them the results of the lab work. Jody's alkaline phosphatase was increased three times normal, and the alanine transferase was now increased to one time the high normal value. It was recommended that Jody have abdominal radiographs and potentially an abdominal ultrasound. Abdominal radiographs showed an enlarged liver silhouette. Jody was referred to an internal medicine specialist, who found a mass on the right lobe of the liver. Jody's parents elected to pursue surgery. The mass was removed and found to be hemangiosarcoma. After recovery from surgery, Jody was weaned off of the gabapentin over three weeks. She slept through the night more nights than not and the pet parents were happy. The supplements and diet were continued.

References

1. Landsberg GM, Nichol J, Araujo JA. Cognitive dysfunction syndrome: a disease of canine and feline brain aging. *Vet Clin North Am: Small Anim Pract.* 2012;42:749–768.

2. Sordo L, Gunn-Moore DA. Cognitive dysfunction in cats: update on neuropathological and behavioural changes plus clinical management. *Vet Rec.* 2021;188:e3. doi:10.1002/vetr.3.

3. Landsberg GM, Denenberg S, Araujo JA. Cognitive dysfunction in cats: a syndrome we used to dismiss as 'old age'. *J Feline Med Surg.* 2010;12:837–848.

4. Colle M-A, Hauw J-J, Crespau F, et al. Vascular and parenchymal beta-amyloid deposition in the aging dog: correlation with behavior. *Neurobiol Aging.* 2000;21:695–704.

5. Rofina JE, van Ederen AM, Touissaint MJ, et al. Cognitive disturbances in old dogs suffering from the canine counterpart of Alzheimer's disease. *Brain Res.* 2006;1069:216–26.

6. Gunn-Moore D, Moffat K, Christie L-A, et al. Cognitive dysfunction and the neurobiology of ageing in cats. *J Small Anim Pract.* 2007;48:546–553.

7. Neilson JC, Hart BL, Cliff KD, et al. Prevalence of behavioral changes associated with age-related cognitive impairment in dogs. *J Am Vet Med Assoc.* 2001;218:1787–1791.

8. Madari A, Farbakova JK, Katina S, et al. Assessment of severity and progression of canine cognitive dysfunction syndrome using the CAnine DEmentia Scale (CADES). *Appl Anim Behav Sci.* 2015;171:138–145.

9. Sordo L, Breheny C, Halls V, et al. Prevalence of disease and age-related behavioural changes in cats: past and present. *Vet Sci.* 2020;7:1–19.

10. Landsberg GM, Madari A, Zika N, et al. eds. *Canine and Feline Dementia. Molecular Basis, Diagnostics, and Therapy.* Cham, Switzerland; 2017.

11. Salvin H, McGreevy PD, Sachdev PS, et al. Growing old gracefully - behavioral changes associated with successful aging in the dog, Canis familiaris. *J Vet Behav.* 2011;6:313–320.

12. Azkona G, Garcia-Beleguer S, Chacon G, et al. Prevalence and risk factors of behavioral changes associated with age-related cognitive impairment in geriatric dogs. *J Small Anim Pract.* 2009;50:87–91.

13. Bain MJ, Hart BL, Cliff KD, et al. Predicting behavioral changes associated with age-related cognitive impairment in dogs. *J Am Vet Med Assoc.* 2001;218:1792–1795.

14. Mariotti VM, Landucci M, Lippi I, et al. Epidemiological study of behavioural disorders in elderly dogs. Abstract. In: Heath S, ed. *Proceedings of the 7th International Meeting of Veterinary Behaviour Medicine.* ESVCE Belgium; 2009: 241–243.

15. Horwitz D. Dealing with common behavior problems in senior dogs. *Vet Med.* 2001;96:869–887.

16. Col R, Day C, Phillips JC. An epidemiological analysis of dog behavior problems presented to an Australian behavior clinic, with associated risk factors. *J Vet Behav.* 2016;15:1–11.

17. Bamberger M, Houpt KA. Signalment factors, comorbidity, and trends in behavior diagnoses in dogs: 1644 cases (1991–2001). *J Am Vet Med Assoc.* 2006;229:1591–1601.

18. Vite CH, Head E. Aging in the canine and feline brain. *Vet Clin North Am Small Anim Pract.* 2014;44(6):1113–1129.

19. Tapp PD, Siwak CT, Gao FQ, et al. Frontal lobe volume, function, and beta-amyloid pathology in a canine model of aging. *J Neurosci.* 2004;224:8205–8213.

20. Milgram NW, Head E, Weiner E, et al. Cognitive functions and aging in the dog: acquisition of nonspatial visual tasks. *Behav Neurosci.* 1994;108:57–68.

21. Studzinski CM, Christie LA, Arauja JA, et al. Visuospatial function in the beagle dog: An early marker of cognitive decline in a model of human cognitive aging and dementia. *Neurobiol Learn Mem.* 2006;86:197–204.

22. Tapp PD, Siwak CT, Estrada J, et al. Size and reversal learning in the beagle dog as a measure of executive function and inhibitory control in aging. *Learn Mem.* 2003;10:64–73.

23. Borras D, Ferrer I, Pumarola M, et al. Age related changes in the brain of the dog. *Vet Pathol.* 1999;36:202–211.

24. Cummings BJ, Head E, Afagh AJ, et al. β-Amyloid accumulation correlates with cognitive dysfunction in the aged canine. *Neurobiol Learn Mem.* 1996;66:11–23.

25. Head E, McCleary R, Hahn FF, et al. Region-specific age at onset of beta-amyloid in dogs: *Neurobiol Aging.* 2000;21:89–96.

26. González-Martínez Á, Rosado B, Pesini P, et al. Plasma β-amyloid peptides in canine aging and cognitive dysfunction as a model of Alzheimer's disease. *Exp Gerontol.* 2011;46:590–596.

27. Heath SE, Barabas S, Craze PG. Nutritional supplementation in cases of canine cognitive dysfunction – a clinical trial. *Appl Anim Behav Sci.* 2007;105:274–283.

28. Fast R, Schutt T, Toft N, et al. An observational study with long-term follow-up of canine cognitive dysfunction: clinical characteristics, survival and risk factors. *J Vet Intern Med.* 2013;27:822–829.

29. Moffat K, Landsberg G. An investigation of the prevalence of clinical signs of cognitive dysfunction syndrome (CDS) in cats. *J Am Anim Hosp Assoc.* 2003;39:512.

30. Osella MC, Re G, Odore R, et al. Canine cognitive dysfunction syndrome: prevalence, clinical signs and treatment with a neuroprotective nutraceutical. *Appl Anim Behav Sci.* 2007;105:297–310.

31. Rosado B, Gonzalez-Martinez A, Pesini P, et al. Effect of age and severity of cognitive dysfunction on spontaneous activity in pet dogs. Part 1- locomotor and exploratory behavior. *Vet J.* 2012;194:189–195.

32. Siwak CT, Tapp PD, Milgram NW. Effect of age and level of cognitive function on spontaneous and exploratory behaviors in the beagle dog. *Learn Memory.* 2001;8(6):317–325.

33. Siwak CT, Tapp PD, Zicker SC, et al. Locomotor activity rhythms in dogs vary with age and cognitive status. *Behav Neurosci.* 2003;117(4):813–824.

34. Siwak CT, Murphey HL, Muggenburg BA, et al. Age-dependent decline in locomotor activity in dogs is environment specific. *Physiol Behav.* 2002;75(1–2):65–70.

35. Cerna P, Gardiner H, Sordo L, Tørnqvist-Johnsen C, Gunn-Moore DA. Potential causes of increased vocalisation in elderly cats with cognitive dysfunction syndrome as assessed by their owners. *Animals.* 2020;10:1092. doi:10.3390/ani10061092.

36. Rème CA, Dramard V, Kern L, et al. Effect of S-adenosylmethionine tablets on the reduction of age-related mental decline in dogs: a double-blind placebo-controlled trial. *Vet Ther.* 2008;9:69–82.

37. Senanarong V, Cummings JL, Fairbanks L, et al. Agitation in Alzheimer's disease is a manifestation of frontal lobe dysfunction. *Dement Geratr Cogn Disord.* 2004;17:14–20.

38. McCurry SM, Gibbons LE, Logsdon RG, et al. Anxiety and nighttime behavioral disturbances. Awakenings in patients with Alzheimer's disease. *J Gerontol Nurs.* 2004;30:12–20.

39. Mongillo P, Pitteri E, Carnier P, et al. Does the attachment system towards owners change in aged dogs? *Physiol Behav.* 2013;120:64–69.

40. Marx A, Lenkei R, Pérez Fraga P, et al. Age-dependent changes in dogs' (Canis familiaris) separation-related behaviours in a longitudinal study. *Appl Anim Behav Sci.* 2021;242:105422.

41. Ray M, Carney HC, Boynton B, et al. AAFP feline senior care guidelines. *J Feline Med Surg.* 2021;23:613–638. https://journals.sagepub.com/doi/10.1177/1098612X211021538.

42. Pan Y, Landsberg G, Mougeot I, et al. Efficacy of a therapeutic diet on dogs with signs of cognitive dysfunction syndrome (CDS): a prospective double blinded placebo controlled clinical study. *Front Nutr.* 2018;5:27.

43. O'Brian ML, Herron ME, Smith AM, Aarnes TK. Effects of a four-week group class created for dogs at least eight years of age on the development and

progression of signs of cognitive dysfunction syndrome. *J Am Vet Med Assoc*. 2021;259(6):637–643.

44. Prpar Mihevc S, Majdic G. Canine cognitive dysfunction and Alzheimer's disease – two facets of the same disease? *Front Neurosci*. 2019;13:604. doi:10.3389/fnins.2019.00604.

45. Stylianaki I, Polizopoulou ZS, Theodoridis A, et al. Amyloid-beta plasma and cerebrospinal fluid biomarkers in aged dogs with cognitive dysfunction syndrome. *J Vet Intern Med*. 2020;34:1532–1540.

46. Salvin HE, McGreevy PD, Sachdev PS, et al. Under diagnosis of canine cognitive dysfunction; a cross-sectional survey of older companion dogs. *Vet J*. 2010;184: 277–281.

47. Pugliese M, Carrasco JL, Andrade C, et al. Severe cognitive impairment correlates with higher cerebrospinal fluid levels of lactate and pyruvate in a canine model of senile dementia. *Prog Neuropsychopharmacol Biol Psychiatry*. 2005;29:603–610.

48. Golini L, Clangeli R, Tranquillo V, et al. Association between neurologic and cognitive dysfunction signs in a sample of aging dogs. *J Vet Behav*. 2009;4:25–30.

49. Quimby J, Gowland S, Carney HC, et al. 2021 AAHA/AAFP Feline Life Stage Guidelines. *J Feline Med Surg*. 2021;23(3): 211–233.

50. Hammerle M, Horst C, Levine E, et al. 2015 AAHA Canine and Feline Behavior Management Guidelines. *J Am Anim Hosp Assoc* 2015;51(4):205–21.

51. Salvin HE, McGreevy PD, Sachdev PS, et al. The canine cognition dysfunction rating scale (CCDR): a data driven and ecologically relevant assessment tool. *Vet J*. 2011;188:331–336.

52. Araujo JA, Studzinski CM, Head E, et al. Assessment of nutritional interventions for modification of age-associated cognitive decline using a canine model of human aging. *Age*. 2005;27:27–37.

53. Zanghi BM, Araujo J, Milgram NW. Cognitive domains in the dog: independence of working memory from object learning, selective attention, and motor learning. *Anim Cogn*. 2015;18(3): 789–800.

54. Head E, Mehta R, Hartley J. Spatial learning and memory as a function of age in the dog. *Behav Neurosci*. 1995;109: 851–858.

55. Adams B, Chan A, Callahan H, et. al. Use of a delayed non-matching to position task to model age-dependent cognitive decline in the dog. *Behav Brain Res*. 2000;108(1):47–56.

56. Milgram NW, Landsberg GM, De Rivera C, et al. Age and cognitive dysfunction in the domestic cat. In: *Proceedings of the ACVB/AVSAB Symposium*. St. Louis; 2011:28–29.

57. Pan Y, Araujo JA, Burrows J, et al. Cognitive enhancement in middle-aged and old cats with dietary supplementation with a nutrient blend containing fish oil, B vitamins, antioxidants and arginine. *Br J Nutr*. 2013;10:1–10.

58. Cotman CW, Head E. The canine (dog) model of human aging and disease: dietary, environmental and immunotherapy approaches. *J Alzheimer's Dis*. 2008; 15(4):685–707.

59. Levine MS, Lloyd RL, Hull CD, et al. Neurophysiological alterations in caudate neurons in aged cats. *Brain Res*. 1987;401: 213–230.

60. Levine MS, Lloyd RL, Fisher RS, et al. Sensory, motor and cognitive alterations in aged cats. *Neurobiol Aging*. 1987;8: 253–263.

61. London ED, Ohata M, Takei H, et al. Regional cerebral metabolic rate for glucose in beagle dogs of different ages. *Neurobiol Aging*. 1983;4: 121–126.

62. Mongillo P, Landsberg GM, Araujo JA, et al. Validation of a cognitive test battery for cats. *J Vet Behav*. 2010;5:32.

63. Milgram NW, Head E, Muggenburg B, et al. Landmark discrimination learning in the dog: effects of age, an antioxidant fortified food, and cognitive strategy. *Neurosci Biobehav Rev*. 2002;26(6): 679–695.

64. Pan Y, Larson B, Araujo JA, et al. Dietary supplementation with medium-chain TAG has long-lasting cognition-enhancing effects in aged dogs. *Br J Nutr*. 2010;103:1746–1754.

65. Araujo JA, Faubert ML, Brooks ML, et al. Novifit (NoviSAMe) tablets improve executive function in aged dogs and cats: implications for treatment of cognitive dysfunction syndrome. *Int J Appl Res Vet Med*. 2012;10:91–98.

66. Milgram NW, Head E, Zicker SC, et al. Long term treatment with antioxidants and a program of behavioural enrichment reduces age-dependant impairment in discrimination and reversal learning in beagle dogs. *Exp Gerontol*. 2004;39:753–765.

67. Araujo JA, Landsberg GM, Milgram NW, et al. Improvement of short-term memory performance in aged beagles by a nutraceutical supplement containing phosphatidylserine, ginkgo biloba, vitamin E and pyridoxine. *Can Vet J*. 2008;49:379–385.

68. Pan Y, Kennedy AD, Jonsson TJ, et al. Cognitive enhancement in old dogs from dietary supplementation with a nutrient blend containing arginine, antioxidants, B vitamins and fish oil. *Br J Nutr*. 2018;119(3):349–358.

69. Adams B, Chan A, Callahan H, et al. The canine as a model of human cognitive aging: recent developments. *Prog Neuropsychopharm Biol Psychiatry*. 2000;24(5):675–692.

70. Head E, Callahan H, Muggenburg BA, et al. Visual-discrimination learning ability and β-amyloid accumulation in the dog. *Neurobiol Aging*. 1998;19: 415–425.

71. Head E, Milgram NW, Cotman CW. Neurobiological models of aging in the dog and other vertebrate species. In: Hof AP, Mobbs C, eds. *Functional Neurobiology of Aging*. San Diego, CA: Academic Press; 2001:457–468.

72. Araujo JA, Nobrega JN, Raymond R, et al. Aged dogs demonstrate both increased sensitivity to scopolamine and decreased muscarinic receptor density. *Pharmacol Biochem Behav*. 2011;98:203–209.

73. Harrison J, Buchwald J. Eyeblink conditioning deficits in the old cat. *Neurobiol Aging*. 1983;4:45–51.

74. McCune S, Stevenson J, Fretwell L, et al. Ageing does not significantly affect performance in a spatial learning task in the domestic cat (Felis silvestris catus). *Appl Anim Behav Sci*. 2008;112(3):345–356.

75. Heckler MC, Tranquilim MV, Svicero DJ, et al. Clinical feasibility of cognitive testing in dogs (Canis lupus familiaris). *J Vet Behav*. 2014;9(1):6–12.

76. González-Martínez Á, Rosado B, Pesini P, et al. Effect of age and severity of cognitive dysfunction on two simple tasks in pet dogs. *Vet J*. 2013;198(1): 176–181.

77. Mongillo P, Araujo JA, Landsberg GM, et al. Assessment of cognitive dysfunction in companion dogs. *J Vet Behav*. 2010;5:153.

78. Watowich MM, MacLean EL, Hare B. et al. Age influences domestic dog cognitive performance independent of average breed lifespan. *Anim Cogn* 2020;23:795–805.

79. Pan Y. Nutrients, cognitive function, and brain aging: what we have learned from dogs. *Med Sci*. 2021;9(4):72. doi:10.3390/medsci9040072.

80. Katina S, Farbakova J, Madari A, et al. Risk factors for canine cognitive dysfunction syndrome in Slovakia. *Acta Vet Scand*. 2016;58:17.

81. Head E, Nukala VN, Fenoglio KA, et al. Effects of age, dietary, and behavioral enrichment on brain mitochondria in a canine model of human aging. *Exp Neurol*. 2009;220:171–176.

82. Milgram NW, Zicker SC, Head EA, et al. Dietary enrichment counteracts age-associated cognitive dysfunction in canines. *Neurobiol Aging*. 2002;23:737–745.

83. Hart BL. Effect of gonadectomy on subsequent development of age-related cognitive impairment in dogs. *J Am Vet Med Assoc*. 2001;219(1):51–56.

84. Salvin HE, McGreevy PD, Sachdev PS, et al. The effect of breed on age-related changes in behavior and disease prevalence in cognitively normal older community dogs, *Canis lupus familiaris*. *J Vet Behav*. 2012;7:61–69.

85. Calderon-Garciduenas L, Mora-Tiscareno A, Ontiveros E, et al. Air pollution, cognitive deficits and brain abnormalities: a pilot study with children and dogs. *Brain Cogn*. 2008;68:117–127.

86. Epstein M, Kuehn N, Landsberg G, et al. AAHA senior care guidelines for dogs and

cats. *J Am Anim Hosp Assoc.* 2005; 41(2):81–91.

87. Willems A, Paepe D, Marynissen S, et al. Results of screening apparently healthy senior and geriatric dogs. *J Vet Intern Med.* 2017;31:81–92.

88. Paepe D, Verjans G, Duchateau L, et al. Routine health screening: results in apparently healthy middle aged and old cats. *J Feline Med Surg.* 2013;15(1):8–19.

89. Chambers JK, Uchida K, Nakayama H. White matter myelin loss in the brains of aged dogs. *Exp Geront.* 2012;47: 263–269.

90. Siwak-Tapp CT, Head E, Muggenburg BA, et al. Neurogenesis decreases with age in the canine hippocampus and correlates with cognitive function. *Neurobiol Learn Mem* 2007;88(2): 249–59.

91. Klug J, Snyder JM, Darvas M, et al. Aging pet cats develop neuropathology similar to human Alzheimer's disease. *Aging Pathobiol Ther.* 2020;2(3):120–125.

92. Dewey CW. Rishniw M, Johnson PJ et al. Canine cognitive dysfunction patients have reduced total hippocampal volume compared with aging control dogs: A comparative magnetic resonance imaging study. *Open Vet J* 2020;10(4): 438–42.

93. Chambers JK, Tokuda T, Uchida K, et al. The domestic cat as a natural animal model of Alzheimer's disease. *Acta Neuropathol Commun.* 2015;3:78. doi:10.1186/s40478-015-0258-3.

94. Zhang C, Hua T, Zhu Z, et al. Age related changes of structures in cerebellar cortex of cat. *J Biosci.* 2006;31:55–60.

95. Uchida K, Tani Y, Uetsuka K et al. Immunohistochemical studies on canine cerebral amyloid angiopathy and senile plaques. *J Vet Med Sci* 1992;54(4): 659–667.

96. Nakamura S, Nakayama H, Kiatipattanasakul W, et al. Senile plaques in very aged cats. *Acta Neuropathol.* 1996;91:437–439.

97. Milgram NW, Ivy GO, Head E, et al. The effect of l-deprenyl on behavior, cognitive function, and biogenic amines in the dog. *Neurochem Res.* 1993;18: 1211–1219.

98. Pugliese M, Cangitano C, Ceccariglia S, et al. Canine cognitive dysfunction and the cerebellum: acetylcholinesterase reduction, neuronal and glial changes. *Brain Res.* 2007;1139:85–94.

99. Zhang JH, Sampogna S, Morales FR, et al. Age-related changes in cholinergic neurons in the laterodorsal and the pedunculo-pontine tegmental nuclei of cats: a combined light and electron microscopic study. *Brain Res.* 2005;1052: 47–55.

100. Insua D, Suárez ML, Santamarina G, et al. Dogs with canine counterpart of Alzheimer's disease lose noradrenergic neurons. *Neurobiol Aging.* 2010;31:625–635.

101. Head E, Moffat K, Das P, et al. β-Amyloid deposition and tau phosphorylation in clinically

characterized aged cats. *Neurobiol Aging.* 2005;26:749–763.

102. Takeuchi Y, Uetsuka K, Murayama M, et al. Complementary distributions of beta-amyloid and neprilysin in the brains of dogs and cats. *Vet Pathol.* 2008;45:455–466.

103. Gunn-Moore D, Mcvee J, Bradshaw J, et al. Ageing changes in cat brains demonstrated by beta-amyloid and AT8-immunoreactive phosphorylated tau deposits. *J Feline Med Surg.* 2006;8: 234–242.

104. Cummings BJ, Satou T, Head E, et al. Diffuse plaques contain c-terminal AB42 and not AB40: evidence from cats and dogs. *Neurobiol Aging.* 1996;17: 4653–4659.

105. Ozawa M, Chambers JK, Uchida K, et al. The relation between canine cognitive dysfunction and age-related brain lesions. *J Vet Med Sci.* 2016;78(6): 997–1006.

106. Bobik M, Thompson T, Russel MJ. Amyloid deposition in various breeds of dogs. *Soc Neurosci.* 1994;20:172.

107. Sordo LS, Martini AC, Houston EF et al. Neuropathology of Aging in Cats and its Similarities to Human Alzheimer's Disease. *Front Aging* 2021;2:684607.

108. Head E, Pop V, Sarsoza F, et al. Amyloid-β peptide and oligomers in the brain and cerebrospinal fluid of aged canines. *J Alzheimers Dis.* 2010;20:637–646.

109. Habiba U, Ozawa M, Chambers JK et al. Neuronal Deposition of Amyloid-β Oligomers and Hyperphosphorylated Tau Is Closely Connected with Cognitive Dysfunction in Aged Dogs. *J Alzheimers Dis Rep.* 2021;5:749–760.

110. Brellou G, Vlennas I, Lekkas S, et al. Immunohistochemical investigation of beta-amyloid (Abeta) in the brain of aged cats. *Histol Histopathol.* 2005;20: 725–731.

111. Poncelet L, Ando K, Vergara C, et al. A 4R tauopathy develops without amyloid deposits in aged cat brains. *Neurobiol Aging.* 2019;81:200–212.

112. Smolek T, Madari A, Farbakova J, et al. Tau hyperphosphorylation in synaptosomes and neuroinflammation are associated with canine cognitive impairment. *J Comp Neurol.* 2016;524: 874–895.

113. Scuderi C, Golini L. Successful and unsuccessful brain aging in pets: pathophysiological mechanisms behind clinical signs and potential benefits from palmitoylethanolamide nutritional intervention. *Animals.* 2021;11(9):2584.

114. Yu CH, Song GS, Yhee JY, et al. Histopathological and immunohistochemical comparison of the brain of human patients with Alzheimer's disease and the brain of aged dogs with cognitive dysfunction. *J Comp Pathol.* 2011;145:45–58.

115. Abey A, Davies D, Goldsbury C, et al. Distribution of tau hyperphosphorylation in canine dementia resembles early Alzheimer's disease and other

tauopathies. *Brain Pathol.* 2021;31(1): 144–162.

116. Dowling AL, Head E. Antioxidants in the canine model of human aging. *Biochim Biophys Acta.* 2012;1822(5):685–689.

117. Cotman C, Head E, Muggenburg BA, et al. Brain aging in the canine: a diet enriched in antioxidants reduces cognitive dysfunction. *Neurobiol Aging.* 2002;23(5):809–818.

118. Fefer G, Khan MZ, Panek WK et al. Relationship between hearing, cognitive function, and quality of life in aging companion dogs. *J Vet Intern Med.* 2022 Aug 6. doi: 10.1111/jvim.16510.

119. Szabó D, Miklósi Á, Kubinyi E. Owner reported sensory impairments affect behavioural signs associated with cognitive decline in dogs. *Behav Process.* 2018;157:354–360.

120. Mills DS, Demontigny-Bédard I, Gruen G, et al. Pain and problem behavior in cats and dogs. *Animals.* 2020;10:318; doi:10.3390/ani10020318.

121. Bognár Z, Piotti P, Szabó D, et al. A novel behavioural approach to assess responsiveness to auditory and visual stimuli before cognitive testing in family dogs. *Appl Anim Behav Sci.* 2020;228. doi:10.1016/j.applanim.2020.105016.

122. Ozawa M, Inoue M, Uchida K, et al. Physical signs of canine cognitive dysfunction. *J Vet Med Sci.* 2019;81: 1829–1834.

123. Eyre R, Trehiou M, Marshall E et al. Aging cats prefer warm food. *J Vet Behav* 2022;47:86–92.

124. Fatjo J, Stub C, Manteca X. Aggression and hypothyroidism. *Vet Rec.* 2002;151: 547–548.

125. Dodman NH, Aronson L, Cottam N, et al. The effect of thyroid replacement in dogs with suboptimal thyroid function on owner directed aggression; a randomized, double-blind placebo-controlled trial. *J Vet Behav.* 2013;8: 225–230.

126. Radosta LA, Shofer FS, Reisner IR. Comparison of thyroid analytes in dogs aggressive to familiar people and in non-aggressive dogs. *Vet J.* 2011;192: 472–475.

127. Carter GR, Scott-Moncrieff JC, Luescher AU, et al. Serum total thyroxine and thyroid stimulating hormone concentrations in dogs with behavior problems. *J Vet Behav.* 2009;4:230–236.

128. Carolina Castilhos da Silva CC, Cavalcante I, de Carvalho GLC, et al. Cognitive dysfunction severity evaluation in dogs with naturally-occurring Cushing's syndrome: a matched case-control study. *J Vet Behav.* 2021;46:74–78.

129. Bécuwe-Bonnet V, Belanger MC, Frank D, et al. Gastrointestinal disorders in dogs with excessive licking of surfaces. *J Vet Behav.* 2012;7:194–204.

130. Frank D, Bélanger M-C, Bécuwe-Bonnet V, et al. Prospective medical evaluation of 7 dogs presented with fly biting. *Can Vet J.* 2012;53:1279–1284.

131. Demontigny-Bedard I, Beauchamp G, Belanger M-C, et al. Gastrointestinal evaluation of cats presented with pica. In: *VBS Proceedings*. San Antonio; 2016: 40–4413.

132. Notari L, Burman O, Mills D. Behavioral changes in dogs treated with glucocorticoids. *Physiol Behav*. 2015;151:609–616.

133. Lopes Fagundes AL, Hewison L, McPeake KJ, et al. Noise sensitivities in dogs: an exploration of signs in dogs with and without musculoskeletal pain using qualitative content analysis. *Front Vet Sci*. 2018;5:17. doi:10.3389/fvets.2018.00017.

134. Overall KL, Dunham AE, Frank DF. Frequency of nonspecific clinical signs in dogs with separation anxiety, thunderstorm phobias, and noise phobia alone or in combination. *J Am Vet Med Assoc*. 2001;219:467–473.

135. Head E. Combining an antioxidant-fortified diet with behavioral enrichment leads to cognitive improvement and reduced brain pathology in aging canines: strategies for healthy aging. *Ann N Y Acad Sci*. 2007;1114:398–406.

136. Snigdha S, de Rivera C, Milgram NW, et al. Exercise enhances memory consolidation in the aging brain. *Front Aging Neurosci*. 2014;6:3.

137. Siwak-Tapp CT, Head E, Muggenburg BA, et al. Region specific neuron loss in the aged canine hippocampus is reduced by enrichment. *Neurobiol Aging*. 2008;29:39–50.

138. Ruehl WW, Neilson J, Hart B, et al. Therapeutic actions of l-deprenyl in dogs: a model of human brain aging. In: Goldstein D, ed. *Catecholamines: Bridging Basic Science with Clinical Medicine, Progress in Brain Research*. vol. 106. NY, USA: Elsevier Press; 1996.

139. Head E, Hartley J, Mehta R, et al. The effects of l-deprenyl on spatial short term memory in young and aged dogs. *Prog Neuropsychopharmacol Biol Psychiatry*. 1996;20:515.

140. Campbell S, Trettien A, Kozan B. A non-comparative open label study evaluating the effect of seleginine hydrochloride in a clinical setting. *Vet Ther*. 2001;2:24–39.

141. Milgram NW, Ivy GO, Murphy MP, et al. Effects of chronic oral administration of l-deprenyl in the dog. *Pharmacol Biochem Behav*. 1995;51:421–428.

142. Carillo MC, Ivy GO, Milgram NW, et al. Deprenyl increases activity of superoxide dismutase. *Life Sci*. 1994;54:1483–1489.

143. Ishii MA, Irimajiri M, Yaoita Y, et al. Efficacy of combined therapy with donepezil, anti-oxidants and behavior modification technique for canine cognitive dysfunction syndrome. In: *Proc ACVB Vet Behav Symposium*. 2021: 16–17.

144. Araujo JA, Greig NH, Ingram DK, et al. Cholinesterase inhibitors improve both memory and complex learning in aged beagle dogs. *J Alzheimers Dis*. 2011;26(1): 143–155.

145. Siwak CT, Gruet P, Woehrle F, et al. Behavioral activating effects of adrafinil in aged canines. *Pharmacol Biochem Behav*. 2000;66:293–300.

146. Martinez-Coria H, Green KN, Billings LM, et al. Memantine improves cognition and reduces Alzheimer's-like neuropathology in transgenic mice. *Am J Pathol*. 2010;176:870–880.

147. Alzheimer drug discovery foundation https://www.alzdiscovery.org/uploads/cognitive_vitality_media/Crisdesalazine.pdf.

148. Zakošek Pipan M, Prpar Mihevc S, Štrbenc M et al. Treatment of canine cognitive dysfunction with novel butyrylcholinesterase inhibitor. *Sci Rep*. 2021;11(1):18098.

149. Landsberg GM. Therapeutic options for cognitive decline in senior pets. *J Am Anim Hosp Assoc*. 2006;42:407–413.

150. Ruehl WW, Griffin D, Bouchard G et al. Effects of l-deprenyl in cats in a one month dose escalation study. *Vet Path*. 1996;33(5):621.

151. Tynes VV, Landsberg GM. Nutritional management of behavior and brain disorders in dogs and cats. *Vet Clin Small Anim*. 2021;51:711–727.

152. Reger MA, Henderson ST, Hale C, et al. Effects of beta-hydroxybutyrate on cognition in memory-impaired adults. *Neurobiol Aging*. 2004;25:311–314.

153. Taha AY, Henderson ST, Burnham WM. Dietary enrichment with medium chain-triglycerides (AC-1203) elevates polyunsaturated fatty acids in the parietal cortex of aged dogs; implications for treating age-related cognitive decline. *Neurochem Res*. 2009;34:1619–1625.

154. Studzinski CM, MacKay WA, Beckett TL, et al. Induction of ketosis may improve mitochondrial function and decrease steady-state amyloid-beta precursor protein (APP) levels in the aged dog. *Brain Res*. 2008;1226:209–217.

155. Kaur H, Singla A, Snehdep S, et al. Role of omega-3 fatty acids in canine health: a review. *Int J Curr Microbiol Appl Sci*. 2020;9(3):2283–2293.

156. Houpt KA, Levine E, Landsberg GM, et al. Antioxidant fortified food improves owner perceived behavior in the aging cat. In: *Proceedings ESFM Feline Conference, Prague, September 21–23*, 2007.

157. Oulhaj A, Jernerén F, Refsum H, et al. Omega-3 fatty acid status enhances the prevention of cognitive decline by B vitamins in mild cognitive impairment. *J Alz Dis*. 2016;50:547–57.

158. Hill AS, Werner JA, Rogers QR et al. Lipoic acid is 10 times more toxic in cats than reported in humans, dogs or rats. *J Anim Physiol Anim Nutr*. 2004;88:150–6.

159. Pero ME, Cortese L, Mastellone V, et al. Effects of a nutritional supplement on cognitive function in aged dogs and on synaptic function of primary cultured neurons. *Animals*. 2019;9(7):393.

160. Araujo JA, Segarra S, Mendes J et al. Sphingolipids and DHA Improve Cognitive Deficits in Aged Beagle Dogs. *Front Vet Sci*. 2022;139(9):646–451.

Resources and recommended reading

Creevy KE, Grady J, Little SE et al. 2019 AAHA Canine Life Stage Guidelines. *J Am Anim Hosp Assoc*. 2019;55(6):267–290.

Geriatric Screening Questionnaire – https://todaysveterinarypractice.com/wp-content/uploads/sites/4/2022/02/Geriatric-Questionnaire-Lap-of-Love.pdf.

International Association for Animal Hospice and Palliative Care - https://iaahpc.org/

Landsberg GM, Madari A, Zika N, et al. eds. *Canine and Feline Dementia. Molecular Basis, Diagnostics, and Therapy*. Cham, Switzerland: Springer International Publishing. 2017.

Purina Institute. Aging brain: https://www.purinainstitute.com/science-of-nutrition/advancing-brain-health/aging-brain.

Quimby J, Gowland S, Carney HC, et al. 2021 AAHA/AAFP Feline Life Stage Guidelines. *J Feline Med Surg*. 2021;23(3):211–233.

Rajapaksha E. Special considerations for diagnosing behavior problems in older pets. *Vet Clin North Am Small Anim Pract*. 2018;48(3):443–456.

Shearer T, (ed). Palliative medicine and hospice care. *Vet Clin North Am*. 2010;41: 477–702.

Sung W, Landsberg G. Nutritional intervention in Canine Cognitive Dysfunction. Today's Veterinary Practice. March/April 2020, 28–31.

Wilhelmy J, Landsberg GM. Cognitive and emotional disorders in the aging pet. In: McMillan F, ed. *Mental Health and Well-Being in Animals*. 2nd ed. Wallingford, Oxfordshire CABI; 2019.

CHAPTER 9

Approach to the diagnosis and treatment

Lisa Radosta, DVM, DACVB

Introduction

Behavioral disorders in dogs and cats are underdiagnosed and undertreated. For example, approximately 17% of dogs in the United States have separation-related disorders and 50% may have noise aversion.[1-3] Undoubtedly, there is a need for veterinarians competent in the diagnosis and treatment of behavior disorders. At the time of this writing, there is a disparity between the level of education received by veterinarians, even those newly graduated, and the level of knowledge necessary to help companion animals with behavioral complaints. From doorknob questions to full behavioral consultations, there are many opportunities to help patients that are suffering from behavioral disorders or that simply have undesirable behaviors, which affect the bond with the family. Historically, the approach to behavior cases included the veterinarian spending 1–3 hours with the pet parent, reviewing a detailed questionnaire, videos, and images. While that may still be the standard of care at referral practices, achieving that in one 20-minute appointment in veterinary practice is unrealistic. Instead, the veterinarian can achieve the same result over three to four appointments without delaying treatment. For those veterinarians who have the time or would prefer to schedule longer initial assessments, the workflow differs, but the approach is the same.

Differing perspectives on the diagnosis and treatment of behavioral changes

As with much of veterinary medicine, there are different, scientifically valid ways to approach the discipline of behavioral medicine. The four most common approaches are behaviorism, neurobiological approach, psychobiological approach, and the French (Pageat) approach. A brief summary of each is below. Recently, the one-medicine approach has been presented, which we espouse in this text and takes elements from the four approaches mentioned above.

Behavioral approach (behaviorism)

The behavioral approach (behaviorism) is commonly regarded as the beginning of modern psychology and is the approach adopted by some scientists and many applied animal behaviorists. By definition, the behavioral approach assesses behavioral changes with an emphasis on the study of objective and observable facts (external stimuli and overt behaviors) rather than subjective and qualitative processes.[4] This is the basis of applied behavior analysis. In this approach, intrinsic processes are not considered as factors affecting behavior. However, intrinsic processes do affect the expression of behavioral clinical signs and those processes are often measurable (e.g., immune response, heart rate, blood pressure, and respiratory rate). The one-medicine approach includes the concepts of applied behavior analysis as a part of the assessment of behavior change with consideration of objective measurement of intrinsic and extrinsic factors affecting behavior change.

Neurobiological approach

The neurobiological approach suggests that behavior problems stem from pathology in the body relating to systemic disease or neurochemical changes, leading to the characterization of behavior changes as disorders. While there may be underlying pathology that can be objectively measured, leading to grouping of clinical signs and final diagnoses, the exploration of behavioral pathology is lacking at this time. Even when pathology in neurochemistry is present, it is unclear if the pathology was present prior to or as a result of the development of the behavioral change. For example, dogs with some forms of aggression have altered 5-HIAA (5-hydroxyindoleacetic acid) concentrations in the central nervous system (CNS).[5] Were these changes caused by epigenetic factors or were they present prior to the behavioral change? At this time, we do not know. Furthermore, some behaviors which are seemingly normal but undesirable must be characterized in order to create a treatment plan. These behaviors are left out of the neurobiological model. The one-medicine model recognizes that pathology is often present, even in behaviors which are normal and undesirable, and that the pathology may be a result of the disorder, a contributing cause, or the etiology. It may also be an intrinsic factor which reinforces or punishes expressed behaviors. Within this model are diagnoses which may simply be descriptions of the behavior (e.g., feline periuria) or may be motivational (e.g., fear-induced aggression). As more evidence is uncovered for biological tests that can elucidate intrinsic processes, veterinarians will better be able to name behavioral changes accurately.

Psychobiological approach

The psychobiological approach combines comparative psychology, evolutionary and behavioral biology, and the neurobiological basis of behavior, considering the context, motivation, and emotion. Motivations are grouped into nine categories: desirables, frustrations, threats, pains, affiliates, attachment figures and objects, dependents, potential sexual partners, and undesirables.[6] More than a few scientifically validated behavior assessments tools have been developed from this approach. See Recommended Reading below. The one-medicine approach, much like the psychobiological approach, looks to find the function, but it differs in that there is more emphasis put on the motivation of the behavior. In the psychobiological approach, the behavioral approach, and the one-medicine approach, the consequences (reinforcement and punishment) are considered in diagnosis and treatment. See Chapter 25 for more information on the psychobiological approach.

French (Pageat) approach

The French approach, like the psychobiological and the one-medicine approaches, considers clinical signs exhibited, accepts that some behavior patterns for which pets are presented and are undesirable are not necessarily associated with physiologic pathology, and considers all inputs (genetic and epigenetic) which might be affecting the behavior. It differs in that the clinical signs are grouped into "psychiatric" syndromes (e.g., sensory deprivation syndrome and hypersensitivity-hyperactivity syndrome), which are clusters of clinical signs statistically occurring together in that species; specific scales are used (e.g., global aggressiveness index, social aggressiveness index and the ratio of those indexes, emotional disorders scale, and ARCAD (Age related cognitive and affective disorders)); behaviors are considered pathologic when they lose their plasticity and adaptive function; medications are selected to treat the neurotransmitter system which may cause these groupings of signs; and treatment is intended to increase the patient's homeostatic threshold.[7]

The one-medicine approach

Historically, behavior disorders in animals have been regarded at least by some as separate from physical (medical) problems. However, recent research supports the one-medicine approach to behavioral disorders, which supports the idea that emotional and physical processes in the body are inextricably linked and both influence behavioral clinical signs.[8-10] For example, otitis externa can cause pain, which can contribute to a dog's threshold for exhibiting aggression when touched. When the otitis is resolved, the dog may not show aggression at any other point in its life, even when put in that situation again. On the other hand, the dog may develop a learned behavior pattern in which the dog shows avoidance or aggression when reaching for the ear or head or when the ear is handled, even if the painful inciting cause is resolved.

In another example, the cat that has painful hip osteoarthritis feels pain when he attempts to climb into the litterbox. For that reason, he urinates outside of the litterbox. When nonsteroidal antiinflammatory medications are administered, the periuria resolves. However, the cat may develop a learned location or litterbox avoidance or a new location or substrate preference where the periuria persists, even if the painful inciting cause is resolved. Instead of approaching situations such as the ones above as physical causes of behavior problems, the one-medicine approach considers all the causes of behavioral clinical signs, not necessarily that behavioral clinical signs can only be caused by behavioral disorders.

Also in the past, veterinarians were encouraged to rule out physical differential diagnoses before considering behavioral differential diagnoses or delay treatment for what were categorized as behavioral clinical signs while physical disease was ruled out. In the one-medicine approach, where behavioral clinical signs are recognized to be caused by diseases of any body system, there is no separation between the emotional and the physical, allowing the pet's pain, fear, and distress to be diagnosed and treated immediately, improving patient welfare. For example, in a cat presented for pruritus, both the welfare (stress) assessment and dermatologic and physical diagnostic evaluation should be evaluated concurrently from the outset both for patient welfare and to accurately diagnose and treat the cause. In veterinary dermatologist's one study of 13 cats with idiopathic ulcerative dermatitis, 12 cats with lesions were healed and welfare improved within 2 weeks with environmental modifications, with one cat also requiring psychotropic medication.[11] Behavior disorders and physical disorders both have a physiologic component. For example, a dog that exhibits signs of a separation-related disorder when the pet parent has departed experiences a similar physiologic stress response as a dog that has just undergone surgery or that has had physical trauma such as would occur with a traumatic injury like a pelvic fracture. Instead of viewing physical and emotional illness as entirely separate, they can be viewed as two parts of the same whole. See Chapter 7 for more information on the stress response associated with behavioral clinical signs.

Inasmuch as possible, objective measures and validated questionnaires are used to measure and characterize behavior. Diagnoses are recognized as labels reflecting the level of knowledge that we have at that moment and are subject to revision as we learn more about the patient and any underlying pathologies. Diagnoses are primarily motivational but can be descriptive and contain the following considerations: extrinsic and intrinsic influences; genetics; punishment and reinforcement; function; and biological parameters.

In the one-medicine approach, the four recognized pillars of treatment are assessment of overall health and wellness; behavioral or cognitive treatments; environmental management, and pharmaceutical treatment. All patients do not need treatments from all four pillars; however, all four pillars should be considered for each patient.

Causes of behavioral pathology

Factors contributing to the development of behavioral clinical signs include genetics, epigenetics (i.e., effect of environment and external factors on the expression of genes), the animal's coping style (affected by intrinsic and extrinsic factors), environmental experience (e.g., extent to which diet, health, living conditions, enrichment, and exercise meet the pet's needs), and learning (intrinsic and extrinsic reinforcement and punishment). Maintenance of behaviors occurs through positive and negative consequences of those behaviors which may be extrinsic (e.g., pet parent dependent) or intrinsic (e.g., dissipation of fear, anxiety, stress, conflict or panic, relief of pain). Behaviors that are reinforced will occur more frequently in the future. For example, if a puppy is being house trained and urinates in the house, the reinforcement is intrinsic (relief of pressure on the bladder). There will be an increased frequency

of that behavior in the future. The pet parent then approaches quickly and scolds (extrinsic punishment) the puppy that is wagging its tail in a friendly way, anticipating the approach of the pet parent. This causes the friendly body language and happy emotional state in response to pet parent approach less likely to be displayed in the future. In another example, a cat is lying on the pet parent's lap as he watches television. The pet parent is absentmindedly petting the cat's head and back. After a couple of minutes, the cat's pupils dilate, it turns its head away from the pet parent, licks its lips, and slightly thrashes its tail. These are disengagement or distance-increasing signals (see Chapter 2). Since the petting is undesirable at that point (the cat is requesting with body language signals for the petting to stop), those body language signals are punished (extrinsic punishment) and they will occur less frequently in that situation in the future. The cat escalates the communication to a bite. When the pet parent is bitten, they pull back their hand (extrinsic reinforcement) and the cat feels less distressed (intrinsic reinforcement). The behavior of biting will occur more frequently in the future in that situation. If these types of interactions occur repeatedly over the course of the pet's life, emotional states such as fear, anxiety, stress, conflict, panic, and frustration are more likely. These emotional states are the foundation on which virtually all behavior disorders and undesirable behaviors are built. This is another argument for the focus to be on prevention in veterinary medicine.

Painful conditions (e.g., abscesses, arthritis, anal sacculitis, and dental disease), conditions affecting neurotransmitter/receptor activity, CNS anatomic abnormalities (genetic, congenital, and acquired), neoplasia (CNS tumors), metabolic disease states (hepatic encephalopathy and endocrine disorders), infections (rabies, feline leukemia virus, and feline immunodeficiency virus), trauma (CNS injury), toxins (lead, pesticides, and illicit drugs), congenital conditions, and cognitive dysfunction in senior pets can all have a direct effect on or be associated with changes in behavior (see Chapters 6 and 8).

Another important reason for physical examination and screening tests is to establish a baseline prior to the use of any pharmacologic therapy and to ensure that there are no contraindications for using the medication(s) being considered. In general, the minimum assessment that should be collected for most behavior problems would be a physical examination, hemogram, biochemical profile, urinalysis, fecal examination with antigen testing including giardia, and thyroid assessment. While there may not be a direct link between a physical problem and a behavioral clinical sign, and while the diagnosis of a physical problem may not be directly contributing to (independent of) the behavioral signs, the pathophysiology of behavior problems is not completely understood. It is widely accepted that any process that causes physiologic stress can cause changes in behavior.

The threshold theory of behavior change

The body is healthiest when it is in homeostasis. Think of this as the perfect, Goldilocks zone of all systems in a healthy place. When an animal encounters a stressor, whether it is physiologic (e.g., acute injury, surgery, inflammatory disease, and chronic disease) or emotional (e.g., anxiety, fear, stress, and panic), a physiologic stress response results, pushing the body away from homeostasis. The stress response can be divided into acute and chronic responses. The acute stress response is immediate after exposure to the threatening stimulus. Consequences include increased blood glucose, tachycardia, tachypnea, and changes in immune function. The chronic response is more dependent on the hypothalamic–pituitary axis (HPA) response. Chronic stress results in chronic exposure to neurotransmitters and neurohormones, which can lead to detrimental changes in heart function, gastrointestinal function, and immune function. Both acute and chronic stress result in behavior changes as the dog or cat attempts to cope and bring the body back into homeostasis. This chronic response is maladaptive and detrimental to the animal (also see Chapter 7). Generally, chronic diseases are regarded as affecting quality of life (e.g., renal disease and osteoarthritis) when in fact, psychological factors have been shown to stimulate the HPA axis more than physical factors. Therefore, addressing mental well-being is essential to both health and welfare.[12–14] Chronic fear, which is prevalent in companion animals, can significantly affect the mental and physical health as well as the welfare of an individual.[15]

Any behavior changes can be and often are reinforced or punished intrinsically by the environment or the people interacting with the animal. Through this process, behavior changes associated with physical disease, psychological pathology, or psychologic trauma become long-term aspects of the animal's behavior pattern. This is one of the reasons that psychologic stress in animals should be evaluated at every veterinary appointment and treated immediately (see Chapters 1, 5, 7, and 14).

Any stimulus can be regarded as a stressor for companion animals, with a broad range of individual variability in response. Each animal has its own life experience and hereditary predispositions which guide that individual's behavior. With that said, some stimuli are known to cause stress in dogs and cats, including social restriction, spatial restriction, veterinary visits, separation from pet parents, sounds, environmental changes, changes in feeding frequency, and travel.

The threshold for behavioral clinical signs resulting in undesirable behaviors can be lowered by medications (e.g., phenobarbital, corticosteroids, benzodiazepines, antidepressants, tramadol, levetiracetam, and gabapentin); gastrointestinal problems (e.g., inflammatory bowel disease and intestinal neoplasia); dermatologic diseases (e.g., atopy, adverse food reactions, and flea allergy dermatitis); orthopedic disease (e.g., neoplasia and osteoarthritis); and any disease that causes pain or discomfort (e.g., chronic disease, diabetes, and hypothyroidism), and by individual variability (sensitivity and reactivity) in response (i.e., genetics and experience) (see Chapter 6).

Undesirable and pathologic behavior

Pathologic behaviors are those that are considered dysfunctional or deviate from the expected function of a behavioral pattern. They may be associated with extreme anxiety, may be out of context or inappropriate with respect to the stimuli, or may be excessive, uninhibited, or impulsive. Compulsive disorders, excessive fear, panic and phobias, aggression arising from dyscontrol or lack of inhibition, and learning deficits associated with hyperactivity are abnormal behaviors,

meaning that they do not have a function in maintaining homeostasis. In these cases, altered neurotransmitter and receptor function may be present, and medical therapy may be a necessary part of the therapeutic program. Undesirable behaviors such as jumping on pet parents or play biting can become dysfunctional due to fear, anxiety, stress, conflict, panic, and frustration resulting from inadvertent reinforcement and punishment through interactions with environmental stimuli or the people in the pet's social group. Families require education as to what is normal canine and feline behavior. They also need to know how these problems can best be managed using behavioral and cognitive therapies, environmental management, treatment of physical comorbidities, and pharmaceutical therapy.

Steps for evaluation, diagnosis, and treatment

Veterinary practice preparation and workflow

Before seeing the first behavior case, workflow should be determined. Who will see patients with primary behavior complaints? Will the pet's primary care veterinarian at the practice see the case initially and then refer within the clinic to the veterinarian who has an interest in behavior? Will the pet parent care representatives automatically schedule all cases with behavioral complaints with one veterinarian? Which technicians are educated in behavior and can assist with behavior appointments? These types of questions and more relating to workflow, appointment fees, and education should be discussed in order to work most effectively and efficiently to help patients with behavioral complaints. Ideally, a veterinary nurse or technician would be a part of the team to participate in education, training, and follow-up. Lists of resources and dog training professionals, as well as the names and contact information of board-certified veterinary behaviorists with whom the pet can be seen, should be easy to access. Chapter 1 outlines practical approaches to behavioral medicine in primary care (see Figure 9.1).

Practice standards and standard operating procedures should be clear to veterinarians and technicians alike to promote a positive, consistent approach to patient care. For example, within the practice electronic medical record, a behavioral set can be made. The set can contain line items for basic handouts (e.g., visitors, aggression, child safety, separation-related disorders, storm phobia, and feline periuria), baseline tests (e.g., complete blood count [CBC], serum chemistry, thyroid evaluation, urinalysis, and fecal evaluation), first-line product recommendations (e.g., behavioral probiotics and pheromone analogs), and appointment charges. In this way, each veterinarian/technician team will be delivering the same standards and consistency of care. Team members can always delete, mark as "not needed" or "declined" those line items which do not apply to that patient. A list of training professionals in the area, vetted and recommended by the hospital, should be readily available. If one veterinarian recommends a trainer who uses shock and another recommends a trainer who uses positive reinforcement, conflict and confusion will ensue within the hospital and potentially for the pet parent. The evidence against aversive methods is overwhelming, with reams of research showing that

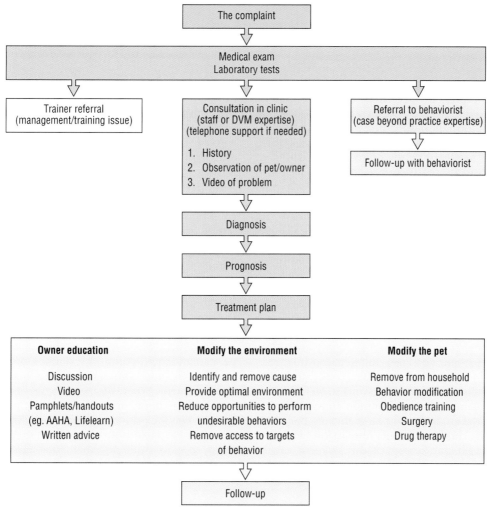

Figure 9.1 Flowchart for a behavior consultation. DVM, Doctor of veterinary medicine; AAHA, American Animal Hospital Association.

methods such as these are less effective, have a high incidence of relapse, are challenging for pet parents to implement, and have a very high likelihood of increasing fear, anxiety, and stress in companion animals. To effectively treat behavioral disorders, the entire team should adhere to best practices when recommending training professionals, meaning that only positive reinforcement trainers should be recommended. With the widespread adoption of telehealth services in veterinary medicine, consultation with a board-certified veterinary behaviorist is only a click away. Setting practice standards for referral can ease the pressure on the veterinary team as to when they should refer cases to a board-certified veterinary specialist. While regulatory and licensing restrictions may limit what and where telehealth services might be available directly to pet parents, teleconsulting with a behaviorist should be offered to support the veterinary team in case counseling. Telehealth services are commonly offered by board-certified veterinary behaviorists.

Gathering history

A complete behavioral and medical history should be gathered on all patients, which can be time-consuming work. However,

as with any skill, it can be developed so that the veterinary team is efficient. What follows are the ideal history collection techniques. Unfortunately, things do not always go as planned. If time is short or the behavioral evaluation is to be split up into several appointments, try to collect as much history as possible about the presenting complaint, overall health and wellness, and any behavior which may cause injury to the pet or the family, including other pets. At subsequent appointments, a more detailed history can be collected.

Utilizing a questionnaire to collect information speeds up the history-taking process. Ideally, a short questionnaire (See Appendix C and Chapter 8) would be filled out by the pet parent at every appointment. That way, undesirable or pathologic behaviors can be caught before they become serious problems. A more detailed questionnaire can be used for a deeper understanding of the presenting complaints and the environment. If a more detailed questionnaire is used, it is best received well before the appointment so that it can be reviewed by the veterinary team. Using a history questionnaire will facilitate and standardize collection of data, keep information together so it can be readily referenced during followups, optimize time for direct interpersonal consultation with the pet parent during the visit, and help the veterinarian avoid overlooking important questions. If you design your own forms, be certain to include questions that address all aspects of the pet's health and behavior, since the primary complaint may be only one sign of a more complex health or behavioral problem.

The veterinarian has to develop the skill of accurate, respectful, and patient yet efficient history taking that allows the pet parent to express their concerns without letting the conversation go awry. Asking closed-ended questions that gather essential information is the best place to start. When multiple family members attend the appointment (which is desired), there may be differing opinions or recounts of situations. Listen to those different recounts, as they will provide clues into how the family interacts with each other and the pet as well as how different members of the family view their interactions. Describing the pet's behavior can be emotional and embarrassing for some families. Some may feel a sense of failure that they are unable to correct the pet's problems without professional help. Oftentimes, the family comes into the consultation a bit apprehensive, not knowing what to expect. Getting the history is important, but so is empathy and being nonjudgmental. Acknowledgement of the family's distress shows that the team cares and can break down barriers to accurate history taking. There is a better chance of gathering a complete history if the team is empathetic and takes an understanding interest in the family's problems, rather than coolly and clinically collecting facts. An indiscreet comment, facial expression, or body gesture can quickly inhibit communication and close your access to important facts. Include the whole family, including children, in the discussion whenever practical, so that all dimensions of the problem can be explored. You will also get a better idea of each family member's emotional investment in the pet as well as their commitment to solving the problem. Additionally, you will have the opportunity to observe the interaction of the pet with each member of the family (provided safety can be ensured) over the course of the consultation. Asking questions about the training methods used and corrections tried can be sticky. Family members often feel embarrassed or may entirely believe what they tried was right (e.g., it has worked with all of my other dogs). Care should be taken to ask closed-ended, nonjudgmental questions to gather information without emotion.

The goal of history taking is to obtain sufficient information to aid in the diagnosis, prognosis, and treatment plan. History collection should include an accurate description of the behavior, health and wellness, environment (prenatal/perinatal, physical, social, and behavioral), comorbidities, and goals and expectations. See Box 9.1 for a complete checklist.

Behavior

Pet parents often have much to share about their pet's behavior, including their assessment of why the behavior occurs. It is easy to spend an inordinate amount of time listening to the pet parent's anthropomorphic opinion of the pet's behavior, resulting in little information that is helpful for diagnosis and treatment. When the pet parents say that the pet was mad, jealous, upset, or spiteful, it is best to ask for a description of what the pet looked like before, during, and after that situation. Pet parents often state that the pet was fine with or happy to see a visitor and then acted aggressively out of the

---

Box 9.1 Checklist for history collection

Behavior
- Description of body language
- Intensity
- Frequency
- Recovery
- Triggers
- Duration
- Latency to arousal (time to gross signs of stress)
- Age when first noted
- How have attempts to alter the behavior been applied and what was the result?

Overall health and wellness
- Signalment
- Baseline laboratory testing prior to presentation
- Historical signs or history of pain or discomfort
- Medications and supplements currently and historically administered
- Diet

Environment
- Prenatal/perinatal
  - Information on dam, sire, and littermates
  - When acquired
  - Where acquired
- Physical
  - Apartment, single-family home, rural, urban
  - Outdoor access
  - Exercise
  - Elimination areas
  - Housing

- Social
  - Family makeup
  - Ages of family members
  - Household schedule
  - At-risk family members
  - Other animals in the family
  - Exposure to unfamiliar people
  - Exposure to unfamiliar pets
- Behavioral
  - Enrichment
  - Training (specific training methods and basic cues)
  - Response to the behavior by the family and the pet's response to their corrections

Comorbidities (if not part of the presenting complaint)
- Sounds
  - Response to storms, thunder, fireworks
  - Response to environmental sounds (indoors, outdoors)
- Separation
  - Response to separation from social group members (animal, human)
  - Response to confinement
  - Response to being left completely alone
- Car
  - Response to car rides

Goals/Expectations
- What is the family's goal?
- What do they expect to happen and when?
- Is there a deadline for treatment to be successful?

blue. However, after a more objective description of the body language of the animal and behavior of the people with whom it was interacting before the bite, it is clear the pet was not fine but was instead fearful, anxious, or stressed. While it is true that pet parents know their pets and they should be listened to, it is also true that if they could accurately assess their pet's behavior, they would not need to bring their pet for a behavioral consultation. For that reason, it is essential that the veterinarian ask for descriptions of what occurred without the pet parent's personal assessment. For each behavior for which the patient is being presented, try to obtain the intensity, frequency, recovery, triggers, latency to arousal, when the behavior was first noted, any attempts to correct the behavior, how those were received by the pet, and the family's response to the pet's reaction to corrections. The intensity of the behavior would include parameters such as the amount of time that the animal stays aroused or exhibits the behavior in one bout or throughout the day. The frequency is how often the behavior occurs, either in one bout or situation on a daily, weekly, or monthly basis. The recovery is the length of time it takes for the pet to return to its behavioral and emotional baseline. The triggers are situation, people, animals, or inanimate objects which trigger the behavior in part or in full. The latency to arousal is the time that passes between exposure to a trigger and the grossly observable signs of fear, anxiety, stress, conflict, panic, or the behavior itself. While taking the history, observe the way that each family member interacts with the pet, the pet's response to those interactions, and the pet's behavior during the visit.

Overall health and wellness

Aside from the signalment of the pet, history should be gathered on any medications or supplements that are currently being administered or were being administered at the time of the first incident, screening for pain or discomfort and knowledge of diet, and previous laboratory testing.

Environment

The environment in which the pet, now lives and previously lived affects current behavioral clinical signs. That will include prenatal, perinatal, physical, social, and behavioral environments. The physical environment includes where the pet lives and the type of housing, where the pet eliminates, the daily or family schedule, the level of exercise provided, the level of ambient sound to which the pet is exposed, and how busy the neighborhood is on any given day. The social environment includes the family makeup, the ages of the social group members and whether or not they are at risk of injury or at greater risk if bitten, other animals in the household and the pet's relationship to those animals, exposure to unfamiliar animals and unfamiliar people, and exposure to wild animals outside.

Behavioral comorbidities

Since it may not be clear of the effect of other behavioral comorbidities on the particular patient's presentation, information on certain key aspects of all behaviors should be collected. Those include the pet's response to sounds, separation, confinement, and car rides.

Goals/expectations

Managing expectations can be the difference between a happy patient and pet parent and relinquishment or euthanasia. At the end of the day, the veterinarian's perception of a positive outcome may be diametrically opposite of the pet parent's perception. For example, in the case of intercat aggression where the veterinarian may view the situation as simplistic and recommend complete separation of the cats for the lifetime of each cat, the pet parent may view that as impossible or impractical to implement. Ask the parents honestly what they would like to have happen and how much time, energy, and finances they can devote to treatment of this problem. Then, the reality of what treatment can achieve must be married with the pet parent's hopes and expectations.

Making a diagnosis

Diagnoses are, at their core, labels. Labels are helpful because they allow us to speak the same language; however, they also can lead to tunnel vision. Behavioral diagnoses can be characterized as functional, motivational, or descriptive. The most common diagnoses in use at this time in North America are either descriptive or motivational. Descriptive diagnoses are as they sound, a description of what is occurring. Examples include noise phobia and separation related disorder. Motivational diagnoses attempt to assess the underlying emotional state or physiologic process causing the behavioral clinical sign. Examples include stress-induced aggression and fear-induced aggression. Functional aggression diagnoses are currently used more infrequently and might include protective aggression and attention-seeking behavior.

Diagnoses reflect the level of our understanding of the problem at the time that the diagnosis is made. At the first appointment, the motivation or function may not be clear; thus the pet is given a descriptive diagnosis. After more information is gathered in follow-up or upon reexamination, a motivational or functional diagnosis can be made. In addition, there are qualifiers which may be applied to any diagnosis, words that modify the meaning of the diagnosis by characterizing it such as redirected and impulsive. A qualifier is not always necessary but can further delineate the characteristics of the diagnosis. The goal should be to describe all behaviors and/or make a list of descriptive, motivational, or functional differential diagnoses at the first appointment. The list most likely will be and should be all inclusive so that all motivations and functions are considered as the case progresses.

Diagnostics

The minimum assessment that should be collected for most behavior problems would be a physical examination, CBC, serum chemistry, urinalysis, fecal examination with antigen testing including Giardia,[16] and thyroid assessment. For cats, include a proBNP. There are also behavioral diagnostics which may prove to be helpful in the future such as hair,[17] nail,[18] salivary[19] and fecal cortisol[20] tests, urine neurotransmitter tests,[21] and potentially, blood neurotransmitters. At this time, they are not widely available.

Diagnostic questionnaires are available as well such as the C-BARQ (Canine Behavioral Assessment and Research Questionnaire),[22] Fe-BARQ (Feline Behavioral Assessment and research questionnaire),[23] Dog Impulsivity Assessment Scale (DIAS),[24] Canine Frustration Questionnaire (CFQ)[25] and Positive and Negative Activation Scale for Dogs (PANAS),[26] the Lincoln Sound Sensitivity Scale (LSSS),[27] and Lincoln Canine Anxiety Scale (LCAS).[28]

Talking to pet parents about their pet's behavior disorder

For whatever reason, the discussion of a behavior disorder or even the pet's behavior in general stirs up more emotions than discussions of disorders of other body systems. There is still a stigma around behavioral disorders which may cause pet parents to feel ashamed, distressed, or a sense of failure. One way to overcome these challenges is to be empathetic when explaining diagnosis, pathology, prognosis, and treatment. Another way is to answer questions before they come up, when the plan is introduced. The most commonly asked questions and answers are in Box 9.2.

Prognosis

The prognosis may determine whether the pet should or will be treated or removed from the home. The way that this topic is approached should be thoughtful and objective. Prognosis is not set for any one animal or diagnosis and depends on many factors. It is impossible to predict the outcome of any particular case. However, in general, pet parents can be counseled that the best prognosis lies with those cases that are predictable and avoidable. Pet parents who are able to adhere to treatment recommendations will generally have better outcomes than those who cannot. Any discussion of predictability should come with a discussion of the obvious triggers for the behavior. Many pet parents will report that their pet has unpredictable or unprovoked aggression when in most cases, thoughtful behavioral history taking reveals that it is in fact chronic, there is a learned component, and/or there are identifiable triggers. The decision to keep an aggressive pet in the family is a personal one. Pet parents need the full picture in order to make a decision as to whether or not to treat their aggressive, fearful, or anxious cat or dog. With that said, there is information from the literature which can be found in the chapters in this text

---

Box 9.2 Common questions and answers

Questions

Did we do something to cause this behavior?	While there may have been something that you did that contributed to the severity of the behavior (e.g., shock collar training, confrontation, punishment-based training, inadvertent reinforcement, boarding and training with aversive techniques, and lack of socialization), it is very unlikely that you caused this behavior in its entirety. Much of behavior is genetic, which of course you have no control over. Whatever happened in the past is the past. Right now, we are working together to improve your pet's behavior. That is what is important.
Will medications make my pet a zombie or change his personality? Will the medications shorten my pet's life? What are the side effects of the medications? How long will my pet be on the medications?	Medications such as the ones that I am recommending for your pet are used all over the world to treat behavior problems in dogs and cats. Medications used for behavior problems help to improve your pet's well-being by reducing fear, anxiety, and stress by normalizing neurotransmission. In essence, they change the neurochemistry of fear, anxiety, and stress so that your pet can be happier and more able to learn how to cope with stressful circumstances. Many patients are treated for a good part of their entire life. Our goal is never for your pet to be a zombie on these medications, although sedation can be a side effect. If your pet gets sedated on these medications, the side effect will go away fairly quickly and we will adjust our dose or discontinue the medication entirely. They will not shorten your pet's life. We are going to run lab work every 6 months to ensure that your pet is healthy and has good kidney and liver function because those organs are primarily responsible for the breakdown and excretion of the medications. Your pet will be treated with these medications as long as you desire. Some pet parents want to wean their pets off and some keep their pets on forever because they have caused such as positive change. That is generally something that we discuss in about 6 months when your pet hopefully is stable.
Is there any hope for my pet?	Yes!! Behavior problems are treatable but not always curable. There are many treatments which can be used.
How long will treatment take?	It depends on your pet's genetics, your ability to work with your pet, whether the entire family cooperates, how well the medications and supplements work for your pet, and your pet's environment. We should expect that if all goes well, your pet is stable (the behavior is tolerable or occurs a lot less frequently) in about 2–3 months. Some cases take longer.
Will he grow out of this?	No, probably not. More often than not, behavior disorders worsen over time when not treated. As a matter of fact, there are studies that show that noise phobia gets worse with time.
What would you do if this was your pet?	That is a really tough question because this is an individual, personal challenge which involves the entire family. I would try to consider my dog's quality of life, the quality of life of my family, and how much we are willing and able to do, and then make a decision.
I cannot live with this dog anymore. I am afraid that he will hurt someone. Do you know of someone who will take him?	I can understand how living with Fido can be really stressful. Unfortunately, now that he has bitten someone, rehoming him has new challenges. How will we find a someone who understands the risks, will treat his behavior disorder, will commit to managing him so that he does not bite again, and will accept liability for living with a dog who has bitten? As you can imagine, this can be a very difficult person or family to find. While sanctuaries for dogs do exist, often "no-kill" facilities keep dogs in crates or runs for their lifetimes if they are not adopted out. Dogs are social animals and that type of living situation is not conducive to a good quality of life.

devoted to specific diagnosis or problems which may help when creating prognoses. If the family has unrealistic goals or if there is poor cooperation, the chances for satisfactory resolution are reduced. The family must have the aptitude to understand the conditions influencing the existence of the problem and the basic principles of the treatment program. Chances for injury are higher (risk assessment) when the family is composed of individuals who are unable to understand or unwilling to comply with safety recommendations (e.g., young children, physically challenged persons, individuals with learning disorders, the elderly, and teenagers). Other factors affecting prognosis include the pet's genetic predispositions, environment, frequency of exposure to triggers, coping strategy (e.g., flight versus fight), and the pet parent's perceived predictability of the behavior and response to management recommendations.

One of the few prognostic factors which is under the control of the veterinarian is the action taken by, the attitude of, and the knowledge level of the veterinarian and the veterinary healthcare team. There is a time to treat the case and a time to refer the case. Parameters which should cause the case to be referred to a board-certified veterinary behaviorist are below.

Treatment

Like many physical problems encountered in veterinary medicine, behavior disorders require immediate treatments as well as long-term treatments in order to achieve positive outcomes. While there is no magic pill, there are recommendations as well as prudent medication choices which can help to alleviate the patient's suffering while long-term treatment is instituted. The treatment of behavioral problems utilizes a variety of approaches to modify either the pet's behavior or the environment to suit the needs of the family and pet.

Therapeutic options for behavioral disorders

The therapeutic options for behavioral disorders are similar to other body systems, including changes to the environment, diet, management of the pet, prevention of future flare-ups, nutraceuticals, and medications. Specifically, options include conscientious (benign) neglect (e.g., no treatment); environmental management (e.g., avoidance, blocking off windows, and basket muzzles); environmental management and neurochemical modulation (e.g., diet, medications, and supplements); environmental management, neurochemical modulation and behavioral treatments, rehoming the pet to a more suitable environment if appropriate, and humane euthanasia. Pet parents should be presented with all applicable options, including the estimated financial and personal (e.g., time, energy, and changes to the schedule) of each. Once the plan is presented, the family then can decide if such a plan is safe, practical for the home, family, and lifestyle, and within their budgets and capabilities. It is critical that the family understands all the options and alternatives. Some families may decide that addressing the problem is more than they can manage, and elect to euthanize the pet. The veterinary healthcare team must be flexible with the recommendations and attempt to

change the plan when possible, while never sacrificing the safety or welfare of the family, pet or the public. See Chapter 10 for more information on environmental management and behavioral treatments. See Chapters 11 and 12 for more information on medications and supplements respectively.

Necessary elements of the behavioral treatment plan

Behavioral treatment plans should include the following recommendation categories:
1. Avoidance of triggers.
2. Modulation of fear, anxiety, stress, conflict, and panic through environmental management, tools (e.g., muzzle, leash, and no-pull harness), medications, diet, and supplements as needed.
3. Management of the environment to provide adequate outlets necessary to address breed-typical needs, increase enrichment, keep the pet and the family safe, and remove reinforcement for undesirable behaviors.
4. Pathways to teach desirable behaviors with positive reinforcement.
5. Education on proper interactions with the pet, species-specific body language, and proper training.
6. Discontinuation of all the positive punishment techniques.
7. Discussion of quality of life of the pet and the family.

There are times when all of these recommendations cannot be made due to time constraints or individual deficits in the veterinarian's abilities and pet parent overwhelm. When that is the case, focus on alleviation of distress and pain and avoidance of triggers.

When to start treatment?

Treatment should start immediately to relieve physiologic and emotional stress and pain. Short-term medications can be started while waiting for the results of diagnostic tests. Environmental management recommendations should focus on changing the behavior through avoidance of triggers. For example, if the pet bites the child, complete separation or boarding at the veterinary hospital can be offered until the house has been modified to allow safe separation. Resources to educate the pet parent and inform them of the options for referral should also be given out at the first appointment.

Implementing a behavioral treatment program

Most veterinarians receive little education in behavior modification. Some practices are fortunate enough to have a veterinary technician who also has behavior modification skills. If that is not the case, an experienced, positive reinforcement dog training professional is essential for the implementation of behavior modification recommendations. Dog training professionals can be great assets because they can help to stop problems before they start, treat unruly behaviors which increase the likelihood of relinquishment, and assist with the implementation of behavior modification plans. Finding a good training professional can be a challenge. Beware of inaccurate claims made of a greater level of knowledge than they actually possess. There is no legal license or certification for trainers at the time of this writing only voluntary certifications. Too often, pets with clinical signs which are outside of normal limits are referred to nonveterinary professionals. Would you refer a patient who had pain due to osteoarthritis to a person who said that they knew about acupuncture but had no formal training and was not certified by a governing body? You would never refer a patient with a medical problem to a nonmedical professional without recognized qualifications. In the same way, you should not refer a patient with abnormal behavioral clinical signs to someone who has no medical experience or education. Keep in mind that the term "behaviorist" can be used by any person, regardless of qualifications. Even when cases are referred away from the practice for implementation of the behavioral treatment plan, veterinarians should still stay involved in the creation of the plan and the progress. Recommendations on how to find a good dog training professional can be found in Chapters 1 and 10.

Approach to prescribing

Acute treatment of behavior problems will involve, at least in some cases, medications. There are many medications to choose from to alleviate stress and anxiety immediately. Drug classes which are commonly used are benzodiazepines, serotonin reuptake inhibitors/antagonists, antihistamines, alpha-2 agonists, gabaminergics, and phenothiazines. First-line recommendations might also include pheromone analogs and behavioral probiotics (see Chapters 11 to 13).

When deciding to institute pharmacologic therapy, the veterinarian should consider these eight questions:
1. Is the environment consistent with a positive outcome?
2. What is the latency to arousal?
3. Is the animal's quality of life affected?
4. Is the animal at risk of injuring itself or others or at risk of euthanasia or relinquishment?
5. Is the behavior predictable?
6. What is the severity of the behavior?
7. What is the recovery time?
8. Would the addition of a medication, supplement, or diet to the plan improve patient welfare, alleviate pet parent distress, improve the likelihood of treatment adherence, or improve the likelihood of positive response to the behavior plan?

See Figure 9.2.

There are four possible outcomes when considering the eight questions above:
1. No medication or supplement;
2. Foundational medication or supplement;
3. PRN medication or supplement;
4. PRN and primary medication or supplement.

Once the veterinarian has determined on the basis of the questions above that the patient does in fact need a medication or supplement to improve significantly, the question becomes which medication to choose. This can be the most difficult part of the process of treatment. First, decide if the patient has acute or urgent needs. If so, an as-needed or quick-acting medication is necessary. If the patient's behavior is entirely predictable, an as-needed medication may be sufficient. If the patient has nonurgent needs or requires long-term support, a foundational or longer-acting medication or supplement is the best choice. Not uncommonly, the patient will have long-term and acute or urgent needs. In those cases, the patient very often needs a short-term and a foundational medication. Once the nature of the medication has been determined, the desired outcome should be considered next.

WHEN TO PRESCRIBE

PARAMETER	PRESCRIBE	DO NOT PRESCRIBE
Time to recovery	Long	Short
Quality of life is poor	Yes	No
Environment conducive to positive outcome	No	Yes
Risk to self or others	Yes	No
Behavior is predictable	No	Yes
Latency (time) to arousal	Short	Long
Severity of the behavior	Mod-sev	Mild
Will the pet's quality of life improve or will treatment adherence improve with pharmaceutical treatment?	Yes	No

Lisa Radosta DVM, DACVB

Figure 9.2 Questions to consider and possible outcomes when prescribing. (*Note:* Predictable behaviors may still need a medication if the pet parent's schedule or home environment does not allow for control of triggers.)

Based on the patient's clinical signs, the veterinarian can choose a desired outcome. For example, if the patient panics when alone and they will not eat, the veterinarian may choose the following outcome: calm behavior and increased appetite when alone. The increased appetite would faciliate pet engagement with a food toy, which is likely to further lower stress. In this case, reasonable options would be benzodiazepines and gabaminergic medications (see Figures 9.3).

Unfortunately, response to medication is not always predictable. It is best to start low and slowly increase the dose over time. In addition, there is no one right medication for any diagnosis or pet. Prepare pet parents by informing them that it may be necessary to try several medications before the right one is found. All too often, veterinarians abandon potentially useful medication because the pet parent reports that there is "no change" in the pet's behavior. Asking closed-ended questions and collecting objective information at follow-up is imperative for effective dosing decisions. To avoid this, veterinarians can apply the 50% rule (see Figure 9.4). The 50% rule is a general guideline for using veterinary psychotropic medications and supplements. The 50% rule states that if there are no side effects and there has been a desirable change in the pet's clinical signs, the dose of the medication generally should be increased through the published dosing range until the point where the medication has had a desirable effect, has caused side effects or the veterinarian has reached the upper limit of the dosing range. Then, if the effect has been to reduce the undesirable clinical signs by at least 50% with no adverse events or side effects, the veterinarian should add in an additional pharmaceutical instead of discontinuing the medication. If the medication has not reached a 50% reduction in undesirable clinical signs, it would be prudent to discontinue that medication and replace it with another one. For example, if medication A has caused a reduction of 50% or more in the pet's undesirable clinical signs, and the dose is at or near the upper end of

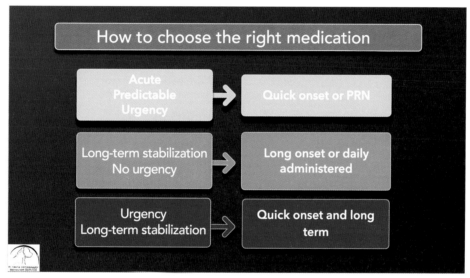

Figure 9.3 How to make medication choices? *(Attribution: Lisa Radosta.)*

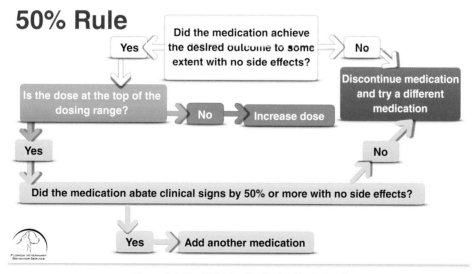

Figure 9.4 The 50% rule. *(Attribution: Lisa Radosta.)*

the accepted published dosing range and there have been no adverse side effects, often it is better to continue to treat the pet with medication A and add in another medication instead of discontinuing medication A entirely.

When prescribing, be sure to check how the medication is eliminated and transformed into its active metabolites; understand the pet's overall health and how that may affect metabolism of the medication or supplement; use caution when combining medications or supplements that affect the same neurotransmitter; and use online interaction checkers to check for interactions between psychotropic medications and any other medications or supplements that the patient is taking.

When should you refer?

Referral to a board-certified veterinary behaviorist should be considered when one of more of the following criteria is present:
1. The owner is considering euthanasia.
2. The case is chronic and thus far, outcomes have been poor.
3. There is a threat of injury to a person.
4. There are immunocompromised, elderly, or very young family members in a household with an aggressive pet.
5. The patient is at risk.
6. The veterinarian has exhausted their comfort level regarding pharmaceutical treatments.
7. Bites are injurious.
8. The pet parent is under threat of legal action.

Follow-up

Another important opportunity for educating and interacting with the family occurs during the follow-up. It is essential that the consultant continues to monitor each case to be sure that the family is correctly following treatment recommendations and that the case is progressing as expected. This also provides an opportunity to gather more information about the situation in general, which is particularly important when there are multiple treatment options and the initial diagnosis was tentative. When medications or supplements have been discussed or dispensed, regular follow-up is essential. In some cases, additional diagnostic tests and owner information will be required following the initial consultation. For most cases, initial follow-up contacts at 1, 3, 5, and 8 weeks in person will provide good assessment of progress. In one study, pet parents who were contacted via phone or email at 10, 30, and 60 days after the behavioral assessment were significantly more likely than pet parents who were not contacted to say that their dog's aggressive, anxious, and fearful behavior had improved; that the veterinary team was accessible after the initial appointment; that such accessibility affected their dog's outcome in a positive way; that they were satisfied; and that they were willing to return if needed despite the fact that there was no significant differences in the numbers of bites after the appointment.[29] The actual frequency and type (e.g., email, phone, text, in person, and telehealth) will depend on the type of problem, the family, and the pet.

Conclusion

Companion animals and their families need the help of the veterinary healthcare team to alleviate pain and suffering, whether emotional or physical. It is entirely possible to be successful at seeing behavior cases in primary care with the right approach to treatment and diagnosis.

References

1. Patronek GJ, Glickman LT, Beck AM, et al. Risk factors for relinquishment of dogs to an animal shelter. *J Am Vet Med Assoc.* 1996;209:572–581.
2. Patronek GJ, McCabe GP, Ecker C. Risk factors for relinquishment of cats to an animal shelter. *J Am Vet Med Assoc.* 1996; 209:582–588.
3. Texeira A, Hall N. Effects of greeting and departure interactions on the development of increased separation related behaviors in newly adopted adult dogs. *J Vet Behav.* 2021;41:22–32.
4. Mazur JE. *Learning and Behavior.* New York and London: Routledge, Taylor and Francis Group; 2017.
5. Reisner IR, Mann JJ, Stanley M, et al. Comparison of cerebrospinal fluid monoamine metabolite levels in dominant-aggressive and non-aggressive dogs. *Brain Res.* 1996;714:57–64.
6. Mills DS. Perspectives on assessing the emotional behavior of animals with behavior problems. *Curr Opin Behav Sci.* 2017;16:66–72.
7. Pageat P. *Pathologie du comportement du chien.* 2nd ed. Paris: Editions du Point Vétérinaire; 1998.
8. Dinwoodie IR, Zottola V, Dodman N. An investigation into the effectiveness of various professionals and behavior modification programs, with or without medication, for the treatment of canine aggression, *J Vet Behav.* 2021;43:46–53.
9. Conzemius MG, Sammarco JL, Perkowski SZ, et al. Correlation between subjective and objective measures used to determine severity of postoperative pain in dogs. *J Am Vet Med Assoc.* 1997;210: 1619–1622.
10. Conzemius MG, Sammarco JL, Perkowski SZ, et al. Correlation between subjective and objective measures used to determine severity of postoperative pain in dogs. *J Am Vet Med Assoc.* 1997;210: 1619–1622.
11. Titeux E, Gilbert C, Amaury B, et al. From feline idiopathic ulcerative dermatitis to feline behavioral ulcerative dermatitis: grooming repetitive behaviors indicators
of poor welfare in cats. *Front Vet Sci.* 2018;5:81. doi:10.3389/fvets.2018.00081.
12. Levine ED. Feline fear and anxiety. *Vet Clin North Am Small Anim Pract.* 2008;38: 1065–1079.
13. Clark JD, Roger DR, Calpin JP. Animal well-being. II. Stress and disease. *Lab Anim Sci.* 2005;57:571–579.
14. Hekman J, Karas AZ, Sharp CR. Psychogenic stress in hospitalized dogs; cross species comparisons, implications for health care, and the challenges of evaluation. *Animals.* 2014;4:331–334.
15. Sarjan HN, Yajurvedi HN. Chronic stress induced duration dependent alterations in immune system and their reversibility in rats. *Immunol Lett.* 2018;197:31–43.
16. Saleh MN. Dissertation submitted to the faculty of the Virginia Polytechnic Institute and State University in partial fulfillment of the requirements for the degree of Doctor of Philosophy in Biomedical and Veterinary Sciences. <https://vtechworks.lib.vt.edu/bitstream/handle/10919/89367/Saleh_MN_D_2017.

pdf?sequence=1&isAllowed=y>. Accessed in 2021.

17. Packer RMA, Davies AM, Volk HA, et al. What can we learn from the hair of the dog? Complex effects of endogenous and exogenous stressors on canine hair cortisol. *PLoS One*. 2018:14:e0216000. doi:10.1371/journal.pone.0216000.

18. Contreras ET, Vanderstichel R, Hovenga C, et al. Evaluation of hair and nail cortisol concentrations and associations with behavioral, physical, and environmental indicators of chronic stress in cats. *J Vet Intern Med*. 2021;1–11. doi:10.1111/jvim.16283.

19. Hekman JP, Karas AZ, Dreschel NA. Salivary cortisol concentrations and behavior in a population of healthy dogs hospitalized for elective procedures. *Appl Anim Behav Sci*. 2012;141: 149–157.

20. Carlisle GK, Johnson RA, Koch CS, et al. Exploratory study of fecal cortisol, weight and behavior as measures of stress and welfare in shelter cats during assimilation into families of children with autism spectrum disorder. *Front Vet Sci*. 2021. doi:10.3389/fvets.2021.643803.

21. Albright JD, Ng Z. Measurement of neurotransmitters excreted in the urine of behaviorally healthy dogs in home and boarding kennel conditions. *J Vet Behav*. 2021. doi:10.1016/j.jveb.2021.09.001.

22. Hsu Y, Serpell JA. Development and validation of a questionnaire for measuring behavior and temperament traits in pet dogs. *J Am Vet Med Assoc*. 2003;223(9):1293–1300.

23. Duffy DL, de Moura RTD, Serpell JA. Development and evaluation of the Fe-BARQ: A new survey instrument for measuring behavior in domestic cats (*Felis s. catus*). *Behav Process*. 2017;141:329–341.

24. Wright HF, Mills DS, Pollux PM. Development and validation of a psychometric tool for assessing impulsivity in the domestic dog (*Canis familiaris*). *Int J Compar Psychol*. 2011;24:210–225.

25. McPeake KJ, Collins LM, Zulch H, et al. The Canine Frustration Questionnaire— Development of a new psychometric tool for measuring frustration in domestic dogs (*Canis familiaris*). *Front Vet Sci*. 2019;6:152.

26. Sheppard G, Mills DS. The development of a psychometric scale for the evaluation of the emotional predispositions of pet dogs. *Int J Compar Psychol*. 2002;15: 201–222.

27. Mills D, Braem Dube M, Zulch H, et al. Appendix B. *The Lincoln Sound-Sensitivity Scale. Stress and Pheromonatherapy in Small Animal Clinical Behavior*. West Sussex, UK: Wiley-Blackwell; 2013: 259–263.

28. Mills DS, Mueller HW, McPeake K, et al. Development and psychometric validation of the Lincoln canine anxiety scale. *Front Vet Sci*. 2020;7:171.

29. Radosta-Huntley L, Shofer F, Reisner I. Comparison of 42 cases of canine fear-related aggression with structured clinician initiated follow-up and 25 cases with unstructured client initiated follow-up. *Appl Anim Behav Sci*. 2007;105:330–341.

Resources and Recommended Reading

Dinwoodie IR, Zottola V, Dodman N. An investigation into the effectiveness of various professionals and behavior modification programs, with or without medication, for the treatment of canine aggression, *J Vet Behav*. 2021. doi:10.1016/j.jveb.2021.02.002.

Koch CS. Veterinary behaviorists should be the first, not the last, resort for optimal patient care. *J Am Vet Med Assoc*. 2018;253:1110-1112.

Lincoln Canine Assessment Scales. https://ipstore.lincoln.ac.uk/products/assessment-tools.

Roshier AL, McBride EA. Canine behaviour problems: discussions between veterinarians and dog owners during annual booster consultations. *Vet Rec*. 2013;172:235. doi:10.1136/vr.101125.

Siracusa C, Provoost L, Reisner IR. Dog- and owner-related risk factors for consideration of euthanasia or rehoming before a referral behavioral consultation and for euthanizing or rehoming the dog after the consultation. *J Vet Behav*. 2017;22:46e56.

CHAPTER 10

Behavioral treatment techniques, behavior modification, and learning theory

Lore I. Haug, DVM, MS, DACVB, CABC

Chapter contents

Introduction

Behavior problems are common in companion animals.[1-3] In many cases, lack of family education and planning contribute significantly to problem behaviors. Often pets are purchased spur of the moment with little thought to the future size, propensities, and behavioral and biological needs of the animal. Additionally, there is a vast body of inaccurate and problematic information available in the media and on the internet. Treatment of behavior problems in dogs and cats combines assessment of overall wellness, environmental management, education of pet parents, behavior modification,

and sometimes neurochemical modulation (e.g., supplements and medications) (see Chapters 11 and 12). In this chapter, the focus is on learning principles and behavior modification techniques or cognitive therapies. Behavior modification techniques can be highly successful and do not have to be complex. For example, in a survey of pet parents regarding treatments for noise aversion, counterconditioning was 70% effective and relaxation training was 69% effective in reducing their dog's fear of fireworks.[4] As the treatment plans become more complex, it is more likely that the veterinarian will need assistance from a training professional or a board-certified veterinary behaviorist.

Foundational concepts

Who should implement the behavioral treatment plan?

Successful behavior modification or cognitive therapy programs are highly correlated with the degree of pet parent comprehension and treatment adherence with appropriate veterinary team recommendations.[5,6] In most cases, family members will be tasked with the implementation of the behavioral treatment plan; therefore, they must understand why something has been recommended, what should be done, and how to do it. It is not necessary for the pet parent to train every step of each behavior in the behavioral treatment plan. However, when a behavior professional implements the plan, the pet parent must still understand why each therapy is important and how to follow through at home. It is acceptable in situations where pet parents are unable or unwilling to implement the behavioral treatment plan themselves to partner with a professional who will then teach the pet the necessary behaviors. However, ideally, this should happen in the home with the pet parent observing. The use of board-and-train facilities where the pet stays overnight or for extended periods of time should be approached with extreme caution. Separation from the home and family can be very traumatic, potentially leading to separation-related disorders, stress colitis, weight loss, and confinement distress. Physiologic stress and emotional stress inhibit the pet's ability to learn new operantly conditioned behaviors. Additionally, in these situations, the pet parent is completely absent from the behavior modification. As noted above, without an understanding of why the behaviors are important, the final criteria for each behavior, and how to continue to reinforce those behaviors at home, it is very unlikely that the behaviors will be retained by the pet over time. Finally, while positive reinforcement board-and-train facilities exist, they are the exception. Often, board-and-train facilities are using positive punishment and negative reinforcement techniques which are detrimental to the pet's welfare, less effective, and more difficult to implement than positive reinforcement and negative punishment (see Figure 10.1). In summary, pet parents should be involved with their pet's training but do not have to train each behavior from the ground up themselves. Board and train should be rarely if ever be recommended and only after careful and thorough vetting of the facility.

Ideally, every person who interacts with the pet should follow the recommendations and share a cohesive goal. Pets with anxiety, fear, or conflict disorders in particular need clarity and consistency during interactions with social group members. Households with members that have differing opinions regarding the severity of the behavior problem(s), philosophies on training, role of the pet in the household, and potential outcomes are likely to demonstrate suboptimal results no matter the type of behavior change plan.

Providing for the pet's needs is essential for success

Blaming behavior problems entirely on pet parent–related factors is unfair and negates the importance that genetic, physiologic, developmental, and environmental factors play in the presentation of undesirable or pathological behavior[3,7-9] (see Chapter 2). Nevertheless, as our societies drive pet ownership more completely into companion roles and further from utilitarian ones, pet parents may gradually lose perspective on the basic emotional and biological needs of our dogs and cats.

Pet parents must understand the physical and emotional needs of their pet so that they can provide them with appropriate outlets for play, exercise, social interaction (both human and conspecific), elimination, chewing, digging, and mental stimulation. This alone may be all that is required to solve some behavior problems such as feline behavioral periuria. For dogs and cats that are afraid of people, helping the pet parent understand that their pet does not desire or need social interaction with certain people or animals can start them on the path to decreasing the problem behavior. Pet parents also benefit from education on how animals communicate and learn. With education, pet parents can understand more clearly which problems are more likely to be completely

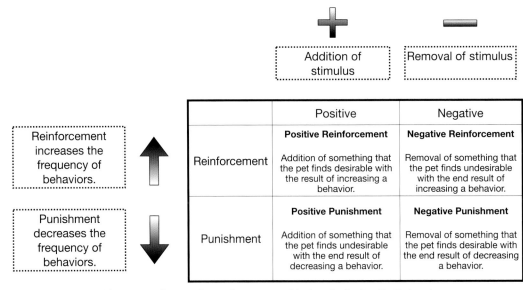

Figure 10.1 Four quadrants of operant conditioning. *(Attribution: Lisa Radosta.)*

eliminated, which are likely to be decreased but require a level of lifelong management, and which will be difficult to change.

Labels—helpful or harmful?

Another foundational concept is the labeling of behavior. As veterinary healthcare team members, we use labeling throughout our day to communicate with each other and pet parents. We label diabetic cats as diabetic ketoacidosis (DKA) and dogs with arthritis as painful. We label disorders by making diagnoses such as fear-induced aggression, separation-related disorders, and noise phobia. The meanings of labels such as those mentioned above are generally well accepted, and devoid of emotional context. They communicate a specific message which is not likely to be easily misinterpreted, although they lack clear information on the specific topography of problem behaviors in any particular pet.

Additionally, it is neither helpful nor accurate to label an animal as dominant, dangerous, "will bite for sure," or stubborn. These are just a few of the commonly used labels which are harmful, doing nothing to help us understand the consequence of or motivation for the animal's behavior. This leads to misinterpretation, offering no value in helping the animal, and typically will undermine treatment. To change behavior, we have to try to understand the "why" of the behavior in scientific and accurate terms. For example, the terms dominant and submissive have been overused and often incorrectly used, particularly in the lay literature. Dominant describes the comparison or relationship between the two individuals, particularly around valuable resources. It is not a personality or character trait. Even when the label of a particular diagnosis is used, the patient's clinical signs and motivation for the behavior should drive treatment, not the diagnosis exclusively. Labeling will not move the treatment plan forward and it may adversely affect the bond between the pet and pet parents. We cannot change "stubborn," but we can change a behavior such as barking at visitors, excessive meowing overnight, or fear of going outside. The clinician should avoid using inaccurate and non-scientific labels when communicating with pet parents.

The impact of fear, anxiety, stress, panic, and conflict on learning

The effect of fear, anxiety, stress, conflict, and panic (FASCP) on learning is powerful. Behaviors learned through trauma, whether physical or emotional, are very resistant to extinction (i.e., termination).[10,11] Once they are acquired, they are more resistant to change compared to behaviors which are learned without excessive sympathetic nervous system (SNS) arousal. Emotional states which involve pronounced SNS activation may be internally reinforcing or punishing. For example, a cat that exhibits fear in the veterinary clinic may have accompanying tachycardia, hypertension, and tachypnea. Those changes in physiology diminish when the cat is put back into the carrier, retreats, or uses aggression to remove the threat prior to being put into the carrier. The diminishing of the emotional and physiologic components of fear can reinforce the behaviors just preceding (e.g., hissing and aggression). This is a good example of why avoidance of situations where emotional responses associated with FASCP are preferred. In addition, it helps to explain how one traumatic incident can change an animal's life entirely.

Learning is a physiologic process

Before embarking on the journey to understand how to alter an animal's behavior through behavior modification (learning) techniques, you must understand the nature of learning itself. Learning is often presented as a passive, conscious, nonphysiologic process, when in fact learning involves activation of many different parts of the brain and body. Learning occurs on a cellular level in the animal's body. Learning also produces changes in physiology and structure of the brain by creating or removing synaptic connections and producing alterations in neurochemistry.[12]

Therapeutic options for behavioral disorders

The therapeutic options for behavioral disorders are similar to other body systems. Changes in lifestyle, diet, medications, supplements, and altering the behavior of the pet and the pet parent can all be employed.

Specific therapeutic options in behavioral medicine include the following:
- Conscientious (benign) neglect (e.g., no treatment)
- Environmental management (e.g., avoidance)
- Environmental management and neurochemical modulation (e.g., diet, medications, and supplements)
- Environmental management, neurochemical modulation, and behavioral treatments
- Rehoming the pet to a more suitable environment, if appropriate
- Humane euthanasia

Once the family is well informed about the situation and treatment options, the family may choose to simply live with the behavior problem. Other families may determine that rehoming or euthanasia is a safer, more appropriate choice for their circumstances.[13]

Environmental management (antecedent arrangements)

Environmental management involves changing or controlling various aspects of the pet's indoor and outdoor environment in order to reduce or eliminate the pet's ability to perform the undesired behavior. Pet parents may erroneously think that behavior is static and that if they are not working to alter the behavior, it will not change. Behaviors that are being repeated are being reinforced in some way; therefore, each time the pet engages in the inappropriate behavior, reinforcement is occurring or the behavior would not be repeated. When the animal is reinforced for a behavior, the likelihood of the pet doing it again increases. In other words, problem behaviors which are not altered with treatment modalities will get worse, not better. As with other medical disorders, treating behavior disorders with a "wait and see" approach is generally unwise.

Several environmental variables can be controlled, including confinement areas, exposure to eliciting stimuli, access to people, access to other animals, and access to targets of the behavior. As noted above, this can be a viable solution for many behavior problems. For example, if an older couple has a dog afraid of children, simply confining the dog away from children is perfectly acceptable, especially if the couple has no grandchildren of their own living with them and no friends who have children. Similarly, dogs that are aggressive at the dog park or day care can simply be removed from these environments. As noted above, pet parents often have preconceived notions or expectations of what should make their dog happy. If their dog is aggressive at the dog park, the dog is not enjoying the experience. If a cat knocks things off the shelves in the child's bedroom at night, confining the cat outside of the bedroom at night can solve the problem. See additional detail on antecedent arrangements in the Behavior Modification section below.

Rehoming the pet

Removing the pet from the home may be an unfortunate but necessary consideration, especially in situations where there is the potential for injury to people or other pets and when the pet parents have unreasonable expectations regarding outcome. Although removal of the pet may seem like a failure, it is desirable if it prevents injury or removes the pet from a situation in which it is subjected to undue distress. However, rehoming may not be an ethical or practical option if the pet would present a similar risk to a new family or the public in the new home. In these cases, euthanasia may be a part of the treatment discussion.[5] With that said, veterinarians should not suggest euthanasia without discussing all other options for treatment.

Behavior modification

Behavior modification is the principal means of changing or controlling undesirable behavior. Therefore, it is critical for practitioners to understand species-typical behavior (see Chapter 2) and the basic principles of learning and motivation if they intend to help pets with behavior problems.

Learning principles

As noted above, veterinarians and pet parents need a working understanding of learning principles in order evaluate how their own behavior influences the animal so they can implement training and behavior modification techniques and exercises effectively. Outlined below are common learning principles, most of which will be critical for formulating a comprehensive behavioral treatment plan for each patient (see Box 10.1).

Box 10.1 Commonly used terminology

- Stimulus: Any animate or inanimate object, event, or situation which elicits a sensory or behavioral response in an organism. A stimulus often precedes or elicits a behavioral response.
- Reinforcement: The consequence that follows a response which causes the behavior to increase in likelihood in the future. This can be play, food, reduction in a negative consequence, petting, or anything else that the pet regards as desirable. Often referred to as reward.
- Punishment: The consequence that follows a response which causes the behavior to decrease in likelihood in the future. This can be a verbal or leash correction, shock from a shock collar, being left alone, stopping something that the pet likes, or anything else that the pet finds aversive.

Habituation

Habituation is the simplest form of learning and occurs in all animals, including invertebrates. The technical definition is the diminishing of a physiological or emotional response to a stimulus due to repeated exposure without any reinforcement or punishment. The animal is repeatedly exposed to the stimulus without the presence of pleasant or unpleasant influences until the response ceases. A classic example is the person who moves to a home near a railroad track. Initially, the sound of the train coming is noticeable, but over time, the person generally learns to ignore the train. Similarly, the animal that has never been in a car may feel comfortable in the car after it takes several car rides. Habituation occurs commonly and without any intervention on the part of the pet parent and is a viable intervention for novel stimuli that do not elicit FASCP or aggression. If the pet shows FASCP or aggression, then merely exposing the pet to the stimulus will cause the behavior to worsen through a process called sensitization (see below).

Sensitization

Sensitization is almost the opposite of habituation—the individual's response to a stimulus increases with repeated exposure. For example, a dog that shows fear, anxiety, stress, conflict, or panic (FASCP) or aggression during a car ride will become more nervous with repeated rides through sensitization. Currently, little is known as to why some individuals habituate to a stimulus while others sensitize. Nevertheless, the intensity of the stimulus, the genetics of the individual, and the level of arousal at the time of exposure may be factors. If a pet parent suspects that their pet is in a situation which may result in sensitization, they should remove the pet promptly and seek professional assistance. In addition, they should avoid that situation until they can receive a proper assessment and therapeutic program.

Classical (Pavlovian or respondent) conditioning

Classical conditioning, also known as respondent or Pavlovian conditioning, is most closely associated historically with the scientist Ivan Pavlov, who conditioned dogs to salivate when they heard a bell. Throughout the rest of the chapter, respondent or Pavlovian conditioning will be referred to as classical conditioning. Classical conditioning involves the conditioning of involuntary responses—reflexes and emotions. For example, when a dog sees a treat training pouch and salivates, or a cat shows fear when the cat carrier is brought out, they are demonstrating the product (salivation and fear) of classical conditioning. Classical conditioning is also responsible for stimulus–stimulus associations such as a cat learning that the sound of the can opener means food or a dog learning that the pet parent putting on certain shoes leads to a walk or play.

Classical conditioning begins with an unconditioned stimulus (US) that elicits a reflex or involuntary behavior called an unconditioned response (UR). Neither the US nor the UR has to be learned—these are innate reactions built into the animal's physiology and behavioral repertoire. For example, a cat does not have to learn to secrete insulin (UR) in response to elevations in blood glucose (US), nor does the heart have to learn to beat faster (UR) when blood oxygen levels are low (US). Similarly, an animal does not have to learn to jerk a limb away (UR) in pain (US) when it steps on something sharp.

Classical conditioning occurs when a neutral stimulus (NS) takes on properties of a US. An NS that has no natural influence on the reflex is repeatedly paired with the US until the NS becomes a conditioned stimulus (CS). This occurs when the CS alone is able to elicit a response similar to the US by itself. The response to a CS is referred to as a conditioned response (CR). It is worthy to note that the UR and the CR are not identical. They may vary in intensity, the CR may include behaviors that the UR does not and vice versa, or they may be complete opposites. For example, the UR to shock in rats is jumping and a rise in heart rate, but the CR to a tone associated with shock is freezing and a lowered heart rate. Any previously neutral stimulus (e.g., location, smell, inanimate object, and animate object), can become a CS (see Table 10.1).

Like anything else in life, how a technique is implemented effects its efficacy. The most effective way to classically condition a stimulus is to present the NS prior to the US. Neutral stimuli predict the presentation of the US. In that way, they become conditioned stimuli. If there is no predictive value of the NS, conditioning is impaired, absent entirely, or may predict the absence of the US. For example, if one was attempting to train a cat to accept insulin injections by pairing the injections with food, the injection should be given first and the food given immediately after. If the food is given first, and the injection just after (backward conditioning), no conditioning will occur. Similarly, if a visitor entered the home and THEN rang the doorbell, dogs would not react to the doorbell because the doorbell would not predict the arrival of the visitor. The various forms of classical conditioning are outlined in Figure 10.2 and Box 10.2.

Classical conditioning occurs all the time in everyday life in relation to wide range of stimuli. Pet parents of storm-phobic dogs can themselves develop a classically conditioned aversion to storms after watching and dealing with their dog's storm panic. Classical conditioning is powerful and pervasive. We cannot stop or eliminate it, but we can control or change certain associations that pets make with proper management and behavior modification exercises. The proper use of classical conditioning for behavior modification is discussed in more detail below.

Operant (instrumental) conditioning

Operant conditioning is the conditioning of voluntary behaviors. The animal has direct control over the consequence that occurs in response to its behavior. This contrasts with classical conditioning, where associations are made between stimuli regardless of how the animal behaves—the doorbell means visitors, no matter whether the dog is sleeping, playing, or barking out the window. Operant conditioning is often referenced by the three-term contingency A–B–C where A refers to the antecedent, B to the behavior, and C to the consequence the animal gains from the behavior.

Consequences involve reinforcement or punishment, and these can be further divided into positive or negative. In the context of learning principles, positive and negative are mathematical terms, not references to the pleasantness or unpleasantness of a stimulus. Reinforcers increase the future probability of a behavior happening and punishers decrease it (see Figure 10.1).

Positive reinforcement is the addition of a desired stimulus or reinforcer following a behavior that results in an increased probability (frequency) of that behavior in the future. If a pet parent gets up and feeds a meowing cat in the middle of the night, the meowing is positively reinforced with food and potentially attention from the pet parent. The behavior of meowing at that time during the night will increase in the future. The time of night and/or the pet parent stirring in bed or getting up to go to the bathroom are the antecedents, B is the cat meowing, and C is the food or attention that the pet parent provides to the cat when the cat meows.

Negative reinforcement is often mistaken for punishment. Negative reinforcement is the removal of an undesirable or aversive stimulus in response to the animal performing a behavior that results in a decreased probability (frequency) of that behavior in the future. The animal is performing a behavior to stop something it does not like. An example of negative reinforcement is an outdated and contraindicated training technique involving pulling up on a choke chain to make a dog sit. The handler applies unpleasant or painful pressure upward with the collar and when the dog sits, the handler releases the pressure on the collar. This makes it more likely that the dog will sit in the future. See below for more information on why this method is contraindicated when training dogs. The application of bug spray is a real-life example of negative reinforcement. We apply bug spray to stop (escape) or prevent (avoid) the unpleasant sensation of bug bites. If you were bitten by bugs in that situation before, it was probably pretty unpleasant. When you applied bug spray, that unpleasant feeling became less likely, increasing the likelihood that you will apply bug spray in the future.

Behavior problems are maintained by negative reinforcement as well. For example, a cat that does not like being petted on its back (A) may bite the pet parent (B), causing the petting to stop (C). The petting (an undesirable or aversive stimulus) stops when the cat bites. The biting in that situation, potentially only with that person, will increase over time via negative reinforcement. When outside during a storm, a dog may learn that seeking shelter under the porch reduces the unpleasantness of the storm. Similarly, if a dog growls or snaps (B) when someone reaches out to pet it (A) and then the person pulls their hand away (C), the dog is reinforced for the growling/snapping. This means the dog is likely to use that strategy to stop people from petting it in the future. This does not mean we should encourage people to keep their hands in the line of fire. Instead, it demonstrates how important prevention of aggression is, as learning occurs whether or not we intend it to be so.

Positive punishment is the addition of an unpleasant or aversive stimulus immediately following a behavior that results in a decrease in the likelihood of that behavior (frequency) being repeated in the future. Spraying a cat with water for scratching the furniture, yelling at the dog for barking out the window, hitting an animal, holding it down, and using a shock collar are examples. Positive punishment is rarely if ever recommended in the treatment of animals with behavior problems. See below for more information.

Negative punishment is the removal of a desirable stimulus after a behavior resulting in a decrease in the probability (frequency) of that behavior in the future. Examples include ignoring a dog that is barking, a cat that is meowing, or

Table 10.1 Common real-life examples of classical conditioning

Subject	US	Possible UR	Possible NS	Possible CS	Possible CR

Dog/Cat	Bite from another animal	• FASCP*
		 • Tachycardia
		 • Tachypnea
		 • Escape attempts
		 • Panic
		 • Stress response
		 • Aggression
			• Characteristics of animal that bit
			 • Characteristics of environment in which the bite occurred
				• Location in which bite occurred
				   • Room inside of house
				   • Neighborhood
				   • Day care
				   • Dog park
				 • Predictors of the activity during which the bite occurred
				   • Leash, collar, treat bag
				 • Dog or cat
				   • Specific colors or sizes of dog or cat
					• FASCP
					 • Refusal
					   • To leave the house
					   • Walk in certain directions
					   • Walk into certain rooms
					 • Attempts to escape
					 • Aggression
					 • Vocalization

Dog/Cat	Thunder	• FASCP • Tachycardia • Tachypnea • Escape attempts • Panic • Stress response • Urination • Defecation • Destruction • Vocalization	• Dark sky • Lightning • Barometric pressure changes • Rain • Wind picking up	• Dark sky • Lightning • Barometric pressure changes • Rain • Wind picking up	• FASCP • Hiding • Trembling • Destruction • Attempts to escape • Aggression • Hypersalivation • Panting • Vocalization • Pacing
Dog/Cat	Separation from a social group member	• FASCP • Hiding • Tachycardia • Tachypnea • Escape attempts • Panic • Stress response • Urination • Defecation • Destruction • Vocalization	• Car keys • Purse • Briefcase/bag • Coffee mug • Alarm (wake up) • Setting house alarm • Shoes • Clothing • Phrases used before separation	• Car keys • Purse • Briefcase/bag • Coffee mug • Alarm (wake up) • Setting house alarm • Shoes • Clothing • Phrases used before separation	• FASCP • Hiding • Trembling • Destruction • Escape attempts • Aggression • Hypersalivation • Panting • Vocalization • Urination • Defecation • Destruction • Tachycardia • Tachypnea • Pacing
Dog/Cat	Pain from veterinary examination	• FASCP • Tachycardia • Tachypnea • Escape attempts • Panic • Stress response • Urination • Defecation • Destruction • Vocalization	• Cat carrier • Veterinary hospital • People in scrubs • Scent of alcohol • Scent of disinfectant • Color of scrubs • Needles/syringes • Stethoscope • Car ride	• Cat carrier • Veterinary hospital • People in scrubs • Scent of alcohol • Scent of disinfectant • Color of scrubs • Needles/syringes • Stethoscope • Car ride	• FASCP • Hiding • Trembling • Tachycardia • Tachypnea • Attempts to escape • Aggression • Hypersalivation • Pacing • Vocalization • Hyperthermia • Mydriasis • Defensive body postures • Urination • Defecation

The extent to which classical conditioning occurs, the associations made, and the responses exhibited are unique to the individual.

*FASCP, Fear, anxiety, stress, conflict, panic.

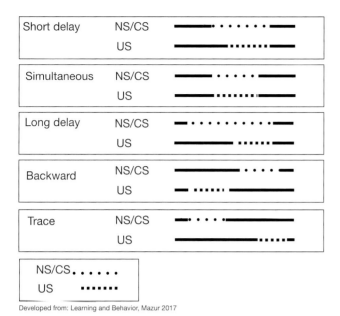

Short delay	NS/CS	
	US	
Simultaneous	NS/CS	
	US	
Long delay	NS/CS	
	US	
Backward	NS/CS	
	US	
Trace	NS/CS	
	US	

NS/CS . . . . . .
US   . . . .

Developed from: Learning and Behavior, Mazur 2017

Figure 10.2 Types of classical conditioning. *(Attribution: Lisa Radosta.)*

turning away from a dog that is jumping up. Denying the animal access to potential reinforcers is also a form of negative punishment—ceasing play or placing the animal in time-out, for example.

Although training is an active way to teach pets which behaviors will receive reinforcers and which ones will be followed by a punisher, a great deal of operant learning occurs independent of pet parent interactions. Pets that knock over a trash can and obtain food are reinforced for knocking over the trash can. Cats that ambush the pet parent and bite their legs are reinforced by a variety of consequences, including the pet parent's movement and the tactile sensation the cat receives through its teeth. Behaviors which are reinforced will increase in the future. While the pet parent may yell at the dog or spray the cat with water, if the reinforcing value of the immediate consequence (e.g., knocking over garbage) is greater than the punishing value of the yelling or water spray, respectively, the undesirable behaviors will persist. In addition, the consequence which immediately follows the behavior will be the most salient and have the most influence on whether the behavior is repeated in the future. For example, if a dog growls when a person reaches toward its bone, the person may pull their hand back to spank the dog. In this sequence, the most immediate consequence is the hand pulling away. This reinforces the dog for growling, even if the pet parent then spanks the dog afterward. The spanking will only serve to negatively reinforce or punish some other behavior the dog did right after growling, which sadly could have been approaching the pet parent or another desirable behavior. This is just one of many pitfalls of positive punishment—the behavior being punished is not always the undesirable behavior.

Avoidance and escape

In avoidance conditioning, the animal learns to avoid an aversive stimulus, while in escape conditioning, the animal performs a behavior to escape or terminate an ongoing aversive stimulus. This is negative reinforcement and the way that most shock collar training is conducted. The trainer applies a level of electric shock to the collar and when the dog does the desired behavior, the shock is terminated. The dog is learning to escape the shock by performing the desired behavior, such as coming when called. Negative reinforcement can easily lead to avoidance conditioning, where the animal attempts to avoid the situation altogether. In this example, the dog may avoid the trainer, run and hide when it sees the shock collar, or try to avoid moving to the actual training location.[14] These responses are maintained by a combination of negative reinforcement and classical conditioning (i.e., the training collar becomes a CS, triggering the CR of fear).

Similar avoidance behavior is frequently seen at the veterinary clinic. A dog with previous negative experience at the veterinary clinic (e.g., vaccinations, procedures, and catheter placement) growls when restrained. The growl is ignored and the patient escalates to biting. The aversive stimulus (e.g., restraint) is removed when the dog bites (negative reinforcement). Since the bite was negatively reinforced, that behavior (biting) will increase in the future. This is not to say that animals that are trying to avoid stressful stimuli should be held more tightly. Instead, these situations should be avoided (see Chapter 16). Avoidance conditioning can prevent an animal from learning that a situation is NOT distressing or painful. For example, a newly adopted cat may be afraid of the new pet parent and continually run away and hide. This behavior is negatively reinforced because the aversive stimulus (pet parent) disappears. In both of the situations above, the animals are showing FASC, which should cause the veterinary healthcare team or pet parent to pause and reassess, not escalate or block escape.

Motion detector alarms, noxious tastes and odors, and unpleasant substrates and surfaces can be used to teach animals to avoid particular objects or areas. A cat that jumps off the counter to avoid a spray of air is escaping the aversive stimulus. However, if an unpleasant event (e.g., taste, alarm, and spray) is paired with a warning stimulus (visual cue such as a warning flag, or audible cue such as a neutral tone), the pet can learn to avoid objects that are paired with the warning stimulus without having to experience the unpleasant event repeatedly. As already mentioned here, the salience of the stimulus is individual to the animal. Some animals will be so frightened by an aversive spray that they will not enter the room again, while some will ignore it entirely.

Avoidance conditioning is most likely to be successful when the desired response from the animal to the aversive stimulus is compatible with the animal's species-specific defensive reaction (i.e., fight, flight, freeze, and fidget). The response of a dog or cat is likely to differ from the reaction of a pigeon or a hedgehog. There is also much within species variation. In practice, most applications for avoidance involve training the pet to avoid or retreat from an object (e.g., couch, garbage can, or snakes) or an area of the home (e.g., windowsill or dining room). However, rather than retreating, the animal may attack the aversive stimulus, especially if the strategy can successfully remove the stimulus. This is a not an uncommon reaction in many cats and dogs. Conditioning associated with fear is powerful and can be life changing for the pet. For the reasons stated here, it is recommended that environmental management and prevention of the behavior is preferred in lieu of avoidance conditioning.

Reinforcement

Whether a particular reinforcer will be effective depends on the individual pet, its temperament, previous experience, current state (e.g., thirsty, hungry, satiated, or tired), and context.[15,16] For example, the pet's sociability, fearfulness, familiarity, and attachment to a person will determine whether affection and attention from that person will be reinforcing. Petting from a nonpreferred person or from a preferred person when it is not wanted may be perceived as punishing. If the pet parent calls a dog and the dog comes, expecting or wanting food but is petted instead, the pet parent may inadvertently punish the dog for coming and make it less likely that the dog will come, when called in the future. The value of a reinforcer is always determined by the receiver, not the giver. Just because the pet parent wants the dog or cat to perform a particular behavior for the reward praise does not mean the pet actually will. As a matter of fact, dogs and cats may work for praise and petting in some situations, but not in others.[17] In addition, petting is a lesser-value reinforcer than food or play.[18]

Pet parents should be encouraged to experiment and make a list of different reinforcers and their values to their pet. While pet parents may feel that they know what their pet likes, at least one study shows that is not the case.[19] Pet parents should test numerous items in each category (e.g., food, toys, play/games, olfactory stimuli, tactile stimuli, different forms of petting in different areas of the body, etc.) For example, in a study examining the reinforcement or enrichment preferences of shelter and owned cats, social interaction with a human was preferred over food, toy, and scent.[20] Generally, having at the ready different values or types of reinforcers can aid in motivating the pet. In one study in dogs, higher-value food rewards altered the speed

at which behaviors were performed when compared with higher quantities of food.[21] In contrast, a recent study in dogs demonstrated no differences in preferences between the two groups of dogs offered variation in reward and identical reward, with 25% of the dogs having no preference at all.[22] What is clear is that animals have preferences which are unique to that individual. To ensure the most effective behavior modification, a list of reinforcers by apparent value to the individual being taught should be made at the start and updated occasionally. See worksheet for Choosing Reinforcement and Reinforcement Choice and Delivery.

Finding the motivational value of any reinforcer in pet dogs and cats can be complicated because pets are often saturated with social attention, petting, and food, which can affect the likelihood of the pet viewing those things as reinforcing. If the pet does not view them as reinforcing, they will not be effective in increasing behaviors. In fact, many dogs and cats receive so much unwanted attention that it may contribute the pet's behavior problem(s) or at minimum, greatly reduce the value of attention from the pet parent as a reinforcer. On the other hand, one study found that dogs that were fed a meal 40 minutes prior to training were more successful than dogs that were fasted.[23] To further complicate matters, food enrichment via a food toy may increase the ability of dogs to learn through reward. For example, in a study of military working dogs, the ability to interact with a food-filled toy regularly increased the ability of dogs to learn via reinforcement and did not negatively affect the likelihood of playing with a toy, acting playful, or motivation to possess or retain toys when compared to control dogs.[24] In this case, the outcome could have been from lowered stress levels in those dogs that received food enrichment, or the food may simply have provided energy for cognitive processes. Finally, the welfare of the pet should be considered when withholding food for behavior modification. If the withholding of food increases the FASCP, it will most likely decrease the learning of desirable behaviors. More information on the pitfalls associated with calorie restriction and food deprivation is available in Chapter 13. As with all of medicine, behavioral medicine and the science of learning must be applied to pets on an individual basis with their motivation and welfare in mind.

For reinforcers to be effective, they must be contingent on the desired behavior. For example, if a dog or cat gets affection without regard for the preceding behavior, the pet may be reinforced for an undesirable behavior or may have difficulty learning when petting is used as the reinforcer. If the pet uses other strategies, such as barking, biting, or jumping up to successfully get attention, these behaviors will have been reinforced and will increase. Pet parents often acknowledge that they should ignore these and then wind up doing so inconsistently, thus putting the behavior on an intermittent reinforcement schedule (see below). This makes the undesirable behavior far more resistant to extinction (see section on Extinction). If attention becomes contingent on desirable behaviors such as sitting or lying down, the animals will exhibit these behaviors more often.

Behavioral health for all animals (including humans) relies in part on the animal feeling a sense of control over its environment. When reinforcers such as attention, treats, walks, or play are given inconsistently, the pet may become increasingly confused and frustrated—that is, unable to determine which behaviors consistently earn those reinforcers. Pets may show progressively more conflicted and anxious behavior, especially if the same behaviors are reinforced during some interactions and punished in others. This could lead to displacement behaviors such as scratching, jumping, mounting, circling, and tail chasing, especially in dogs that are genetically predisposed. Conflict and frustration can exacerbate or lead to aggression as well.

Effective reinforcers are also contiguous (i.e., closely follow the target behavior). If the reinforcement occurs too long after the desired behavior, the animal will have difficulty learning that the behavior and the behavior exhibited between the desired behavior and the reinforcement will increase instead. The more closely the reinforcer occurs in relation to the target behavior, the more effectively the animal will learn the desired response. Rapid reinforcement is particularly important in the early phases of training, so the animal gets swift feedback when it performs a desirable behavior. For example, pet parents often give their pets a treat after they come inside from eliminating, thinking they are reinforcing the act of eliminating when in truth they are reinforcing the behavior of running back into the house. This means some dogs will go outside and then try to get back inside as quickly as possible since this is the behavior the pet parent reinforced which can lead to incomplete voiding of the bladder or evacuation of the colon and eventual housetraining problems.

As noted above, the pet determines whether something is reinforcing (or punishing). Just because we think it should be does not mean it is. Family members must be cautioned that sometimes their attempts to scold a pet actually reinforces the pet's behavior. If a dog jumps up and the pet parent verbally reprimands the pet and pushes it down, this attention and physical contact may reinforce the jumping behavior. However, if the physical reprimand is then increased in intensity, the pet could learn not to exhibit the behavior, to enjoy rougher handling, or become fearful and conflicted about greetings.

Rather than use punishment techniques to decrease the performance of those behaviors that the pet parent considers undesirable, it is much more practical and humane to provide appropriate outlets for chewing, play, feeding, and elimination, and then reinforce any behavior that the pet parent wants the animal to repeat. In this way, little if any punishment or correction will ever be required (see Boxes 10.3 and 10.4).

Primary reinforcers

Primary reinforcers are those stimuli that animals find inherently reinforcing—no learning is required. These generally include food, water, sexual behavior, shelter/safety, sensory feedback, and some aspects of social companionship. Contrary to popular mindset, verbal praise is NOT a primary reinforcer in animals.[25] It is also a grave misconception that petting and human attention are primary reinforcers in all dogs or cats. Although there are individual differences, overall most dogs prefer food to petting and work harder and faster for food than social interaction.[16,26]

Box 10.3 Pitfalls of positive punishment

- Increases FASCP
- Very difficult to apply correctly.
- Must occur 1–2 seconds after the undesirable behavior and before ANY other behaviors are exhibited.
- Must be aversive or undesirable enough to outweigh any potential reinforcement or motivation for the behavior, but not so aversive to cause FASCP.
- Accompanying FASCP and pain can unintentionally cause classically conditioned associations with almost any other stimulus present in the environment.
- Exacerbates anxiety disorders and increase/produce conflict and aggression.
- When applied incorrectly, can physically injure pet.
- When applied incorrectly, serious welfare issues can arise.

Box 10.4 Foundational concepts of reinforcement

- Reinforcement value is determined by the animal being reinforced.
- Reinforcement value will vary by individual animals, even within the same species and breed.
- Reinforcement must be delivered immediately after the desired behavior but before another behavior occurs.
- Reinforcement value or preferences may vary with time.
- Reinforcement value or preferences will be affected by their relative accessibility by the pet.
- Petting and praise are usually less motivating than food and play.

However, the dog's response to petting can vary with context, familiarity with the person, and relative deprivation of social contact.[20] While many dogs and cats do find petting reinforcing, many do not. In fact, they may find such contact aversive, leading to biting or scratching behaviors or avoidance of people altogether.

One of the most powerful primary reinforcers is actually control—the animal's ability to influence its environment and control outcomes based on its behavior. Everyone behaves to produce desirable outcomes or avoid undesirable ones. Control is essential for behavioral health; lack of control indicates a serious welfare situation for the individual. Behavior treatment programs should be devised to give animals as much control over reinforcers in their lives as possible.

Conditioned or secondary reinforcers

Conditioned reinforcers are established through classical conditioning by pairing a previously neutral stimulus (e.g., verbal praise, a clicker, or a leash) with a primary reinforcer (e.g., food, play, or going for a walk). Dogs become excited when they see their harness or leash because these previously neutral items have been repeatedly paired with something desirable and fun (going for a walk). The leash has become a conditioned reinforcer. This has implications for how applying the leash can shape a dog's behavior without the pet parent realizing it. For example, a dog may get excited and jump and bark before a walk. The pet parent then struggles to get the leash on quickly so that she can get the dog outside for the walk. Over time, the prewalk excitability will increase because it is being reinforced by application of the leash and the subsequent walk.

Money is the penultimate example of a conditioned reinforcer. It has no inherent value—you cannot eat or drink it and it does not generally provide much companionship. However, by pairing it with a variety of primary and other secondary reinforcers, it has gained incomparable reinforcement power in our society. Thus, secondary reinforcers can sometimes be extremely powerful. If the functional outcome of a behavior is unclear, it is important to evaluate which secondary reinforcers may be playing a role in maintaining the behavior.

Bridging stimulus

By repeatedly pairing an NS such as a clicker with the delivery of a food treat or toy, the clicker becomes predictive of the treat and therefore becomes a CS or conditioned (secondary) reinforcer. This type of conditioned reinforcer is also called a *marker signal* or *bridging stimulus* because it is used to "mark" the moment the animal does the correct or desired behavior and it "bridges" the time between the behavior and the delivery of the primary reinforcer. Marker signals ideally are short, unique sounds that the animal hears primarily only during training, hence the popularity of whistles or mechanical clickers. Words can be used as marker signals, but ideally should be unique and short, such as "boop," "zip," "dot," "click," etc. This reduces the likelihood that the trainer injects varying emotional connotations. Additionally, common words such as "yes" may lose conditioning if the animal hears them frequently throughout the day (during casual conversations) in the absence of pairing with the primary reinforcer. Training specifically with a clicker (a plastic box which makes a sound when the button is pressed) has been shown to speed the acquisition of new behaviors but also may decrease the ability of the animal to discriminate in more complex processes which require assessment and decision making[27,28] (see Figures 10.3 and 10.4). However, in a recent study in shelter

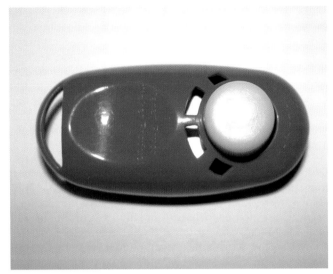
Figure 10.4 The i-click emits a softer click and may be more appropriate for sound-sensitive dogs or cats. *(Attribution: Lisa Radosta.)*

puppies, the use of a marker such as a clicker or verbal praise did not improve training progress or rate of training compared to the effective use and timing of primary reinforcement alone.[29] This may seem contradictory; however, the efficacy of any device as a teaching aid will depend to some extent on the user's ability to manipulate it effectively.

Schedules of reinforcement

Reinforcement schedules refer to the pattern in which a behavior is reinforced. Behaviors may be reinforced continuously, intermittently, or over some time interval.

Continuous reinforcement occurs when each correct behavioral response is reinforced. This schedule promotes the most effective and fastest learning. When a new behavior is being trained, continuous reinforcement is ideal. If a cat is being trained to come, the pet parent should reinforce the cat every single time it comes when called.

With intermittent reinforcement schedules, the target behavior is reinforced only sporadically. Intermittent reinforcement can be either fixed or variable on a ratio or interval schedule. Either the ratio can be fixed (a response is reinforced after a fixed number of repetitions) or the interval can be fixed (the first response after a fixed interval of time is reinforced). Similarly, the ratio can be variable (a response is reinforced after a variable number of repetitions) or the interval can be variable (the first response after a variable length of time is reinforced). Variable ratio and interval schedules produce behavior that is more resistant to extinction. Unfortunately, many undesirable behaviors (e.g., begging, jumping up, vocalization, and lunging at dogs on walks) are reinforced variably and intermittently so that they are highly resistant to extinction, making them more challenging to modify.

Schedules of reinforcement can become quite complicated in laboratory or applied behavior settings, but pet parents should be encouraged to keep their pets on a continuous reinforcement schedule for most behaviors. Invariably, pet parents will miss reinforcement opportunities and thus unintentionally put the pet on a variable schedule

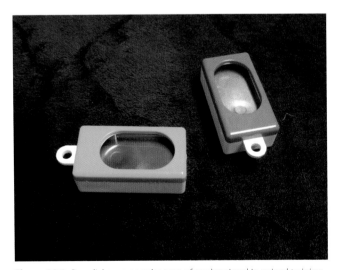
Figure 10.3 Box clickers, a popular type of marker signal in animal training. *(Attribution: Lore Haug.)*

anyway. If pet parents are "given permission" to skip reinforcement for some behaviors, then the reinforcement rate is likely to fall so low that the desirable behavior will go into extinction and eventually fade. Pet parents often ask when they can stop giving treats for desirable behaviors. The short answer is most likely never. Behaviors that are not reinforced will stop occurring. It is unlikely that pet parents will be successful at reinforcing every single correct attempt, effectively putting their pet on a variable reinforcement schedule anyway. Finally, problem behaviors may have competing motivations which are not adequately controlled, such as petting when a dog jumps up. If the pet parent stops reinforcing alternate behaviors such as sitting or lying down with a more valuable reinforcer such as food, for example, the behaviors of sitting or lying down will be reinforced less than jumping and they will decrease in frequency over time. A real-life example is an employee's paycheck. Employees perform behaviors at work which are neither natural nor innate but may be stressful, such as staying calm with a disgruntled pet parent. What would happen to the employee's behavior at work if we decreased or eliminated entirely their pay? It would be very likely that their performance would decrease in the future or they would leave their job for another better-paying job. The same is true for all animals. The most salient reinforcer will have the greatest effect on the pet's behavior (see Box 10.5).

Punishment

As stated earlier, punishment, by definition, results in the reduced probability of a behavior being repeated in the future. Negative punishment and positive punishment are defined above and in Figure 10.1. As with reinforcement, the receiver determines whether something is punishing or not. Some cats find petting punishing while others find it

---

> **Box 10.5** Answers to the common question: When can I stop giving my pet treats in training?
>
> - Behaviors which are not reinforced will stop being offered. If you stop giving your pet something that he or she finds rewarding when he or she does what you like, your pet will no longer perform those behaviors that are so important to you.
> - Your pet is unlikely to do what you want him to do for praise alone. In most dogs and cats, praise or petting is not enough to motivate them to learn and perform new behaviors.
> - Even though your pet loves you, love is not enough to motivate him or her to overcome his fear. Food and play are more powerful motivators. They also can change the way that your dog or cat feels, making them less afraid.
> - Since your dog or cat is praised so much throughout the day, which is not necessarily a bad thing, praise does not necessarily act as a reward anymore. Instead, food is more powerful.
> - Your pet is scared and stressed. What you are asking him to do is hard work. For that work, he needs a paycheck, just like you and me. How long would you continue to go to work if your boss no longer paid you?
> - Your pet is scared and stressed. Those are what is called competing motivations. Those in particular happen to be really powerful competing motivations. If we do not use equally powerful reinforcers, it will be very challenging to change your pet's behavior.

---

reinforcing. For punishment to be effective in decreasing a behavior, a sufficiently unpleasant stimulus needs to be presented during or within 1–2 seconds following that behavior and must be intense enough to reduce the pet's desire to repeat the behavior without causing physical or emotional harm. When positive punishment is applied incorrectly, whether in the timing or intensity (which is very common when it is implemented by pet parents), serious welfare issues can arise. Positive punishment can exacerbate anxiety disorders and/or produce conflict and aggression. In a survey of 354 dog pet parents, dogs that were trained with positive reinforcement techniques were rated by their pet parents as more obedient than dogs that were trained with mixed positive- and punishment-based training and dogs trained with solely punishment-based techniques. Furthermore, dogs that were trained with punishment-based techniques were more likely to exhibit problematic behaviors such as separation-related disorders and overexcitement.[30] Finally, agility dogs exposed to play (e.g., tug of war and chase) showed decreased salivary cortisol levels compared with those that were exposed to punishment-based techniques (e.g., yelling and pushing) after agility competition.[31]

Positive punishment is difficult to implement correctly without psychological and physical harm in some dogs, leading to conflict and problematic behaviors, and is not more effective than positive reinforcement techniques. Before positive punishment is used, consultation with skilled behavior professionals is indicated (see Box 10.3).

While some forms of punishment can be useful in some situations to reduce undesirable behaviors, it must be used as part of a comprehensive behavior treatment plan and should never be the sole intervention. In fact, even if positive punishment is effective at stopping unwanted behavior, it often leads to a negative (fearful) classically conditioned association with the stimulus or punisher. It is therefore important that the form of punishment be tailored to each pet and problem. If the punishment is timed incorrectly or of the wrong intensity, the animal may habituate to it, leading to failure in modifying the problem behavior. It will also inflict unnecessary pain and discomfort on the pet and cause repercussions such as defensive aggression and/or fear and avoidance. In some circumstances, it might inadvertently reinforce the undesirable behavior by providing attention. It certainly can erode the human animal bond.

Positive punishment and aversive training methods negatively impact welfare and have been associated with increased fear and aggression and both behavioral signs (e.g., tenseness and lower body posture) and physiological signs (e.g., panting and elevated cortisol) of stress.[32–34] Studies show that training with positive punishment, including hitting, prong collars, hanging by choke collars, shock, physical methods such as alpha rolls, and even yelling "no" is associated with increased aggression and avoidance.[35–37] On the other hand, dogs trained solely with reward-based training had fewer behavior problems than dogs that had punishment as part of their training.[27] In addition, when positive punishment-based techniques were/are used in training, the dogs were less likely to approach a stranger, less playful, less trainable, more fearful, and at increased risk of aggression toward family members, unfamiliar people, and in the veterinary clinic.[24,26,32,38–40] By comparison, dogs trained with positive reinforcement techniques had greater playfulness, higher training scores, performed better when taught a new task, and had fewer behavior problems including fear, aggression, and attention seeking.[27,32,33] In a study in military service dogs, positive reinforcement training was associated with higher closeness, increased attachment behavior, and more playfulness, while more fear and less closeness was associated with the greater use of punishment.[34] Positive punishment is difficult to apply effectively, can increase fear, anxiety, and aggression, and is less effective than positive reinforcement when training animals.

One might anticipate that the more aversive the stimulus, the more effective the punishment will be, but this is not necessarily true. For example, many dogs continue to hunt porcupines and skunks even after they have experienced the ill effects of such a meeting. This is an example of how the reinforcing effects of chasing a skunk and the timing of positive punishment are critical for learning. In this case, chasing the skunk is inherently and highly reinforcing. The punishment follows the chase, but the reinforcement is not negated. It is unfair and potentially damaging to punish a pet for a behavior when steps have not been taken to teach the pet what response IS appropriate.

Shock or electronic stimulation

Shock devices marketed to pet parents fall into several categories:
- electronic avoidance devices (e.g., mats) used to keep pets out of smaller areas;
- outdoor containment systems;
- indoor containment systems;
- pet parent–activated shock collars;
- remote-activated collars; and
- collars that emit a shock when a dog barks.

Shock collars

The use of shock, remote training, or electronic stimulation collars at any level of intensity for any length of time is never recommended as a part of a behavior modification plan for pets. The risk far outweighs any potential benefits. In fact, shock collars are considered inhumane and are illegal to use in many countries and regions including Scotland, Denmark, Norway, Sweden, Austria, Switzerland, Slovenia, Germany, Québec, Wales, and parts of Australia. Many organizations have published position statements advising against the use of electronic collars, including the European Society of Veterinary Clinical Ethology (ESVCE), American Veterinary Society of Animal Behavior (AVSAB), Association of Professional Dog Trainers (APDT), Pet Professional Guild (PPG), Humane Society of the United States, and the United Kingdom Kennel Club, to name a few.

Why have so many countries and organizations spoken out against and legislated the ban of shock collars? Most arguments against their use center on animal welfare. As the primary protectors of the welfare of companion animals, we should be aware of the arguments for and against the use of shock collars and the peer-reviewed literature on the subject. Before reviewing the controversy surrounding shock collars, a quick review of the use of reinforcers and

punishers is in order. To ensure proper learning regardless of technique, punishment and reinforcement should follow the target behavior immediately and before any other behavior is exhibited (good timing); the training method should not increase FASCP; and the stimulus (punishment or reinforcement) should be salient enough to act as intended—either as a punisher or a reinforcer. Deviation from the science of learning theory will cause less effective learning to occur. Despite the published scientific evidence against the use of shock (discussed below) in the training of companion animals, this type of training is still prevalent in the United States. In order to properly educate pet parents, veterinarians should be aware of the common reasons for use, the questions posed by the pet parents, and the conclusions which can be drawn from peer-reviewed literature (see also Box 10.6).

Intensity variability One of the guidelines for using punishment effectively is the control of the intensity of the punishment. Too high an intensity can cause pain, FASCP, and aggression,[41,42] while too low of an intensity can cause habituation. Unfortunately, when using a shock collar, regardless of whether it is remote activated, bark activated, containment, or user activated, the intensity of the shock and subsequent pain experienced by the animal cannot be fully controlled by the user due to tissue impedance. According to the Merriam-Webster dictionary, impedance is the resistance electricity encounters to complete a circuit. The conductivity of electricity through the tissues (experience of shock intensity) varies indirectly with the tissue impedance and is affected by the degree of humidity, hair length, hydration of the dog, location of the electrodes on the tissue during the training session, position of the head, dirt and debris on the hair coat, and subcutaneous fat.[43] In summary, pain is highly subjective to the individual, so no trainer can determine that a certain level of shock is or is not painful to that individual animal. Trainers commonly test shock collars on their own hands or arms to try to convince pet parents that the shock is not actually painful, but this is a fallacious argument. In addition, pet parents often start with a low-intensity shock and gradually increase the shock, which increases the likelihood of welfare degradation (due to inability to control the actual intensity) and habituation to the punisher. Finally, unlike other electrical devices such as coffee makers, in many countries there is no regulation or standardization of quality, consistency, or intensity levels of shock collars, meaning that a pet parent can purchase without prior knowledge a device which can potentially harm their pet, even on a low setting.

Associations with unintended stimuli As noted in Table 10.1, any previously neutral stimulus can be associated with any emotional state or involuntary response through classical conditioning. Dogs and cats can associate the pain of shock with anything in the environment, including animals, people, locations, scents, or auditory stimuli, that is salient to them at the time—even unconsciously perceived stimuli.[42,44] This can lead to aggression to animals and people, refusal to walk outside, refusal to go into areas of the home, unexplained or "unpredictable" panic (e.g., animal exposed to scent previously paired with shock), and FASCP

Box 10.6 Answers to pet parent queries about the use of shock collars

Question/challenge	Answers
Do you think that I should use a shock collar to train my dog?	No. We do not recommend the use of shock collars. They have been extensively studied in dogs and have been found to increase signs of fear and anxiety, cause physiologic stress along the lines of a panic attack, and can cause physical pain and injury. When shock collars are used, the dog's emotional state is not taken into consideration; when you add physical harm to stress, anxiety or fear, you see an increase in those things. An obedient dog can still be stressed and fearful. Also, studies show that they are not more effective than positive reinforcement techniques. Why would we use something that is not more effective and can hurt your dog?
I am super-busy. I need something simple and quick.	I get it! We all want that. Unfortunately, to reach your goals for your dog, we do not have a quick fix. The good news is that if we manage your dog's environment and change your goals a little bit, we can stop him from performing the behavior until you can implement a complete treatment plan. Let us talk about some quick fixes for your dog.
I need a permanent fix.	I agree. The most permanent fix for behavior problems comes from addressing all four aspects of treatment: systemic disease, management of the environment, cognitive therapies with positive reinforcement training, and medications or supplements to change the neurochemistry which may be driving the behavior.
Electric fencing is not really shock.	I can understand why you might feel that way. I want to tell you why we do not recommend electronic fencing. When dogs are sufficiently motivated to leave the property, they may do so whether they are shocked or not. Many times, dogs will choose to leave the property to access some exciting stimuli (to chase a cat, for example), but once they are off-property, do not want to reenter for risk of being shocked. Shock collars are not an effective way to keep any dog on the property, especially one that has shown aggression to other animals or people. In fact, one study shows that dogs contained with electric fences are almost twice as likely to escape as dogs contained with solid fences. I would not want to recommend anything that jeopardizes your dog's safety. In addition, they do not keep other animals, adults, or children off of your property.
I only had to shock my dog once. He responds to the beep now.	While it is true that dogs that are trained using shock collars respond to the beep, studies in dogs show that the beep sound produces a stress response in the dog, including increases in cortisol (a stress hormone) and increases in heart rate. Even the beep is scary to your dog and causes his body to have a stress response, as he would during any scary situation.
The shock collar does not hurt my dog.	If the shock did not cause pain of some sort, the collar would not work to change behaviors, plain and simple. If the shock did not elicit pain from the dog, it would not be punishing and the behavior would not decrease.

associated with previously neutral stimuli (e.g., type of clothing worn by the handler when shock training was conducted). While it is true that poorly timed reinforcement can also cause inaccurate associations made by the animal, there is a much smaller chance that positive reinforcement training will lead to undesirable associations when compared to avoidance learning and aversive methods.

No room for error Because of the salience of the aversive stimulus (pain), the user's timing must be perfect, otherwise the likelihood of increased aggression and fear is amplified.[41,45] It cannot be emphasized enough that most pet parents are not professional animal trainers. The likelihood that timing of shocks will be incorrect in the hands of an inexperienced trainer without professional education is high, increasing the risk of the negative outcomes listed above.[46]

Risks to welfare The potential for abuse, especially in the hands of an unskilled trainer or pet parent, is quite high. If the pet parent is frustrated or angry, they may be tempted to shock several times or increase the intensity of the shock, doing irreparable damage to the pet emotionally and potentially physically (see Figure 10.5A and B). In addition, there are physiologic ramifications of using shock, including increases in salivary cortisol (indicator of physiologic stress), heart rate,[47] and physical injury.

No greater efficacy than positive reinforcement methods
There are no studies showing increased acquisition or retention of new behaviors when shock collars are used compared to positive reinforcement training.[48] However, while there is no difference in efficacy, there is a difference in the welfare of the dogs being trained as evidenced by stress-related body language.[49] In clinical practice, when evaluating treatment modalities for any disorder, veterinarians consider the risks to the patient compared to the benefits which may be derived. In the case of shock, the risks to welfare are much higher than the potential benefits.

The quick fix Many pet parents try using a shock collar on their own or in the hands of a trainer before coming to their veterinarian or seeking out other methods. Behavior modification plans can seem daunting unattainable, and lengthy to pet parents. As with any other aspect of life, people may seek out what seems easy and quick. Learning to use an electronic collar without damage to the pet is neither quick nor easy, if attainable at all. In fact, studies have shown that dogs trained using shock show more stress behaviors than and to allow dogs the freedom to run free on a large unfenced property. However, in reality, most of these problems can be prevented, managed, or improved without the need for pain or discomfort. In addition, since these products deter behaviors by causing varying levels of fear and pain, they can condition new fear responses and further intensify underlying anxiety. This may lead to further emotional issues for the pet and the development of new behavior problems (e.g., defensive or redirected aggression or intense avoidance responses). Some dogs, despite the level of discomfort, continue to engage in the undesirable behavior despite even high-intensity shock.

One and done Pet parents often comment that after one shock, they only need to use the tone to get their dog to behave. As explained above, an NS (tone) can become a CS, eliciting a CR via classical conditioning. In fact, dogs that are conditioned to the tone/shock sequence show increases in heart rate from 82 to 150 BPM after the presentation of the tone and before the shock. While the heart rate at baseline was lower when a person was present, the increase in heart rate to 150 BPM still occurred before the shock was administered.[52]

Is electronic fencing different? Electronic fencing is often regarded by pet parents as less harmful than a handler-activated or bark-activated collar. In reality, the literature does not support this claim. This type of fencing does not keep people or other animals off the dog's property or keep the dog on the property. Dogs contained on electric fences are more likely to have escaped (44%) than dogs that are confined with a physical fence.[53] If the dog does escape, it will get shocked if it tries to return, which can inhibit the return to property and cause an association between entering the property and shock. Is this the association that we want dogs to make? Additionally, this author feels that the idea of an *invisible* "foe" that attacks the dog out of the blue presents a particularly egregious detriment to the animal's welfare.

Where the products are legal, practitioners should advise pet parents of the potential harm these products might cause to the pet and its welfare, and provide alternative options that can effectively address the pet parents' concerns. Under no circumstances should shock collars be used to train dogs and cats.

Conditioned punisher

By repeatedly pairing a neutral cue (e.g., a verbal "no" or "stop," duck call, or buzzer) with punishment (whether positive punishment such as a scentless air spray or negative punishment such as the removal of food or affection), the neutral cue becomes a classically conditioned stimulus predictive of punishment. The pet then may learn to retreat or cease a behavior with the cue alone, reducing the need for the actual punishment. The primary punishment need not be applied if the conditioned punisher achieves its goal.

Discriminative stimulus (command or cue)

A discriminative stimulus is a learned stimulus that informs an animal that reinforcement is attainable if a certain behavior is performed. These stimuli are generally called cues when they are purposely given by a human to trigger a

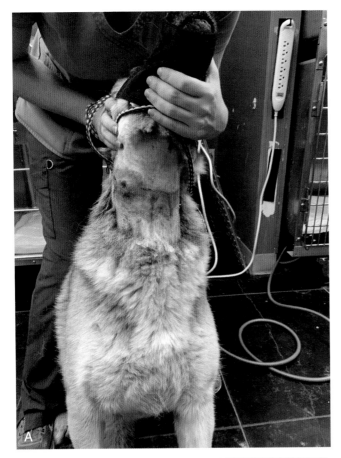

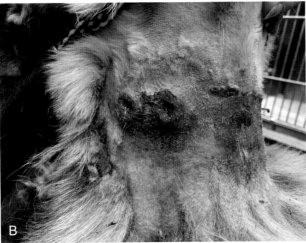

Figure 10.5 (A and B) Injuries due to a shock collar use. *(Courtesy of Jamie R. Bishop, DVM.)*

those trained in other ways, even when training is done by an experienced handler, while positive reinforcement training was found to be more effective in teaching target behaviors without the risks to welfare and quality of life.[50,51] Unfortunately, the effects are often long lived and difficult to overcome.

The last option Pet parents may feel that while not a good option, shock collars can be used in situations where safety is a factor, the problem might otherwise lead to relinquishment,

Current training practices focus on giving animal's choice and reinforcing appropriate behaviors. Therefore, the term "cue" is preferred over the term "command," as the latter implies that the animal must comply rather than inferring choice and voluntary cooperation.

response in the animal. For example, we say "sit" when we want the dog to put is rear end on the ground. Discriminative stimuli can be environmental cues as well. For example, the sound of the pantry opening may become a cue for the cat to run to the kitchen, jump on the counter, and meow for food. The sound of a plastic bag may be the cue for a dog to come to the kitchen (see Box 10.7).

A discriminative stimulus could also predict something the animal wants to avoid. If a pet parent frequently picks up a water bottle and sprays the cat when it has done something unacceptable, then the cat may learn to run and hide when it sees the pet parent pick up the bottle. Similarly, some dogs run away or cower when they see a prong collar or the shock collar remote as the dog has learned to avoid these stimuli. Note that classical conditioning is also occurring since the dog has developed a conditioned fear response to these stimuli.

A cue can be any stimulus in any sensory modality that the animal can perceive and find salient. Dogs actually focus better on visual cues versus auditory ones; thus, it is easier to teach them hand signals versus verbal cues. In one study where two new behaviors were taught using both a verbal cue and a visual cue, once the behaviors were learned the verbal cue for one behavior was given at the same time as the opposing visual cue for the other behavior. In all cases, the dogs responded to the visual cue over the contradictory verbal cue.[54] However, the response to a combination of congruent verbal and visual cues may be even quicker and more effective.[55] Therefore, in training, care should be taken to ensure that visual signals do not overshadow verbal cues. Additionally, pet parents must be cautious that they do not accidentally give conflicting verbal or visual cues. While the pet parent may be focusing on the behavior for the verbal cue, the dog will respond to the visual cue potentially resulting in the pet parent scolding the dog for being "wrong." This decreases the potential learning that could occur and can increase the conflict.

Extinction

Extinction occurs when a previously learned behavior is no longer reinforced. Both classically and operantly conditioned behaviors can undergo extinction. With classical conditioning, this involves separating the CS from the US. Using Pavlov's salivation example, this means ringing the bell without ever presenting food again. This breaks the contingency between the two stimuli, making the bell no longer predictive of the presentation of food. This can also happen when pet parents or trainers use a clicker without the subsequent presentation of a primary reinforcer, leading to the pet parent reporting that the clicker did not work for their dog. Each unpaired trial serves to break the level of conditioning. If this only happens a few times, little effect will be seen, but if it happens frequently, the marker may lose some or all of

its reinforcing power. If a pet parent trains a dog to come using food treats and then once the behavior is learned stops giving food altogether when the dog comes on cue, the dog will stop coming when called. This is an example of operant extinction.

Using extinction to resolve behavior problems can be difficult as we cannot always control the pet's access to all the potential reinforcers; nevertheless, extinction is an important part of behavior modification. Both desirable and undesirable behaviors that have been reinforced intermittently are much more resistant to extinction. Once extinct, it takes only an occasional reinforcement for the behavior to resurface. In some cases, spontaneous recovery can occur after a rest period between extinction trials.

If pet parents are asked to ignore or withdraw reinforcement for certain nuisance behaviors, they must be educated regarding the extinction burst. Extinguishing a behavior by withdrawing reinforcement which was previously given for that behavior produces some level of frustration in the learner—why is this behavior no longer working? This frustration leads to an intensification of the behavior—the animal tries harder. This is the classic "kicking the dispensing machine" behavior. You put in money, expecting what was selected, and nothing happens. So you bang on the machine, try more money, stick your arm up inside, etc. to try to get reinforcement. Eventually, you give up and go away. Pet parents must be instructed to ignore this escalation of behavior or the new and more intense behavior will be reinforced.

Motivation

Motivation is an animal's drive or desire to perform a behavior. The pet's level of motivation is a key consideration in training and in trying to reduce behaviors through behavior modification. Motivation is dependent on the attractiveness of the reinforcer or the power of the aversive the animal is trying to escape or avoid. Motivating operations are environmental variables or internal states that influence the reinforcing or punishing quality of a consequence. For example, withholding part of a dog's meal prior to a training session may increase the reinforcing power of that food. In another subject, food which is delayed significantly from the scheduled time may decrease learning. Taking a dog for a long walk before introducing the dog to visitors may reduce the dog's arousal during the greeting. A dog in pain will be less motivated to play ball because the pain makes fetching less enjoyable (or more punishing). Motivating operations can be manipulated to enhance behavior modification exercises and to reduce the appearance of undesirable behaviors (by reducing the effectiveness of the reinforcement for the problem behavior). Nevertheless, severe deprivation is unacceptable as a training tool, as it compromises the animal's welfare and control over its own environment. Effective behavior change programs can be designed such that harsh deprivation is unnecessary.

Taste aversion

Taste aversion is a specific form of aversive conditioning in which the animal develops an aversion to a particular odor or taste that is associated with illness. This is generally a single-event learning experience, although taste aversion can occur gradually, with some repeated exposure causing lower level nausea. Taste aversion is likely an innate defense mechanism, so that the animal learns to avoid potentially toxic substances. Taste aversion differs from other forms of aversion therapy or avoidance conditioning in that it can occur after a single event and the illness may take place hours after the ingestion of the substance.

Taste aversion can occur in animals that have intermittent chronic gastrointestinal upset and could be one reason they appear to develop "finicky" eating habits. Dogs that have gastrointestinal disease may become more and more resistant to accepting various food reinforcers, thus making behavior modification difficult. Addressing the underlying gastrointestinal disease is crucial to a successful outcome.

Observational learning

Observational learning refers to learning that occurs passively by watching others.[56] There is some question as to how effectively pets can learn by observation, although there are now a few studies of kittens and puppies learning from their mothers.[57,58] In one study, puppies that observed their mother learn to sit with food rewards were significantly better at learning the task than puppies that had not observed their mother during the initial learning phase.[59] In another study, dogs that observed a group of dogs undergo clicker training were then able to learn a new task using a secondary reinforcer, while dogs that had not observed the clicker training could not learn the task.[60] In each of these examples, the critical issue appears to be the observation of the learning itself rather than the end result (the behavior). However, it is likely that in most cases of apparent observational learning in dogs, social or group facilitation of behavior is at work. Examples include cooperative hunting, group-facilitated barking, and socially facilitated eating. In addition, dogs and cats are likely to attend to the same cues as other pets in the household, but their responses may be the same or different based on individual motivation and previous experience.

One-event (trial) learning

One-trial learning occurs when an animal learns after a single pairing of a stimulus and response. This may relate to either operant or classical conditioning (or both at the same time). Single-event learning is particularly likely with aversive events. If the pet is shocked when it bites into an electrical cord, it is unlikely that it will chew on a cord again. Single-event learning is most likely to occur when something unexpected happens, as the surprise factor makes the experience more salient. Single-event learning sometimes is an effective way to teach the pet to avoid particularly dangerous or undesirable activities. For example, the use of a highly noxious taste may deter chewing of electrical cords. However, care must be taken any time significant aversive stimuli are going to be employed to avoid causing emotional damage and worsening of behavior (see section on Punishment).

Overlearning

This involves the continued practice and reinforcement of a behavior that appears to be completely mastered. While continued practice does not change the observable behavior, studies show that it does improve retention and make the behavior more resistant to extinction. So, pet parents should be encouraged to continue to practice behaviors even after they think the pet "knows" the behavior.

Premack principle and response deprivation

The Premack principle states that high probability behaviors can reinforce low probability behaviors. That is, behaviors that an individual performs at a higher baseline rate can reinforce behaviors that occur at a lower baseline rate. For example, if a dog "prefers" playing tug versus fetching a ball, then tugging can be used to reinforce fetching. A dog that likes to jump on people could be trained to sit for greetings by then giving the dog permission to jump up as reinforcement. Over time, sitting occurs more frequently and the cue to jump can be reduced in frequency or omitted. The Premack principle is based in part on the concept of relative value of behaviors as reinforcers; however, in some cases, low probability behaviors have been observed to reinforce high probability behaviors. The response deprivation theory (RDT) serves to address some of the problems with the Premack principle.[61] Every behavior an individual does occurs at some baseline rate. The RDT states that a behavior becomes reinforcing when the animal (or person) is prevented from engaging in the behavior at its normal, desired frequency. Being permitted to perform this behavior can then become contingent on the animal engaging in a different behavior. For example, if a dog spends 40% of its time in the yard barking and running along the fence and only 5% of the time lying quietly on the patio, then the former behavior can be used to train the dog to rest quietly more often. If the high baseline behavior can be controlled (e.g., putting the dog on a leash), then the dog can be given permission to engage in fence running after resting quietly on the patio for a certain time frame. As training progresses, the resting behavior is shaped for longer duration before the dog is given permission to engage in fence running. Similarly, dogs can be trained to walk quietly at heel by then giving them permission to sniff, explore, and eliminate (especially urine marking for males). The Premack principle and RDT are powerful behavior modification tools, especially for situations where traditional reinforcers such as food and praise are unavailable or rejected by the animal.

Behavior modification techniques and protocols

Introduction

While protocols are available detailing how to treat certain behavior problems, behavior treatment plans should be tailored to each individual animal with consideration of their sex, hereditary influences, socialization history, environment, the influence of other animals in the environment, and the people who live with them. When other pets in the household are involved (e.g., barking, eliminating, and aggression), all pets need to be treated for successful outcome. Behavioral treatment is intended to address the animal's response to certain stimuli in the environment and starts with a functional analysis.

Functional analysis

Functional analysis evaluates the antecedents (i.e., stimuli, cues, and situations) and consequences (i.e., reinforcement and punishment) that maintain problem behavior. The clinician should try to establish an A–B–C for each problem behavior the pet parent reports or that the clinician identifies. This ensures that we understand specifically what triggers the behavior (e.g., the dog bit the toddler because the toddler hugged the dog) and what the dog obtains from the behavior (when the dog bit the toddler, the toddler let go of the dog—and then was removed entirely by his parents). Identification of the functional consequence is ideal but is not always possible because much of the information gleaned about the animal's behavior will be via pet parent report. When the functional consequence (what continues to fuel the behavior) is identified, it can be removed, shifted, or avoided by devising a protocol that allows the pet to obtain the same consequence with a different, more acceptable behavior. For example, if the dog mentioned above barks as the toddler approaches, the parent can remove the toddler before it hugs the dog. The functional consequence in both cases is identical—removal of the toddler. In the latter example, barking has been reinforced instead of biting. A cat that is uncomfortable being picked up bites and the pet parent puts the cat down. The functional consequence is that the cat is put down (not carried). In this example, picking the cat up can be avoided and instead the cat can be taught to jump up onto the couch to sit with the pet parent.

In cases where the functional consequence is not clear, the practitioner should write out the possible functional consequences similar to a differential diagnosis list, then start a protocol based on one of the consequences and observe whether the behavior is increasing or decreasing in frequency over time. If the former is occurring, the protocol should be changed and centered on one of the other possible functional outcomes. One noteworthy value in using functional analysis is that it avoids labeling the animal or behavior. As noted above, labels do nothing to help us understand the consequence of the animal's behavior and why the animal persists in doing it. A functional analysis allows the practitioner to understand the reason for the behavior.

Hierarchy of behavior change procedures[62]

Once the clinician has established a problem list and a functional analysis for each problem behavior, then the clinician devises a management and behavior modification program. In cases where there are multiple problems, the behaviors should be triaged to allow for more rapid and effective change. Behaviors that cause a danger to the pet or others, may increase relinquishment or euthanasia, cannot be easily avoided, pose a welfare risk, and/or cause the pet parent the most distress should be addressed first (see Box 10.8).

Behavioral treatment programs should use the least intrusive method possible, should not include positive punishment, and should be centered on the animal's welfare and ability to engage willingly in the training protocols. Effective and humane treatment plans can be constructed using two

Box 10.8 Behaviors that should be addressed first in behavior treatment plans

Behavior	Examples
Behaviors causing daily danger or significant disruption to the household.	Dog growling at child, cat biting child or other immunosuppressed individual.
Behaviors not easily avoided.	Dog barks at other dogs on walks and the pet parent lives in an apartment that requires multiple daily walks for elimination.
Behaviors which cause the most distress to the pet parent, even if they do not pose a notable public risk or welfare risk to the animal.	Cat exhibits nocturnal vocalization, disrupting the pet parent's sleep.
Situations that pose a moderate to severe welfare risk to the animal.	Dog with storm phobia or separation-related disorder that panics and tries to escape the house or crate.

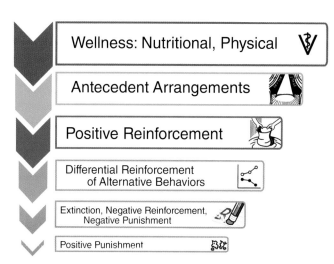

Figure 10.6 Hierarchy of behavior change protocols (HoBCP). *(Courtesy of Dr. Susan Friedman, PhD.)*

sources: the hierarchy of behavior change procedures (HoBCP) (see Figure 10.6) and the Five Freedoms of Welfare (see Chapters 1 and 7). The following paragraphs will touch on each of the intervention levels outlined in the HoBCP, created by Dr. Susan Friedman.[51]

Providing for biological needs

An individual's physical health and mental health are intimately tied together. For a behavior change program to be most successful, we must be working with an animal that is physically healthy. Careful evaluation of veterinary care, exercise programs, and nutrition are part of a behavior change program (see Chapters 6 and 7).

Animals evolved to interact with their environment and evolution has honed certain behaviors so that there is a strong biological drive to perform them. For example, hunting behavior in cats occurs independent of hunger.[63] This means even well-fed cats have an instinctual drive to hunt. Indoor cats are almost completely deprived of the ability to perform this behavior and this contributes to the development of behavior problems. Similarly, most dog breeds were bred for certain functions and therefore have a high "drive" to do these behaviors (e.g., digging, retrieving, hunting, guarding, etc.). If the dogs are not given access to these outlets or acceptable substitutes, there is a negative impact on their welfare and an increased likelihood of behavior problems. A well-designed behavior change program includes finding ways to meet the animal's needs for exercise, mental stimulation, social contact, good nutrition, etc. Environmental enrichment for captive and companion animals is not an option; it is an obligation. As noted earlier in the chapter, pet parents may not fully understand their pet's basic needs. As a result, many dogs and cats are receiving inadequate amounts or inappropriate types of mental and physical stimulation. Aerobic exercise is essential for most dogs and a 15-minute walk around the neighborhood while the pet parent talks on the cell phone is not adequate. Exercise should not only be aerobic but also constructive, meaning that running the fence line and barking, while aerobic, is not constructive.

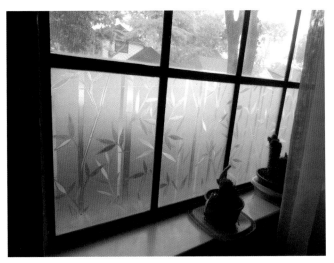

Figure 10.7 Opaque decorative window film can significantly reduce barking at outside stimuli. *(Attribution: Lore Haug.)*

Environmental management (antecedent arrangements) prevention rehearsal of the problem behavior

Practice makes perfect. This applies to desirable and undesirable behaviors. Pet parents may work very hard to reinforce positive and alternate behaviors. However, if the pet is still practicing and being reinforced for the undesirable behavior, the outcome will be unsatisfactory.

Preventive techniques (i.e., avoidance) are some of the most valuable, essential, and effective tools in behavior therapy. Animals exhibit behaviors in response to environmental cues—see a dog out the window and bark. If they do not see the dog, then they may not bark. These cues are the behavioral antecedents. By changing access to the antecedents (i.e., the things that trigger the behavior), the pet parent can often eliminate or diminish the expression and rehearsal of the problem behavior. This also reduces reinforcement of the problem behavior, which makes reinforcement of competing behaviors more effective.

For example, if a dog barks out the window in response to people walking by, the pet parent can block the dog from accessing the front part of the house or cover the windows with opaque window film to prevent the dog from seeing outside (see Figure 10.7). This intervention often significantly reduces nuisance or territorial barking in dogs. Walking dogs at different times of day or in different locations allows the pet parent to avoid the sight of other dogs that cause barking and lunging from their own dog. If necessary, pet parents can (for a time) stop walking the dog altogether and exercise them inside or play only in the back yard. If the cat jumps on the counter to steal food, the pet parent should avoid leaving food out on the counter. Territorial dogs should be confined to a bedroom or crate in a back bedroom when visitors are in the house.

Denying the pet the opportunity to perform unacceptable behaviors may help shift the pet's behavior to something more acceptable, assuming acceptable alternatives are provided. These behaviors can then be reinforced. Prevention may also be the most practical way to prevent injury and avoid damage to the pet parent's possessions. In some cases, antecedent arrangements alone will accomplish the pet parent's goal or provide an acceptable level of improvement without the pet parent investing potentially scarce resources into an intensive behavior modification program.

This type of environmental management is one of the most important but overlooked aspects of a treatment plan for behavior problems. Eliminating antecedents for problem behavior should be the first intervention outlined for pet parents. Pet parents often feel this is somehow cheating or detrimental, so most are grateful when they are given permission to just avoid problem situations altogether. While antecedent management will not "cure" the problem behavior (the dog will still lunge at other dogs on walks if the pet parent does encounter one), it does prevent the pet from continuing to rehearse (and therefore be reinforced) for the undesirable behavior.

Positive reinforcement

The next level of intervention in the HoBCP is the use of positive reinforcement. As stated before, animals behave to achieve reinforcement. Many animals with behavior problems are unknowingly subjected to poor welfare because their day is devoid of adequate opportunities to achieve reinforcement in an acceptable way. When animals engage in undesirable behaviors to achieve reinforcement, the pet parents expend considerable energy trying to stop the pet, usually with some type of punishment or aversive interaction. This erodes the human–animal bond and puts the pet's goal and the pet parent's goal at odds—conflict becomes the norm. For example, if a high-energy dog does not get adequate exercise, it is likely to engage in other stimulating behaviors such as barking, digging, running the fence line, or pestering the pet parent to play. Instead of focusing on enrichment and the reinforcement of other (alternate and incompatible) behaviors, if the pet parent yells at or otherwise punishes the dog, the relationship between the dog and the pet parent breaks down. By the time the aforementioned dog is presented for treatment, the behavior problem may be severe and the pet parent is likely to be very frustrated.

How do you feel when your day goes really well? When pet parents are not upset with you, your partner takes you to a surprise dinner, and your teenager gives you a surprise hug? Who does not want a more joyful and positive day? Animals are no different. Positive reinforcement-based interactions with family members should grossly outbalance aversive interactions. For every one aversive interaction (e.g., the pet parent scolds the pet), the pet parent should have at least 30–50 positive interactions (e.g., the pet parent praises the dog for lying quietly on its bed) every day. Implementing some simple daily training tasks using positive reinforcement allows the pet to achieve desired reinforcers (e.g., food, play, and attention) in a predictable and acceptable way. Pet parents should learn to actively observe the pet throughout the day to capture desirable behavior and reinforce the pet any time they see the pet performing such behaviors. Examples include the pet playing with its own toys, resting calmly on its dog bed or cat tree, socializing in an acceptable manner, looking quietly out the window (rather than whining or barking), scratching on appropriate surfaces, etc. It is not infrequent for aggressive dogs to become much more social and compliant just in response to the pet parents spending time practicing sitting for food treats each day. The value of implementing a simple positive reinforcement-based training program cannot be overemphasized.

Positive reinforcement is also used to train skills that are necessary or useful in the behavior modification program. For example, relaxation training for separation-related disorder is sometimes easier if the pet has previously been trained to lie down (see the Foundation Skills section below).

Reinforcer assessment

Since an individual pet's response to any specific reinforcer may vary, it is essential that the family determines which reinforcers are most likely to motivate the pet. Reinforcers of each type (e.g., food, play/toys, social contact, or activities) can be categorized in a hierarchy, (i.e., most to least favorite). See Reinforcement Choice and Delivery and Motivating Operations above. This allows the pet parent/trainer to choose reinforcers most appropriate for the training situation. For example, in general, higher value reinforcers are preferred for challenging behaviors and higher distraction situations.

The effectiveness of the reinforcer might be enhanced by withholding it at times rather than giving the animal free access. As noted above, it is unacceptable to actually deprive the animal of essential reinforcers in order to increase motivation. Pets should not be ration restricted or starved in order to try to enhance training effectiveness.

Differential reinforcement of alternative behaviors

Differential reinforcement protocols are commonly used. Three of the most common include the differential reinforcement of alternative behaviors (DRA), as well as differential reinforcement of incompatible behaviors (DRI) and differential reinforcement of other behavior (DRO). Other less commonly used protocols include DR of low rate responding, DR of high rate responding, and DR of higher or lower intensity responding. Each of the principal differential reinforcement protocols focuses on reinforcing the animal for some desirable behavior while letting the undesirable behavior extinguish. An example of a DRI protocol is to reinforce a dog for sitting when it greets people rather than jumping. Sitting is incompatible with jumping. If the dog jumps, the behavior is ignored, putting jumping on an extinction schedule, while sitting is heavily reinforced. Training a cat to sit on a chair in the kitchen during feeding time prevents the cat from chasing the other cats out of the area. Training a dog to sit and look at the pet parent on walks rather than lunging and barking at dogs is an example of a DRA protocol. Sitting is incompatible with lunging, but sitting dogs can still bark. An example of a DRO protocol for dogs that bark at environmental stimuli when out in the backyard involves instructing pet parents to go outside with the dog at all times and reinforce the dog for all appropriate behaviors (other) that do not involve barking. So, the dog is reinforced for sniffing, eliminating, looking at the pet parent, playing with another household dog, lying calming in the grass, wandering around, playing with toys, etc. By doing this, the rate of these behaviors increases and the rate of barking decreases.

The rate of reinforcement in DR schedules should be high, at least initially. Since DR schedules include a degree of extinction for the problem behavior, the animal may experience frustration and an extinction burst if the pet parent is not adequately reinforcing the competing desirable behavior(s).

Extinction and negative punishment

Extinction is best utilized for attention-seeking behaviors and those where ignoring the problem behavior will not lead to a safety risk for the animal or anyone around it. For example, if the dog barks at the pet parent for attention, the pet parent ignores the dog (extinction) and later reinforces the dog for a more appropriate behavior (DRA) such as resting on its bed or playing with a toy. In this situation, no one is going to get injured if the pet parent ignores the dog. In contrast, if a dog is growling at and advancing on a visitor to the home, having the visitor and pet parent ignore the dog is not an appropriate response. Rather, the dog should be redirected away and then a more appropriate plan devised for introducing the dog to visitors.

Negative punishment is a common intervention and often used for problems in which the reinforcement can be easily controlled or removed such as barking, jumping, or pulling on leash in dogs and vocalization and play biting in cats. One example is of a dog that jumps on people. The dog jumps and the person turns away from the dog, removing attention. In this case, the jumping is negatively punished and will decrease over time. Alternatively, consider the cat that bites during play. If, as soon as the cat bites, the pet parent removes all chance of play, which can include exiting the room themselves, the biting will be punished and should be performed less in that situation in the future. As these two examples demonstrate, timing is crucial. In both cases, if the dog or cat receives attention, even in the way of yelling, the behavior is potentially being reinforced, not punished, causing the behavior to increase.

Negative reinforcement

This operant technique involves the utilization of an aversive intervention and is recommended only if appropriately chosen and implemented positive techniques have failed or are deemed to be detrimental to the animal's situation and welfare. These protocols should be implemented in the most benign manner possible and the animal's body language and motivation to willingly engage in the training evaluated. If the animal shows signs of stress and/or appears reluctant to willingly continue in a training session, then the level of aversive is too high. The plan should be reevaluated and adjustments made for a less aversive experience. Even knowledgeable, experienced, and skilled behavior professionals and veterinarians can feel like they are at a loss as to how to proceed with a certain case. This may lead to the use and misuse of aversive techniques when they are not necessary. Consultation with behavior professionals, veterinarians, and board-certified veterinary behaviorists can elucidate non-aversive treatments that have not yet been tried or identify implementation problems with current protocols which may have resulted in their failure.

Negative reinforcement is the most controversial intervention on this level of the hierarchy because it does involve the purposeful application of an aversive to the animal. In fact, in a comparison of positive reinforcement and negative reinforcement in teaching the same behavior (sit) to dogs, dogs trained with negative reinforcement showed more signs of fear and dogs trained with positive reinforcement were more attentive to the handler.[26] Head collars (e.g., Walk With Me, Halti, and Comfort Trainer) (see Figures 10.8 and 10.9) and no-pull harnesses (e.g., Freedom, Sensible, and Balance) (see Figures 10.10 and 10.11) cause their effect via negative reinforcement. When the dog pulls, the head collar or harness tightens, which is an unpleasant sensation. When the dog

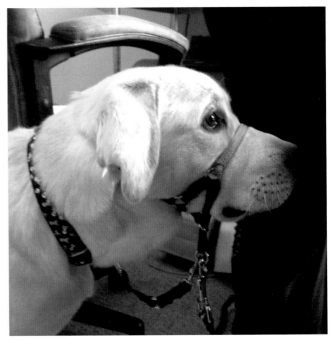

Figure 10.9 The Comfort Trainer head collar. *(Attribution: Lisa Radosta.)*

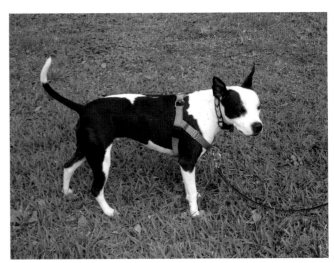

Figure 10.10 The Freedom harness is one example of a front clip harness. Front clip harnesses can provide better physical control, especially for large and/or unruly dogs. *(Attribution: Lore Haug.)*

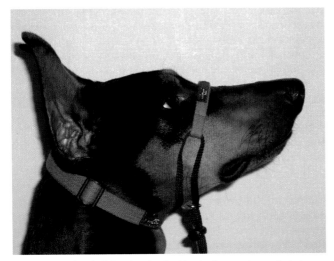

Figure 10.8 The Black Dog head collar. Head collars can be particularly useful for pet parents with certain physical limitations and also for dogs that tend to redirect aggression toward their handler in the presence of triggering stimuli. *(Attribution: Lore Haug.)*

stops pulling, the tension is released automatically by the device. The behavior of walking at the pet parent's side on a loose leash is reinforced because the unpleasant sensation disappears when the dog is not pulling.

Constructional aggression treatment (CAT)[64] and behavior adjustment training (BAT)[65,66] are techniques which use negative reinforcement to decrease aggression in dogs. Both techniques involve allowing the aggressive dog to visualize the stimulus to which it is aggressive (e.g., dog and person) at a distance where the dog shows little to no signs of arousal. The decoy is removed or the dog is moved away from the decoy, depending on the method being employed, when the dog shows a more appropriate reaction, such as

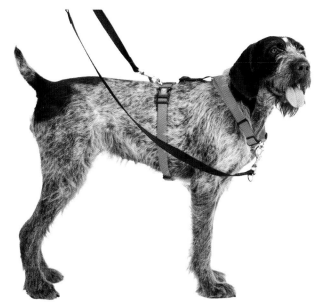

Figure 10.11 Blue-9 no pull harness. *(Attribution: Blue9 Pet Products; www. blue9.com.)*

turning away and lying down (see Figure 10.12). In this way, calmer, more ritualized behaviors (lower rungs on the stress ladder) are reinforced because the arousing stimulus is removed when those signs are exhibited. Over time, the calmer body language will be exhibited when the dog encounters the stimulus if the procedure was done correctly. CAT and BAT are only successful if the functional consequence reinforcing the aggressive behavior is the disappearance of the trigger stimulus. For example, if a dog barks at dogs on walks to keep the other dog away, then using CAT or BAT can teach the patient dog that turning away is now the most successful behavior at keeping the other dog at bay. These techniques, while often quite successful, require considerable skill, careful coaching, and good control

of the environment, stimulus, and pet to implement. In addition, if done incorrectly, they can increase fear and aggression. Only skilled practitioners should attempt these techniques.

As noted earlier, it is critical to evaluate the animal's stress level during any training. With negative reinforcement techniques in particular, there is risk of punishing whatever behavior the animal is doing at the time the aversive is applied. In the example above of the dog walking on the leash on a head collar or no-pull harness, if the pet parent continues to keep the leash tight after the dog stops pulling (a common mistake), the dog will not learn that pulling is undesirable because the unpleasant sensation continues regardless of whether the dog is pulling or not. At minimum, this leads to an inhibition of learning and at worst, it leads to conflict and aggression. When a deficit in pet parent handling is noted, it indicates the need for immediate change in the training plan.

Positive punishment

Positive punishment (PP) is the lowest level on the HoBCP and is almost always avoided. Positive punishment has been discussed in detail earlier in this chapter. With proper information and a skilled enough behavior practitioner, positive punishment is not warranted. All too frequently, practitioners resort to PP techniques, even though proper application may be beyond their level of skill or knowledge. Practitioners should consult with colleagues and/or refer to a board-certified veterinary behaviorist before resorting to positive punishment techniques. An example of PP is the use of remote location repellents such as compressed air devices, uncomfortable mats, carpet runner pointy side up, double-sided sticky tape, and physical repellents that make it uncomfortable but not painful for the cat to step on the surface to keep cats off of the kitchen counter. Aversive sound-making devices such as bark breakers, penny cans, or audible location alarms should never be used in multipet homes! These devices punish all the animals, no matter what they are doing at the time the device is activated.

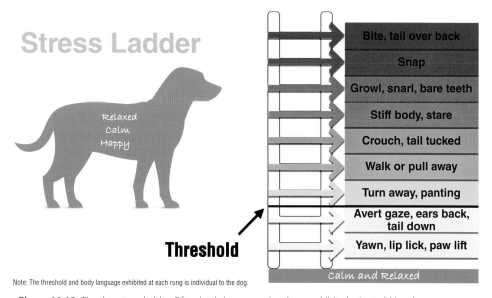

Note: The threshold and body language exhibited at each rung is individual to the dog.

Figure 10.12 The dog stress ladder. Often body language signals are exhibited prior to biting, but go unnoticed by pet parents. *(Attribution: Lisa Radosta. Modified from Shepherd, K 2009. BSAVA Manual of Canine and Feline Behaviour, 2ⁿᵈ edition.)*

Classical conditioning (Pavlovian-based behavior modification)

The techniques outlined in the HoBCP section are operantly based protocols, meaning that the animal is being trained to exhibit voluntary behaviors. The behavior modification techniques listed in this section are designed primarily around a classical conditioning paradigm. These are chosen when the primary goal is to manipulate the pet's emotional or physiological state with less regard to the specific behavior being performed (e.g., whether it is sitting or lying down). It is critical to remember that classical and operant conditioning are always happening together, even if the intent is to utilize only one methodology. While the behavior change practitioner may focus on creating a conditioned emotional response to a stimulus, the animal will also be reinforced for operant responses and this must be monitored as the process proceeds.

Conditioned arousal

Problem behaviors in pets often manifest as behaviors with elevated activity and autonomic arousal—conditioned arousal. This is particularly true in dogs, as much of their daily structure and activity is a feeding ground for rehearsal and reinforcement of over aroused behaviors. Examples include jumping around when the pet parent picks up the leash, barking at dogs outside, lunging at squirrels, barking as people pass the home, and jumping on visitors. What starts as excitement, frustration, or nervousness can escalate into massive eruptions of arousal and aggression. Many forms of aggression are heightened when the animal is in a high state of arousal. This is very akin to mob or riot behavior in humans. Overarousal can be in response to one situation, or a pet may be overstimulated much of the day. Some dogs are so aroused or anxious that their pet parents do not understand the gravity of the problem because they never see the contrast with their pet being truly relaxed. Some pets maintain above average autonomic arousal even when they are sleeping. Education about body language is critical for enlightening pet parents.

As an example, consider a pet parent who is working on teaching their leash-reactive dog an "engage–disengage" exercise (dog is reinforced for looking at the dog and then back at the pet parent). This is a form of differential reinforcement. If this new behavior is trained when the dog is in a state of high arousal, then the dog will learn to do the new behavior in a state of high arousal as well. This limits the effectiveness of the process because this sympathetic elevation keeps the dog close to the reactive threshold, no matter what the dog is being trained to do. Hence, the dog never actually learns to relax around other dogs.

Arousal reduction interventions should occur early in the behavior modification program and definitely before controlled exposure sessions to problematic stimuli. Spending time teaching pet parents how to reinforce calm behavior may be necessary even before teaching new foundation skills (see below) so the pet learns the new skills while in a relaxed state.

It is worth restating that animals work to achieve behavioral outcomes—they work for reinforcers and to avoid punishers. Individuals are biologically wired to seek reinforcement, so for behavioral health, animals need to achieve a certain level, or number, of reinforcements per day. While there is no scientifically specified number, in this case, more is likely better. Once pet parents are educated about reading body language, they should be taught to "capture" their pet behaving in a calm and relaxed manner and reinforce the pet for these moments at least 30 times per day. This means learning to observe the pet's behavior as the pet parent goes about their daily routine, so the pet parent is actively searching and finding even brief moments when the pet is quiet and relaxed. These moments are then reinforced with social attention, treats, or other reinforcements. Aroused or undesirable behaviors are ignored whenever that can be done safely. If praise disrupts the pet's quiet demeanor and triggers arousal, then the pet parent immediately ignores the pet again until the pet once again calms. This way the pet is gradually taught that praise means, "I like what you are doing, keep doing it."

Pet parents often inadvertently reinforce conditioned arousal in contexts such as their arrival home, feeding time, or preparing for walks. For example, the cat that is over-aroused at mealtime, biting the pet parent as she prepares the food, is reinforced for biting when the pet parent sets the food down. The biting and associated overarousal will increase over time. In the future, the cat may be conditioned to exhibit overarousal when it is hungry because that physiologic state has been associated with reinforcement.

Reducing arousal in these contexts requires gradually shaping the pet to exhibit calmer behavior to gain the desired reinforcer (e.g., put the leash on to go for a walk). Addressing arousal during these interactions requires the pet parent to plan extra time to accomplish the task. If the pet parent is always in a hurry when prepping for a walk, then they will end up rushing the process and continuing to put the dog's leash on when the dog is excitable and hyperaroused. As an example, the pet parent may set a subjective criterion level of acceptable arousal (and associated behavior) that is 10% less than the dog's current average when the pet parent picks up the leash. When the dog becomes aroused, the pet parent stands and ignores the dog until the dog's arousal has reduced by 10%. This may mean that the dog can now sit, but is still vocalizing. When this criterion is met, the pet parent praises the dog calmly and then starts to lean to put the leash on. If the dog cycles up to 100% arousal, then the process stops and the pet parent stands and waits again until the dog's arousal has reduced by 10%, then the pet parent tries again. This process is repeated, thus giving the dog rapid "yes" (we continue) and "no" (we stop doing what you want) feedback. Clearly changing the process can be frustrating for the dog and the pet parent, so every effort is made to set up the situation to maximize the dog's success and reduce failure. This may include changing where the leash is stored, leashing the dog up alone rather than with another dog in the household, altering which person leashes the dog, etc. Having food treats to reinforce some behaviors (e.g., sitting) may help some dogs but contribute to the arousal of other dogs.

Changing the process can be frustrating for the animal and the pet parent, so every effort should be made to set up the situation to maximize the animal's success and reduce failure. Strategies to maximize success include reducing opportunities for reinforcement of negative behavior (e.g., using automatic feeders for cats and letting dogs exercise in a fenced back yard), changing the environment where the behavior occurs (e.g., moving where the cat is fed or where the dog is leashed), and reinforcing alternative behaviors throughout the day (e.g., sitting quietly for both cats and dogs). A discussion of behavioral treatments in pets would not be complete without the mention of medications to lower arousal and facilitate learning. Treatment plans often include medications or supplements as well as behavior modification. See Chapters 9 and 11 for more detail.

As noted above, new behaviors should be taught when the pet is calm so the pet learns to perform these in a relaxed emotional state. If a cat learns to station on a mat in a physiologically relaxed state, then when that cat is cued to do that behavior in the presence of another cat in the home, the mat behavior will facilitate better introduction.

Response blocking (flooding)

Response blocking (RB) is an escape extinction process. It involves exposing the subject to a full-intensity, fear-evoking stimulus and "blocking" the subject's escape until the physiologic (fear) response to the stimulus ceases. If the animal is permitted to escape the fear-evoking stimulus, the animal is negatively reinforced for the escape and never learns not to fear the stimulus. While RB is considered a classical conditioning technique, it is a clear example of the tight link between the classical and operant conditioning. Blocking the animal's escape response (operant) allows the classically conditioned response (emotional) to extinguish, resulting in reduced fear of the stimulus. Since the process must be in place for as long as necessary for the physiologic fear response to dissipate, RB sessions are often of long duration—potentially hours. If the sessions are too short, the animal might be released from the situation too soon, which will reinforce and strengthen the fear response. A common (often unintentional) example occurs when people hold and pet fearful animals, thinking the animal will see how nice they are and no longer fear them. In situations where these pets are briefly petted and then released, the fearful behavior generally persists or worsens. If the person tends to hold the pet for long periods (generally hours), then effective flooding may occur and the animal may become less fearful. Another example is a practice called umbilical cording, where a fearful dog is tethered to a person by a long leash, forcing the dog to always remain in the person's presence until the dog no longer shows fear and tries to escape.

In practice, flooding is stressful and potentially dangerous to the pet and nearby individuals. Exposure of a pet to a strong fear-eliciting stimulus may severely traumatize it and/ or trigger the animal to attack the fear-evoking stimulus or anyone nearby. While flooding may be useful for low-level fear if carefully done (e.g., some cases of umbilical cording), it is a technique that is largely discouraged, as it eliminates all of the learner's control and poses a serious risk to the animal's welfare.

Systematic desensitization

Systematic desensitization (SD) is a common behavior modification technique to reduce fear and anxiety. It is different from RB in that the subject is exposed to the fear-evoking stimulus in small gradients to allow Pavlovian extinction to occur—breaking the contingency between the CS (e.g., nail clippers, thunder, new person, and new pet) and the CR (fear). Common protocols for introducing new cats into homes are based on SD. The new cat is confined away from the resident cats so they cannot see each other. The cats are allowed to acclimate to the smell and sound of each other and then they are allowed to see each other in small exposures (e.g., through a crack in a door, then across a gate, or through a window). When the cats are no longer showing any aversive response to each other, they may be allowed out in the same room together for short periods as long as they are able to remain relaxed.

SD is most successful if the behavior practitioner first devises a "fear hierarchy." This is a list of the fearful situations from least to most intense. For example, a dog afraid of people may be least fearful of short women met at home and most fearful of tall, loud, and bearded men met out in public. As many stages as possible are put into the list so there may be, for example, 20 gradients between the least and most fearful stimulus situations. The animal is then exposed to those situations in order and trained to relax or engage in low arousal behaviors until the animal shows no fear of short women met at home. The animal is then exposed to the next level on the list until it no longer shows fear in that situation, and so on. Systemic sensitization is quite effective when done properly; nevertheless, SD is frequently combined with classical and/or operant counterconditioning to speed the process. In some situations, SD is not realistic as a treatment tool because pet parents cannot control the environment enough to allow for small, graduated exposures to the problematic stimulus.

Counterconditioning (classical counterconditioning)

Classical counterconditioning (CC) alters the animal's emotional (involuntary) response to a stimulus and is used to modify the behavior of fearful and anxious pets. When CC is conducted properly, the CS that incites the fearful response (e.g., unfamiliar person) is paired with a US (e.g., food), resulting in a contingency where the appearance of an unfamiliar person (CS) predicts food (US) and evokes the opposite emotional response (e.g., happiness).

Success with CC is dependent on several factors. First is the relative strength of the competing stimuli. If the level of the animal's fear is more salient than the value of the food, effective conditioning will not occur, even if the animal eats the food during training. Thus, the training trials should be constructed such that the intensity or proximity of the fear-evoking stimulus is reduced, thereby giving the competing "pleasant" stimulus greater saliency. For this reason, counterconditioning is often used in conjunction with SD (see above where the animal is exposed to the stimulus at increasing levels over time).

The second critical factor for successful CC is that the fear-evoking CS must predict the appearance of the new US (e.g., food) and these pairings should occur consistently—each time the dog sees a person on the walk, the dog is presented with high-value food. If the dog sees people on walks and sometimes does not get food, then a phenomenon called degraded contingency occurs, where the sight of the person is not adequately predictive of food. This results in poor or no conditioning. Pet parents must be ready to commit to implementing the training consistently.

Third, for the new US (e.g., food) to produce the most effective conditioning, that particular US should be given to the dog only in the presence of the CS the pet parent is trying to change (e.g., seeing people on walks). If the pet parent walks the dog and gives the dog a lot of food rewards for leash walking skills, for example, and then gives the dog more of the same food rewards when the dog sees people, conditioning will be less effective or ineffective. One way to counter this is to have pet parents carry two different reinforcers, one type of treat they give to reinforce other good behavior and one type (of higher value) that is reserved for pairing with the sight of people.

The fourth and fifth factors to consider for efficacy are the number of trials and the total training time. Generally, more conditioning occurs with more total training time; however, longer intertrial intervals produce better conditioning.[36,67] This means that it is helpful for pet parents to give the pet frequent and potentially lengthy breaks between the exposure trials. In other words, walking in areas where the dog sees people only sporadically will be more effective than walking where the dog is constantly seeing people.

The most effective CC will occur if exposure sessions are scheduled and structured rather than opportunistic. With the former, the pet parent or trainer arranges to have decoy people help with training trials that allow the decoy to move in and out of sight, beginning with minimal intensity, at threshold exposures. When the decoy is in sight, the dog is fed and when the decoy leaves, feeding stops. Again, longer and variable intertrial intervals can enhance conditioning.

If a pet parent is unable to set up structured exposure sessions, then they can find places where the stimulus will move in a predictable path and set up exposures opportunistically. This type of trial risks more unexpected outcomes (e.g., someone suddenly moving toward the dog), which can reduce efficacy of the process. When working with a dog-reactive dog, the pet parent may set up training off the side of the parking lot to a veterinary clinic, grooming shop, or pet store, where they can anticipate dogs will move from the cars to the building entrance and back again. This allows the pet parent to control the distance their dog is from the path of travel. Recreational and dog parks are NOT good locations because people may turn dogs loose or wander in variable, less predictable, patterns around the area.

As with many things in medicine, practical behavior therapy does not always match the textbook ideal. Often, some of the five criteria above for maximum success with counterconditioning cannot be achieved realistically. For example, if a pet is at the veterinary hospital for an appointment and is fearful, food can be used to distract, engage, and occupy the pet with something pleasant and allow a physical examination or procedures to be completed. While this violates some of the criteria for maximum success such as presenting the CS prior to the US (the food is presented in this case prior to examination), counterconditioning should still be attempted, as some effective learning may occur. At minimum, the food distraction may help prevent further aversive conditioning. Another example involves thunderstorm-phobic dogs. Counterconditioning (e.g., giving food toys, feeding, and playing) has been shown to be 70% effective at reducing signs of fear even

though the stimulus is many times at maximum intensity, the pet is already aroused, and the training session is not structured.[4] Even small advances can be made when situations cannot be perfectly orchestrated.

Counterconditioning can be used alone or to augment other techniques in a variety of situations such as reducing fear of procedures at the veterinary clinic, changing how dogs feel about visitors to the house, integrating cats together, and helping pets be less fearful of noise events such as storms and fireworks.

Aversion therapy

Aversion therapy is a classical conditioning procedure for eliminating undesirable behavior by pairing the unwanted behavior with a sufficiently unpleasant stimulus. This is basically a type of counterconditioning where the goal is to change the stimulus from something the animal desires (or finds reinforcing) to something the animal wants to avoid. For example, one might pair an aversive stimulus such as bitter taste with the behavior of chewing on or eating valuable or dangerous items (furniture or rocks).

In humans, associating an unpleasant outcome (e.g., noise, taste, odor, nauseant, or even pain) with smoking, gambling, drinking, drug use, or even nail biting may successfully stop the undesirable habit. To be successful, the degree of noxiousness or discomfort must outweigh the motivation to perform the behavior. However, humans have the choice to participate in these protocols. This is not the case with pets, so pet parents and behavior practitioners should carefully consider the ethical and welfare repercussions of implementing such an approach before doing so.

Establishing new behaviors

Teaching new skills or teaching the pet to behave in a different manner in the presence of a problematic stimulus means that the pet parent/trainer must be able to create, or generate, the desired behavioral response. The first step in training is to get the animal to offer a behavior that can be reinforced. Reinforceable behavior can be obtained in four general ways, each with its pros and cons: capturing, prompting, luring, and shaping.

Capturing involves waiting for the animal to exhibit the desired behavior in its final, complete format. For example, if trying to teach a dog to lie down, the trainer simply waits until the dog lies down on its own and reinforces this. Capturing works best for behaviors that the animal performs frequently in the desired form so that reinforcement occurs often enough to strengthen the behavior. The more the pet is reinforced for lying down, the more often the pet will offer to lie down. The likelihood of the pet offering the desired behavior can be maximized by setting up the environment to encourage performance of the behavior. For example, the pet parent can take the dog into a small room without toys or other distractions, then sit and read and wait for the dog to lie down. The dog is reinforced with food or a toy that is tossed on the ground so the dog has to stand up to get it. Then the pet parent waits until the dog lies down again and repeats the sequence. Eventually the dog will be lying down predictably right after consuming the reinforcer. At this time, the cue for the behavior (e.g., "down") can be introduced right after the pet consumes the reinforcer but before the dog performs the behavior again. Because cues are learned via classical conditioning, the cue must occur before the behavior and before delivery of the reinforcer.

Capturing is not a good technique to use for behaviors that occur infrequently, as reinforcement cannot occur often enough to build the strength and frequency of the behavior fast enough without causing the animal frustration. Additionally, if the behavior is put on extinction, the pet parent or trainer must resume the capturing process all over in order to "recover" the behavior (although learning will occur faster than it did during the initial establishment of the behavior). Capturing is obviously beneficial for behaviors that are difficult or impossible to shape or lure, such as training a pet to eliminate on cue.

Prompting involves using some stimulus or handler body movement to encourage the animal to exhibit a desired behavior that can be reinforced. For example, one could prompt a dog to get on the couch by patting the seat cushion. A pet parent could prompt a cat to go to a certain room by walking there themselves and see if the cat follows (and then reinforcing the cat). These behaviors are then reinforced and when the animal starts to show the behavior on its own, the prompts are quickly faded. Some prompts can be turned into a cue (e.g., patting the seat cushion) or a different verbal or auditory cue can be conditioned.

Luring is a form of prompting and a common training technique for novice trainers and pet animals. It generally involves using food to lure the animal into a desired position or to a desired location. For example, a common method for teaching puppies and dogs to sit is to hold a food treat near their nose (allowing them to nibble on it, if necessary) and then slowly raise the treat up in the air while also moving it slightly back over the pet's head. As the puppy follows the treat with its nose and head, the rear end often naturally sinks until the puppy is in a sitting position. As soon as the puppy sits, the treat is released into its mouth. The process is repeated until the puppy sits immediately when the lure is presented. At this point, a verbal cue can be introduced just before beginning the luring process.

Luring is a desirable method for behaviors that naturally occur at low frequency. Luring also has the advantage of establishing a hand signal (nonverbal cue) during the luring process. As related to the example above, the puppy will learn to respond to the motion of the hand in the air above its head by sitting, and the food (or toy) lure can then be faded out. Lured behaviors are sometimes easier to recover after extinction by quickly repeating the luring process and once again reinforcing the desired response. Since the dogs are more likely to respond to hand signals compared to verbal cues, when they are given in a conflicting fashion, lures should be faded and the dog trained to respond fluently to the verbal cue alone.

Shaping is a technique whereby the animal is reinforced for tiny, successive approximations toward the goal behavior. For example, the animal is first reinforced for even the most vague version of the goal behavior. When the pet has performed this version successfully for several trials, then the reinforcement criterion is changed to a version that is a slightly closer approximation of the final behavior. This process is repeated until the final behavior is obtained.

Shaping is often used in conjunction with luring or prompting. Alternatively, a behavior can be "free shaped," without the use of any external prompt or lure. While free shaping does allow the pet to explore the learning process unimpeded, it is not appropriate for every animal or situation. Pets that are behaviorally inhibited, either due to temperament or previous (usually punitive) training experiences, will offer low rates of behavior. This may result in such a low reinforcement rate that the pet becomes further discouraged or frustrated. In these situations, using lures or prompts may give the pet more information, leading to better reinforcement rates. Alternatively, some pets have had such bad experience with previous training that any interaction with a person that appears too "training-like" results in avoidance, inhibition, or aggression. In these cases, setting up a free shaping protocol for some simple behavior can begin to recondition the pet that training interactions are fun and equitable.

Foundation training skills

Reducing problem behavior is best accomplished by teaching the animal what behavior we want them to do instead (see Table 10.2). If a dog sitting with its pet parent on the couch attacks other dogs that approach, the pet parent may want the pet to stop the biting, but that goal does not tell the dog how it should behave instead. A more specific and achievable goal is to train the dog to rest quietly on a designated spot on the couch or floor near the pet parent when the other dog approaches. Counterconditioning augments this strategy by also changing how the dog feels about the other dog approaching. Clearly, for this to be a viable strategy, the dog in question first needs to know how to lie down on cue and to lie down in the designated area. Basic cue training may not itself alter anxious or aggressive behavior, but these skills are important precursors to starting Controlled Exposures (see section below). There are multiple ways to teach any behavior, but the HoBCP and the Five Freedoms should always be kept in mind so that the most positive, least intrusive methods are chosen. So, rather than electing to use a shock or vibration collar to teach a dog to come when called, the pet parent or trainer should elect methods based on positive reinforcement. This maximizes on the philosophy of giving the animal as much choice and control as feasible while also piggybacking on the desirable adjunctive classical conditioning that will occur by pairing

Table 10.2 Foundational skills for pets

Skill	Dogs	Cats
Sit	X	x
Come	X	x
Name orientation	X	x
Targeting (stick or hand)	X	x
Down	X	x
Stationing/go to your spot	X	x
Loose leash walking	X	
Muzzle training	X	
Relaxation	X	x
Independence/confinement training	X	x

the training with desirable outcomes. In addition, as stated above, research shows that animals acquire new behaviors (learn) more effectively and efficiently when positive reinforcement is used and positive punishment is avoided. For each foundational skill, one method is presented here. There are many humane and effective methods for teaching behaviors. What is provided below are examples of one method of training each behavior.

Targeting

Targeting behaviors inarguably are the most commonly taught skills in the modern animal training community. Targeting involves training the animal to place part or all of its body in contact with some designated environmental object or location. Teaching a dog to go to its bed or teaching a cat to bunt to signal when petting is desired are forms of targeting. Animals are frequently trained to touch their noses (or beaks) to the end of a target stick (see Figure 10.13). Target sticks are useful for moving animals from one location to another or to train other behaviors. For example, a target stick can be used to train a cat to sit on a cat tower or a bear to stand up vertically on its enclosure fence so the veterinarian can examine its ventrum.

In addition to target sticks, dogs are commonly taught to touch their nose to an outstretched palm or fist. This behavior can be used to direct the dog's focus from another animal on a walk or in the veterinary clinic lobby. Hand targeting is also an excellent way to countercondition a dog to having hands reach out toward it—rather than this now meaning someone will touch the dog, it now means the dog gets to play a fun game. This makes targeting a good "ice breaker" for introducing dogs to new people. For many dogs, this is an easy starter behavior to get the dog interested in training in general (see Box 10.9).

Relaxation protocols

As noted in the section on Conditioned Arousal, shaping calmer behavior and relaxation is an overarching theme for most behavior modification programs. Rarely does a pet parent come to a practitioner asking for help in making their pet more active or excitable. Relaxation protocols are common exercises in the dog and cat training community. These are generally accomplished by training the pet to lie down and relax on a specified training mat or pet bed. Mat

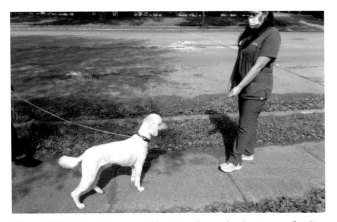

Figure 10.13 Using the target stick to introduce a shy dog to an unfamiliar person. *(Attribution: Lore Haug.)*

- The pet parent finds a low distraction area to train and has desirable reinforcers (usually food, although toys can be effective reinforcers later in the training process).
- The pet parent presents an open palm, fingers toward the dog, as though handing the dog a treat. The fingers are presented about 2–4 inches from the dog's nose with the palm facing up, then the pet parent waits for the dog to stretch forward to sniff.
- The moment the dog sniffs the fingers or palm, the behavior is marked (see section on conditioned reinforcers above), the hand is withdrawn, and the dog given a food treat.
- Once the dog consumes the treat and is focused again, the process is repeated.
- When the dog has touched the fingers with his nose consistently for 5–10 trials in a row, the pet parent can then present the hand so the fingers are now 4–6 inches (10–15 cm) from the dog's nose. This gradually extends how far the dog must reach to touch the palm or fingers. Over training sessions, the distance between the palm and the dog's nose is extended to the desired goal range, generally a minimum of 10–30 feet (3–9 m).
- When the dog is touching consistently at a distance of 12 inches (30 cm), the verbal cue (e.g., "touch") is attached by saying the cue right before the hand is presented for the dog to touch. The behavior then is still marked and reinforced as usual.
- The behavior is then generalized to other locations and distraction levels.
- As with any behavior, the animal should be well conditioned to the targeting game and be under good stimulus control before trying to use the targeting in a real-life distracting situation (e.g., to get the leash-reactive dog to stop focusing on another dog in sight or to introduce the dog to a new person).

relaxation exercises are somewhat different than just teaching a pet to go to its bed as a stationing spot. The relaxation mat should be portable so that it may be used to facilitate the pet learning relaxed behavior in a variety of situations and locations (e.g., veterinary clinic, the local park, or in the car).

Relaxation exercises are invaluable in helping pets learn better coping strategies in stimulus trigger situations. They are a mainstay for working on graduated absence training with dogs with separation-related disorder. Mat relaxation exercises are also instrumental in helping pets overcome car ride anxiety, fear at the veterinary clinic, and for visitor introductions with fearful or territorial pets. As with other behaviors, there are several ways to teach mat relaxation exercises. The method outlined in Box 10.10 may be best suited for patient pet parents and dogs with moderate to low activity or anxiety level. For dogs with high excitability or those with low frustration tolerance, this method may prove to be too stressful and other methods may be required.

Focus

The focus or "look" behavior involves teaching the animal to focus on the pet parent's face on cue. Arguably, this same behavior could be accomplished by merely calling the pet's name. However, because the pet's name is used throughout the day in many contexts, it is worthwhile to have a separate cue when the pet parent/trainer intends to add long duration to the behavior (i.e., name means glance at me whereas "look" means focus on me until specifically released to do something else) (see Box 10.11).

Box 10.10 Teaching relaxation

- The pet parent finds a low distraction area to train where the dog is comfortable training. Training may be more effective if the pet has been exercised or walked prior to reduce excessive energy.
- The dog is placed on leash and the pet parent has some moderate-value food treats.
- The pet parent sits in a chair with the dog's mat on the floor close by.
- A few treats are dropped on the mat to draw the dog's attention to the mat. The pet parent continues to drop treats on the mat while the dog is standing, sitting, or lying on the mat but otherwise ignores the dog.
- The pet parent continues to periodically drop treats on the mat and gradually focuses on timing the treats when the dog shows any increased sign of relaxation, such as sitting or lying on the mat, sighing, etc.
- Over training sessions, the dog should learn to lie down on the mat. This allows the pet parent to continue to gradually shape increased signs of relaxation such as placing the head down or the dog rolling over onto its side.
- Once the pet is consistently lying down and relaxing on the mat, the pet parent then repeats the training process in other locations and situations of gradually increasing distraction level to generalize the response.

Box 10.11 Teaching focus

The simplest way to teach the behavior is as follows:
- Find a small, low-distraction area in which to train.
- Have moderate-value reinforcers available. It is often helpful to hold the treats or toy behind the handler's back so the pet does not become fixated on looking at the hands.
- Stand quietly with the pet nearby and wait for the pet to glance at the handler's face. Mark this and reinforce. Repeat.
- At first, even partial glances are reinforced and the pet may not even look entirely at the handler's face, but over training sessions, the pet is shaped to focus on the handler's face and hold the eye contact until it hears the marker signal or the release word.
- In some cases, the pet responds more quickly if the handler holds the treat out away from their body at arm's length and waits for the pet to glance back at their face.
- Some trainers suggest gaining the pet's focus by holding a treat up near the handler's eyes. This can be successful for many pets, but does often just teach the pet to stare at the treat rather than focusing on the handler. If this technique is used, the food lure near the face should be faded early in the training process.
- Gradually increase the amount of time you require eye contact to last and then start adding distractions in the background, like people playing or a fridge door opening. The dog only gets reinforced for holding the eye contact. Note that there are no corrections if the dog looks away; the dog merely does not get reinforced. If the dog is verbally or physically corrected for looking away, the dog will become more anxious.
- Once the dog is consistent in giving the correct response even when there are distractions, go to other places (outside) and add mild distractions, such as another dog nearby or children playing. After each successful session, gradually increase the distractions and work in busier environments.
- The goal is for the dog to maintain calm and steady eye contact for several minutes regardless of the amount of distraction and background activity.

Go to place

Go to place (or bed) is a form of targeting and is often referred to as station training. The animal is trained to go stand, sit, or lie in a certain location that is generally marked by a bed, platform, shelf, bench, or mat. This behavior is useful for preventing or treating a variety of problems such as pestering visitors and intercat aggression. Animals that pace around or scuffle with each other during meal preparation can be trained to sit or lie on their respective stations while their meals are prepared. Similarly, stationing can prevent a dog or cat from begging at the table or crowding infants playing on their floor play mats (see Box 10.12).

Loose leash walking

Leash walking can be divided into actual heeling and loose leash walking. With the former, the dog is trained to walk in a designated spot at the handler's left or right side and match the handler's pace and position. When the handler stops, the dog should stop and wait at the handler's side. With loose leash walking, the dog is expected to walk politely within the confines of the leash but is not restricted to a certain area near the handler nor necessarily a certain side of the handler's body. The criterion of keeping the leash loose (no pulling) is still in place as it is with true heeling. Heeling may not be much fun for the dog, but it is a control position that is useful or necessary for some dogs with overreactive and aggressive behavior.

Loose leash walking is the dog's part of the walk, as it allows the dog to sniff, explore, eliminate, and have some freedom of choice during the walk. However, this freedom may present a greater public danger for dogs with certain forms of aggression when in certain situations, hence the benefit of being able to move the dog back and forth between these two behaviors. Both behaviors can also be

Box 10.12 Teaching go to place/station

- Start in a low distraction location.
- Have the dog bed or station nearby.
- It is acceptable to lure the pet onto the station initially by dropping some food treats on it. As soon as the pet steps on the bed, mark and reinforce again by dropping a treat on the bed. Continue to reinforce the pet when it is on the station and stop reinforcing if it steps off.
- When the pet is consistently staying on the station with the handler immediately nearby, the handler can move 1–2 feet (30–60 cm) away and repeat the process.
- Teaching the pet to actually GO to the bed occurs by creating a "behavior loop" where the pet is marked for stepping on the bed, the pet is marked and treated on the bed with a high-value treat, and then a lower-value treat it tossed off the bed to "reset" the pet for the opportunity to move to the bed again.
- When the dog is moving back to the bed consistently from the 1–2 foot (30–60 cm) mark, the handler can move another 2 feet (60 cm) away and repeat.
- A cue such as "go to bed" or "place" is added as the dog is moving to the bed. The dog is then marked and reinforced as before.
- Over training sessions, the handler can move further away from the bed and practice from different orientations in the room to be able to send the pet to the bed from the desired distance.

taught to cats and other animals. There are a variety of good resources for teaching heeling (see Appendix A).

Controlled exposure to problematic stimuli

Once effective antecedent arrangements are in place and the pet has been taught a set of foundation skills, the pet parent is then ready to put these to use in controlled stimulus exposures. With these sessions, the pet is exposed in a structured fashion to the problematic stimulus or situation. Controlled exposure techniques are intended to expose the pet to a muted or reduced intensity of the stimulus where an acceptable alternate response can be conditioned. These protocols generally use a combination of systematic desensitization/counterconditioning (DS/CC) and differential reinforcement. Exposure begins below threshold, the point at which the animal starts to show some reaction to the stimulus. Controlled exposures ideally are started after the pet has learned foundations skills and conditioned arousal has been reduced. While in some cases starting DS/CC immediately can be effective, many pets, especially dogs, have so much conditioned arousal and are so generally out of control, starting DS/CC right away poses a much higher risk of the pet parent losing control of the pet or the situation and something unfortunate or tragic happens.

During exposures, the pet parent or trainer chooses ONE stimulus to address at a time. So, if the dog is barking and lunging at joggers, dogs, bicycles, etc., only one of these stimuli is used during the training sessions. When the pet has improved response to that stimulus, then sessions can be devised to address the others, one at a time. If the pet parent attempts to go out and expose the dog to all of these in one session, there is a high likelihood of overstimulation and failure.

Controlled exposure sessions ideally are structured setups. The time, location, and decoy are all arranged and staged to maximize success. This means if the pet parent is working on addressing a dog's response to visitors, they should arrange to have a friend come over specifically to help train the dog, rather than trying to train the dog when the cable repair technician happens to be in the house. Certainly, there are situations where staged setups are very difficult or impossible (e.g., working with storm-phobic dogs or a pet parent who does not have any friends with decoy dogs). In these instances, opportunist exposure sessions might be successful with careful planning, but they always have an element of unpredictability, which makes them riskier.

Exposure sessions are scheduled for times and locations where extraneous stimuli can be best controlled or eliminated. For example, if a pet parent of a leash-reactive dog is working on exposure to decoy dogs, choosing a location relatively free of squirrels will help the dog focus on the salient stimuli during the session. Ambient and surface temperatures are important. In areas with warm climates, there is high risk of pad burns from dogs working on asphalt or concrete during training sessions. Humans wear shoes and therefore often are not cognizant of how hot the sidewalks or streets have become. Similar care should be taken when working around ice or snow. Sessions can be up to 1 hour in duration, but any session over 30 minutes should include frequent and relatively prolonged breaks (up to 5–10 minutes each). Exposures are aligned along one axis of the "3 D's" of training: distance, duration, and distraction. Distance is the distance between the pet and the problematic stimulus. When introducing cats together into a new home, the cats should be as far apart as possible during the first exposures. Based on their response in training sessions, they are then gradually moved closer together. Similarly, if a dog is being trained to accept having its ears handled, the training may start with the pet parent placing their hand in the air above the dog's ear and then gradually moving closer over many training sessions until the dog will calmly accept having the ear actually touched (and then handled). Duration refers to the time that the pet is exposed to the problematic stimulus. When working with a dog that is afraid of motorcycle engines, the dog is first exposed to a short—perhaps 1–2 seconds—burst of sound (at a low volume). Over sessions, the dog is gradually exposed to longer-duration playbacks. Distraction can refer to the stimulus itself or to the local competing distractions in the environment. These also are introduced one at a time and gradually over sessions. Stimulus distraction has several subfactors that are manipulated. These include the number of stimuli (how many dogs the leash-reactive dog sees at once) and the intensity of the stimulus (how loud, how energetic or active is the decoy dog, etc.). A dog being counterconditioned to children may be able to stay under threshold if the child is sitting quietly but then become too aroused and fearful if the child starts talking or laughing loudly and waving their arms around.

While the goal is to stay below the threshold, if the pet shows a low-level reaction, the trial may continue until an acceptable response is obtained and reinforced. The inappropriate response is allowed to extinguish by waiting quietly until the behavior stops and then reinforcing the pet once a desirable behavior is exhibited. The trainer must remain relaxed and calm, as agitation in the handler and punishment of the pet will further aggravate the problem.

Maintaining the response

Once the desired operant or classically conditioned response has been established, the challenge then is to maintain it across time and contexts. Many pet parents cease reinforcing a behavior (e.g., come or loose leash walking) once the pet's response is acceptable, thinking that because the pet now "knows" the behavior, the pet will just continue to do it. But knowing a behavior and being motivated to do it (to achieve desirable outcomes) are two different things. Always remember that individuals perform behaviors to obtain or avoid certain consequences. If these consequences are withdrawn, the behavior is put on an extinction schedule and will eventually disappear. Pet parents should continue to reinforce trained skills and other desirable behaviors forever. Once a behavior is established, the behavior may be put on an intermittent reinforcement schedule, but if the reinforcement rate drops too low, the behavior will diminish. If a pet parent notices that the dog's response to come is waning or the cat no longer holds its station on the cat tower during feeding time, then the pet parent needs to evaluate the reinforcement rate and value and adjust so the behavior sharpens again.

As noted in the learning section above, continuous reinforcement schedules generally are appropriate and recommended for the majority of behaviors and situations. To reduce reliance on food, pet parents can begin to substitute other "life" reinforcers for a variety of behaviors. For example, when the dog walks nicely on leash for a while, the pet parent may release the dog from heel to go sniff in the grass. An indoor/outdoor cat can be trained to ring a bell to get the pet parent to open the door. Ringing the bell first may have been trained with food, but then the reinforcer was transitioned to door opening once the bell was put into that context.

One pitfall of using food (or toys) for reinforcers is that the sight of the reinforcer may become part of the discriminative stimulus for the behavior (i.e., the animal only responds to the cue if it sees that the pet parent has food or toys present). This occurs because the pet parent actually only reinforces the pet when the pet parent has food visibly present! The solution is to start keeping food out of sight during training, especially once the animal is clear on the behavior expected. The pet parent may have hidden food earlier in the day in their pocket, in a nearby drawer, or in a container on a shelf. Food stashes can be placed in areas outside the house as well so the pet learns that food can be delivered, even if it does not see or smell food on the pet parent or handler. Similarly, toys can be stashed away and then once the animal performs the cued behavior, the behavior is marked and the pet parent quickly gets the toy. As noted above, gradually replacing some of the food with other reinforcers also helps to reduce the risk of food becoming part of the discriminative stimulus.

Classically conditioned behaviors also need continued reinforcement to maintain the desired CR. If a cat's tolerance for petting was increased by pairing petting with food, the cat should continue to periodically receive food in conjunction with petting. Marker signals must continue to be followed by primary reinforcers if they are to maintain their power as a training tool.

Disruption and redirection

Some stimuli will interrupt a behavior the pet is performing without affecting the future frequency of the behavior. These stimuli are called disrupters or interrupters; they are not true punishers. Dog whistles, squeakers, ultrasonic trainers, non-punishing sounds such as shaking a treat bag or jar, and a single word in a sharp tone might be effective for disrupting the undesirable response but may not reduce the likelihood the pet does the behavior again in the future.

Interrupters can be useful in some situations, but their use should be carefully evaluated with the HoBCP in mind. For behaviors that are easily reinforced by social attention, pet parent-emitted interrupters (e.g., verbal scolding) may result in reinforcement of the behavior. Interrupters are most useful in situations where the problem behavior cannot be ignored safely. If ignoring the behavior will put the pet, a person, another animal, or the behavior program at risk, then an interrupter may be used to abort the current episode of behavior so the pet can be redirected to a safer location and/or more appropriate behavior. Interrupters should get the animal's attention but should not be so aversive as to trigger fear or defensive aggression from the animal. Any stimulus can cause fear and be viewed as punishment by the pet. As always, prevention of undesirable behaviors through manipulation of the environment and reinforcement of positive behaviors is the safest and most efficacious course.

For intrahousehold interdog aggression, a pet parent might try to abort an ongoing fight by making a loud noise or spraying the pets with water. This intervention is unlikely to punish the fighting behavior effectively, but it may break the dogs apart long enough that the pet parent can get them separated. For a dog that charges the door when the doorbell rings, the dog can wear a harness and drag leash that can be used to calmly and quickly interrupt the charge and move the dog to another location before the door is opened. For a cat that is aggressive toward another cat in the household, a clap of the hands can get the cat's attention so that they can be redirected to a cat tree or a safe space.

Pet parents are often instructed to use previously trained cues (e.g., targeting and come when called) to redirect pets when they exhibit problematic behavior. Cues can be effective as interrupters, but there is some risk to using them too frequently when the pet is displaying objectionable behavior. If these behaviors are trained with positive reinforcement, there is a classically conditioned association between the behavior, the cue, and the reinforcer. Positively reinforced behaviors (and their associated cues) serve as secondary reinforcers. In practice, this means that a pet parent can actually reinforce the unwelcome behavior by repeatedly redirecting the dog with a cue for a different behavior. If a dog was taught "off" or "leave it" with food and the pet parent uses this cue to interrupt the dog every time it jumps on the counter, the pet parent may reinforce the counter jumping. Keeping data on the frequency of the behavior over time will allow the practitioner to determine if this is occurring.

Punishment techniques

Other more appropriate interventions should always be used before resorting to positive punishment. Cats and dogs can become fearful of the person, stimulus, or environment associated with the punishment, leading to avoidance, increasing uncertainty, and even severe aggression toward the punisher. Even something as benign as a squirt bottle can cause fear of bottles, the location where the bottle is kept, and the person who most often uses the bottle.

Remote punishments can have some utility in certain situations. These are devices that produce an aversive experience that is independent of the pet parent's presence, such as contact paper with the sticky side up. These are most useful for keeping animals off furniture or countertops. For outdoor use, motion-activated alarms, motion-activated water sprinklers, or pet repellents might also help to keep the pet parent's pet out of selected areas on the property or stray animals off the property.

Time-out

Reduction in some behaviors may be achieved through negative punishment such as time-outs.

The goal of time-out is for the pet to learn that misbehavior leads to temporary isolation and the removal of opportunity to earn reinforcement. Shortly after the time-out, the pet must be given the opportunity to engage in appropriate behavior to earn reinforcement. Since this is an aversive intervention, the process should be implemented carefully. Time-outs should only be employed after other more positive interventions have been attempted. Additionally, it is recommended to use the procedure for ONE specific problem behavior, rather than the pet ending up in time-out frequently for a long list of annoyances.

Perhaps the time-out is used to reduce some residual cat chasing in the home. When the dog focuses on the cat, the dog is given a verbal cue such as "leave it." If the dog responds appropriately, it is reinforced. If the dog begins to advance on the cat anyway, the behavior of advancing on the cat is marked with a "time-out!" phrase and then the dog is promptly but calmly taken to the predesignated time-out area. Efficiency getting the dog to the time-out area generally requires that the dog be wearing a harness and light drag leash so the process can occur quickly. Time-outs will not be effective if the pet parent has to chase the dog around the house for a few minutes before finally catching it to drag (or carry) it to the time-out area. Time-out locations ideally are small areas where the dog can neither hurt itself nor engage in any type of reinforcing activity. Bathrooms are often ideal, as they are also conveniently located in most homes. The dog should not be put in time-out in its crate or any other location where the dog enjoys hanging out. The pet is left in the time-out area for 30–120 seconds and then let out if it is quiet. At the very least, the time-out will remove the pet from the stimulus and location of the undesirable behavior, and prevent the continuation of the problem. The pet parent can then simply open the door, walk away, and let the pet resume normal activity, or if the problem might resume, direct the pet into an alternate desirable behavior and location. If the time-out procedure does not reduce the frequency of the problem behavior (e.g., cat chasing) within several trials or days, then the process should be reevaluated.

Products to augment behavior modification

While good management and behavior modification are the backbone of every successful treatment program, this process can be augmented by a variety of useful behavior-related products. Choosing the right equipment for the right situation can make the difference between pet parents getting early positive reinforcement or not. The earlier pet parents feel they are making headway, the more likely they are to commit further energy and other resources to the rest of the process.

Collars, harnesses, and leads

For reactive and aggressive dogs, the most important decision likely involves the training/walking equipment. Pet parents should not use choke or slip chains and pinch or prong collars. While some dogs may walk fine on a regular buckle collar, many dogs will pull excessively in these (note that dogs will learn to pull in any piece of equipment without proper training). Most dogs will do best in a well-fitted front clip or front/back clip combo harness such as the Freedom, Balance, or Perfect Fit harnesses (see Figures 10.9 and 10.10). Some dogs will do best if fitted with a head collar such as a Walk with Me, Black Dog, Halti, or Comfort Trainer (see Figures 10.7 and 10.8). Specific indications for head collars include dogs that exhibit pet parent redirected

aggression on walks and dogs that can easily physically overpower their pet parents (e.g., large, powerful dogs with smaller or unstable pet parents). Unlike most harnesses, the use of head collars generally requires acclimatation training, similar to muzzle training, before the dog can be effectively walked in the product.

All collars and harnesses should be paired with an appropriately sized 6-foot (2 m) cotton or leather leash (see Figure 10.13). Pet parents of small to medium dogs almost invariably purchase leads that are much too large and heavy for the size of their dog. This is particularly problematic if the dog is wearing a head collar, as the weight of the clip and the lead is hanging on the dog's head and face. During training, pet parents should avoid putting extraneous items (such as dog waste bag holders and keys) on the leash, as these often end up swinging into the dog's face at some point during training or walking (see Figure 10.14). With rare exceptions, retractable leashes are inappropriate for training and behavior modification. Bungee-type leashes should be avoided, especially in dogs that have a history of lunging at dogs, people, or objects (e.g., cars and bicycles).

Cats also benefit from harness and leash training. Some cats do well in small padded dog harnesses. Other popular harnesses include the Kitty Holster harness. These again should be paired with lightweight leashes fitting the cat's small size.

Remote-activated treat dispensers

These devices deserve special mention related to behavior modification. Remote treat dispensers allow pet parents to reinforce pets from a distance, either within in the home or from a distant location. The Manners Minder (see Figure 10.15) can be set to dispense treats on a frequency schedule or activated by a hand-held device from another location in the home. Newer models such as the Furbo Cube and Pet Tutor (see Figure 10.16) function with a smartphone-compatible application that can allow pet parents to reinforce pets from any location that has a cell phone signal. These treat dispensers are

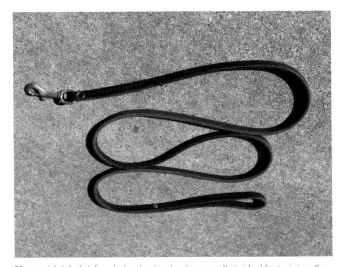

Figure 10.14 A 6-foot latigo leather leash generally is ideal for training. For safety and long-term strength, this author prefers leads that are stitched and riveted versus braided. With simple proper care, leather leads become soft and pliable during handling and can last longer than the lifespan of the dog. *(Attribution: Lore Haug.)*

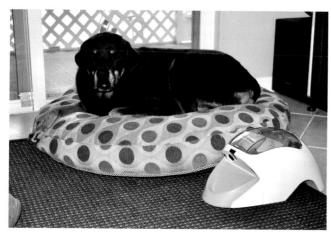

Figure 10.15 Remote treat dispensers and improve timing and aid in learning. The Manners Minder. *(Attribution: Lisa Radosta.)*

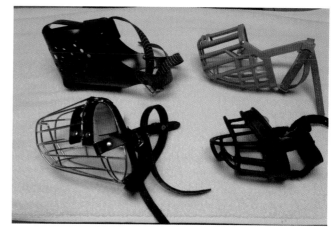

Figure 10.17 Examples of basket-style muzzles. Clockwise from top left: Jafco, Italian plastic, Baskerville Ultra, and Morocco heavy-duty wire. *(Attribution: Lore Haug.)*

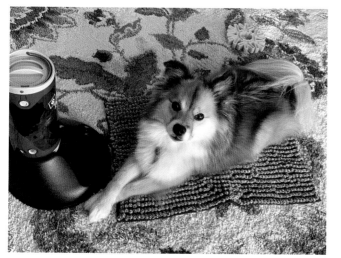

Figure 10.16 Remote treat dispensers and improve timing and aid in learning. The Pet Tutor. *(Courtesy of Colleen Koch.)*

beneficial in myriad contexts, some of which include reinforcing crated dogs in another room (e.g., when visitors are in the house), reinforcing calm behavior during car rides, training pets to station in a certain location when the front door opens, and reinforcing pets for relaxed behavior during pet parent separations or noise events. Remote treat dispensers also allow single-pet parents to train two pets at the same time, which is particularly helpful for introduction protocols between new pets or pets with a previous fighting history. One pet can be tethered or confined near the treat dispenser while the pet parent handles the other pet on leash or behind another gate.

Muzzles

Muzzle training is essential for any dog or cat with a biting history or a probability of future biting. Training will go more smoothly if the muzzle is properly sized and fitted to the particular dog's or cat's head and muzzle conformation. Muzzles may be basket style or nylon "sleeve" style. The latter type is only appropriate for short duration use in climate-controlled situations, as they are too restrictive to limit biting risk while simultaneously allowing for appropriate thermoregulation.

Nevertheless, nylon-style muzzles are more appropriate for certain dogs and situations and allow for easier treat delivery compared to basket-style muzzles (see Figure 10.17).

The Baskerville Ultra muzzle is likely the most widely used basket muzzle for many dogs and tends to fit dogs with moderate length snouts and medium width skull shape (e.g., Pit Bull–type dogs, Rottweilers, Labradors, and Beagles). Dogs with longer snouts and more slender heads (e.g., Doberman Pinschers, German Shepherd Dogs, Belgian Malinois, Whippets, etc.) may be better served by a plastic Italian basket muzzle. Dogs with excessive flews can be particularly challenging to fit but some companies offer custom-fitted muzzles (Bumas, Dean and Tyler). There are also muzzles now available specifically designed for brachycephalic dogs such as Pugs and French Bulldogs (see Appendix A).

Muzzles should be long enough to avoid rubbing on the end of the dog's nose and should have enough vertical clearance that the dog can open its mouth to pant, eat treats, and drink some water. Additionally, during routine wear, the muzzle should stay clear of the dog's eyes and avoid rubbing on the masseter muscles and zygomatic arches.

There are a wide variety of other products that can be useful in the prevention and management of undesirable behavior in pets. These include calming music, ThunderShirt, Calmz Vest, and the Assisi Calmer Canine Loop. A list of some of the product manufacturers can be found in Appendix A. Additionally, such products are discussed in more detail in Chapter 12.

Conclusion

Learning results in the acquisitions of new behaviors. Those behaviors are associated with neurochemical and anatomical changes in the brain. Behavioral treatment, a powerful tool which can make a lasting change in the pet's life, can potentially lower the need for medications. Training may be widely regarded as easy when in fact it takes a great deal of skill. Dogs and cats that have behavior problems rooted in anxiety, fear, and stress require even more skill and knowledge of learning theory and the physiology of behavior. The information in this chapter lays a solid foundation of knowledge on which the veterinary team can build skill.

References

1. Patronek GJ, Glickman LT, Beck AM, et al. Risk factors for relinquishment of dogs to an animal shelter. *J Am Vet Med Assoc*. 1996;209(3):572–581.

2. Voith VL. Attachment of people to companion animals. *Vet Clin North Am Small Anim*. 1985;2:289–295.

3. Dinwoodie IR, Dwyer B, Zottola V, et al. Demographics and comorbidity of behavior problems in dogs. *J Vet Behav*. 2019;32:62–71.

4. Riemer S. Effectiveness of treatments for firework fears in dogs. *J Vet Behav*. 2020; 37:61–70.

5. Casey RA, Bradshaw JWS. Owner compliance and clinical outcome measures for domestic cats undergoing clinical behavior therapy. *J Vet Behav*. 2008;3(3):114–124.

6. Pineda S, Anzola B, Olivares A, et al. Fluoxetine combined with clorazepate dipotassium and behaviour modification for treatment of anxiety-related disorders in dogs. *Vet J*. 2014;199:387–391.

7. Appleby D, Bradshaw JWS, Casey RA. Relationship between aggressive and avoidance behavior by dogs and their experience in the first six months of life. *Vet Rec*. 2002;150:434–438.

8. Salonen M, Sulkama S, Mikkola S, et al. Prevalence, comorbidity, and breed differences in canine anxiety in 13,700 Finnish pet dogs. *Nature*. 2020;10:2962. doi:10.1038/s41598-020-59837-z.

9. Overall KL, Hamilton SP, Chang ML. Understanding the genetic basis of canine anxiety: phenotyping dogs for behavioral, neurochemical and genetic assessment. *J Vet Behav*. 2006;1:124–141.

10. Gwinn GT. The effects of punishment on acts motivated by fear. *J Exp Psychol*. 1949; 39:260–269.

11. Johnson LR, McGuire J, Lazarus R, et al. Pavlovian fear memory circuits and phenotype models of PTSD. *Neuropharmacology*. 2012;62(2):638–646. doi:10.1016/j.neuropharm.2011.07.004.

12. Eichenbaum H. Learning from LTP: a comment on recent attempts to identify cellular and molecular mechanisms of memory. *Learn Mem*. 1996;3:61–73.

13. Haug LI. Treat or euthanize: helping owners make critical decisions regarding pets with behavior problems. *Vet Med*. 2011;106:11:564–569.

14. Cooper J, Cracknell N, Hardiman J, et al. The welfare consequences and efficacy of training pet dogs with a focus on positive reinforcement. *Front Vet Sci*. 2020;7:508. doi:10.3389/fvets.2020.00508.

15. Killeen PR, Jacobs KW. Coal is not black, snow is not white, food is not a reinforcer: the roles of affordances and dispositions in the analysis of behavior. *Behav Anal*. 2016;40:1–22.

16. Schultz W, Dayan P, Montague PR. A neural substrate of prediction and reward. *Science*. 1997;275:1593–1599.

17. Cook PF, Prichard A, Spivak M, et al. Awake canine fMRI predicts dogs' preference for praise vs food. *Soc Cogn Affect Neurosci*. 2016;11: 1853–1862.

18. Feuerbacher EN, Wynne CDL. Most domestic dogs (*Canis lupus familiaris*) prefer food to petting: population, context and schedule effects in concurrent choice. *J Exp Anal Behav*. 2014;101:385–405.

19. Waite MR, Kodak TM. Simple food preference assessments for companion dogs. In: *Vet Beh Symposium Proceedings*. 2021:21.

20. Vitale Shreve KR, Mehrkam LR, Udell MAR. Social interaction, food, scent or toys? A formal assessment of domestic pet and shelter cat (*Felis silvestris catus*) preferences. *Behav Proc*. 2017;141; 322–328.

21. Riemer S, Ellis SLH, Thompson H, et al. Reinforcer effectiveness in dogs—the influence of quantity and quality. *Appl Anim Behav Sci*. 2018; 2016,87–93.

22. Bremhorst A, Butler S, Wurbel H, et al. Incentive motivation in pet dogs— preference for constant vs varied food rewards. *Sci Rep*. 2018;9:9756.

23. Miller HC, Bender C. The breakfast effect: dogs (*Canis familiaris*) search more accurately when they are less hungry. *Behav Proc*. 2012;91:313–317.

24. Gaines SA, Rooney NJ, Bradshaw JWS. The effect of feeding enrichment upon reported working ability and the behavior of kenneled working dogs. *J Forensic Sci*. 2008;53:6. doi:10.1111/j.1556-4029. 2008.00879.x.

25. Feuerbacher EN, Wynne CDL. Shut up and pet me! Domestic dogs (*Canis lupus familiaris*) prefer petting to vocal praise in concurrent and single-choice alternative choice procedures. *Behav Proc*. 2015; 110:47–59.

26. Feuerbacher EN, Wynne CDL. Relative efficacy of human social interaction and food as reinforcers for domestic dogs and hand reared wolves. *J Exp Anal Behav*. 2012; 98:105–129.

27. Paredes-Ramos P, Diaz-Morales JV, Espinosa-Palencia M. Clicker training accelerates learning of complex behaviors but reduces discriminative abilities of Yucatan miniature pigs. *Animals*. 2020; 10:959. doi:10.3390/ani10060959.

28. Wood LA. *Clicker Bridging Stimulus Efficacy*. 2015. [PhD thesis].

29. Dorey NR, Blandina B, Udell MAR. Clicker training does not enhance learning in mixed-breed shelter puppies (*Canis familiaris*). *J Vet Behav*. 2020;39: 57–63.

30. Hiby EF, Rooney NJ, Bradshaw JWS, et al. Dog training methods; their use, effectiveness and interaction with behavior and welfare. *Anim Welf*. 2007; 13:63–69.

31. Jones AC, Josephs RA. Predicting canine cortisol response from humane affiliative and punitive behaviors. In: *Current Issues and Research in Veterinary Behavioral Medicine, Papers presented at the 5th International Behavior Meeting*. West Lafayette, IN: Purdue University Press; 2005:194–197.

32. Vieira de Castro AC, Fuchs D, Morello GM, et al. Does training method matter? Evidence for the negative impact of aversive-based methods on companion dog welfare. *PLoS ONE* 2020;15(12): e0225023.

33. Horváth Z, Dóka A, Miklósi Á. Affiliative and disciplinary behaviour of human handlers during play with their dog affects cortisol concentrations in opposite directions. *Horm Behav*. 2008;54:107–114.

34. Casey R, Loftus Be, Bolster C, et al. Human directed aggression in domestic dogs (*Canis familiaris*): occurrence in different contexts and risk factors. *Appl Anim Behav Sci*. 2014;152:52–63.

35. Herron F, Shofer F, Reisner I. Survey of the use and outcome of confrontational and non-confrontational training methods in client-owned dogs showing undesirable behaviors. *Appl Anim Behav Sci*. 2009;117:47–54.

36. Hsu Y, Sun L. Factors associated with aggressive responses in pet dogs. *Appl Anim Behav Sci*. 2010;123:108–123.

37. Blackwell EJ, Twells C, Seawright A, et al. The relationship between training methods and the occurrence of behaviour problems as reported by owners, in a population of domestic dogs. *J Vet Behav*. 2008;3: 207–217.

38. Rooney NJ, Cowan S. Training methods and owner-dog interactions: links with dog behaviour and learning ability. *Appl Anim Behav Sci*. 2011;132:169–177.

39. Stellato AC, Flint HE, Dewey CE, et al. Risk-factors associated with veterinary-related fear and aggression in owned domestic dogs. *Appl Anim Behav Sci*. 2021;241:105374. doi:10.1016/j. applanim.2021.105374.

40. Follette MR, Rodriguez KE, Ogata N, et al. Military veterans and their PTSD service dogs: Associations between training methods, PTSD severity, dog behavior, and the human-animal bond. *Front Vet Sci*. 2019;6:23. doi:10.3389/fvets.2019. 00023.

41. Schalke E, et al. Clinical signs caused by the use of electric training collars on dogs in everyday life situation. *Appl Anim Behav Sci*. 2007;105:369–380.

42. Polsky, RH. Can aggression in dogs be elicited through the use of electronic pet containment systems? *J Appl Anim Welf Sci*. 2000;3:345–357.

43. Jacques J, Myers S. Electronic training devices: a review of current literature. *Anim Behav Consult: Theor Pract*. 2007;3: 22–39.

44. Blackwell E, Casey R. *The Use of Shock Collars and Their Impact on the Welfare of Dogs*. University of Bristol; 2006.

45. Schilder MBH, Van der Borg JAM. Training dogs with the help of the shock collar: short and long term behavioural effects. *Appl Anim Behav Sci*. 2004;85:319–334.

46. Salgerli Y, Schalke E, Boehm I, et al. Comparison of learning effects and stress between 3 different training methods (electronic training collar, pinch collar and quitting signal) in Belgian Malinois Police Dogs. *Rev Méd Vét.*. 2012; 163(11):530–535.

47. Beerda B, Schilder MBH, van Hooff JARAM, et al. Behavioural, saliva cortisol and heart rate responses to different types of stimuli in dogs. *Appl Anim Behav Sci*. 1998;58:365–381.

48. Hiby EF, Rooney NJ, Bradshaw JWS. Dog training method: their use, effectiveness and interaction with behaviour and welfare. *Anim Welf*. 2004;13:63–69.

49. Cooper JJ, Mills D. The welfare consequences and efficacity of training pet dogs with remote electronic training collars in comparison to reward based training. *PLoS One*. 2014;9:e102722.

50. Deldalle S, Gaunet F. Effects of two training methods on stress related behaviors of the dog (*Canis familiaris*) and on the dog–owner relationship. *J Vet Behav*. 2014;9(2):58–65.

51. China L, Mills DS, Cooper JL. Efficacy of dog training with and without electronic collars vs. a focus on positive reinforcement. *Front Vet Sci*. 2020;7:508. doi:10.3389/fvets.2020.00508.

52. Lynch JJ, McCarthy JF. The effects of petting on classically conditioned emotional response. *Behav Res Ther*. 1996;5:55–62.

53. Starinsky NS, Lord LK, Herron ME. Escape rates and biting histories of dogs confined to their owner's property through the use of various containment methods. *JAVMA*. 2017;250:297–302.

54. Skyrme R, Mills DS. Pairing of vocal and visual commands during training. Does one overshadow the other? In: *Proceedings of the 7th International Veterinary Behaviour Meeting*. Belgium: Edinburgh, ESVCE; 2009:95–96.

55. Scandurra A, Alterisio A, Aria M, et al. Should I fetch one or the other? A study on dogs on the object choice in the bimodal contrasting paradigm. *Anim Cogn*. 2018;21:119–126.

56. Adler L, Adler H. Ontogeny of observational learning in the dog (*Canis familiaris*). *Dev Psychobiol*. 1977;10:267–272.

57. Chesler P. Maternal influence in learning by observation in kittens. *Science*. 1969;166:901–903.

58. Slabbert JM, Rasa OAE. Observational learning of an acquired maternal behavior pattern in working dogs' pups; an alternative training method? *Appl Anim Behav Sci*. 1997;53:309–316.

59. Mayoral N, Masy ED, Ruiz J, et al. Are puppies capable of learning through observational learning? In: *Proceedings of the 2010 European Veterinary Behaviour Meeting*. Belgium: Hamburg, ESCVE; 2010:186–188.

60. Tomlinson J, Zulch HE. Observational learning of secondary reinforcement in the domestic dog. Is it possible? In: *Proceedings of the 7th International Veterinary Behaviour Meeting*. Belgium: Edinburgh, ESVCE; 2009:62–63.

61. Mazur JE, *Learning and Behavior*. 6th ed. New Jersey: Pearson Prentice Hall; 2006: 215–216.

62. Friedman SG. What's wrong with this picture? Effectiveness is not enough. *J Appl Comp Anim Behav*. 2009;3:41–45.

63. Turner DC. Social organization and behavioural ecology of free-ranging domestic cats. In: Turner DC, Bateson P, eds. *The Domestic Cat. The Biology of Its Behaviour*. 3rd ed. Cambridge: Cambridge University Press; 2014.

64. Miller P. Build better behavior. Constructional aggression treatment, a promising new approach to modifying canine aggression. *Whole Dog J*. 2008; 17–23.

65. Stewart G. BAT 2.0: upgrades to behavior adjustment training require second look. In: *The APDT Chronicle of the Dog*. Spring; 2014.

66. Stewart G. Behavior adjustment training (BAT). <https://grishastewart.com/bat-overview/>.

67. Gottlieb DA, Begej EL. Principles of Pavlovian conditioning. In: McSweeney FK, Murphy ES, eds. *Wiley Blackwell Handbook of Operant and Classical Conditioning*. West Sussex: Wiley Blackwell; 2014:4–25 [Ch. 1].

Resources and recommended reading

American College of Veterinary Behaviorists. *Decoding Your Dog*. New York: Houghton Miflin Harcourt; 2015.

American College of Veterinary Behaviorists. *Decoding Your Cat*. New York: Houghton Milfin Harcourt; 2020.

Bradshaw J, Ellis S. *The Trainable Cat*. New York: Basic Books; 2016.

Howell A, Feyrcilde M. *Cooperative Veterinary Care*. Hoboken, NJ: Wiley-Blackwell; 2018.

Mills DS. Training and learning protocols. In: Horwitz DF, Mills DS, eds. *BSAVA Manual of Canine and Feline Behavioural Medicine*. 2nd ed. Gloucester, UK: BSAVA; 2009: 49–64.

Pryor K. *Don't Shoot the Dog. The New Art of Dog Training*. Gloucester: Ringpress; 2002.

Pryor K. *Reaching the Animal Mind: Clicker Training and What It Teaches Us About All Animals*. New York: Scribner; 2009.

Reid P. *Excel-Erated Leaning. Explaining in Plain English How Dogs Learn and How Best to Teach Them*. Berkeley: James and Kenneth; 1996.

Shaw J, Martin D, eds. *Canine and Feline Behavior for Veterinary Technicians and Nurses*. Ames, Iowa: Wiley-Blackwell; 2014.

VanArendonk Baugh, L. *Fired Up, Frantic, and Freaked Out: Training Crazy Dogs from Over the Top to Under Control*. Indianapolis: Aeclipse Press; 2013.

CHAPTER 11

Pharmacologic intervention in behavioral therapy

Leticia M. S. Dantas, MS, PhD, DVM, DACVB and Lisa Radosta, DVM, DACVB

Chapter contents

Introduction

The timely and appropriate use of medications may allow the pet parent an opportunity to resolve the pet's behavior problem successfully, modify its behavior sufficiently to allow the pet to remain in the home, and positively affect the pet and pet parent's quality of life. Veterinary behavior and psychiatric problems can be very disruptive for the family and the people within the pet's social group, often to the point of severely affecting the human–animal bond. Thus, the quick and effective control of clinical signs is usually one of the main goals of behavioral treatment protocols. Medications can take effect very quickly, within 20 minutes in some cases; therefore, treatment should not be delayed, barring any physical illness which would cause medical treatment to be contraindicated. Failure to identify and suggest potentially helpful pharmacological agents may mean the difference between a safe and healthy pet–pet parent relationship and the pet's relinquishment and/or euthanasia. Medication selection ideally requires an accurate diagnosis of the behavioral or psychiatric condition and a comprehensive knowledge of which medication(s) would be the safest and most effective for resolving the problem at hand (Box 11.1). With that said, there are times when a diagnosis cannot be made. In those cases, a medication plan can still be created by observing and recording the clinical signs displayed by the patient and focusing on medications which alleviate those clinical signs (see Chapter 9).

Medication prescribing must proceed in agreement with local, and federal regulations, approved use and licensing requirements. Since most medications used in canine and feline behavior therapy are not approved for use in pets, they should be used with care and attention to potential interactions and side effects. Whenever possible, medications approved for use in the species and for the intended purpose should be used and to meet the requirements of the regulatory body for dispensing. For off-label use (use not specifically indicated on the product label) or compounded medications, the hospital should ensure full disclosure and the pet parent should sign a release where appropriate, indicating informed consent for the use of a product not approved for this purpose. However, a release does not absolve the practitioner from liability, particularly if the rationale for selection and use of the medication cannot be medically justified. Caution should be taken to assess carefully whether any concurrent medication, supplements, or diet is being utilized that in any way interacts with the medication that has been selected. Of course, pet parent compliance, including ability to administer the medication, may also impact the choice of medication and whether compounding might be necessary (see below). Pet parents should be advised as to what behaviors are likely to be improved (i.e., intensity, frequency, severity) and over what time frame, and what side effects or adverse events might be expected. Although the family should be advised to report any unexpected change in health or behavior immediately, the veterinary clinic should be proactive in regularly contacting the pet parent to assess progress or potential problems. Veterinary literature should be regularly reviewed for reports of adverse effects or changes in dosage recommendations. Although human studies cannot necessarily be extrapolated to animals, it is also advisable to consult the human literature and manufacturers' data to determine areas of potential concern, including but not limited to disease and organ function, contraindications, and drug interactions. Ideally, blood and urine tests should be performed before any behavioral medication is dispensed to rule out underlying medical problems and establish a baseline against which future tests can be measured (see Chapters 1, 6, and 9). Testing should be repeated at regular intervals (minimally once a year) based on the pet's age and health and the potential side effects of the medication being used. When there is more than one potentially effective treatment regimen, the safest course of action should be followed.

Prescribing norms may vary geographically. In the United Kingdom, the prescription cascade requires that the first step in dispensing medications be those authorized for a specific condition for a specific species and that, if there is no suitable medication authorized in the United Kingdom, the veterinarian can treat the animal in the following order. Step 2 would be medications approved for a different application or another species; Step 3 for a human medication authorized in the United Kingdom; and the final step would allow for formulation and compounding. In the United States, off-label use is not uncommon. Prescribing choices are generally presented under the umbrella of the best choice, risk-based decision making for the patient while considering the approved purpose of a medication.

In current clinical behavioral medicine, medications that are nonaddictive, relatively free of potential organ toxicity, and cause minimal or no sedation have gradually replaced the use of older medications with lower rates of efficacy, less specific effects, and higher potential for side effects (such as acepromazine and the progestins).

Evidence-based medicine and veterinary behavioral and psychiatric pharmacology

Most available information on medication therapy for behavior and mental health problems in companion animals comes from clinical experience of board-certified veterinary behaviorists as well as from inferred comparisons between psychiatric conditions in humans and behavior problems of pets. According to the Oxford Centre for Evidence-Based Medicine scoring system (www.cebm.net), the weakest levels of evidence for measuring therapeutics (levels 4 and 5) are attributed to case-based studies, in vitro research, or expert opinion without crucial appraisal. A systematic review of case-controlled studies with homogeneity or individual case-controlled studies would receive a higher rating in terms of evidence (level 3), while a systematic review of cohort studies, individual cohort studies, and lower-quality randomized control trials (RCTs) would receive level 2 ratings. The gold standard (level 1) would be a systematic review with homogeneity of RCTs.[1] However, with few published trials for most veterinary behavioral therapeutics, veterinarians have little access to such rigorous research. Whenever possible, it is clear that RCTs should be the standard way to assess efficacy of medication therapy in behavioral medicine, particularly regarding the placebo effect, which may be responsible for 50% or more of the effects in some behavioral studies. For instance, in a study in which fluoxetine was compared to placebo in the treatment of separation-related disorders, the effect of treatment on global improvement ranged from 58.6% to 65.1%, while the placebo group had improvements ranging from 43.4% to 51.3%.[2] In two studies in which a homeopathic remedy for firework phobias was compared to placebo for the treatment of noise sensitivities, both treatment groups reported a significant level of change over the course of treatment, but there was no evidence that the homeopathic remedy had any effect above the control group.[3,4] In addition, knowledge of participating in a placebo-controlled trial appeared to have no effect on the pet parent's perception of treatment effect.[4]

In prior periods, the amount of published independent clinical trials on psychopharmacology of behavior problems in companion animals was sparse. One of the main limitations for conducting proper controlled clinical trials is the ethical concern of setting up a pure placebo group on a population of owned animals presented for behavior problems. Fortunately, over the past few years, more and more clinical trials have been conducted on medication treatment of behavior problems of dogs and cats. For example, the vast majority of available studies on the use of fluoxetine to treat canine behavior problems have been published since the year 2000. A systematic review of RCTs examining the effects of therapeutic agents on urine marking in cats has been published, representing the highest level of evidence for the use of those medications to treat that particular condition.[5]

Recently, laboratory models have been developed for a variety of behavior problems, allowing for the assessment of medications, natural supplements, and behavior products in a controlled environment, including minimal subject variability, validated measures of behavior, and removal of pet parent bias. An example of this approach is the work done by CanCog Inc. (cancog.com) to develop a variety of validated models for: (1) learning and memory tasks in dogs and cats with specific applications for cognitive dysfunction and brain aging (see Chapter 8); (2) fear of noises[6]; (3) fear of humans[7]; and (4) travel anxiety.[8,9] These models have proven invaluable in validating the efficacy of a number of diets, natural supplements, and medications that are now approved for use in dogs and cats. Nevertheless, while laboratory models are an effective means of supporting the efficacy of a product over a placebo or control group, clinical trials in affected pets are necessary to support the efficacy of the product for specific behavioral applications in a real domestic environment.

Many recommended medications in behavioral medicine have been widely used in humans to treat psychiatric conditions. Nevertheless, while disposition and metabolism for some of these medications have been determined for dogs and cats, this is not always the case. Therefore, direct extrapolation of dosages of human psychotropic medications to animal use may not be accurate, as medication metabolism including metabolites, half-life, and routes of excretion as well as neurotransmitter and receptor effects, may vary between species.[10] In fact, for some medications, the active metabolites in humans may not be produced in the same amount and routes of excretion may vary.

Compounding might be considered when dose, compliance, or availability is an issue. However, solubility, stability, absorption, and potency are potential concerns. In addition, transdermal medications, while a particularly convenient way to administer psychotropic medications in cats, have been shown to lack efficacy in that species. Several studies have been conducted to assess the effect of transdermal fluoxetine in cats. In one study, the serum levels of fluoxetine and norfluoxetine (the active metabolite of fluoxetine) were significantly different and varied in individual cats that received oral versus transdermal medication, with the oral recipients showing higher serum levels.[11] In another study, the bioavailability of transdermal fluoxetine was approximately 10% of oral dosing.[12] Systemic absorption after administration of transdermal amitriptyline and buspirone has also been found to be negligible (compared to oral dosing).[13] In one study, transdermal gabapentin was found to have poor bioavailability in the cat;[14] however, in another, transdermal gabapentin was found to be effective at reducing pain in cats.[15] In one clinical study comparing buspirone at 1 mg/kg orally to 4 mg/kg transdermally for five weeks for feline urine marking, a significant improvement was seen in both groups.[16] The absorption of transdermal medications depends on the vehicle, the health of the skin, whether the medication is lipophilic or lipophobic, hydrophilic or hydrophobic, and the molecular weight of the medication. Because there is more evidence to discourage the use of transdermal psychotropic medications in animals, when compared to oral administration, and because the evidence points to a high variability in absorption, transdermal medications are not currently considered an effective method to administer psychotropic medications in dogs and cats.

Medication dosage information is provided in Appendix B.

Considerations before prescribing

In order to decide if medication is needed to treat a particular patient and what medication(s) can be most effective, the clinician needs to consider the following questions:

1. What is the presenting clinical condition or clinical signs?
2. What elements of that particular behavior condition could be modified or improved with medications?
3. What is the overall health and wellness of the patient? Are there any underlying conditions which might change the medication choices?
4. Is the medication plan reasonable for the pet parent and the patient (e.g., ease of dosing, dosing schedule, cost)?
5. What are the available safe, efficacious medications and what are their pharmacological profiles?

Factors specific to psychotropic medications

Clinical trials usually refer to the use of specific medications to treat a specific diagnosis, like canine separation-related disorders, noise sensitivities, or urine marking in cats. When conducting clinical trials, it is advantageous for analysis of the results and approval of the medication to limit the animals in the study to one diagnosis or specific clinical signs. It can be challenging to translate that information into clinical decisions. Because a medication is approved for use for a specific behavioral diagnosis, that is not to say that the medication cannot be used to treat other diagnoses. One of the most effective ways to prescribe is to consider the underlying motivational states, functions, emotions (e.g., fear, anxiety, stress, conflict, panic and impulsivity), neurochemistry and overt clinical signs (e.g., reactivity, barking, lunging, hiding, panting, pacing). This is one of the reasons that understanding the clinical signs being exhibited by the patient is so very important.

The most important neurotransmitters in psychiatric medicine are serotonin, norepinephrine, dopamine, acetylcholine, gamma-aminobutyric acid (GABA), and glutamate. While these are discrete neurotransmitters, their effects certainly are not discrete. Instead, they are intertwined so that when one neurotransmitter in this group is modulated, others are also modulated in a downstream effect due to projections and receptors throughout the brain. To magnify this effect further, there are some neurotransmitters that when increased cause far-reaching effects on neurons in other parts of the brain, causing a consequent increase in a completely different neurotransmitter. For example, stimulation of the cortical pyramidal neurons (glutamate pathway) stimulates dopamine (substantia nigra), serotonin (ventral tegmental area), and norepinephrine (locus coeruleus) neurons to release their respective neurotransmitters. This is just one of many examples. Variations occur based on where neurons originate and terminate, and their function (e.g., norepinephrine manufacture versus glutamate manufacture), among other things. Just as behavior does not occur in a vacuum, the modulation of neurotransmitters has effects reaching far beyond that neurotransmitter, receptor, or neuron.

The aforementioned neurotransmitters act as modulators of broad aspects of behavior control, including motivation and emotional states, which can be the same across different behavior conditions. For this reason, the same medication is often prescribed to treat different diagnoses. As an example, the array of conditions that can be treated with fluoxetine includes urine marking in cats,[17] separation-related disorders in dogs,[18] acral lick dermatitis in dogs,[19] and aggression.[20] The reason is that fluoxetine affects the turnover of serotonin, a neurotransmitter involved in the regulation of wide aspects of behavior, from fear and anxiety to aggression and impulse control.

To complicate things, some psychotropic medications act on more than one neurotransmitter system. For instance, clomipramine inhibits the reuptake of serotonin and norepinephrine but also has actions on acetylcholine and histamine. Furthermore, medications acting on the same modulatory system can do so by acting on different mechanisms or receptors for that particular neurotransmitter. Thus, different medications can be used to treat the same condition and the same condition can be treated with different medications.

The current research in humans suggests that some of the patient's individual response to a particular medication or potentially a medication class is dependent at least in part on that particular patient's genetic makeup, especially regarding the P450 enzymes.[21] This is one reason why two patients who on the surface appear to present in the same way with the same clinical signs and diagnoses will respond differently to the same medication. Practitioners should be ready for this eventuality with several options for medical treatment for each patient.

Pet parents may approach the treatment of psychiatric disorders in animals as they do a urinary tract infection – the medication is the cure. Behavior disorders have multifactorial etiologies and as such, need multimodal treatment, much like atopy or food allergies, in order to resolve. Medication is a piece of the puzzle of resolution. Pet parents should be informed that a 50% positive change in the behavioral clinical signs is considered successful as a treatment. There is evidence that medications can decrease behavioral clinical signs

in some disorders such as noise aversion by as much as 91% in some patients,[22] and certainly when medications are prescribed for single events such as plane travel, they may be 100% effective.

When should a medication be added to the behavioral treatment plan?

From a clinical perspective, there are several situations where medication therapy might be indicated for behavioral and psychiatric conditions: (1) when the pet's welfare and quality of life are compromised by the situation or the psychiatric disorder; (2) the presence of factors associated with a poor outcome; (3) to decrease fear, anxiety, stress, and arousal and facilitate behavioral treatment; (4) medication desensitization; (5) when medication is necessary as the primary mode of treatment; and (6) when an underlying pathology is present.

When the patient's welfare and quality of life are compromised

The patient's welfare and quality of life are often affected by psychiatric and behavior disorders. Cats that eliminate in the house are relegated to a life outdoors. Dogs that destroy the house because they are panicking during a thunderstorm are relinquished to shelters. Medications can be an immediate treatment, improving quality of life and welfare by decreasing the animal's stress and the outward expression of that stress that the pet parent sees as the behavioral clinical signs (see Chapter 7). The veterinarian's assessment of patient welfare may differ from the pet parent's assessment. The veterinarian's charge in this situation is to marry those two viewpoints to make an overall assessment of welfare and quality of life. If the quality of life and welfare of the patient are compromised, the veterinarian should create a treatment plan which includes consideration of medications.

Factors are present which are associated with a poor outcome

When discussing the diagnosis and treatment with pet parents who present their pets for behavior disorders, there is no room for judgment and assumptions. An honest conversation should be held with the pet parent about their expectations and what will be necessary to improve their pet's behavior to meet that expectation. If there are risk factors in the household for a poor outcome, those should be considered. If those risk factors cannot be abated, a medication or pharmaceutical should be considered. For example, one study found that one of the factors associated with a poor outcome in interdog aggression cases was two dogs of the same sex.[23] Pet parents in this situation should be counseled that there may be a likelihood of a poor outcome and a medication could be helpful in treatment of their pets' behavior problem. In other cases, the environment is not conducive to a postiive outcome or change in the target behavior(s). For example, if there is a child in the home who needs to be separated from the dog and the dog is unable to be separated from the family without panicking, a medication can be immediately helpful to relax the dog in confinement, keeping the child safe and reducing the risk of relinquishment.

To decrease fear, anxiety, stress, and arousal and facilitate behavioral treatment

Psychotropic medications are commonly used as an adjunct to behavior therapy. Some patients are not able to learn new coping tools or modify their behavior without first lowering fear, anxiety, stress, conflict, panic, impulsivity and arousal. Patients that rise to these emotional states or cannot recover from stressors quickly are good candidates for medication. The treatment of separation-related disorders, fears, phobias, and aggression are examples of conditions in which a medication might help facilitate the initiation and implementation of behavior therapy. For example, studies on the use of clomipramine for separation-related disorders showed that there was greater and faster improvement in the group with medications and behavior modification compared with the group with behavior modification alone (i.e., placebo group).[17] Choosing an appropriate medication may provide an opportunity to resolve the problem in a quicker or safer manner. However, without concurrent behavioral modification, the problem may not improve significantly and is likely to recur when the medication is removed. Pet parents must be made aware that the the medication will only help while the patient is receiving the medication unless other treatment modalities are employed.

Medication desensitization

Medication desensitization is a technique that can be applied when the stimulus cannot be effectively controlled or reduced, or when there are multiple stimuli that lead to fear, anxiety, stress, conflict, panic, impulsivity or aggression. The medication should be given at a sufficient dosage so that the pet is relaxed and calm when exposed to the stimulus. By pairing exposure to the stimulus with favored treats, a positive association can be made (counterconditioning). Even if the medication alone does not completely calm the pet, it may still be possible to reduce its arousal enough to get the pet to respond to a cues for alternate behaviors such as focus, sit/stay, or settle, and this response can then be reinforced (i.e., differential reinforcement of an alternate behavior). Medication-aided desensitization should be combined with other behavioral treatment techniques such as systematic desensitization, counterconditioning, and differential reinforcement (see Chapter 10) so that behavioral techniques, rather than the medication itself, are the principal methods of altering behavior. As soon as the successful response (and mood) can be consistently achieved in the presence of the stimulus, the medication can be gradually reduced at subsequent training sessions.

Medication is necessary as the primary mode of treatment

Another indication for medication use is when a behavior problem is unlikely to be resolved by behavioral therapy techniques alone. Some behavior disorders require medications to help control the condition, and it may not be possible to withdraw the medications without the condition recurring.

Underlying pathology present

A final indication for medication use is when underlying pathology, whether physical or behavioral, is present. Systemic disease of other body systems can cause and intensify behavioral clinical signs (see Chapter 6). Similarly, behavioral pathology and psychiatric conditions (i.e., where behavioral changes may be due to altered neurotransmitter function) may only improve with appropriate medication therapy. There are times where it is appropriate to use a medication to alleviate the signs of systemic disease which is concurrently being treated. For example, a dog that has osteoarthritis may have difficulty walking on slick floors. While a complete plan is being implemented for the osteoarthritis, including rehabilitation, weight loss, joint support, pain relief, and environmental changes, the fear of walking on slick floors will compromise the patient's quality of life and may lead to undesirable problems such as elimination in the house. Alleviation of the patient's fear and anxiety regarding walking on slick floors can circumvent entirely the development of behavior problems, improve quality of life, and maintain the human–animal bond. In this way, behavioral medications can be a part of a complete treatment plan for many systemic diseases.

Classification and selection of psychotropic medications

A psychotropic medication can be named and classified according to different criteria, including the chemical structure, the main pharmacological action, and the most common clinical use. For instance, alprazolam can be referred to as benzodiazepine, a medication acting on GABA, or an antianxiety agent.

Labeling a medication for its therapeutic value might seem clear and self-explanatory, but it could create some confusion for both the clinician and the pet parent. Many conditions in human beings, like anxiety or panic, have a clear counterpart in veterinary medicine. However, others, like depression or schizophrenia, do not. Since most psychotropic medications used in veterinary behavioral medicine are only approved for humans, clinicians must emphasize to their pet parents that information contained on the package insert (or from books, brochures, or web sites) refers to use in humans and does not necessarily apply to animals.

To add to the confusion, paroxetine, for example, is classified as an antidepressant, but is FDA approved for use in humans to treat generalized anxiety disorder, panic disorder, and posttraumatic stress disorder, among other things. This disparity between the medication class or the lay language used around a medication and the approved use, or in veterinary behavioral medicine, the off-label use of a medication, confuses pet parents, often causing them to ask why an antidepressant is being used if their pet is not depressed. Veterinary healthcare teams can easily answer this question or preempt it by knowing the neurotransmitters targeted by the medication to be prescribed and the medication's target effect.

It is becoming more and more clear in veterinary behavioral medicine and human psychiatry that very few, if any, psychotropic medications can be considered diagnosis specific. Thus, the current trend in human psychiatry is to abandon the terminology based on indications in favor of that referring to the primary effects on neurotransmission or to the chemical structure.[24] Before considering the different categories of psychotropic medications, it is best to understand the neurophysiology of the main neurotransmitters involved in their action.

Neurotransmitters

Neurotransmission is a complex process, basically resulting from a dynamic interaction between the neurotransmitter, the presynaptic and postsynaptic receptors, the reuptake pump, and the degradation enzymes. Psychotropic medications act at varying sites, presynaptically, postsynaptically, and within the synapse to enhance the production and release of the neurotransmitter, block the effects of the neurotransmitter at the postsynaptic receptor, affect receptors on the presynaptic neuron as well as on the postsynaptic neuron, and block the reuptake of neurotransmitter into the presynaptic neuron. Medications may also act by inhibiting the breakdown of neurotransmitters within the presynaptic neuron or within the synapse. After being released by the presynaptic neuron, the neurotransmitter interacts with both presynaptic and postsynaptic receptors, resulting in major biological changes within the presynaptic and the postsynaptic neurons. Activation of these sites may influence a variety of physiological activities, including ion movement across the cell membrane, changes in cell membrane potential, and activation of intracellular enzymes, mostly through G-proteins.

Medications that have molecular conformations similar to that of the primary neurotransmitter can attach to the receptor sites and either mimic neurotransmitter activity (agonists) or block normal neurotransmitter activity (antagonists), depending on the specific character of the molecule. Different receptor subtypes may exist for an individual neurotransmitter, which can have different functions and may be differentially expressed in different brain regions. Many psychotropic medications are able to target one or more specific subtypes of receptors.

Many presynaptic receptors have a self-regulatory function on the neurotransmitter (autoreceptors). Activation of these sites following attachment of neurotransmitter molecules diffusing through the intercellular space provides negative feedback by having an inhibitory influence on neurotransmitter synthesis and release. Thus, pharmacological blockage or desensitization at these sites results in less inhibition and increased synthesis and release of neurotransmitter molecules.

After detaching from receptor sites, the neurotransmitter molecules are either enzymatically degraded or diffuse to reuptake receptor sites on the presynaptic neuron, where they attach and are transferred into the cell. The reuptake pump decreases the neurotransmitter's interneural concentration by physically removing molecules from the interneural space but also indirectly by increasing the intracellular storage pool. This occurs because an intracellular feedback system inhibits neurotransmitter synthesis as the concentration of neurotransmitter increases within the neuron. Thus, the reuptake receptor site provides an excellent target for medication action by effectively increasing the amount of neurotransmitter available to interact with the postsynaptic cell. Many psychotropic medications exert their action by either blocking the degrading enzyme or blocking the reuptake pump (Figure 11.1).

Up to a certain point, neurons are able to self-regulate neurotransmitter function by controlling the expression of

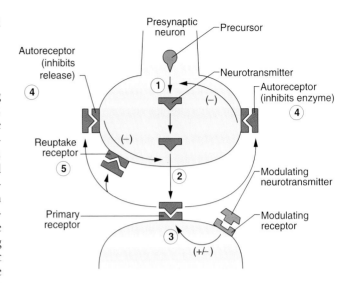

Stages of neurotransmission

1. Synthesis of neurotransmitter in the prejunctional neuron
2. Release of neurotransmitter in response to an action potential
3. Interaction of neurotransmitter with the receptor
4. Autoregulation
5. Reuptake

Figure 11.1 The stages of neurotransmission and receptor.

its receptors. When neurotransmitter levels in the synaptic cleft are kept high and sustained, a process called downregulation reduces the number of receptors. If neurotransmitter levels are low, an opposite mechanism of upregulation results in an increase in the number of receptors.

From a clinical perspective, understanding the complexity of neurotransmission is necessary to explain some of the characteristics of medication action. For instance, when a serotonin reuptake inhibitor such as fluoxetine is given, blocking the reuptake of serotonin into the neuron results in an increase in serotonin in the synaptic cleft, which stimulates the postsynaptic receptors. This accumulation of serotonin also activates autoreceptors, which decreases the release of neurotransmitter from the presynaptic neuron. With time, the overstimulated autoreceptors become hyposensitized and inhibition of serotonin synthesis and release wanes, so that the net effect is increased serotonin transmission. This sequence of biochemical changes, including the downregulation of receptors, takes time, is the likely reason that the effects of fluoxetine and other medications in the antidepressant category take four to six weeks to have an effect on clinical signs. As is explained above, there are changes in the neurochemistry of the brain and expression of receptors immediately, which explains why side effects can be seen with the very first dose of many antidepressants.

The influence of the primary neurotransmitter on the effector cell may be modulated by secondary neurotransmitters, such as polypeptides, as they interact at separate modulator receptor sites on the postsynaptic cell membrane. Attachment of modulatory neurotransmitters at these sites can result in the inhibition or facilitation of the effect of a primary neurotransmitter on the postsynaptic cell. Medications with a correct fit can also work at these sites to regulate neurotransmitter effect.

As noted above, the neurotransmitters that are altered by medications in veterinary behavioral medicine are primarily serotonin, norepinephrine, dopamine, acetylcholine, GABA, and glutamate. It is important to realize that the mechanisms of action of most psychotropic medications have not been fully elucidated. This could be an additional factor to explain the different clinical responses to medications apparently belonging to the same category (see Table 11.1).

The cholinergic system

Acetylcholine

Acetylcholine's main involvement in behavior is linked to its action within the CNS, supporting mnemonic function through the activation of different structures of the cortex and the limbic system. A defect in central cholinergic transmission may lead to learning and memory deficits and has been found in human patients with Alzheimer's disease.[25] Some of the adverse effects of tricyclic antidepressants such as clomipramine (Clomicalm) and amitriptyline (Elavil) are derived from their action as muscarinic acetylcholine receptor antagonists and include sedation, dry mouth, and constipation. At the time of this writing, there are no medications used in veterinary behavioral medicine which are prescribed for their effects on acetylcholine; however, there may be potential applications for cholinesterase inhibitors in improving learning and memory in cognitive dysfunction in senior dogs.[26]

Chemistry and pharmacology

Acetylcholine is synthesized from the union of acetyl coenzyme A and choline in the axonal boutons and is stored in the synaptic vesicles. Acetylcholine action is rapidly terminated by the enzyme acetylcholinesterase and most of the choline necessary for the production of acetylcholine is obtained through reuptake from the synaptic cleft. It is the only major neurotransmitter not derived directly from an amino acid. In vertebrates, acetylcholine is the neurotransmitter at all neuromuscular junctions and is involved in preganglionic to postganglionic neurotransmission for both the sympathetic and parasympathetic nervous systems (nicotinic synapses). Nicotinic receptors are excitatory. There are both N-m nicotinic receptors, which are located at the neuromuscular junction leading to muscle contraction, and N-n receptors, which are found in the brain, adrenal medulla, and autonomic ganglia. Acetylcholine is also the postganglionic neurotransmitter of the parasympathetic nervous system (muscarinic synapses). Muscarinic stimulation leads to a decrease in heart rate, cardiac output, and arteriole vasodilation, and an active digestive system. Five subtypes of muscarinic receptors have been identified, each acting on a different secondary messenger system. Acetylcholine is present in subcortical structures above the brainstem, especially in the area of the lower part of the basal ganglia named the nucleus basalis of Meynert, which is deeply involved in the neurophysiology of learning. Atropine blocks muscarinic synapses and therefore the effect of the parasympathetic system at the target organs, while curare blocks nicotinic synapses, thereby paralyzing skeletal muscles. Acetylcholinesterase inhibitors, such as some organophosphate compounds, potentiate the effects of cholinergic activity, while atropine acts as an antidote by blocking cholinergic receptors in the brain.

Monoamines

This neurotransmitter group is divided into catecholamines, indoleamines, and histamine. The catecholamines norepinephrine (noradrenaline), epinephrine (adrenaline), and dopamine are all synthesized from the amino acids tyrosine and phenylalanine, and share a common chemical structure. The indoleamines serotonin (5-hydroxytryptamine) and melatonin are synthesized from tryptophan.

Catecholamines are the neurotransmitters associated with the arousal of the autonomic nervous system. Catecholamine depletion in the brain results in mood changes and locomotor deficits. During states of physiologic and emotional stress, the catecholamines dopamine and norepinephrine are released, resulting in CNS stimulation and anxiety. Chronic stress might lead to exhaustion and depletion of norepinephrine and dopamine and resultant depression. Almost all classes of psychotropic medications interact in one way or another with the monoamine system.

Dopamine

Dopamine is involved in the regulation of many aspects of behavior, including motivation, social bonding, reward-based

Table 11.1 Pharmaceuticals and their effects on neurotransmitters

Neurotransmitter	Increased action	Decreased action
Acetylcholine	Cholinesterase inhibitors	Atropine, tricyclic antidepressants
Dopamine	L-DOPA, methylphenidate, apomorphine, bromocriptine, selegiline, MAO inhibitors	Acepromazine
GABA	Benzodiazepines, gabapentin	Flumazenil
Norepinephrine	Alpha-adrenergics (ephedrine, phenylpropanolamine), MAO inhibitors, tricyclic antidepressants, serotonin/norepinephrine reuptake inhibitors	Beta-blockers (pindolol, propranolol), alpha-2 agonists (clonidine; dexmedetomidine, guanfacine)
Serotonin	Tryptophan, selective serotonin reuptake inhibitors, MAO inhibitors, buspirone, trazodone, tricyclic antidepressants	Cyproheptadine

GABA, γ-aminobutyric acid; MAO, monoamine oxidase.

learning, attention, and the control of voluntary movements. Excessive dopamine may be associated with stereotypies. Glutamate and GABA (see below) play a role in regulation of the release of dopamine from dopaminergic neurons. Altered dopamine transmission may lead to behavioral changes such as decreased alertness, cognitive decline, anxiety, depression, extrapyramidal signs, Huntington's chorea in humans, and parkinsonian-like tremors, and may be a contributory factor in certain forms of pituitary-dependent hyperadrenocorticism. There are five dopaminergic receptors (D1–D5). Single nucleotide polymorphisms of the DRD2 gene, which encodes the dopamine 2 receptor, have been correlated with increased social fear in Havanese and noise reactivity in Soft-Coated Wheaten Terriers and Collies (See Chapter 3).[27]

In veterinary medicine, medications blocking the inactivation of dopamine are used to treat clinical conditions like cognitive dysfunction, stereotypies, fear, and anxiety. The most commonly used veterinary behavioral medicine which affects dopamine directly is the monoamine reuptake inhibitor selegiline (Anipryl), labeled for the treatment of canine cognitive dysfunction.

Chemistry and pharmacology

Dopamine is a neurotransmitter that is synthesized from tyrosine by dopaminergic neurons. Tyrosine is converted to levodopa and then dopamine. It is stored in prejunctional vesicles. After release, dopamine interacts with dopaminergic receptors. This is followed by reuptake by the prejunctional neuron. Levels are held constant by changes in tyrosine hydroxylase activity and not by levels of tyrosine. Therefore, medications that reduce the activity of the enzyme will lead to a reduction in catecholamine production. Dopamine is inactivated by the enzymes monoamine oxidase (MAO), primarily MAO B, and by catechol-O-methyltransferase (COMT) into dihydroxyphenyl acetic acid and homovanillic acid (HVA). HVA is used as a measure of dopamine turnover in the CNS of dogs.[28] Urinary HVA has been used as a measure of adrenergic stimulation in dogs.[29] There is evidence that impulsive dogs have lowered levels of 5-HIAA/HVA ratio when compared to dogs that are not impulsive.[30] Dopamine neurons in the midbrain extend into the limbic system and cortex. Increases in dopamine, such as might be caused by amphetamines or apomorphine, are associated with stereotypic behaviors. The neurotoxin 1-methyl-4-phenyl-1,2,3,6-tetrahydropyridine (MPTP), which depletes the brain of dopamine, will cause irreversible parkinsonian signs in humans and alterations in circadian rhythms and increased cortisol output in dogs.

Norepinephrine and epinephrine

Norepinephrine and epinephrine are closely related and bind at the same receptors, although affinity varies. For this reason, they will be discussed together. Norepinephrine, also known as noradrenaline, is the primary catecholamine neurotransmitter in the CNS and is involved in the regulation of mood, learning, memory, sleep–wake cycles, anxiety, attention, vigilance, pain, and arousal. Epinephrine, also known as adrenaline, is directly involved in the autonomic response of the acute stress response. Together, they cause sympathetic effects, for example, pupillary dilation, piloerection, tachycardia, glucose release, and vasoconstriction.

Adrenergic receptors generally stimulated by norepinephrine and epinephrine are divided into alpha [α_{1a}, α_{1b}, α_{1d}, α_2 (autoreceptor), α_{2a}, α_{2b}, α_{2c}] and beta (β_1, β_2, β_3). Activation of alpha-receptors leads to vasoconstriction, increased cardiac contractile forces, iris dilation, intestinal relaxation, pilomotor contraction, contraction of the intestinal and bladder sphincters, and inhibition of the parasympathetic nervous system. Stimulation of beta 1 (β_1) receptors leads to an increase in cardiac output, while β_2 receptor stimulation causes vasodilation, intestinal relaxation, uterine relaxation, and dilation of coronary vessels as well as bronchodilation. Epinephrine and norepinephrine have equal affinity for α_1 and α_2 receptors, however, epinephrine has greater affinity for the β_2 receptor when compared to the α_1 receptor until concentration exceeds a threshold at which the affinity switches to α_1 receptors. Medications which affect adrenergic receptors are widely used in veterinary medicine. While all are not prescribed for behavior disorders specifically, their administration can affect a pet's behavior and cause behavioral side effects because of their modulation of norepinephrine effect. Clonidine, dexmedetomidine, guanfacine, and tasipimidine are α_2 receptor agonists. Each has their own affinities for specific receptors within the alpha class. In addition, tricyclic antidepressants (amitriptyline, clomipramine) and serotonin/norepinephrine reuptake inhibitors (venlafaxine) inhibit the reuptake of norepinephrine at the norepinephrine reuptake transporter. Terbutaline, a medication prescribed in veterinary medicine for asthma, is a β_2 agonist. Propranolol and sotalol are beta adrenergic antagonists. Medications that block beta-receptors for norepinephrine and epinephrine, such as propranolol, may therefore block some of the physiological signs associated with fear.

Chemistry and pharmacology

Norepinephrine is synthesized from tyrosine in noradrenergic neurons. Tyrosine enters the neuron via an active transport pump. Tyrosine hydroxylase (TOH) converts tyrosine to DOPA. Next DOPA decarboxylase (DDC) converts DOPA into dopamine (DA). Finally, dopamine beta-hydroxylate (DBH) converts DA to norepinephrine. As with all monoamine neurotransmitters, norepinephrine is stored in vesicles in specialized neurons until an action potential causes release into the synapse and its action is terminated by MAO A, COMT and reuptake into the neuron. The locus coeruleus, which is located in the gray matter of the pons, is the principal noradrenergic nucleus. Noradrenergic neurons in the locus coeruleus send their processes into the thalamus, cerebral cortex, cerebellum, and spinal cord. Norepinephrine is also the neurotransmitter of the sympathetic postganglionic neurons. Epinephrine is also produced from tyrosine in the adrenal medulla. The enzyme phenylethanolamine N-methyltransferase facilitates the methylation of norepinephrine to epinephrine in the chromaffin cells. In response to stress, epinephrine is secreted from the adrenal gland and is one of the key neurotransmitters in the acute stress response. One study found no correlation between epinephrine and norepinephrine in the urine of dogs and an acute stressor.[31] However, in another study, urinary catecholamine:creatinine ratios (i.e., epinephrine:creatinine and norepinephrine:creatinine) were increased in dogs postveterinary visit compared to at home (previsit), while epinephrine:creatinine ratios were increased postexamination in the clinic compared to examination in the home.[32]

Serotonin

Serotonin (5-hydroxytryptamine; 5HT) is probably the most relevant neurotransmitter in behavioral medicine, with many medications exerting their primary action on serotonin pathways. The effects of serotonin on behavior are direct and also related to its role as regulator of other neurotransmitters. The role of serotonin in behavior is very complex and includes the regulation of mood and emotional states, like fear and aggression, arousal, impulse control, sleep–wake cycle, food intake, and pain. There are 14 different classes of serotonin receptors. Review of all receptors is outside of the scope of this text. There are several of interest in veterinary behavioral medicine, such as $5HT_{1A}$ receptors, which are located in high concentrations the hippocampus (memory), amygdala (emotion) hypothalamus (maintains homeostasis) and neocortex (cognition). High concentrations of the $5HT_{2A}$ receptors are found in the frontal cortex (executive function). Significant changes were found in $5HT_{2A}$ receptor binding in impulsive/aggressive (increased binding) and anxious dogs (decreased binding) in the frontal, temporal, and occipital cortices when compared to normal dogs.[33] In addition, aggressive dogs had modifications in the adrenergic and serotonergic receptor and increased serotonin receptors in the frontal cortex, thalamus, hippocampus, and hypothalamus.[34] Mice lacking the $5HT_{1B}$ receptor were more aggressive, while mice lacking $5HT_{1A}$ receptors were more anxious.[35,36]

A decrease in serotonin may lead to depression, increased anxiety, aggression, and decreased food intake. In humans, altered serotonergic system function is associated with hyperaggressive states, schizophrenia, affective illness, major depressive illness, and suicidal behavior. Increasing or normalizing serotonin levels may be useful in the treatment of depression in people, compulsive and stereotypic disorders, and some forms of aggression and anxiety. Selective serotonin reuptake inhibitors (SSRIs), serotonin/norepinephrine reuptake inhibitors (SNRIs), and tricyclic antidepressants (TCAs) increase serotonin availability by decreasing reuptake, and MAO inhibitors (MAOIs) increase serotonin by decreasing serotonin breakdown. Trazodone (a serotonin reuptake inhibitor/antagonist) inhibits reuptake and also antagonizes the $5HT_{2A}$ receptor.

Serotonin may act to inhibit aggression, at least in part by antagonizing the aggression-promoting effects of vasopressin. It has also been suggested that there is a relationship between dopamine and serotonin levels in that higher levels of 5HT may inhibit dopamine release.

Chemistry and pharmacology

Serotonin is synthesized from tryptophan by serotonergic neurons and is found mainly in cells in the midline raphe. Serotonin levels are controlled by cellular uptake of tryptophan and the action of tryptophan hydroxylase, which is involved in the rate-limiting step in serotonin synthesis. Tryptophan is discussed in detail in Chapter 12. Inactivation is by reuptake or by breakdown by MAO. Impulsivity

(disinhibition, unpredictability, prolonged arousal) may be correlated with the presence of low serotonin metabolites in the cerebrospinal fluid (5-HIAA).[12] Urinary 5-hydroxyindoleacetic acid (5-HIAA) excretion in the urine may be indicative of serotonin turnover. Attempts to correlate serum serotonin and behavioral clinical signs, specifically aggression, have yielded mixed results. Several studies have shown an inverse relationship between specific behavioral clinical signs (aggression, fear) and serum serotonin levels in dogs.[37–40] Alternatively, several studies found no correlation between serum serotonin levels and behavioral clinical signs (aggression, impulsivity, fear, reaction to stressful events).[41,42] Analysis and interpretation of results is challenging, as there is evidence that certain breeds have different baseline levels of serum serotonin, there is variation between sexes and with laterality, serotonin changes with pleasurable interactions,[43–45] and reference ranges have yet to be validated.[46]

Histamine

Histamine is found in low quantities in the brain. It may help to regulate body rhythms, thermoregulation, and neuroendocrine functions. Histamine activity is high during the waking state, reduced during slow-wave sleep, and nearly absent during rapid eye movement (REM) sleep.

Chemistry and pharmacology

The precursor to histamine is histidine. Histamine receptors are found primarily in the hypothalamus and initiate secondary messenger systems. Tricyclic antidepressants are histamine antagonists, which explains in part the side effects (sedation, dry mouth).

Amino acids

Amino acids are the most prevalent of the CNS neurotransmitters and are involved in rapid point-to-point communication at most nerve synapses. Glycine, glutamate, and GABA are three of the most important of the 20 amino acids that function as neurotransmitters. Glycine is an inhibitory neurotransmitter of the hindbrain and spinal cord. There are no veterinary psychiatric medications that directly affect glycine at the time of this writing.

Glutamate

Glutamate (glutamic acid) is the major excitatory neurotransmitter in the brain, affecting virtually all neurons and indicated in aggression, depression, and impulse control disorders in humans. Glutamate receptors can be inotropic, ligand-gated ion channels (NMDA) and metabotropic, G protein-linked receptors. N-methyl-D-aspartic acid (NMDA) receptor antagonists used in veterinary medicine include amantadine, ketamine, memantine, and dextromethorphan. Increased plasma glutamine has been linked to fearfulness in dogs.[47]

Anxitane, Composure Pro, and Solliquin all contain l-theanine, which functions as a glutamate antagonist. Glutamate has become an important neurotransmitter of recent interest for medications and supplements alike. See Chapter 12 for more information on supplements.

Chemistry and pharmacology

Glutamate originates from glutamine. Glutamate is stored in synaptic vesicles in glutaminergic neurons and is recycled into glial cells (and other types of cells) via an excitatory amino acid transporter (EAAT). Once glutamate has been taken up into the glial cell, it is broken down by glutamate synthetase into glutamine. Glutamine may exit the glia via a specific neutral amino acid transporter (SNAT) to be taken up into another neuron for conversion back into glutamate by mitochondrial glutaminase. It is then stored again in vesicles until triggered for release.

Gamma-aminobutyric acid

GABA is the most widespread inhibitory neurotransmitter in the brain, with concentrations in up to 1000 times greater than monoamines in some parts of the brain, and is an important mediator of aggression, anxiety, sleep disorders, vigilance, muscle tension, and pain. GABA's receptors include $GABA_A$ (ligand-gated ion channel, inotropic) and $GABA_B$ (G protein-linked, metabotropic). The $GABA_A$ receptor is very important in veterinary behavioral medicine and has benzodiazepine and nonbenzodiazepine subtypes. Seizure activity and Parkinson's disease may be associated with GABA decreases or disorders, so GABA agonists such as benzodiazepines can be useful in the treatment of these conditions. GABA agonists may also be helpful in the treatment of anxiety disorders. The most commonly used medications in veterinary behavioral medicine which modulate GABA are benzodiazepines, gabapentin, phenobarbital, pentobarbital, imepitoin, and pregabalin. L-theanine and alpha-casozepine are widely available in supplement form. Both modulate GABA.

Chemistry and pharmacology

Much like glutamate, GABA is conserved after excretion by the neuron through reuptake, packaging in vesicles, and storage until needed again by the neuron. GABA is synthesized from glutamate by glutamic acid decarboxylase (GAD), which is only found in cells which use GABA as a neurotransmitter. The action of GABA is terminated by reuptake into glial cells and presynaptic nerve terminals. GABA, which is taken back up into GABA neurons, is recycled as above. The remaining neurotransmitter is taken up into glial cells and by GABA transferase (GABA-T).

Neuropeptides

Endorphins and neurokinins (substance P and NK1)

This group is composed of molecules that are short-chain amino acids. They mainly function as modulators of other neurotransmitters, evoking facilitation or inhibition of neurotransmitter activity at the postneuron receptor site. The opioid system plays an important role in mediating both physical pain and social affective disorders.[48] Endogenous brain opioids may be involved in the development and maintenance of social behavior and social attachments.[49] Opioids have been shown to reduce crying and motor agitation in puppies during

social isolation.[50] Opioid administration in socially deprived kennel dogs has also been shown to ameliorate chronic emotional distress through opioid blockade. Administration of morphine increases social interactions but decreases tail wagging when dogs are in a deprived state, while naloxone increases tail wagging following nondeprivation.[51] Because opioids play a role in distress related to social isolation and modulate social interactions, it is very likely that they also play a role in the development and treatment of fear and anxiety. CNS endorphin release has been implicated in some stereotypic behaviors which also presumably have a pain or local illness component, such as feather damaging behavior and acral lick dermatitis. The most commonly used medications in veterinary behavioral medicine which modulate endogenous opioids are butorphanol, naloxone, and naltrexone.

Substance P is a neuropeptide that is found in the spinal cord and CNS; it is a modulator of nociception involved in signaling the intensity of noxious stimuli. Along with neurokinin 1 (NK1), substance P is likely involved in the body's response to stress, anxiety, invasion of territory, and noxious or aversive stimuli. Substance P is present in the limbic system, including the hypothalamus and amygdala, and may play a role in emotional behavior. NK1 is present in the hypothalamus, pituitary, and amygdala, which play a role in affective behavior and response to stress. In cats, NK1 substance P receptors in the midbrain periaqueductal gray potentiate defensive rage and suppress predatory aggression.[52] Substance P is one of the primary neurotransmitters released during tissue and mast cell damage.[53] Blocking substance P might reduce inflammation, pain, nausea, and neuropathic pain.[54] Therefore, as a substance P inhibitor (NK1 antagonist), maropitant citrate (Cerenia: Zoetis Animal Health) may reduce neurogenic inflammation, and substance P inhibitors have potential applications for inflammatory conditions in humans.[55] In cats with nonflea-, nonfood-induced hypersensitivity dermatitis, pruritus and lesions were reduced in all but one cat after four weeks of administration at a dose of 2 mg/kg PO q24.[56] Maropitant is approved for use in dogs for the prevention and treatment of emesis at a daily dose of 2 mg/kg orally or 1 mg/kg subcutaneous or IV, and for motion sickness at 8 mg/kg daily given at least 2 hours before travel with a small amount of food on an empty stomach.[57] Peak concentrations in dogs are reached 1 hour following subcutaneous administration with a half-life of 8.8 hours, and less than 2 hours after oral administration with a half-life of 4.2 hours.[55] In dogs, maropitant administered preoperatively has been shown to prevent the vomiting associated with opioids, promotes a faster return to normal feeding, and improve the quality of recovery.[58] In cats, maropitant is approved for the treatment of vomiting at a dose of 1 mg/kg subcutaneously or IV daily and is also used extralabel for the prevention of vomiting and motion sickness at 1 mg/kg oral or subcutaneously. It has a peak effect 2 to 3 hours after oral administration and 0.5 hours after subcutaneous administration and a half-life of 15.5 hours.[55,59] Maropitant could cause depletion of substance P, potentially leading to depletion in dopamine and resultant parkinsonian-like tremors, although in a study of daily injections of maropitant citrate in cats at up to 5 mg/kg for 15 days, it was well tolerated with no adverse effects except for one cat that developed mild tremors during sleep; there were no adverse events.[57]

Other neurotransmitters

There are numerous other mediators of neurotransmitter release (e.g., encephalins, nitric acid), but further discussion is beyond the scope of this text.

Hormones

Endogenous compounds such as hormones or other substances are not commonly used in veterinary behavioral medicine with the exception of melatonin (see Chapter 12). Although some may consider that using substances already found in the body is somehow safer, hormone excess can lead to serious medical problems.

Vasopressin and oxytocin

Vasopressin and oxytocin are pleotropic peptides with similar structures. They are often discussed together, as their effects can be manifested through combined activity. Both are synthesized in the supraoptic nucleus, paraventricular nucleus, and hypothalamus. Nonetheless, they are distinct molecules with their own actions. In addition, each neurotransmitter can bind to the receptors of the other.

Oxytocin is widely referred to as the "love" hormone. It facilitates social bonding, inhibits the sympathoadrenal axis, and reduces anxiety, fear, and immobilization when frightened. Dogs have high levels of oxytocin, which may be essential for the formation of stable social groups,[60] and exhibit an increase in oxytocin after pleasurable interactions with a familiar person.[61] Oxytocin administration appears to enhance learning in dogs, decrease aversion to training signals which might be intimidating such as direct gaze, and increase social interactions.[62] Vasopressin's nonbehavioral effects include antidiuresis cardiovascular regulation, and antipyresis. Its behavioral effects include mobilization when threatened (enhanced self-defense), increased sympathoadrenal activity, and arousal; decreased anxiety, and improved memory.

One study found no significant changes in vasopressin between dogs with separation-related disorders and nonseparation-related disorders.[63] Differences in serum oxytocin and vasopressin have been found between aggressive and nonaggressive dogs. There is evidence that aggressive dogs may have a different biochemical profile than nonaggressive dogs. One study showed that aggressive dogs had lower free and higher total plasma vasopressin than control dogs, and assistance dogs bred for lack of aggression had higher free and total plasma oxytocin than control dogs.[3,64]

In hamster and rat studies, injections of vasopressin in multiple CNS sites led to offensive aggression, while vasopressin receptor antagonists inhibited aggression. It has been hypothesized that at least in the hamster, serotonin inhibits fighting by antagonizing the aggression-promoting action of vasopressin.

Main classes of psychotropic medications

Adrenergic receptor agonists and antagonists

Clonidine is a selective alpha-2 agonist that blocks norepinephrine release on presynaptic neurons in the locus coeruleus, reducing sympathetic outflow from the brain. Although originally developed as an antihypertensive agent, it has been used in both human psychiatry and veterinary behavioral medicine since it reduces sympathetic outflow from the brain, thereby blocking autonomic responses to anxiety (fight or flight). It may also offer centrally acting analgesic effects by blocking pain signal transmission to the brain.[65] In human psychiatry, it has been used for the treatment of hypervigilance, ADHD, posttraumatic stress disorder, and impulsivity. Clonidine administration has been shown to inhibit firing of the locus coeruleus noradrenergic neurons in cats. According to the results of an open-label trial, it has been used in conjunction with serotonin reuptake inhibitors and/or buspirone for fear and territorial aggression and for anxiety disorders such as separation-related disorders, noise and storm phobias, and nocturnal barking that have been unresponsive to other therapeutic strategies in dogs.

It is generally dosed approximately 1.5–3 hours prior to an event, up to TID. It has also been used as adjunctive therapy in the treatment of inflammatory bowel disease in dogs and cats. Other than hypotension, at higher doses it can cause sedation and incontinence in dogs and has been reported to cause sleep disturbances, excitation, and decreased concentration in humans. Clonidine should be used cautiously in pets with cardiac disease and medications that might increase norepinephrine levels.

Dexmedetomidine oromucosal (OTM) gel form is FDA approved for the treatment of noise aversion in dogs at a dose of 0.125 $\mu g/m^2$ given 20–60 minutes in advance of the event.[66] It has also been demonstrated to be effective for use in situations of anxiety, including car travel and veterinary visits.[8,67–69] Time to maximum concentration and bioavailability for dexmedetomidine OTM gel (Sileo) is 0.6 hours and 28%, respectively, and with an elimination half-life of 0.5–3 hours. It is contraindicated in dogs with shock, severe debilitation, and stress due to extreme heat, cold, or fatigue, and it should not be given to patients with a history of sensitivity to dexmedetomidine or other alpha-2 agonists. Patients with severe cardiovascular, respiratory, liver, or kidney disease can be potentially overdosed, so caution is warranted. The most common adverse reaction published is sedation.[70]

Dexmedetomidine OTM gel is not approved for cats, but one dot (0.25 mL or 0.025 mg dexmedetomidine hydrochloride) of Sileo per cat has demonstrated efficacy in decreasing clinical signs of anxiety related to travel and postcar ride cortisol.[9] However, in another recent placebo-controlled study, administration of dexmedetomidine OTM gel in 30 cats, resulted in no significant reduction in travel or veterinary clinic anxiety in cats.[71]

For fearful and aggressive dogs and cats, effective sedation for situational use (e.g., veterinary visits, procedures, and preoperative use) may be achieved with transmucosal doses of 10–40 μg/kg, alone or in combination with narcotics such as butorphanol, buprenorphine, and methadone.[72–74] Tasipimidine (Tessie) is an alpha-2 agonist and has been shown to alleviate the clinical signs of separation-related disorders, noise anxiety and travel phobia in dogs; and some anxiolytic effect during the veterinary physical exam.[75–77] A canine version is approved in Europe for "Short term alleviation of situational anxiety and fear triggered by noise or owner departure" at a dose of 30 μg/kg 1 hour in advance. See resources and recommended reading below.

Beta-adrenergic receptor antagonists

Because fear leads to the release of the neurotransmitter norepinephrine, beta-blockers such as *propranolol* have been used successfully to treat some forms of anxiety. By blocking beta-adrenergic activity, the physical signs of anxiety (tachycardia, tachypnea, muscle tremors, palpitations, sweating, trembling, gastrointestinal upset) are decreased. Without these signals, the fear response can be diminished. By reducing tone in muscle spindles, beta-blockers might reduce effects on the reticular activating system that lead to reactivity and vigilance. In addition, propranolol might act centrally to increase 5HT release. In humans, they are seldom effective for generalized anxiety or panic situations; however, beta-blockers have been used successfully in people with situational or performance anxiety (e.g., stage fright), sometimes referred to as fight or flight situations. In veterinary medicine, propranolol has been used in combination with buspirone, SSRIs, TCAs, phenobarbital, benzodiazepines, and selegiline in dogs and cats for the treatment of fears, anxiety, and phobias (especially when there are strong somatic signs).[78] Beta-blockers are contraindicated in pets with bradycardia, congestive heart failure, diabetes, or pulmonary diseases, including asthma.

Pindolol is a beta-adrenoreceptor antagonist and 5-HT$_{1A}$ antagonist. As with propranolol, anxiety may be reduced by blocking some of the autonomic signs of fear and anxiety. However, because pindolol has an additional effect on the 5-HT$_{1A}$ receptor, it may also have direct effects on those clinical signs attributable to serotonin dysregulation. In addition, by blocking presynaptic autoreceptors, the initial downregulation associated with reuptake inhibitors may be prevented, resulting in augmentation and acceleration of the antidepressant effect of the serotonin reuptake inhibitor. Studies in humans have shown a faster SSRI response when combining pindolol with an SSRI (especially paroxetine) compared to the SSRI alone.[79] Some studies have also demonstrated an improved response to depression with pindolol plus fluoxetine versus fluoxetine alone.[80] Potential side effects of pindolol are panting, increased anxiety, and urinary incontinence.

Anticonvulsants

Anticonvulsants have applications in clinical veterinary behavior, particularly in cases where a forebrain lesion might be responsible for the behavioral signs. There also may be comorbidity between seizures and behavioral disorders[81,82] (also see Chapter 6). The use of anticonvulsants for the treatment of seizures are beyond the scope of this text. For more information on the correlation between neurologic disease and behavioral disorders, see Chapter 6.

Phenobarbital and other barbiturates were used in the past as antianxiety agents in both humans and animals. In fact, a combination of phenobarbital and propranolol has previously been suggested for the treatment of noise phobias.[83] However, for the most part, benzodiazepines have replaced barbiturates for the treatment of anxiety-related disorders. On the other hand, some benzodiazepines, such as clonazepam and diazepam, have been shown to be useful as adjunctive therapy in the control of seizures.[84] Although the elimination half-life is approximately 1 to 2 hours at low doses, with higher doses and long-term therapy, seizure control might be maintained with BID to TID therapy.[85] *Clonazepam* has a slower onset of action and may be safer for pets with compromised hepatic function since it has no active intermediate metabolites. Due to the possibility of physical dependence with anticonvulsants, withdrawal should be gradual. Signs of abrupt withdrawal might include "wet dog shakes," increased temperature, listlessness, and seizures.

Carbamazepine is a tricyclic compound, similar to imipramine in structure, that has been used for adjunctive anticonvulsant therapy and for neuropathic pain, specifically trigeminal neuritis in humans. Carbamazepine may also act as a mood stabilizer and antidepressant. In humans, it has been used for epilepsy-related aggression and aggression with agitation, anxiety, and irritability, and has been used in dogs with irritable and explosive types of aggression, compulsive behaviors, and for behavior changes associated with seizures.[86] It has been used alone or in combination with medications such as fluoxetine. In animals, carbamazepine is slightly sedating, mildly anticholinergic, and does not cause significant muscle relaxation. In cats, carbamazepine has been found to reduce some forms of fear-induced aggression and may make individual cats more affectionate toward people.[87] The medication is contraindicated in patients with known renal, hepatic, cardiovascular, or hematological disorders, and should not be used in pets kept for reproductive purposes. It has a short elimination half-life and dosing can be further complicated by the fact that in humans the medication induces CYP3A4, which metabolizes carbamazepine itself (as well as other medications metabolized by CYP3A4); therefore, higher doses may be required to maintain effect over time. In humans, there is a risk for agranulocytosis and aplastic anemia, so regular blood monitoring is recommended.

Levetiracetam is an antiepileptic medication that was the first medication in humans approved for partial seizures and is also used for other psychiatric disorders, including anxiety, stress, panic, mood disorders, Tourette's, and behavioral signs such as aggression that might be associated with seizures.[88,89]

Antidepressants

This category includes the TCAs, SNRIs, and the SSRIs in veterinary behavioral medicine at the time of this writing. The main pharmacological action of these psychotropic medications is on serotonin pathways. Antidepressants have been used in veterinary behavioral medicine to treat compulsive behavior, stereotypical behavior, aggression, fear, anxiety, stress, phobias, generalized anxiety, and panic. For generalized and recurrent fears and anxieties, antidepressants may be preferable to anxiolytics since they are nonaddicting and less sedating. However, for the immediate control of anxiety, phobias, and panic, quicker-acting medications such as benzodiazepines, gabapentin, pregabalin, or alpha-2 agonists may also be needed. These medications could also be used concurrently or on an as-needed basis during antidepressant therapy. As with any medication which alters the neurochemistry, antidepressants as a group can increase irritability, which may increase aggression (see Table 11.2).

While antidepressants reach peak plasma levels within hours, this does not reflect their therapeutic effect since over

Table 11.2 Comparative effects of antidepressants[85,124]

Most anticholinergic	Moderately anticholinergic	Least anticholinergic
Amitriptyline	Clomipramine, paroxetine, nortriptyline, imipramine, doxepin	Fluoxetine, fluvoxamine, sertraline, citalopram, trazodone, venlafaxine, buspirone
Most hypotensive	**Moderately hypotensive**	**Least hypotensive**
Imipramine, amitriptyline	Clomipramine, doxepin	Nortriptyline, SSRIs
Most sedating	**Moderately sedating**	**Least sedating**
Doxepin, amitriptyline	Clomipramine, imipramine, nortriptyline, paroxetine, trazodone	Fluoxetine, citalopram, sertraline, fluvoxamine, venlafaxine, buspirone
Most antihistaminic	**Moderately antihistaminic**	**Least antihistaminic**
Doxepin*, amitriptyline	Imipramine, clomipramine, nortriptyline	SSRIs, trazodone (mild), venlafaxine
Most serotonergic	**Moderately serotonergic**	**Least serotonergic**
SSRI, clomipramine	Imipramine, amitriptyline, trazodone, venlafaxine	Nortriptyline, doxepin
Most noradrenergic	**Moderately noradrenergic**	**Least noradrenergic**
Desipramine, nortriptyline,	Amitriptyline, imipramine, clomipramine, doxepin, venlafaxine**	SSRIs, paroxetine (weak)
Most seizure potential	**Moderate seizure potential**	**Lowest seizure potential**
Amitriptyline, clomipramine, imipramine, doxepin	Desipramine, nortriptyline	SSRIs, SNRIs, trazodone

SSRIs, Selective serotonin reuptake inhibitors.
*Greatest effect.
**Dose related (at higher doses).

time, reuptake inhibition may induce changes in the expression of receptors, including downregulation of postsynaptic receptors. Therefore, while effects may be seen within the first two weeks, at least four to eight weeks of therapy is generally recommended to assess therapeutic effects fully.[90] The behavioral effects of chronic administration of antidepressants may lead to stimulation of neurogenesis in the hippocampus.[91] Side effects may include gastrointestinal signs, inappetence, lethargy, paradoxical agitation, and neurological signs such as tremors or seizures. However, because antidepressants affect neurotransmitters in slightly different ways, there is some variability in indications, effects, and side effects between antidepressants.

Tricyclic antidepressants

The primary mechanism of action of TCAs such as clomipramine and amitriptyline is to block the reuptake of serotonin and, to a lesser extent, norepinephrine. The degree of serotonin and norepinephrine reuptake blockade, as well as anticholinergic, antihistaminic, and alpha-adrenergic effects, varies between TCAs and account for differences in TCA effects and side effects. TCAs are contraindicated with glaucoma and cardiac disease or where urine retention is a concern. Most TCAs are well absorbed from the gastrointestinal tract and metabolized by the liver to an active intermediate metabolite before excretion through the kidneys. Therefore, they should be used cautiously in the elderly or when there is compromised hepatic metabolism. Amitriptyline has moderate effects in inhibiting both serotonin and norepinephrine reuptake, and strong antihistaminic

and anticholinergic effects. Doxepin has marked antihistaminic effects but minimal effects on serotonin reuptake and moderate effects on noradrenergic reuptake. The alpha-adrenergic effects of imipramine may aid in improving sphincter control in pets with enuresis or conflict, excitement, or submissive (fear induced) urination, while also ameliorating anxiety. However, while doxepin, imipramine, and amitriptyline have all been used to varying degrees in veterinary behavioral medicine, there is little evidence of their efficacy in pets. In one study, approximately 50% of separation-related disorder cases showed some improvement, which is far below the levels of improvement reported with clomipramine or fluoxetine.[92] No significant improvement was seen in canine aggression cases treated with amitriptyline.[93] In a retrospective study of compulsive disorders in dogs and cats, clomipramine was significantly more efficacious than amitriptyline.[94] Amitriptyline has been replaced by more efficacious medications that are more selective for serotonin reuptake and as such is used for the most part as an adjunctive treatment.

Clomipramine blocks serotonin reuptake and desmethylclomipramine (the active metabolite) blocks norepinephrine reuptake into the presynaptic neuron, thereby increasing the concentration of each in the synapse. Clomipramine is metabolized in the liver to an active metabolite, desmethylclomipramine. Peak levels for both clomipramine and desmethylclomipramine are reached in 1–3 hours and terminal half-lives were 4 hours or less. With increasing dosage, mean residence times and terminal half-lives of both compounds are increased.[95] A steady state is achieved in about one to four days. In humans, clomipramine has mild anticholinergic effects, is moderately antihistaminic, and is a potent alpha-1 antagonist. These effects likely account for much of the medication's side effects, including sedation, dry mouth, retained urine or stool, tachycardia, hypotension, and dizziness. However, in dogs, clomipramine is associated with less urinary stasis, cardiac disease, and anticholinergic effects compared to humans, possibly because of a shorter half-life and rapid elimination.[94] In addition, in dogs the ratio of clomipramine to desmethylclomipramine is higher (3:1) than in humans (1:2.5) and it is the desmethylclomipramine that is responsible for most of the anticholinergic properties.[89] At therapeutic doses, neither clomipramine nor amitriptyline altered cardiac rate or rhythm in dogs.[96]

On electrocardiogram, there was also no effect of clomipramine after 28 days in cats, although thyroid levels were suppressed.[97] Clomipramine can suppress iodine uptake in the thyroid gland in dogs. For this reason, dogs starting clomipramine or any TCA should have thyroid levels checked at baseline and every six months thereafter.

Because clomipramine is the most selective inhibitor of serotonin reuptake of all of the TCAs, its indications and applications, including the treatment of compulsive disorders in dogs and humans, more resembles that of the SSRIs. Clomipramine in combination with a behavior modification plan is an effective treatment for separation-related disorders and reduction of clinical signs such as vocalization, contact seeking, destruction, and pacing in dogs with anxiety disorders.[16,98,99] In a follow-up of 76 cases of dogs with separation-related disorders that were treated with clomipramine, 12 dogs remained on treatment for over 13 months with no adverse effects or relapse, and 10 of the dogs showed further improvement. Of 22 dogs with complete resolution, 13.6% relapsed when the medication was ceased.[100] Clomipramine has been shown to be effective for compulsive and anxiety disorders in dogs and cats, feline hyperesthesia (0.5–1.0 mg/kg PO q24h)[101–105] and feline urine marking.[16,106,107] Urine retention may be a concern at higher doses.[108] One RCT found no significant differences between dogs with separation-related disorders treated with behavior modification plus clomipramine and dogs treated with behavior modification alone.[109] Clomipramine was found to be ineffective in the treatment of cases of pet parent-related aggression.[110]

TCAs may also be used in combination with other anxiolytic agents. For example, benzodiazepines may be used on an as-needed basis along with the ongoing use of a TCA, for stress-evoking events such as pet parent departures, thunderstorms, or veterinary visits. In one study, clomipramine in combination with behavior modification and alprazolam as needed was effective for the treatment of storm phobias.[111] TCAs may also be used in combination with medications such as gabapentin for the treatment of neuropathic pain.[112] TCA should be used in young animals and those that need the calming effect of the antihistamine qualities of a TCA. Older patients may not be able to tolerate the side effects. Care should be exercised in cats and dogs that have urinary tract disease because of the risk of urinary retention.

In summary, TCAs are widely used in dogs and cats historically. They have moved into the second choice column for many patients due to age and side effects. Nonetheless, they should be utilized when their action matches the clinical signs of the patient being treated. Like any other psychotropic

medication, the metabolism and response is individual to that patient. Multiple doses or medications may have to be tried before finding that perfect fit. They are best chosen in young, healthy animals with no urinary retention or urinary tract disease and in which calming or sedation is desired.

Selective serotonin reuptake inhibitors

SSRIs are selective in their blockade of the reuptake of serotonin into the presynaptic neurons. Because they are selective for serotonin reuptake, they generally have fewer side effects than TCAs, including fewer cardiac effects and hypotension and perhaps greater safety in pets with seizures.[113] In fact, one study found that fluoxetine may have anticonvulsant activity in humans.[114] They may also be preferable where urine retention, increased intraocular pressure, sedation, or anticholinergic effects might be a concern, although urinary retention and fecal retention have been reported in cats that are under treatment with fluoxetine. Side effects with SSRIs particularly include reduced appetite, weight gain, agitation, urinary retention, urinary incontinence, lowering of seizure threshold, and sedation.[115,116] Side effects which are intolerable or reduce the patient's quality of life should result in a reduction of dose by one-half. If the patient's side effects do not resolve within three days, the medication should be discontinued. If the patient's clinical signs resolve in three days, it is reasonable to keep the patient on the lower dosage of the SSRI for two weeks. If the patient continues to do well after that time, the dose can be increased again, more slowly than previously done.

The most commonly used antidepressants in behavioral medicine at this time are fluoxetine, paroxetine, sertraline, fluvoxamine, and escitalopram. While each medication in this class generally has the same function, there are small differences in action which may be clinically helpful (see Figure 11.2 and Table 11.2). For example, paroxetine is mildly anticholinergic. Side effects may therefore include urine or fecal retention. In dogs, SSRIs are used for disorders having clinical signs associated with fear, anxiety, and stress which require long term treatment (greater than one month) or where signs are generalized, unpredictable or global, prohibiting treatment with only a premedication. A complete discussion of the approach to diagnosis, treatment, and prescribing is found in Chapter 9.

Fluoxetine is very commonly used in cats and dogs. In an eight-week RCT with a chewable fluoxetine tablet combined with a behavior modification plan, a significantly greater improvement was seen in the fluoxetine group.[84] In a second multicenter six-week RCT of dogs with separation-related disorders, overall severity scores were improved for dogs on fluoxetine and no behavior therapy compared to placebo.[2] Although there was a significant medication effect, greater improvement was achieved using the combination of fluoxetine plus behavior modification.[89] Studies indicate that fluoxetine has a T_{max} of 1.8 hours and 12.8 hours for its active intermediate metabolite norfluoxetine, and reaches a steady state in approximately 10 days.[117] Since the clearance half-life of fluoxetine is 6.2 hours and 49 hours for norfluoxetine, the start of new medications that might be contraindicated when used in combination may need to be delayed.

In addition to the approved use of fluoxetine for the treatment of separation-related disorders in dogs, SSRIs may also be useful for a wide variety of other extra-label applications,

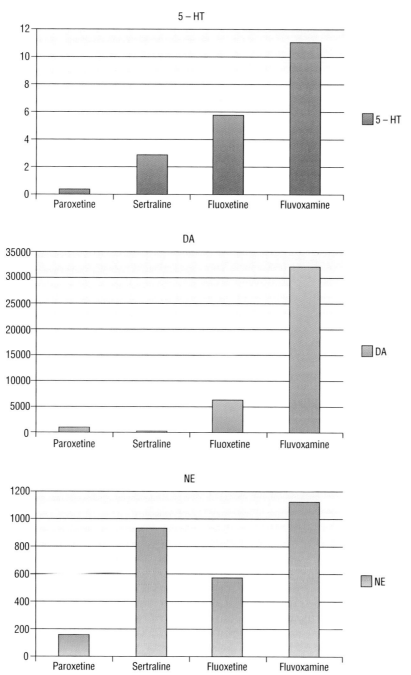

Figure 11.2 Reuptake inhibition profiles of SSRIs. Mean concentration of drug (nmol/L) required to inhibit reuptake by 50%. The higher the value, the smaller the reuptake inhibition potency. The low values of these drugs for 5HT compared with DA and NE show how selective they are for 5HT. *5-HT*, Serotonin; *DA*, dopamine; *NE*, norepinephrine (*Reproduced from Sussman N, Selective serotonin reuptake inhibitors. In: Sadock BJ, Sadock VA, Ruiz P, eds. Kaplan and Sadock's Comprehensive Textbook of Psychiatry. 9th ed. Philadelphia: Wolters Kluwer – Lippincott Williams & Wilkins; 2009:3193.)*

including compulsive disorders, stabilizing mood, reducing impulsivity, and some forms of aggression.[118] In a study of generalized anxiety disorders, fluoxetine and paroxetine in combination with behavior modification were effective,[119] and fluoxetine has been useful in some forms of canine aggression.[19,120] Fluoxetine has also been effective in the treatment of compulsive disorders in dogs,[18,121] as have sertraline[55,101] and citalopram.[122] Fluoxetine may also be effective in the treatment of feline urine marking.[16,123] Fluvoxamine

can be effective in the treatment of anxiety disorders in dogs with a low incidence of side effects.[124] In the aforementioned study and in clinical experience, finding an effective dose which is likely to be unique in any particular animal is paramount to resolution of minimization of clinical signs.

The differences in the applications and efficacy of SSRIs may be related to minor differences in the way they affect neurotransmitters. Based on human studies, Figure 11.2 demonstrates the relative potencies of SSRIs with respect to serotonin reuptake blockade and their effects on dopamine and norepinephrine. Although there have been no studies in pets to demonstrate any difference as to which SSRI would be most suitable for a particular problem, some guidelines have been recommended for applications in dogs and cats based on human studies and anecdotal evidence to date. It has been suggested that sertraline is effective for panic, generalized anxiety, anxious, irritable, and inhibited dogs as well as for compulsive disorders; fluoxetine and fluvoxamine for hyperactivity and aggression as well as fears and phobias, generalized anxiety, and compulsive disorders; and paroxetine for social anxiety, agitation, and panic disorders.[57,85,125] For cats, paroxetine has been used in the treatment of urine marking, compulsive disorders, and aggression toward people and cats; sertraline for compulsive disorders, anxiety, and inappropriate urination, and fluoxetine for the treatment of elimination disorders, anxiety, aggression, compulsive disorders, and self-trauma.[57,85] Escitalopram is widely used in human medicine for depression.[126] It is a potent inhibitor of serotonin reuptake at the presynaptic neuron. At the time of this writing, there is only one study examining dosing in dogs; however, it did not examine efficacy at that dose.[127] For this reason, it should not at the time of this writing be a first choice for treatment.

SSRIs have been combined with other psychotropic medications and supplements to enhance their clinical effects, such as with the use of benzodiazepines for calming prior to specific events (e.g., separation-related disorder departures, noise phobias); with clonidine, either prior to specific events or as adjunctive therapy for fear and territorial aggression or for anxiety disorders such as separation-related disorders, noise and storm phobias, and nocturnal barking[66]; and with trazodone for generalized anxiety, separation-related disorders, and thunderstorm phobias on an as-needed basis (prior to events) or up to two to three times daily or prior to bedtime for sleep disturbances.[128] Benzodiazepine levels may be increased when used with SSRIs that inhibit CYP2C19 or 3A4 including but not limited to fluvoxamine and fluoxetine, and trazodone levels increase with SSRIs that inhibit CYP2D6 or 3A4 including but not limited to fluoxetine, fluvoxamine, and paroxetine. Buspirone levels may be elevated by medications that inhibit CYP 3A4 including but not limited to fluvoxamine. When using any medications concurrent with SSRIs that might further increase serotonin, pets should be more closely monitored for any signs of serotonin syndrome. SSRIs have also been combined in humans with gabapentin for refractory anxiety disorders, or hypnotics, trazodone, or mirtazapine for agitation or insomnia.

In summary, SSRIs are used for disorders of fear, anxiety, and stress which need long-term treatment or are more generalized. While they all have individual effects and side effects, in general this class of medications behaves in the same way. Because of the individual way that these medications are metabolized and the genetic nature of behavioral disorders, it is not uncommon to try two or three SSRIs before the right one is found for any given patient. These medications are generally safe medications in healthy animals. In light of the differences in terminology and metabolism between humans and companion animals, it is best to treat clinical signs and their presumptive neurotransmitter dismodulation instead of first focusing on diagnosis. For a more complete discussion of this topic, see Chapter 9.

Selective serotonin reuptake/norepinephrine reuptake inhibitors

The SNRIs block the reuptake of both norepinephrine and serotonin at the reuptake transporter on the presynaptic neuron.[129] The most well-known medications in this class for use in animals are duloxetine and venlafaxine. Venlafaxine may be useful in the treatment of misdirected play, impulse aggression, and behavioral periuria in cats.[130-132] It acts as a serotonin reuptake inhibitor at low doses and inhibits norepinephrine reuptake only at higher doses. Duloxetine, on the other hand, inhibits norepinephrine and serotonin approximately equally throughout the dosing range. Duloxetine is used in women to reduce urine leakage due to stress incontinence and has been shown to increase external urethral sphincter EMG activity and bladder capacity in cats.[133,134]

Serotonin antagonists/reuptake inhibitors

Trazodone is a serotonin receptor antagonist (5-HT2A, 5-HT2C) and a serotonin reuptake inhibitor. It is often classified as a SARI (serotonin antagonist/reuptake inhibitor). It also is an α-adrenoceptor and histaminergic (H1) antagonist. In humans, it has been used as an antidepressant, anxiolytic, and sleep aid, and for the treatment of obsessive-compulsive disorders. When used with an SSRI or TCA, the effects may be additive, although when combining serotonergic medications, the risk of serotonin syndrome is always present. The clinical effect of trazodone in cats and dogs is primarily sedation and mild stress relief. Trazodone may be useful for treating many types of fears and phobias, including generalized anxiety, separation-related disorders, noise aversion, thunderstorm phobia, situational anxiety (e.g., car rides, veterinary visits),[126] and some types of aggression when sedation or calming is desired or until long-term treatments can be employed. Additionally, it can be useful to enhance sedation in hospitalized pets or postorthopedic surgery, and in reducing signs of stress (panting, lip licking, whining) in hospitalized dogs.[135,136] When administered 2 hours prior to induction at doses ranging from 5–7 mg/kg PO, no differences were seen in anesthetic needed for induction or cardiovascular parameters when compared to acepromazine administered IM 30 minutes prior to induction.[137] Trazodone can be used on an as-needed basis or up to two to three times daily in dogs.[126,133] In dogs, the oral bioavailability is adequate when given at a dose of 8 mg/kg, however, the time to peak plasma concentration is highly variable (445 ± 271 minutes).[138] This may explain why in some dogs trazodone takes several hours to take effect.

It has been used in cats as a single dose ranging between 10.6 and 33.3 mg/kg, 90 minutes prior to veterinary examination. The cats in the aforementioned study showed signs of sedation as measured by an accelerometer, as would be expected, but their stress scores were not lower than controls with hypersalivation, immobility, open mouth breathing, aggression, and struggling no different between treatment and control groups.[139] Trazodone was well tolerated and caused sedation at all doses used with a peak effect for 100 mg observed at 2.5 hours.[137] A more recent study used a single dose with the dose range of 7.7–15.2 mg/kg 60–90 minutes prior to the cats being put into their carriers and being driven to the clinic. Cats were examined by a veterinarian

1.5–2 hours after administration. Trazodone significantly improved the cats' anxiety and stress levels during transport (compared to placebo) and were easier to handle by their veterinarians.[140] In dogs, at a dose of 9–12 mg/kg given 90 minutes prior to travel, while pet parents reported a lower dog stress score (DSS) during the physical examination and video analysis showed decreased stress, there were no significant differences in aggression, sedation, cortisol levels, or compliance based on pet parent or researcher scoring.[141]

In summary, trazodone is a very useful medication for inducing behavioral calm or sedation and reducing arousal in dogs and cats. It may relieve stress in some situations, but it is not a potent stress reliever nor anxiolytic in these species. It may take several hours to take effect. The time to effect is variable, as is the clinical effect at a specific dose in an individual dog.

Tetracyclic antidepressants

Mirtazapine is a tetracyclic antidepressant which has serotonergic, noradrenergic, and mild antihistaminic effects. It is an antagonist at central presynaptic alpha-2 autoreceptors, 5HT2, 5HT3, and histamine (H1) receptors.[57,142] It is used in pets primarily for its antiemetic, antinausea, and appetite-stimulating effects, although it has been used in the treatment of anxiety disorders in dogs and cats. In humans, it has been used for depression, panic disorders, generalized anxiety disorders, posttraumatic stress disorders, and insomnia. It is dosed at 1.88 mg/cat daily in cats and 0.5–1 mg/kg daily in dogs. Alternate day therapy is recommended for cats with chronic kidney disease and compromised hepatic function.[57,143] In cats with chronic kidney disease, a longer half-life and prolonged clearance was demonstrated with alternate day therapy, resulting in increased appetite and activity and decease in vomiting.[144,145] The most common adverse effects are vocalization, agitation, vomiting, ataxia, restlessness, and tremors; however, only one cat was reported to have adverse effects at a dose of 1.88 mg/cat compared to 25 cats at 3.75 mg/cat.[146] An FDA-approved 2% mirtazapine transdermal gel for appetite stimulation has been approved for use in cats, for which a 1.5 inch strip is applied on the ear pinna (2 mg/cat).[147]

Mirtazapine can be used alone or in conjunction with SSRIs, gabapentin or benzodiazepines for fearful, anxious, and stressed dogs and cats, and to increase appetite and as an aid in counterconditioning and reinforcement-based training.[148] Cautious dosing is recommended in small dogs and cats, pets with hepatic or renal failure, and when combining with other medications that might increase serotonin. In addition, since it is a substrate for CYP2D6, 1A2, and 3A4, it should be used cautiously with SSRIs, particularly fluoxetine, paroxetine, and fluvoxamine. As mirtazapine acts as an alpha-2 antagonist, its use should be avoided in combination with alpha-2 agonists due to competing mechanisms.

Antihistamines

Antihistamines may be useful for the treatment of pruritus, self-trauma, sleep disorders, and anxiety. Those antihistamines that have sedative CNS effects (hydroxyzine, chlorpheniramine, diphenhydramine, cetirizine, trimeprazine) may also be useful in situations of mild anxiety or overactivity, or to help induce sleep. However, compared to acepromazine, diphenhydramine did not cause clinical appreciable sedation in healthy dogs.[149] Anxiety associated with car rides, excessive vocalization, and undesirable nighttime activities are conditions that may respond to antihistamine therapy. They may also be useful postoperatively and for anxiety associated with pruritus. TCAs such as clomipramine, doxepin, and amitriptyline may also have potent antihistaminic effects and may therefore be more suited for anxiety with self-trauma. Since antihistamines are anticholinergic, pet parents should be warned that they may cause a dry mouth and constipation, and are contraindicated in patients with glaucoma, urine retention, or hyperthyroidism. Cyproheptadine, an antihistamine with antiserotonergic effects, may also be an effective appetite stimulant in cats and dogs and may be useful for inducing sleep. It has also been used with variable success to treat urine spraying in cats.[150]

Azapirones

The only azapirone applicable to veterinary behavioral use is *buspirone*, a partial serotonin ($5HT_{1A/B}$) receptor agonist, serving to regulate the neurotransmission of serotonin.[151] Buspirone has not proven to be particularly effective in veterinary practice for pets with intense fears, anxiety, phobias, compulsive disorders, or canine aggression. Buspirone is unique among serotonergic medications in that it appears to increase boldness and sociability, making it useful in reducing fear in an overly fearful pet in its relationship with people or other pets. However, those same effects can increase pushy behavior, counter surfing, jumping, and aggression. In general, buspirone is best used in pets that do not show aggression upon presentation. In one study, it was found to be effective in reducing feline urine marking in over 50% of cases, with less recurrence after withdrawal than medications such as diazepam.[152] Buspirone might also be combined with benzodiazepines for the treatment of some anxiety disorders, although both medications can increase boldness and sociability, making the combination best for nonaggressive, apathetic, withdrawn patients. Although some effect may be seen after a single treatment (e.g., pretravel) with higher doses of 2 mg/kg, it is more commonly dispensed for ongoing use at doses of 0.5–1 mg/kg BID and several weeks might be needed to achieve clinical efficacy. It may also be effective at reducing motion sickness in cats.[153] Combining buspirone with drugs that increase serotonin, such as SSRIs, may increase risk of serotonin syndrome.[57,84]

In summary, buspirone has a unique mode of action among veterinary psychotropic medications. Because of its clinical effect (increased boldness and sociability), it is best used in patients that are nonaggressive, apathetic, and fearful. As with most serotonergic medications, it takes several weeks to have a clinical effect.

Benzodiazepines

Benzodiazepines can be considered for the treatment of any condition that may have an underlying component of fear or anxiety, including separation-related disorders, noise phobias, specific phobias, behavioral periuria (stress or anxiety etiology), and urine marking. They potentiate the effects of

GABA. This acts to mute the effects of glutamate, the excitatory neurotransmitter from which GABA is made.

In general benzodiazepines cause decreased anxiety, hyperphagia, muscle relaxation, decreased locomotor activity, and varying degrees of sedation. Benzodiazepines act as mild sedatives at low doses, as antianxiety agents at moderate doses, and as hypnotics at high doses. They may also act as anticonvulsants. Studies of animal models of anxiety have shown that the inhibition related to fear and anxiety can lead to a decrease in eating, drinking, and exploratory behaviors and an increase in avoidance or aggression, while treatment with benzodiazepines leads to disinhibition, resulting in increased exploration, resumption of appetite, and a decrease in avoidance and aggression.[81,154] However, in some instances, such as where the fear response is one of avoidance, disinhibition could lead to an increase in aggression. In humans and laboratory animals, the aggression-heightening effect of benzodiazepines seems to be dose dependent, with lower doses enhancing aggression; however, in clinical practice this is not always the case. Some evidence from studies on laboratory rodents indicates that certain benzodiazepines such as oxazepam and clorazepate might be safer in terms of their potential aggression-heightening effect.[155]

Benzodiazepines can cause paradoxical excitability, which can be particularly problematic in situations where a calming effect is desired and is also a concern if the medication is to be administered during periods when there is no pet parent supervision, such as in separation-related disorders. In those situations, it is advised before beginning the treatment to test the medication in the pet parent's presence. Benzodiazepines may cause a variable degree of anterograde amnesia, which is an inability to create new memories. Amnesic effects of benzodiazepines can have positive or negative consequences, depending on how they are integrated in the overall treatment scheme. It is not clear if this effect is present with clinical dosing.

In one study examining the effects of *diazepam* in dogs with behavior problems, it was very effective or somewhat effective in 67% of anxiety-related behavior cases.[156] Reasons for discontinuation of diazepam included: either lack of efficacy or adverse effects ranging from sedation to increased appetite, ataxia, agitation, activity, and aggression. Pet parents reported greater success when using diazepam for fear of thunderstorms than for separation-related disorders. When doses of 0.8 mg/kg were used, there were greater reports of increased activity.[156] Therefore, when side effects are seen, dose adjustments should be considered or alternative benzodiazepines selected.

Benzodiazepines are often used on an as-needed basis for the treatment of situational anxiety, panic, and phobias such as with thunderstorms, fireworks, car rides, visits to veterinary clinics, return home from the clinic for aroused cats, or the anxiety associated with departures in dogs with separation-related disorders. With that said, they can also be used up to four times daily, depending on which benzodiazepine is being used. Long-term use of benzodiazepines in dogs is regarded as generally safe. Dogs that receive benzodiazepines daily for greater than two weeks should be weaned off to avoid rebound clinical signs. Most reach peak effect within 45–90 minutes after each dose and can be used alone or in combination with other medications on an as-needed basis.[85,143,158,159] Time to maximum serum concentrations in dogs after oral dosing has been reported as 0.75–1 hours for diazepam, 0.5 hours for lorazepam, 1–3 hours for oxazepam and clonazepam, and 1 to 2 hours (0.75–6 hours) for clorazepate.[85,160–162] Benzodiazepines might be useful to facilitate desensitization and counterconditioning in animals showing intense fear since they decrease anxiety and increase appetite. However, since they can impair learning and it is unclear at which dose this occurs in any given patient on any specific medication, the dose should be gradually adjusted. The amnesic effects of benzodiazepines can be useful for unavoidable exposures to the stimuli causing fear or anxiety, for they might reduce the long-term impact of those negative experiences.

All of the benzodiazepines act as anxiolytic medications and have similar therapeutic effects. But onset of action, duration of effect, intensity of effects, and metabolism differ, so a particular benzodiazepine might be more suited to a particular application.

Benzodiazepines may be classified based on onset of action, duration of action, and target action. Most frequently, they are classified as short-, intermediate-, or long-acting, based on the half-life of the medication. These types of classifications can be misleading, as the effect of benzodiazepines is dose dependent and most studies leading to characterization are single-dose studies; the active metabolites may have longer clearance times than the parent compound; duration of action may be incongruent with half-life as a result of differences in distribution from blood into fatty tissues; onset is dependent on rate of absorption; and accumulation in tissues may cause a longer duration of action than predicted by the half-life.[152] For example, diazepam has a long elimination half-life in humans, but a short duration of action because of the rapid distribution to fatty tissues, whereas lorazepam, which has a shorter half-life, has a longer duration of action because it is not distributed as quickly into fatty tissues.[162] For these reasons, it may be challenging to know which benzodiazepine to choose under which circumstances for individual patients. Factors considered in selection should be based on half-life in the species for which the veterinarian is prescribing, elimination, distribution, and absorption (see Boxes 11.2–11.5).

Benzodiazepines are absorbed unchanged from the gastrointestinal tract, with the exception of clorazepate, which is

---

Box 11.2 Factors affecting onset of action, duration of action, and clinical effect of benzodiazepines

- Absorption rate
- Rate of distribution (parent and active metabolites)
- Extent of distribution (parent and active metabolites)
- Elimination half-life (parent and active metabolites)
- Number of doses (single versus multiple)
- Clearance (parent and active metabolites)
- Accumulation in the brain, plasma, and fatty tissues (parent and active metabolites)
- Individual variation in absorption, half-life, clearance, rate of distribution

From Greenblatt DJ, Shader RI, Divoll M, et al. Benzodiazepines: a summary of pharmacokinetic properties. *Br J Clin Pharmac*. 1981;11:11S-16S.

Box 11.3 Classification of benzodiazepines based on single-dose half-life of the parent compound or active metabolite(s)

Classification	Half-life of parent compound and/or metabolite
Long acting	>24 hours
Intermediate acting	5–24 hours
Ultra-short/immediate	<5 hours

From Greenblatt DJ, Shader RI, Divoll M, et al. Benzodiazepines: a summary of pharmacokinetic properties. *Br J Clin Pharmac.* 1981;11:11S-16S.

Box 11.4 Classification of benzodiazepines based on half-life or parent compound and active metabolites by species

	Long-acting (half-life >24 hours)	Intermediate-acting (half-life 5–24 hours)	Short-acting (half-life <5 hours)
Humans	Diazepam Chlordiazepoxide Clorazepate Clonazepam	Clonazepam Alprazolam Lorazepam Oxazepam	Midazolam Triazolam
Dogs		Diazepam Chlordiazepoxide Clonazepam Clorazepate Oxazepam	Lorazepam
Cats		Lorazepam Diazepam	

If not listed, published information is lacking in that species. From Greenblatt DJ, Shader RI, Divoll M, et al. Benzodiazepines: a summary of pharmacokinetic properties. *Br J Clin Pharmac.* 1981;11:11S-16S.
Crowell-Davis SL, Murray TF, Dantas LMS. *Veterinary Psychopharmacology.* 2nd ed. Hoboken, NJ: Wiley-Blackwell; 2019.
Koechlin B, D'Arconte L. Determination of chlordiazepoxide (Librium) and of a metabolite of lactam character in plasma of humans, dogs, and rats by a specific spectrofluorometric micro method. *Anal Biochem.* 1963;5:195-207.

Box 11.5 Benzodiazepine (onset of action, active metabolites)

Benzodiazepine	Active metabolites
Alprazolam	Alpha-hydroxy-alprazolam-1/2 the biologic activity as alprazolam
Chlordiazepoxide	Desmethylchlordiazepoxide, oxazepam, desmethyldiazepam (nordiazepam), demoxepam
Clonazepam	No
Clorazepate	Desmethyldiazepam (nordiazepam)
Diazepam	Desmethyldiazepam (nordiazepam), oxazepam
Lorazepam	No
Oxazepam	No
Midazolam	No

From Greenblatt DJ, Shader RI, Divoll M, et al. Benzodiazepines: a summary of pharmacokinetic properties. *Br J Clin Pharmac.* 1981;11:11S-16S.

converted to its intermediate metabolite nordiazepam (desmethyldiazepam) in the gastrointestinal tract prior to its absorption. Most benzodiazepines, such as diazepam, are metabolized by the liver and some have active intermediate metabolites that may be more active than the parent compounds. The metabolites are then conjugated by the liver and excreted in the urine. For instance, nordiazepam, which in turn is converted to the active metabolite oxazepam, is an active metabolite of chlordiazepoxide, diazepam, and clorazepate. Alprazolam and triazolam have short-lived metabolites with minimal activity. Diazepam and particularly its active metabolites have been reported to cause rare cases of hepatotoxicity in cats and for this reason is no longer considered the benzodiazepine of choice in that species.[163] Anorexia can be a sign that the cat is having a hepatic reaction and should be cause for immediate cessation of the medication and assessment of serum liver tests. Clonazepam is metabolized in several inactive metabolites. Oxazepam and lorazepam have no intermediate metabolites and therefore may be safer for obese or elderly pets, or those with liver disease, and have less chance of residual or cumulative effects (see Boxes 11.2–11.5).

In cats, diazepam has been used successfully for spraying, anxiety-motivated undesirable elimination, anxieties, and fears (including fear aggression). It has also been used successfully to stimulate appetite, to control seizures, and to treat feline hyperesthesia. Diazepam may also decrease predation through its inhibitory effect on acetylcholine. Because of the relatively short half-life in dogs (1–3.2 hours compared with 3.5–5.5 hours in cats) as well as the short half-life of its active metabolite nordiazepam (2–10 hours in dogs compared with 21 hours in cats), its primary use in dogs is alone or in combination with SSRIs or TCAs as an adjunct to desensitization programs for fears and fear aggression, and prior to fear-evoking and anxiety-evoking events such as pet parent departures, fears and phobias including thunderstorms or fireworks, fear-based urination, and fear of people.[85,57,123] However, with continued oral dosing of 1 to 2 mg/kg TID, steady-state plasma concentrations might be achieved.[144]

Because of its short duration of action and high potency, *alprazolam* is most useful for acute fears and panic of short duration.[77,106] At low doses, it may successfully reduce fear and aggression with less effect on motor function than diazepam. In a study evaluating the effectiveness of treatments for fireworks fears, where prescription drugs were dispensed, the highest reported effectiveness was with alprazolam (91% of 32 dogs).[164]

Clonazepam has a slower onset of action and may be safer for pets with compromised hepatic function since it has no active intermediate metabolite. A mean elimination half-life of 4.75 hours has been reported after a single dose and 6–9 hours after multiple doses.[85,144] Given twice daily, the average half-life in the first week is about 2 hours while after 3 weeks this increases to 8 hours.[85] Clorazepate reaches peak concentrations in 2 hours with no prolongation in absorption or serum concentrations for the sustained release compared to the regular release formulations with an elimination half-life of approximately 9 hours.[85,156,157]

Oxazepam is an effective appetite stimulant for cats and provides a longer duration of action than diazepam. The time to peak maximum concentration of oxazepam in dogs is 1–3 hours with a half-life of about 2.5 hours.[148] After administration of diazepam as the parent compound, the half-life of oxazepam was 4.2–6 hours.[144] Oxazepam has been used to treat feline hyperesthesia syndrome at a dose of 0.20–0.50 mg/kg PO q12–24h.[105]

Lorazepam provides more sustained release in people, but has a slower onset of action. In dogs, with oral dosing, it has been reported to reach peak plasma levels in 0.5 hours with a half-life of approximately 1 hour, although brain levels may persist longer.[57,85] In cats, peak plasma concentrations are achieved in 12 hours with a half-life of 17 hours.[85] Lorazepam has been used to treat feline hyperesthesia syndrome at a dose of 0.125–0.50 mg PO q8–24h.[105]

Long-term use of benzodiazepines may lead to physiologic dependence, with least intense physical dependence of the benzodiazepines reported with lorazepam and oxazepam in dogs.[57] In humans, benzodiazepines also pose a risk of dependency and abuse; therefore, while medication use by pets can be responsibly controlled by the pet parent, veterinarians should exercise some caution in dispensing and monitoring of benzodiazepine use if they suspect that there might be a potential for human abuse. All benzodiazepines, particularly those of high potency, should be withdrawn slowly (e.g., 25% per week). Behavior problems may recur when the medication is withdrawn. In one study, 91% of cases of behavioral periuria in cats recurred when the diazepam was discontinued.[165]

Although medications such as SSRIs and TCAs may be more appropriate for chronic anxiety situations such as separation-related disorders, shorter-acting medications that do not require several weeks to reach a therapeutic state, such as benzodiazepines, may be better suited to treat anxieties of shorter duration, such as a boarding situation, thunderstorms, fireworks, or for a few days after a move or other changes in the household.

Combination therapy of benzodiazepines and TCAs, SSRIs, beta-blockers, alpha-2 agonists, or phenothiazines have also been used in veterinary medicine (e.g., separation-related disorders, thunderstorm phobias). In an open trial, alprazolam in conjunction with clomipramine and behavior modification was effective in controlling noise phobia in dogs.[109] In an open trial treatment with clorazepate at 1 mg/kg daily for four weeks in combination with behavior modification and fluoxetine for 10 weeks at 1 mg/kg per day, was effective in 69.4% of dogs with a greater improvement in clinical signs of anxious nonaggressive dogs than anxious aggressive dogs.[145] In another open trial with diazepam at 0.3 mg/kg daily for four weeks in combination with behavior modification and fluoxetine at 1 mg/kg daily for 10 weeks, 76% of dogs were improved with no significant difference in dogs with aggression and anxiety without aggression.[166] Disinhibition-related aggression was not observed with either diazepam or clorazepate treatment.[145,162] Intranasal midazolam has been shown to be efficacious in humans for modulation of panic attacks.[167] For immediate control of panic or phobic states, intranasal lorazepam or oromucosal midazolam or intrarectal diazepam may be an option for some pet parents where oral dosing is impractical and immediate effects (5–10 minutes) are needed.[57,168,169]

Benzodiazepines marketed for anxiety can also be used for sleep induction. Clonazepam has also been reported to be effective for some REM sleep movement disorders.[170] Oxazepam may help to sustain sleep but is not an effective sleep inducer. In people, the primary use for hypnotic benzodiazepines such

as flurazepam and triazolam is for the treatment of insomnia. Flurazepam has rapid absorption and a long half-life, and may sedate during the next day in people. At low doses, it may not affect REM sleep in humans. Triazolam has slower absorption and a very short half-life. When used for pets that wake during the night, flurazepam may be preferable if pets wake too early on triazolam or alprazolam. Triazolam has also been reported to be effective in some cases of aggression in cats.

Imepitoin is a partial low-affinity GABA-A agonist that is approved in the European Union and in the United States for use in dogs with noise aversion, although at the time of this writing, the medication is not yet marketed in the United States. It is approved for the treatment of canine epilepsy in the United Kingdom and in several European countries. In a randomized, placebo-controlled trial, imepitoin has demonstrated efficacy in decreasing signs of noise aversion in dogs.[171] Although it may be effective within 2 hours after administration, it is recommended for use at 30 mg/kg twice daily beginning two days prior to the aversive event. In another recent randomized, placebo-controlled trial over 28 days, pet parents reported significantly reduced fear and anxiety during storms and other noise events with imepitoin treatment at a dose of 30 mg/kg twice daily over 28 days.[172] Studies have also demonstrated a reduction in signs of distress in a series of clinical cases of fear- and anxiety-related behavior problems at a dose of 10–30 mg/kg BID, a reduction in cortisol in a laboratory thunderstorm model, and a reduction in serum cortisol in dogs with generalized anxiety disorder at a dose of 20 mg/kg BID for three days.[173–175] However, in dogs with epilepsy under treatment with imepitoin, no improvement in anxiety-related behaviors were noted as measured in an online survey (C-BARQ).[176] The most common reported side effect is ataxia, followed by increased appetite, lethargy, emesis, hyperactivity, and somnolence.[158] In cats, a dose of 10–30 mg/kg twice daily beginning 5–10 days prior to the triggering event has been recommended[177]; however, imepitoin is not approved for cats and controlled studies have not been published to date.

In summary, benzodiazepines are very useful in the treatment of disorders in which fear, anxiety, and stress without aggression are present. As with all psychotropic medications, each medication within this class has slightly different effects, metabolism, and duration of effect.

CNS stimulants

In some cases of overactivity disorders, learning deficits, and aggression in dogs, stimulants may have a paradoxical calming effect in much the same way as they do for attention deficit disorders (ADD) in humans. Of course, these stimulants would generally have an activating effect and are therefore contraindicated in dogs that are displaying overactivity or aggression from other causes. Stimulants enhance the release of dopamine and block dopamine and norepinephrine reuptake. This might then help to enhance inhibitory output from the frontal lobe to improve concentration and impulse control and decrease motor activity. Occasionally, the less serotonergic antidepressants such as the TCAs or selegiline may also be useful in cases of ADHD. Most cases of hyperactivity are not due to physiological disorders. In humans, ADD may or may not be associated with hyperactivity (ADHD). ADD in humans is associated with lack of impulse control, overactivity, and lack of attention which interferes with ability to learn. Hyperkinetic dogs have been reported to exhibit overactivity (barking, chewing, pacing), tachycardia, panting, salivation, lack of trainability, aggression, and failure to calm down in neutral environments.[178] However, it has been speculated that dogs without hyperactivity that show signs of repetitive behavior, anxiety, aggression, poor learning or inattention and perhaps gastrointestinal signs might also have ADD. Historically, diagnosis was made by administering 0.2–0.5 mg/kg *dextroamphetamine* orally and then observing the dog every 30 minutes for 1 to 2 hours to determine if the dog's heart or respiratory rate decreased or the dog became calmer.[164] However, this is most likely not a good assessment for hyperactivity in dogs. Alternatively, *methylphenidate* can be prescribed for three days at 0.5 mg/kg in the morning and early afternoon. Target behaviors (repetitive behaviors, aggression, anxiety, overactivity) and somatic signs (respiratory and cardiac rates, salivation) should be assessed to determine if there is any significant improvement. If there is no improvement, the dose can be increased by 0.25 mg/kg BID every three days to assess efficacy to a maximum dose of 2 mg/kg BID.[179] While this is not diagnostic for hyperactivity, it will serve to assess the effect of the medication as a therapeutic option. However, if there is aggravation in the condition at any dose, the medication should be considered ineffective. In one European trial of dogs with hypersensitivity–hyperactivity disorders, about 55% of the dogs improved with methylphenidate therapy. Some of the dogs improved on fluvoxamine, selegiline, or sertraline therapy. CNS stimulants might also be indicated for narcolepsy. In a recent retrospective study of 89 dogs diagnosed by French veterinary behaviorists with hypersensitivity–hyperactivity syndrome (as defined by the French veterinary psychiatry community), an ADHD-like disorder with signs of motor activity, reduced sleep, and lack of satiety, fluoxetine at a dosage of 2–4 mg/kg PO q24 provided improvement in 68 of 89 dogs depending on sign assessed. Adverse effects were reported in 61% of dogs, the most common of which was decreased appetite, followed by fatigability, sedation, weight loss, and tremors. While most adverse events were mild, six dogs required reevaluation, all of which remained on a dosage of 2 mg/kg per day.[180]

Dopamine agonists

Dopamine agonists such as *bromocriptine* directly stimulate dopaminergic postsynaptic receptors in the brain, which inhibits prolactin release from the anterior pituitary. In cats, bromocriptine has been reported to reduce urine spraying. Side effects include increased affection, prolapsed nictitating membranes, and inappetence for 24–48 hours. Oral tablets are available, but exact dose rates have not been determined. It is thought that steady-state plasma levels are reached in 10 days and that the medication should be given twice daily for four to eight weeks. In humans, the medication may cause dizziness, hypotension, and nausea (so should be taken with food), and transient elevations in alanine aminotransferase, creatine phosphokinase, blood urea nitrogen, aspartate aminotransferase, and serum alkaline phosphatase. Bromocriptine may also be useful in the treatment of false pregnancy in dogs and in occasional cases of pituitary-dependent hyperadrenocorticism.

Vomiting, diarrhea, hypotension (especially with the first dose), and behavior changes such as sedation and fatigue have been observed in dogs.

Gabaminergic medications

GABA modulators such as gabapentin and pregabalin are widely used in veterinary behavioral medicine. *Gabapentin* is structurally similar to GABA, but unlike GABA, it has been formulated to cross the blood–brain barrier and does not appear to have any effect on GABA receptors. One suggested mode of action is enhancement of neuronal GABA synthesis. In addition to its anticonvulsant effect, gabapentin is widely used in the treatment of neuropathic pain and chronic pain management, generalized anxiety disorders and social phobia, impulsivity, mood disorders, phobias, panic disorder, feline hyperesthesia, as a situational medication for veterinary visits, and as adjunctive therapy in compulsive disorders. Gabapentin is metabolized to *N*-methyl gabapentin in the liver in dogs. The parent compound and intermediate metabolite are excreted in the kidneys, so dose adjustments might be needed in renal patients. The mean elimination half-life in dogs is 2–4 hours and the time to achieve steady-state concentration is less than a day.[57] Since self-mutilatory disorders, hyperesthesia, and interstitial cystitis in cats have a pain component, gabapentin should be considered for these conditions. In cats, peak effect is reached in 1–3 hours with a mean elimination half-life of approximately 3 hours.[81,181] A study by Hudoc and Griffin (2019) showed that gabapentin used preemptively (25–30.5 mg/kg) decreased signs of stress in cats subjected to intradermal allergy testing.[182] Other studies also showed decreased stress signs when a single dose of gabapentin was used in cats prior to trap-neuter-release procedures and veterinary visits.[183,184] In a comparative study of the effects of gabapentin on postsurgical (ovariectomy) food intake, gabapentin-treated and mirtazapine-treated cats ate significantly more than placebo-treated cats at 2–8 hours postsurgically.[185] The dosing range for gabapentin is wide, which may be due to the dependency of transport on a saturable amino acid transporter at least in dogs and presumably in cats.[186] In a study examining the absorption of transdermal gabapentin in cats, gabapentin was detected in the serum and pain scores decreased in cats dosed with 5 and 10 mg/kg TD q8 for five days. This study did not compare transdermal dosing to oral dosing and for that reason it is unclear if the serum levels with transdermal dosing are comparable to oral dosing.[187] In a study of 10 healthy cats administered 21–36 mg/kg at a single dose orally, 70% of the cats exhibited mild sedation within 120 minutes of administration. Of those that exhibited sedation, over half did so within 1 hour. In that same study, there were no differences found between placebo and gabapentin groups regarding blood pressure and heart rate; however, while echocardiographic changes were noted between the two groups, none were outside of the reference range.[188] In placebo-controlled studies in dogs, treatment with gabapentin at a single dose of 50 mg/kg 2 hours prior to veterinary visits reduced lip licking,189 while a dose of 25-30 mg/kg at least 90 minutes in advance reduced fear responses during thunderstorms (See resources and recommended reading).[189]

Pregabalin is an anticonvulsant antineuralgic which binds to the α2 delta subunit at voltage-sensitive calcium channels, reducing neurotransmitter release and decreasing neuronal activity. Pregabalin is structurally similar to GABA but has no known effects on GABA. It has a peak effect in 1.5 hours and a half-life of 6.9 hours in dogs, and a peak level at 0.5-2.9 hours and a half-life of 10.4-14.7 hours in cats.[57,85] Like gabapentin, pregabalin may be used as adjunctive therapy for refractory or focal seizures, treating neuropathic and chronic pain, and for the treatment of fear, anxiety, and night waking.[57] It has recently been approved in Europe for the treatment of acute anxiety and fear associated with transportation and veterinary visits in cats at a dose of 5 mg/kg 1.5 hours in advance. See resources and recommended reading below.

In summary, gabaminergic medications have been shown to be useful in the treatment of disorders involving anxiety, fear, stress, muscle tension, and pain. Gabapentin is safe to use long term and more information is needed on long term use of pregabalin in animals.

Hormonal therapy

Synthetic *progestins* have been used to treat behavioral periuria and some forms of anxiety and aggression. They are antiandrogenic and cause an increase in appetite and nonspecific depression of the CNS. This latter effect explains why progestins cannot be used to assess the potential effects of castration on behavior. Because of their effects on the endocrine system, numerous unacceptable side effects may result. High doses or long-term use may lead to diabetes mellitus, adrenocortical suppression, bone marrow suppression, acromegaly, endometrial hyperplasia, pyometra, and mammary hyperplasia and carcinomas. Behavioral use of progestins should be avoided as there are many options which are both more efficacious and have fewer side effects.

Since the presence of male hormones can lead to an increase in sexually dimorphic behaviors (such as mounting, mating, masturbation, roaming, urine marking, and perhaps some forms of aggression), there is some question as to whether medications that might reduce the effects of androgens could also have an effect on behavior. *Finasteride* inhibits the conversion of testosterone into dihydrotestosterone (DHT) so that both intraprostatic and circulating DHT levels are reduced. However, in clinical trials in males treated with finasteride for benign prostatic hypertrophy, there was little or no decline in libido and in canine studies, there was no effect on serum testosterone.[190] *Delmadinone* is an androgen antagonist that leads to suppression of secretory activity of the prostate gland, but it does not lead to lower serum DHT levels. Since neither of these medications appears to lower circulating testosterone levels, they are not likely to have any significant effect on reduction of androgen-influenced behaviors. *Deslorelin* is also a gonadotropin-releasing hormone agonist in the form of a subcutaneous implant for the induction of temporary infertility in healthy, intact, sexually mature male dogs. An initial rebound effect in testosterone production is observed, followed by a downregulation of pituitary gonadotropin-releasing hormone receptors, leading to a loss of gonadal activity. Deslorelin has proven to be an effective alternative to surgical castration in both dogs and cats. Sexually dimorphic behaviors such as mounting and urine marking, are initially unaffected or even increased,

but they progressively show a significant reduction after the first weeks of treatment.[191]

Diethylstilbestrol is used for the treatment of estrogen-responsive incontinence in spayed female dogs by increasing sphincter tone. Estrogens, however, can be toxic to the bone marrow and cause blood dyscrasias, so the lowest effective dose should be utilized and complete blood counts should be monitored regularly. Incontinence in neutered male dogs has been successfully treated with repository parenteral treatment of *testosterone propionate*, since most oral testosterone is rapidly broken down by the liver. The prostate should be regularly assessed in dogs undergoing testosterone therapy. Potential side effects are the development, aggravation, or recurrence of sexually dimorphic male behaviors. Testosterone and estrogen depletion may also be related to cognitive decline and possibly mood disorders (see Chapter 8). It is as yet undetermined whether hormone replacement therapy might help to prevent or slow the progress of cognitive decline or would lead to an improvement of clinical signs. However, in old dogs with cognitive decline, estrogen-treated females made significantly fewer errors in size-reversal learning tasks but made more errors in spatial memory tasks.

Recent research has shown the utility of oxytocin in the formation of bonds and social behavior. For oxytocin to be effective at modifying behavior, it has to be given intranasally, as it is not effective when given orally. It is being used sporadically in dogs for anxiety, fear, and aggression toward specific people.

In summary, hormones are very rarely if ever used to treat psychiatric problems in animals due to side effects (with the exception of oxytocin). Oxytocin shows promise in increasing sociability and bonding in dogs, but due to mode of administration, it has not been widely used.

Monoamine oxidase inhibitors (MAOIs)

MAO is an enzyme that metabolizes norepinephrine, dopamine, and serotonin. MAOIs (e.g., phenelzine, isocarboxazid, tranylcypromine) inhibit both MAO A and MAO B and are irreversible in their actions. Since MAOIs prevent the breakdown of epinephrine, norepinephrine, and serotonin, they cause elevations of these monoamines for the treatment of depression, social phobias, anxiety, eating, and panic disorders in humans. They are less anticholinergic and less sedating than TCAs, but have the potential for greater side effects and may interact with a number of medications that enhance the serotonin system (such as SSRIs and some TCAs), as well as foods that are rich in tyramine (such as cheese and wine) to precipitate a hypertensive crisis. Tyramine is normally inactivated by MAO in the gut. However, when nonselective irreversible MAOIs are administered, tyramine may not be inactivated. This may lead to an increase in norepinephrine release, leading to vasoconstriction and an increase in blood pressure. Adverse reactions include CNS stimulation, hepatoxicity, dizziness, hypertension or hypotension, dry mouth, blurred vision, and constipation. A variety of nutraceuticals can also contain or influence MAOIs, including resveratrol, goldenseal (berberine), turmeric (curcumin), ginkgo biloba, and perhaps St. John's wort (*Hypericum perforatum*).

As with other antidepressants, a therapeutic effect may not be achieved for up to four weeks. Newer selective reversible inhibitors of MAO are far less likely to precipitate a hypertensive crisis and may therefore be a safer and more practical treatment option. However, they can lead to insomnia at night and daytime lethargy. Most MAOIs nonselectively inhibit both MAO A and B and have few animal applications.

Selegiline (also known as L-deprenyl) selectively inhibits MAO B in the dog at therapeutic levels. Although no increase in brain dopamine levels has been demonstrated in the dog, it may enhance dopamine transmission by inhibiting dopamine reuptake and by increasing levels of phenylethylamine, which is a facilitator of dopamine activity. Selegiline may also enhance the release of norepinephrine.[196] It increases free radical elimination by enhancing superoxide dismutase and catalase activity and may be a potent free radical scavenger.[79] Because free radicals cause cell injury and may contribute to brain pathology and signs of aging, selegiline may decrease nerve damage and degeneration. Selegiline also exhibits "rescue" of CNS and peripheral neurons damaged by trauma or neurotoxins. In fact, pretreatment with selegiline has been shown to prevent the damage caused by dopaminergic, serotonergic, and cholinergic toxins.

In both laboratory studies and field trials, selegiline has been found to improve cognitive function in aging dogs and may be useful in the treatment of disrupted sleep–wake cycles, indifference to the environment, decreased responsiveness to verbal cues, decreased attentiveness and activity, weakness or stiffness, and geriatric-onset house soiling with no concurrent organic disease. Selegiline may also be effective in the treatment of some forms of pituitary-dependent hyperadrenocorticism, which may result from hypothalamic dopamine depletion, although its effects are inconsistent and variable.[197] It may also be effective in suppressing cataplexy in cases of canine narcolepsy. Selegiline is approved in North America for the treatment of canine cognitive dysfunction and pituitary-dependent hyperadrenocorticism. There is also anecdotal evidence of improvement of signs of cognitive dysfunction in cats with selegiline, and one small study found no toxicity in cats up to 10 mg/kg.[198] Additional details on selegiline and its application for geriatric behavior problems are discussed in Chapter 8.

In some European countries, selegiline is approved for the treatment of emotional disorders, as diagnosed in part by the EDED scale. Improvement has been reported in feeding, drinking, and sleeping disorders, physical signs such as tachycardia, diarrhea, and acral lick dermatitis, and to a lesser extent, learned and exploratory behavior. Regarding generalized phobia, selegiline could be effective for the treatment of fearful dogs, particularly those showing a strong behavioral inhibition. Selegiline may also improve incentive learning, decrease the effects of distraction, and improve exploration.[199] To date, there have been no published studies on the efficacy of selegiline in geriatric cats, although there have been reports of its efficacy for cognitive dysfunction and for emotional disorders in cats.[200] Signs of cognitive dysfunction that might be improved include disorientation, increased anxiety, decreased responsiveness to pet parents and other stimuli, decreased nocturnal activity and vocalization, and decreased grooming and appetite. It has also been advocated by European behaviorists for the treatment of emotional disorders in cats, including productive signs (such as aggression, insomnia, and bulimia) and deficit signs (such as anorexia and increased sleep). Improvement has been reported in cats with territorial aggression, fear or fear aggression, reduced appetite, compulsive licking, night waking, house soiling and spraying, excessive vocalization, and overactivity. There was little effect on hyperattachment or predatory aggression, and no side effects were noted.[201]

In healthy laboratory dogs, spontaneous behavior was unaffected by once-daily oral doses below 3 mg/kg while at higher doses, there was stereotypical responding characterized by increased locomotion and decreased exploratory behavior (sniffing). These behavioral effects were thought to be due to increased levels of phenylethylamine resulting from inhibition of MAO B and/or dopaminergic enhancement by L-amphetamine metabolites of selegiline. It is important to note that the amphetamine that is a metabolite of selegiline is L-amphetamine and not D-amphetamine, which is a much more potent inducer of stereotypy. Gastrointestinal upset is occasionally seen but usually improves when the medication is discontinued for a few days, or it may be avoided by using a lower starting dose. Hyperactivity and restlessness have also occasionally been reported. Toxicity has been reported on rare occasions in humans when selegiline is used concurrently with antidepressants, ephedrine, phenylpropanolamine, narcotics, or other MAOIs (including amitraz). Therefore, these combinations should also be avoided in dogs.

Neuroleptics/antipsychotics

Neuroleptics (antipsychotics) are medications that are dopamine antagonists in the brain, causing a nonspecific depression of the CNS with a reduction of motor function and reduced awareness of external stimuli. Neuroleptics include phenothiazines (acepromazine, chlorpromazine, promazine, thioridazine) and atypical antipsychotics (haloperidol). Neuroleptics have been widely used in veterinary medicine as tranquilizers and also to control motion sickness. They are not considered first-line medications for any behavioral disorder but can be appropriate adjunctive treatments.

Phenothiazine tranquilizers, such as *acepromazine, chlorpromazine,* or *promazine*, have been used for rapid tranquilization and also to treat the clinical signs associated with fearful, anxious, and phobic behaviors as an adjunctive treatment with antianxiety medications. Tranquilized pets should be cautiously assessed, as phenothiazines have a variable effect on aggression, and some patients may be more reactive to noises and may easily startle. Antipsychotics may also be useful in controlling productive signs of canine anxiety such as destruction, escape, and agitation, as in thunderstorm phobias and separation-related disorders. However, they are not true antianxiety agents. Their use is limited as adjuncts for behavior modification therapy for patients already on arousal and anxiety-reducing medications for which sedation or calming is desired. The potential side effects of neuroleptics include hypotension (due to alpha-adrenergic blockade), decreased seizure threshold, bradycardia, ataxia, and extrapyramidal signs such as muscle tremors, muscle spasms, muscle discomfort, and motor restlessness. The so-called high-potency neuroleptics, such as perphenazine and haloperidol, are less sedating but have the highest potential for extrapyramidal effects. For these reasons, they are rarely used in veterinary behavioral medicine. Caution should be taken in patients with liver disease because of slow hepatic clearance.

Due to their antiemetic properties, antipsychotics have been also extensively used for motion sickness in the past. However, the NK1 antagonist maropitant citrate (Cerenia) offers a better alternative to acepromazine for this purpose without remarkable sedative effects. The administration of neuroleptics, particularly acepromazine, is still common practice for tranquilizing pets in transit. Nevertheless, it should be emphasized that neuroleptics may impair normal balance, thus increasing the risk of injury as well as causing air obstruction due to abnormal postures. For these reasons, among others, the International Air Transport Association discourages the use of medication, particularly neuroleptics, to control panic attacks during travel.

On the other hand, acepromazine might be particularly beneficial as part of a complete medical plan in the sedation of dogs that are too fearful or aggressive to handle or restrain safely and effectively. Oral combinations with benzodiazepines, gabapentin, or trazodone might be effective prior to veterinary visits, grooming, or other potentially fear-evoking events.

N-methyl-D-aspartic acid antagonists

Altered glutaminergic neurotransmission may be a factor in the pathogenesis of compulsive disorders, in which case blocking glutamate-sensitive NMDA with medications such as memantine, amantadine, or dextromethorphan may be an effective treatment option, often in conjunction with SSRIs.[202–204] Memantine is an NMDA receptor antagonist that is used in human medicine for moderate to severe cases of dementia. In rodent studies, it has been shown to improve cognition and reduce anxiety.[205] In one case series, memantine reduced the severity of compulsive disorders, including light and shadow chasing, spinning and circling, and tail chasing in 64% of 11 treated dogs within two weeks of treatment.[194] Memantine may be effective alone or when combined with fluoxetine, may have a synergistic effect. Dextromethorphan may also be useful because of its NMDA antagonist properties.[195] However, due to its short half-life, rapid clearance, and variable absorption in dogs, it may not be a reliable form of therapy.[206]

Opiate antagonists and agonists

Since *opioids* such as *morphine* have been shown to reduce social need and social solicitation, there may be theoretical indications for their use in socially deprived individuals and those with separation-related disorders. Conversely, *naloxone* increases solicitive behavior, including tail wagging and face licking.[192] Opiate peptides are released during stress and conflict. The activation of narcotic receptors may lead to some stereotypic behaviors. In addition, opioids activate the dopamine system, which may also contribute to compulsive or stereotypic behaviors. Release of opioids may further serve to reinforce these behaviors. Endogenous opioids may also induce analgesia, reducing the pain that might otherwise inhibit self-mutilation. Thus, opiate (endorphin) receptor blockers may be effective in reducing some compulsive stereotypic behaviors, especially those that have been ongoing for a relatively short time. The resultant increase in pain perception may further reduce self-mutilation. Narcotic antagonists have been variably effective in the treatment of a number of compulsive and stereotypic disorders, such as self-mutilation, acral lick dermatitis, tail chasing, and flank sucking in Doberman Pinschers.[193,194] *Naltrexone* can be given orally, but most other opiate antagonists or mixed agonists–antagonists are only available in injectable form. A trial with naltrexone would indicate its effectiveness; however, the medication may not be practical for long-term therapy because of its expense. It has also been found that supplying an exogenous source of opioids, such as *hydrocodone*, may be successful in the treatment of some self-mutilatory behaviors such as acral lick dermatitis.[195]

Psychotropic medications and P450 enzyme inhibition

Most medications are converted into metabolites either in the gut wall or in the liver (phase 1), followed by glucuronidation or sulfation prior to excretion by the kidneys. Most phase 1 metabolism is mediated by these P450 enzymes. These metabolites may or may not be pharmacologically active; in addition, those that are active can have a different pharmacological profile from the parent compound. Therefore, SSRIs that inhibit cytochrome enzymes can cause increased toxicity or an altered therapeutic effect when used with medications that are metabolized by these enzymes. P450 enzymes can also be induced, such as the effects of phenobarbital, St. John's wort, or carbamazepine on CYP3A, leading to a faster clearance of medications metabolized by these enzymes and resulting in reduced clinical effect or a need for higher dosing.

Since there are well-documented genetic polymorphisms in these enzyme systems in humans, responses between populations and individuals can range from extensive metabolizers to poor metabolizers. While evaluation of human data may provide some insight about potential medication interactions in pets, there may be significant species differences between humans and other species. In addition, genetic polymorphisms in pets between breeds as well as individuals in how medications are metabolized undoubtedly exist.

In humans, of the SSRIs, fluvoxamine is the strongest inhibitor of CYP1A2 and CYP3A4; fluvoxamine and fluoxetine are the strongest inhibitors of CYP2C19; and paroxetine and fluoxetine have the greatest inhibition CYP2D6 (with a less potent effect of fluvoxamine, citalopram, and sertraline). Therefore, caution should be exercised when combining fluvoxamine with CYP1A2, CYP2C19, and CYP3A4 substrates tricyclic antidepressants (amitriptyline, clomipramine, imipramine), theophylline, benzodiazepines (diazepam, alprazolam, triazolam, midazolam), buspirone, mirtazapine, propranolol, theophylline, omeprazole, and venlafaxine; and fluoxetine and paroxetine with CYP2D6 substrates tricyclic antidepressants (amitriptyline, clomipramine, doxepin, imipramine), amphetamines, tramadol, venlafaxine, clonidine, and trazodone[79,81,207,208] In dogs, two CYP2C enzymes have been identified: CYP2C21, which is the predominant CYP identified to date in canine liver, and CYP2C41, which is not present in all dogs. The canine ortholog (comparable enzyme) to CYP2D6 is CYP2D15, which metabolizes dextromethorphan, propranolol, imipramine, and celecoxib, while the ortholog of CYP3A4 is CYP3A12, which metabolizes benzodiazepines, erythromycin, testosterone, and progesterone. There has been little published work on CYP450 enzymes in cats[209,210] (see Table 11.3).

Table 11.3 Potential inhibitors, inducers, and substrates of CYP enzymes commonly used in veterinary medicine with an emphasis on psychiatric medications in humans, dogs, and cats

P450	Inhibitor	Inducer	Substrates
CYP1A2	Fluvoxamine* Cimetidine	Carbamazepine Phenobarbital Omeprazole	Amitriptyline Clomipramine Doxepin Imipramine Fluvoxamine Mirtazapine Propranolol Theophylline
CYP2C9	Fluconazole Ketoconazole Fluoxetine* Fluvoxamine Metronidazole	St. John's wort Carbamazepine Phenobarbital	Amitriptyline Doxepin Fluvoxamine Fluoxetine Meloxicam Piroxicam Venlafaxine
CYP2C19	Fluoxetine* Fluvoxamine* Fluconazole Ketoconazole Omeprazole	Carbamazepine St. John's wort	Amitriptyline Citalopram Clomipramine Diazepam Doxepin Imipramine Omeprazole Propranolol Sertraline
CYP2D6	Cimetidine Citalopram (weak) Escitalopram (weak) Clomipramine (weak) Fluoxetine* Paroxetine Sertraline (weak) Diphenhydramine	None	Amitriptyline Amphetamines Clomipramine Clonidine Desipramine Doxepin Fluoxetine Fluvoxamine Imipramine Mirtazapine Nortriptyline Paroxetine Propranolol Tramadol Trazodone Venlafaxine Hydrocodone
CYP3A	Clarithromycin Erythromycin Fluconazole Itraconazole Ketoconazole Fluvoxamine Norfluoxetine Sertraline	Phenobarbital Carbamazepine St. John's wort	Alprazolam Amitriptyline Buspirone Carbamazepine Citalopram Escitalopram Clomipramine Clonazepam Corticosteroids Cyclosporine Diazepam Erythromycin Fentanyl Imipramine Itraconazole Ketoconazole Midazolam Mirtazapine

P450	Inhibitor	Inducer	Substrates
			Opioids Sertraline Tacrolimus Trazodone Venlafaxine Vinblastine Vincristine Zonisamide

Human cytochrome P450 enzyme inhibitors, inducers, and substrates of behavioral drugs.[84,123,201,202]
*Greatest inhibition.

Serotonin syndrome

Serotonin syndrome is a serious and potentially fatal concern which may arise when antidepressants that inhibit serotonin reuptake are used at high doses or in combination with other medications, and dietary supplements that may increase serotonin. TCAs and SSRIs should not be used concurrently with MAOIs such as selegiline or amitraz. In addition, combination with other antidepressants should generally be avoided, although there may be situations in which prudent and cautious use might be considered – see Combination/Augmentation Therapy below. Caution should also be used when combining with St. John's wort (*H. perforatum*), amphetamines, and possibly tramadol, tryptophan (i.e., tryptophan supplements or commercial diets supplemented with tryptophan), metoclopramide, S-adenosylmethionine (SAMe), or dextromethorphan, as well as serotonin receptor agonists such as buspirone and bromocriptine. The serotonin syndrome results mainly in mental, neuromuscular, and autonomic signs including restlessness, mental confusion, agitation, anxiety, hyperesthesia, shivering, shaking, ataxia, hyperthermia, tachycardia, hypertension, hypotension, tachypnea, abdominal pain, diarrhea, vomiting, hypersalivation, muscle twitching, tremors, nystagmus, seizures, coma, and death.[84] With mild clinical signs, treatment merely requires stopping the administration of medications, herbal remedies, or dietary supplements that enhance serotonin. In severe cases, serotonin blockers (such as cyproheptadine at 1.1 mg/kg every 6 hours) can be administered, as well as other medications to control signs like agitation, seizures, and hyperthermia. Diazepam, lorazepam, or phenobarbital may help to control seizures and tremors. Fluid therapy might be required to maintain cardiovascular function, and fans and cold baths could be applied to control excessive body temperature.[57,84] Phenothiazines should be used with caution since they may lower the seizure threshold. With proper veterinary care, cases that survive appear clinically normal within 36 hours. Nevertheless, until the complete remission of symptoms, affected dogs should be closely monitored. Having pet parents take a baseline heart rate and reporting any significant increase may help to identify a problem before more noticeable clinical side effects appear.

Combination/augmentation therapy

Combining medications may be the best way to achieve efficacy for refractory, chronic or complex problems and those patients with comorbidities. Another common reason for combination therapy is that most of the medications approved for veterinary behavioral medicine can take several weeks or longer to achieve therapeutic effect; therefore, for immediate or situational use, quick-acting or bridging medications may also be required. Bridging medications bridge the gap between initiation of treatment and the onset of action of longer-acting medications. They can often but not always be discontinued or reduced when the long-acting medication is taking effect.

When medications are used for augmentation therapy, extreme caution and close monitoring should be exercised since enhancing the effects of a medication could also increase side effects or have adverse effects. When combining medications that might inhibit or induce CYP450 enzyme systems, be cautious of potential increased or decreased levels of the substrates. In addition, if medication combinations might increase serotonin, cautious monitoring is necessary for possible signs of serotonin syndrome. Caution is also needed when combining medications that might have hypotensive or hypertensive effects. Psychotropic medications can also be combined with complementary therapeutics (see Chapter 12). However, knowledge of where these complementary modalities might exert their therapeutic effect should be considered for any potential contraindications; for example, medications that enhance serotonin transmission, such as clomipramine or fluoxetine, should be used cautiously with natural products that might also affect serotonin, such as SAMe, tryptophan, or St. John's wort (see Table 11.4 and Box 11.6).

Prescribing psychotropic medications can be stressful, especially when not exposed while in veterinary school. Pets that suffer with behavioral disorders suffer deeply and medications are a way to help them to have a better quality of life. Slow entry into prescribing and monotherapy will help the practitioner gain confidence with these medications.

Table 11.4 Common medication combinations

Medication 1	Medication 2	Notes
SSRI, SNRI, TCA, azapirone	Benzodiazepines, mirtazapine, alpha-2 agonists, beta blockers, phenothiazines, gabaminergic medications, melatonin	Bridging medication is used until antidepressant takes effect, trazodone [observe for serotonin syndrome, phenothiazines (use with anxiolytic medication)]
Gabapentin	Benzodiazepines	

Box 11.6 Medications for fear, anxiety, and stress

Quick onset	Long onset (prolonged use to effect)
Acepromazine **always use with anxiolytic medication, never as a sole agent**	Amitriptyline
Alprazolam	Clomicalm (clomipramine)
Chlordiazepoxide	Escitalopram
Clonazepam	Fluoxetine
Clonidine	Fluvoxamine
Clorazepate	Paroxetine
Diazepam	Sertraline
Gabapentin	Venlafaxine
Guanfacine	
Imepitoin	
Lorazepam	
Pregabalin	
Propranolol	
Dexmedetomidine oromucosal gel (Sileo)	
Tasipimidine	

References

1. *OCEBM Levels of Evidence Working Group.* "The Oxford Levels of Evidence 2". Oxford Centre for Evidence-Based Medicine. https://www.cebm.ox.ac.uk/resources/levels-of-evidence/ocebm-levels-of-evidence – accessed July 1, 2021.
2. Landsberg GM, Melese P, Sherman-Simpson B, et al. The effectiveness of fluoxetine chewable tablets in the treatment of canine separation anxiety. *J Vet Behav.* 2008;3:11–18.
3. Cracknell NR, Mills DS. A double-blind placebo-controlled study into the efficacy of a homeopathic remedy for fear of firework noises in the dog (Canis familiaris). *Vet J.* 2008;177:80–88.
4. Cracknell NR, Mills DS. An evaluation of pet parent expectation on apparent treatment effect in a blinded comparison of 2 homeopathic remedies for firework noise sensitivity in dogs. *J Vet Behav.* 2011;6:21–30.
5. Mills DS, Redgate SE, Landsberg GM. A meta-analysis of studies of treatments for feline urine spraying. *PLoS One.* 2011;6:e18448.
6. DePorter TL, Landsberg GM, Araujo JA, et al. Harmonease reduces noise-induced fear and anxiety in a laboratory canine model of thunderstorm simulation: a blinded and placebo-controlled study. *J Vet Behav.* 2012;7(4):225–232.
7. Araujo JA, de Rivera C, Ethier JL, et al. Anxitane tablets reduce fear of human beings in a laboratory model of anxiety-related behavior. *J Vet Behav.* 2010;5:268–275.
8. Landsberg G, Mougeot I, Kosziwka W, et al. Development and validation of a dog travel anxiety model. In: *Proc 12th International Veterinary Behaviour Meeting.* Washington, D.C. IVBM, Upton, UK; 2019:21–23.
9. Landsberg G, Dunn D, Korpivaara M. Anxiolytic effect of dexmedetomidine oromucosal gel (Sileo) and gabapentin in a feline travel anxiety model. In: *Proc. 12th International Veterinary Behaviour Meeting.* Washington, D.C. IVBM, Upton, UK; 2019:94–95.
10. Boxenbaum, H. Comparative pharmacokinetics of benzodiazepines in dog and man. *J Pharmacokinet Biopharm.* 1982;10:4.
11. Eichstadt LR, Corriveau LA, Moore GE, et al. Absorption of transdermal fluoxetine compounded in a lipoderm based compared to oral fluoxetine in client-owned cats. *Int J Pharm Compd.* 2017;21:242–246.

12. Ciribassi J, Luescher A, Pasioske KS, et al. Comparative bioavailability of transdermal versus oral fluoxetine in healthy cats. *Am J Vet Res.* 2003;64: 994–998.

13. Mealey Kl, Peck KE, Bennett BS, et al. Systemic absorption of amitriptyline and buspirone after oral and transdermal administration to healthy cats. *J Vet Intern Med.* 2004;18:43–46.

14. Adrian D, Papich MG, Baynes R, et al. The pharmacokinetics of gabapentin in cats. *J Vet Intern Med.* 2018;32:1996–2002.

15. Slovak JE, Costa AP. A pilot study of transdermal gabapentin in cats. *J Vet Intern Med.* 2021:1–7. doi:10.1111/jvim.16137.

16. Chavez G, Pardo P, Ubilla MJ, et al. Effects on behavioural variables of oral versus transdermal administration in cats displaying urine marking. *J Appl Anim Res.* 2016;44:454–457.

17. Hart BL, Cliff KD, Tynes VV, et al. Control of urine marking by use of long-term treatment with fluoxetine or clomipramine in cats. *J Am Vet Med Assoc.* 2005;226:378–382.

18. King JN, Simpson BS, Overall KL, et al. Treatment of separation anxiety in dogs with clomipramine: results from a prospective, randomised, double-blind, placebo-controlled, parallel-group multicenter clinical trial. *Appl Anim Behav Sci.* 2000;67:255–275.

19. Wynchank D, Berk M. Fluoxetine treatment of acral lick dermatitis in dogs: a placebo-controlled randomized double blind trial. *Depress Anxiety.* 1998;8:21–23.

20. Dodman NH, Donnelly R, Shuster L, et al. The use of fluoxetine to treat dominance aggression in dogs. *J Am Vet Med Assoc.* 1996;209:1585–1587.

21. He W, Mei Y, Yuan Z, et al. Effects of cytochrome P450 2C19 genetic polymorphisms on responses to escitalopram and levels of brain-derived neurotrophic factor in patients with panic disorder. *J Clin Psychopharm.* 2019;2: 117–123.

22. Reimer S. Effectiveness of treatments for fireworks fears in dogs. *J Vet Behav.* 2020;37:61–70.

23. Sherman CK, Reisner IR, Taliaferro LA, et al. Characteristics, treatment and outcome of 99 cases of aggression between dogs. *Appl Anim Behav Sci.* 1996;47:91–108.

24. Sussman N. Biological therapies. In: Sadock BJ, Sadock VA, Ruiz P, eds. *Kaplan and Sadock's Comprehensive Textbook of Psychiatry.* 9th ed. Philadelphia: Lippincott Williams & Wilkins; 2009: 965–3334.

25. Francis P. The interplay of neurotransmitters in Alzheimer's disease. *CNS Spectr.* 2005; 10:6–9.

26. Araujo JA, Greig NH, Ingram DK, et al. Cholinesterase inhibitors improve both memory and complex learning in aged beagle dogs. *J Alzheimer's Dis.* 2011;26:143–155.

27. Bellamy KKL, Storengen LM, Handegard KW. DRD2 is associated with fear in some dog breeds. *J Vet Behav.* 2018;27: 67–73.

28. Dockx R, Baeken C, Bundle DD, et al. Accelerated high-frequency repetitive transcranial magnetic stimulation positively influences the behavior, monoaminergic system, and cerebral perfusion in anxious aggressive dogs: a case study. *J Vet Behav.* 2019;33:108–113.

29. Durocher LL, Hinchcliff KW, Williamson KK, et al. Effect of strenuous exercise on urine concentrations of homovanillic acid, cortisol, and vanillylmandelic acid in sled dogs. *Am J Vet Res.* 2007;68: 107–111.

30. Wright HF, Mills DS, Pollux PMJ. Behavioural and physiological correlates of impulsivity in the domestic dog (Canis familiaris). *Physiol Behav.* 2012;105: 676–682.

31. Albright JD. Measurement of neurotransmitters excreted in the urine of behaviorally healthy dogs in home and boarding kennel conditions. In: *Proceedings Veterinary Behavior Symposium.* Indianapolis: ACVB; 2017:20.

32. Hoglund K, Hanas S, Carnabuci C, et al. Blood pressure, heart rate and urinary catecholamines in healthy dogs subjected to different clinical settings. *J Vet Intern Med.* 2012;26:1300–1308.

33. Dockx R, Baeken C, Vermier S, et al. Brain SPECT in the behaviourally disordered dog. In: Dierckx RA, Otte A, de Vries EFJ, et al. *PET and SPECT in Psychiatry.* Cham: Springer; 2021:817–839. doi:10.1007/978-3-030-57231-0_25.

34. Badino P, Odore R, Osella MC, et al. Modifications of serotonergic and adrenergic receptor concentrations in the brain of aggressive Canis familiaris. *Comp Biochem Physiol A Mol Integr Physiol.* 2004;39:343–350.

35. Saudou F, Amara DA, Dierich A, et al. Enhanced aggressive behavior in mice lacking 5-HT1B receptor. *Science.* 1994;265: 1875–1878.

36. Matsumoto M, Yoshioka M. Possible involvement of serotonin receptors in anxiety disorders. *Nippon Yakurigaku Zasshi.* 2000;115.39 44.

37. Rosado B, Garcia-Belenguer S, León M. Blood concentrations of serotonin, cortisol and dehydroepiandrosterone in aggressive dogs. *Appl Anim Behav Sci.* 2010;123:124–130.

38. Çakiroglu D, Meral Y, Sancak AA, et al. The relationship between the serum concentrations of serotonin and lipids and aggression in dogs. *Vet Rec.* 2007; 161:59–61.

39. Leon M, Rosado B, Garcia-Belenguer S, et al. Assessment of serotonin in serum, plasma, and platelets of aggressive dogs. *J Vet Behav.* 2012;7:348–352.

40. Alberghina D, Rizzo M, Piccione G, et al. An exploratory study about the association between serum serotonin concentrations and canine-human social interactions in shelter dogs (Canis familiaris). *J Vet Behav.* 2017;18:96–101.

41. Riggio G, Mariti C, Sergi V, et al. Serotonin and tryptophan serum concentrations in shelter dogs showing different behavioural responses to a potentially stressful procedure. *Vet Sci.* 2021;8. doi: 10.3390/vetsci8010001.

42. Rayment DJ, Peters RA, Marston LC, et al. Relationships between serum serotonin, plasma cortisol, and behavioral factors in a mixed-breed, -sex, and -age group of pet dogs. *J Vet Behav.* 2020;38:96–102.

43. Amat M, Mariotti VM, Le Brech S, et al. Differences in serotonin levels between aggressive English cocker spaniels and aggressive dogs of other breeds. *J Vet Behav.* 2010;5:46.

44. Höglund K, Häggström J, Hanås S, et al. Interbreed variation in serum serotonin (5-hydroxytryptamine) concentration in healthy dogs. *J Vet Cardiol.* 2018;20: 244–253.

45. Karpinski M, Ognik K, Garbiec A, et al. Effect of stroking on serotonin, noradrenaline, and cortisol levels in the blood of right- and left-pawed dogs. *Animals.* 2021;11. doi: 10.3390/ani11020331.

46. Alberghina D, Tropia E, Piccione G, et al. Serum serotonin (5-HT) in dogs (Canis familiaris): preanalytical factors and analytical procedure for use of reference values in behavioral medicine. *J Vet Behav.* 2019;32:72–75.

47. Puurunen J, Tiira K, Vapalahti K, et al. Fearful dogs have increased plasma glutamine and γ-glutamyl glutamine. *Sci Rep.* 2018;8:15976. doi:10.1038/s41598-018-34321-x.

48. Stein DJ, van Honk J, Ipser J, et al. Opioids: from physical pain to the pain of social isolation. *CNS Spectr.* 2007;12:669–674.

49. Kubinyi E, Bence M, Koller D, et al Oxytocin and opioid receptor gene polymorphisms associated with greeting behavior in dogs. *Front Psychol.* 2017;8: 1520. doi: 10.3389/fpsyg.2017.01520.

50. Panksepp J, Herman BH, Vilberg T, et al. Endogenous opioids and social behavior. *Neurosci Biobehav Rev.* 1980;4:473–487.

51. Knowles PA, Conner RL, Panksepp J. Opiate effects on social behavior of juvenile dogs as a function of social deprivation. *Pharmacol Biochem Behav.* 1989;33: 533–537.

52. Gregg TR, Siegel A. Differential effects of NK1 receptors in the midbrain periaqueductal gray upon defensive rage and predatory attack in the cat. *Brain Res.* 2003;994:5–66.

53. Baluk P. Neurogenic inflammation in skin and airways. *J Invest Dermatol Symp Proc.* 1997;2:76–81.

54. Duffy RA. Potential therapeutic targets for neurokinin-1 receptor antagonists. *Expert Opin Emerg Drugs.* 2004;9:9–21.

55. O'Connor TM, O'Connell J, O'Brien DI, et al. The role of substance P in inflammatory disease. *J Cell Physiol.* 2004;201:167–180.

56. Maina E, Fontaine J. Use of maropitant for the control of pruritus in non-flea, non-food-induced feline hypersensitivity dermatitis: an open-label, uncontrolled pilot study. *J Feline Med Surg.* 2019;21: 968–972.

57. Plumb DC. Plumbs Veterinary Drugs – app.plumbs.com – accessed July 06, 2021.

58. Ramsey D, Fleck T, Berg T, et al. Cerenia prevents perioperative nausea and vomiting and improves recovery in dogs undergoing routine surgery. *Int J Appl Res Vet Med.* 2014;12:228–237.

59. Hickman MA, Cox SR, Mahabir S, et al. Safety, pharmacokinetics and use of novel NK-1 receptor antagonist maropitant (Cerenia) for the prevention of emesis and motion sickness in cats. *J Vet Pharmacol Ther.* 2008;31:220–229.

60. Kramer KM, Cushing BS, Carter CS, et al. Sex and species differences in plasma oxytocin using an enzyme immunoassay. *Can J Zool.* 2004;82:1194–1200.

61. Odendaal J, Meintjes R. Neurophysiological correlates of affiliative behaviour between humans and dogs. *Vet J.* 2003;165:296–301.

62. Oliva J, Rault J-L, Appleton B, et al. Oxytocin enhances the appropriate use of human social cues by the domestic dog (Canis familiaris) in an object choice task. *Anim Cogn.* 2005;18:767–775.

63. Pirrone F, Pierantoni L, Bossetti A. Salivary vasopressin as a potential non-invasive biomarker of anxiety in dogs diagnosed with separation-related problems. *Animals.* 2019;9:1033. doi:10.3390/ani9121033.

64. MacLean EL, Gesquiere LR, Gruen ME, et al. Endogenous oxytocin, vasopressin and aggression in domestic dogs. *Front Psychol.* 2017;27. doi:10.3389/fpsyg.2017.01613.

65. Ogata N, Dodman NH. The use of clonidine in the treatment of fear-based behavior problems in dogs: an open trial. *J Vet Behav.* 2011;6:130–137.

66. Korpivaara M, Laapas K, Huhtinen M, et al. Dexmedetomidine oromucosal gel for noise-associated acute anxiety and fear in dogs—a randomised, double-blind, placebo-controlled clinical study. *Vet Rec.* 2017;180:356. doi:10.1136/vr.104045.

67. Hauser H, Campbell S, Korpivaara M, et al. In-hospital administration of dexmedetomidine oromucosal gel for stress reduction in dogs during veterinary visits: a randomized, double-blinded, placebo-controlled study. *J Vet Behav.* 2020;39:77–85.

68. Amat M, Le Brech S, Garcia-Marato C, et al. Preventing travel anxiety using dexmedetomidine hydrochloride oromucosal gel. In: Denenberg S, ed. *Proc 11th International Veterinary Behaviour Meeting.* Oxfordshire, UK: CABI; 2017:20–21.

69. Korpivaara M, Huhtinen M, Aspergren J, et al. Dexemedetomidine oromucosal gel for alleviation of fear and anxiety in dogs during minor veterinary or husbandry procedures. In: Denenberg S, ed. *Proc 11th International Veterinary Behaviour Meeting.* Oxfordshire, UK: CABI; 2017:22–23.

70. Orion Corporation (2015). Sileo® (dexmedetomidine oromucosal gel). www.sileodogus.com. Accessed on August 25, 2020.

71. Carson MA, Pankratz KE, Messenger KM, et al. Efficacy of dexmedetomidine oromucosal gel to attenuate anxiety in client owned cats presented for routine veterinary care. In: *Proc Vet Behav Symposium.* 2020:5.

72. Cohen A, Bennett SL. Oral transmucosal administration of dexmedetomidine for sedation in 4 dogs. *Can Vet J.* 2015;56: 1144–1148.

73. Porters N, Bosmans T, Debille M, et al. Sedative and antinociceptive effects of dexmedetomidine and buprenorphine after oral transmucosal or intramuscular administration in cats. *Vet Anaesth Analg.* 2014;41:90–96.

74. Dent BT, Aarnes TK, Wavreille VA, et al. Pharmacokinetics and pharmacodynamic effects of oral transmucosal and intravenous administration of dexmedetomidine in dogs. *Am J Vet Res.* 2019;80:969–975.

75. Korpivaara M, Huhtinen M, Pohjanjousi M, et al. Tasipimidine, a novel orally dosed alpha-2 adrenoreceptor agonist, alleviates canine acute anxiety and fear associated with travel-a pilot study. In: *Proceedings of the ACVB Veterinary Behavior Symposium.* 2021:12.

76. Korpivaara M, Huhtinen M, Pohjanjousi M, et al. Tasipimidine, a novel orally dosed alpha-2 adrenoreceptor agonist, alleviates separation anxiety in dogs-a 5 week study. In: *Proceedings of the ACVB Veterinary Behavior Symposium.* 2021:14.

77. Korpivaara M, Huhtinen M, Pohjanjousi P, et al. Tasipimidine, a noveral orally active alpha-2 adrenoceptor agonist, alleviates signs of anxiety shown during veterinary examination- a pilot study. *Proc European Veterinary Congress of Behavioural Medicine and Animal Welfare.* 2021:96–97.

78. Notari L. Combined use of selegiline and behaviour modifications in the treatment of cases in which fear and phobias are involved: a review of 4 cases. In: Mills D, Levine E, eds. *Current Issues and Research in Veterinary Behavioral Medicine.* West Lafayette, Indiana: Purdue University Press; 2006:267–269.

79. Plegne P, Mellerup ET. Pindolol and the acceleration of the antidepressant response. *J Affect Disord.* 2003;75:285–289.

80. Pérez V, Gilaberte I, Faries D, et al. Randomised, double-blind, placebo-controlled trial of pindolol in combination with fluoxetine antidepressant treatment. *Lancet.* 1997;349:1594–1597.

81. Elliott B, Joyce E, Shorvon S. Delusions, illusions and hallucinations in epilepsy: part 1, 2. *Epilepsy Res.* 2009;85:162–186.

82. Dodman NH, Knowles KE, Shuster L, et al. Behavioral changes associated with suspected complex partial seizures in Bull Terriers. *J Am Vet Med Assoc.* 1996;208: 688–691.

83. Walker R, Fisher J, Neville P. The treatment of phobias in the dog. *Appl Anim Behav Sci.* 1997;52:275–289.

84. Lane SB, Bunch SE. Medical management of recurrent seizures in dogs and cats. *J Vet Int Med.* 1990;4:26–39.

85. Crowell-Davis SL, Murray TF, de Souza Dantas LM. *Veterinary Psychopharmacology.* 2nd ed. Hoboken, NJ: John Wiley and Sons; 2019.

86. Carter GR. Carbamazepine for the treatment of canine aggression; seven case studies. *New Orleans: ACVB/AVSAB Proceedings.* 2008:50.

87. Schwartz S. Carbamazepine in the control of aggressive behavior in cats. *J Am Anim Hosp Assoc.* 1994;30:515–519.

88. Farooq MU, Bhatt A, Majid A, et al. Levetiracetam for managing neurologic and psychiatric disorders. *Am J Health Syst Pharm.* 2009;66:541–561.

89. Moore SA, Munana KR, Papich MG. Levetiracetam pharmacokinetics in healthy dogs following oral administration of single and multiple doses. *Am J Vet Res.* 2010;71:337–341.

90. Sherman-Simpson B, Landsberg GM, Reisner IR, et al. Effects of Reconcile (fluoxetine) chewable tablets plus behavior management for canine separation anxiety. *Vet Ther.* 2007;8: 18–31.

91. Santarelli L, Saxe M, Gross C, et al. Hippocampal neurogenesis contributes to the behavioral effects of antidepressants. *Science.* 2003;301: 805–809.

92. Takeuchi Y, Houpt KA, Scarlett JM. Evaluation of treatments for separation anxiety in dogs. *J Am Vet Med Assoc.* 2000;216:342–345.

93. Virga V, Houpt KA, Scarlett JM. Efficacy of amitriptyline as a pharmacologic adjunct to behavioral modification in the management of aggressive behaviors in dogs. *J Am Anim Hosp Assoc.* 2001;37: 325–350.

94. Overall KL, Dunham AE. Clinical features and outcome in dogs and cats with obsessive compulsive disorder; 126 cases (1989–2000). *J Am Vet Med Assoc.* 2002;1445–1452.

95. King JN, Maurer MP, Altman B, et al. Pharmacokinetics of clomipramine in dogs following single-dose and repeated-dose oral administration. *Am J Vet Res.* 2000;61:80–85.

96. Reich MR, Ohad DG, Overall KL, et al. Electrocardiographic assessment of antianxiety medication in dogs and correlation with serum medication concentrations. *J Am Vet Med Assoc.* 2000;216:1571–1575.

97. Martin KM. Effect of clomipramine on the electrocardiogram and serum thyroid concentrations of healthy cats. *J Vet Behav.* 2010;5:123–129.

98. Petit S, Pageat P, Chaurand JP, et al. Efficacy of clomipramine in the treatment of separation anxiety in dogs: clinical trial. *Rev Med Vet*. 1999;150:133–140.

99. Volonte L, Michelazzi M, Cavallone E. Effects of a behavioral and pharmacological therapy on dogs with an anxiety-related disorders: a pilot clinical study. In: *Proceedings of the 6th International Veterinary Behaviour Meeting and European college of veterinary behavioural medicine-companion animals European society of veterinary clinical ethology*. 2007:121–123.

100. King JN, Overall KL, Appleby BS, et al. Results of a follow-up investigation to a clinical trial testing the efficacy of clomipramine in the treatment of separation anxiety. *Appl Anim Behav Sci*. 2004;89:233–242.

101. Hewson CJ, Luescher UA, Parent JM, et al. Efficacy of clomipramine in the treatment of canine compulsive disorder. *J Am Vet Med Assoc*. 1998;213:1760–1765.

102. Rapaport JL, Ryland DH, Kriete M. Medication treatment of canine acral lick, an animal model of obsessive-compulsive disorder. *Arch Gen Psychiatry*. 1992;49:517–521.

103. Seksel K, Lindeman MJ. Use of clomipramine in the treatment of anxiety-related and obsessive-compulsive disorders in cats. *Aust Vet J*. 1998;76:317–321.

104. Goldberger E, Rapaport JL. Canine acral lick dermatitis: response to the antiobsessional medication clomipramine. *J Am Anim Hosp Assoc*. 1991;27:179–182.

105. Hartung M, Michniewicz A. Feline hyperesthesia syndrome and its affect on cats. In: *The Book of Articles National Scientific Conference "Second Summer Scientific On-line School"*. August 07, 2021.

106. Landsberg G, Wilson AL. Effects of clomipramine on cats presented for urine marking. *J Am Anim Hosp Assoc*. 2005;41:3–11.

107. King JN, Steffan J, Heath SE, et al. Determination of the dosage of clomipramine for the treatment of urine spraying in cats. *J Am Vet Med Assoc*. 2004;225:881–887.

108. Pfeiffer E, Guy N, Cribb A. Clomipramine-induced urinary retention in a cat. *Can Vet J*. 1999;40:265–267.

109. Podberscek AL, Hsu Y, Serpell JA. Evaluation of clomipramine as an adjunct to behavioural therapy in the treatment of separation-related problems in dogs. *Vet Rec*. 1999;145:365–369.

110. White MM, Neilson JC, Hart BL, et al. Effects of clomipramine hydrochloride on dominance-related aggression in dogs. *J Am Vet Med Assoc*. 1999;215:1288–1291.

111. Crowell-Davis SL, Seibert LM, Sung W, et al. Use of clomipramine, alprazolam and behavior modification for the treatment of storm phobias in dogs. *J Am Vet Med Assoc*. 2003;222:744–748.

112. Gilron I, Bailey JM, Tu D, et al. Nortriptyline and gabapentin, alone and in combination for neuropathic pain: a double-blind, randomized controlled crossover trial. *Lancet*. 2009;10:1252–1261.

113. Steinberg MI, Smallwood JK, Holland DR, et al. Hemodynamic and electrocardiographic effects of fluoxetine and its major metabolite norfluoxetine in anesthetized dogs. *Toxicol Appl Pharmacol*. 1986;82:70–79.

114. Robinson RT, Drafts BC, Fisher JL. Fluoxetine increases GABA-A receptor activity through a novel modulatory site. *J Pharmacol Exp Ther*. 2003;304:978–984.

115. Movig KLL, Leufkens HGM, Belitser SV, et al. Selective serotonin reuptake inhibitor-induced urinary incontinence. *Pharmacoepidemiol Drug Saf*. 2002;11:271–279.

116. Cascade E, Kalali A, Kennedy S. Real-world data on SSRI antidepressant side effects. *Psychiatry*. 2009;2:16–18.

117. Reconcile prescribing information. https://www.reconcile.com/ accessed: July 5, 2021.

118. Chutter M, Perry P, Houpt K. Efficacy of fluoxetine for canine behavioral disorders. *J Vet Behav*. 2019;33:54–58.

119. Reisner I. Diagnosis of canine generalized anxiety disorder and its management with behavioral modification and fluoxetine or paroxetine; a retrospective summary of clinical experience (2001–2003). *J Am Anim Hosp Assoc*. 2003;39:512.

120. Dodman NH. Pharmacologic treatment of aggression in veterinary patients. In: Dodman NH, Shuster L, eds. *Psychopharmacology of Animal Behavior Disorders*. Malden, MA: Blackwell Science; 1998:41–63.

121. Irimijami M, Luescher AU, Douglass G, et al. Randomized, controlled clinical trial of the efficacy of fluoxetine for treatment of compulsive disorders in dogs. *J Am Vet Med Assoc*. 2009;235.705–709.

122. Stein DJ, Mendelsohn I, Potocnik F, et al. Use of the selective serotonin reuptake inhibitor citalopram in a possible animal analogue of obsessive-compulsive disorder. *Depress Anxiety*. 1998;8:39–42.

123. Pryor PA, Hart BL, Cliff KD, et al. Effects of a selective serotonin reuptake inhibitor on urine spraying behavior in cats. *J Am Anim Hosp Assoc*. 2001;219:1557–1561.

124. Bazin I, Desmarchelier M. Retrospective study on the use of fluvoxamine in 72 dogs with anxiety disorders. *J Vet Behav*. 2022;50:60–69.

125. Overall K. Behavioral pharmacotherapeutics. In: Mealey KL, ed. *Pharmacotherapeutics for Veterinary Dispensing*. Hoboken, NJ: Wiley Blackwell; 2019:377–402.

126. Culpepper, L. Escitalopram: a new SSRI for treatment of depression in primary care. Primary care companion. *J Clin Psychiatry*. 2002;4:6.

127. Taylor O, Laeken NV, Polis I, et al. Estimation of the optimal dosing regimen of escitalopram in dogs: a dose occupancy study with DASB. *PLoS One*. 2017;12(6):e0179927. doi:10.1371/journal.pone.0179927.

128. Gruen ME, Sherman BL. Use of trazodone as an adjunctive agent in the treatment of canine anxiety disorders: 56 cases (1995–2007). *J Am Vet Med Assoc*. 2008;233:1902–1907.

129. Celikyurt IK, Mutlu O, Ulak G. Serotonin Noradrenaline Reuptake Inhibitors (SNRIs). www.intechopen.com.

130. Pflaum K, Bennett S. Investigation of the use of venlafaxine for treatment of refractory misdirected play and impulse-control aggression in a cat: a case report. *J Vet Behav*. 2021;42:22–25.

131. Bjorvatn B, Fornal C, Martin F, et al. Venlafaxine and its interaction with WAY 100635: effects on serotonergic unit activity and behavior in cats. *Eur J Pharmacol*. 2000;404:121–132.

132. Hopfensperger MJ. Use of oral venlafaxine in cats with feline idiopathic cystitis or behavioral causes of periuria. In: *Proceedings of the ACVB Veterinary Behavior Symposium*. 2016;19–23.

133. Thor KB, Katofiasc MA. Effects of duloxetine, a combined serotonin and norepinephrine reuptake inhibitor, on central neural control of lower urinary tract function in the chloralose-anesthetized female cat. *J Pharmacol Exp Ther*. 1995;274(2):1014–1024.

134. Norton P, Zinner NR, Yalcin I, Bump RC. Duloxetine versus placebo in the treatment of stress urinary incontinence. *Neurourol Urodyn*. 2001;20(4):532–534.

135. Gruen ME, Roe SC, Griffith E, et al. Use of trazodone to facilitate postsurgical confinement in dogs. *J Am Vet Med Assoc*. 2014;245:296–301.

136. Gilbert-Gregory SE, Stull JW, Rice MR, et al. Effects of trazodone on behavioral signs of stress in hospitalized dogs. *J Am Vet Med Assoc*. 2016;249(11):1281–1291.

137. Murphy LA, Barletta M, Graham L. Effects of acepromazine and trazodone on anesthetic induction dose of propofol and cardiovascular variables in dogs undergoing general anesthesia for orthopedic surgery. *J Am Vet Med Assoc*. 2017;250:408–416.

138. Jay AR, Krotscheck U, Parsley E, et al. Pharmacokinetics, bioavailability, and hemodynamic effects of trazodone after intravenous and oral administration of a single dose to dogs. *Am J Vet Res*. 2013;74:1450–1456.

139. Orlando JM, Case BC, Thomson AE, et al. Use of oral trazodone for sedation in cats: a pilot study. *J Feline Med Surg*. 2016:1–7.

140. Stevens BJ, Frantz EM, Orlando JM, et al. Efficacy of a single dose of trazodone hydrochloride given to cats prior to veterinary visits to reduce signs of transport- and examination-related anxiety. *J Am Vet Med Assoc*. 2016;249: 202–207.

141. Kim S, Borchardt MR, Lee K, et al. Effects of trazodone on behavioral and physiological signs of stress in dogs during veterinary visits: a randomized double-blind placebo-controlled crossover clinical trial. *J Am Vet Med Assoc*. 2022;260(8):876–883.

142. Benjamin S, Doraiswamy PM. Review of the use of mirtazapine in the treatment of depression. *Expert Opin Pharmacother*. 2011;12:1623–1632.

143. Quimby JM, Gustafson DL, Samber BJ, et al. Studies on the pharmacokinetics of mirtazapine in healthy young cats. *J Vet Pharmacol Ther*. 2011;34:388–396.

144. Quimby JM, Gustafson DL, Lunn KF, et al. Pharmacokinetics of mirtazapine in cats with chronic kidney disease and in age matched controls. *J Vet Intern Med*. 2010;24:768.

145. Quimby JF, Lunn KF. Mirtazapine as an appetite stimulant and antiemetic in cats with chronic kidney disease: a masked placebo controlled crossover clinical trial. *Vet J*. 2013;197:651–655.

146. Ferguson LE, McLean MK, Bates JA, et al. Mirtazapine toxicity in cats: retrospective study of 84 cases (2006–2011). *J Feline Med Surg*. 2016;18:868–874.

147. Poole M, Quimby JM, Hu T, et al. A double-blind, placebo-controlled, randomized study to evaluate the weight gain drug, mirtazapine transdermal ointment, in cats with unintended weight loss. *J Vet Pharmacol Ther*. 2019;42(March 2):179–188.

148. Argüelles J, Enriquez J, Bowen J, et al. Mirtazapine as a potential drug to treat social fears in dogs: five case examples. In: *Proceedings of the 11th International Veterinary Behaviour Meeting*; 2017 September 14–16. Samorin, Slovakia: 2017:84–86.

149. Hoffmeister EH, Egger CM. Evaluation of diphenhydramine as a sedative for dogs. *J Am Vet Med Assoc*. 2005;226: 1092–1094.

150. Schwartz S. Use of cyproheptadine to control urine spraying in a castrated male domestic cat. *J Am Vet Med Assoc*. 1999;215:501–502. 482.

151. Hart BL, Eckstein RA, Powell KL, et al. Effectiveness of buspirone on urine spraying and inappropriate urination in cats. *J Am Vet Med Assoc*. 1993;203: 254–258.

152. Greenblatt DK, Shader RI, Divoll M, et al. Benzodiazepines: a summary of pharmacokinetic properties. *Br J Clin Pharmacol*. 1981;11:11S-16S.

153. Lucot JB, Crampton GH. Buspirone blocks motion sickness and xylazine induced emesis in the cat. *Aviat Space Environ Med*. 1987;58: 989–991.

154. Cryan JF, Dev KK. Animal models of anxiety. In: Blanchard RJ, Blanchard DC, Griebel G, et al., eds. *Handbook of Anxiety and Fear*. Amsterdam: Academic Press; 2008:276–278.

155. Miczek KA, Fish EW. Monoamines, GABA, glutamate and aggression. In: Nelson RJ, ed. *Biology of Aggression*. Oxford: Oxford University Press; 2006:114–149.

156. Herron M, Shofer FS, Reisner IR. Retrospective evaluation of the effects of diazepam in dogs with anxiety-related behaviour problems. *J Am Vet Med Assoc*. 2008;233:1420–1424.

157. Brown SA, Forrester SD. Serum disposition of oral clorazepate from regular-release and sustained-delivery tablets in dogs. *J Vet Pharmacol Ther*. 1991;14:426–429.

158. Frey HH, Löscher W. Pharmacokinetics of anti-epileptic drugs in dogs: a review. *J Vet Pharm Ther*. 1985;8:219–233.

159. Pineda S, Anzola B, Olivares A, et al. Fluoxetine combined with clorazepate dipotassium and behaviour modification for treatment of anxiety-related disorders in dogs. *Vet J*. 2014;199:387–391.

160. Brown SA, Forrester SD. Serum disposition of oral clorazepate from regular-release and sustained-delivery tablets in dogs. *J Vet Pharmacol Ther*. 1991;14(December 4):426–429.

161. Sanders S. *Seizures in Dogs and Cats*. Ames, Iowa: John Wiley and Sons; 2015:329.

162. Wala EP, Sloan JW, Martin WR, et al. The effects of flumazenil-precipitated abstinence on the pharmacokinetics of chronic oxazepam in dogs. *Pharmacol Biochem Behav*. 1990;35:347–350.

163. Center SA, Elston TH, Rowland PH, et al. Fulminant hepatic failure associated with oral administration of diazepam in 11 cats. *J Am Vet Med Assoc*. 1996;209:618–625.

164. Riemer S. Effectiveness of treatments for firework fears in dogs. *J Vet Behav*. 2020;37:61–70.

165. Hart BL. Behavioral and pharmacologic approaches to problem urination in cats. *Vet Clin North Am Small Anim*. 1996;26: 651–656.

166. Ibáñez M, Anzola B. Use of fluoxetine, diazepam, and behavior modification as therapy for treatment of anxiety-related disorders in dogs. *J Vet Behav*. 2009;4: 223–229.

167. Hollenhorst J, Munte S, Friedrich L, et al. Using intranasal midazolam spray to prevent claustrophobia induced by MR imaging. *AJR*. 2001;176:865–888.

168. Mariani CL. A comparison of intranasal and intravenous lorazepam in normal dogs. In: *Proceedings of the 21st ACVIM Forum*. Charlotte, NC; 2003.

169. Musulin SE, Mariani CL, Papich MG. Diazepam pharmacokinetics after nasal drop and atomized nasal administration in dogs. *J Vet Pharm Ther*. 2011;34: 17–24.

170. Hendricks JC, Lager A, O'Brien D, et al. Movement disorders during sleep in cats and dogs. *J Am Vet Med Assoc*. 1989;194: 686–689.

171. Engel O, Muller HW, Klee R, et al. Effectiveness of imepitoin for the control of anxiety and fear associated with noise phobia in dogs. *J Vet Intern Med*. 2019;33: 2675–2684.

172. Perdew I, Emke C, Johnson B, et al. Evaluation of Pexion® (imepitoin) for treatment of storm anxiety in dogs: a randomised, double-blind, placebo-controlled trial. *Vet Rec*. 2021:e18. doi:10.1002/vetr.18.

173. Engel O, Masic A, Landsberg G, et al. Imepitoin shows benzodiazepine-like effects in models of anxiety. *Front Pharmacol*. 2018;9:1225. doi: 10.3389/fphar.2018.01225.

174. McPeake K, Mills D. The use of imepitoin (Pexion) on fear and anxiety related problems in dogs—a case series. *BMC Vet Res*. 2017;13:173.

175. Forster B, Engel O, Erhard M, et al. Short-term imepitoin treatment reduces stress level in dogs with generalized anxiety disorder. *J Vet Behav*. 2020;38: 67–73.

176. Packer RMA, De Risio L, Volk HA. Investigating the potential of the anti-epileptic durg imepitoin as a treatment for co-morbid anxiety in dogs with idiopathic epilepsy. *BMC Vet Res*. 2017;13:90. doi:10.1186/s12917-017-1000-0.

177. Denenberg S, Dube MB. Tools for managing feline problem behaviors: psychoactive medications. *J Feline Med Surg*. 2018;20:1034–1045.

178. Luescher UA. Hyperkinesis in dogs: six case reports. *Can Vet J*. 1993;34: 368–370.

179. Burghardt W. Repetitive and self traumatic behaviors. In: *San Antonio: Presentation to the American Veterinary Society of Animal Behavior specialty meeting AAHA*. 1996.

180. Bleuer-Elsner S, Muller G, Beata C, et al. Effect of fluoxetine at a dosage of 2–4 mg/kg daily in dogs exhibiting hypersensitivity-hyperactivity syndrome, a retrospective study. *J Vet Behav*. 2021;44:25–31.

181. Siao KT, Pypendop BH, Ilkiw JE. Pharmacokinetics of gabapentin in cats. *Am J Vet Res*. 2010;71:817–821.

182. Hudec CP, Griffin CE. Changes in the stress markers cortisol and glucose before and during intradermal testing in cats after single dose administration of pre-appointment gabapentin. *J Feline Med Surg*. 2020;22:138–145.

183. van Haaften KA, Forsythe LRE, Stelow EA, et al. Effects of a single preappointment dose of gabapentin on signs of stress in cats during transportation and veterinary examination. *J Am Vet Med Assoc*. 2017;251:1175–1181.

184. Pankratz KE, Ferris KK, Griffith EH, et al. Use of single-dose oral gabapentin to attenuate fear responses in cage-trap confined community cats: a double-

blind, placebo-controlled field trial. *J Feline Med Surg*. 2018;20:535–543.

185. Fantinati M, Trnka J, Signor A, et al. Appetite-stimulating effect of gabapentin vs mirtazapine in healthy cats post-ovariectomy. *J Feline Med Surg*. 2020;22: 1176–1183.

186. Grubb T. https://todaysveterinarypractice. com/gabapentin-and-amantadine-for-chronic-pain/. Accessed December 18, 2021.

187. Slovak JE, Costa AP. A pilot study of transdermal gabapentin in cats. *J Vet Intern Med*. 2021;35(4):1981–1987.

188. Allen ME, LeBlanc NL, Scollan KF. Hemodynamic, echocardiographic, and sedative effects of oral gabapentin and healthy cats. *J Am Anim Hosp Assoc*. 2021;57:278–284. doi:10.5326/ JAAHA-MS-7081.

189. Stollar O, Moore GE, Mukhopadhyay A, et al. Effects of a single dose of oral gabapentin in dogs during a veterinary visit: a double-blinded, placebo-controlled study. *J Am Vet Med Assoc*. 2022;260(9):1031–1040.

190. Sirinarumitr K, Johnston SD, Kustritz MVR, et al. Effects of finasteride on size of the prostate gland and semen quality in dogs with benign prostatic hypertrophy. *J Am Vet Med Assoc*. 2001;218:1275–1280.

191. Goericke-Pesch S, Georgiev P, Antonov A, et al. Clinical efficacy of a GnRH-agonist implant containing 4.7 mg deslorelin, Suprelorin, regarding suppression of reproductive function in tomcats. *Theriogenology*. 2011;75: 803–810.

192. Knowles PA, Conner RL, Panksepp J. Opiate effects on social behavior of juvenile dogs as a function of social deprivation. *Pharmacol Biochem Behav*. 1989;33:533–537.

193. White SD. Naltrexone for treatment of acral lick dermatitis in dogs. *J Am Vet Med Assoc*. 1990;196:1073–1076.

194. Brown SA, Crowell-Davis S, Malcolm T, et al. Naloxone-responsive compulsive tail chasing in a dog. *J Am Vet Med Assoc*. 1987;190:884–886.

195. Brignac MM. Hydrocodone treatment of acral lick dermatitis. In: *Montreal: Proceedings of the 2nd World Congress of Veterinary Dermatology*. 1992.

196. Milgram NW, Ivy GO, Head E, et al. The effect of l-deprenyl on behavior, cognitive function, and biogenic amines in the dog. *Neurochem Res*. 1993;18: 1211–1219.

197. Bruyette D, Ruehl WW, Smidberg TL. Canine pituitary-dependent hyperadrenocorticism: a spontaneous animal model for neurodegenerative disorders and their treatment with l-deprenyl. *Prog Brain Res*. 1995;106: 207–215.

198. Ruehl WW, Griffin D, Bouchard G, et al. Effects of l-deprenyl in cats in a one month dose escalation study. *Vet Pathol*. 1996;33:621.

199. Mills D, Ledger R. The effects of oral selegiline hydrochloride on learning and training in the dog: a psychobiological interpretation. *Prog Neuro-Psychopharmacol Biol Psychiatry*. 2001;25:1597–1613.

200. Landsberg GM. Therapeutic options for cognitive decline in senior pets. *J Am Anim Hosp Assoc*. 2006;42:407–413.

201. Dehasse J. Retrospective study on the use of Selgian in cats. In: *New Orleans: Presentation to the American Veterinary Society of Animal Behavior*. 1999.

202. Schneider B, Dodman NH, Maranda L. Use of memantine in treatment of canine compulsive disorders. *J Vet Behav*. 2009;4:118–126.

203. Wald R, Dodman N, Shuster L. The combined effects of memantine and fluoxetine on an animal model of obsessive-compulsive disorder. *Exp Clin Psychopharmacol*. 2009;17:191–197.

204. Dodman NH, Shuster L, Nesbitt G, et al. The use of dextromethorphan to treat repetitive self-directed scratching, biting or chewing in dogs with allergic dermatitis. *J Vet Pharmacol Ther*. 2004;27:99–104.

205. Minkeviciene R, Banerjee P, Tunila H. Cognition-enhancing and anxiolytic effects of memantine. *Neuropharmacology*. 2008;54:1079–1085.

206. Kukanich B, Papich MG. Plasma profile and pharmokinetics of dextromethorphan after intravenous and oral administration in dogs. *J Vet Pharmacol Ther*. 2004;27:337–341.

207. Indiana University Division of Pharmacology. Flockhart Table. Available online at: https://drug-interactions. medicine.iu.edu/MainTable.aspx – accessed July 6, 2021.

208. UMN drug interaction table: https:// www.d.umn.edu/~jfitzake/Lectures/ DMED/TAA/Q_A/CYP450Interaction Table.htm – accessed July 6, 2021.

209. Trepanier LA. Cytochrome P450 and its role in veterinary drug interactions. *Vet Clin Small Anim*. 2006;36:975–985.

210. Okamatsu G, Komatsu T, Ono Y, et al. Characterization of feline cytochrome P450 2B6. *Xenobiotica*. 2017;47: 93–102.

Resources and recommended reading

Bleuer-Elsner S, Medam T, Masson S. Effects of a single oral dose of gabapentin on storm phobia in dogs: A double-blind, placebo-controlled crossover trial. *Vet Rec*. 2021;189(7):e453. doi:10.1002/ vetr.453.

Craven AJ, Pegram C, Packer RMA, et al. Veterinary drug therapies used for undesirable behaviours in UK dogs under primary veterinary care. *PLoS One*. 2022;17(1):e0261139.

Crowell-Davis SL, Murray TF, Dantas LMS. *Veterinary Psychopharmacology*. 2nd ed. Hoboken, NJ: Wiley-Blackwell; 2019.

Imepitoin – https://todaysveterinarypractice. com/imepitoin-in-behavioral-and-neurobehavioral-medicine/.

Korpivaara M, Huhtinen M, Pohjanjousi P, et al. Tasipimidine, a novel orally administered alpha-2 adrenoceptor agonist, alleviates canine acute anxiety associated with owner departure—a pilot study. *J Vet Behav*. 2022. https://doi. org/10.1016/j.jveb.2022.11.003

Korpivaara M, Pohjanjousi P, Huhtinen M. Tasipimidine, a novel orally dosed alpha-2 Adrenoceptor agonist, alleviates canine acute anxiety and fear associated with noise – a pilot study. *Proc 3rd European Veterinary Congress of Behavioural Medicine and Animal Welfare*. 2021:148.

Lamminen Terttu, Korpivaara M, Suokko M, et al. Efficacy of a single dose of pregabalin on signs of anxiety in cats during transportation-a pilot study. *Front Vet Sci*. 2021;8:711816. doi: 10.3389/fvets. 2021.711816.

Lamminen T, Doedée A, Hyttilä-Hopponen M, et al. Pharmacokinetics of single and repeated oral doses of pregabalin oral solution formulation in cats. *J Vet Pharmacol Ther*. 2022;45: 385–391.

Maropitant in cats – https://todaysveterinary practice.com/maropitant-use-in-cats/.

Plumb's Veterinary Drugs: https://plumbs.com/.

Pregabalin (Bonqat) – European Medicines Agency. https://www.ema.europa.eu/en/ medicines/veterinary/EPAR/bonqat..

Stahl SM. *Stahl's Essential Psychopharmacology*. 4th ed. Cambridge: Cambridge University Press; 2021.

Stahl SM. *The Prescriber's Guide*. 6th ed. Cambridge: Cambridge University Press; 2020.

Tasipimidine (Tessie). European Medicines Agency. https://www.ema.europa.eu/en/ medicines/veterinary/EPAR/tessie.

CHAPTER 12

Treatment – integrative medicine

Megan Petroff, DVM, Gary Landsberg, DVM, MRCVS, DACVB, DECAWBM, and Lowell Ackerman, DVM, DACVD, MBA, MPA, CVA, MRCVS

What is integrative medicine?

Integrative medicine incorporates both conventional and complementary medicine in an holistic approach to caring for the emotional and physical health and well-being of the patient. This approach to medicine is designed to examine and treat the whole pet, including both physical and behavioral clinical signs, taking into account the environment, the disease and the relationship of pet and the pet parent, and to develop an integrative medical plan based on the findings. Treatment modalities focus on the most efficacious, least invasive, least expensive, and least harmful path to successful outcomes, combining both conventional and complementary forms of therapy.

Complementary and alternative medicine (CAM) refers to healthcare practices that are not part of conventional medical care. Current modalities include acupuncture, Chinese herbal medicine, chiropractic, homeopathy, aromatherapy, pheromones, Bach flower remedies, massage, sound healing therapy (e.g., music), magnetic field therapy, vibration therapy, and natural supplements including vitamins, minerals, phytotherapy (herbal medicine), cannabinoids, probiotics, nutraceuticals, and functional foods. Comprehensive discussion of complementary and alternative veterinary medicine (CAVM) is beyond the scope of this book, but a brief overview related to behavioral medicine will be provided. The National Center for Complementary and Integrative Health (nccih.nih.gov) provides resources and a research database on complementary and alternative therapies.

Is integrative medicine safer and more effective?

In conventional (sometimes referred to as "Western") medicine, those therapeutic modalities that have not been tested or proven effective using established scientific principles are viewed cautiously or skeptically. Ideally, all medications and therapeutic modalities used in animals should be subject to the same stringent criteria for safety and effectiveness. While many complementary therapeutics are purported to have behavioral therapeutic effects, very few have been studied or tested.

Any drug or supplement that has not been tested against placebo in controlled trials, has the potential for toxicity, or is used as an alternative to a proven effective drug, may pose a greater risk to the pet and lead to higher expense for the pet parent. This is by no means a condemnation of complementary medicine therapies. Practitioners should remain cognizant and informed of the potential benefits, science, and evidence for integrative medical therapies. In time, some will prove to be effective while others will prove to be ineffective or even harmful.

Placebo-controlled studies are generally lacking to prove the efficacy of many alternative products and therapies available. In the field of behavioral medicine, placebo effects of 50% or higher are not unusual (see Chapter 11). Therefore, any treatment, whether supplement or medication, that has not been subjected to an objective validated scoring system or has not been proven superior to placebo should be considered unproven with respect to efficacy.

In behavioral medicine, the treatment program should include behavioral treatment or modification and environmental management techniques that identify and address both the underlying cause of behavior problems as well as perpetuating factors. Therefore, regardless of whether a drug or complementary form of treatment is utilized, an holistic approach is needed to address all the issues that impact the pet's behavior and well-being (i.e., health, nutrition, environment, and behavioral management).

Dietary supplementation

Dietary supplementation is a popular topic among pet parents, breeders, and veterinarians. One of the reasons for supplementing diets is that the published nutritional requirements are not necessarily the same as actual requirements. Some dogs and cats respond to supplements even if there is no dietary deficiency. This is because some nutrients have positive pharmacologic benefits apart from their nutritional claims.[1]

We are rediscovering some basic facts about nutritional therapy – fiber can help prevent colon cancer; fresh vegetables can help prevent heart disease; melatonin may be helpful for sleep problems and jet lag. We may forget that aspirin (acetylsalicylic acid) was originally derived from the bark of willow trees, or that digitalis comes from the foxglove plant. Many popular drugs used today were originally isolated from nature.

Veterinary drugs must be proven to be safe and efficacious by law in order to achieve licensing by government regulatory agencies. Toxicity, contraindications, drug interactions, and potential side effects must be established.

Products that are sold as supplements or natural remedies that do not make claims with respect to health or disease can be sold in most countries in the absence of these safeguards. However, when botanical and nutraceutical products are used to treat physical or behavioral ailments, they are indeed being used with therapeutic intent. Many people put a great deal of trust in products that are "natural," yet, while variable between countries, there are few to no regulatory controls or requirements regarding quality, efficacy, tolerance, side effects, or contraindications.

With botanicals and nutraceuticals, there may also be no protection against substandard products and no standardization of active ingredients between competitive products, and there may even be variation between batches of the same product. The different species and different plant parts vary considerably in their biochemistry and effectiveness, even on a seasonal basis. Independent studies continue to find great ranges in active ingredients from well below to none to well above the manufacturer claims. Therefore, unless equivalency has been established between products, any evidence of efficacy might only apply to the specific product that has been tested.

Toxic contaminants are another concern. For example, eosinophilia-myalgia syndrome has been reported in humans due to contaminants in commercially available 5-hydroxytryptophan, which was being promoted for insomnia, depression, and headaches after tryptophan was banned. A number of Canadians developed nausea and vomiting when their dandelion root product was found to contain buckthorn bark. In 2007 the FDA (www.fda.gov) recalled 12 Chinese herbal products containing ephedra, aristolochic acid, and human placenta, so natural does not equate to safe.

Finally, the issue of how to dose and how much to dose has yet to be established for most herbal medicines in animals, and trial and error will be needed to find correct dosages. Even if a dose were to be established, the environment in which the plant grows, the part of the plant used, the age of the plant at harvest, and the method of administration may all affect dose and efficacy of individual batches. Greater study on the pharmacognosy of these plants is needed. Expect that some complementary and alternative products will eventually become mainstream medications once their active ingredients have been determined and safe doses established.

Herbal therapy (phytotherapy) and nutraceuticals

Most "natural" therapeutics lack evidence of efficacy beyond case reports and anecdote (lowest level of evidence). More recently, however, a number of veterinary products with nutraceutical or herbal ingredients have been tested in either clinical or laboratory trials or both. Unlike pharmaceuticals, nutraceutical and herbal products can be brought to market as long as they demonstrate little or no toxicity and make no label claims of efficacy. Therefore, even those "natural" products that have data to support their efficacy are unlikely to have been subjected to the rigors required for pharmaceutical licensing.

Practitioners will need to examine the quality of evidence, indications, contraindications, mode of action, and dosing recommendations before prescribing or recommending these supplements. Products that have not yet been assessed using acceptable scientific methods should be used only with pet parent consent and full disclosure of the evidence or lack thereof.

Veterinary nutraceuticals and therapeutic supplements

Cognitive enhancement

There are several supplements and diets that may support brain aging and executive function in dogs and cats. Although some products, such as S-adenosyl-L-methionine

(SAMe) may contain a single active ingredient, many of the cognitive supplements and diets are combinations of antioxidants, mitochondrial cofactors, fatty acids, and other ingredients that might collectively improve the signs or slow the progression of cognitive dysfunction. Products and diets for enhancement of cognitive function in senior pets are discussed in more depth in Chapter 8.

Medium chain triglycerides

Medium chain triglycerides (MCT) are fats made of a glycerol molecule and three fatty acids in a chain. High levels of MCTs can result in higher levels of ketone bodies in dogs, which may provide an alternative energy source for the aging brain as glucose metabolism declines.[2,3] They may be most useful for adjunctive treatment of seizure conditions and support for canine cognitive dysfunction (CCDS or CDS).[4-6] More detailed discussion and current products and diets containing MCTs can be found in Chapter 8.

L-theanine

L-theanine is an amino acid found in green tea. It binds the excitatory glutamate receptors to block transmission and increases GABA, resulting in inhibitory and relaxing effects. It may increase serotonin and dopamine in specific brain areas.[7] L-theanine can be found in many human, canine, and feline products used for the treatment of fear, anxiety, and stress (FAS). The most commonly used veterinary supplements containing L-theanine are Anxitane (Virbac Animal Health), Solliquin (Nutramax Laboratories), and Composure Pro (VetriScience). More information about these products can be seen in Table 12.1.

Anxitane contains 99.95% purified L-theanine (Suntheanine) that may be useful in the treatment of FAS in dogs and in urine marking and avoidance behaviors in cats. Several studies in dogs support an effect of L-theanine in reducing noise fears and phobia, storm-related anxiety, and fear of unfamiliar people over 4-8 weeks of twice-daily treatment.[8-11] Anxitane tablets are palatable, with no apparent sedative or adverse health effects.

In an open label clinical study in cats, treatment with Anxitane for 30 days significantly improved stress-related signs including hypervigilance, nervousness, fear, and undesirable elimination, and reduced stress scores in 91% of cats. Tablets were palatable in 94% of the cats and no side effects were reported.[7] Doses of up to 25 mg/kg/day in dogs for up to two months and up to four times the label dose in cats for 14 days were well tolerated.[12,13] Dosing L-theanine 5-10 mg/kg twice daily has been considered safe in dogs and cats for long term use. Some clinicians reportedly use L-theanine situationally, dosing every 12 hours as well as 2 hours prior to the stressful event.

Solliquin contains L-theanine, extracts of *Magnolia officinalis* and *Phellodendron amurense*, and dried whey protein concentrate. In a case series of 18 dogs and 2 cats with signs of fear and anxiety, 14/19 pet parents reported an effective response.[14] A combination of magnolia and phellodendron has been shown to reduce noise-induced anxiety in a laboratory study in dogs.[15]

Composure Pro contains L-theanine, thiamine, and C3 Colostrum Calming Complex. In a study assessing the effect of a single dose on noise aversion in dogs, it appears that it may have a positive effect in as little as 30 minutes, lasting at least 4 hours.[16] It has also been used to maintain positive behavior patterns in dogs and cats presented for aggression once initial medications for treatment had been discontinued.[17]

Alpha-casozepine

Alpha-casozepine is a naturally occurring trypsin hydrolysate of alpha S1-casein, a protein found in cows' milk which binds at the GABA-A receptor,[18] resulting in benzodiazepine-like anxiolysis, without the reported side effects or sedation. It is presently available in the United States as Zylkene (Vetoquinol) and as a supplement in several diets (Royal Canin Canine and Feline Calm Diets, and Hill's Prescription Diets Feline Urinary Stress and Canine i/d Stress). The recommended starting dose is 15 mg/kg once daily with efficacy expected in 2-4 weeks, although higher doses (up to 30 mg/kg) and longer treatment might be required to achieve maximal effect. See Table 12.2 for more dosing information.

Several studies have demonstrated an improvement in stress-related behavior problems with alpha-casozepine treatment in dogs and cats. In a study in dogs comparing the effects of alpha-casozepine to selegiline hydrochloride over two months, both treatments were equally effective in reducing emotional disorder scores.[19] In an eight-week feeding trial, dogs fed a diet supplemented with alpha-casozepine had a significant reduction in cortisol compared to a control diet.[20] In an eight-week feeding trial, anxious dogs fed a diet containing alpha-casozepine had significantly decreased plasma cortisol compared to controls. In cats, alpha-casozepine treatment combined with

Table 12.1 Summary of behavior problems for which there is evidence to support calming supplements may be effective

Supplement	Ingredients	Research showing efficacy in dogs	Research showing efficacy in cats
Anxitane[7-13]	• L-theanine	• Noise fears/phobia • Storm-related anxiety • Fear of unfamiliar people	• Stress-related signs including hypervigilance, nervousness, fear • Inappropriate elimination
Solliquin[14]	• L-theanine • *Magnolia officinalis* • *Phellodendron amurense* • Dried whey protein concentrate	• Noise-induced anxiety • Fear • Anxiety	• Fear • Anxiety
Composure Pro[16]	• L-theanine • thiamine a • C3 colostrum calming complex	• Noise aversion • Maintaining positive behavior patterns	• Maintaining positive behavior patterns

Table 12.2 Doses for therapeutic supplements

Active ingredient	Label dose	Recommended initial dose	Recommended target dose
L-Theanine	2.5–20 mg/kg PO SID	5 mg/kg PO BID	10 mg/kg PO BID
Alpha-casozepine	15–30 mg/kg PO SID	15 mg/kg PO SID	30 mg/kg PO SID
BLL-9	1 packet once daily	1 packet once daily	

This table summarizes the dosing recommended by various manufacturers for each product, as well as the dosing the author has found to be generally safe and effective. It is recommended to start at the initial dose for 7–14 days to ensure patient tolerance, prior to increasing to the target dose

behavior modification significantly improved fearful and anxious behavioral scores compared to placebo after 56 days.[21] Alpha-casozepine can be dosed at higher dosages for situational FAS. In a study in cats evaluating the effects of alpha-casozepine on stress during veterinary visits, 75 mg/kg q24 administered for three successive days prior to the veterinary visit reduced paw sweating (a sign of physiologic stress),[22] implying that this could be useful as a previsit pharmaceutical and/or useful for situational FAS.

Diets supplemented with both alpha-casozepine and L-tryptophan have also demonstrated an effect in reducing behavioral and physiological measures of anxiety and stress in both dogs and cats, and in reducing signs of idiopathic cystitis in cats.[23-26]

Probiotics

There is currently great interest in the role of the microbiome and gastrointestinal health in behavioral disorders of humans and animals. The parasympathetic and sympathetic nervous systems allow bidirectional communication between the gastrointestinal and central nervous system.[27] Along with the gut microbiome, this is referred to as the gut–brain axis. Because the communication is bidirectional, when there is emotional stress, the brain can cause gastrointestinal upset, nausea, hypermotility, and inappetence. Conversely, when there is disease in the gut, signals are sent to the brain which can contribute to anxiety, stress, and fear. In dogs, the gut microbiome has been associated with changes in aggression, anxiety, and memory performance.[28,29] In addition, the gut microbiome plays a role in the production of monoamine neurotransmitter precursors and GABA, which modulate fear, anxiety, aggression, hypervigilance, muscle tension, and stress.[30] See Chapters 6 and 14 for more information on the gut–brain axis. Gastrointestinal microbiome differences have been found between dogs with conspecific aggression and dogs without aggression,[28] with anxiety and without anxiety,[31] and in working dogs exposed to 2.5 hours of cabin air travel compared to working dogs that did not travel.[32]

A veterinary probiotic supplement (Calming Care, Purina) containing the bacterial strain *Bifidobacterium longum* 999 (BL999), has been shown to reduce anxious behaviors in dogs. In a placebo-controlled blinded, cross over study of 24 anxious Labrador Retrievers over six weeks of treatment, dogs treated with BL999 had a significant reduction in anxious behaviors including barking, jumping, spinning, and pacing; reduced salivary cortisol levels; a decrease in heart rate; and increased heart rate variability.[33] In a study evaluating the effects of the feline product in a shelter environment, cats were significantly less likely to have sneezing associated

with FHV-1, to have abnormal serum cortisol levels, and to pace in cages compared to placebo when exposed to mild stress from change in housing.[34]

Relaxigen, a supplement containing *Griffonia simplicifolia*, *Camellia sinensis*, conjugated linoleic acid-CLA, krill oil, *L. reuteria* NBF1 inactivated, glyceryl tribuyrate, fructo-oligosaccharides, and vitamin E was investigated in a placebo-controlled study in dogs to assess its effect on stress and anxiety. Dogs in the treatment group had a probability of improving >50% when compared to dogs in the placebo group.[31]

Cannabidiol

Currently, there are no FDA-approved products containing cannabinoids, and veterinary recommendation of cannabidiol (CBD) in the United States is illegal at the federal level without a schedule I DEA license. State and federal laws that legalize the medicinal use of CBD for humans do not apply to veterinary use (AVMA).[35] Despite this, numerous nutraceutical products containing CBD are readily accessible to pet parents. Significant concerns relate to safety and efficacy due to the lack of evidence of anxiolytic effect of CBD, possible side effects, drug interactions, and effective dosing ranges for animals. In addition, consumers must be aware of the potential lack of quality control. One study assessing three formulations of CBD available found that all three contained less CBD than what was indicated on the label.[36]

There are currently no evidence-based studies to support an effect of CBD in reducing anxiety in dogs and cats, although preliminary studies have demonstrated potential effects as adjunctive therapy in dogs for seizure control and for reducing osteoarthritis pain.[37,38] Of two published behavioral studies to date, CBD chews did not have an anxiolytic effect on dogs exposed to storm sounds when dosed at 1.4 mg/kg in one study, and the second did not find a significant difference between CBD-treated dogs and controls in reducing aggression towards humans in shelter dogs.[39,40] Doses, and associated side effects in pets have not yet been established. Studies currently published have ranged from 0.3 to 2.0 mg/kg bid (up to 10 mg/bid) with a peak effect of 1.4–5.8 hours in dogs and 2-3 hours in cats.[36-43] While CBD is generally well tolerated, mild and transient, gastrointestinal upset and hypersalivation have been reported with increasing doses up to 30.5 mg/kg in cats and 62 mg/kg in dogs.[36,41,42,43] In cats, liver markers including alkaline phosphatase, ALT, bilirubin and GGTP remained within the normal range at all doses,[43] except one cat with an elevated ALT over the course of the 12 week study.[41] In dogs, elevation in alkaline phosphatase, particularly with increase duration and higher dose has been reported in some dogs across several studies with no concomitant increase in ALT, GGT, bilirubin or bile acids.[36-38,42] Also see recommended reading and resources below.

Melatonin

Melatonin is an indolamine derivative of serotonin that may inhibit dopamine. Production is primarily within the pineal body. The hormone is secreted into the blood and cerebrospinal fluid at high levels during the night and at low levels during the day. Melatonin has a time-keeping function in many mammals. A true physiologic role for melatonin in humans has yet to be clearly established. It may decrease free radical production, reduce central nervous system excitability, and potentiate GABA.[44]

Although controlled and long-term studies are lacking, case reports suggest that melatonin may be useful in the treatment of anxiety, fear of fireworks and thunder, and sleep cycle disorders in dogs and cats. In one case report, melatonin in conjunction with amitriptyline was used to treat noise phobia successfully at a dose of 0.1 mg/kg daily, and up to every 8 hours during firework and storm events. Dosing of 1.5 mg for small dogs, 3 mg for dogs 15–50 kg, and 3–6 mg for large dogs given every 8–24 hours has been suggested.[44] Few toxic effects have been reported.

Tryptophan

Tryptophan is an amino acid precursor of serotonin. Lower levels of tryptophan in the diet have been associated with a decrease in serotonin levels, which might be associated with impulsivity, sleep disturbances, and mood and memory alterations. While supplementation with tryptophan might result in increased serotonin synthesis, it is unlikely that this is the case. Tryptophan competes with other large neutral amino acids (LNAAs) for a common carrier to cross the blood–brain barrier. Therefore, a higher ratio of tryptophan relative to other LNAA would be required to increase availability to the brain.[45,46] Without crossing into the brain, the tryptophan cannot be used for serotonin synthesis and has no effect on neurotransmitters. Studies thus far assessing tryptophan supplementation in dogs and cats for reducing anxiety have been limited to small group sizes and short duration, with equivocal effects.[45,46] For example, in one study, dogs were fed either a control diet with added tryptophan or one of three other diets with successively higher levels of tryptophan for 24 weeks and no change was seen in behaviors when approached by a person, whether unfamiliar or familiar.[45]

Current widely used products supplemented with tryptophan are Composure Pro by VetriScience, the Royal Canin Veterinary Canine and Feline Calm diets, and Hill's c/d Multicare Stress. Diets supplemented with tryptophan and alpha-casozepine have demonstrated evidence of effect in in the treatment of anxiety in dogs and cats and in reducing signs of feline interstitial cystitis.[23-26] In another study in cats, a diet supplemented with a combination of lemon balm, fish peptides, oligofructose, and L-tryptophan resulted in a lower average 24-hour urinary cortisol/creatinine ratio compared to tryptophan alone.[47] More information on diets supplemented with tryptophan can be found in Chapter 13. Supplementation with tryptophan should be used with caution if combining with medications that increase serotonin

due to potential adverse effects of serotonin syndrome (see Chapters 6 and 11).

Tyrosine

Tyrosine is a nonessential amino acid which acts as the precursor to dopamine, epinephrine, and norepinephrine. In one study of Labrador Retrievers, Toy Poodles and German Shepherd Dogs, supplementation with tyrosine decreased the time needed to acquire a new behavior and the reaction time to the cue given.[48]

Herbal therapeutics

Valerian

Valerian, an herb derived from the roots of *Valeriana officinalis* and *V. wallichii*, has been used for its sedative, anxiolytic, and hypnotic effects in people. The GABA-A receptor has been identified as the major target of the active ingredient valerenic acid, resulting in anxiolysis.[49] However, because it can potentiate the effects of barbiturates and benzodiazepines, it should be avoided in patients undergoing anesthesia. No other drug reactions or toxicities have yet been reported. Valerian may improve quality of sleep for humans, but several weeks may be required to achieve effect.[50] Evidence is available to support the use of valerian in providing olfactory enrichment for cats and dogs. In one study of 100 cats living in a sanctuary, 47% responded positively to olfactory enrichment with valerian root, compared to 68% for catnip and 79% to silver vine.[51] In a shelter study, dogs provided with a cloth impregnated with valerian spent more time resting and had reduced vocalization behavior compared to controls.[52] Though evidence is lacking, valerian may help pets to sleep through the night and might be useful alone or in combination with other psychotropic drugs in reducing fear and anxiety in dogs and cats.

Catnip

Catnip (*Nepeta cataria*) produces allomones which result in an apparent euphoric reaction in some cats in response to its smell. The active compound in catnip responsible for causing "the catnip effect" is an oil, nepetalactone. It is available as a leaf, but liquid and aerosol forms are also available. Both catnip and silver vine appear to activate the opioid system, resulting in increases in beta endorphins.[53] Catnip produces an active response in about 50–80% of cats. These cats may sniff, lick, shake their head, or rub their head, chin, or cheek against the catnip, and then twitch, salivate, and roll over it for 5–15 minutes.[51,53] The response resembles elements of playful, predatory, and sexual behaviors. Catnip responsiveness is reported to be an autosomal dominant trait, beginning at about eight weeks of age. Catnip may provide olfactory environmental enrichment, increase play and exploration in both shelter and home environments, stimulate scratching post use, and be used as a reinforcer for behavior modification and training.[54-56]

In a shelter study in which cats were exposed to cloths impregnated with different olfactory stimuli, cats spent more time interacting with the catnip cloth compared to lavender, prey scent (rabbit), or control, although interest significantly decreased over the second and third hours of presentation.[57] In another study comparing four different types of enrichment in both shelter and pet cats, social interaction with people was preferred compared to food, toys, and scent. However, in the scent category, catnip was preferred by significantly more cats than prey scent or the scent of another cat.[55]

Catnip is not toxic; however, adverse effects of gastrointestinal upset and lethargy have been reported. In addition, catnip should be used cautiously in group housing, as it may cause too much conflict.[57]

Silver vine (*Actinidia polygama*)

Like catnip, silver vine has allomone properties affecting many cats. It has six active components, including nepetalacol, with a similar mode of action and producing similar behavioral effects to catnip.[51,53] Silver vine has applications for olfactory enrichment and to encourage scratching post use in cats.[54,58] In one study of 100 domestic cats, 79% had a positive behavioral response to silver vine compared to 68% with catnip, and cats responded more intensely to silver vine than catnip. The most reliable response was to the powder of dried fruit galls and less frequently to silver vine.[51] Silver vine is considered safe, nontoxic, and not addictive.[58] As is clear from the review of catnip and silver vine research above, cat preferences first and foremost should be considered when using olfactory enrichment, as some will prefer catnip and some will prefer silver vine.

Pheromone therapy

Pheromones are chemical substances that influence social and sexual behavior between members of a species. Compared to other natural substances, there are extensive data on the applications and efficacy of pheromones in veterinary behavior therapy. Semiochemicals are substances used in intra- and interspecific communication, while pheromones are semiochemicals secreted for communication between members of the same species.[59] Appeasing pheromones, produced by the mother in the first few days after birth, play a role in the attraction and attachment of newborn to mother. Synthetically produced appeasing pheromones can have a relaxing effect for both young and adults of a species.

Pheromones are detected in the vomeronasal (VNO) or Jacobson's organ, an accessory organ of the olfactory tract found along each side of the nasal septum. In some species, including cats, the flehmen or gape response enhances the perception of sexual pheromones. In dogs, tonguing (flicking tongue against incisive papilla) and panting likely aid in the perception of pheromones. Pheromones bind to pheromone-binding proteins in the VNO, stimulating structures in the limbic system to alter the pet's emotional state (primers) or activate physiologic effects. Receptors are generally found only in the species that produces the pheromones. See Chapter 2 for more information about chemical/olfactory communication.

In clinical applications, they can be used alone or safely with any other medication or supplement. While synthetic pheromones have no known toxicity, side effects such as local skin irritation and agitation have been reported. Synthetic

pheromones are available in several applications, including plug-in diffusers, sprays, wipes, and collars.

While there are extensive studies demonstrating the efficacy of pheromone therapy in helping pets cope with stress-evoking situations and in reducing anxiety, not all findings have been significant or strong, with variability in effects depending on the individual, the environment, the application, and the level and intensity of the response.[60-69] For this reason, pet parent expectations should be managed upon recommendation, meaning that veterinarians should explain that in general, supplements and natural products will cause less of a change in behavioral clinical signs when compared to medications.

Feline facial pheromone – F3 fraction

The F3 fraction of the feline facial pheromone serves to mark boundaries of passageways and provide for emotional stability, perhaps by indicating known objects from unknown.[59]

Synthetic F3 analogs such as Feliway Classic (Ceva Santé Animale) may aid in the prevention, control, and treatment of behavioral and physical signs of fear, anxiety, and stress including urine marking, territorial scratching, and loss of appetite, and reduced exploration, interest in play, and social interactions. Synthetic F3 pheromones can be applied directly on surfaces such as a hospital cage, household surfaces, cat carriers, and bedding 15 minutes prior to the cat's exposure to the surface and repeated after 4–5 hours.

Synthetic F3 pheromones have demonstrated efficacy in reducing marking and anxiety when introducing new cats to the home, adapting to changes in the home, or moving to a new environment by increasing appetite, reducing spraying and roaming, and in reducing stress and anxiety associated with travel, veterinary visits, and in shelters.[70-79]

In a meta-analysis of 10 studies that evaluated pharmacotherapy or pheromone therapy for urine marking in cats, there was a significant ($P < .001$) association between the use of any intervention and the number of cats that ceased or reduced urine spraying by at least 90%. Analysis by intervention type indicated that fluoxetine, clomipramine, and pheromonatherapy (pheromone therapy) may each assist in managing urine spraying beyond a placebo-based intervention.[76] In the veterinary hospital, F3 pheromone spray has been shown to reduce stress associated with veterinary examination and procedures, increase food intake in hospitalized cats when sprayed in the cat's carrier, and increase calming in acepromazine-sedated cats.[71,78,79] For preventing and reducing stress in the veterinary setting, pheromones should be integrated into a multimodal approach that includes cat-friendly health care, gentle handling, and a calming environment. In addition, F3 pheromone might also be useful as adjunctive therapy in preventing and reducing the effects of stress on physical health such as in feline interstitial cystitis.[69,80]

Cat-appeasing pheromone

A synthetic form of cat-appeasing pheromone produced by the mammary sebaceous glands of the lactating queen (Feliway MultiCat in the United States and Feliway Friends in Europe; Ceva Santé Animale), has demonstrated efficacy in the management of aggression between housemates.

A 2019 randomized, double-blind, placebo-controlled pilot trial of 42 multicat households treated with Feliway Multicat diffuser or placebo resulted in a decrease in aggression scores over one month.[81] The most significant clinical effect occurred within the first 14 and 21 days. In a study comparing treatment with either a Feliway Multicat diffuser or Adaptil diffuser over four weeks, both products improved the dog–cat relationship, including a reduction in dog chasing, barking, and staring at the cat and in the cat running away, hiding, and staring at the dog. Cat pet parents perceived greater relaxation with Feliway.[82]

New pheromone complex

Feliway Optimum a new pheromone complex by Ceva Santé Animale is a synthetic pheromone marketed to improve vertical scratching, spraying, excessive fears, and intercat relationships within the same home. The active ingredient in the product is Feline Pheromone Complex. The mechanism of action is yet to be elucidated. Strong evidence to support the claims of the product are not yet available at the time of publishing, but preliminary studies suggest it may be a promising adjunctive therapy. One initial open-label uncontrolled trial has shown improvement after 28 days of treatment in urine spraying, furniture scratching, fear, and intercat relationships.[83]

Dog-appeasing pheromone

Adaptil is a synthetic version of the dog-appeasing pheromone secreted by the sebaceous glands in the mammary chains of the lactating female during nursing. Its function is to calm and reassure (appease) the offspring.[59] Dog-appeasing pheromone (DAP) has demonstrated effect in reducing fear, anxiety, and stress in veterinary clinics, shelters, and during travel, for helping puppies adjust to a new home, reducing arousal in puppy classes, calming and reducing anxiety during maternal care and weaning, and in the treatment of noise phobias and separation-related disorders (in combination with behavior modification).[65,65,68,84–94] In a placebo-controlled study in the veterinary hospital, treatment with DAP spray improved postsurgical alertness and visual exploration and decreased the decline in serum prolactin, a hormone which modulates the stress response.[84] The DAP diffuser has been shown to increase relaxation during veterinary visits in the examination and consultation rooms and during hospitalization.[84,85]

When used in puppy classes, the pheromone collar has been shown to reduce fear and anxiety and improve learning and long-term socialization compared to placebo.[95] In newly adopted puppies, dogs wearing pheromone collars displayed fewer nuisance behaviors, fear, and distress after the first two weeks of adoption compared to placebo collars.[96,97] DAP may also improve relationships between dogs and cats in a home. Both Adaptil and Feliway Multicat diffusers significantly reduced chasing, barking, and staring at cats, and cats hiding from dogs, while the Adaptil increased friendly greetings and times spent relaxed in the room together. Dog pet parents perceived greater relaxation with Adaptil.[82] New pheromone products for modifying behavior are also now available but efficacy studies have yet to be published. A new semiochemical derived from cat anal glands has developed that has been shown to reduce feline elimination in the location where it is sprayed.[98]

Aromatherapy

Aromatherapy is the practice of using natural plant extracts such as volatile oils to heal the mind and body (NAHA.org). Oils can be administered by aerosolization, topical application, and less commonly, orally. Essential oils are obtained from the flowers, buds, fruits, leaves, bark, roots, or seeds of plants. The aromatic plant with the most significant evidence in treatment of animal behavior conditions is lavender. Though the mode of action by which it affects animals is unclear, there is evidence that lavender may have calming effects on humans, pigs, dogs, and cats.[99–106]

Aromatherapy with lavender might be effective in reducing travel-induced excitement in dogs during car rides. In one placebo-controlled study, dogs spent significantly more time resting and less time vocalizing when lavender oil was applied to a cloth in the car.[107] Aromatherapy may be beneficial in shelter housing in dogs.[88,103–105] Simultaneous exposure to vanilla, valerian, coconut, and ginger resulted in a reduction of vocalization and overall activity, while exposure to coconut and ginger alone resulted in increased sleep.[52] Diffused chamomile and lavender resulted in increased resting and decreased vocalization, suggesting relaxation.[52]

Aromatherapy may also provide olfactory enrichment. In kenneled dogs exposed to various scented (rabbit or lavender) and unscented toys, stress-related behaviors were reduced and dogs played more and for longer with the scented toys compared to unscented toys.[105] Lavender aromatherapy may reduce anxiety and stress during hospitalization. In one study in cats, exposure to lavender oil via inhalation over 30 minutes in a veterinary hospital resulted in significant reduction in stress scores compared to a control group.[106] Lavender may have less potential for olfactory enrichment than catnip in cats. In a shelter study exposing cats to various scented cloths, they spent more time interacting with catnip scent than lavender or control.[56]

Homeopathy

Homeopathy works on the principle of like cures like – that clinical signs are purportedly cured by a remedy prepared by repeatedly diluting a substance that caused the disease process. The remedy is said to contain the "energy" or "life force" needed to heal the patient. Homeopathic remedies are commonly diluted to the point that likely not a single molecule still exists and may fail to contain detectable levels of the "active" ingredient, yet are reported to have an increase in "potency" with increased dilution.

Scientifically validated evidence of efficacy in the treatment of canine and feline behavior problems with homeopathic remedies is lacking, as is a scientifically plausible biochemical mechanism of action.[108–110] Two placebo-controlled studies in dogs with noise phobias have failed to show any efficacy.[111,112] Though homeopathic remedies may be safe and nontoxic because of their extreme dilution, they may cause harm if an ill or suffering patient is deprived or delayed in receiving a most efficacious treatment.[110]

Bach flower remedies

A physician, Edward Bach, developed homeopathic remedies in the 1930s to improve the emotional state of the human or pet using minute dilutions of plant essences. Rescue Remedy is a combination of five of Bach's flower essences that has been sold for the immediate or acute treatment of FAS. Despite the lack of any data to support the efficacy of these products, they continue to experience popularity.

Acupuncture

Acupuncture is said to stimulate the vital force (Qi) within the animal to bring about homeostasis and healing. Stimulation of acupuncture points is intended to bring about balance along lines of energy called meridians and may lead to alteration in neurotransmitter pathways. Brain-mapping studies have revealed correlation between acupuncture point stimulation and cortical activation. In a study in laboratory Beagles assessing the effects of 20 minutes of acupuncture on dogs exposed to thunder recordings, stress behaviors including hiding, restlessness, bolting, and running around were significantly reduced in the acupuncture group; however, there was no effect on heart rate or serum cortisol.[113] High-quality, randomized controlled trials are needed to evaluate the role and efficacy of acupuncture in clinical veterinary behavioral medicine.

Therapeutic touch

The Tellington Touch Equine Awareness Method (TTEAM) is a physical manipulation technique originally developed by Linda Tellington-Jones to modify behavior in horses. It was eventually modified for all animals (TTouch) to reduce stress and relax animals by increasing the animal's body awareness and balance. Some described uses are to decrease pain, restore intestinal function following surgery, or relax a fearful pet. Although there are numerous anecdotal reports of its effectiveness, there are no experimental data to support effectiveness in treatment of behavior disorders of dogs and cats.

Magnetic field therapy

In this form of therapy, magnets are used to alter the energy fields of the individual. There is no documented mechanism of action, although transcranial stimulation is said to enhance serotonin metabolism. There are no published placebo-controlled studies in the treatment of behavior disorders with magnetic field therapy in humans or pets, but transcranial magnetic stimulation (TMS) has been effective in treating depression in humans.

The Calmer Canine has been designed to deliver targeted pulsed electromagnetic field (tPEMF) signals to the brain. In an open label pilot study with the Calmer Canine Assisi Loop in nine dogs with separation-related disorders, 56% of pet parents reported that their signs had resolved after six weeks of twice-daily treatments, while video observation showed that 80% of dogs had at least one clinical sign improve after one month of treatment.[114]

Veterinary chiropractic

Chiropractic manipulation is intended to correct mechanical imbalances related to the neuromuscular consequences of subluxation and is purported to improve a variety of other physiologic conditions. No studies have demonstrated that chiropractic is effective in the management of behavior problems in dogs and cats.

Vibrational therapy

The Calmz Anxiety Relief System uses a combination of tonal and vibrational therapy with the intent of reducing anxiety. In one laboratory study of 24 dogs, signs of noise (thunder)-induced anxiety was significantly reduced compared to control.[115]

Music therapy

Music has been a major focus of study for its potential to help to maintain a relaxed state in animals in a variety of environments. Several studies have shown both classical music and cat-specific music to have calming benefits for cats compared to no music and other genres. In a study of 14 cats during ovariohysterectomy (spay) surgery, cats required less anesthesia and had lower respiratory rates and lower pupillary diameter when exposed to classical music compared to pop music or heavy metal.[116] In dogs, a recent study did not find that classical music improved sedation.[117]

Species-specific music is produced with a frequency range and similar tempo to those used in typical communication of that species.[118] Cat-specific music significantly lowered stress-related behaviors in cats visiting veterinary clinics for physical exams.[119] Another study showed a preference in cats for cat-specific music compared to classical music in the home environment.[118]

In dogs, a systematic review of nine studies on the effects of music on canine behavior found strong evidence that classical music can have a calming effect in stressful environments including kennels and shelters.[120-124] Unlike cats, there is no current evidence to support dog-specific music providing calming benefits to dogs.[124] Heavy metal music increased the likelihood of barking and standing.[121,122] Audiobooks have been demonstrated to have a calming effect in shelter dogs.[128] In another recent study in shelter dogs comparing enrichment with music to appeasing pheromones, lavender, and control, music caused the greatest reduction in vocalizations and increase in calm body postures.[88] However, dogs exposed to the same music over a longer period of time may habituate to it, suggesting that a variety of music may be optimal.[120]

Music may also reduce anxiety and stress for pets, pet parents and veterinary personnel in the veterinary hospital.[126-128] A systematic review demonstrated that classical music had a significant positive impact on canine behavior and physiological parameters (heart rate variability, vocalizations, and time spent resting), and some supportive but equivocal evidence to support a reduction in stress in hospitalized dogs.[126]

Pressure garments

Various garments have been marketed to reduce anxiety by swaddling with balanced pressure. While one study supports an effect of reducing anxiety in limited circumstances in dogs that are not on behavioral medications, in most studies there are no other significant findings to support efficacy of pressure wraps. The lack of effect when used with medications could be because the effect of the garment is so negligible that it is not statistically significant if other modalities are used. One study showed that when the pressure wrap is applied incorrectly, which certainly could be the case with a pet parent applying the garment, there was no difference between the pressure wrap and placebo. Pressure wraps should not be applied too tightly, as one dog in one study died after application, and the pet should be monitored closely to ensure that it is more settled rather than exhibiting an inhibited or passive fear response.[129-133]

Conclusion

Integrative medicine has its place in the treatment of behavioral disorders in companion animals. Review of literature and diligent research is a must before prescribing any product, whether medication, nutraceutical, supplement, or products such as pressure wraps. In addition, managing pet parent expectations so that they anticipate subtle or variable changes in the pet's clinical signs is essential. That will help pet parents to know what to expect and to understand that if a "natural" product is recommended, they will likely need to layer in other products in order to achieve the same effect as a medication.

References

1. Ackerman L. *Canine Nutrition – What Every Owner, Breeder and Trainer Should Know*. Loveland, Colorado: Alpine Publication; 1999.
2. London ED, Ohata M, Takei H, et al. Regional cerebral metabolic rate for glucose in beagle dogs of different ages. *Neurobiol Aging*. 1983;4:121–126.
3. Pan Y, Larson B, Araujo JA, et al. Dietary supplementation with medium-chain TAG has long-lasting cognition-enhancing effects in aged dogs. *Br J Nutr*. 2010;103:1746–1754.
4. Larsen JA, Owens TJ, Fascetti AJ. Nutritional management of idiopathic epilepsy in dogs. *J Am Vet Med Assoc*. 2014;245:504–508.
5. Berk BA, Law TH, Packer RMA, et al. A multi-center randomized (CDS): a prospective double blinded placebo controlled clinical trial. *Front Nutr*. 2018;5:127. doi:10.3389/fnut.2018.00127.
6. Pan Y, Landsberg G, Mougeot I, et al. Efficacy of a therapeutic diet on dogs with signs of cognitive dysfunction syndrome (CDS): a prospective double blinded placebo controlled clinical trial. *Front Nutr*. 2018;5:127. doi:10.3389/fnut.2018.00127.
7. Dramard, V, Kern L, Hofmans J, et al. Effect of l-theanine tablets in reducing stress-related emotional signs in cats: an open-label field study. *Irish Vet J*. 2018.
8. Michelazzi M, Berteselli G, Minero M, et al. Effectiveness of l-theanine and behavior modification for treatment of phobias in dogs. *J Vet Behav*. 2010;5:34–5.
9. Michelazzi M, Berteselli G, Talamonti Z, et al. Efficacy of l-theanine in treatment of noise phobias in dogs; preliminary results. *Veterinaria*. 2015;29:1–7.
10. Pike A, Horwitz DL. An open label prospective study of the use of l-theanine (Anxitane) in storm sensitive client owned dogs. *J Vet Behav*. 2015;10:324–331.
11. Araujo JA, de Rivera C, Ethier JL, et al. Anxitane tablets reduce fear of human beings in a laboratory model of anxiety-related behavior. *J Vet Behav*. 2010;5:268–75.
12. Specific safety trial in dogs: clinical impact. Virbac Animal Unit internal study no. 691.05/70001.
13. Doig, A. *Safety Assessment Study for Anxitane® in Cats*. 2009.
14. DePorter TL, Bledsoe DL, Conley JR, et al. Case report series of clinical effectiveness and safety of Solliquin® for behavioral support in dogs and cats. In: *Proc Vet Behav Sympos*. San Antonio; 2016:27–28.
15. DePorter TL, Landsberg GM, Araujo JA, et al. Harmonease chewable tablets reduces noise-induced fear and anxiety in a laboratory canine thunderstorm simulation: a blinded and placebo-controlled study. *J Vet Behav*. 2012;7: 225–232.
16. Vetriscience White Paper. Assessment of anxiolytic properties of a novel compound in Beagle dogs with a noise induced model of fear and anxiety. 2016. Available at: https://www.vetriproline.com/techpieces/Composure2016StudySummary.pdf.
17. Kulluck E, Sayilkan BU, Dalgin D, et al. Complementary nonpharmaceutical therapy efficience in canine and feline aggressive behavior-clinical observation. In: *Proceedings of the 2nd International and 13th National Veterinary Internal Medicine Congress*. 2019.
18. Miclo L, Perrin E, Driou A, et al. Characterization of alpha-casozepine, a tryptic peptide from bovine αs1-casein with benzodiazepine-like activity. *FASEB J*. 2001; doi:10.1096/fj.00-0685fje.
19. Beata C, Beaumont-Graff E, Diaz C, et al. Effects of alpha-casozepine (Zylkene) versus selegiline hydrochloride (Selgian, Anipryl) on anxiety disorders in dogs. *J Vet Behav*. 2007;2:175–83.
20. Palestrini C, Minero M, Cannas S, et al. Efficacy of a diet containing caseinate hydrolysate on signs of stress in dogs. *J Vet Behav*. 2010;5:309–17.
21. Beata C, Beaumont-Graff E, Coll V, et al. Effect of alpha-casozepine (Zylkene) on anxiety in cats. *J Vet Behav*. 2007;2:40–46.
22. Makawey A, Iben C, Palme R. Cats at the vet: the effect of alpha-s1 casozepin. *Animals*. 2020;10:2047. doi:10.3390/ani10112047.
23. Kato M, Miyaji K, Ohtani N, et al. Effects of prescription diet on dealing with stressful situations and performance of anxiety-related behaviors in privately owned anxious dogs. *J Vet Behav*. 2012; 7:21–6.
24. Meyer H, Becvarova I. Effects of a urinary food supplement with milk protein hydrolysate and l-tryptophan on feline idiopathic cystitis – results of a case series in 10 cats. *Intern J Appl Res Vet Med*. 2016; 14:59–65.
25. Landsberg GM, Milgram NW, Mougeot I, et al. Therapeutic effects of an alpha-casozepine and l-tryptophan supplemented diet on fear and anxiety in the cat. *J Fel Med Surg*. 2017;6:594–602.
26. Miyaji K, Kato M, Ohtani N, et al. Experimental verification of the effects on normal domestic cats by feeding prescription diet for decreasing stress. *J Appl Anim Welf Sci*. 2015;18: 355–362.
27. Goyal RK, Hirano I. The enteric nervous system. *N Engl J Med*. 1996;334: 1106–1115.
28. Kirchoff NS, Udell MAR, Sharpton TJ. The gut microbiome correlates with conspecific aggression in a small population of rescued dogs (*Canis familiaris*). *PeerJ*. 2019;7:e61-e63.
29. Kubinyi E, Bel Rhali SB, Sándor S, et al. Gut microbiome composition is associated with age and memory performance in pet dogs. *Animals*. 2020;10:1488.
30. Mondo E, Barone M, Soverini M, et al. Gut microbiome structure and adrenocorticoal activity in dogs with aggressive and phobic disorders. *Heliyon*. 2020; 6(1):e03311.
31. Cannas S, Tonini B, Bela B, et al. Effect of a novel nutraceutical supplement (Relaxigen Pet dog ®) on the fecal microbiome and stress-related behaviors

in dogs: a pilot study. *J Vet Behav.* 2021; 42:37–47.

32. Venable EB, Bland SD, Holscher HD, et al. Effects of air travel stress on the canine microbiome: a pilot study. *Int J Vet Sci.* 2016;4:132–139.

33. McGowan RTS, Barnett HR, Czarnecku-Maulden G, et al. Tapping into those "gut feelings": impact of BL99 (Bifidobacterium longum) on anxiety in dogs. In: *Proceedings of the ACVB Behav Sympos.* Denver, CO, July 11–12, 2018.

34. Davis H, Franco P, Gagné J, et al. Effect of Bifidobacterium longum 999 supplementation on stress associated findings in cats with feline herpesvirus 1 infection. In: *ACVIM Forum 2021 Proceedings.*

35. AVMA online resources and tools. Cannabis Use and Pets. American Veterinary Medical Association. Available at: https://www.avma.org/resources-tools/veterinarians-and-public-health/cannabis-use-and-pets (Accessed October 2, 2020).

36. McGrath S, Bartner LR, Rao S, et al. A report of adverse effects associated with the administration of cannabidiol in healthy dogs. *J Am Holist Vet Med Assoc.* 2018;52:34–38.

37. McGrath S, Bartner LR, Rao S, et al. Randomized blinded controlled clinical trial to assess the effect of oral cannabidiol administration in addition to conventional antiepileptic treatment on seizure frequency in dogs with intractable idiopathic epilepsy. *J Am Vet Med Assoc.* 2019;254:1301–1308.

38. Gamble LJ, Boesch JM, Frye CW, et al. Pharmacokinetics, safety, and clinical efficacy of cannabidiol treatment in osteoarthritic dogs. *Front Vet Sci.* 2018;5. doi:10.3389/fvets.2018.00165.

39. Morris EM, Kitts-Morgan SE, Spangler DM, et al. The impact of feeding cannabidiol (CBD) containing treats on canine response to a noise-induced fear response test. *Front Vet Sci.* 2020;7. doi:10.3389/fvets.2020.569565

40. Corsetti S, Borruso S, Malandrucco L, et al. Cannabis sativa L. may reduce aggressive behaviour towards humans in shelter dogs. *Sci Rep.* 2021;11:2773. doi:10.1038/s41598-021-82439-2.

41. Deabold KA, Schwark WS, Wolf L, et al. Single-dose pharmacokinetics and preliminary safety assessment with use of CBD-rich hemp nutraceutical in healthy dogs and cats. *Animals.* 2019;9. 10:832.

42. Vaughn DM, Paulionis LJ, Kulpa JE. Randomized, placebo-controlled, 28-day safety and pharmacokinetics evaluation of repeated oral cannabidiol administration in healthy dogs. *Am J Vet Res.* 2021;82(5):405–416.

43. Kulpa JE, Paulionis LJ, Eglit GM, Vaughn DM. Safety and tolerability of escalating cannabinoid doses in healthy cats. *J Feline Med Surg.* 2021;23(12):1162–1175.

44. Aronson L. Animal behavior case of the month. A dog was evaluated because of extreme fear. *J Am Vet Med Assoc.* 1999; 215:22–24.

45. Templeman JR, Davenport GM, Cant JP, et al. The effect of graded concentrations of dietary tryptophan on canine behavior in response to the approach of a familiar or unfamiliar individual. *Can J Vet Res.* 2018;82:294–305.

46. Bosch G, Beerda B, Beynen AC, et al. Dietary tryptophan supplementation in privately owned mildly anxious dogs. *Appl Anim Behav Sci,* 2009;121:197–205.

47. Jeusette I, Tami G, Anna Fernandez A, et al. Evaluation of a new prescription diet with lemon balm, fish peptides, oligofructose and L-tryptophan to reduce urinary cortisol, used as a marker of stress, in cats. *J Vet Behav.* 2021;42:30–36.

48. Kano M, Uchiyama H, Ohta M, et al. Oral tyrosine changed the responses to commands in German Shepherds and Labrador Retrievers, but not in toy poodles. *J Vet Behav.* 2015;10:194–198.

49. Benke D, Barberis A, Kopp S, et. al. GABA A receptors as in vivo substrate for the anxiolytic action of valerenic acid, a major constituent of valerian root extracts. *Neuropharmacology.* 2009;56:174–181.

50. Fernandez-San-Martin MI, Masa-Font R, Palacaios-Soler L. Effectiveness of valerian in insomnia: a meta-analysis of randomized placebo controlled trials. *Sleep Med.* 2010;11:505–511.

51. Bol S, Caspers J, Buckingham L, et al. Responsiveness of cats (Felidae) to silver vine (*Actinidia polygama*), tatarian honeysuckle (*Lonicera tatarica*), valerian (*Valeriana officinalis*) and catnip (*Nepeta cataria*). *BMC Vet Res.* 2017;13:70.

52. Binks J, Taylor S, Wills A, et al. The behavioural effects of olfactory stimulation on dogs at a rescue shelter. *Appl Anim Behav Sci.* 2018;202:69–76.

53. Uenoyama R, Miyazaki T, Hurst JL, et al. The characteristic response of domestic cats to plant iridoids allows them to gain chemical defense against mosquitoes. *Sci Adv.* 2021; 7(4):eabd9135. doi:10.1126/sciadv.abd91.

54. Zhang, L, John JM. Scratcher preferences of adult in-home cats and effects of olfactory supplements on cat scratching. *Appl Anim Behav Sci.* 2020;227:104997.

55. Shreve KR, Vitale LR, et al. Social interaction, food, scent or toys? A formal assessment of domestic pet and shelter cat (Felis silvestris catus) preferences. *Behav Process.* 2017;141:322–328.

56. Ellis, SLH, Wells DL. The influence of olfactory stimulation on the behaviour of cats housed in a rescue shelter. *Appl Anim Behav Sci.* 2010;123:56.

57. Myatt, AE. *An olfactory enrichment study at the Ashland Cat Shelter. Diss.* Ashland University; 2014. https://etd.ohiolink.edu/apexprod/rws_etd/send_file/send?accession=auhonors1399629978&disposition=inline. Accessed August 7, 2021.

58. Abramson CI, Lay A, Bowser TJ, et al. The use of silver vine (*Actinidia polygama* Maxim, family Actinidiaceae) as an enrichment aid for felines: Issues and prospects. *Am J Anim Vet Sci.* 2012;7(1):21–27.

59. Mills DS, Braem-Dube M, Zulch H. *Stress and Pheromonatherapy in Small Animal Clinical Behavior.* Chichester: Wiley-Blackwell; 2013.

60. Frank D, Beauchamp G, Palestrini C. Systematic review of the use of pheromones for treatment of undesirable behavior in dogs and cats. *J Am Vet Med Assoc.* 2010;236:1308–1316.

61. Chadwin RM, Bain MJ, Kass PH. Effect of a synthetic feline facial pheromone product on stress scores and incidence of upper respiratory infection in cats. *J Am Vet Med Assoc.* 2017;251:413–420.

62. Conti LM, Champion T, Guberman UC, et al. Evaluation of environment and a feline facial pheromone analogue on physiologic and behavioral measures in cats. *J Feline Med Surg.* 2015;19(2):165–170.

63. Broach, D, Dunham, A. Evaluation of a pheromone collar on canine behaviors during transition from foster homes to a training kennel in juvenile military working dogs. *J Vet Behav.* 2016;14:41–51.

64. Taylor S, Webb L, Montrose T, et al. The behavioral and physiological effects of dog appeasing pheromone upon canine behavior during separation from owner. *J Vet Behav.* 2020;40: 36–42.

65. Grigg EK, Piehler M. Influence of dog appeasing pheromone (DAP) on dogs housed in a long-term kennelling facility. *Vet Rec Open.* 2015;2(1). doi:10.1136/vetreco-2014-000098.

66. Sheppard G, Mills, DS. Evaluation of dog-appeasing pheromone as a potential treatment for dogs fearful of fireworks. *Vet Rec.* 2003;152:432–436.

67. Tod E, Brander D, Wran N. Efficacy of a dog appeasing pheromone in reducing stress and fear related behaviour in shelter dogs. *Appl Anim Behav Sci.* 2005;93:295–308.

68. Taylor K, Mills DS. A placebo controlled study to investigate the effect of dog appeasing pheromone and other environmental and management factors on the reports of disturbance and house soiling during the night in recently adopted puppies (*Canis familiaris*). *Appl Anim Behav Sci.* 2007;105:358–368.

69. Da Silva, BPL, Knackfuss FB, Labarthe N, et al. Effect of a synthetic analogue of the feline facial pheromone on salivary cortisol levels in the domestic cat. *Pesqui Vet Bras.* 2017;37(3):287–290.

70. Contreras ET, Hodgkins E, Tynes V, et al. Effect of a pheromone on stress-associated reactivation of feline herpesvirus-1 in experimentally inoculated kittens. *J Vet Int Med.* 2017;32(1)406–417.

71. Cerissa A, Griffith CA, Steigerwald ES, et al. Effects of a synthetic facial pheromone on behavior of cats. *J Am Vet Med Assoc.* 2000;217:1154–1156.

72. Pageat P, Tessier Y. Usefulness of the F3 synthetic pheromone Feliway in

preventing behaviour problems in cats during holidays. In: *Proc. 1st Int Conf Vet Behav Med*. Birmingham: 1997:231.

73. Hunthausen W. Evaluating a feline facial pheromone analogue to control urine spraying. *Vet Med*. 2000;95: 151–156.

74. Ogata N, Takeuchi Y. Clinical trial of a feline pheromone analogue for feline urine marking. *J Vet Med Sci*. 2001;63: 157–161.

75. Mills DS, Mills CB. Evaluation of a novel method for delivering a synthetic analogue of feline facial pheromone to control urine spraying by cats. *Vet Rec*. 2001;149:197–199.

76. Mills DS, Redgate SE, Landsberg GM. A meta-analysis of studies of treatments for feline urine spraying. *PLoS One*. 2011;6:e18448.

77. Gaultier E, Pageat P, Tessier Y. Effect of a feline appeasing pheromone analogue on manifestations of stress in cats during transport. In: *Proceedings of the 32nd Congress of the International Society of Applied Ethology*. Clermont-Ferrand: 1998:198.

78. Kronen PW, Ludders JW, Erb HN, et al. A synthetic fraction of feline facial pheromones calms but does not reduce struggling in cats before venous catheterization. *Vet Anaesth Analg*. 2006;33:258–265.

79. Pereira JS, Fragoso S, Beck A, et al. Improving the feline veterinary consultation: the usefulness of Feliway spray in reducing cats' stress. *J Feline Med Surg*. 2016;18:959–964.

80. Gunn-Moore DA, Cameron ME. A pilot study using synthetic feline facial pheromone for the management of feline idiopathic cystitis. *J Feline Med Surg*. 2004;6:133–138.

81. DePorter T, Bledsoe D, Beck A, et al. Evaluation of the efficacy of an appeasing pheromone diffuser product vs placebo for management of feline aggression in multi-cat households: a pilot study. *J Feline Med Surg*. 2019;21:293–305.

82. Prior, MR, Daniel SM. Cats vs. dogs: the efficacy of Feliway Friends™ and Adaptil™ products in multispecies homes. *Front Vet Sci*. 2020;7:399.

83. De Jaeger X, Meppiel L, Endersby S, et al. An initial open-label study of a novel pheromone complex for use in cats. *Open J Vet Med*. 2021;11:105–116.

84. Siracusa C, Manteca X, Cuenca R, et al. Effect of a synthetic appeasing pheromone on behavioral, neuroendocrine, immune, and acute-phase perioperative stress responses in dogs. *J Am Vet Med Assoc*. 2010;237:673–681.

85. Mills DS, Ramos D, Estelles MG, et al. A triple blind placebo-controlled investigation into the assessment of the effect of dog appeasing pheromone (DAP) on anxiety related behaviour of problem dogs in the veterinary clinic. *Appl Anim Behav Sci*. 2006;98:114–126.

86. Kim Y-M, Lee J-K, Abd el-Aty AM, et al. Efficacy of dog-appeasing pheromone (DAP) for ameliorating separation-related behavioral signs in hospitalized dogs. *Can Vet J*. 2010;1:380–384.

87. Gaultier E, Bonnafous L, Bougrat L, et al. Comparison of the efficacy of a synthetic dog-appeasing pheromone with clomipramine for the treatment of separation-related disorders in dogs. *Vet Rec*. 2005;156:533–538.

88. Amaya V, Paterson MJA, Phillips CJC. Effects of olfactory and auditory enrichment on the behaviour of shelter dogs. *Animals*. 2020;10(4):581.

89. Levine, ED, Ramos, D, Mills, DS. A prospective study of two self help CD based desensitization and counter-conditioning programmes with the use of dog appeasing pheromone for the treatment of firework fears in dogs (*Canis familiaris*). *Appl Anim Behav Sci*. 2007;105:311–329.

90. Landsberg GM, Beck A, Lopez A, et al. Dog appeasing pheromone collars reduce sound-induced fear and anxiety in Beagle dogs: a placebo-controlled study. *Vet Rec*. 2015;10:391–398.

91. Graham D, Mills DS, Bailey G. Evaluation of the effect of temporary exposure to synthetic dog appeasing pheromone (DAP) on levels of arousal in puppy classes. In: Landsberg G, et al. ed. *Proc the 6th IVBM/ECVBM-CA*. Fondazione Iniziative Zooprofilattiche e Zootecniche: Brescia, IT; 2007:133.

92. Gaultier E, Pageat P. Effects of a synthetic dog appeasing pheromone (DAP) on behaviour problems during transport. In: Seksel K, Perry G, Mills D, et al. eds. *Proceedings of the 4th IVBM, Caloundra, Australia*. Post Graduate Foundation in Veterinary Science: Sydney; 2003: 33–35.

93. Estelles MG, Mills DS. Signs of travel-related problems in dogs and their response to treatment with dog-appeasing pheromone. *Vet Rec*. 2006;159:140–148.

94. Santos NR, Beck A, Maenhoudt C, Fontbonne A. Influence of ADAPTIL® during the weaning period: a double-blinded randomised clinical trial. *Animals*. 2020;10:2295.

95. Denenberg S, Landsberg GM. Effect of dog-appeasing pheromones on anxiety and fear in puppies during training its effects on long term socialization. *J Am Vet Med Assoc*. 2008;233:1874–1882.

96. Gaultier E, Bonnafous L, Vienet-Legue D, et al. Efficacy of dog-appeasing pheromone in reducing stress associated with social isolation in newly adopted puppies. *Vet Rec*. 2008;163:73.

97. Gaultier E, Bonnafous L, Vienet-Legue D, et al. Efficacy of dog appeasing pheromone in reducing behaviours associated with fear of unfamiliar people and new surroundings in newly adopted puppies. *Vet Rec*. 2009;164:708–714.

98. Kasbaoui N, Marcet-Rius M, Bienboire-Frosini C, et al. A feline semiochemical composition influences the cat's toileting location choice. *Animals*. 2022;12(7):938. doi.org/10.3390/ani12070938.

99. Lehrner J, Marwinski G, Johren P, et al. Ambient odors of orange and lavender reduce anxiety and improve mood in a dental office. *Physiol Behav*. 2005;86 (1–2):92–95.

100. Atsumi T, Tonosaki K. Smelling lavender and rosemary increases free radical scavenging activity and decreases cortisol level in saliva. *Psychiatry Res*. 2007;150(1): 89–96.

101. Bradshaw RH, Marchant JN, Meredith MJ, et al. Effects of lavender straw on stress and travel sickness in pigs. *J Altern Complement Med*. 1998;4(3):271–275.

102. Wells DL. Aromatherapy for travel-induced excitement in dogs. *J Am Vet Med Assoc*. 2006;229:964–967.

103. Binks J, Taylor S, Wills A, Montrose VT. The behavioural effects of olfactory stimulation on dogs at a rescue centre. *Appl Anim Behav Sci*. 2018;202:69–76.

104. Graham D, Wells DL, Hepper PG. The influence of olfactory stimulation on the behaviour of dogs housed in a shelter. *Appl Anim Behav Sci*. 2005;91:143–153.

105. Murtagh K, Farnworth MJ, Brilot BO, et al. The scent of enrichment: exploring the effect of odour and biological salience on behaviour during enrichment of kennelled dogs. *Appl Anim Behav Sci*. 2020;223:104917.

106. Goodwin, S, Reynolds, H. Can aromatherapy be used to reduce anxiety in hospitalised felines. *Vet Nurse*. 2018: 9(3):167–171.

107. Wells, DL. Aromatherapy for travel-induced excitement in dogs. *J Am Vet Med Assoc*. 2006;229:964–967.

108. Overall KL, Dunham AE. Homeopathy and the curse of the scientific method. *Vet J*. 2009;180:141–148.

109. Bausell RB. *Snake oil science. The Truth About Complementary and Alternative Medicine*. New York: Oxford University Press; 2007.

110. Lees P, Pelligand L, Whiting M, et al. Comparison of veterinary drugs and veterinary homeopathy: Part 2. *Vet Rec*. 2017;181(8):198–207.

111. Cracknell NR, Mills DS. A double-blind placebo-controlled study into the efficacy of a homeopathic remedy for fear of firework noises in the dog (*Canis familiaris*). *Vet J*. 2008;177: 80–88.

112. Cracknell NR, Mills DS. An evaluation of owner expectation on apparent treatment effect in a blinded comparison of two homeopathic remedies for firework noise sensitivity in dogs. *J Vet Behav*. 2011;6:21–30.

113. Maccariello CEM, de Souza CCF, Morena L, et al. Effects of acupuncture on the heart rate variability, cortisol levels and behavioural response induced by thunder sound in beagles. *Physiol Behav*. 2018;186:37–44.

114. Pankratz K, Korman J, Emke C, et al. Randomized, placebo-controlled

prospective Clinical trial evaluating the efficacy of the Assisi anti-anxiety device (calmer canine) for the treatment of canine separation anxiety. *Veterinary Behavior Symposium Proc.* Austin, Tx: 2022:27–28.

115. Milgram NW, Landsberg GM, Snow B. Anxiety reducing effectiveness of Calmz® Anxiety Relief System in beagle dogs in a modified thunderstorm model. *ACVB/AVSAB Vet Behav Sympos Denver.* 2014:29–30.

116. Mira F, Costa A, Mendes E, et al. Influence of music and its genres on respiratory rate and pupil diameter variations in cats under general anesthesia; contribution to promoting patient safety. *J Feline Med Surg.* 2016;18:673–678.

117. Albright JD, Sedigghi RM, Ng Z, et al. Effect of environmental noise and music on dexmedetomidine-induced sedation in dogs. *Peer J.* 2017;5.

118. Snowdon CT, Teie D, Savage M. Cats prefer species appropriate music. *J Appl Anim Behav Sci.* 2015;166:106–110.

119. Hampton A, Ford A, Kox RE. Effects of music on behavior and physiological stress response of domestic cats in a veterinary clinic. *J Feline Med Surg.* 2020;22(2):122–128.

120. Bowman A, Scottish SPCA, Dowell FJ, et al. 'Four seasons' in an animal rescue centre: classical music reduces environmental stress in kenneled dogs. *Physiol Behav.* 2015;143:70–83.

121. Wells DL, Graham L, Hepper PG. The influence of auditory stimulation on the behaviour of dogs housed in a rescue shelter. *Anim Welf.* 2002;11: 385–393.

122. Kogan LR, Schoenfeld-Tacher R, Simon AA. Behavioral effects of auditory stimulation on kenneled dogs. *J Vet Behav.* 2012;7:268–275.

123. Bowman A, Scottish SPCA, Dowell FJ, et al. The effects of different genres of music on the stress level of kenneled dogs. *Physiol Behav.* 2017;171:207–215.

124. Lindig AM, McGreevy P, Crean A, et al. Musical dogs: a review of the influence of auditory enrichment on canine health and behavior. *Animals.* 2020;10(1):127.

125. Brayley C, Montrose VT. The effects of audiobooks on the behavior of dogs in kennels. *Appl Anim Behav Sci.* 2016; 174:111–115.

126. Koster LS, Sithole F, Gilbert GE, et al. The potential beneficial effects of classical music on heart rate variability in dogs used in veterinary training. *J Vet Behav.* 2019;30:103–109.

127. McDonald C, Zaki S. A role for classical music in veterinary practice: does exposure to classical music reduce stress in hospitalised dogs? *Aust Vet J.* 2020;98(1–2):31–36.

128. Engler W, Bain M. Effect of different types of classical music played at a veterinary hospital on dog behavior and owner satisfaction. *J Am Vet Med Assoc.* 2017;251:195–200.

129. King C, Buffington L, Smith TJ, et al. The effect of pressure wrap (ThunderShirt™) on heart rate and behavior in cgruanines diagnosed with anxiety disorder. *J Vet Behav.* 2014;9:215–221.

130. Cottam N, Dodman NH Ha JC. The effectiveness of the anxiety wrap in the treatment of canine thunderstorm phobia: An open-label trial. *J Vet Behav.* 2013;8(3):154–161.

131. Damon M, Rozanski E, Spagnoletti C, et al. Use of the thundershirt to control anxiety in the ICU. *J Vet Emerg Crit Care.* 2014; S5–S6 (abstract). doi:10.1111/vec.12227.

132. Pekkin A, Hänninen L, Tiira K, et al. The effect of a pressure vest on the behavior, salivary cortisol and urine oxytocin of noise phobic dogs in a controlled test. *Appl Anim Behav Sci.* 2016;185:86–94.

133. Buckley LA. Are pressure vests beneficial at reducing stress in anxious and fearful dogs? *Vet Evid.* 2018;3. Available at: https://www.veterinaryevidence.org/index.php/ve/article/view/152.

Resources and recommended reading

Ackerman, L. *Proactive Pet Parenting. Anticipating pet health problems before they happen.* Problem Free Publishing; 2020.

Berk, BA, Packer, RMA, Law, TH, et al. Medium-chain triglycerides dietary supplement improves cognitive abilities in canine epilepsy. *Epilepsy Behav.*, 2021;114:107608. doi:10.1016/j.yebeh.2020.107608.

Buckley, LA. Is alpha-casozepine efficacious at reducing anxiety in dogs? *Vet Evid.* 2017;2(3). doi:10.18849/ve.v2i3.67.

Dramard V, Kern L, Hofmans J, et al. Effect of L-theanine tablets in reducing stress-related emotional signs in cats: an open-label field study. *Irish Vet J.* 2018;7(1). doi:10.1186/s13620-018-0130-4.

Johnson KA. Complementary and alternative veterinary medicine: Where things stand for feline health. *Sci Technol Libr.* 2018;37(4):338-376.

Schwartz S. *Psychoactive Herbs in Veterinary Medicine.* Ames, Iowa: Blackwell; 2005.

Tynes VV, Landsberg GM. Nutritional management of behavior and brain disorders in dogs and cats. *Vet Clin Small Anim.* 2021;51:711–727.

Vaughn D, Kulpa J, Paulionis L. Preliminary investigation of the safety of escalating cannabinoid doses in healthy dogs. *Front Vet Sci.* 2020;7:51. doi:10.3389/fvets.2020.00051.

Vitale, KR. Tools for managing feline problem behaviors: pheromone therapy. *J Feline Med Surg.* 2018;20(11): doi:10.1177/1098612X18806759.

Wakshlag JJ, Schwark WS, Deabold KA, et al. Pharmacokinetics of Cannabidiol, Cannabidiolic Acid, Δ9-Tetrahydrocannabinol, Tetrahydrocannabinolic Acid and Related Metabolites in Canine Serum After Dosing With Three Oral Forms of Hemp Extract. *Front Vet Sci.* 2020;7:505. doi:10.3389/fvets.2020.00505.

CHAPTER 13

Feeding and diet-related problems

Meaghan Ropski, DVM and Amy L. Pike, DVM, DACVB

Introduction

Some pets eat to live and some live to eat. For all animals, food is a primary reinforcer, meaning that it naturally strengthens any response that it follows. See Chapter 10 for a discussion of primary reinforcers. As such, animals do not need to be taught that food is valuable or be exposed to it to find it reinforcing. The importance of food goes beyond what is needed for life or its nutritional value. Eating behavior is one of the first clinical signs noted by pet parents when their pet is ill and is widely regarded by most pet parents as an indicator of quality of life. What, where, and how a pet eats affects its overall wellness and its overall wellness affects its behavior. On a molecular level, individual nutrients can affect pain, neurochemistry, and inflammation, all potentially changing behavioral clinical signs. On the microscopic level, the microbiome is affected by stress and through the gut–brain axis, can increase feelings of stress. The behavior of dogs and cats is influenced by the activities and circumstances associated with eating.

Normal ingestive behavior

It is important to understand the species-typical behavior surrounding the apprehension and ingestion of food in order to create treatment plans for pets which consider welfare and behavior as well as other physical signs. The innate feeding instincts of dogs and cats include both hunting (comprised of prey seeking, stalking, chasing, and killing) and scavenging. These activities utilize energy and are a significant component of an animal's daily time budget.

Studies have found that cats living exclusively outdoors may capture up to 10–20 small prey items per day to satisfy their caloric requirements and that less than half of the capture events are successful.[1,2] Like their wild cousins, domestic cats eat up to 12 small meals over a 24-hour period in darkness and during daylight.[3] The act of hunting or apprehending food is so important to cats that they will even hunt following a meal fed at double the minimum daily requirement.[4] Kittens that watch their mother eat novel foods or are exposed to novel foods with their mother present are more likely to eat novel foods when exposed to them later in life.[5] Kittens that grow up in human households eating one type of food and not being exposed to different foods early in life may be less amenable to diet changes and possibly administration of medication of different flavors or hidden in food. Cats do not appear to be as susceptible to dogs to the influence of other animals on the speed or the amount of food they consume.[6]

Dogs, on the other hand, might spend a large proportion of the day exploring, scavenging, hunting, and catching. Like cats, dogs will eat many small meals throughout the day; however, they generally eat only in the daylight[3] and their ingestive behavior is affected by social facilitation.[7] In addition, humans have selectively bred dogs such as pointers, retrievers, terriers, and setters that can find, track, contain, retrieve, or hunt down prey. These behaviors are innate in many breeds and will be performed even when satiated. Due to the importance of these behaviors to the dog's welfare, behavior problems arise if sufficient attention is not paid to the feeding and hunting requirements that are natural for the species and breed. For more on development of puppies and kittens, see Chapter 2.

The impact of feeding strategy and diet on welfare

What, how much, and the way in which the food is delivered all affect the welfare of the pet. Dogs and cats can be free fed or meal fed. In some cases of possessive aggression in dogs and cats, the recommendation is made to create an environment of plenty by free feeding instead of meal feeding. In this way, anxiety around feeding can be reduced because the animal has control over when it eats and the resource is not scarce. To support that, in one study dogs that are fed free choice displayed less food-related aggression when compared with meal-fed dogs.[8]

Training prior to meals or reserving a part of a meal for training is not an uncommon practice. While this can increase the value of that particular food as a reinforcer for the dog or cat, it can also inhibit learning in some animals and increase irritability and possessive aggression. When calorie reduction is prescribed, care should be taken to also recommend enrichment; low-fat, high-fiber or high-water-content treats (e.g., fruits, vegetables); addition of water or broth to the meal; frequent, smaller feedings; and food toys. In this way, behavior problems and deterioration of the pet's quality of life can be avoided.

The physiological influence of diet on behavior

The nutrients ingested by an animal can have an impact on its behavior. For example, the synthesis of neurotransmitters depends on the availability of circulating precursors which are derived from the diet (tryptophan for serotonin, choline for acetylcholine, and tyrosine for catecholamines – see Chapters 11 and 12) and the ratios of those precursors to other neutral amino acids which may compete for transport into the brain (e.g., serotonin). However, the amount of nutrient ingested, the concentration reaching the brain, and its effect on nerve transmission are not linearly correlated. In fact, in one study in cats comparing the effect on neurotransmission in the dorsal raphe (high concentration of serotonin-containing cells) after feeding various meals with differing amounts of tryptophan and neutral amino acids, there was no increase in neurotransmission regardless of diet.[9]

Dietary ingredients and behavior

It is not unreasonable to assume that some dogs and cats might have behavioral problems related to the ingredients in their diet, and that a change in diet might be a consideration when they display abnormal behavior patterns such as fear, anxiety, stress, aggression, or difficulty training. In dogs, behavior changes alone can be the sole clinical sign of food intolerance such as nonceliac gluten hypersensitivity;[10] however, they can often accompany more common gastrointestinal signs such as vomiting.[11] An elimination diet (i.e., one that does not contain the suspected offending ingredients) or a hydrolyzed diet (i.e., one that breaks the proteins into such small molecules that they are unrecognizable to the immune system) could be used to test this hypothesis. A pet parent simply changing their pet's diet to test their suspicions will likely not be successful if they are not properly educated as to what diet to choose and how it must be the sole source of food and treats for the duration of the trial in order to eliminate the potential offending ingredients.

Protein and tryptophan

Most concerns regarding diet and behavior focus on the role of protein, including quantity, quality, and processing. High-protein diets could conceivably result in lowered levels of the neurotransmitter serotonin in the brain due to the high level of amino acids competing with tryptophan (the serotonin precursor) for the carrier that transports amino acids across the blood–brain barrier. Low serotonin levels have been associated with aggression in some animals.[12] In dogs, a low-protein diet with concurrent tryptophan supplementation may reduce territorial aggression, while a high-protein diet with supplementation or a low-protein diet may reduce dominance aggression.[12] However, when interpreting the results of the aforementioned study, it should be noted that by today's diagnostic standards, most if not all cases previously designated as dominance aggression, would be characterized as fear, conflict, stress induced, impulsive or possessive aggression. See Chapter 23. In a separate population of dogs, low (17%) and medium (25%) protein diets were shown to decrease territorial aggression, but not other forms of aggression.[13] In a series of case reports, a low-protein diet (15–18% protein) reduced aggressive behavior; however, there were no controls or statistical analysis.[14] Studies that measure serotonin metabolites in the cerebrospinal fluid after ingestion of diets with a variety of protein levels in dogs have found no differences regardless of diet fed.[15] Most recently, no measurable impact of dietary protein levels was found on the behavior of Golden Retrievers.[16] In a preliminary placebo-controlled study, supplementation with L-tryptophan led to a reduction of stress-related behaviors and a decrease in anxiety signals in both dogs and cats.[17] In another study, dogs were fed either a control diet with 0.18% tryptophan or one of three other diets with successively higher levels of tryptophan for 24 weeks, and no change was seen in behaviors when approached by a person, whether unfamiliar or familiar.[18]

Several diets containing L-tryptophan are available, including Royal Canin Calm Canine and Feline, Hill's Pet Nutrition Prescription Diet c/d Multicare Urinary Stress, and Hill's Pet Nutrition Prescription Diet i/d Digestive Care (see Chapter 12). The Royal Canin Calm diet contains vitamin B_6 and alpha-casozepine as well as L-tryptophan (in an increased ratio to other large amino acids). In one canine study, feeding for seven weeks resulted in significant reductions in four anxiety-related behaviors when compared with a group which was fed a control diet. In addition, dogs that were exposed to a stressor (toenail trim) while being fed the diet showed reduced stress response (as measured by urine cortisol creatinine ratio).[19] Further studies are needed to determine the cause of the observed reduction in stress (whether tryptophan supplementation, protein reduction, supplementation of casozepine, or a combined effect). In a second study, where dogs were fed a diet with caseinate hydrolysate as the only additive, there were no significant changes on anxiety scores, lysozyme, neutrophil:lymphocyte ratio, or heart rate in dogs fed the diet for four weeks when compared to dogs fed a control diet, although dogs fed the treatment diet had significantly decreased cortisol levels.[20] See Chapters 11 and 12 for more information on tryptophan.

Carbohydrate

Carbohydrates have not been as widely investigated in dog and cat diets as they relate to behavioral clinical signs when compared with protein; however, there are several studies which have attempted to examine the effect in dogs. As tryptophan competes with other large neutral amino acids (LNAA) (leucine, isoleucine, valine, tyrosine, and phenylalanine) for the transport across the blood–brain barrier, the ratios of those proteins to tryptophan will affect the amount of tryptophan crossing into the brain and therefore available for synthesis of serotonin. In rats, a large-carbohydrate, protein-free meal increases tryptophan concentrations in the brain and increases subsequent serotonin synthesis.[21] It has been suggested that this effect is due to insulin secretion shunting the LNAAs into the muscle, leaving tryptophan to enter the brain unencumbered by competition.

In one study comparing an isoenergetic diet (vegetable protein, higher in carbohydrates) and isonitrogenous diet (animal protein, lower level of carbohydrates) fed to dogs for 40 days, no significant differences were found between the groups regarding aggressive and nonaggressive reactions.[22] In a smaller study of three dogs, blood was collected 8 hours after carbohydrate meal and serum levels of cortisol, tryptophan, and serotonin were measured. No differences were found after ingestion of a carbohydrate meal in any of the parameters measured.[23] While observed experimentally in rodents, there appears to be an effect on levels of tryptophan and serotonin; that has not been shown in dogs. There have been no published studies on the effects of carbohydrate ingestion and behavioral clinical signs in cats.

Preservatives, additives, and natural diets

"Natural" diets with no artificial preservatives are popular with many pet parents. Additionally, there is speculation on how preservatives and food additives affect behavior. However, the evidence is lacking in dogs and cats that preservatives have significant impact on behavior. A study published in 1980 examined the behavior of "hyperactive" Beagle crosses when fed hydroxyanisole and Food, Drug and Cosmetic red dye number 40 and found no relationship between the ingestion of the additives and level of activity.[24] At present, there is no published evidence that preservatives or food coloring have any effect on the behavior of dogs and cats.

Fatty acids

While the essential fatty acids (*cis*-linoleic acid in the dog and *cis*-linoleic acid and arachidonic acid in the cat) are, by definition, essential for life, attention has been focused recently on the long-chain omega-3 fatty acids, specifically docosahexaenoic acid (DHA) and to a lesser extent eicosapentaenoic acid (EPA). DHA, while technically not considered essential, is important in neural and retinal development, neurotransmission, immune function and cognitive function. Also see Chapter 8.[25-28] EPA is an important antiinflammatory agent used in the treatment of atopic dermatitis and degenerative joint disease.[25,26] Supplementation with DHA-rich dietary oils results in higher circulating levels of DHA,[26,27] which cannot be easily achieved with shorter-chain omega-3 fatty acids such as alpha-linolenic acid, especially after weaning.[26] Due to the inefficiency in converting alpha-linolenic acid to EPA and DHA, supplementing with the preformed dietary long-chain fatty acids, typically derived from marine oils, is preferred.[28] DHA is especially important for neuronal development and health. Throughout life, it is concentrated in the membranes of neurons and affects the activity of the structures reliant on the health of the membrane such as membrane-bound proteins, receptors, and enzymes.[29] It is hypothesized that the behavior (e.g., binding, reuptake, metabolism, catabolism) of neurotransmitters such as catecholamines (e.g., norepinephrine, dopamine) could be affected by deficiencies in DHA because their activities are dependent on a healthy neuronal membrane.

Omega-3 and omega-6 fatty acids have been extensively investigated in adults with depression,[29] children with attention deficit-hyperactivity disorder,[30] bipolar disorder, posttraumatic stress disorder, and schizophrenia.[29] In some studies, supplementation is successful in alleviating clinical signs, while in others it appears that only certain individuals who have a deficit in fatty acids will respond. In still others, the ratio of the fatty acids is paramount to successful treatment with supplementation. One current hypothesis is that humans who respond have a genetic predisposition to alterations in fatty acids. More investigation is needed.

In addition to retinal function and brain development, an improvement in the performance of memory and learning tasks, trainability, cognitive function, psychomotor function, immunologic function, and problem-solving skills has been demonstrated in puppies with DHA supplementation.[25,26,28] Therefore, there may be benefits for supplementing pet diets with DHA-rich fatty acids during gestation, lactation, and the immediate postweaning period to 16 weeks of age, as well as in senior pets with cognitive dysfunction. Aggressive German Shepherd Dogs may have a lower DHA concentration and higher omega-6/omega-3 ratio when compared to nonaggressive dogs.[31] In another study of German Shepherd Dogs with attention deficit-hyperactivity disorder-like behaviors, they were found to have lower serum phospholipid levels and higher arachidonic acid levels.[32] Older Beagles fed a diet with DHA supplementation showed improved initial learning on contrast discrimination tests but not improved long-term recall of the task.[33] Currently, there are no published studies investigating the effects of fatty acid supplementation in cats. Ratios of omega-3 to omega-6 may be just as important as individual levels of DHA and EPA. The ratio of omega-3 to omega-6 has been investigated in humans with acute stress (oral examination), depression, hyperactivity, and schizophrenia with mixed results.[34]

Probiotics and the role of the gut microbiome

The gut microbiome is made up of the trillions of bacteria within the gastrointestinal tract that work to protect against pathogens, synthesize vitamins, support the immune system, and modulate the central nervous system. The parasympathetic and sympathetic nervous systems allow bidirectional communication between the gastrointestinal and central nervous systems.[35] Along with the gut microbiome, this is referred to as the gut–brain axis. As the communication is bidirectional, the brain can, when there is emotional stress, cause gastrointestinal upset, nausea, hypermotility, and inappetence. Conversely, when there is disease in the gut, signals are sent to the brain which can contribute to anxiety, stress, and fear. In dogs, the gut microbiome has been associated with changes in aggression, anxiety, and memory performance.[36,37] A study comparing the gut microbiome of aggressive and nonaggressive dogs, although limited by sample size, demonstrated a difference in the bacterial clades between the two groups and indicated a link between aggression and gut microbiome.[36] In addition, the gut microbiome plays a role in the production of monoamine neurotransmitter precursors and gamma aminobutyric acid (GABA), which modulate fear, anxiety, aggression, hypervigilance, muscle tension, and stress.[38]

Probiotics are living bacteria that are ingested to confer health benefits to the host. Calming Care (Purina) contains *Bifidobacterium longum* (BL999), which has been shown to reduce the clinical signs associated with anxiety in dogs. In a study of 24 anxious Labrador Retrievers, those treated with Calming Care displayed less anxious behavior, decreased salivary cortisol concentration, decreased heart rate, and increased heart rate variability [a measure of decreased sympathetic nervous system (SNS) activation] when exposed to stressful stimuli.[39] In a study evaluating the effects of the feline product in a shelter environment, cats were significantly less likely to have sneezing associated with feline herpes virus (FHV-1), to have abnormal serum cortisol levels, and to pace in cages compared to placebo when exposed to mild stress from change in housing.[40] See Chapter 12.

Vitamins

The eight B vitamins are B_1 (thiamine), B_2 (riboflavin), B_3 (niacin), B_5 (pantothenic acid), B_6 (pyridoxine), B_7 (biotin), B_9 (folate), and B_{12} (cobalamin). They are not synthesized in the body of dogs and cats and must be supplied in the diet. Neurotropic B vitamins include B_1, B_6, and B_{12}, which act specifically in the central and peripheral nervous systems. Vitamin B_1 plays a part in the maintenance of nerve membrane function, energy metabolism in nerve cells, and the synthesis of myelin, acetylcholine, serotonin, and amino acids.[41] Vitamin B_3 (nicotinamide) increases the affinity of GABA for its receptors. GABA is the most prevalent modulator of excitatory neurotransmission in the brain. Vitamin B_6 (pyridoxine) aids in the production of serotonin, GABA, and norepinephrine, and has neuroprotective qualities.[18,42] It has been investigated in rats as an adjunctive treatment for depression and obsessive-compulsive behavior when administered with clomipramine, venlafaxine, and fluoxetine. In this study, there were no significant differences in behavior when supplemented with B_6.[43] Vitamin B_{12} acts as a cofactor in biochemical processes intended to maintain nervous system health. Supplementation with B vitamins with direct measurement of behavioral effects is lacking and may be a promising focus of study in the future.

Commercial diets with efficacy in behavioral medicine

High-quality commercial diets have been shown to decrease the incidence of cognitive dysfunction.[44] See Chapter 8. Other commercial diets with published behavioral effects are mentioned above and in Chapter 12.

Diagnosis of diet-related behavior problems

Behavioral assessment should include an evaluation of whether the pet has sufficient outlets to display its natural repertoire of behaviors, including the time and activities that would normally be spent in food acquisition. Treatment might require more stimulating, time-consuming, and natural ways for pets to feed. Although feeding live prey or dead carcasses is impractical and likely undesirable from the human perspective, providing toys and feeders that require physical manipulation to release the food, utilizing search games where the pet has to find its food, conditioning the pet to receive pieces of its food as a reinforcement for a desirable behavior (i.e., training), or stuffing food in toys and freezing can increase the work, mental enrichment, and daily time budget required to obtain food rewards (see Chapters 5 and 10).

If diet is implicated as a contributing factor to behavioral clinical signs, a diet trial can be prescribed, monitoring for changes in behavioral clinical signs. Diets with single novel protein sources, novel protein and carbohydrate sources, and hydrolyzed diets are commercially available.[45] Diet trials to assess for behavioral effects may not be as simple as novel ingredient or hypoallergenic diets because the inciting factor may be the relative concentration of ingredients (e.g., protein, carbohydrate). Commercially available diets may not be adequate, and the pet may need a homemade diet trial. Any homemade diet should be nutritionally balanced by a board-certified veterinary nutritionist (https://acvn.org/nutrition-consults/) to ensure adequate nutrition and appropriate selection of the elimination diet. If the behavioral clinical signs are consistent with those which are responsive to changes in protein (see above), it may be an option to test the response to protein levels by feeding a reduced protein-canned diet with ratios matching published evidence in that species (e.g., prescription formulas designed for renal disease), which would provide a balanced restricted protein diet.

In the studies referenced in the sections above, dogs were fed the same diet for 40 days to 24 weeks. While improvements may be seen in a shorter time frame, these studies may be used as a guide for the amount of time needed for a behavioral diet trial; however, evidence is lacking at this time regarding the length of trial necessary for determination of the contribution of ingredients to behavioral clinical signs. To assess the effect of diet on behavior, diet trials can be conducted by referencing current recommendations regarding length for other body systems such as dermatological, nutritional, and gastrointestinal. Prior to a trial with any new diet as a part of a behavioral assessment, the patient should receive a complete physical examination, complete blood count (CBC), serum chemistry, $fT4_{ED}$ (free T4 by equilibrium dialysis), and urinalysis to assess overall health and wellness.

Pet parents often express that they have tried hypoallergenic or elimination diets in the past. Unfortunately, some retail pet foods marketed as hypoallergenic have been found to contain known food allergens.[46] In addition, behavioral clinical signs are not necessarily attributable to the presence of the nutritional substance, but instead may be caused by the ratios of those substances. Therefore, if an adverse food reaction is still a consideration, a completely novel protein source from a prescription diet with verified ingredients that the pet has never been fed should be recommended. When performing an elimination diet trial, strict pet parent compliance is paramount and must be emphasized.

Treatment of diet-related behavior problems

If there is a positive response to the elimination diet trial, the pet parent can be given the option of challenging with specific ingredients (e.g., individual protein sources, additives, preservatives) to assess their effect on the pet's behavior rather than continuing to feed the test diet indefinitely. For animals that respond to a diet trial and the pet parent elects to challenge with ingredients or ratios of ingredients, it should be made clear that at this time there is no published best practice for length of trial. Following with the recommendations made for patients with adverse food reactions, challenges should last 7–10 days at minimum before considering items tolerable (items causing issues at any time after feeding can be considered problematic); however, as above, it is unclear if longer or shorter time periods are necessary when assessing behavioral clinical signs. If pet parents are selecting their own foods from a pet supply outlet, they must look for diets which substantially match the formulation of the trial food or that are devoid of the items determined to be problematic.

If it is suspected that the behavioral clinical signs are a result of an additive such as a preservative, canned foods may be an option and there are also preservative-free diets commercially available. Although it is unlikely that a pet's behavior is affected by preservatives (e.g., ethoxyquin, butylated hydroxyanisole, butylated hydroxytoluene), canned diets contain the least amount of preservatives. Home-delivered, preservative-free, and home-prepared pet foods are all options with which veterinarians should become familiar. However, as discussed above, current regulations make it almost impossible to be assured that there are actually no preservatives in preservative-free diets. Manufacturers only need to list on the label those preservatives that they add themselves during ration preparation. Therefore, there is no guarantee that the manufacturer did not purchase the raw ingredients already preserved. If the pet improves when placed on a homemade diet, then the role of additives must also be considered. If the decision is made to maintain the pet on a homemade diet, a diet recipe prepared by a veterinary nutritionist is highly recommended; computer software is available so that customized diets can be formulated by practitioners, and web-based options are also available. See American College of Veterinary Nutrition (acvn.org) for more information.

Prevention of diet-related behavior problems

Aside from studies investigating specific vitamins and essential fatty acids, there is little research from which to glean preventive strategies regarding nutrition as it applies to behavior disorders. Nutrition as it relates to behavior appears to be linked somewhat to the genetic makeup of that particular dog or cat. Epigenetics is the study of heritable changes in phenotype or gene expression due to mechanisms other than DNA mutations (see Chapter 3). The interaction of nutrients with genetic and epigenetic traits is sometimes referred to as nutritional genomics or nutrigenomics. Nutrients may affect the expression of a certain genetic trait, make a pet more or less susceptible to disease processes, and have a variety of other positive or negative effects. This will become progressively more important in veterinary medicine as researchers find links between genetic profiles and disease, the impact of diet on epigenetic inheritance, and the effects of diet on gene transcription and translation rates.[47]

There may be genetic factors associated with diet and there is some anecdotal evidence that behavior problems due to some dietary ingredients may be familial. It has been suggested that some breeds seem to react to preservatives (e.g., Cavalier King Charles Spaniels), some to exorphins (Golden Retrievers), and others to serotonin-influencing factors of different meat proteins.[48] In addition, mutations of the proopiomelanocortin (POMC) gene in some Labrador Retrievers has been shown to mediate increased appetite and obesity, which could have significant impact on behavior, including food stealing and begging behavior.[49] Continued research is needed to confirm these possibilities. Neutering animals with these dietary idiosyncrasies and gene abnormalities will lessen the contribution of any hereditary factors to the breed gene pool. See Chapter 3 for an in-depth discussion of the role of genetics in behavior.

Presentation

James, a neutered male 12-year-old, 24-kg English Springer Spaniel, had become increasingly anxious and aggressive in the past year.

History

When familiar relatives and friends visited the home, he greeted them at the door by wagging his tail level with his back, with a loose body posture, ears in neutral position, and his mouth hanging open softly. When they reached for him, he had growled and snapped. When resting on the couch, the pet parents' bed, or his bed, and someone reached for him, he growled. The pet parents reported that behavior previously and that it continues occasionally, even though James appeared to enjoy resting on the couch. Even when he seemed happy, if they reached to pet him, he would growl and/or get up and move away. When they tried to remove food items or his food, he growled but would eventually let them take it. He had been chewing and licking both front feet and carpi for a duration of about a year. In addition, he had developed otitis externa about 1.5 years earlier, which had become chronic. At the time of his third otitis externa flare-up, about nine months earlier, James was placed on a daily prednisone/antihistamine combination, which had been weaned down to every other day for the past six months. This prevented further ear flare-ups, although some of the skin chewing persisted. The pet parents had tried a commercial fish-based diet (for sensitive skin), an organic beef-based preservative-free commercial food, and a bones and raw food (BARF) diet, with no success.

Workup

The diagnostic workup included skin scraping, tape prep, ear cytology, physical examination, CBC, serum chemistry, fT4$_{ED}$, and urinalysis. No primary lesions were found. Malassezia were found on cytology in both ears. All blood parameters were within normal limits. No pain was found on physical examination; however, salivary staining was present on both front paws and carpi.

Differential diagnoses

Dermatologic differential diagnoses included yeast otitis externa, atopic dermatitis, adverse food reactions, or other inflammatory dermatologic disease. While atopic dermatitis is less likely to be first detected in older pets, it remained a consideration because of the presenting signs. Differential diagnoses for aggression to familiar people included: iatrogenic (prednisone), pain-induced aggression (associated with otitis externa), stress-induced aggression (underlying systemic disease such as dermatologic disease), conflict-induced aggression (familiar people only), fear-induced aggression, and attention-seeking behavior.

Treatment

James was placed on a novel protein diet for eight weeks to investigate the role of diet further. As the pet parents also needed treats for training

(e.g., to give up toys and greet visitors), a hydrolyzed protein treat was also dispensed. The yeast otitis was treated with systemic medication to avoid any potential conflict involved with manipulating the ears. The behavioral plan included avoiding interactions which induced aggression (e.g., reaching for him, James greeting people at the door, allowing him on the couch or bed, people approaching him when he was on his bed), behavioral treatments focused on functional behaviors to help the pet parents interact with him safely (e.g., leave it/drop it, off, go to your spot), and slow discontinuation of the oral corticosteroids. The use of psychotropic medications and supplements were discussed with the pet parents; however, they were not recommended at the first appointment because of the strong suspicion of a component of pain (otitis externa) and discomfort pruritus.

Follow-up

At the eight-week reexamination visit, the otitis externa had resolved and the foreleg licking had ceased. The pet parents were not keeping him from the front door or off of the couch and bed. They had, however, asked visitors to stop reaching for him and had themselves stopped reaching for him when he was lying down. They had taught drop it, but no other behaviors. James had not showed aggression in four weeks when visitors came into the home or when the pet parents tried to take things from him (they used the drop it cue). By this time, the corticosteroids had been discontinued.

The diet was continued for four more weeks, at which point the pet parents indicated that the aggression around food items had disappeared entirely even when they did not use the drop it cue. They had allowed familiar visitors to the home to reach for him with no aggression in four weeks. They continued to avoid reaching for him when he was sleeping. A presumptive diagnosis of adverse food reaction was made, and the pet parents elected to continue a maintenance form of the elimination diet indefinitely.

Discussion

The causes in this case are multifactorial. This patient's behavioral clinical signs may have been entirely due to the pain and discomfort of dermatologic disease and otitis externa, and the use of prednisone. See Chapters 6 for more information on how prednisone can affect behavior. In addition, there are most likely genetic reasons that this particular dog responded to discomfort and prednisone with aggression instead of retreat, for example. See Chapter 3 for more information on how genetics affect behavior. The most likely behavioral diagnoses in this case are stress induced aggression and pain-induced aggression. In this case, because the diet change and treatment of the otitis externa appeared to control the aggression or at least contributed significantly, dietary management should be continued indefinitely. Also, because of the probability of this patient showing aggression as a side effect of prednisone, this medication should be avoided, if possible, in the future.

Ingestive behavior problems

Unlike many of us, dogs and cats usually eat less when they are stressed. However, some stressed animals have an increased appetite, eat nonfood items, eat grass, or have a change in eating speed. Appetite changes can be a result of systemic disease or emotional stress. For this reason, it is important that the overall health of the pet be assessed including a physical examination and any indicated tests.

Ingestive behavior problems may be related to management issues (e.g., obesity), undesirable but normal behaviors (e.g., food stealing/garbage raiding), medication or physical illness-induced ingestive disorders (polyphagia due to corticosteroid administration or hyperadrenocorticism; environmental licking due to gastrointestinal upset), and

abnormal ingestive behaviors such as pica. In cats, ingestive problems were the third most common reason for referral at one behavior practice, comprising 4.3% of 736 referral cases (of which 40% were Siamese cats with pica).[50] In dogs, abnormal ingestive behaviors (e.g., pica, coprophagia, hyperphagia, anorexia, excessive chewing and licking) represented 1.4% of 1644 referral cases.[51] More recent studies have reiterated the importance of a full medical workup and the likelihood that pica may be a primary medical diagnosis.[52,53]

Ingestive behavior as a measure of stress

As most animals eat less when they are stressed, level of appetite can be used to measure stress. For example, if in general the dog or cat has a good appetite at home but does not eat when in the car or at the veterinarian's office, those situations are most likely stressful. Stress can often be reduced (if there is no nausea component) by using foods which are very enticing in those situations. Appetite stimulants can also be used (see below) to increase the pet's appetite, enticing them to eat and potentially lowering stress. For situations such as car rides, motion sickness must be ruled out if there are any clinical signs associated with car rides (see Chapters 6 and 9).

Some dogs and cats are fearful and will not approach the food bowl or area where they are fed. This can be due to a traumatic incident in that area or with the food bowl itself. Pet parents can vary where the food bowl is placed and try different types of bowls or plates for feeding.

Obesity

Obesity is the most common companion animal nutritional disorder in North America.[54] A sad statistic is that over half of all dogs are overweight.[55] This is a worldwide problem with an estimated 60% of cats in the United States and 48% of cats in the United Kingdom qualifying as overweight or obese.[56,57] Initially, body fat was thought of as a rather inert substance, but it is now known to be an important endocrine organ and initiator of inflammation. White adipose tissue, the accumulation of adipocytes referred to as "fat," secretes a variety of adipokines (such as leptin, adiponectin, resistin, interleukin-6) that have metabolic and endocrine functions. As adipocytes enlarge by storing increasing amounts of free fatty acids, there are a variety of systemic effects, including the release of proinflammatory cytokines. Due to these wide-ranging effects, obesity is sometimes referred to as a "disease" rather than a "condition" – one that warrants aggressive treatment.[58]

Obesity is a disease that directly affects the animal's welfare and quality of life. Dogs and cats are more likely to suffer from osteoarthritis, tracheal collapse, respiratory distress, diabetes mellitus, hepatic lipidosis (cats), hypertension, decreased heat tolerance, some forms of cancer, reduced longevity, and increased anesthesia and surgical risks.[59,60] Obesity may also be associated with feline urinary tract disease, canine urinary tract infections, altered cardiorespiratory function, and liver dysfunction. Overweight pets are less active and may be less social.[60] Pets that are uncomfortable due to systemic disease or osteoarthritis are more likely to exhibit pain-induced aggression and irritable aggression. In addition, they may show anxiety and aggression in circumstances where they anticipate pain, such as the approach of a housemate or walking across a slick floor. Finally, cats that are in pain and overweight often have trouble getting into the litterbox, leading to elimination disorders such as feline periuria.

Obesity becomes more common as pets get older. Females are more prone to obesity than males, and neutered pets are more likely to become obese than intact pets.[59,60] Genetic factors are also contributory.[59] Labrador Retrievers, Cocker Spaniels, Collies, Dachshunds, Cavalier King Charles Spaniels, Beagles, Basset Hounds, Miniature Schnauzers, Shetland Sheepdogs, and some terriers are more prone to obesity than other breeds.[59,61,62] Labrador Retrievers may also carry the deletion mutation of the POMC gene in some which has been shown to mediate increased appetite and obesity.[60] Some breeds, most notably the German Shepherd Dog, Boxer, Whippet, and Greyhound, actually have a lower incidence of obesity.

Although genetics play a role, so does caloric intake and physical activity.[59,60] The pet food industry markets highly palatable, energy-dense, high-calorie diets with a focus on the consumer.[59] The supplement market contributes biscuit treats and fatty acid supplements that are usually calorie dense. The pet parent, with a strong emotional bond to the pet, wants to provide a healthy, tasty meal that the pet readily devours. Food is love to many pet parents. The veterinarian must counsel the pet parent about what is in the best interest of the pet while also considering the risks to the welfare and behavioral risks to the pet (e.g., decreased obedience from less reinforcement with food, increased aggression), which can accompany calorie restriction and reducing diets.

Prevention

Unfortunately, once excess weight is gained, calorie restriction and changing feeding practices can be challenging for pet parents to implement successfully. As always, preventing weight gain in pets is more desirable than assisting in weight loss. Understanding of predisposing factors in the development of unhealthy weight gain allows the veterinarian to design a preventative plan, educate pet parents with accurate information, and engage the pet parent in proper treatment. The family should be educated on proper feeding guidelines based on the veterinarian's assessment (not the pet parent's) of the pet's body condition, spay/neuter status, breed predispositions, lifestyle, and actual activity level. Pet parents should understand that the feeding guidelines on the label of their pet's food are suggestions, not necessarily the ideal amount of food for their pet. In addition, warning pet parents of the side effects of gonadectomy such as decreased activity and weight gain.

In cats, the most common predictors of being overweight were being neutered, middle-aged (over three years), mixed breed, pet parents underestimating body condition, primarily dry diet (cats 12 to 13 months), and apartment dwelling[63–66] (see Box 13.1). Some factors appear to protect against obesity in cats, such as the presence of a dog or other cats, in the household, presence of a sanctuary space, elimination outside (this may be due to increased exercise when outside), being outdoors, and less time alone in the house (half day as opposed to all day)[67] (see Box 13.2).

Box 13.1 Factors predisposing to obesity in cats

- Apartment dwelling
- Indoor only
- Mixed breed
- Pet parents underestimating body condition
- Primarily dry diet (especially in cats 12 to 13 months)
- Gonadectomized
- Middle-aged

Box 13.2 Factors protecting against obesity in cats

- Presence of a dog or other cats
- Access to outdoors
- Presence of a sanctuary space
- Less time alone

A preventative plan for cats should include canned food as a part of the daily ration, feeding from food toys to increase exercise and enrichment and decrease rate of eating and spread the food over multiple small meals throughout the day, safe catio or outdoor time, adding another pet to the house (ideally adopting two bonded cats at the same time), using small treats, creation of a sanctuary space, and play time with family (see Box 13.3, Figures 13.1–13.5).

Box 13.3 Preventative plan for obesity in cats

- Educate
  - Prepare pet parents that weight gain and decreased energy are likely after gonadectomy.
  - The ration amount on the pet food package is a suggestion which is likely to be too many calories for the average pet.
- Food type
  - Canned food as a part of the daily ration.
- Lifestyle
  - Play regularly.
  - Allow access to a safe catio, enclosure, or walk on leash.
  - Consider adding another cat or a dog to the household.
  - Create a sanctuary space as soon as possible after adoption.
- Food delivery
  - Feed all food from food toys if possible from the day of adoption to facilitate movement and increasing calorie expenditure. Food toys will also slow the rate of eating, leaving pets satiated when eating less food.
  - Consider recommending multiple small meals and automatic feeders.
- Treats
  - One treat should be given for each positive behavior.
  - Breaking treats in half is acceptable so that the treat is 1/8 of an inch.
  - Treats should be calculated into the total daily calorie count and should not exceed more than 10% of daily nutrition.

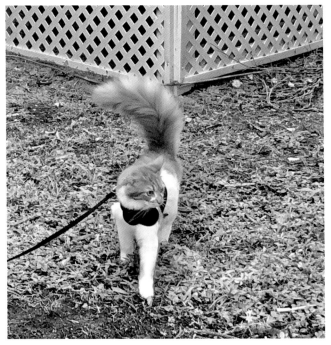

Figure 13.2 Cats can be trained to walk on leash. *(Attribution: Alison Gerken, DVM.)*

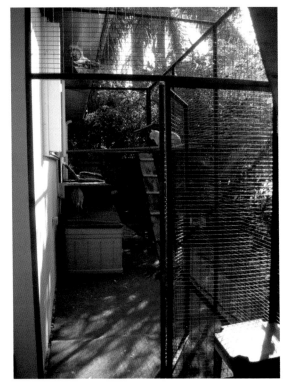

Figure 13.1 A "catio" or safe, enclosed outdoor area, provides enrichment and encourages exercise. *(Attribution: Lisa Radosta.)*

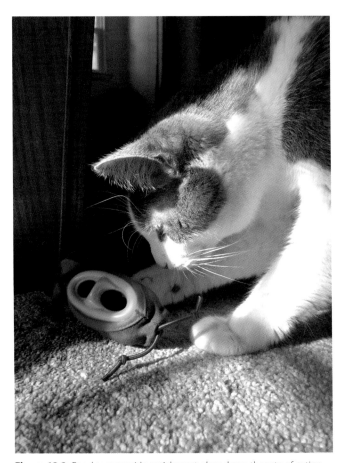

Figure 13.3 Food toys provide enrichment, slow down the rate of eating, mimic more "natural" eating patterns, and encourage exercise. *(Attribution: Meaghan Ropski.)*

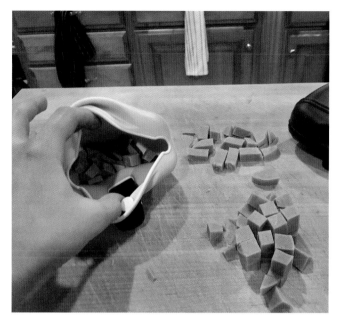

Figure 13.4 Food rewards should be about 1/8 of an inch in size. *(Attribution: Meaghan Ropski.)*

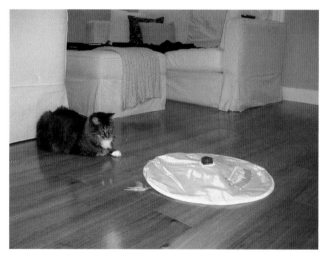

Figure 13.5 Predatory toys encourage exercise and provide environmental enrichment. *(Attribution: Lisa Radosta.)*

Box 13.4 Contributing factors for obesity in dogs

- Lack of exercise
- Lower income-earning pet parent
- Feeding table scraps
- Pet parent age
- Excess number of treats given
- Breed
  - Decreased risk: German Shepherd Dog, Boxer, Whippet, and Greyhound
  - Increased risk: Cocker Spaniel, Golden Retriever, Labrador Retriever, Cairn Terrier, Scottish Terrier, Cavalier King Charles Spaniel, Beagle, Dachshund, Basset Hound, Collie, Rottweiler, Bernese Mountain Dog, Newfoundland, Saint Bernard
- Neutered
- Female
- Age over eight years

Edney AT, Smith PM. Study of obesity in dogs visiting veterinary practices in the United Kingdom. *Vet Rec.* 1986;118:391–396.

Box 13.5 Preventative plan for obesity in dogs

- Educate
  - Prepare pet parents that weight gain and decreased energy are likely after gonadectomy.
  - The ration amount on the pet food package is a suggestion which is likely to be too many calories for the average pet.
- Food type
  - Reducing diets should be considered when significant weight gain is noted.
- Lifestyle
  - Play regularly.
  - Increase exercise.
- Food delivery
  - Feed all food from food toys if possible from the day of adoption to facilitate movement and increasing calorie expenditure. Food toys will also slow the rate of eating, leaving pets satiated when eating less food.
- Treats
  - One treat should be given for each positive behavior.
  - Treat calories should be calculated into the total daily calorie count and should not exceed more than 10% of daily nutrition.
  - Use small, low-calorie treats.
  - Breaking treats in half is acceptable so that the treat is 1/4 of an inch for medium to large dogs and 1/8 of an inch for smaller dogs.

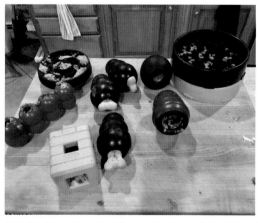

Figure 13.6 Food toys slow down the rate of eating and provide enrichment. *(Attribution: Meaghan Ropski.)*

In dogs, contributing factors in obesity include sex (female), breed (Cocker Spaniel, Golden Retriever, Labrador Retriever, Cairn Terrier, Scottish Terrier, Cavalier King Charles Spaniel, Beagle), neuter status (neutered), age (over eight years), pet parent's age and income, treats given, exercise, and eating table scraps[60,68] (see Box 13.4).

A preventative plan for dogs should include increasing exercise within the limits of the dog's overall health, feeding from food toys to increase exercise, providing environmental enrichment, decreasing the rate of eating, following diets after spay/neuter, and having play time with family (see Box 13.5, Figures 13.6–13.8).

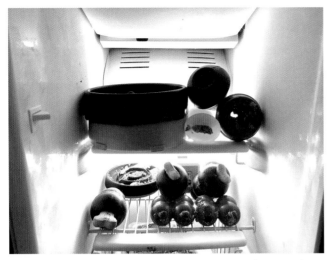

Figure 13.7 Freezing food toys can further slow the rate of eating and provide much needed mental stimulation. *(Attribution: Meaghan Ropski.)*

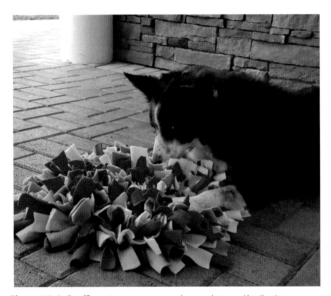

Figure 13.8 Snuffle mats are easy-to-make puzzle toys. *(Attribution: Mindy Cox, CPDT-KSA.)*

Diagnosis and prognosis

The diagnosis and treatment of obesity in cats and dogs is described more fully elsewhere. The discussion of these topics here will be the behavioral strategies to minimize welfare and worsening of behavior problems with caloric restriction and behavior modalities which can facilitate the treatment of obesity.

Pets are considered overweight when they are 15% above their ideal weight and obese when they are 30% more than their ideal weight, although there is quite a bit of variability in how the terms are defined.[69,70] This can be assessed by visual inspection (fat covering of ribs) and palpation. Body condition scoring (BCS) uses a scale to evaluate body fat subjectively and semiquantitatively by visual assessment and

palpation. The 9-point numeric scoring system for BCS is commonly used (see Figure 13.9 and WSAVA global nutrition guidelines https://wasava.org/global-guidelines/global-nutrition-guidelines/). BCS should be evaluated and appropriate dietary recommendations discussed at each visit. Using the BCS is just one of the ways that body condition is evaluated. There is a fair chance that individual veterinarians may score the same dog differently. This is impossible to avoid, considering the subjective nature of the BCS. Most important when using BCS is that individual veterinarians are consistent in their own scoring.

The first step of weight management is to determine the reason for the obesity and calculate the amount of calories/joules the pet needs per day. All obese pets should have a thorough physical examination and laboratory profile, including complete blood count, chemistry panel, urinalysis, thyroid profile, blood pressure, and if indicated, imaging to rule out physical causes.

The second step is education. Pet parents may not be aware that they or certain members of the household are overfeeding the pet. Other times, there is a family dynamic which will prohibit changes such as an elderly parent who feeds the pet or a child who tosses food. The family dynamics around feeding can be complicated. Providing calorically dense treats and leftovers from the dinner table is an important interaction for many pet parents but adds additional energy to the pet's daily total about which most pet parents are unaware. Many over-the-counter supplements such as fish oil and fatty acids are also calorie dense and are most often not accounted for in the total daily intake.

Third, determine how and where the pet is fed as well as any potential behavioral fallout to the changes that are being recommended. For example, if food is left available all day, many pets will not limit themselves to the appropriate number of calories. On the other hand, anxious or fearful dogs may only eat when alone, when the pet parent is present, or when fed free choice. Pet parents of obese animals are commonly overweight themselves, making this an awkward and emotionally sensitive topic that veterinarians must address accordingly.[59,60] Veterinarians counseling pet parents of obese pets must be prepared to determine the animal's caloric needs, all calorie contributors in the pet's diet, and the amount of energy-burning activities in the pet's lifestyle. Most pet parents are able to manage the problem effectively with proper guidance, and prognosis is favorable in these cases. Pet parents in denial or who are noncompliant with the plan will set the pet up for a poor prognosis.

Treatment

When obesity is confronted from a scientific and health-conscious standpoint, with the commitment of the pet parent, a pet can achieve successful weight loss. Weight loss at a cost to welfare and behavioral health is not ideal. Veterinarians should stress the balance between tasty rewards for good behavior and risks of obesity. All weight reduction programs should be performed under the supervision of a veterinarian to achieve the desired goal safely and effectively. A healthy weight loss goal is a loss

⊞ Nestlé PURINA

BODY CONDITION SYSTEM

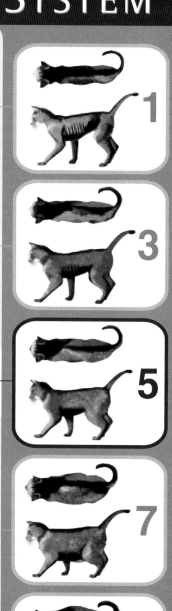

1 Ribs visible on shorthaired cats; no palpable fat; severe abdominal tuck; lumbar vertebrae and wings of ilia easily palpated.

2 Ribs easily visible on shorthaired cats; lumbar vertebrae obvious with minimal muscle mass; pronounced abdominal tuck; no palpable fat.

3 Ribs easily palpable with minimal fat covering; lumbar vertebrae obvious; obvious waist behind ribs; minimal abdominal fat.

4 Ribs palpable with minimal fat covering; noticeable waist behind ribs; slight abdominal tuck; abdominal fat pad absent.

IDEAL

5 **Well-proportioned; observe waist behind ribs; ribs palpable with slight fat covering; abdominal fat pad minimal.**

TOO HEAVY

6 Ribs palpable with slight excess fat covering; waist and abdominal fat pad distinguishable but not obvious; abdominal tuck absent.

7 Ribs not easily palpated with moderate fat covering; waist poorly discernible; obvious rounding of abdomen; moderate abdominal fat pad.

8 Ribs not palpable with excess fat covering; waist absent; obvious rounding of abdomen with prominent abdominal fat pad; fat deposits present over lumbar area.

9 Ribs not palpable under heavy fat cover; heavy fat deposits over lumbar area, face and limbs; distention of abdomen with no waist; extensive abdominal fat deposits.

Call 1-800-222-VETS (8387), weekdays, 8:00 a.m. to 4:30 p.m. CT

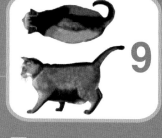

⊞ Nestlé PURINA

Figure 13.9 Purina BCS scale. *(From: Purina.)*

of 0.5–2% of body weight a week.[59,60,71] Having a dedicated paraprofessional in the practice that guides and encourages the pet parents through the weight loss process, monitoring the dog's weight and behavior through weekly phone check-ins and periodic weigh-ins, will likely result in the most successful outcome.

Once the total energy requirement is calculated, the veterinarian can divide those calories among dog food, supplements, and food rewards. Treat size should be about 1/4 of an inch for most medium- to large-sized dogs and smaller for smaller dogs. Treats about 1/8 of an inch wide will suffice for cats. Pet parents should be instructed to use low-calorie treats such as apples and carrots for everyday activities, and higher-value treats for those harder to maintain behaviors. Low-fat cheese, yogurt pops, or white meat chicken and turkey are good examples of higher-value, low-fat foods which can be used as treats.

Placing the pet on a reduction diet may help them feel satiated, hopefully reducing begging and distress to the pet and pet parent.[72] In addition, this will allow the pet parent to give more healthy, small treats. There are a variety of weight reduction diets, each marketed to reduce the intake of energy while maintaining optimum nutrition. Unfortunately, there can be wide variation in recommended energy intake on the packaging, kilocalories/joules, and costs for diets marketed for weight loss in pets.[73] Higher-protein diets may facilitate the maintenance of lean body mass during weight loss and improve weight loss success rates.[74] High-protein, low-carbohydrate diets have also been advocated to enhance weight loss in dogs.[75] Additional caution must be taken to restrict calories more gradually and to monitor food intake when beginning a weight reduction program in cats to prevent hepatic lipidosis.[76] High-fiber diets resulted in greater weight loss in an eight-week study of cats compared to an equicaloric and high-protein diet with diet not affecting the appetitive and satiated behaviors of the cats.[77] For the most up-to-date science-based recommendations on nutrition and weight loss in animals, consult an appropriate specialist in veterinary nutrition (www.acvn.org, https://www.esvcn.eu/college).

Physical exercise and other forms of activity such as play will increase calorie expenditure while providing additional enrichment opportunities. However, no evidence exists to suggest how much exercise to prescribe (qualitative and quantitative) to effect weight loss in dogs and cats.[55] While longer walks and more play activities might be good general suggestions for dogs, pet parents should be encouraged to focus on activities that are most appropriate for the age, health, breed, and individual needs of the dog and most practical for the family and household.

Behavioral and physical benefits can be achieved through an increase in social activities, including:
- Reward-based training sessions (ensuring caloric intake is calculated with daily calorie needs)
- Interactive games such as tug or fetch
- Agility, competitive flyball, or disc dog (Figure 13.10)
- Play sessions with other dogs
- Activities such as herding trials, pulling carts, retrieving, swimming, or even a treadmill

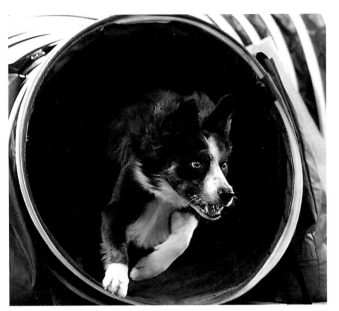

Figure 13.10 Dog sports provide enrichment and physical exercise. *(Attribution: Mindy Cox, CPDT-KSA.)*

For older pets or those with physical limitations, short walks for a sniff around the environment can help. Cats can also benefit from reward-based training, walking outdoors on a leash, or time outdoors in a cat enclosure. As mentioned above, feeding from food toys encourages movement on the pet's part, provides environmental enrichment, and also slows the rate of eating. For pets just adopted, all meals can often be given out of food toys in place of the bowl entirely; however, some pets may be stressed by this. If that is the case, most of the meal can be fed from a food toy followed by a very small meal from a bowl.[78] Games of search and seek for food (e.g., nosework) can help to increase physical activity by encouraging stair climbing, jumping, and perching for cats, or exploration and scavenging for dogs. Toys that stimulate chase such as dangled wand toys with feathers or cardboard prey, or small toys that the cat can roll and bat, provide an outlet for predatory activity while expending calories. The exploratory nature of cats can be further encouraged by providing novelty in the form of paper bags, cardboard boxes, and locations for climbing, scratching, and perching, which might include small food treats to further encourage and reward these activities.[79]

Weighing portions and intake in grams will be significantly more accurate than measurement using cups. The family should also learn how to control the provision of food better to be able to last through the entire day in order to reduce begging behavior. Automated feeders might be used to measure and deliver smaller portions of food throughout the day, to dissociate the feeding from the pet parent, and to provide food at times such as during sleep when the pet might be most disruptive.[59] Pet parents should be cautioned that providing food when a pet is begging further reinforces that behavior. Demands for food should be met with complete inattention, which will serve to extinguish the behavior. If pet parents provide food in a regular and predictable way (e.g., from food bowls or feeding toys or as rewards for training and cease giving food for attention-seeking behaviors), food solicitation should cease. Stimulus control modification can also be used to regulate the cues that trigger feeding; in other words, stimuli that may become paired with feeding need to be carefully managed. Stimuli where the pet might expect food or a treat include the pet parent's arrival home, entering the kitchen, opening cupboards, drawers, or the refrigerator, or eating a meal. Occupying the pet in other activities at these times (e.g., play, taking for walk, placing outdoors) can change the meaning of these cues. Alternately, a small measured portion of calories/joules can be provided in a food manipulation puzzle at each of these times as part of the overall feeding program. By sticking to predictable feeding routines, times, and places, the pet should soon learn when and where to expect food.

The efficacy of any program should be measured by regularly scheduled follow-up visits to reassess BCS, weigh the pet, behavior and make adjustments where sufficient improvement is not being achieved. Once the weight has been safely lost, it is important not to resort to the old behaviors that resulted in obesity to begin with. The continued use of reduced-calorie foods with a target of 90% of requirements is usually recommended, as increased nonmeal food items and a decrease in activity are common missteps following weight loss.[80] Regardless of whether the approach is diet, increased activity, or medical therapy, managing feeding behavior and education of the pet parent are ultimately the keys to success.

It is possible that some pets that eat voraciously and perhaps display concurrent food-related aggression may have a pathologic "compulsive" eating disorder. This is extremely rare and should only be considered if there are no other physical causes (see Chapter 6). These cases would be treated as with other compulsive disorders (see Chapter 18) by identifying and reducing stressors, environmental and behavior management, and potentially with medications (see Chapters 9 and 11).

CASE EXAMPLE

Signalment

Sheldon, a 19-kg, 6-year-old neutered male terrier mix, presented for his annual physical examination.

History

Sheldon ate one cup of food twice daily as recommended by the pet food manufacturer. The pet parents thought that perhaps he might have problems with his metabolism because he also was not very "spunky." Both of the pet parents worked, leaving Sheldon alone most of the day. They left food available for him at all times and some of it was still in his bowl when they got home at night. He got three biscuit snacks in the morning when they left for work, three when they returned, and three before bedtime. When eating or snacking themselves, they gave Sheldon "a small portion" from the table. The pet parents did not view Sheldon as overweight and were not convinced that Sheldon was being overfed, but agreed to explore the situation further.

Workup

His physical examination was unremarkable except for obesity (BCS 8/9). A worksheet was used to determine everything that Sheldon ate on a typical day as well as his usual exercise schedule.

Routine hematological and biochemical tests, including a thyroid profile, urinalysis, and fecal antigen + Giardia were within normal limits.

Treatment

It was determined that Sheldon should be receiving no more than 850 kcal daily based on an ideal weight of 14 kg. However, his nine biscuits alone amounted to 810 kcal, not to mention the few "extras" he received when the pet parents were eating or snacking. The pet parents were instructed to either divide each treat into three pieces of roughly 30 kcal each and to provide Sheldon with no more than four of these (or 120 kcal/day) or give lower-calorie treats and give more treats per day. The pet parents were given lists of acceptable treats that they could make at home (carrots) and low-calorie, commercially available treats. The treats were only to be given for positive behaviors captured throughout the day and training sessions. To decrease begging, the pet parents were given a recommendation for a positive reinforcement trainer to assist with impulse control behaviors such as down and stay. The pet parents were educated on how to use food toys to increase the amount of time that it took Sheldon to eat and help him feel more satiated. Resources for food toys, including types and how to use them, were given to the pet parents, with the instructions to slowly over two to three weeks wean him onto feeding exclusively out of those toys. He was put on a commercial weight loss diet and the pet parents were instructed how much to feed each day. Additional instructions included adding water, steamed vegetables, or low-sodium broth to his meals to help him feel full. Exercise instructions included two 10-minute walks a day when it was not too hot, and fetch inside of the house for 5 minutes twice daily. The pet parents were given guidelines for assessment of how well he was tolerating the exercise.

Follow-up

Regular follow-ups weekly were conducted by the veterinary technician. On reexamination 12 weeks later, Sheldon was a svelte 16 kg and much more energetic. The pet parents had difficulty not showing Sheldon love by giving him table scraps, but they had agreed to decrease the amount of table scraps and put those scraps in food toys. They reported that Sheldon was "brilliant" because he was able to figure out any food toy. They loved watching him move the levers and open slots to get to his food. While the walks had not progressed past 10 minutes each, they were playing fetch and tug in the house for up to 15 minutes at a time. As the pet parents were unable to stop giving table scraps and Sheldon appeared to be maintaining his weight, a recheck was recommended for a weigh-in with the technician in one month. If he continued to maintain his weight on this plan, Sheldon could continue this way indefinitely.

Discussion

Part of the key to success in Sheldon's case is the addition of exercise, training, and enrichment. These activities bond pet parents to their pets around food in a healthy way. Also, the pet parents, while not completely compliant, followed most recommendations.

Pica

Pica is an abnormal craving or appetite for ingesting non-food substances. Many animals, especially young animals, may chew on a variety of objects that might also be ingested as a part of exploratory behavior. These might include cable and telephone cords, carpeting, leather objects, pet parent clothing, toys, plastic bags, and plants.[53] Both dogs and cats can display pica. While stress can be a component of this disorder, diseases of the gastrointestinal tract should be ruled out as well as attention-seeking behavior, innately reinforcing behavior (garbage raiding or counter surfing), and lack of enrichment (see Chapter 6).

The cause of pica in pets is unknown, although exploratory behavior of puppies and kittens, inadvertent pet parent reinforcement, gastrointestinal or endocrine disease, stress, and persistence of infantile oral behavior could all contribute. In one study, pica in cats was associated with gastric reflux and delayed gastric emptying.[53] In addition, genetic factors have been identified that contribute to pica associated with object sucking (blanket sucking and other picas in Doberman Pinschers and wool sucking in Oriental breeds of cats).[81-83] Although woolen items are most commonly chosen (93% of cases), affected cats also may chew on cotton, synthetics, rubber, plastic, paper, shoelaces or threads, various fabrics, and cardboard.[53,82] In dogs, rock and stone eating is a problem that appears to be of particular concern, especially due to the sequelae of this behavior to the dog's teeth and gastrointestinal tract.

Grass eating is normal in dogs and cats, although each species consumes grass for seemingly different reasons.[6,84] The ingestion of plants has been reported in 79% of dogs. Of plant-eating dogs, 68% ate plants on a daily or weekly basis with grass being the most common plant ingested. Nine percent of dogs were reported to be ill before ingestion and 22% were reported to vomit following ingestion.[85] Cats may eat grass because they are seeking fiber, like the taste, like the texture, or as a normal part of exploring their environment.[6,85] Pet parents should be aware of which plants are toxic and which are cat safe before giving the cat access to any plants or cut flowers. Dogs might eat grass because they are nauseated, bored, hungry, or as a displacement behavior.[86] A displacement behavior may be exhibited when a dog or cat is anxious or conflicted.

Prevention

As the underlying causes of pica are varied and not well understood, the prevention of this disorder is equally mysterious. Potential strategies would include varied food types and textures, environmental enrichment in the way of food toys, exercise and outdoor exposure (cats), rotating foods to maintain interest, decreasing access to unacceptable chew items, providing safe grasses for chewing and ingestion, muzzle training (dogs), teaching a drop it or leave it cue in puppyhood (dogs), avoiding all punishment for picking up items, and education of pet parents as to their breed's predisposition.

Diagnosis and prognosis

Pica is diagnosed by observing the abnormal behavior. A full medical workup is essential, as medical conditions that lead to nutritional deficiencies or electrolyte imbalances, gastrointestinal disturbances, conditions that lead to polyphagia, and central nervous system disturbances should all be ruled out. The prognosis is variable, but most cases can be improved through diligent management and appropriate treatment of any underlying contributions.

Treatment

The problem can generally be managed by keeping the ingested objects away from the pet (or vice versa) and ensuring that the pet's behavioral and enrichment needs are adequately addressed. In addition, providing alternate feeding activities (e.g., food puzzle toys, durable and appealing chew toys) and other forms of oral stimulation such as dental chews or cat grass, or diets that might better meet the pet's nutritional and behavioral needs (e.g., increased bulk, nutritional balance) might reduce pica. Medication may be helpful for true compulsive disorders (see Chapters 11 and 18).

Coprophagia

Coprophagia is an ingestive behavior involving the consumption of feces. It is normal in nursing bitches in order to keep the den clean[6,87] and briefly in puppies, presumably to help establish gut flora and meet certain nutritional needs.[88] While it is considered normal in dogs, it is rare in cats. In one study, four weeks after adoption from an animal shelter, about 10% of dogs were reported to eat feces.[89] In an internet survey, 16% of dogs were frequent stool eaters, engaging in the behavior at least six times, while an estimated 23–49% of domestic dogs have been reported to exhibit the behavior at some point.[90-92] Coprophagic dogs were more likely to be described as greedy, with minimal reported success from the use of commercial products or behavior modification.[90] Ingestion was directed at fresh stools, supporting the hypothesis that coprophagy is an inherited tendency to keep the den area clean and free of fecal parasites.[90]

Dogs may first eat fecal matter out of exploration and curiosity; mimicry of other dogs; attraction to the smell and taste; increased appetite, including medical conditions causing or contributing to polyphagia or pica (poor absorption, malnutrition);[87] and iatrogenic polyphagia (e.g., benzodiazepines, phenobarbital, corticosteroids).[87,88,93] Pets that are underfed or placed on an overly restricted diet may have a voracious appetite, which may result in ingestion of stool.[87] Perpetuating factors include pet parent reinforcement (e.g., attention, yelling), environmental reinforcement (e.g., competition with other dogs, desirable taste), dietary insufficiency (e.g., thiamine insufficiency), gastrointestinal disease (e.g., exocrine pancreatic insufficiency, malabsorption), and continued treatment with medications causing polyphagia.

Prevention

Risk factors include purchase from pet store,[94] history of starvation or a poor diet,[92] anxiety disorders, prolonged confinement or insufficiently stimulating environment (enrichment),[87,88,95] oral disorders (e.g., pica, plant eating),[92] greedy eating, households with <2 dogs/household, eating dirt and eating cat fecal matter, and living with a coprophagic cohabitant.[87,88,96] In one study, the terrier and hound breed groups were most common, with Shetland Sheepdogs overrepresented and poodles underrepresented.[90] No differences were found between age, sex, neuter status, habits, lifestyle, habitat, diet, number of meals, nutritional background, diet, ease of house training, compulsive disorders, or lack of normal mothering.[90,92] The risk of developing coprophagia has not been correlated with height, body weight, canine cephalic index,[97] frequency of feeding, presence or absence of toys, time spent outside, frequency of fecal matter removal from yard, feeding schedule, vitamin or enzyme supplement, time spent alone, time spent with people, amount of exercise, amount of training, body condition score,[92] level of house training, or compulsive disorders.[94] While no studies have examined prevention specifically, examination of the risk factors associated with coprophagia can at minimum inform the recommendations to the pet parent. A preventative plan for dogs might include puzzle and food toys to slow down eating, a nutritionally balanced diet, surveillance of the health of all pets in multidog households, avoidance of punishment-based techniques when the dog picks up items, teaching leave it/drop it, environmental enrichment, exercise, and muzzle training.

Diagnosis

One of the most important aspects of diagnosis is the medical history:

- What feces are being ingested (own stools, family dogs, unfamiliar dogs, other animals)?
- Signalment: sex, neuter status, stage of estrous cycle
- Diet: eating habits, changes in diet prior to onset
- Physical health, especially as it pertains to appetite, weight, metabolic rate, and digestion
- Concurrent medications, including those that might have an effect on appetite
- Feces consistency, volume, appearance, frequency, and any evidence of tenesmus
- Description of the problem, including when it began, and when and where it takes place
- Pet parent's response and attempts at correction
- Any changes in household, diet, or health prior to onset of problem
- Other behavioral clinical signs, including pica
- House training status, including where and when the pet eliminates and how often the area is cleaned
- Health of other pets in the household
- Housing, including daily schedule for play, exercise, attention, training, and elimination

Potential behavioral diagnoses include attention-seeking behavior,[95,98] lack of stimulation/enrichment,[95] learned behavior from other dogs in the household,[93] learned behavior through pet parent reinforcement, self-reinforcing behavior (presumed attractive smell/taste),[96] hunger, play, environmental stress,[99] and anxiety.[87,92,94] Potential dietary causes include thiamine deficiency,[100] intestinal parasites, and hunger. Potential gastrointestinal causes include chronic pancreatic insufficiency[87,101] and malabsorption.[102] Potential endocrine causes include those that cause hyperphagia, such as Cushing's disease. Potential iatrogenic causes include treatment with medications which increase appetite such as benzodiazepines, gabapentin, corticosteroids, Entyce, mirtazapine, and phenobarbital. Energy-restricted diets, especially those that are not balanced or do not adequately satiate the

dog, may also lead to coprophagia. In addition, pets that are prone to hyperphagia and overeating may be at risk. See Chapters 6 and 9 for more information on causes of coprophagia and medications which can increase appetite.

The minimum database includes physical, behavioral, and fecal examination. Ideally, a CBC, serum chemistry, thyroid profile, fecal PCR for Giardia and other internal parasites, and urinalysis would be performed to complete the evaluation. Pancreatic and gastrointestinal function tests should be performed when gastrointestinal involvement is suspected.

Treatment

Physical problems must first be diagnosed and treated. If the dog is eating its own feces, the focus should be on evaluation of the pet for any health issue that might lead to poor digestion or increased appetite. Changing the diet to one with greater digestibility or one with more bulk or fiber to satiate the dog better may help. Dietary supplements containing proteolytic enzymes might increase protein absorption and decrease the appeal of the feces. For dogs that prefer to eat feces of a more solid consistency, fiber or vegetable oil may alter the texture to reduce its appeal. Extending dinner time by placing food in puzzle toys or through seek-and-search games might help. A number of commercial or homemade products containing monosodium glutamate, capsicum, yogurt, pineapple, or spinach have been suggested to make the food more digestible and the stools less appealing. However, while there may be anecdotal reports of efficacy, a recent survey of 11 different products reported cure rates of 0–2%.[90,103,104]

The most effective behavioral treatments are (1) avoidance, (2) redirection, (3) differential reinforcement (differential reinforcement of alternative behavior [DRA], differential reinforcement of incompatible behavior [DRI], differential reinforcement of other behavior [DRO], see Chapter 10),[89] and (4) environmental enrichment.[87,88,92] Preventing access to feces has been shown to be the most common and effective way of stopping the behavior, followed by rewarding desirable behavior and distracting the pet from the feces, while ignoring the behavior, punishment, and food additives are least effective.[92]

Discontinue, if possible, all medications which increase appetite. Preventing and denying access to feces is the first step. The dog should be closely observed outdoors and remain on leash until the feces are removed. After each elimination, the dog can be taught to come and sit before the pet parent cleans up. After all dogs in the family have eliminated and the feces have been removed, the dog can be allowed to roam in the yard. Keeping the dog on leash in areas with feces and/or using a basket muzzle can be helpful. Some dogs will push the basket muzzle into the feces to eat it. This is part of the reason that the best plan is one of avoidance.

Punishment of coprophagia is not indicated and is not effective.[92,94] While verbal reprimands, chasing the dog away, yelling, grabbing the dog, or using a citronella collar may reduce the frequency of the behavior initially, the long-term outcome with these types of treatments is poor, often resulting in fear of the pet parent (hindering further treatment) and "sneaking away" from the pet parent to ingest feces. As noted above, products relying on taste aversion to lessen the likelihood of coprophagia can be applied directly to the feces or added to the diet depending on the specific product instructions. However, pet parents must treat all dogs in the household and dogs are likely to continue eating stools that are untreated. The aversive taste does not address the underlying motivation and appeal of ingesting stools, and anecdotally, some dogs may even develop a taste for the flavored feces, thereby increasing the undesirable behavior.

Pet parents should eliminate the opportunity to eat feces by keeping the dog on leash or indoors when not directly monitored; putting the dog in the yard or taking the dog on walks alone; picking fecal matter up immediately; and basket muzzle training.[96,101] To avoid variable reinforcement (a powerful type of reinforcement in which a response is reinforced after an unpredictable number of responses) of the coprophagia,

the affected dog cannot eat untreated feces even once during treatment until the behavior has been extinguished.[105] A toy or treat to redirect the dog's attention can be used if they see the dog sniffing the ground in areas where feces have likely been deposited. Pet parents can teach the dog an alternative behavior (DRA) (e.g., sitting, making eye contact) when the dog discovers fecal matter and then consistently reinforce the alternative behavior with a high-value reward. The environment should be enriched in case the dog is understimulated, paying close attention to oral enrichment devices (e.g., food toys). The rate of eating should be decreased during meal times by using food toys and puzzle toys.

CASE EXAMPLE

Signalment

Phineas, a 4-year-old neutered male Labrador Retriever, presented for coprophagia of five to six months' duration.

History

Phineas was adopted from a pet store at 12 weeks of age. When he was adopted, the pet parents noted that he and other puppies were in an enclosure where there was feces on the floor. After changing his diet to a high-quality puppy food and adding a commercial monosodium glutamate supplement (Forbid), the behavior resolved. He seemed excessively destructive to them, destroying toys quickly and ingesting them. He had been hospitalized at six months of age for a suspected foreign body. After the hospitalization, the emergency veterinarian recommended that the pet parents remove all toys, which they did. When Phineas was one year old, he developed recurrent, chronic, superficial yeast infections under his chin and on his chest. At that time, on the recommendation of the veterinarian, they stopped letting him swim in the pool. Ferb, a 2-year-old female spayed Golden Retriever, had been obtained at four months of age from the same pet store. Phineas and Ferb had a backyard which was fenced and they were taken for at least two walks a day, primarily by the teenage son. Usually, the dogs were let out into the fenced yard unsupervised. About three months ago prior to presentation, the pet parents noticed while Phineas was licking them that he had putrid-smelling breath. About a month ago prior to presentation, Phineas vomited overnight, and the vomitus smelled like feces. The pet parents became suspicious and observed Phineas outside in the yard eating feces. At that time, it was unclear whether he was eating his own feces, Ferb's feces, or both.

The pet parents had tried a change to a dental diet with higher fiber, a trial with a monosodium glutamate supplement, and a variety of internet-suggested additives, including adding pineapple, a probiotic, and even a breath mint with Retsyn. Lacing the stool with cayenne pepper and intermittent yelling at him, grabbing him by the collar, and pushing his face into the remaining feces had also been ineffective. They noticed that recently when they went into the yard, he ran from them and was hard to catch.

Workup

A complete history was obtained, including environmental changes over the course of Phineas' life, diet, eating habits, and general wellness. Health problems in both dogs were ruled out through physical exam, fecal antigen including Giardia, and blood and urine testing.

Treatment

The pet parents were instructed to stop yelling at, hitting, or grabbing for Phineas, as it was causing him to run away from them out of fear. Instead, they were given a referral to a positive reinforcement dog trainer for muzzle training, relationship repair (between the pet parents and the dog), sit, down, stay, and leave it. The end goal would be for him to sit when he saw feces so that the pet parent could reinforce him. They were instructed as to how to safely enrich his life with toys and physical

activity such as walks and occasional swimming. Dog sports such as nosework and tracking were recommended as well because he apparently enjoys sniffing things out. They were given instructions as to how to feed him and Ferb from food toys exclusively. They were to clean up the yard immediately after each dog eliminated. Then they could let the dogs off leash. When they needed to get Phineas into the house, they were to use high-value treats to lure him in.

Follow-up

The veterinary technician followed up by phone every two weeks for four weeks. Phineas was seen back for a recheck with the doctor in six weeks. There had been no incidents of coprophagia when the pet parents were present, but they reported that their teenage son was not watching the dogs outside in the yard when he was responsible for their care. They were working with the dog trainer and seeing progress with both dogs. Phineas was "surprisingly smart" and was able to sit when asked when there was feces to be cleaned up. At that point, basket muzzle training was recommended so that he would not engage in coprophagia when the son was watching the dogs. The pet parents had invested in toys which spilled food and squeaky "indestructible" toys. They reported that the toys were in fact not indestructible and Phineas tore through them in "5 minutes." They were given resources for tough toys, how to sew toys back together, and reminded that he always must be monitored whenever he had a toy. In addition, all previous recommendations were to be continued. At the 10-week recheck, Phineas was alerting to feces to the point where the pet parents called him the "poop alert dog." Phineas would see the feces and alert the pet parents by sitting so that he could be reinforced. They had not muzzle trained him and were trying to motivate their son to comply with the recommendations. He was being fed all meals from food toys. They reported that he no longer ran from them in the yard but instead, followed them around waiting for treats. The pet parents were satisfied with the outcome and planned to continue with the recommendations.

Discussion

In this case, the pet parents thought that this was an acute problem when in fact, Phineas had several predisposing factors combined with poor management and recommendations made, which further increased the likelihood of this behavior progressing. This case highlights the importance of considering behavior, no matter the presenting complaint. For example, the emergency doctor who noted that Labrador Retrievers are predisposed to pica and foreign bodies could have referred the pet parent to a board-certified veterinary behaviorist for a preventive plan for foreign body ingestion. The veterinarian who recommended that Phineas stop swimming could have recommended other ways or given resources to keep him occupied and enriched to reduce the likelihood of aberrant behaviors. As veterinarians, we should approach animals with the "one health" foundational concept, looking at the entire animal and how our recommendations will affect other body systems, behavior, and welfare (See Chapter 9).

Hyporexia: the "fussy" or "picky" eater

Both dogs and cats can be finicky eaters. In most cases where the appetite decrease causes weight loss, there is an underlying physical cause. A common one is nausea. Any medical problem, even if short term, that leads to nausea can incite a food aversion. The causes of most feeding idiosyncrasies are unknown. What is known is that odor, taste, texture, and temperature can be adjusted to tempt the problem feeder to eat, and that novel foods may increase appetite.

A pet may also be reluctant to eat a commercial diet because it has learned that if it waits long enough, it will receive more palatable food from the pet parent. It may develop a negative-conditioned emotional response to a food when paired with a frightening stimulus such as sounds, people, or locations. In addition, if the food is paired with something that is distasteful, such as administration of medication, the pet can develop a negative-conditioned response to that food or the food receptacle.

Many pet parents will state that their pet is inappetent or hyporexic when, in fact, they not only did not lose weight but are gaining weight. This can be elucidated with a careful history.

Prevention

Normal, healthy pets rarely try to starve themselves. Most finicky pets actually receive adequate nutrition on a daily basis. Veterinarians should make dietary recommendations from the outset to avoid the development of unbalanced and unhealthy dietary preferences. Discussing the types of treats that would be most healthy and how and when they might be given is recommended. Be certain that the family counts any treats or human foods into the daily caloric calculations and limits them to a small proportion of the diet to ensure that they do not have an impact on nutritional balance. Some variety in protein source, flavor, and texture (canned versus dry) might be considered when feeding young pets, especially cats, to avoid the development of a narrow range of food preferences.

Diagnosis and prognosis

If the pet parent complains of a finicky eater or one that occasionally skips meals, first determine if the pet's weight is in the normal range. In many cases, these pets are of normal weight (or even overweight) and are already consuming all the calories needed on a daily basis. Some dogs may even skip an occasional day with no ill effects. This may be a normal mechanism for maintaining optimal weight. If the pet has an acceptable body weight, it is important to rule out the possibility that the pet is obtaining food elsewhere, either from a neighbor or by hunting or scavenging. Inquire about biscuits, treats, or table scraps the pet might obtain from family members or visitors.

For pets that are hyporexic and underweight, a complete history and thorough medical evaluation need to be completed to rule out underlying disease processes. Pancreatic, dental, gastrointestinal, renal, and hepatic disease can all account for dietary discrimination. If the pet is on any medication, determine if it might have any effect on reducing appetite and discontinue as a test if not contraindicated.

Evaluate the pet for signs of chronic or recurrent anxiety, which can suppress appetite. Anorexia of acute onset, especially in cats, can be due to stressors such as the addition of a new cat or other significant changes in the home, family, or schedule, and can have serious sequelae such as hepatic lipidosis if not attended to immediately. Olfaction is the key to palatability, and lack of olfaction, (i.e., anosmia) can decrease the ability to both locate food and satisfy appetite.[93] Anosmia can be seen secondary to upper respiratory tract infections, neoplasia, use of chemotherapeutics, and cognitive dysfunction.[106]

Treatment

Underlying physical problems should be addressed. One of the most insidious causes of dietary discrimination is dental disease. In cats, it is the second most common disease after obesity. Therefore, some dogs and cats may have dental pain that could interfere with feeding. With gastrointestinal disturbances, concurrent signs such as abnormal bowel movement frequency or consistency, abdominal pain, flatulence, or environmental licking might be expected; alternately, some degree of improvement might be seen with a change in food to a bland or novel protein diet, or gastric medications such as H_2 antagonists, proton pump inhibitors, sucralfate, or an antinauseant. Gastrointestinal causes were found in 74% of dogs exhibiting excessive licking of surfaces.[107] Following treatment, improvement was noted in the frequency and duration of the licking behavior and resolution in 53%.[107]

For healthy animals that continue to turn up their noses at mealtime, there are some alternatives. First, an assessment of fear, anxiety, stress, and conflict around the food bowl should be made. Potentially, the pet parents have punished the dog by yelling out of frustration when the dog did not eat. Another possibility is that the pet is wearing an indoor or outdoor shock collar and has been shocked in that room, near the bowl, or while eating. Another possibility as mentioned above is that the pet could have a negative-conditioned emotional response as a result of being in a frightening situation during eating.

Commonly, pet parents do not realize how much their pet should be eating from a caloric standpoint. Educating pet parents regarding the appropriate caloric intake for their pet can allay their concerns about their pet's appetite. Rewards (such as special treats) can be given each time the pet voluntarily eats its designated food. Clicker training can be used to shape the pet's behavior around the food bowl.

There are often taste preferences among dogs and cats and switching protein source or food offered can sometimes help the hyporexic patient. Dogs have been shown to prefer meat to a higher-protein nonmeat diet and have preference for one meat over others. Order of preference are typically beef, pork, lamb, chicken, and horsemeat.[108,109] Canned food is most often preferred over dry food, and a novel flavor is preferred over a known flavor.[109] Cats will show a preference for fish and novel diets.[110] In addition, warming canned foods may improve food consumption in cats with decreased interest in eating.[111]

Appetite stimulants

Drugs such as cyproheptadine, and benzodiazepines such as diazepam, oxazepam, or flurazepam may be useful as appetite stimulants on a short-term basis. Mirtazapine, a human anti-depressant with serotonergic and noradrenergic effects, has been found to be an effective appetite stimulant and nausea treatment for dogs and cats and is now available as a transder-mal ointment for cats.[112] Entyce (capromorelin oral solution), another appetite stimulant, is a ghrelin receptor agonist that signals the hypothalamus and causes a feeling of hunger.[113] See Chapter 11 for more information about medications.

References

1. Fitzgerald DM, Turner DC. Hunting behaviours of domestic cats and their impact on prey populations. In: Turner D, Bateson P, eds. *The Domestic Cat; the Biology of its Behaviour.* 3rd ed. Cambridge: Cambridge University Press; 2014.

2. Members of the Panel on Feline Behavior Guidelines. Feline behavior guidelines from the American Association of Feline Practitioners. *J Am Vet Med Assoc.* 2005; 227:70–80.

3. Mugford RA. External influences on the feeding of carnivores. In: Kare MR, Maller O, eds. *The Chemical Senses and Nutrition.* New York, NY: Academic Press; 1977.

4. Turner DC. Social organisation and behavioural ecology of free-ranging domestic cats. *The Domestic Cat; the Biology of its Behaviour.* 3rd ed. Cambridge: Cambridge University Press; 2014.

5. Bateson P. Behavioral development in the cat. In: Turner D, Bateson P, eds. *The Domestic Cat; the Biology of its Behaviour.* 3rd ed. Cambridge: Cambridge University Press; 2014.

6. Houpt KA. Ingestive behavior: food and water intake. In: *Domestic Animal Behavior for Veterinarians and Animal Scientists.* 6th ed. Ames: Iowa State University Press; 2018.

7. James WT, Gilbert TF. The effect of social facilitation on food intake of puppies fed separately and together for the first 90 days of life. *Br J Anim Behav.* 1955; 3: 131–133.

8. Mariotti VM, Hervera M, Fatjo J, et al. Review of pet dog feeding habits in Spain. *Supplement to Compendiu.* 2008; 30:87.

9. Trulson ME. Dietary tryptophan does not alter the function of brain serotonin neurons. *Life Sci.* 1985;37:1067–1072.

10. Sunol A, Perez-Accino J, Kelley M, et al. Successful dietary treatment of aggression and behavioral changes in a dog. *J Vet Behav.* 2020;37:56–60.

11. Kang BT, Jung DI, Yoo JH, et al. A high fiber diet responsive case in a poodle dog with long-term plant eating behavior. *J Vet Med Sci.* 2007;69:779–782.

12. DeNapoli JS, Dodman NH, Shuster L, et al. Effect of dietary protein content and tryptophan supplementation on dominance aggression, territorial aggression, and hyperactivity in dogs. *J Am Vet Med Assoc.* 2000;217:504–508.

13. Dodman NH, Reisner I, Shuster L, et al. Effect of dietary protein content on behaviour in dogs. *J Am Vet Med Assoc.* 1996;208:376–379.

14. Mugford RA. The influence of nutrition on canine behavior. *J Small Anim Pract.* 1987;28:1046–1055.

15. Annunziata C, Shell L, Thatcher C, et al. Effects of a low protein diet on levels of serotonin in canine cerebrospinal fluid. Behavioral abstract. *Am Vet Soc Anim Behav Newslett.* 1996;18:3.

16. Davis GM, Labadie JD, Swafford BM, et al. Relationship between dietary protein content and behavior in Golden Retrievers. *Vet Behav Symp Proc.* Austin, TX, 2022, 24.

17. Da Graca Pereira G, Fragoso S. L-tryptophan supplementation and its effect on multi-housed cats and working dogs. In: *Proceedings of the 2010 European Veterinary Behaviour Meeting.* Hamburg; 2010:30–35.

18. Templeman JR, Davenport GM, Cant JP, et al. The effect of graded concentrations of dietary tryptophan on canine behavior in response to the approach of a familiar or unfamiliar individual. *Can J Vet Res.* 2018;82:294–305.

19. Kato M, Miyaji K, Ohtani N, et al. Effects of prescription diet on dealing with stressful situations and performance of anxiety-related behaviors in privately owned anxious dogs. *J Vet Behav.* 2012;7: 21–26.

20. Palestrini C, Minero M, Cannas S, et al. Efficacy of a diet containing caseinate hydrolysate on signs of stress in dogs. *J Vet Beh.* 2010;5:309–317.

21. Fernstrom MH, Massoudi MS, Fernstrom JD. Effect of 8-hydroxy-(di-n-propylamino)-tetralin on the tryptophan-induced increase in 5-hydroxytryptophan accumulation in rat brain. *Life Sci.* 1990;47:283–289.

22. Pellegrini O, Casini L, Mariotti V, et al. Effect of different dietary protein sources and carbohydrate content on canine behavior. *Supplement to Compendium.* 2008;30:77.

23. Gazzano A, Ogi A, Macchioni F. Blood serotonin concentrations in phobic dogs fed a dissociated carbohydrate-based diet: a pilot study. *Dog Behav.* 2019;2:9–17.

24. Barcus R, Schwebel A, Corson S. An animal model of hyperactive-child syndrome suitable for the study of the effects of food additives. *Pavlov J Biol Sci.* 1980;15:183–187.

25. Kaur H, Singla A, Snehdep S, et al. Role of omega-3 fatty acids in canine health: A review. *Int J Curr Microbiol Appl Sci.* 2020; 9(3):2283–2293.

26. Bauer J. Responses of dogs to omega-3 fatty acids. *J Am Vet Med Assoc.* 2007; 231(11):1657–1661.

27. Filburn CR, Griffin D. Effects of supplementation with a docosahexaenoic acid-enriched salmon oil on total plasma and plasma phospholipid fatty acid composition in the cat. *Intern J Appl Res Vet Med.* 2005;3:116–123.

28. Zicker SC, Jewell DE, Yamka RM, et al. Evaluation of cognitive learning, memory, psychomotor, immunologic, and retinal functions in healthy puppies fed foods fortified with docosahexanoic aced-rich fish oil from 8 to 52 weeks. *J Am Vet Med Assoc.* 2012;241:583–594.

29. Perica MM, Delas I. Essential fatty acids and psychiatric disorders. *Nut Clin Prac.* 2011;26:409–425.

30. Johnson M, Ostlund S, Fransson G, et al. Omega-3/omega-6 fatty acids for attention deficit hyperactivity disorder: a randomized placebo-controlled trial in children and adolescents. *J Atten Disord.* 2009;12:394–401.

31. Re S, Zanoletti M, Emanuele E. Aggressive dogs are characterized by low omega-3 polyunsaturated fatty acid status. *Vet Res Commun.* 2008;32:225–230.

32. Puurunen J, Sulkama S, Tiira K, et al. A non-targeted metabolite profiling pilot study suggests that tryptophan and lipid metabolisms are linked with ADHD-like behaviours in dogs. *Behav Brain Funct.* 2016;12: doi:10.1186/s12993-016-0112-1.

33. Hadley KB, Bauer J, Milgram NW. The oil-rich alga Schizochytrium sp. as a dietary source of docosahexaenoic acid improves shape discrimination learning associated with visual processing in a canine model of senescence. *Prostaglandins Leukot Essent Fatty Acids.* 2017;118:10–18.

34. Haag M. Essential fatty acids and the brain. *Can J Psychiatry.* 2003;48:195–203.

35. Goyal RK, Hirano I. The enteric nervous system. *N Engl J Med.* 1996;334;1106–1115.

36. Kirchoff NS, Udell MAR, Sharpton TJ. The gut microbiome correlates with conspecific aggression in a small population of rescued dogs (Canis familiaris). *Peer J.* 2019;7:e61–e63.

37. Kubinyi E, Bel Rhali S, Sándor S, et al. Gut microbiome composition is associated with age and memory performance in pet dogs. *Animals.* 2020;10:1488. doi:10.3390/ani10091488.

38. Mondo E, Barone M, Soverini M, et al. Gut microbiome structure and adrenocorticol activity in dogs with aggressive and phobic disorders. *Heliyon.* 2020;7:e03311.

39. McGowan RTS, Barnett HR, Czarnecki-Maulden G, et al. Tapping into those 'gut feelings' impact of BL999 (*Bifidobacterium longum*) on anxiety in dogs. In: *Proc*

ACVB Vet Behav Symp. Denver, CO, July 11–12. 2018.

40. Davis H, Franco P, Gagné J, et al. Effect of Bifidobacterium longum 999 supplementation on stress associated findings in cats with feline herpesvirus 1 infection. In: *ACVIM Forum 2021 Proceedings.*

41. Expert Group on Vitamins and Minerals. *Covering Note for EVM 00/14/P-Review of Thiamine.* 2000.

42. Calderon-Ospina CA, Nava-Mesa MO. B vitamins in the nervous system: current knowledge of the biochemical modes of action and synergies of thiamine, pyridoxine and cobalamin. *CNS Neurosci Ther.* 2020;26;5–13.

43. Mesripour A, Hajhashemi V, Kuchack A. Effect of concomitant administration of three different antidepressants with vitamin B6 on depression and obsessive compulsive disorder in mice models. *Res Pharm Sci.* 2017;12:46–52.

44. Madari A, Farbackova J, Katina S, et al. Assessment of severity and progression of canine cognitive dysfunction syndrome using the Canine Dementia Scale (CADES). *Appl Ani Behav Sci.* 2015;171: 138–145.

45. Ackerman L. Adverse reactions to foods. *J Vet Allergy Clin Immunol.* 1993;1:18–22.

46. Raditic DM, Remillard RL, Tater KC. ELISA testing for common food antigens in four dry dog foods used in dietary elimination trials. *J Anim Physiol Anim Nutr.* 2011;95:90–97.

47. Swanson KS. Nutrient–gene interactions and their role in complex diseases in dogs. *J Am Vet Med Assoc.* 2006;228: 1513–1520.

48. Ballarini G. Animal psychodietetics. *J Small Anim Pract.* 1990;31:523–532.

49. Raffan E, Dennis RJ, O'Donovan CJ, et al. A deletion in the canine POMC gene is associated with weight and appetite in obesity-prone Labrador Retriever dogs. *Cell Metab.* 2016;23:893–900.

50. Bamberger M, Houpt KA. Signalment factors, comorbidity, and trends in behaviour diagnosis in cats; 736 cases (1991–2001). *J Am Vet Med Assoc.* 2006;229:1602–1606.

51. Bamberger M, Houpt KA. Signalment factors, comorbidity, and trends in behaviour diagnosis in dogs; 1644 cases (1991–2001). *J Am Vet Med Assoc.* 2006;229:1591–1601.

52. Demontigny-Bédard I, Bélanger MC, Hélie P, et al. Medical and behavioral evaluation of 8 cats presenting with fabric ingestion: an exploratory pilot study. *Can Vet J.* 2019;60(10): 1081–1088.

53. Demontigny-Bédard I, Beauchamp G, Bélanger MC, et al. Characterization of pica and chewing behaviors in privately owned cats: a case-control study. *J Feline Med Surg.* 2016;18(8):652–657.

54. Kallfelz FA, Dzanis DA. Overnutrition: an epidemic problem in pet animal practice? *Vet Clin North Am.* 1989;19:433–445.

55. Courcier EC, Thomson RM, Mellor DJ, et al. An epidemiological study of environmental factors associated with canine obesity. *J Small Anim Pract.* 2010;51: 362–367.

56. Courcier EA, O'Higgins R, Mellor DJ, et al. Prevalence and risk factors for feline obesity in a first opinion practice in Glasgow, Scotland. *J Feline Med Surg.* 2010;12:746–753.

57. Association for pet obesity prevention. 2018; petobesityprevention.org. Accessed August 30, 2021.

58. German AJ, Ryan DH, German AC, et al. Obesity, its associated disorders and the role of inflammatory adipokines in companion animals. *Vet J.* 2010;185:4–9.

59. Shepherd M. Canine and feline obesity management. *Vet Clin Small Anim.* 2021;51:653–667.

60. Raffan E. Obesity. In: Tilley LP, Smith Jr. FWK, Sleeper MM, et al., eds. *Blackwell's 5 Minute Veterinary Consult. Canine and Feline.* 7th ed. Hoboken, NJ: Wiley-Blackwell; 2021:986–987.

61. Edney AT, Smith PM. Study of obesity in dogs visiting veterinary practices in the United Kingdom. *Vet Rec.* 1986;118: 391–396.

62. Mason E. Obesity in pet dogs. *Vet Rec.* 1970;86:612–616.

63. Scarlett JM, Donoghue S, Saidla J, et al. Overweight cats – prevalence and risk factors. *Int J Obesity.* 1994;18(Suppl 1):S22–S28.

64. Sloth C. Practical management of obesity in dogs and cats. *J. Small Anim Pract.* 1992;33:178–182.

65. Allan FJ, Pfeiffer DU, Jones BR, et al. A cross-sectional study of risk factors for obesity in cats in New Zealand. *Prev Vet Med.* 2000;46:183–196.

66. Rowe E, Browne W, Casey R. Risk factors identified for owner reported feline obesity at around one year of age: dry diet and indoor lifestyle. *Prev Vet Med.* 2015;121:273–281.

67. Arena L, Menchetti L, Diverio S, et al. Overweight in domestic cats living in urban areas of Italy: risk factors for an emerging welfare issue. *Animals.* 2021;11: 2246.

68. Preet GS, Turkar S, Gupta S, et al. Dog obesity: epidemiology, risk factors, diagnosis and management: a review paper. *Pharma Innov Jl.* 2021;10:698–705.

69. Burkholder WJ. Use of body condition scores in clinical assessment of the provision of optimal nutrition. *J Am Vet Med Assoc.* 2000;217:650–654.

70. Bjornvad CR, Nielsen DH, Armstrong PJ, et al. Evaluation of a nine-point body condition scoring system in physically inactive pet cats. *Am J Vet Res.* 2011;72:433–437.

71. Byers CG, Wilson CC, Stephens MB, et al. Treating excess weight with a multiple-modality approach. *Vet Med.* 2011;106: 193–200.

72. Buffington CAT. Management of obesity – the clinical nutritionist's experience. *Int J Obesity.* 1994;18(Suppl 1):S29-S35.

73. Linder DE, Freeman LM. Evaluation of calorie density and feeding directions for commercially available diets designed for weight loss in dogs and cats. *J Am Vet Med Assoc.* 2010;236:74–77.

74. German AJ, Holden SL, Bissot T, et al. A high protein high fibre diet improves weight loss in obese dogs. *Vet J.* 2010; 183:294–297.

75. Bierer TL, Bui LM. High-protein low-carbohydrate diets enhance weight loss in dogs. *J Nutr.* 2004;134:2087S-2089S.

76. Butterwick RF, Wills JM, Sloth C, et al. A study of obese cats on a calorie-controlled weight-reduction programme. *Vet Rec.* 1994;134:372–377.

77. Levine ED, Erb HN, Schoenherr B, et al. Owner's perception of changes in behaviors associated with dieting in fat cats. *J Vet Behav.* 2016;11:37–41.

78. Davies K. The effects of a novel feeding device on the behaviour of domestic cats. In: Heath S. ed. *Proceedings of the 7th International Veterinary Behavior Meeting.* Lovendegem, Belgium: ESVCE; 2009.

79. Neilson JC, Forrester SD. Multimodal management of feline obesity. *NAVC Hill's Feline Symposium.* 2011.

80. Roudebush, P, Schoenherr, WD, Delaney, SJ. An evidence-based review of the use of therapeutic foods, owner education, exercise, and drugs for the management of obese and overweight pets. *J Am Vet Med Assoc.* 2008;233:717–725.

81. Tynes V, Sinn L. Abnormal repetitive behaviors in dogs and cats: a guide for practitioners. *Vet Clin North Am Small Anim Pract.* 2014;44.3:543–564.

82. Bradshaw JWS, Neville PF, Sawyer D. Factors affecting pica in the domestic cat. *J Appl Anim Behav Sci.* 1997;52:373–379.

83. Moon-Fanelli A, Dodman NH, Cottam N. Blanket and flank sucking in Doberman Pinschers. *J Am Vet Med Assoc.* 2007;231:907–912.

84. Overall K. *Manual of Clinical Behavioral Medicine for Dogs and Cats.* 2nd ed. St Louis, MO: Elsevier; 2013.

85. Sueda KLC, Hart BL, Cliff KD. Characterization of plant eating in dogs. *Appl Anim Behav Sci.* 2008;111:120–132.

86. Bjone SJ, Brown WY, Price IR. Grass eating patterns in the domestic dog, Canis familiaris. In: *Recent Advances in Animal Nutrition in Australia.* 2007;16:45–49.

87. Tynes V. Coprophagia and pica. In: Tilley LP, Smith Jr. FWK, Sleeper MM, et al., eds. *Blackwell's 5 Minute Veterinary Consult. Canine and Feline.* 7th ed. Hoboken, NJ: Wiley-Blackwell; 2021:332–333.

88. Beaver B. Canine ingestive behavior. In: *Canine Behavior: Insights and Answers.* 2nd ed. St. Louis: Saunders Elsevier; 2009.

89. Wells DJ, Hepper PG. Prevalence of behavior problems reported by owners of dogs purchased from an animal rescue shelter. *Appl Anim Behav Sci.* 2000;69: 55–65.

90. Hart BL, Hart LA, Thigpen AP, et al. The paradox of canine conspecific coprophagy. *Vet Med Sci.* 2018;4:106–114.

91. Amaral AR, Porsani MYH, Martins PO, et al. Canine coprophagic behavior is influenced by coprophagic cohabitant. *J Vet Behav.* 2018;28:35–39.

92. Boze B. A comparison of common treatments for coprophagy in Canis familiaris. *J Appl Compan Anim Behav.* 2008;2(1):22–28.

93. Rogers VP, Hartke GT, Kitchell RL. Behavioral technique to analyze a dog's ability to discriminate flavors in commercial food products. In Hayaski Y, ed. *Olfaction and Taste II.* Oxford, England, Pergamon; 1967:353–359.

94. McMillan FD, Serpell JA, Duffy DL, et al. Differences in behavioral characteristics between dogs obtained as puppies from pet stores and those obtained from noncommercial breeders. *JAVMA.* 2013;242(10):1359–1363.

95. Hart BL, Hart LA, Bain MB. *Canine and Feline Behavior Therapy.* 2nd ed. Ames: Blackwell Publishing; 2006.

96. McKeown D, Luescher A, Machum M. Coprophagia: food for thought. *Can Vet J.* 1988;29(10);849–850.

97. McGreevy PD, et al. Dog behavior co-varies with height, body weight and skull shape. *PLoS One.* 2013:8(12); e80529. doi:10.1371/journal. pone.008529.

98. Hart BL, Kart LA. *Canine and Feline Behavioral Therapy.* Philadelphia: Lea & Febiger; 1985.

99. Houpt KA, Wolski TR. Ingestive behavior problems of dogs and cats. *Vet Clin North Am.* 1982;12:683–690.

100. Read DH, Harrington DD. Experimentally induced thiamine deficiency in beagle dogs: clinical observations. *Am J Vet Res.* 1981;42(6):984–991.

101. Overall K. How to stop even well-trained dogs from ingesting foreign objects. *DVM.* 1996;27(1):65.

102. Hill F, Malabsorption syndrome in the dog: a study of thirty-eight cases. *J Small Anim Pract.* 2008;13(10):575–594.

103. Hart BL, Tran AA, Bain MJ. Canine conspecific coprophagia; who, when and why dogs eat stools. In: *Proc ACVB/ AVSAB Behavior Symposium.* San Diego: 2012;8.

104. Wells DL. Comparison of two treatments for preventing dogs eating their own faeces. *Vet Rec.* 2003;153:51–53.

105. Hutchins R, Messenger H, Vaden S. Suspected carprofen toxicosis caused by coprophagia in a dog. *JAVMA.* 2013:243(5).

106. Johnson LN, Freeman LM. Recognizing, describing, and managing reduced food intake in dogs and cats. *J Am Vet Med Assoc.* 2017;251.11:1260–1266.

107. Becuwe-Bonnet V, Belanger MC, Frank D, Parent J, Helie P. Gastrointestinal disorders in dogs with excessive licking of surfaces. *J Vet Behav.* 2012;7: 194–204.

108. Houpt KA, Hintz HF, Shepherd P. The role of olfaction in canine food preferences. *Chem Senses.* 1979;3.3: 281–290.

109. Lohse CL. Preferences of dogs for various meats. *J Am Anim Hosp Assoc.* 1974;10:187–192.

110. Gershoff SN, Hegsted DM, Lentini E. The development of palatability tests for cats. *J Vet Res.* 1956;17.65:733.

111. Eyre R, Trehiou M, Marshall E, et al. Aging cats prefer warm food. *J Vet Behav.* 2022;47:86–92.

112. Poole M, Quimby JM, Hu T, et al. A double-blind, placebo-controlled, randomized study to evaluate the weight gain drug, mirtazapine transdermal ointment, in cats with unintended weight loss. *J Vet Pharmacol Ther.* 2019;42(2):179–188.

113. Zollers B, Wofford JA, Heinen E, et al. A prospective, randomized, masked, placebo-controlled clinical study of capromorelin in dogs with reduced appetite. *J Vet Intern Med.* 2016;30.6:1851–1857.

Recommended Reading

Heinemann KM, Bauer JE. Docosahexaenoic acid and neurologic development in animals. *J Am Vet Med Assoc.* 2006;228:700–706.

Raditic D, Gaylord L. Fish oil dosing in pet diets and supplements. *Today's Veterinary Practice.* 2020;10(3):30–34.

Tynes VV, Landsberg GM. Nutritional management of behavior and brain disorders in dogs and cats. *Vet Clin Small Anim.* 2021;51:711–727.

CHAPTER 14

Fears, phobias, and anxiety disorders

Carlo Siracusa, DVM, PhD, DACVB, DECAWBM

Chapter contents

Introduction

Fear is a primary emotion normally experienced by animals, including humans, and is part of self-defense mechanisms that are responsible for the survival of individuals and the propagation of a species. For this reason, fear represents one of the main motivations behind animal behaviors. Therefore, it is not surprising that fear and related emotions, anxiety and phobia, are associated with a majority of canine and feline behavior disorders.

While fear is readily apparent as the primary motivation behind some disorders such as storm phobia, noise phobia, social avoidance, fear-induced aggression, and submissive urination, almost all clinical behavior problems of companion animals can be exacerbated or complicated by fear. This is the case in urine marking, territorial aggression, possessive aggression (resource guarding), and compulsive, abnormal repetitive disorders, just to name a few examples. Therefore, understanding the behavioral and physiologic aspects of anxiety and the fear response, as well as how to choose and coach the pet parent patiently through conditioning exercises, become important aspects of working with a wide variety of behavior problems (see Box 14.1).

> **Box 14.1** Behavior disorders which may have a fear component or be complicated by fear
>
> - Storm fear and phobia
> - Noise aversion, fear and phobia
> - Global fear and phobia
> - Neophobia
> - Specific fears and phobias (people, places, objects)
> - Aggression (fear induced, conflict induced, territorial, possessive, stress induced)
> - Conflict and fear-induced urination
> - Urine marking
> - Separation-related disorders (isolation fear, isolation phobia, separation fear, separation phobia)

Clinical presentations of fear-induced behaviors: sensitivity, fear, anxiety, and phobia

In feral or semiferal conditions, most fear-related behaviors are adaptive and allow an individual animal to avoid predators and other potential threats. When fear is triggered in these contexts, it is short-lived, as the animal either manages

- Sensitivity
- Fear
- Phobia
- Anxiety

- Hypervigilance, scanning
- Increased motor activity (restlessness, pacing, circling, barking, jumping)
- Vocalization/whining
- Displacement behaviors – out-of-context grooming and scratching, yawning, lip licking, whining, barking, destructive, digging
- Changes in social soliciting behavior – increase or decrease in attention seeking
- Hiding, escape attempts
- Physiologic signs (trembling, dilated pupils, hypersalivation, ↑ respiratory rate, ↑ heart rate, urination, defecation, vomiting) increased blood pressure
- Decreased appetite

For additional body language signs, see Chapter 2 and Appendix A.

to avoid, escape, or fight against or perishes from the threat. In captive conditions however, fear-induced behaviors can be maladaptive because the animal often is not able to control the outcome, or avoid or escape a threat due to the presence of environmental constraints (e.g., physical barriers, pet parent behavior). In such conditions, fear can be long lasting and magnified, resulting in chronic stress and poor welfare (see Chapter 7).

Based on the intensity and adaptive value of the fear-induced behaviors displayed, we can distinguish four types of clinical presentations in no particular order (see Box 14.2).

Sensitivity: Sensitivity describes the lowest intensity of fear in response to a perceived threat. This is an adaptive response that is often displayed as orienting toward the perceived threat and/or startling. The clinical significance of this fear-related display is low, and most animals habituate to the stimuli that trigger a startling response. Nevertheless, this behavior should always be noted and monitored because some dogs and cats may further sensitize to the perceived threat and transition to a more intense fear response if individual (e.g., high arousability and emotional dysregulation) and environmental (e.g., confinement) characteristics allow.

Fear: An emotional response due to the presence or proximity of a specific stimulus (e.g., object, noise, individual, social situation) that the pet perceives as a threat or danger. It is a psychological and physiological state characterized by somatic, emotional, cognitive, and behavioral components. It can be a normal adaptive response. The appropriateness of the fear response is determined by its magnitude and the context in which it occurs.

Phobia: A profound, excessive, abnormal fear response that occurs without the presence of a true threat or is out of proportion to the needs for dealing with an actual threat. While fears may be adaptive responses, phobias are maladaptive and interfere with normal function. With repeated exposure, the extreme fear persists or intensifies.

Anxiety: A reaction of apprehension or uneasiness to an anticipated danger or threat. The absence of an identifiable fear-eliciting stimulus differentiates it from fear. Signs are physiologic (e.g., autonomic arousal, increased heart and respiratory rate, trembling, salivation, gastrointestinal, and hypervigilance) and behavioral (e.g., freezing, lip licking, yawning, pacing, stress vocalizations, restlessness). Anxiety may be displayed in the absence of an identifiable stimulus. It may become generalized in some pets or may be specific to situations of perceived threat. Animals exposed to contexts in which they experienced intense fear in the past can develop anxiety in anticipation of the potential upcoming threat. For example, a dog that with fear of thunderstorms that had negative experiences during walks outside in rainy days may develop anticipatory anxiety and refuse to go out for walks. Another example is a cat that anticipates that being put in the carrier will be followed with a visit to the veterinarian, which is frightening, and therefore hides from the pet parent when it sees the carrier (see Box 14.3).

Diagnoses related to fear, anxiety, and phobia

Clinical presentations can be associated with diagnoses; however, dogs and cats can be anxious or fearful in a certain situation, for example, without having a fear or anxiety disorder. Fear or anxiety displayed in certain situations may be precursors to a fear or anxiety disorder and it may not. In other words, the presence of fear or anxiety does not mean that the pet has a pathologic problem. Anxiety and fear can become pathologic when they progress intrinsically without environmental justification and do harm to the individual's quality of life and welfare. Anxiety and fear underly most behavioral problems seen by veterinarians. See Chapter 13 for ingestive disorders, Chapter 15 for noise aversion, Chapter 17 for separation-related disorders, Chapter 18 for repetitive disorders, Chapters 21 and 22 for urination disorders, and Chapters 23 and 24 for aggression disorders.

Specific or situational anxiety

Situational or specific anxiety occurs when an animal shows signs of anxiety such as hypervigilance, scanning, somatic physiologic response, increased reactivity, vocalizations, trembling, hypersalivation, increased motor activity, and muscle tension in distinct situations without the presence of the triggering stimuli.[1] This may be expressed when anticipating car or plane travel, veterinary visits, certain types of people or people in general, certain species, dogs or cats of a certain coat color or size, or any triggering stimulus that the pet views as a threat. Diagnoses such as noise sensitivity/aversion, separation-related disorders, and isolation anxiety all fall into this category, though pets with those specific diagnosis would be diagnosed as such, not with specific or situational anxiety.

Generalized anxiety

Generalized anxiety occurs when a dog or cat is persistently, excessively, and/or chronically anxious, hyperreactive, and/or hypervigilant in three or more environments or distinct circumstances outside of the presence of an obvious stimulus.[2,3] It can be characterized by increased anxiety-related activity interfering with daily activities (e.g., social interaction, species-typical behavior), increased motor activity, constant or frequent reactivity, alertness, lack of focus, and hypervigilance in the absence of a triggering stimulus.[4] Additional clinical signs may include trembling, increased heart rate, changes in appetite, changes in social interaction, and muscular tension.[1,3] Not all diagnostic criteria fit each patient. For example, some dogs with generalized anxiety show hypervigilance but not increased motor activity. The behavioral phenotype depends to some extent on the environment and the pet's genetic predisposition. Generalized anxiety comorbidities include almost any behavioral diagnoses, including separation-related disorders, noise fear/aversion/phobia, fear-induced aggression, conflict-induced aggression, stress-induced aggression, attention-seeking behaviors, displacement behaviors, territorial aggression, interdog aggression, and panic attacks.[3,5] Noise aversion, fear, or phobia can contribute to the development of generalized anxiety.

Specific or situational fear

A specific or situational fear is exhibited when there is a fearful response to a triggering stimulus. Clinical signs include tachycardia, tachypnea, hypertension, mydriasis, lowered tail and body, ears back, panting, pacing, vocalizing, attempts to escape or hide, aggression (pet would also be diagnosed with an aggression diagnosis), and increased nonproductive motor activity. Specific or situational fears could be triggered by any stimulus, including but not limited to car travel, veterinary visits, sounds, objects, people, animals, and environments.

Generalized fear

Generalized fear may have a genetic component, as is likely with other behavioral clinical signs and disorders.[6] Generalized fear occurs when a dog or cat shows signs of fear or stress in several environments or distinct circumstances (usually three or more) outside of the presence of the fear-inducing stimulus (e.g., person, animal, place, scent, auditory stimuli, object). It is characterized by signs of fear interfering with daily activities (e.g., social interaction, species-typical behavior), increased or decreased motor activity, constant or frequent reactivity, trembling, tachycardia, tachypnea, increased muscle tension, hypertension, mydriasis, lowered tail and body, ears back, panting, pacing, vocalizing, attempts to escape or hide, aggression (pet would also be diagnosed with an aggression diagnosis), and increased nonproductive motor activity when the stimulus is present. This diagnosis is difficult at times to distinguish from generalized anxiety because the triggering stimulus may not be apparent to the observer (e.g., scent) but is apparent to the dog and the signs of fear and anxiety are very similar. Furthermore, fear can lead to anxiety without the dissolution of fear, meaning that both may very well be present in the same patient.

Generalized phobia

Generalized phobia is an irrational, profound, excessive, out-of-context fear response that occurs without the presence of the triggering stimulus or is out of proportion to the threat caused by the triggering stimulus. The signs of general phobia are similar to those listed for fear and anxiety above except that the response is more profound, out of context, and can include signs of anxiety and fear. The qualifier "generalized" is used when the clinical signs occur in several environments or distinct circumstances (usually three or more). Clinical signs interfere with daily activities (e.g., social interaction, species-typical behavior) and can include increased or decreased motor activity, constant or frequent reactivity, trembling, increased heart rate, and muscular tension when the stimulus is presented.

Neophobia

Neophobia is diagnosed when a dog or cat has an intense, profound, out-of-context fear, anxiety, or stress response when in the presence of any new stimuli.[3] The clinical signs are similar to those listed above for situational fear and generalized fear. Patients that are neophobic do not habituate to new items, as would be expected in a behaviorally appropriate dog. This can be distinguished from generalized fear or global phobia by its limitation to new items in the environment. It can be distinguished from nonpathologic fear of new items by the absence of productive recovery (reduction of physiologic arousal back to baseline) or habituation to the item (becoming accustomed to it). It can be distinguished from global phobia and generalized fear by the limitation to new objects in the environment.

Neurobiology of fear: the stress response

Fear is considered a basic emotion, which is an emotion associated with hard-wired neurobiological systems selected by evolution for the survival of a species. The experience of fear is controlled by the fear-defense system. This is an innate system that organizes species-typical defensive behaviors to threats that promote survival. Experiencing short-lived fear is, therefore, adaptive for animals and helps them survive dangerous threats, such as predators.[7]

The perception of fear is associated with the activation of the biological stress response. This response prepares the body to cope with a perceived threat or challenging stimulus. Four components can be distinguished in the stress response: the behavior component, the autonomic component, the neuroendocrine component of the hypothalamic–pituitary–adrenal (HPA) axis response, and the immune component.[8] These four components are connected and integrated.

The behavior display associated with the activation of the stress response can greatly vary. An animal that perceives a threat can display an aggressive behavior (fight), an avoidance behavior (flight), tonic immobility (freeze), or displacement activities (fidget). Although fearful behavior is often represented as a flight or freeze display, it is extremely important to keep in mind that aggressive behaviors and displacement behaviors also can be motivated by the perception of threats.[9,10]

Regarding the autonomic response, the two branches of the autonomic nervous system (ANS), sympathetic and parasympathetic, reciprocally contrast their actions to determine the prevalent type of coping response that we observe in an animal. The changing balance between the sympathetic and parasympathetic branches of the ANS will determine the behavioral display. The sympathetic system releases norepinephrine (noradrenaline) and epinephrine (adrenaline) from the subcortical areas of the brain and adrenal gland. The physiologic response is an almost instantaneous, immediate increase in heart rate, blood pressure, respiratory rate, and vasoconstriction to internal organs. Epinephrine also stimulates breakdown of glycogen and fat (lipolysis) and increases glucose production (gluconeogenesis) to provide immediate energy to fuel fight or flight.

Stimulation of the HPA axis provides cortisol release, which aids in the immediate response; however, chronic stimulation may lead to the medical and behavioral consequences associated with chronic stress (see Chapter 7). Studies have shown that psychological factors may stimulate the HPA axis more than physical factors; therefore, addressing mental well-being is essential to both health and welfare.[11–13]

A proinflammatory immune response is activated by acute stress to prepare the body for possible injuries caused by the perceived threat. This early response is therefore adaptive and will subside once the threat is removed with no injuries occurred. However, when the stress persists and the threat is not removed, the immune response causes a depletion of inflammatory resources with immune suppression. This chronic response is maladaptive and detrimental to the animal. Chronic fear can significantly affect the mental and physical health as well as the welfare of an individual.[14]

Neuroanatomy of fear

The activation of the stress response and the associated perception of fear is triggered by the activation of the amygdala. The amygdala is an almond-shaped structure located deep within the temporal cortex; it is considered part of the limbic system. The amygdala is considered to be the primary site responsible for processing external and internal stimuli, both pleasant and unpleasant, that are relevant to the animal. Inputs run from the sensory organs through the thalamus.[15] When an animal perceives the stimulus, the amygdala triggers an immediate physiologic fear or startle response, priming the body for immediate action. A second, slower pathway travels through the cortex to analyze the signal to determine if the threat is real, but once the emotional stage is triggered, it may be difficult to inhibit. The amygdala signals the cells of the paraventricular nuclei of the hypothalamus to release corticotrophin-releasing hormone, thus stimulating the hypothalamic–pituitary axis and the release of norepinephrine from the locus ceruleus.[9] In addition, the more anxious or aroused the individual, the less the ability to make a voluntary cognitive response (i.e., the cortical response or high road) before the immediate or subconscious response (low road) is triggered.[16] The amygdala is also the central site for fear conditioning; it integrates prior learning and memory to stimulate other brain centers to initiate the autonomic threat response.[17] Fear conditioning is thought to play a role in the development of fear and anxiety disorders such as phobias, panic, and posttraumatic stress.

The hippocampus is another major nucleus of the limbic system and is involved in memory storage.[18] It has anatomical connections with the amygdala and hypothalamus. It is also considered to be responsible for processing contextual information and differentiating between safe and dangerous; dysfunction may lead to an anxiety response to an otherwise benign stimulus as a result of overestimation of the potential threat, as in posttraumatic stress disorder in humans.[19] The hippocampus can normally suppress the HPA axis. However, chronic stress and cortisol can damage the hippocampus, resulting in dysregulation of the HPA axis.[20] A reduction in hippocampal volume has been identified in posttraumatic stress disorders and in animals exposed to chronic stress.[21] The individual is thought to be less able to draw on memory to evaluate the nature of the stressor when hippocampal function is compromised.

A brain structure which is particularly relevant for the regulation of the neuroendocrine fear response is the locus ceruleus. The locus ceruleus is a brainstem nucleus located in the gray matter of the pons.[22] The locus ceruleus contains the highest concentration of norepinephrine neurons in the brain and sends projections to many brain regions, including the cortex, hypothalamus, hippocampus, and the median and dorsal raphe nuclei.[23] Stimulation of the locus ceruleus triggers the release of norepinephrine. Inputs to the locus ceruleus arrive via sensory and visceral stimuli and from afferent projections from the central nucleus of the amygdala. Corticotrophin-releasing factor resulting from amygdala stimulation has an excitatory effect on the locus coeruleus.[24] Dysregulation of the locus ceruleus may be associated with sudden and intense fear responses (paniclike) that cause an animal to be unable to focus and unresponsive to verbal cues for behavior modification. This may explain why many pet parents report that their leash-aggressive dog is very obedient except when it sees another dog.

The dorsal and medial raphe nuclei are two functional neuron clusters located in the centromedial portion of the brainstem and considered part of the reticular formation.[25] Together, these nuclei provide virtually all serotonin input to the forebrain.[26] It is hypothesized that the limbic projections of the medial raphe nucleus help modulate fear and anxiety, including autonomic responses, while the dorsal raphe nucleus modulates cognitive and motor components that inhibit flight or fight responses.[26] The forebrain is also involved in the fear response in that it has some influence in modulating the limbic system and hypothalamus, and a functioning forebrain is necessary to unlearn fear responses. Dysregulation of fear pathways appears to be important in manifestation of the clinical signs associated with phobias and anxiety disorders. This dysregulation involves alterations in the activity of a number of neurotransmitters, including serotonin, norepinephrine, and gamma-aminobutyric acid (GABA). Of these neurotransmitters, serotonin and GABA are inhibitory and typically quiet the stress response (see Box 14.4).

Development of fearful behavior

Fearful behavior can be directed toward different targets: people, other dogs, animals, and environmental stimuli in general. Regardless of the target, however, fearful behavior has a common origin and development. Similarly, the same

Box 14.4 The nature of fear

Determinants of fear

Genetics
- Species: unconditioned stimuli for fear such as predators, environmental danger, novel situations, and social threats
- Individual: temperament

Environmental
- Inadequate socialization, habituation
- Sensory isolation/nutritional deprivation/illness during development
- Traumatic/aversive experiences (conditioning)
- Consequences/learning (negative reinforcement by stimulus retreat)
- Systemic illness, pain, discomfort at any stage of life

Components of fear

Physiology
- Activation of autonomic and neuroendocrine systems with influence on the cardiovascular system, pupils, piloerection, and glucose metabolism

Behavior
- The type of fearful behavior that is exhibited is determined by genetics (species, breed, individual), experience, environment, type and intensity of stimulus, and presence/absence of conspecifics, family
- The function of fear-related behavior is to remove the stimulus (threats) or remove the animal from the fearful situation (escape)

Emotion
- Observation of the emotional state of stimulus, family members, or other pets

foundational principles of behavior modification can be applied to all presentations of fearful behavior.

Ontogeny of fear

Excessive fear responses may be due to genetics and epigenetics, inadequate early environmental experiences, inadequate early socialization, a conditioned fear due to one or more unpleasant experiences, medical or behavioral pathology, or a combination of these factors (see Chapter 2 and Box 14.4).

Many fearful behaviors can be linked to experiences in the first year of development. Proper handling, nutritional, and maternal care during the first few weeks of life in the breeder's environment, exposure during the socialization period to a variety of people, places, animals, objects, and sensory stimuli (e.g., sights, sounds, odors, surfaces, handling) with which the pet will be interacting in the future can set the pet up for success. Conversely, a lack of exposure can contribute to fearful behaviors that might be difficult, if not impossible, to resolve (see Chapters 2 and 5). Together with adequate early exposure, maintaining a long-term positive exposure to appropriate social and environmental experiences is necessary for preventing excessive fear.[27] This seems to be particularly important around the age of sexual maturity, when there may be a second phase of heightened sensitivity.[27,28]

Unpleasant and stressful experiences during early adolescence, including punishment-based training, may also

contribute to fear conditioning and increased avoidance[29-35] (see Chapters 2, 5, and 10). Attendance at puppy classes and use of pheromones may to some degree be preventive[36-38] (see Chapters 2, 5, and 12). When dogs and cats are exposed to new stimuli, their response will depend on their genetics, epigenetics, stage of development, previous experience with similar stimuli, and the emotional and medical health of the pet at the time of exposure.[11] If the outcome is positive, then the fear may decrease with further exposure. If the stimulus has no consequence, the pet may ignore the stimulus with further exposure. However, pets that have an unpleasant experience or perceive that the stimulus might be harmful will avoid or become increasingly fearful of the stimulus. The perception of impending harm or threat is in the eye of the beholder. Many pet parents are not aware of the subtle signs of fear and anxiety or may be misinformed or inappropriately counseled to ignore them. For this reason, they may continue to expose their pet to the stimulus, inducing more intense fear. Pet parents may bring their pet to the veterinarian at a later date reporting a sudden change in behavior when in fact, the onset was insidious. Increasing the frequency of exposure to fear-evoking stimuli has been shown to increase the risk of inducing further fear and phobias.[39] An intensely unpleasant or aversive event can lead to an intensely fearful and lasting memory of the stimulus (one-event or single-event learning) (see Chapter 10). Although the pet may only become fearful of specific stimuli such as a noise (e.g., gunfire), place (e.g., veterinary clinic), or person (e.g., neighbor's child), some pets may generalize to many similar stimuli (e.g., all children). In addition, the pet may become fearful or anxious when exposed to stimuli associated with events which precede or predict the unpleasant situation (e.g., the car ride that precedes the veterinary visit). Emotional dysregulation and/or high emotional arousal place the dog in a state of hypervigilance, where fear responses are sudden and intense, and preclude the possibility of conscious decisions as to how to respond to environmental stimuli. Therefore, only if the pet's level of emotional arousal is sufficiently low can it review options and make conscious decisions as to whether a stimulus is positive, aversive, or of no consequence. Arousal can be reduced by ensuring that the pet has a good control of the environment. This can be achieved through selection of an appropriate environment and stimuli that will keep the animal under its fear threshold and through behavior modification that will help manage challenging contexts and stimuli. Medication therapy may also be useful.

Regardless of the cause, each fear-eliciting event that does not end with a positive outcome is likely to aggravate the problem further.[39] Any response from the pet parent or the same fear-inducing stimulus that might lead to an unpleasant consequence will further increase the fear and anxiety. Therefore, punishment and other aversive correction techniques must be entirely avoided, and the stimuli should be muted, minimized, or avoided until controlled and successful exposure training can be implemented. If the pet escapes from the situation or aggression results in retreat of the stimulus, then the behavior might be negatively reinforced because the threatening stimulus has been removed. See Chapter 10 for a discussion of negative reinforcement. This is not to say that pets that are showing signs of anxiety and fear should be made to endure frightening stimuli instead of retreating in order to avoid negative reinforcement of escape behavior. This type of treatment is called flooding. Flooding (response blocking) can be very difficult to implement without doing harm to the pet and should be avoided.

It is oft heard in veterinary hospitals that the pet parent's anxiety causes the pet's anxiety to increase. While the pet's anxiety is not likely to be caused by the pet parent's emotional state, it may be influenced by it. There is evidence that dogs are sensitive to the emotional states of others and may show empathy to humans and other dogs by changing their behavior.[40-42] This may occur even when the subject is not part of the dog's social group[43] and in situations with only auditory stimuli.[44]

There is in fact evidence that emotional contagion (changes in one individual's emotional state causing the same emotional state in another individual) exists in dogs toward humans and other dogs within their social group, specifically, if dogs' emotional states were positively correlated with the emotional valence of the sounds to which they were exposed.[45] Chemosignals may play a part in the transmission of emotional state from humans to dogs.[46] In summary, if the pet parent displays any emotions of anger, fear or anxiety, this is likely to increase the pet's anxiety, while calm and happy visual, olfactory and auditory expressions and responses can help to reduce it.[44-47]

Clinical signs associated with fear, phobia, and anxiety in pets

The fearful response could include aggression, cowering, shaking, freezing, or escape. Signs of emotional conflict that suggest a pet is becoming uncomfortable in a situation include displacement behaviors such as yawning, lip licking, whining, out-of-context grooming, or circling. Other changes in the body language of an animal associated with fear include: tail held low or tucked, ears held back, avoidance of eye contact, lowered body position, leaning away, lateral recumbency, and submissive urination. In fearful situations, the animal will attempt to perform behaviors to disengage from the threatening interaction. The innate behavior patterns typical of the species, the personality of the individual animal, its learning and conditioning, the nature of the stimulus (e.g., adult versus child) and the location where the interaction happens, will determine the coping response of the pet (i.e., whether the animal freezes, flees, fidgets, or fights). Fear may result in aggression by some pets, while others respond by cowering, remaining motionless, or attempting to escape. These behaviors may be associated with autonomic signs, including trembling, hypersalivation, elimination, and dilated pupils.

Prevention

Appropriate socialization can help prevent fear of people (see Chapters 2 and 5). The young animal should be exposed to a wide variety of people during its socialization period in the early months of life, taking care that it is not so overwhelmed as to become fearful. Treats, play, and upbeat social interaction will facilitate socialization. Animals that are excessively fearful should not be used for breeding, as fear has been shown to have a heritable component.[48] Fear of animals can often be prevented with healthy neonatal care and adequate socialization with other animals. Puppy socialization classes

and kitty kindergarten can be particularly beneficial. Adequate supervision and control are important when introducing the pet to other animals in order to ensure that the interaction is amicable. See the case of Ron below. Play that is too rough or leads to fear can be counterproductive; therefore, be prepared to separate the animals with verbal cues, treats, and/or removing the animal from the context if arousal becomes excessive or anxiety is noted. For this reason, busy dog parks may not be the ideal environment for socialization of puppies. Continued ongoing reward training and positive exposure to other pets should be continued into adulthood.

The veterinarian should be instrumental in reinforcing these notions for all pet parents. In spite of ample opportunities for socialization and in the absence of abuse, some cats and dogs may still exhibit fear and timidity of people. There are likely underlying genetic problems in these animals. Genetic fears may be evident in the first 2–3 months, although some fears do not become evident until later in adolescence (e.g., sexual maturity). See Chapter 3 for a more detailed discussion of the genetics of behavior.

Foundational treatment concepts

Behavior disorders are treated with four modalities: (1) evaluation of systemic wellness; (2) management of the environment to reduce or eliminate interactions with fear-eliciting stimuli; (3) neurochemical modulation through supplements, medications, diet, and pheromone analogs; and (4) behavioral therapies (behavior modification). This is discussed extensively in Chapters 9–12 and Box 14.5. Not every pet will need a treatment from every modality listed above; however, all modalities should be considered for their potential usefulness in each case. Behavioral therapies for treating fear are based on two important principles: (1) avoidance of any stimuli or situations that evoke a fear response and (2) controlled exposure to stimuli in such a way that the pet becomes tolerant and comfortable with their presence and they no longer elicit a fear response (see Box 14.6).

Punishment must not be used with fearful pets even when it can successfully suppress undesirable behaviors, as it actually conditions further fear (see the case of Harry below). For example, if a pet is playfully lunging, chasing, or overly rambunctious with another pet, pet parents may try to suppress the behavior with punishment or corrections instead of teaching, encouraging, and reinforcing appropriate play, resulting in the perpetuation and negative progression of the behavior at least. At worst, the pet could develop a fear response to the pet parent. As noted above, any fear, frustration, or anger on the part of the pet parent, or fear and aggression by the other

---

> **Box 14.5** Four modalities used in treating behavioral disorders
>
> - Evaluation of systemic wellness
> - Management of the environment to reduce or eliminate interactions with fear-eliciting stimuli
> - Neurochemical modulation through supplements, medications, diet, pheromone analogs
> - Behavioral therapies (behavior modification)

Box 14.6 Considerations in creation of a behavioral therapy plan for fearful, phobic, and anxious pets

- List of stimuli to which the pet shows fear or anxiety
- Identification of the specific body language signals associated with fear and anxiety
- Identification of the functional reward associated with the performance of any behaviors associated with fear or anxiety
- Identification of the threshold for fear
- Controlled exposure
- Teaching the pet coping tools or alternate behaviors
- Modifying the behavior performed by the pet by modifying the emotional state
- Avoidance of any aversive training techniques
- Utilization of desensitization, counterconditioning, differential reinforcement of alternative or incompatible behaviors (see Chapter 10).

animal, will further fuel the fear response. On the other hand, trying to reassure a fearful pet will contrast the emotional experience of fear and contribute to change the mood state of the animal, thereby decreasing the chance that the pet is further sensitized. If the level of arousal of the fearful pet is low enough to engage or direct the pet to focus onto an operantly conditioned alternate behavior, then the pet parent can ask the pet to perform a previously trained verbal cue that has been associated with a positive outcome. If the animal is too aroused to be successful, the pet parent should not be afraid to attempt comforting and calming the dog or cat because the fear will not be positively reinforced by the pet parent's affection. Instead, the pet will be calmer and feel safer. On the other hand, the best option when a pet is too stressed to learn is to leave the situation. Comforting and calming a pet may include gentle verbal measurements, invitations to engage in positive behaviors ("let's go play"), and high-value treats. Techniques for behavior modification should always be positive reinforcement based.[49-53]

Creation of a behavior therapy plan should include the following: (1) list of stimuli to which the pet shows fear or anxiety; (2) identification of the specific body language signals associated with fear and anxiety; (3) identification of the functional reward associated with the performance of any behaviors associated with fear or anxiety; (4) identification of the threshold for fear; (5) controlled and gradually escalating intensity of exposure (desensitization) with or without counterconditioning (CC) (DS/CC); (6) teaching the pet coping tools or alternate behaviors (differential reinforcement) (7) modifying the behavior performed by the pet by modifying the emotional state (counterconditioning); and (8) avoidance of any aversive training techniques. Pets that exhibit fear from an early age (8–12 weeks or younger) with no known exposure to traumatic environmental events may be very difficult to treat successfully.

The prognosis is better for cases in which:

- the pet was adequately socialized to stimuli such as people, animals, sounds, and environments;
- the problem started during adulthood;
- the fear is of appropriate duration and intensity for the specific fear-evoking stimulus;
- the pet does not have other concurrent fears;
- the pet parent can successfully control the environment and the pet to improve its relationship with other animal(s) gradually.

Desensitization and counterconditioning can be effective, especially if the intensity of the fear-evoking stimulus can be controlled for the training session. Conversely, this training strategy may difficult to implement, takes a substantial amount of time to complete, is best done with a highly skilled animal training professional, and less likely to succeed if the location has been associated with fear-evoking events before the training can be started, if the fear is intense, if there are signs of aggression, and if the intensity of the fear-evoking stimulus cannot be controlled (e.g., invasive medical procedures). Pet parent compliance (willingness and ability) is also an issue with respect to effectively implementing a desensitization and counterconditioning program.

Management of the environment can reduce fear and anxiety significantly, even without other treatments. As discussed in Chapters 2, 5, and 10, environmental enrichment and the creation of a sanctuary space for dogs and cats that are anxious and fearful can decrease fear, anxiety, and stress, improving welfare. Enrichment, whether toys, exercise, auditory, or olfactory, can provide the pet with useful displacement activities to redirect fear and anxiety. For example, some dogs carry toys around and/or chew on them when scared or nervous as a self-soothing activity. Depending on the nature of the fear, sanctuary spaces and hiding places may be enhanced with other features such as a physical barrier to protect a fearful cat from the household dogs. Failing to provide fearful pets with the possibility to avoid fear-eliciting stimuli in an uncontrolled environment may result in further sensitization to the fear-evoking stimulus, with worsened fear and potentially an onset of fear-related aggression.

Although behavioral modification and environmental management are the two main components of fear treatment, medication, supplements, diet, and pheromone analogs can be useful or even necessary for a positive outcome. Neurochemical modulation is discussed in detail in Chapters 9, 11, and 12. Fearful pets with emotional dysregulation that causes them to overreact to mild stimuli and prevents them from easily calming down once the stimulus is removed may benefit from medication. Sometimes, even pets with a moderate fear may need the help of medication. This may be the case, for example, when the fear-evoking stimulus cannot be removed because the environment does not allow it or because the stimulus itself is necessary (e.g., an unfamiliar person needs to handle a dog or cat with fear of people).

Finally, all patients that present with behavioral disorders should receive a full physical examination and screening lab work at minimum. Even if the pet parent believes that the patient's clinical signs are due to purely psychiatric disease, there is overwhelming evidence that behavioral clinical signs can and often are linked to systemic or painful disease processes. In addition, physical examination and laboratory screening should be considered an essential baseline prior to dispensing of any psychotropic medication (see Chapters 6 and 9).

Prognosis

Prognosis is somewhat dependent of the pet parent's goals for the pet, their ability to complete the treatment, and their tolerance of the pet's clinical signs. Pet parents who are more tolerant, have reasonable welfare centered goals, and can implement at minimum the management and medication plans will generally achieve positive outcomes. Conversely, pet parents with unrealistic goals or that do not have the ability to treat the pet properly may experience poor and unsatisfactory outcomes. The prognosis may be better if the onset of the fear-related behavior is recent and its duration is proportional to the intensity of the stimulus, if the pet has a stable temperament and was adequately socialized to people, and if the pet parent can control further interactions to ensure safety and success. The prognosis may be more negative for pets with a strong genetic component and intense emotional dysregulation, with an early age of fear onset, or that have had grossly inadequate early socialization. The prognosis is also worse in environments where control of fear-eliciting stimuli is difficult or when safety cannot be ensured. In these cases, prevention may be the only practical way to ensure safety and minimize stress for the pet. Regardless, many pets can do very well with proper treatment and realistic expectations.

Fear of people

Fear of people can be toward unfamiliar people in general, specific persons (either unfamiliar or familiar), or people with certain physical and behavioral characteristics (e.g., children, babies, or males with beards or in uniform). Fear of people can progress to phobia, and can lead to aggression. It can also generalize to all people, or to people of a certain ethnicity, or possessing similar characteristics (visual, auditory, olfactory). It is essential that the pet parent has reasonable goals. If the pet is intensely fearful or has the potential for aggression, interactions, especially with children or the elderly, may need to be limited or entirely avoided.

If a pet is afraid of guests visiting the house, the pet is usually (or will become) reactive also to stimuli that predict the visitor coming in (e.g., doorbell). In this case, desensitization and counterconditioning to these stimuli may need to precede the controlled exposure to people. Dogs may bark and run toward the door while cats may run away from the door and hide. Dogs that are fearful may hide as well and may not always bark. Sanctuary spaces can be very helpful in situations where the pet is afraid of visitors to the home. Using reward-based training, the pet can be taught to stay in the sanctuary space calmly. Very fearful or aggressive pets can stay in that space while the visitors are present and be let out when they leave the home. Visitors should be told to call and refrain from knocking or ringing the doorbell. For pets that are ready to interact with visitors (i.e., have foundational behaviors and can perform them calmly), controlled exposures can begin on leash.

Common mistakes in treating fear, anxiety, or phobia of people are (1) forcing the pet to interact with a person who the pet views as threatening; (2) lack of awareness of body language signals indicative of fear; (3) leaving the pet loose instead of keeping the pet confined on leash; (4) unrealistic goals requiring the pet to interact with all visitors in a friendly manner; (5) moving too quickly through the controlled exposures; and (6) treatment with confrontation or punishment.

When the dog or cat appears entirely relaxed with the visitors and there is no history or potential for aggression, the question then becomes how much interaction with the stranger the pet would enjoy. It is important to note that some pets will find interactions with unfamiliar people undesirable or potentially threatening. In fact, dogs and cats often show limits in how much affection they will tolerate, even from familiar people and family members. Therefore, it is essential for pet parents to know their pet and read its facial expressions, body language, and posturing to determine how far to proceed with each stranger and the pet's limits of comfort. For some pets, it will never be safe nor appropriate for them to interact with the people or types of people of whom they are afraid. Especially when severe fear-based aggression is a possible outcome, keeping a pet entirely away from visitors is often the safest option.

If the pet enjoys physical contact from known individuals and the pet parent can evaluate the situation and determine that the dog or cat is relaxed and willing to engage in further interaction, the pet parents should proceed to structured interactions with the visitors. Most cat pet parents will not engage in this activity, as cats may be less likely to lunge and bite in this situation than dogs, making the pet parent less concerned about fear of unfamiliar people. However, if the person who is unfamiliar will be a part of the family's social group, introduction may be important and the instructions here will apply to both dogs and cats.

It is optimal to instruct visitors to interact with the animal using an operantly conditioned verbal cue. For example, they may ask the dog to "high five" or "give the paw" or "target/touch" and then reward the dog. This does several things to help make the situation safe. By using a cue that the animal has learned will consistently end with a reward, the pet controls the outcome, lowering anxiety and stress. If, for some reason, the pet shows signs of fear and is too anxious to eat, the interaction should not yet progress to physical interaction. Therefore, if it does not respond with focusing and settling, the dog or cat may be indicating that it is not comfortable with taking the reward from the stranger. When the pet does take the treat from the visitor, it is building a positive relationship with the stranger.

CASE EXAMPLES

Case 1

Harry

Presentation

Harry, a 2-year-old intact male 5 kg Pomeranian, was presented for barking and escape attempts whenever someone on a bike approached during a walk.

History

Harry was adopted at five months from a Pomeranian rescue. History prior to five months of age included adoption from a breeder at eight weeks of age by a previous family. Because of a global pandemic, he was not socialized but instead kept on the pet parent's property. He was relinquished to the rescue at four-and -a-half months of age because the previous pet parents said that they

CASE EXAMPLES—cont'd

didn't have time for him. The current family noticed that when he walked in their neighborhood, his tail was tucked, he scanned the environment, and he panted heavily, even when the environment was not warm. They had worked with a trainer who rode a bike back and forth while the pet parent corrected Harry by pulling on a leash attached to a pinch collar each time that he barked or tried to escape. The pet parent initially thought that this process was working, as Harry eventually would lie on the sidewalk. However, over the next year and a half, his behavior had gotten worse. Sometimes, he refused to walk outside altogether for 24 hours after seeing a bike.

Workup

A physical examination, CBC, chemistry, U/A, fT4 (ED), fecal antigen test + Giardia were unremarkable. Harry was tentative but ate treats readily and approached the veterinary healthcare team to solicit attention.

Differential diagnoses

The differential diagnoses for Harry included specific (situational) anxiety, specific (situational) fear, and fear-induced aggression specific (situational) phobia. He was diagnosed with specific (situational) phobia and fear-induced aggression (barking).

Treatment

Because his clinical signs were chronic and started at a young age, he had not been socialized well, had experienced trauma during training sessions, and had a long recovery time, indicating that the autonomic response associated with the response was prolonged, a short-term medication, clonidine, was dispensed for walks at a dosage of 0.01 mg/kg PO 1.5 hours prior to walks up to TID. The pet parents were given resources for body language, training tools, environmental modification, and behavior modification. In addition, they were given a referral to a positive reinforcement animal training professional. The plan included: (1) avoidance of walks at times when they were likely to see bikes; (2) identification of his favorite rewards; (3) differential reinforcement of all calm behaviors outside; (4) discontinuation of all aversive training (e.g., pinch collar); (5) teaching an alternate behavior (DRA) which he could perform when he saw bikes; (6) reinforcing all calm behaviors in the presence of the stimulus (counterconditioning); and (7) eventually, if desired by the pet parents, desensitization and counterconditioning.

Follow-up

The veterinary nurse followed up by phone in one week. The pet parent noted no difference in frequency, intensity, or recovery with the clonidine. The pet parent was instructed to increase the clonidine to 0.02 mg/kg PO 1.5 hours prior to walks up to TID. If needed, they could go up to 0.03 mg/kg PO 1.5 hours prior to walks up to TID. They were reminded of the side effects of clonidine. They had yet to call the trainer, however they had stopped using the pinch collar, were spending most of their time in the backyard, and had enriched the indoor environment with toys. The veterinary nurse reminded them that working with the trainer was essential if they were going to reach their goals of happily walking him in the neighborhood.

The veterinary nurse followed up in three weeks by phone. The pet parents had two sessions with the trainer. Harry was in the process of learning to make eye contact with the pet parents on cue and the pet parents were using a clicker and treats when outside to reinforce any attention to them and any calm behavior. They noted that when he saw a bike through the fence, he glanced over at them. The veterinary nurse reminded them that they should always click and treat for those glances, as reinforced behaviors are offered more frequently.

Harry came in for a recheck examination with the veterinarian six weeks after the original appointment. He was receiving 0.025 mg/kg

clonidine PO 1.5 hours prior to walks. They had noted no side effects. They had four sessions with the trainer. Harry was now a "master" at looking at them. They demonstrated in the exam room how he could look at them even when the veterinary nurse shook a treat jar to try and distract him. They were taking five-minute walks outside of the house. The pet parents noticed that he was calmer and scanning less when he was outside. When he did get scared, he looked at them immediately. They had been doing what the trainer had said, giving him a treat for this behavior and then turning away from the stimulus, moving in the opposite direction. They felt like he recovered quickly enough with this method that they could within a block turn and go back in the original direction. The veterinarian instructed them to continue with the trainer.

Twelve weeks from the first appointment, the veterinary nurse checked in by phone. The pet parents were still giving the clonidine. They were able to take 45-minute walks in the neighborhood using the look cue and a new cue, "see that." The "see that" cue was intended to reinforce Harry for looking directly at the bikes. The pet parents were very pleased with the progress. Systematic desensitization and counterconditioning was discussed; however, the pet parents felt that significant progress had been made with the skills taught and that no further behavior modification was necessary.

Discussion

Harry's behavior could be genetic in origin. However, he could also have started showing fear of bikes due to trauma at his first home or while in foster or due to a lack of socialization (positive exposure to bikes) during the socialization period. The training which was done initially with the pinch collar most likely contributed in a negative way to his behavior (classically condition an unpleasant association with the stimulus). While the pet parent interpreted his behavior of lying down as improvement, it was more likely to be learned helplessness. Learned helplessness is an emotional state where the animal doesn't clearly understand how to escape the painful or frightening stimulus and essentially gives up, enduring the pain and refraining from offering any behavior in that situation. This is damaging to the relationship between dog and pet parent, breaking down the trust bond, inhibiting learning and negatively affecting welfare. This pet needed medication as well as behavior modification to improve. The pet parents didn't begin the systematic desensitization and counterconditioning program because they had reached their goals and the time commitment with that type of program is substantial.

Case 2

Hermione

Presentation

Hermione, a 1-year-old spayed 4 kg female DSH, cat presented for fear of people.

History

Hermione lived in a household with two adults. She was rescued from under a car when she was six weeks old. She would not come closer than about 2.5 meters to family members and scurried away when approached. She hid under the bed when visitors were in the home. She was very shy when adopted and friends suggested that the family catch her daily, hold her, and attempt to pet her to show her they were friendly. Upon returning home from work, they would chase her, pull her out from under furniture, and attempt to pet her, but she always became frantic and quickly escaped. The family soon stopped the interaction as they noticed that the pet's avoidance was getting worse.

Workup

At presentation, Hermione displayed signs of intense fear, attempting to escape and hide under a chair in the consult room. The

continued

physical examination was unremarkable, but blood could not be drawn nor could urine be collected due to her level of fear, anxiety, and stress.

Differential diagnoses

Differential diagnoses include generalized anxiety, generalized fear, and specific (situational) fear or phobia. She was diagnosed with situational fear.

Treatment

Previsit pharmaceuticals were discussed with the family and a plan was made for them to bring Hermione back after they had given 100 mg of gabapentin three hours prior to their scheduled time of arrival at the veterinary hospital.

They were given resources on feline body language, cat training, environmental enrichment for cats, and how to properly interact with fearful pets. They learned that they had been too assertive in trying to befriend her. They were told to begin ignoring her, especially avoiding eye contact. Additional recommendations included creating a sanctuary space in an area of the house where she tended to find refuge, making sure that all her resources (water, food, litterbox, toys, comfortable bedding) were available without the need to leave the sanctuary space. Finally, they were given the name of a cat training professional who could work with them via video conference on clicker training Hermione to approach them.

During quiet times, when she was at the periphery of the family room, the pet parents were instructed to click and calmly toss small pieces of shrimp just behind her (treat–retreat). They were to shape her to come closer and closer, all the while ignoring her. The home environment was to be kept as calm and quiet as possible. The veterinarian also discussed that she may need a supplement or medication to be a social cat with people.

Follow-up

When Hermione came in for the blood draw, the veterinary nurse spoke to the pet parents about her behavior. They had set up the sanctuary space and she was coming around the corner into the living room, giving them opportunities to work with her regularly. The lab work and fecal examination were within normal limits.

Three weeks from the first appointment, the veterinary nurse followed up with the pet parents by phone. They reported that she would jump up on the couch to eat shrimp from their hands. They had met with the cat training professional, who had taught them how to teach Hermione to target so that they could know when she wanted to be petted.

Five weeks from the original appointment, the veterinary nurse followed up by phone. The pet parents reported that Hermione was sitting next to them on the couch while they watched movies. As long as they didn't get up, she stayed on the couch with them. They were very pleased. They asked how they could introduce them to visitors. The veterinary nurse discussed that she most likely didn't want to be introduced to visitors, based on her behavior and the assessment of the veterinarian. If they wanted to introduce her to visitors, they could work with the cat training professional for 2–6 months. They would need to have regular visitors over in order to achieve a meaningful result. Alternatively, they could work with one particular person if there was someone that she just had to get to know. The pet parents felt that she had to get to know their adult child who visited frequently. They decided to work on this with the cat training professional, using the same clicker training exercises that they used themselves. For visitors other than their adult child, they decided to let Hermione go to her sanctuary space and stay there if she wanted.

Because Hermione remained very fearful when outside of her home (e.g., during veterinary visits or when boarded), gabapentin was used for all veterinary visits, as described previously. To minimize the use of boarding facilities as much as possible, the pet parents arranged to have a family friend come to their home and take care of Hermione when they needed to travel.

Discussion

Hermione's family certainly loved her, however by forcing their love on her, she became more fearful of them. For the best outcome, families should, as Hermione's family did, accept that their cat may not need to meet every person who visits the house.

Fear of animals

Dogs and cats may be fearful of members of the same or of other species. Also, as is the case with all behavior disorders, the origin of fear is very likely to be multifactorial and is influenced by genetics, epigenetics, and early experience. Early positive exposure to different species and breeds can determine if the pet is fearful and to which stimuli that fear is directed (e.g., species, specific breeds). Poor maternal behavior and lack of social experience with other members of one's own species during neonatal development (e.g., hand rearing) and sensitive period for socialization (see Chapter 2) can result in a pet that is fearful of other animals of its species or unable to communicate effectively. This can be dangerous if the fearful pet responds with aggression. Effective socialization, including puppy or kitten classes at a young age as well as ongoing positive interactions through adulthood, may prevent problems. Because the brains of young individuals are very plastic and shaped by learning and experience, early intervention with behavior modification and potentially medications or supplements is essential. Early onset of moderate to severe fear may be refractory to treatment, especially if treatment is delayed.

On occasion, a single traumatic event can lead to fear of another animal. This is a particular concern in cats, which do not have a good repertoire of reconciliation behaviors once problems arise. For example, if one cat in the household hears a sudden, frightening noise while another pet is nearby, it may redirect its arousal and aggression to that pet, and the relationship may be altered by the single event. Pet parents that try to suppress behaviors directed toward other pets (exuberance, lunging) by using harsh punishment techniques may classically condition further fear and anxiety. See above for diagnosis and treatment.

CASE

Presentation

Ron, a 2-year-old, 6 kg, neutered male DSH cat was presented for fear of the family dog.

History

Ron was recently adopted from a shelter by a family with a 6-year-old female Labrador Retriever, Luna. The medical record from the shelter indicated that Ron was in good physical health and did not exhibit any problem behaviors during his stay at the shelter. When Ron was brought home, Luna ran up to the carrier, sniffing and wagging her tail. Ron was brought into another room, where he was let out of the carrier. Later that night, Luna was let into the room with him. She walked up and play bowed, pushing her nose toward him. Ron became piloerect, his pupils dilated, he hissed and ran under the bed. Since that time, when the two were out together, Ron was under the bed. When Luna goes to daycare or for a walk, Ron comes out into the house and "acts as if he owns the place."

Workup

Ron's physical examination, lab work, and fecal PCR showed evidence of Giardia and hookworms. Other than that, it was unremarkable.

Differential diagnoses

The differential diagnoses included specific (situational) fear or phobia. Ron was diagnosed with specific fear and intestinal parasites.

Treatment

The pet parents were given instructions on how to properly treat the intestinal parasites. In addition, they were given resources on cat and dog training, cat and dog body language, and the name of a positive reinforcement dog trainer. The plan consisted of impulse control training for Luna (e.g., go to your place, stay, leave it), creation of sanctuary spaces for Ron and Luna, clicker training Ron to go to a spot on top of a cat tree, environmental enrichment for Luna and Ron, including high spaces for Ron in the main living areas and food toys for Luna, and settle exercises for both pets when they were together. In addition, the pet parents were instructed to separate the pets at all times except during training sessions. Neurochemical modulation was discussed with the pet parents in the way of supplements, medications, and diet. They were reluctant because they had just adopted Ron.

Follow-up

Two weeks after the initial appointment, the veterinary technician followed up with the pet parents by phone. They were working on the training on their own and hadn't called the trainer. They felt that the resources that they were given by the veterinary healthcare team such as websites, books, online courses, and videos had given them enough information to be successful. Twice daily, Luna received a 10-minute reward training session to learn relaxed behaviors ("go to your spot," "lie down," and "wait") before exposure to the cat. Ron was trained in his sanctuary space to go to a spot on a cat tree. So far, they were pleased with the process.

Four weeks after the initial appointment, the veterinary technician followed up with the pet parents. Luna and Ron had both been successful at learning their respective tasks; however, the pet parents could not get Ron to come out of his room when Luna was out, no matter how calm she was. The veterinary technician recommended a recheck with the veterinarian.

At the recheck examination, the pet parents relayed the same information that they had told the veterinary technician on the phone. At this time, a physical examination was completed, which was unremarkable, and a fecal antigen was repeated, which was also unremarkable. The veterinarian suggested that they use Zylkene (a commercial diet containing alpha-casozepine could have also been used), a supplement to decrease fear, anxiety, and stress so that Ron would come out of the sanctuary space long enough to work with Luna. See Chapter 12 for more information on Zylkene. The pet parents were told that the supplement could take six weeks to work.

In four weeks, the veterinary nurse followed up with the pet parents by phone. They reported that about three weeks after starting the Zylkene, Ron was more social and affectionate with everyone in the house, including Luna. While he wouldn't bunt her, he was able to be in the room and stay on top of the cat tree while she was on her bed. The pet parents were happy with this and agreed to continue to reinforce these behaviors with food.

Fear of places

Pets can become anxious and fearful about locations and surfaces, in much the same way they can about people, animals, and noises, and the principles of treatment are much the same. Every veterinarian is familiar with the pet that is fearful of the veterinary clinic. Many pet parents report that their pet loves to ride in the car but becomes anxious when it approaches the clinic. Other animals are afraid to be kept in a crate or confined to a room at home. Pets may also become fearful of a particular environment or a particular type of flooring. Some pets may be fearful of travel in moving vehicles and some may even have a fear of certain neighborhoods, parks, or even going to the pet parent's backyard.

Prevention

Frequent exposure to all types of environments should be employed in a controlled, positive way during the early months of the pet's life so that the pet habituates to a variety of environments and situations.

CASE

Presentation

Dobby, a 6-year-old, 6 kg spayed female Toy Poodle was presented for fear at the groomer's office. She lived in a family of five – two adults and three children.

History

Dobby shook uncontrollably and crouched against the back of her cage during each visit to the grooming shop. She had previously been "great" at the groomer's office, but in the past year, she had started to show fear.

continued

Workup

Dobby did not approach the veterinary healthcare team, trembled and kept her tail tucked throughout the visit. The physical examination was unremarkable with the exception of pain (yelping) upon manipulation of the right stifle. The veterinarian diagnosed her with medial patellar luxation. The pet parent did not report any sign of limping or acute pain; however, radiographs were recommended to rule out any pain component to the fear at the groomer's office. In addition, screening lab work and a fecal antigen test was recommended. The lab work and fecal were unremarkable. Because Dobby showed fear at the veterinarian's office, trazodone was prescribed at a dosage of 5 mg/kg PO three hours prior to the veterinary visit where she was to have the radiographs completed.

Dobby returned in one week for radiographs of her stifles and hips, which showed mild osteoarthritis in the right stifle and right hip. The veterinarian prescribed a nonsteroidal antiinflammatory for daily use for 14 days, discontinued the trazodone for visits to the veterinarian and groomer, and instead instructed the pet parent to give gabapentin 20 mg/kg PO three hours prior to veterinary or grooming visits.

Follow-up

The veterinary technician followed up in two weeks by phone. The pet parents reported that Dobby was now jumping up on the couch. They hadn't noticed that she had stopped doing that in the past year. The veterinary technician recommended that they get steps for the couch, gave them websites at which to shop, and told them briefly how to train the behavior. They hadn't been to the groomer yet, but they were planning to go the following week. They were told to continue the NSAID per the veterinarian's recommendations. In addition, they were given resources for body language and training as well as living with fearful pets. The pet parent was instructed to visit the grooming shop two to three times each week for food and play; however, they expressed that this was not possible with their schedule. They wanted to do what they could for Dobby, of course. With that said, they were a busy family and this would not be possible. The veterinary technician advised them to continue

with all recommendations and let them know how the visits to the groomer progressed.

The veterinary technician checked in with the pet parent in four weeks from the initial appointment. The pet parents had gone to the groomer and tested the gabapentin, and stated that the groomer said that it didn't work. When pressed, they said that they had given the gabapentin only one hour prior to the grooming visit. The veterinary technician reminded them that they should try this medication three hours prior to the appointment and to do a "test run" to see the effect before Dobby needed grooming. In addition, if they could watch the grooming when it did take place, either in person or on video, or if the groomer could send videos, that would be helpful in determining the extent to which the medication was working. She also discussed that there was behavior modification which would result in a more permanent positive change and reduce the medication burden for Dobby, but the pet parents declined.

The veterinary technician checked in with the pet parent eight weeks from the initial appointment. The pet parent had completed one test run with the gabapentin given three hours prior. They reported at 25% change in her behavior while at the groomer's office. She was calmer and didn't tremble, but she was still in the back of the cage with her tail tucked and didn't want to enter the office. The veterinary technician instructed the pet parents to increase the dosage of gabapentin to 30 mg/kg PO three hours prior to the grooming visit as per the veterinarian's instructions. Also, they were instructed to use food throughout the waiting process, ask the groomer to give food during grooming, and ask for Dobby to be done first so that they could pick her up immediately. They agreed to try these things.

The veterinary technician checked in with the pet parent 12 weeks from the initial appointment. The pet parent had completed a grooming visit with the gabapentin given three hours prior at the prescribed dose. They reported a 75% change in her behavior while at the groomer's office. Not only was she calmer, but she was able to eat in the waiting room and during grooming. The veterinary technician instructed them to continue with this plan indefinitely. She again offered behavior modification and they declined. They were happy with the outcome of treatment.

Conclusion

Fears, anxieties, and phobias are extremely common in companion animals. Ideally, all four modalities of treatment would be included in every plan. As was demonstrated by the case examples, while all modalities are considered for every case, pet parents are inevitably in the driver's seat and will decide what is reasonable for their pet and their family. Regardless treatment for fears and phobias can be very rewarding, improving the quality of life of pets and their families.

References

1. Piotti P, Uccheduu S, Alliani, et al. Management of specific fears and anxiety in the behavioral medicine of companion animals: punctual use of psychoactive medications. *Dog Behav.* 2019;23–30: doi:10.4454/db.v5i2.109.
2. Denenberg S. Problem behaviors and management in cats and dogs. In: *Small Animal Veterinary Psychiatry.* Oxfordshire, UK: CAB International; 2021.
3. Overall KL. *Manual of Clinical Animal Behavioral Medicine for Dogs and Cats.* St. Louis MO: Elsevier; 2013.
4. Talegon MI, Delgado BA. *Anxiety Disorders in Dogs.* www.intechopen.com. 262–280.
5. Bamberger M, Houpt KA. Signalment factors, comorbidity, and trends in behavior diagnosis in dogs: 1,644 cases (1991–2001). *J Am Vet Med Assoc.* 2006;229:1591–1601.
6. Sarviaho R, et al. Two novel genomic regions associated with fearfulness in dogs overlap human neuropsychiatric loci. *Transl. Psychiatry.* 2019;9:18.
7. Panksepp J. *Affective Neuroscience:* The Foundations of Humans and Animal Emotions. New York: Oxford University Press; 1998:206–222.
8. Russell PA. Fear-evoking stimuli. In: Sluckin W, ed. *Fear in Animals and Man.* New York: Van Nostrand Reinhold; 1979:86–124.
9. Carlson NR, Birkett MA. *Physiology of Behavior.* 12th ed. Essex, England: Person Education; 2017:344–379.
10. Rushen J. Some issues in the interpretation of behavioural responses to stress. In: Moberg GP, Mench JA, eds. *The Biology of Animal Stress. Basic Principles and Implications for Animal Welfare.* Wallingford, UK: CABI; 2000: 23–42.
11. Levine ED. Feline fear and anxiety. *Vet Clin North Am Small Anim Pract.* 2008;38: 1065–1079.

12. Clark JD, Roger DR, Calpin JP. Animal well being. II Stress and disease. *Lab Anim Sci.* 2005;57:571–579.

13. Hekman J, Karas AZ, Sharp CR. Psychogenic stress in hospitalized dogs; cross species comparisons, implications for health care, and the challenges of evaluation. *Animals.* 2014;4:331–334.

14. Sarjan HN, Yajurvedi HN. Chronic stress induced duration dependent alterations in immune system and their reversibility in rats. *Immunol Lett.* 2018;197:31–43.

15. Carlson NR, Birkett MA. *Physiology of Behavior.* 12th ed. Essex, England: Person Education; 2017.

16. Fung BJ, Qi S, Hassabis D, et al. Slow escape decisions are swayed by trait anxiety. *Nat Hum Behav.* 2019;3:702–708. doi:10.1038/s41562-019-0595-5. https://www.apa.org/monitor/nov02/synaptic.

17. Phelps EA, LeDoux JE. Contributions of the amygdala to emotion processing: from animal models to human behavior. *Neuron.* 2005;48:175–187.

18. McEwen BS, Magarinos AM. Stress effects on morphology and function of the hippocampus. *Ann NY Acad Sci.* 1997; 821:271–284.

19. Shin LM, Rauch SL, Pitman RK. Amygdala, medial prefrontal cortex, and hippocampal function in PTSD. *Ann N Y Acad Sci.* 2006;1071:67–79.

20. Mizoguchi K, Ishige A, Aburada M, et al. Chronic stress attenuates glucocorticoid negative feedback: involvement of the prefrontal cortex and hippocampus. *Neurocscience.* 2003;119:887–897.

21. Apfel B, Ross J, Hlavin J, et al. Hippocampal volume differences in Gulf War veterans with current versus lifetime posttraumatic stress disorder symptoms. *Biol Psychiatry.* 2011;69:541–548.

22. Benarroch EE. The locus ceruleus norepinephrine system: functional organization and potential clinical significance. *Neurology.* 2009;73: 1699–1704.

23. Hsiao JK, Potter WZ. Mechanisms of action of antipanic drugs. In: Ballenger JC, ed. *Clinical Aspects of Panic Disorder.* New York: Alan R Liss; 1990:239–317.

24. Bouret S, Duvel A, Onat S, et al. Phasic activation of locus ceruleus neurons by the central nucleus of amygdala. *J Neurosci.* 2003;23:3491–3497.

25. Briley M. Neurobiological mechanisms involved in antidepressant therapies. *Clin Neuropharmacol.* 1993;16:387–400.

26. Grove G, Coplan JD, Hollander E. The neuroanatomy of 5-HT dysregulation and panic disorders. *J. Neuropsychiatry Clin Neurosci.* 1997;9:198–207.

27. Serpell J, Duffy DL, Jagoe AJ. Becoming a dog: early experience and the development of behavior. In: Serpell J, ed. *The Domestic Dog.* Cambridge: Cambridge University Press; 2017.

28. Dehasse J. Sensory, emotional and social development in the young dog. *Bull Vet Clin Ethol.* 1994;2:6–29.

29. Fox MW. *Understanding Your Dog.* New York: McCann and Geoghegan; 1972.

30. Hilby EF, Rooney NJ, Bradshaw JWS. Dog training methods; their use, effectiveness and interaction with adult behavior and welfare. *Anim Welf.* 2004;13:63–69.

31. Herron M, Shofer F, Reisner I. Survey of the use and outcome of confrontational and non-confrontational training methods in client-owned dogs showing undesirable behaviors. *Appl Anim Behav Sci.* 2009;117:47–54.

32. Blackwell EJ, Twells C, Seawright A, et al. The relationship between training methods and the occurrence of behaviour problems as reported by owners, in a population of domestic dogs. *J Vet Behav.* 2008;3:207–217.

33. Hsu Y, Sun L. Factors associated with aggressive responses in pet dogs. *Appl Anim Behav Sci.* 2010;123:108–123.

34. E, Loftus B, Richards G, et al. How do people train their dogs? A survey of training techniques used and training class attendance by UK dog owners. In: *Proceedings of the 2010 European Behaviour Meeting.* Hamburg, Belgium: ESVCE; 2010:179–181.

35. Roll A, Unshelm J. Aggressive conflict amongst dogs and factors affecting them. *Appl Anim Behav Sci.* 1997;52: 229–242.

36. Denenberg S, Landsberg GM. Effect of dog-appeasing pheromones on anxiety and fear in puppies during training its effects on long term socialization. *J Am Vet Med Assoc.* 2008;233:1874–1882.

37. Sterry J, Appleby D, Bizo L. The relationship between measures of problematical behaviour in adult dogs and age of first exposure outside the first owners' home and attendance at puppy classes. In: *Proceedings of the 2005 CABTSG Annual Study Day.* CABTSG; 2005:21–23.

38. Thompson KF, McBride EA, Redhead E. Training engagement and the development of behaviour problems in the dog. In: *Proceedings of the 7th International Veterinary Behavior Meeting.* Edinburgh, Belgium: ESVCE; 2009: 77–84.

39. Corridan CL, Mills DS, Pfeffer K. Predictive models for dogs with fears and phobias. In: *Proceedings of the 2010 European Behaviour Meeting.* Hamburg, Belgium: ESVCE; 2010:63–65.

40. Romero T, Konno A, Hasegawa T. Familiarity bias and physiological responses in contagious yawning by dogs support link to empathy. *PLoS One.* 2013; 8(August):1–8. pmid:23951146.

41. Van Bourg, J, Patterson, JE, Wynne CDL. Pet dogs (Canis lupus familiaris) release their trapped and distressed owners: individual variation and evidence of emotional contagion. *PLoS One.* 2020;15(4):e0231742. doi:10.1371/journal.pone.0231742.

42. Albuquerque N, Guo K, Wilkinson A, et al. Dogs recognize dog and human emotions. *Biol Lett.* 2016;12:20150883. doi:10.1098/rsbl.2015.0883.

43. Custance D, Meyer J. Empathic-like responding by domestic dogs (Canis familiaris) to distress in 9 humans: an exploratory study. *Anim Cogn.* 2012;15(May):851–859. pmid:22644113.

44. Silva K, Bessa J, de Sousa L. Auditory contagious yawning in domestic dogs (Canis familiaris): first evidence for social modulation. *Anim Cogn.* 2012;15:721–724.

45. Huber A, Barber ALA, Faragó T, et al. Investigating emotional contagion in dogs (Canis familiaris) to emotional sounds of humans and conspecifics. *Anim Cogn.* 2017;20:703–715.

46. D'Aniello B, Semin GR, Alterisio A, et al. Interspecies transmission of emotional information via chemosignals; from humans to dogs (Canis lupus familiaris). *Anim Cogn.* 2018;21:67–68.

47. Muller CA, Schmitt K, Barber ALA, Huber L. Dogs can discriminate emotional expressions of human faces. *Curr Biol.* 2015;25:601–605.

48. Goddard ME, Beilharz RG. Genetic and environmental factors affecting the suitability of dogs as Guide Dogs for the Blind. *Theor Appl Genet.* 1982;62: 97–102.

49. Baum M. Veterinary use of exposure techniques in the treatment of phobic domestic animals. *Behav Res Ther.* 1989;27:307–308.

50. Hothersall D, Tuber DS. Fears in companion dogs: characteristics and treatment. In: Keehn JD, ed. *Psychopathology in animals.* New York: Academic Press; 1979:239–255.

51. Tuber DS, Hothersall D, Peters MF. Treatment of fears and phobias. *Vet Clin North Am Small Anim Pract.* 1982;12: 607–623.

52. Voith VL, Borchelt PL. Fears and phobias in companion animals. In: Voith VL, Borchelt PL, eds. *Readings in Companion Animal Behaviour.* Trenton, NJ: Veterinary Learning Systems; 1996:140–152.

53. Walker R, Fisher J, Neville P. The treatment of phobias in the dog. *Appl Anim Behav Sci.* 1997;52:275–289.

Noise aversion

Kelly C. Ballantyne, DVM, DACVB

Introduction

Noise aversion is a term used in veterinary medicine to describe an animal's negative emotional and behavioral response(s) to noise. While commonly referred to as noise phobia, noise sensitivity, and noise reactivity, noise aversion may be a more appropriate term to describe the problem, as not all responses meet the criteria for phobia.[1-3] Noise and thunderstorm aversion are among the most common emotional disorders of dogs, ranging in prevalence from 17% to as high as 50% of the pet dog population.[4-9] While cats can also have noise aversions, their behavioral responses of freezing or hiding may be overlooked by pet parents, or not deemed as problematic or necessitating treatment unless the noise aversion results in more troublesome responses such as unacceptable elimination. In addition, noise aversion is one of the most common triggers of redirected aggression in cats toward people, other cats, and dogs.[10] Genetic sensitivity, trauma associated with noise, lack of socialization, and poor maternal care may contribute to the development and progression of the problem.[2,7,8,11,12] Fearful dogs have been shown to have greater noise sensitivity than nonfearful dogs.[4,7] One study suggested social transmission may play a role, whereby the dog learns its fear from another dog in the household,[10] but additional empirical data on this phenomenon are lacking. Noises that trigger an aversion include fireworks, thunder, gunshots, vacuum cleaners, or loud vehicle noises,[3,4,11] and dogs averse to one noise are not always averse to all noises.[2,5] Prevalence of noise aversion varies with study populations (e.g., behavior referral cases versus pet parent surveys) and with location, perhaps due to differences in geography, genetics and breed distribution, environment and upbringing, and cultures. In a web-based survey of over 4000 dog owners, 75% of whom were from the United States, 25% were fearful of noises (including storms) while in a UK postal survey of almost 4000 UK pet parents, 49% of dogs were reported to have noise fears. One study showed approximately 90% of dogs with storm phobias have noise phobias, but only 75% of dogs with noise phobias have storm phobias.[1] Some studies suggest a comorbidity with separation-related disorders and other fear and anxiety disorders.[1,7,8,9] However, one study found that about 50% of dogs with separation-related disorders were afraid of loud noises, while 23% of dogs with noise sensitivity had signs of anxiety.[7] In yet another study, fear of gunshots, thunder, and fireworks commonly co-occurred, but there was low association with other fearful and anxious behaviors including separation-related disorders, fear of people, and attention seeking.[4] Yet dogs with fear of less salient noises such as traffic, loud sounds on TV, and vacuum cleaners were more likely to have a comorbidity with separation-related disorders, fear of people, and fear of animals.[5] Similarly, Tiira et al. found a correlation between thunder, fireworks, and gunshots but not with other loud noises such as vacuums and leaf blowers.[7] This may indicate an association between fear of less salient noises with more fearful personalities (sensitivity, reactivity), while fear of more salient noises occurs in a wider range of dogs due to the nature of these stimuli.[4,13] Noise aversions typically develop around one to two years of age,[5,11] with prevalence[4,8,11] and severity[5,6] increasing with age. The aversion may generalize to the location where the noise was experienced and/or the conditions that co-occur with the noise (e.g., rain, wind, dark skies); therefore, animals may demonstrate signs of distress when exposed to these stimuli without the noise. Dogs that generalize their noise aversion to associated locations or develop signs later in life should be carefully evaluated for chronically painful conditions such as osteoarthritis.[14]

Exposure to fireworks, engine noises, banging doors, vacuum cleaners, and loud voices before six months of age[12] and proactive training prior to the onset of noise aversions may have protective effects.[5]

The best way to prevent fears and phobias is to carefully expose pets to as many different stimuli as possible while they are still young. As early as two weeks of age, puppies and kittens should be exposed to a wide variety of mild stimuli, including noises, lights, surface textures, and odors. The goal is to habituate them to a variety of stimuli during the socialization period and through the first year of life. Proactive counterconditioning to stimuli that are known to evoke fear, such as the sound of thunder or fireworks, using the animal's favorite reinforcer should begin as soon as possible.[5] See Chapters 2 and 5 for a discussion of socialization and prevention of behavior problems and Chapter 10 for a discussion of behavior modification, including desensitization and counterconditioning (DSCC).

Diagnosis and potential outcomes

Signs of noise aversion can include trembling, hiding, vocalization, attention seeking, crouching, pacing, freezing, panting, hypersalivation, destruction, escape attempts, decreased appetite or anorexia, vocalization, and urination or defecation in response to a noise or throughout the duration of a noise event.[3,4,6,15,12] (see Figure 15.1). The intensity of the clinical signs can range from mild signs of anxiety to intense panic. Return to normal baseline behavior following the end of the noise event may be delayed in some dogs, with approximately 12% taking 3–7 days to recover from the event, and approximately 3% taking several weeks to months.[5] In most cases, the fear-eliciting sound is loud and quite distinct (e.g., fireworks, thunder, gunshots) and difficult to localize. The diagnosis is straightforward if the pet parent is present at the time of the noise event to observe the pet's response; however, noise aversions may mimic separation-related

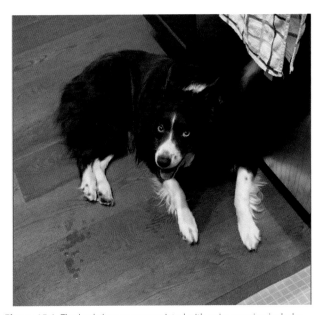

Figure 15.1 The body language associated with noise aversion includes ears back, panting, hiding, lying down, not moving, head down, and dilated pupils. *(Attribution: Kelly C. Ballantyne.)*

disorders if the pet's distress is more intense when home alone during a noise event.[16] Some pets may display aggression toward humans and other animals during or following noise events, either as redirected aggression or if attempts are made to force the frightened animal out of a hiding spot.

As with all behavior disorders, noise aversion is treated with four modalities in mind: systemic wellness, management of the environment, behavior modification, and neurochemical modulation (i.e., medications, supplements, diet). Many noise aversions can be managed successfully with a combination of environmental management, behavioral modification, and neurochemical modulation. The prognosis varies greatly depending on the individual, the duration and intensity of the problem, the ability to control stimuli during treatment, the household, and pet parent expectations. Successful resolution of noise aversions is possible for some dogs,[5] but management and medication may be necessary for many dogs throughout their lives.

We know that noise aversions can have a genetic component, which might explain why treatment of some dogs can be such a challenge. Other factors lending to a negative prognosis include the presence of concurrent fears and phobias and the inability to completely avoid fear-eliciting stimuli outside of controlled behavior modification sessions, which makes DSCC less effective. Complete avoidance of noise stimuli, especially thunderstorms and fireworks, is not possible for many animals. Thunderstorm season can last several months in some parts of the world and fireworks may occur daily for several weeks surrounding major holidays in some regions. In addition, thunderstorms have multiple stimuli, including sounds of rain, thunder, lightning, and possibly barometric pressure and static charges that are difficult to reproduce for DSCC sessions. In comparison, gunshots, cars, trucks, or other noises that might cause noise aversions can be more practically reproduced for DSCC. Another issue is that DSCC takes time and commitment, and treatment adherence is variable.[17,18] Therefore, management, rather than resolution, might be a more reasonable goal.

Management

An important initial step in the treatment of noise aversions is management of the pet and environment to minimize or prevent exposure until behavior modification can be effectively implemented (Box 15.1). As the problem is often a serious concern for the pet parent (e.g., concern over the pet's well-being, disturbing sleep, household damage) and further exposure generally worsens the problem, some method of avoiding, masking, muting, or reducing the intensity of the sights and sounds should be the initial focus. During noise exposure, the pet parent should develop strategies for helping the pet to calm, such as taking it to an area where it feels most secure and attempting to engage the pet in a pleasant activity such as feeding or play. Retreat to a safe hiding place is a normal, appropriate, and adaptive response to storms. It is not uncommon for pet parents to be told to ignore their pet when they are showing signs of fear or panic during a noise event. This recommendation is outdated, ineffective, and inhumane. Fear cannot be positively reinforced. In other words, if the pet parent hugs their cat if it is afraid of a storm, they will not be more afraid of the storm. However, the pet parent

Box 15.1 Management of pets with noise aversions

1. Protect from overwhelming exposures to fear-evoking noises or thunderstorms
   a. Avoid situations where the pet may encounter the sound if possible.
      i. Walk at different times of day
      ii. Don't bring the pet to areas where they may encounter the sound (e.g., fireworks display, baseball games)
2. Make a sanctuary space (Figures 15.2 and 15.3)
   a. Room, area of the home, crate, or carrier.
   b. Follow the pet's lead. If the pet has already chosen a space, try to make it work.
   c. If necessary, condition the pet to accept a new sanctuary space.
   d. Choose a room with small or no windows.
   e. If windows are present, draw the curtains, blinds, or shades.
   f. Prepare the space with food, toys, litterbox (cats) or pee pads (dogs) if applicable, litterbox (cats) or pee pads (dogs) if applicable, reduction of sound, etc. before any event where it might be needed. For storm-phobic dogs in southern states, it will need to be prepared each day.
   g. Train the pet to settle and relax in the area and enter the area voluntarily and on cue using positive reinforcement.
3. Reduce the sound
   a. Provide sound reduction by nesting cardboard boxes, blankets, or covers made of acoustic foam. Be certain to maintain sufficient air circulation.
   b. Use white noise, brown noise, classical music, a fan, or the television. Note: background noise such as white or brown noise is best.
4. Countercondition whenever possible
   a. Give favored chews, companionship
   b. Offer favored reinforcers (food, play) immediately following loud noises
   c. Throw a storm party by running around the home, excitedly tossing treats and toys
   d. Offer a food-filled toy for the pet to enjoy throughout the noise event

5. Use commercially available products if helpful and the pet has been positively conditioned to wearing them.
   a. Wearables to mute auditory stimuli such as Mutt Muffs (Figure 15.4), Happy Hoodies and noise-canceling headphones for dogs
   b. Wearables to mask visual stimuli such as Doggles, Rex Spex, and ThunderCaps
   c. Pressure wraps, including the Anxiety Wrap and ThunderShirt, may have small but beneficial effects. Habituation to the wrap and repeated use may improve the likelihood of any benefit.[18,30]
6. Keep it positive
   a. Do not punish.
   b. Redirect the pet immediately to the sanctuary space or a safety behavior when fearful if the pet can recover from the fearful event spontaneously
   c. Offer contact and comfort if that decreases the pet's distress
7. Desensitize and countercondition
   a. Select a calm location with few distractions for training.
   b. Desensitize with a reproduction of the noise (or a masked, muted, reduced, or sufficiently distanced presentation of the noise (e.g., gunshots) and countercondition with favored reinforcers reserved exclusively for associating with the noise recording.
   c. Desensitization and counterconditioning is only effective if complete avoidance of the fear-inducing stimuli is possible until the entire process is complete. This rarely works for thunderstorms, but may work for more discrete stimuli.
8. Neurochemical modulation/anxiolytic support
   a. Use an SSRI, TCA, or SNRI on an ongoing basis year-round or through the time of year when distress-inducing noises might be expected.
   b. Use an as-needed medication for storms either initially until the antidepressant is effective (4–6 weeks) or consistently (e.g., orotransmucosal dexmedetomidine gel, imepitoin, a benzodiazepine, clonidine, trazodone, or gabapentin).

also isn't teaching the pet any coping tools in order to self-soothe. Nor are they ensuring that the disorder doesn't progress. Don't tell pet parents to ignore their pets during a panic attack. Tell them to distract, redirect, move their pet into the sanctuary space, or countercondition their pets.

Treatment

One of the most effective ways to treat noise aversion is to provide the patient with a sanctuary space (see Chapters 5 and 14). A sanctuary space is a room, crate, or another space where the pet can get away from frightening sounds (see Figures 15.2 and 15.3). The room should be comfortable with all that the pet needs including water, a comfortable bed and if for a cat, a litterbox (see Box 15.1). It should have no windows, or the windows should be able to be closed and covered so that the lightning and dark sky is not seen by the pet. It is notable that pets often choose their own sanctuary spaces. While ideally we would train them to move to a more appropriate space if the one that they have chosen is less than ideal, that isn't always practical. Sometimes, we need to make the space that they have chosen safe using the techniques below. The purpose of the sanctuary space is not to necessarily confine the pet there, as many pets that have noise aversion may also have confinement distress. Instead, the room is open to them. They are taught to go there when

they are stressed. The room should be prepared for storms beforehand with background noise (e.g., white, brown) or classical music, a bed, water, pheromone analogs, potentially aromatherapy, and a toy filled with food. The pet can be conditioned to go there using hide-and-seek games or a go to your mat cue. In the latter, the pet is taught to go a mat and stay there in the sanctuary space. Products that drown out sound such as Mutt Muffs noise-canceling headphones or a small amount of cotton in the outside of the ear may help as well (see Figure 15.4). For both dogs and cats, toys filled with food can be used to help condition a calm response. In a multipet household, one of the pets may need to be confined if they are likely to fight over resources.

DSCC is a commonly recommended treatment for noise aversions in dogs; in two studies that utilized sound recordings and a written DSCC protocol for treatment of fireworks fears, pet parents reported improvement in their dogs' firework fears and high satisfaction with the treatment.[19,20] This treatment is most effective when fear-inducing stimuli are avoidable. In addition, the stimuli used for DSCC will need to be modified and controlled. For example, controlling the volume or distance from the stimulus to the subject can be used to set up a gradient of stimuli. Audio recordings and camera flashes can be used for dogs that are afraid of storms or fireworks. Recordings are available for most noises that might be aversive, including fireworks, gunshots, cars, trucks, motorcycles, vacuum cleaners, hot air balloons, and more. For sources of noise

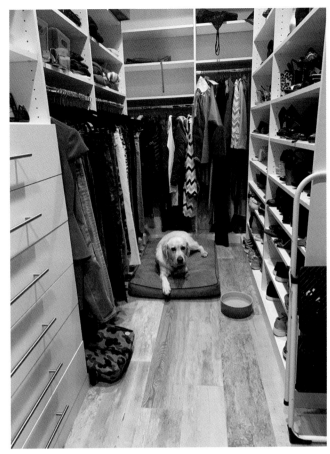

Figure 15.2 A sanctuary space can be made anywhere and is the foundation of improvement for storm and fireworks treatment. *(Attribution: Lisa Radosta.)*

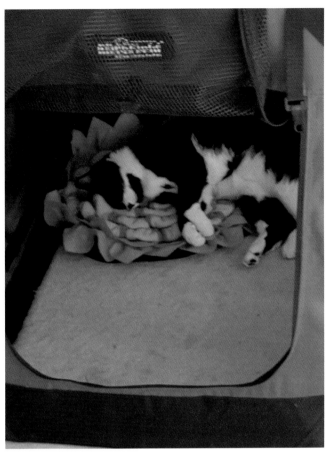

Figure 15.3 Sanctuary spaces can be made for cats as well. *(Attribution: Erica Grier, DVM.)*

desensitization audio recordings, see Appendix A. It should be noted, however, that not all noise-averse dogs may respond to a recording of the noise.[20]

Before starting DSCC, the pet should be trained to go to a site to relax and settle using positive reinforcement (see Chapter 10 for details). Desensitization is intended to expose the pet to a low enough level of the fear-evoking stimulus (in this case the recording) while the pet remains relaxed. The dog's most preferred reinforcers, such as food or play, should be identified and then paired with the sounds (counterconditioning). By identifying and pairing the pet's preferred reinforcers with each desensitization session, the dog develops a positive emotional response to the recorded sounds. An enthusiastically positive emotional response to gradually increased levels of sound intensity might then transfer to actual storms or fireworks. Stimulus reduction and products that might further help to reduce noise aversion might be used concurrently (Box 15.1). While counterconditioning is paired with desensitization during planned training sessions, counterconditioning can be used exclusively during an actual noise event. This can be achieved by offering the dog's favorite reinforcers (e.g., food or play) immediately after each loud noise or throughout the noise event. This technique is simple and easy to learn, and focusing pet parent efforts on easy-to-implement strategies may improve treatment adherence. A recent study reported that counterconditioning and relaxation training were the

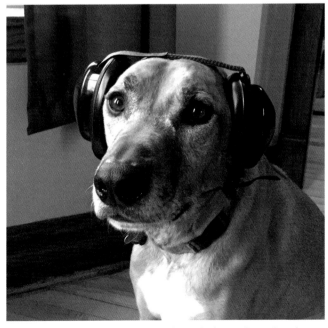

Figure 15.4 Mutt Muffs and other products which cancel sound can be helpful management tools. *(Courtesy Dr. Kelly C. Ballantyne.)*

most effective training strategies for treating fireworks fears, while DSCC had a lower success rate as rated by dog owners.[21]

If the noise aversion is intense, medication will most likely be needed. The frequency of noise events, the intensity of the dog's noise aversion, and the refractory period after exposure to return to an unstressed baseline will determine the type of medication selected. For example, dogs that experience noise events infrequently and have mild to moderate noise aversions may respond well to situational treatment with rapidly acting anxiolytic drugs. Orotransmucosal dexmedetomidine (Sileo) is FDA approved for the treatment of noise aversions in dogs and can be administered as needed 30–60 minutes prior to the fear-evoking event, at the first loud noise, or first signs of fear.[22] Tasipimidine, an alpha-2 agonist, is approved in Europe for alleviation of situational anxiety and fear triggered by noise or owner departure in dogs at a dose of 30 µg/kg 1 hour in advance. See resources and recommended reading. Imepitoin (Pexion) is FDA approved for the treatment of noise aversion in dogs and has demonstrated efficacy in alleviating storm anxiety; however, at the time of writing it is distributed in Europe but not yet in the United States. It is administered twice daily starting two days before an expected noise event.[23,24] Benzodiazepines such as alprazolam or diazepam can be given on an as-needed basis one to two hours prior to a fear-evoking event.[25,26] They might even have some value during or after the storm to speed recovery and in theory to possibly induce amnesia of the event.[27] In addition, there is also some supportive evidence that repeated dosing with an anxiolytic such as dexmedetomidine gel over a series of noise events may decrease the need for medication administration over time.[28] Clonidine, trazodone, or gabapentin may be useful as well in the treatment of storm phobia and noise aversion.[29-32] In a double-blinded, placebo-controlled crossover study, storm-phobic dogs were treated with a single dose of gabapentin ranging from 25 to 30 mg/kg PO 90 minutes prior to exposure. Dogs in the study were less fearful when treated with gabapentin and side effects were rare. As with other studies, a common side effect was ataxia.[32] When treating dogs that experience frequent noise events, have severe noise aversions, or have comorbidities such as separation-related disorders, use of selective serotonin reuptake inhibitors (SSRIs) (e.g., fluoxetine, paroxetine, sertraline) or tricyclic antidepressants (TCAs) (e.g., clomipramine) in combination with situational anxiolytics is indicated. The SSRI or TCA is given daily and may take four to six weeks to become effective. Selegiline is sometimes used for noise aversions associated with chronic anxiety and can be used concurrently with benzodiazepines but only after complete withdrawal of any SSRI or TCA. Other drugs that might be added or combined are phenobarbital or acepromazine (for sedation but not anxiety), or pindolol and propranolol (see Chapter 11). Natural therapeutics such as dog-appeasing pheromones (Adaptil)[19] or supplements such as Solliquin,[33,34] alpha-casozepine (Zylkene or in calm and stress therapeutic diets), L-theanine,[35] melatonin, or aromatherapy might also be considered as part of the treatment regime (see Chapter 12). Extralabel drug use and drug combinations should be used cautiously, with informed pet parent consent and under close supervision by the pet parents to monitor for efficacy or potential side effects.

CASE EXAMPLE

Presentation

Thor, a 7-year-old, 30-kg neutered male mixed-breed dog, was presented for fear during storms, heavy rain, fireworks, and every evening after sunset.

History

Thor would hide in the bathtub, tremble, pant, whine, and sometimes dig or force himself into tight spaces during thunderstorms, heavy rain, fireworks, and every evening after sunset. These signs developed following an event when he was caught outdoors with his pet parents during a severe thunderstorm.

Workup

Thor's physical examination, fecal antigen test, and lab work were within normal limits. He was found to have uneven nail wear on the right hind foot when compared to the left hind foot. The veterinarian elicited pain upon extension of the right hip. For these reasons, radiographs were recommended and completed. Radiographs showed moderate osteoarthritis in the right hip and mild osteoarthritis in the left hip.

Differential diagnoses

The differential diagnoses included hip dysplasia, osteoarthritis, noise phobia, storm phobia, and generalized anxiety. Thor was diagnosed with hip dysplasia, osteoarthritis, noise phobia, and storm phobia.

Treatment

NSAIDs were dispensed for use daily for 14 days. In addition, Thor was given fatty acid and joint supplementation. The pet parents were given instructions as to how to set up a sanctuary space in a windowless bathroom. Thor should have access to the space at all times. The sanctuary space should be as comfortable and sound proof as possible using soft bedding and white noise. They were given resources for dog body language, dog training, and best practices for living with a fearful dog. Finally, they were counseled to avoid forcing Thor out of his hiding space. There was concern that he would injure himself in attempts to hide in tight spaces, so it was recommended that these areas be proactively blocked off using closed doors and baby gates. During quiet times of the day, the pet parents were to practice short sessions of relaxation training with Thor in the sanctuary space.

As Thor experienced distress daily regardless of the weather and storms and fireworks were frequent around Thor's home, treatment with the SSRI fluoxetine was initiated in addition to nightly administration of gabapentin 10–20 mg/kg PO two hours prior to sunset and the onset of a noise event up to every 8–12 hours if needed. When there was a noise event, the pet parents were to take him to the bathroom, where white noise was turned on. Thor was offered his favorite food in a long-lasting chew toy during the event.

Follow-up

The veterinary technician followed up with the pet parents in two weeks from the initial appointment. They reported that Thor continued to hide nightly but did not tremble, whine, or pant, at which point the frequency of hiding decreased to only during storms and fireworks. During storms and fireworks, he continued to hide, pant, whine, and tremble, and showed no interest in the food-filled toy. They were giving the fluoxetine,

continued

supplements, NSAIDs, and gabapentin as directed. They noted that he was able to get up more quickly and fetch the ball for longer periods of time in the yard. In addition, they reported that the fluoxetine "wasn't doing anything." The veterinary technician reminded the pet parents that the fluoxetine may take up to six weeks to have an effect. They reported no side effects from any of the treatment except a mild decrease in appetite. Because he was still eating 75% of his daily food ration and was eating treats, the veterinary technician instructed them to continue with the fluoxetine. Because the pet parents were seeing a difference in his behavior, but it wasn't at least a 50% change, per the veterinarian's recommendations, the veterinary technician instructed them to increase the gabapentin to 30 mg/kg PO two hours prior to stressful events and bedtime. They had set up the sanctuary space and were practicing relaxation training using the instructions in the books and videos which were recommended.

The veterinary technician followed up by phone four weeks after the appointment. Thor continued to improve. He was tolerating the gaba-pen-tin and fluoxetine well. He had regained his normal appetite. In addition, he was going to the sanctuary space on his own. When he went to the sanctuary space during a storm, he was able to lie down and eat out of the food toy without any other overt signs of panic. However, the pet parents were concerned about the upcoming fireworks.

Six weeks after the original appointment, Thor was seen for a follow-up to evaluate his pain level and discuss the upcoming

fireworks holiday. The pet parents were very concerned and expressed that they would prefer that he be more "out of it" than he was on gabapentin. The veterinarian recommended orotransmucosal dexmedetomidine (Sileo) given 30 minutes prior to fireworks and repeated in two to three hours as needed for up to five doses. They were to put him into the sanctuary space one hour prior to when they anticipated that the fireworks would start and keep him there until they were completely over. The gabapentin was to be continued for storm events.

The veterinary technician followed up with the pet parents in two weeks. Thor had gotten his medications as directed for the holiday and he had slept in his sanctuary space. The pet parents stayed with him for the entire fireworks display. He was calmer but was not too sedated, which made the pet parents happy.

He continued to go to his sanctuary space during severe storms, but would not pant, tremble, or whine, and would eat food out of his chew toy. DSCC using an audio recording was discussed, but Thor did not demonstrate signs of distress in response to audio recordings when tested. The pet parents elected to continue daily fluoxetine year-round, given the frequency of storms and fireworks near their home, and continue to use oromucosal dexmedetomidine gel and counterconditioning as needed during noise events.

Discussion

Thor presented in middle age, which is a common signalment for dogs with noise aversion that also have pain or systemic disease. Even though there was an inciting incident in his past which fit nicely with a behavior-only cause, the veterinarian still took the time to do a complete physical examination and follow through with appropriate diagnostics. For all behavior disorders, disorders of all body systems must be considered. It is typical for pets to need more than one medication for the treatment of noise aversion or phobia. In addition, fireworks are such stressful events that they may need an add on medication. Trazodone would have

been a good option instead of gabapentin if Thor did not have osteoarthritis.

Conclusion

Noise aversion is common in dogs and with future study is likely to be found to be common in cats. It can contribute to generalized anxiety, elimination in the house and separation-related disorders as well as severe negative effects on the quality of life of the patient and the pet parent. The good news is that treatment is available, and most pets can be helped.

References

1. Overall KL, Dunham AE, Frank D. Frequency of nonspecific clinical signs in dogs with separation anxiety, thunderstorm phobia, and noise phobia, alone or in combination. *J Am Vet Med Assoc.* 2001;219:467–473.
2. Overall KL, Dunham AE, Juarbe-Diaz SV. Phenotypic determination of noise reactivity in 3 breeds of working dogs: a cautionary tale of age, breed, behavioral assessment, and genetics. *J Vet Behav.* 2016;16:113–125.
3. Sherman BL, Mills DS. Canine anxieties and phobias: an update on separation anxiety and noise aversions. *Vet Clin North Am Small Anim.* 2008;38: 1081–1106.
4. Blackwell EJ, Bradshaw JWS, Casey RA. Fear responses to noises in domestic dogs: prevalence, risk factors and co-occurrence with other fear related behaviour. *Appl Anim Behav Sci.* 2013; 145:15–25.
5. Riemer S. Not a one-way road—severity, progression and prevention of firework fears in dogs. *PLoS One.* 2019;14:e0218150.
6. Dale AR, Walker JK, Farnworth MJ, et al. A survey of owners' perceptions of fear of fireworks in a sample of dogs and cats in New Zealand. *N Z Vet J.* 2010;58:286–291.
7. Tiira K, Lohi H. Early life experiences and exercise associate with canine anxieties. *PLoS One.* 2015;10:e0141907. doi:10.1371/journal.pone.0141907.
8. Tiira K, Sulkama S, Lohi H. Prevalence, comorbidity, and behavioral variation in canine anxiety. *J Vet Behav.* 2016;16: 36–44.
9. Dinwoodie IR, Dwyer B, Zottola V, et al. Demographics and comorbidity of behavior problems in dogs. *J Vet Behav.* 2019:32,62–71.
10. Amat M, Manteca X, Ruiz de la Torre JL, et al. Evaluation of inciting causes, alternative targets, and risk factors associated with redirected aggression in cats. *J Am Vet Med Assoc.* 2008;233: 586–589.
11. Storengen LM, Lingaas F. Noise sensitivity in 17 dog breeds: prevalence, breed risk and correlation with fear in other situations. *Appl Anim Behav Sci.* 2015; 171:152–160.
12. Iimura, K. The nature of noise fear in domestic dogs. Master's Thesis - The Lincoln Repository. 2006. Available at: http://eprints.lincoln.ac.uk/id/eprint/4513/. Accessed September 8, 2020.
13. Handegard KW, Storengen LM, Lingaas F. Noise reactivity in standard poodles and

Irish soft coated wheaten terriers. *JVB*. 2020;36:4–12.

14. Fagundes ALL, Hewison L, McPeake KJ, et al. Noise sensitivities in dogs: an exploration of signs in dogs with and without musculoskeletal pain using qualitative content analysis. *Frontiers Vet Sci*. 2018;5:1081–1085.

15. Mills DS, Mueller HW, McPeake K, et al. Development and psychometric validation of the Lincoln Canine Anxiety Scale. *Frontiers Vet Sci*. 2020;7:171.

16. Horwitz DF. Separation-related problems in dogs and cats. In: Horwitz DF, Mills DS, eds. 2nd ed. *BSAVA Manual of Canine and Feline Behavioural Medicine*. British Small Animal Veterinary Association, 2010;146–158.

17. Ballantyne KC, Buller K. Experiences of veterinarians in clinical behavior practice: a mixed-methods study. *J Vet Behav*. 2015; 10:376–383.

18. Levine ED, Mills DS. Long-term follow-up of the efficacy of a behavioural treatment programme for dogs with firework fears. *Vet Rec*. 2008;162: 657–659.

19. Levine ED, Ramos D, Mills DS. A prospective study of two self-help CD based desensitization and counter-conditioning programmes with the use of Dog Appeasing Pheromone for the treatment of firework fears in dogs (Canis familiaris). *Appl Anim Behav Sci*. 2007; 105:311–329.

20. Overall KL, Dunham AE, Scheifele P, et al. Fear of noises affects canine problem solving behavior and locomotion in standardized cognitive tests. *Appl Anim Behav Sci*. 2019;221: 104863.

21. Riemer S. Effectiveness of treatments for firework fears in dogs. *J Vet Behav*. 2020; 37:61–70.

22. Korpivaara M, Laapas K, Huhtinen M, et al. Dexmedetomidine oromucosal gel for noise-associated acute anxiety and fear in dogs-a randomised, double-blind, placebo-controlled clinical study. *Vet Rec*. 2017;180:356–357.

23. Perdew, I, Emke, C, Johnson, B, et al. Evaluation of Pexion® (imepitoin) for treatment of storm anxiety in dogs: a randomised, double-blind, placebo-controlled trial. *Vet Rec*. 2021. doi:10.1002/vetr.18.

24. Engel O, Müller HW, Klee R, et al. Effectiveness of imepitoin for the control of anxiety and fear associated with noise phobia in dogs. *J Vet Intern Med*. 2019;33:2675–2684.

25. Herron ME, Shofer FS, Reisner IR. Retrospective evaluation of the effects of diazepam in dogs with anxiety-related behavior problems. *J Am Vet Med Assoc*. 2008;233:1420–1424.

26. Crowell-Davis SL, Seibert LM, Sung W, et al. Use of clomipramine, alprazolam, and behavior modification for treatment of storm phobia in dogs. *J Am Vet Med Assoc*. 2003;222:744–748.

27. Dantas LM, Crowell-Davis SL. Benzodiazepines. In: Crowell-Davis SL, Murray TF, Dantas LM, eds. 2nd ed. *Veterinary Psychopharmacology*. 2019;67–102.

28. Gruen M, Case BC, Robertson JB, et al. Evaluation of repeated dosing of a dexmedetomidine oromucosal gel for treatment of noise aversion in dogs over a series of noise events. *Vet Rec*. 2020;187(12):489. doi:10.1136/vr.106046.

29. Gruen ME, Sherman BL. Use of trazodone as an adjunctive agent in the treatment of canine anxiety disorders: 56 cases (1995–2007). *J Am Vet Med Assoc*, 2008;233:1902–1907.

30. Ogata NN, Dodman NH. The use of clonidine in the treatment of fear-based behavior problems in dogs: an open trial. *J Vet Behav*. 2011;6:130–137.

31. Orlando JM. Animal behavior case of the month. *J Am Vet Med Assoc*. 2017;251: 1011–1014.

32. Bluer-Elsner S, Medam T, Masson S. Effects of a single oral dose of gabapentin on storm phobia in dogs: a double-blind, placebo controlled crossover trial. *Vet Record*. 2021. doi:10.1002/vetr.453.

33. DePorter TL, Landsberg GM, Araujo JA, et al. Harmonease Chewable Tablets reduces noise-induced fear and anxiety in a laboratory canine thunderstorm simulation: a blinded and placebo-controlled study. *J Vet Behav*. 2012;7:225–232.

34. Landsberg G, Huggins S, Fish J, et al. The effects of a nutritional supplement (Solliquin) in reducing fear and anxiety in a laboratory model of thunder-induced fear and anxiety. Proceedings of the 11th International Veterinary Behaviour Meeting, 14–16th September 2017, Samorin, Slovakia. 2017;94–97.

35. Pike AL, Horwitz DF, Lobprise H. An open-label prospective study of the use of l-theanine (Anxitane) in storm-sensitive client-owned dogs. *J Vet Behav*. 2015;10: 324–331.

Resources and recommended reading

Albright JD, Ballantyne KC. Can anxiolytic medications induce long-term improvement in dogs with noise aversion? *Vet Rec*. 2020;187: 486–488.

Ballantyne KC. Separation, confinement, or noises: what is scaring that dog? *Vet Clin North Am Small Anim Pract*. 2018;48: 367–386.

Fear free happy homes – Fear of Thunder or Fireworks. https://www.fearfreehappy homes.com/kit/fear-of-thunder-fireworks/.

Keep your pets stress-free during fireworks season. https://todaysveterinarypractice. com/pet-owner-resources/pets-noise-aversion-fireworks-handout/

Korpivaara M, Pohjanjousi P, Huhtinen M. Tasipimidine, a novel orally dosed alpha-2 Adrenoceptor agonist, alleviates canine acute anxiety and fear associated with noise – a pilot study. Proc 3rd European Veterinary Congress of Behavioural Medicine and Animal Welfare, 2021:148.

Tasipimidine (Tessie) European Medicines Agency https://www.ema.europa.eu/en/ medicines/veterinary/EPAR/tessie.

CHAPTER 16

Reducing fear, anxiety, and stress in veterinary clinics

Amy Learn, VMD, DACVB and Gary Landsberg, DVM, MRCVS, DACVB, DECAWBM

Chapter contents

The problem with the status quo

It is natural that we would consider our veterinary hospital to be a welcoming environment for pets and pet parents may even agree, based on their own perceptions, and yet animals might have a very different perspective. For them, the veterinary clinic can be a terrifying place. There are unfamiliar and fear-evoking sights, sounds, odors, and surfaces. A typical exam might include being held in close contact by an unfamiliar person who most likely carries smells of unfamiliar animals, a bright light gets shined in the eyes, a cold, stiff otoscope placed in the ears, a thermometer inserted rectally, not to mention the pain and discomfort associated with injections and sample collection. A sick or injured pet may also need wound treatment, intravenous therapy, or surgery (as well as what we refer to as "hospitalization"), which all

contribute to negative experiences that further condition fear. To make matters worse, pet parents often do not properly condition their pets to the experiences that take place at a veterinary examination.

A 2014 American Animal Hospital Association-American Veterinary Medicine Association white paper found that 51% of pets dislike going to the veterinarian, an increase from 45% just four years earlier.[1] Furthermore, pet parents report impaired welfare at some point during the veterinary visit in over 77% of dogs and 85% of cats.[2,3] Up to 87% of pet parents reported that their dogs were fearful during veterinary visits (of which 22.4% were severe), 70% were unwilling to enter the veterinary hospital,[4] 78% were fearful on the exam table, 55% were fearful during veterinary examination, 84% pulled to leave,[5] and 31% of dogs had shown aggression (of which 8.2% were reported as severe).[6,7] The picture is not any prettier for cats. Up to 77.8% of cat pet parents report that their cats knew that they were going to the veterinary hospital before arriving, 51.5% recognized signs of stress before leaving their home, and 59.3% were stressed by travel, which is a primary factor in why cat parents avoid veterinary visits.[3,8] In fact, cats that are not familiar with carriers and car rides were more fearful and stressed at the veterinary visit.[9]

Therefore, positive carrier acclimation and travel training should be essential first steps for the prevention and alleviation of veterinary stress to ensure a positive experience during their first visit.[9] See Chapter 5 and Appendix A resources for more information on cat-carrier training. In the waiting room, only 26.8% of cats were judged to be calm by their pet parents.[3] As cats pass through the hospital and into the exam room, the number of cat pet parents who rated their pet as calm decreased to 20.8%, and on the exam table, the amount of cats rated as calm decreased to 15%.[3] What may be most disturbing is that cats may stay stressed for hours and some remain stressed for days (the physiologic stress response and all of its ramifications) after they returned home from a veterinary visit.[8] Pet parents recognize their pet's stress, feel stressed themselves, and often wait to bring their pets to the clinic when they are ill.[8] If 85% of your cat patients were affected by a disorder, wouldn't you want to know as much as possible about that disorder and how it could be successfully managed? Up to 85% of your patients are suffering from fear, anxiety, stress, conflict, and panic (FASCP) so powerful that it affects them before they arrive and for hours or even days after they leave. It is imperative that we understand how to prevent stress in the veterinary clinic. The good news is that there is evidence to show that even when the pet has a history of negative veterinary experiences, stress can be decreased with consistent, patient-centric handling techniques that allow us to lower stress in our patients with just one visit.[10]

Most of our patients are already feeling physiologically stressed, anxious, confused, or afraid, yet we might (unrealistically) expect them to be calm and cooperative for procedures. If the patient struggles, there might be a tendency to call for assistance, using more forceful restraint to make sure that we win the battle, forgoing the most simple, kind, and safe ways to help everyone involved – changing our own behavior, whether the way that we restrain or the use of sedation. In this chapter, you will find the foundation of creating a better experience for your patients (and pet parents). Readers are encouraged to further their knowledge with the recommended reading at the end of this chapter and in Appendix A.

It is no longer acceptable to interact with patients in a way that may have been permissible previously (or even advocated in earlier textbooks). One of the highest priorities for veterinary healthcare team members and our patients is safety. Bites and scratches are often some of the leading causes of injury to veterinary team members. When using force-based restraint, injuries from bites, scratches or even sprain, strains, or blunt force trauma are not uncommon. All veterinarians have taken an oath to "first do no harm," yet when we struggle with a patient, we are causing emotional anguish which is associated with a physiologic response, negatively affecting the patient's wellness and directly affecting heart rate, respiratory rate, core body temperature, response to palpation, and immune response (see Chapter 7). This would directly violate our oath in a significant way. Even just one negative experience at a veterinary hospital may lead to progressive anxiety and fear with each subsequent visit,

possibly culminating in aggression toward the veterinary staff. In fact, almost 3/4 of pet parents complained that their cat's association with the veterinarian changed after the first visit, and over 1/3 of cats had a worse perception of all further car travel.[3] The most alarming possibility is that a pet could associate that emotion with other contexts or even generalize their behavior in such a way that they act more aggressively to all unfamiliar people. With the knowledge that fear-based aggression is meant to be protective or defensive, we can see how generalizing that experience may contribute to more drastic unwanted behavior and even behavioral euthanasia. Another harmful sequel to careless, rushed, or forceful handling at the veterinary office is the negative impact on credibility, reputation, and pet parent perception of the veterinary healthcare team and the hospital.

Emotionally, we are not necessarily that different from our patients, even with superior cognition and the ability to discuss and better understand the circumstances of an intervention. If you had an appointment with your dentist and you expressed your fear and concern about what was going to happen, you would expect the dentist to be accommodating. If the dentist denied you pain-relieving or stress-relieving medications, and instead had staff members hold you in the chair while you struggled, how would you feel? You may very well not return for your next checkup. You may be so upset that you decide not to see a dentist ever again. Would you be more likely to visit a dentist who provided the same level of care but prescribed medications to alleviate pain and fear, had televisions mounted on the ceiling so that you could watch television during the visit, kept you comfortable during interventions, and checked in with you periodically to make sure you were fine? Of course, you would! Animals are no different. Having positive experiences increases the likelihood of cooperation with treatment. The physiologic parameters on which we rely to diagnose and treat our patients, such as blood pressure, heart rate, body temperature, blood glucose, and respiratory rate, are significantly elevated from an individual dog's or cat's baseline at home compared to values measured at the hospital, with the biggest variability potentially in those who are already compromised.[10–13] Urinary catecholamines (a measure of stress) increased in dogs after examination, which explains the increase in heart rate, respiratory rate, and blood pressure.[14] Heart rate increases and heart rate variability goes down (high heart rate variability correlates with low stress) in dogs that are caged in the hospital and not directly being handled, indicating that the environment itself is frightening enough to ignite the stress response.[15]

Fear, anxiety, stress, conflict, panic, phobia, pain, and nausea

Fear is an emotional response to a threat (as perceived by the animal) due to the presence or proximity of a specific stimulus (e.g., object, noise, individual, social situation), which results in physiologic and psychologic responses characterized by somatic, emotional, cognitive, and behavioral components, most frequently fight, flight, freeze, or fidget. More subtle body language signs may include lip licking, yawning, or circling. See Chapter 2 for a more detailed discussion of body language. The response may vary with the situation or type and intensity of stimulus, previous experience, and personality of the individual. Each fearful event may condition a negative conditioned emotional response (CER) with the stimulus.

Anxiety is a state of apprehension or uneasiness to an anticipated danger or threat in the absence of an identifiable fear-eliciting stimulus. As with fear, there is a physiologic and psychologic component. Scanning or hypervigilance, inability to relax, and nervous responses are signals that indicate anxiety. A phobia is a profound, excessive, abnormal fear response that occurs without the presence of a true threat or is out of proportion to the needs for dealing with an actual threat. See Chapter 14 for a more detailed discussion of fear, anxiety, and phobia.

Stress is an emotional response in which there are physiologic and psychologic changes that arise in the face of a real or perceived threat to the individual's well-being.[16] Stressors are initially perceived, and responses transmitted, through sensory pathways (e.g., visual, auditory, olfactory, or somatic) to the hypothalamus. See Table 16.1 for a list of visual, auditory, and olfactory stimuli commonly found in veterinary hospitals, which may be paired with a negative CER. Communication with the hypothalamus activates behavioral, endocrine, and sympathetic nervous system responses, such as increased epinephrine, norepinephrine, cortisol, blood glucose, body temperature, blood pressure, heart rate, and respiratory rate and neutrophil counts, mydriasis, and decreased pain perception, to deal with the threat. The amygdala (the emotional decision-making center of the brain), the locus coeruleus (the primary norepinephrine nucleus of the brain), and the hippocampus are recruited to make split-second decisions, initiate a sympathetic nervous system response, and lay down memories to aid in learning. Associational learning occurs in the hippocampus with connections to the cortex, which controls executive function. Memories that are formed during a stress response when triggered are more easily retrieved than those which are not formed during a stress response. When they are triggered (e.g., repeat visit to the veterinary hospital), the response is often immediate, with a release of catecholamines that increases hypervigilance and overrides conscious decision making and new learning.

While reactions to stressors may ultimately be immune suppressing, the initial response may be immune enhancing and proinflammatory to cope and prepare the immune system for challenge.[17,18] Timing, duration, intensity and type of stressor, and the degree of cortisol secretion are critical factors in the direction of the immune response. Acute, short-term stressors, at the early stages of immune activation and in advance of the immune challenge, can enhance immune activity. However, with stress that is excessive, frequent, prolonged, or chronic, the immune response may be suppressed, leading to delayed wound healing, increased susceptibility to infection, and further fear sensitization.[17,19-21] In addition, chronic stress can result in mental, immune, endocrine, and metabolic disorders, affecting behavior (e.g., repetitive, anxiety, reactivity, phobia) as well as cardiovascular, respiratory, renal, urinary, dermatologic, reproductive and gastrointestinal health, exacerbation of pain, and even a shortened life span,[16,17,22] while pain and illness will further contribute to fear, anxiety, and stress.[23,24]

Table 16.1 Sensory stimuli that may affect a patient

Sensory stimuli	Considerations – enhance positive, prevent/eliminate negative
Visual environment and social	• Lighting – natural /dimmable, colors, avoid animal pictures • Hiding areas in cages, towels, e-collar, ThunderCap • Veterinary and pet parent body language/emotions/demeanor; considerate approach • Attention to movement – gradual • Elevated surfaces and perching areas (heights) for cats • Unfamiliar animals, unfamiliar people, previous negative associations (white coat) • Pet parent
Olfactory environment and social	• Odors and pheromones (same species) that communicate alarm or distress • All surfaces (and air) – disinfectants and odor counteractants • Avoid harsh, strong, nasal irritants • Appeasing pheromones and aromatherapy might help to calm • Pet parent – fear versus happy
Auditory environment (activities, equipment) and social (people, animals)	• Intensity – noise, sound baffling/muting – walls, door, between cages – other animals • Cover carrier, white noise, fan, water fountain, texting, avoid knocking • Isolate mechanical/equipment • Classical music for dogs – also reggae, soft rock, audio books – classical or species-specific for cats • Sounds – minimize, soft/calming voice, staff, pet parent, gradient of intensity
Tactile balance/pressure/pain	• Clean, comfortable, secure – walkways, floors – avoid cold, slippery, wet • Examination/treatment surfaces – stable, mats, warm, fleece, own bedding • Temperature • Gentle control – pet control (less is more, handle versus restrain/clutch) • Petting or grooming if solicits/positive • Pet parent – contact • Gradient of intensity • Small gauge, warm, oral versus nasal (avoid visual anticipation) • Pain management – oral/topical/regional/systemic – nausea management

The stress response is a normal process meant to help an individual cope with the physiologic or psychological triggers of daily life. Physiologic stress arises when internal or external environmental factors alter the body's physiologic homeostasis, while psychogenic stress refers to altered psychological well-being. Negative psychogenic stressors might be social or nonsocial and may be controllable (e.g., choosing to retreat to the back of a cage) or noncontrollable (e.g., an outside force applying physical restraint). Normally, after the cause for the stress response has been removed, the body returns to physiological homeostasis. However, stress can be harmful when it is triggered too intensely, repeatedly, or is prolonged. As such, distress is when the body is unable to return to physiological homeostasis and/or mental well-being.[17] The stimulus, duration, and intensity of the response to a trigger, previous experience, as well as personality of the individual, all contribute to the psychological and physiological impact of stress. Two factors may activate the stress response more strongly: lack of control and lack of predictability. In human medical care, people have control over scheduling and participation in medical care; know the benefits, reasons, and the help they will receive; know what, when, and how long the procedure and any associated FASCP will last; and can verbally communicate their level of FASCP, before and during procedures. Pets have no control to participate or to decline; do not know what, when, or how long the procedure or visit will last, or what might be yet to come (unpredictable); do not know the benefits, rationale, or help they will receive (why); and their levels of FASCP are solely based on recognition and alleviation by the pet parents and veterinary personnel. In short, a pet's experience will be one of FASCP (negative associations), enjoyment or pleasure (positive associations), or indifference (net neutral). Yet even indifferent outcomes with the veterinary visit can increase the risk for further fear and aggression.[7] This most likely results from a negative association which was made and went unnoticed by the veterinary team. In reality, it is unlikely that most pets have a net-neutral experience. It is more likely that some pets are able to cope with and recover from the negative experience more aptly than others. In addition, while individual stimuli might not be sufficiently intense or prolonged to cause distress, when an individual is exposed to multiple simultaneous triggers or to consecutive triggers without the opportunity to habituate in between, the additive effect (cumulative stress) may lead to longer, more intense, and harmful distress.[2,6,14] An example might be if a pet that is fearful of carrier and car rides is brought into a previously fear-evoking veterinary environment and is further frightened by sounds, sights, odors, or social interactions, with no opportunity to settle or return to baseline between each fear-evoking event or trigger. This prolonged exposure and increasingly more intense stress may push the pet beyond the threshold for distress. The emotional or behavioral response of the pet parents and that of the veterinary team may further increase the pet's stress through the process of social referencing and emotional contagion including sights, sounds, and scents.[25-27] Indeed, pet parent nervousness has been identified as a risk factor for veterinary-related fear and aggression.[7] The concept of emotional contagion is not an excuse to take pets from their pet parents. Studies have shown that pets are more tractable and have lower heart rate and blood pressure measurements with the pet parent present than without them.[14] Instead, the knowledge of emotional contagion

should be a jumping-off point to counsel pet parents on their behavior in the examination room. See Chapter 14 for a more detailed discussion of emotional contagion and Chapters 6 and 7 for detail on the stress response.

Pain and discomfort in the past may have been viewed as completely separate from FASCP. In reality, they are intimately linked in a cycle of development and feedback. Pain increases stress, which subsequently exacerbates pain and negatively impacts emotional health. Preventing, identifying, and treating pain is essential to pet welfare. Pain plays a role in behavioral signs of fear and anxiety, including noise sensitivities and aggression.[23,24] Pain scores should be recorded in the medical records for all pets for veterinary visits, procedures, surgery, and hospitalization. Standardized pain scales should be used for consistency in scoring pain within the hospital. These scales can be used for assessment, recording, and for monitoring response to pain management. See Chapter 6 and Appendix A.

Identifying, managing, and alleviating pain (acute and chronic) is essential to physical and emotional well-being. Any stimuli (e.g., experiences, locations) that are paired with pain (e.g., veterinary hospital, exam table, hospital cages, white coat, scrubs, scrub color, scent of cleaners or perfumes, sounds of animals recovering from anesthesia, handling, and procedures) may condition a negative CER to those stimuli. This additional fear and stress prior to procedures can further exacerbate pain and increase the need for analgesia.[28]

Consideration should be given to alleviate pain based on the presenting signs, medical history, emotional records, planned and required procedures, and physical examination. These can include oral medications, injectable analgesics, local nerve blocks, and topical medications. Several studies have demonstrated that the application of topical lidocaine/prilocaine (EMLA) cream 20–30 minutes prior to jugular venipuncture or cephalic catheter placement in cats significantly reduces stress and reactivity.[29,30]

Nausea is a common sequela of car travel, medical conditions, anesthesia, and some pharmacologic interventions. Preventing or treating nausea and gastrointestinal discomfort may prevent or reduce the stress associated with these circumstances, and improve postsedation recovery and return to normal eating following sedation and veterinary care.[31,32] Maropitant (NK1 receptor antagonist), a frequently used and effective antiemetic drug, can be used to relieve motion sickness in dogs and cats. In dogs, it should be dosed at 8 mg/kg PO at least 2 hours prior to car rides on an empty stomach but administered with a small bite of food for the treatment of motion sickness and 2 mg/kg PO once daily at least 2 hours in advance, or 1 mg/kg subcutaneously or slow IV 45 minutes to 1 hour in advance for the treatment and prevention of vomiting such as in advance of emetogenic medications. Premedicating dogs with 1 mg/kg subcutaneously 45 minutes in advance or 2–4 mg/kg orally 120 minutes in advance of opioid administration has been demonstrated to reduce vomiting and hasten return to normal feeding.[31,32] In cats, dosing ranges from 0.6 to 2.9 mg/kg PO once daily for the treatment of nausea for up to two weeks.[33]

Learning and associations are continually being made (see Chapter 10). As a result of classical conditioning, a pleasant or positive experience or outcome immediately following a stimulus creates a pleasant or positive emotional association with the stimulus or event. Alternatively, a negative experience or outcome, including fear, pain, and discomfort, creates a negative CER with the stimulus or event. Therefore, if the physical (e.g., veterinary hospital, equipment) or social (e.g., procedures, handling, people, other pets) experiences are associated with positive responses and outcomes, a positive CER is created with the veterinary experience for the pet, the pet parents, as well as the veterinary team. However, unpleasant experiences and outcomes, such as with car travel and veterinary visits, create a negative CER and can sensitize the pet to fear future exposure to the same or similar experiences.[3] While CERs can intensify with repetition, even a single aversive event can cause a conditioned fear of the stimulus (single-event or one-trial learning). This can be explained from a basic survival instinct: the responses given to a fear-invoking acute stressor emanate from predatory avoidance behaviors. Due to the immediate and powerful conditioning associated with fear-inducing situations and stimuli, every interaction with every veterinary healthcare team member at every appointment matters.

Any response which involves a physiologic stress response (e.g., fear, anxiety, stress, panic, phobia, conflict) has the potential to lower the threshold for clinical signs due to other physiologic diseases and disorders, shorten life span, and contribute to the development of disorders of other body systems such as gastrointestinal, cardiovascular, urinary tract (e.g., feline interstitial cystitis), and dermatologic.[16,17,34] In addition, the physiologic stress response is associated with immune changes, impaired wound healing, increased susceptibility to sepsis, and changes in blood glucose.[16,17,19] As mentioned above, each veterinarian desires to "first do no harm." To follow this tenet, we must reduce FASCP at the veterinary hospital at each visit, every time. The effects of FASCP are discussed in more detail in Chapters 6, 7, and 14.

It should be clear that the emotional stress response and the physiologic stress response are one and the same; these responses alter physiological and laboratory measures necessary for proper diagnosis and treatment of physical and emotional disorders; the effects on the body are immediate and have serious long-term implications for the quality of life, health, and life expectancy of the pet, and are triggered by any perceived threat, including veterinary visits. Similarly, nausea and emesis associated with motion sickness and the use of medications such as narcotics will further condition fear of travel and veterinary visits. Pain, nausea, and the associated distress can slow and impede recovery and a return to normal behavioral and physical health and appetite. For the veterinary team, reducing patient's FASCP creates more manageable, cooperative patients; a safer, more efficient work environment; strengthens pet parent relationships and increases pet parent retention and patient visits; improves veterinary professional and staff job satisfaction; and may increase pet parents who seek out more compassionate care for their pets.[6,35-37]

Hospital strategies to maximize patient comfort and safety

Hospital teams that previously had resorted to overpowering pets to get them to accept interventions may find it difficult to appreciate that there is a better way – that such interventions can be achieved without resorting to wasting time or elaborate procedures – but it is true. However, it is also true that it can feel overwhelming to change the approach to handling and restraint that has become an integral part of what veterinary healthcare teams do each day. The good news is that when broken down into digestible steps within the practice, the transition to lower-stress patient interactions does not have to be painful for the team. There is a learning curve associated with any new skill, but any inconvenience is transitory. This was true, for example, when you first learned how to spay a pet. However, just as with spay surgery, you soon became proficient. Changes to handling and restraint are no different. With proper training and practice, competence in handling will become second nature and will not take more time.[36,38,39] Occasionally, there are extra-special patients that do require more time. We can use medications in the short term and schedule future appointments to work on building skills, tolerance, and cooperation, and do so at an additional charge to the pet parent to keep such approaches cost effective. In addition, many pet parents will need education on the reasoning behind this new way of managing their pet. Pet parents often do not recognize FASCP. They may feel personally offended or defensive when more or different care is needed with their pet than they perceive is necessary or that has been used in the past. Explaining what is being done and why at each stage of the visit at every visit, but especially the first vist will help pet parents to feel comfortable and buy in to this new approach (see Table 16.2).

This chapter highlights ways to increase hospital efficiency while also reducing patient stress. The focus is on providing a comfortable and safe environment as well as clear guidance for the pet and parent, with the goal of reducing fear and stress in our patients and allowing the veterinary team to reduce the time needed during the visit and make each future visit easier for all involved (see Box 16.1).

At-home preappointment preparation

Preparation starts with the pet parent care representative (receptionist). When the phone rings, it is the first opportunity to plan the best visit possible for that pet. Each call is the start of a new relationship, and pet parent care representatives should take advantage of getting to know that pet parent and pet for the first time. They can determine if the pet is comfortable riding in the car or getting in a carrier so that the pet's trip to the hospital is as calm as possible. This is also a good time to provide guidance to help the pet parents condition the pet to the carrier or restraint device and car ride prior to veterinary visits, including resources on carrier training and travel (www.catvets.com, www.fearfreepets.com www.fearfreehappyhomes.com, www.catfriendly.com). See Carrier training – Reading and Resources Chapter 5 and Appendix A.

The next consideration is the pet's safety and comfort level on the way to the veterinary clinic. If the pet is fearful, stressed, anxious, panicked, or nauseous in the car, they will arrive at the practice having already been under the influence of the stress response. If the pet is stressed before entering the clinic, it will be more challenging to alleviate that stress as the visit proceeds. For this reason, stress minimization during preparation and travel is essential.

Table 16.2 Pet parent concerns and suggested responses regarding low-stress hospital management

Preemptive conversation with pet parent	Pet parent statement/ questions	Veterinary healthcare member response
We are using small treats today to give Fido the most comfortable experience while he is here.	My dog is very good at the Vet. He does not need treats.	You are right, he is very good while he is here. We are giving him treats so that he will not be afraid and in the future be happy when he is here. Think of it as a happiness insurance policy.
We are using really yummy food today so that Fluffy will love coming to see us.	I do not want my dog to have any people food.	I completely understand. Dr. Smith does not want Fluffy to have a lot of people food either. That is why today, we are using freeze-dried chicken, which is low in fat and calories. Dogs and cats really love it, and it is good for them, too.
We are using really yummy food today so that Fluffy will love coming to see us.	My pet needs to behave without food.	I understand what you are saying. Fluffy's behavior today is not a matter of behaving. It is about making our office less scary and hopefully fun so that she will love coming to see us! The small, low-calorie treats work really well for that, but if your pet has a favorite toy that would work, feel free to bring that next time.
We are using really yummy food today so that Fluffy will love coming to see us.	My dog needs to do "insert command here" to get any treats.	I love that you taught your dog a way to say please. At our office, we have to do things that a lot of dogs find uncomfortable or scary. We are using the treats as a distraction, so they do not need to perform a cue before getting them, just while they are here.
We are going to offer your pet something really yummy and smelly to eat while we do this procedure.	My pet never eats anything while at the vet.	I would like to offer something anyway. You never know, we might find your pet's new favorite! Even if your pet does not eat, the yummy smell can distract them from what we are doing.
We are going to collect the blood here in the room with you, if you are okay with needles.	Why don't you just take him to the back and get it done?	We could do that, but your pet is comfortable here and we have all the things that we need in the exam room. If you are uncomfortable with needles, we can have you wait right outside while we collect the blood.
My nurse is going to hold your pet for the physical examination.	I can just hold him still. Let me do it.	We would appreciate your help. We need you where your pet can see you. He trusts you, so we want you to be feeding him. I would like you to use this food and lots of praise to get your pet in position and keep them distracted throughout the procedure.
We are going to place a muzzle on Fluffy.	He does not need to be muzzled! He is not aggressive!	Fluffy is exhibiting body language that tells us he is fearful (describe body language here). He is already uncomfortable, and it is likely that me reaching over him to examine him will make him more uncomfortable. We need to take every precaution to keep everyone safe. Muzzling is like a seatbelt – we hope to never need it, but we are grateful it is there in the rare instances we do.
We are using food to position Fluffy for his exam/procedure.	Why can't you hold his collar to position him and hold him like you used to?	You are right, we used to do it that way. We know more now, and we have learned more about the emotional health of pets and how it can affect their lives in the long term. Scientific research has shown that veterinary visits are very stressful for pets. Your pet will come here many more times over the course of his life. I want him to love it here so that I can give him the very best health care possible. We use food and gentle handling techniques like this so Fluffy has positive emotions about his visit and about us so that he is happier to see us next time.

> **Box 16.1** The animal-centric approach to reducing fear, anxiety, stress, conflict, and panic in the veterinary hospital
>
> 1. At home preparation that the pet parent can implement at home
> 2. Hospital flow and location set up to make movement through the hospital less stressful
> 3. Animal-centric approach
> 4. Cooperative care for the fearful pet
> 5. Use of previsit pharmaceuticals

Crates, carriers, and car rides

Carriers that are most successful are designed for easy access, comfort, and security; a top that can be easily and quietly removed for patient examination in the carrier, ventilation, and bedding. For most pets, these criteria would be satisfied by a hard plastic carrier with an easily removable top. With the top half removed, these carriers can also allow for examination and procedures while the cat remains in the bottom half of the carrier (Figures 16.1 and 16.2). As with most of veterinary medicine, one size does not fit all. If the pet cannot be handled and will need sedation for the veterinary visit, soft mesh carriers are best to facilitate administering injections (see Figure 16.3). Some carriers are hybrids of mesh and harder materials. For example, the Sleepypod carrier, which has been independently crash tested (www.sleepypod.com), can be used as a bed and a carrier (see Figure 16.4). Covering the carrier with a blanket or towel will prevent exposure to visual and some auditory stimuli to reduce stress. Carriers can be lined with a blanket, towel, or fleece with the household scent for comfort and familiarity (see Box 16.2). Carriers should be secured in the car. Sitting carriers flat instead of on the slanted seat of the car can help pets feel more secure. Not all carriers and seatbelts are

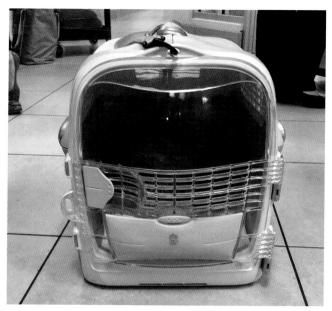

Figure 16.1 For most pets, the best carriers can easily be disassembled like this one. The pet parent should cover the cat carrier with a towel if the sides are clear, such as this one. *(Attribution: Lisa Radosta.)*

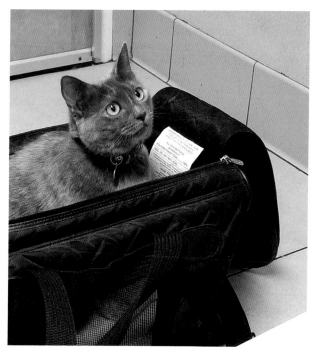

Figure 16.3 Soft carriers can work best for cats that need to be sedated within the carrier. *(Attribution: Amy Learn, VMD.)*

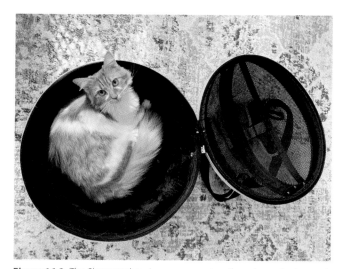

Figure 16.2 The Sleepypod carrier comes apart easily and can also be used as a bed. *(Attribution: Alison Gerken, DVM.)*

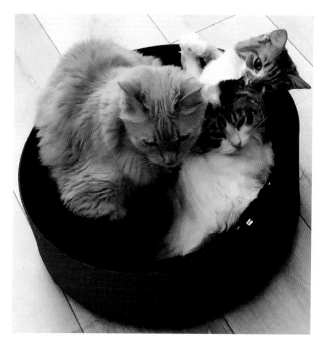

Figure 16.4 Sleepypod. *(Attribution: Alison Gerken, DVM.)*

created equal. Pet parents can be directed to independent crash test organizational web sites to view which seatbelts and carriers have scored the highest during crash tests. Carriers which are easily disassembled allow the pet to be accessed in multiple ways, allowing physical exams and most blood draws to be done within the carrier. When transporting a pet in the carrier, be certain to provide support from underneath for balance and security, instead of using the handle. Swinging back and forth like a pendulum does not set the pet up for a less stressful visit! For dogs that do not ride in a carrier or crate, a seatbelt is recommended for safety and security. Many pets may need previsit pharmaceuticals in order to ride without FASCP in the car (see Chapters 9, 11, and 12). Anything that causes fear, anxiety, pain, nausea, or discomfort can be negatively associated with the veterinary visit. This includes pinch, choke, and shock collars. There is

Box 16.2 Characteristics of ideal pet carriers

1. Easily taken apart
2. Easily cleaned
3. Well ventilated
4. Soft bedding
5. Secure
6. Hard sided with the exception of cats that need to be sedated in the carrier

no place for these tools when training pets, and there is a risk that the discomfort associated with them will be linked with the veterinary visit. The best advice is to advise pet parents to refrain from using those products. Aversive tools do not relieve fear or improve emotional well-being and have no place in a veterinary office. In fact, dogs that have been positively punished in training or during veterinary visits are at greater risk of aggression at the veterinary visit, while negative punishment (i.e., ignoring unwanted behaviors) reduced the risk.[7]

Some dogs and most cats have a negative association with the carrier. When this is the case, the carrier triggers a stress response, which can negatively affect the pet's response to the veterinary visit. For those pets, carrier training can be very helpful. The slow, systematic exposure of the pet to the stimulus of which it is afraid while conditioning a new, positive response with food is called desensitization and counterconditioning (DS/CC). From this point on, it would be counterproductive to continue to use the crate for travel to an unpleasant veterinary visit. Most pets that have an underlying fear of the travel crate or carrier will not get used to it over time; however, the frequent exposures will cause an increase in fear and often a progression from fear to panic. For that reason, the process of DS/CC should be initiated at a level at which the pet does not show any outward signs of stress. The starting point for many pets is simply the sight of the crate in the house. Difficulty can be increased slowly and systematically while monitoring for any signs of fear or stress. While for some patients DS/CC takes months, others with little historical negative experience may only take days to reduce fear and stress.

The process starts with feeding the dog or cat their regular meal in the crate or carrier. The pet parent may have to place the bowl at the front of or just outside of the crate or carrier to encourage them to approach. The top can be taken off of the carrier to make it less frightening. When the dog or cat is reliably, over several sessions, approaching the carrier without fear, the bowl can be moved inside of the carrier. It is important to structure the steps so that the bowl is moved slowly and only when the pet is comfortable proceeding without hesitation on at least three consecutive occasions. Some dogs and cats will go into the crate or carrier on their own, which might be facilitated by placing an appealing and elevated (for cats) location with bedding and some favored rewards inside. An alternative solution is to put the behavior on cue and reinforce the response of entering the kennel. Chapter 10 has a more detailed discussion of DS/CC. Detailed instructions on carrier training for cats and crate training for dogs can be found in the Reading and Resources of Chapter 5 and in Appendix A. DS/CC can also be used to condition the pet to riding in the car. As with carrier and travel crate training above, this should be done slowly and systematically. The steps might include reinforcement for visualizing the car in the driveway, approaching the car, entering the car with the engine turned off, sitting in the car with the engine running and in park, riding in the car for a couple of minutes, and finally taking gradually longer trips. Safely securing the pet is also important. Carriers can be seat belted in place and many dog harnesses have seat belt connectors.

Some pet parents will not be able to complete carrier training with their cat or dog. The pet may be too fearful, anxious, or stressed to complete the conditioning, or the pet parent may not be able for whatever reason to follow through. For those pets, previsit pharmaceuticals may be necessary. If the pet shows any sign of FASCP in the car, even if they do not have hypersalivation, vomiting, or diarrhea, motion sickness should be on the differential diagnosis list as contributing to the behavior in the car. For that reason, a motion sickness treatment trial should be completed with maropitant at the dose mentioned above. If there is any improvement, even if the behavior pattern does not resolve, motion sickness should be treated before each car ride.

A certain subset of pets, potentially more dogs than cats, will simply need distraction in the car. This is an easy technique which should be used as a first resort for most pets. This can be accomplished with food-stuffed puzzle toys or treat dispensers. See Chapters 2, 10, and 13 and Appendix A for more information on how to use food and puzzle toys to distract dogs and cats (see Figure 16.5).

Other strategies which help to decrease stress prior to departure and through travel include ensuring that the pet feels secure in the car (e.g., secure footing, level surface), adding a bed, blanket, or towel, use of a pressure wrap, blocking vision if external stimuli are contributing to the anxiety (e.g., covering the crate, ThunderCap), calming music, tossing treats inside of the carrier or crate throughout the day for the pet to find, an automated or remote treat dispenser, playing chase or fetch with a toy in and out of the crate, practicing obedience cues in and around the crate, playing games like nosework in the crate, and using pheromone analog sprays in the car or carrier 15–30 minutes prior to travel (see Box 16.3).

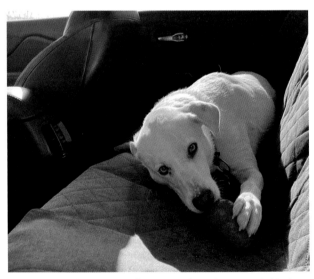

Figure 16.5 Food toys are excellent ways to keep dogs occupied in the car on the way to the veterinary hospital. *(Photo courtesy of Kong Company.)*

Box 16.3 Strategies to ease stress during travel

1. Carrier or crate training
2. Bed or blanket to lie on
3. Pressure wraps
4. Blocking visual stimuli (e.g., towel, ThunderCap)
5. Calming music
6. Pheromone analogs

Hospital flow and location setup

The hospital environment and flow can either contribute to or diminish patient stress. Have you ever walked into a restaurant for the first time and had a negative experience? Maybe the hostess was rude or the restaurant looked or smelled unclean, or was too noisy. Perhaps it took too long for you to receive service. How did you feel about eating at that restaurant? How did that affect your enjoyment of your meal? Did you give that restaurant a good review? Maybe you turned and left to go find a meal elsewhere. If you have experienced this feeling or something similar, you know how an environment and first impressions can change our experiences. The veterinary environment is similar with the added factor of patient's FASCP. Once the pet parent brings their pet to the hospital, hopefully happy and calm, the rest is up to the veterinary healthcare team. If the pet is stressed in anticipation of going to the veterinarian or is fearful in the waiting room, this is a predictor that the pet will be stressed entering the exam room, on the examination table, and when approached by the veterinarian.[2,3,6,14]

Situational predictability and control are factors that reduce FASCP. One of the ways that we can give the pet control and predictability over their experience at the veterinary hospital is to keep an emotional record. An emotional record is a permanent note in the patient's file, describing the preferred reinforcement, distractor, or reward, positioning and location of the physical examination, blood draws and other procedures, notes about the patient's body language, and response to handling or procedures and any other observations, including what the pet finds unpleasant or aversive, and where and when medication and behavior modification products may be helpful or necessary for future visits to the hospital (see Figure 16.6; also available as an online resource – see Appendix C). The note does not have to be long. It can have checkboxes filled out on paper and then added or scanned into the file or as a separate entry in an electronic medical records system. Once preferences are found, the note need only be updated if something changes. When the CCR and/or technician/nurse prepares the clinic and room for the pet's arrival and procedures, and food is offered that is preferred by the pet, it is noticed, and most pet parents truly appreciate the care taken to make their pet comfortable.

The lobby and entrance

Evaluate the lobby for overall sound, smell, visualization of other animals and animals of different species, and layout with patient and pet parent safety in mind. One pet may not like others staring at them in the face (especially different species). All pets should be in carriers or on nonretractable leashes held within 1–2 feet (30–60 cm) of the pet parent. Many pet parents are distracted on their smartphones or using inappropriate tools (e.g., prong collar, choke collar). To assist the pet parent, a notice can be posted on the door requesting that all pets be on leash (if retractable, it should be locked) or in carriers and thanking them for their courteous preparation. If possible, separate entries or waiting spaces in the lobby to segregate cats from dogs with visual (and preferably sound) barriers. In addition, the veterinary team's behavior should be respectful of patient and pet parent needs. CCRs should be

Previsit protocol	
This helps the pet arrive to the clinic in a calm mood.	• Antinausea • Oral anxiolytic • Analgesia • Sedation • Music • Pheromones • Blanket/bed/garment
Health team preference	
Some pets have person preferences, and we want to support them.	• Technician _____ • Doctor preference _____ • No preference • White-coat trigger
Entrance plan	
Especially nervous friends may prefer a separate quiet entrance or waiting in the car.	• No preference • Lobby • Side or back door • Parking lot/wait in car
Motivators	
Consider what helps that pet feel most comfortable and distracts them best.	• Food _____ • Toys _____ • Brushing • Praise
Stressors	
Evaluate what previous experiences have been most stressful.	• Restraint • Extra person • Petting • Body part _____ • Other _____
Comfort zone location	
Pets may prefer a certain location to help them stay calm. Not all pets want to be up on a table.	• Car • Floor • Lap • Table • Carrier • Baby scale • Shelf/tree • Other _____
Calming tools	
Other tools may be necessary but should not be relied upon without considering the medication protocol as well.	• Towel • Blanket • Calming cap • Basket muzzle • Comfy cone • Other _____
Adjustments for next visit	
What was successful and what needs to be changed-being proactive is better than being reactive.	• Change meds: • Add _____ • Preplan _____ • Behavior modification _____

Figure 16.6 An emotional record provides predictability for the pet, reducing fear, anxiety, stress, panic, and conflict. *(Attribution: Amy Learn, VMD.)*

educated on patient body language so that they can adjust their behavior to suit the patient. It also involves the flow from the parking area, and smells, sounds, and sights along the way. The waiting room may not be the ideal space to wait for many patients, especially cats. Many hospitals are moving to a protocol that allows pets to move from the car directly into the exam room, possibly by staggering appointment times to minimize numbers of people arriving and departing at the same time. When the appointment is made, CCRs should assess the level of stress of the patient via a few questions asked of the pet parent. In addition, by reviewing the pet's emotional record (see Figure 16.6) at the time of scheduling, the clinic can prepare for the pet's arrival, knowing what the pet (and pet parent) likes and dislikes. If the pet is stressed, the pet parent can be told at that time to call or text when they get to the hospital. The technician/nurse can go to the car and get them, or call/text them when the room is ready. This will keep the pet's stress level down and avoid congested waiting rooms and confrontations with other patients.

If possible, "cat only" days or times can be scheduled to reduce the stress around veterinary visits. Pheromone analog diffusers and calming music used in the waiting room and throughout the hospital in the waiting area and exam rooms may also help calm pets (see Chapter 12).

The Scale

The weight-determining scale is potentially frightening for cats and dogs alike. These devices can be slippery and can move in unpredictable ways.[5] In one study, dogs were found to be notably more stressed on the scale than in the waiting room.[40] Whenever possible, a baby scale in the exam room should be used for small dogs and cats. The scale can be put on the floor and the pet can be allowed to acclimate. Treats can be used to entice them to go onto the scale and reward them when they are on it. Accurate weights can be captured in this way while the history is taken, or pet parent education is completed. For larger pets, a rug with rubber backing or yoga mat can be used on top of the scale so that the surface is nonskid. Adding a blanket or towel over the rug or mat, draping it over the sides of the scale to further disguise it, can be helpful. Blankets and towels alone should not be used, as they do not make the surface less slippery. Using food to lure the pet onto the scale either by hand or by using a treat trail can be very effective. When using a treat trail, drop small food rewards about 2–3 inches (5–7.5 cm) apart so that the pet has to take no more than one-half to one step to get to the next treat (see Figure 16.7). It is not uncommon for a pet to eat several bits of food and then stop because the next piece is farther away than they dare to go. When luring a pet, keep the treat very close to the mouth if it is safe. Very fearful, stressed, and all aggressive animals should not be lured but instead should use the treat-trail technique above. Keep food rewards handy by keeping them on a wall-mounted shelf or

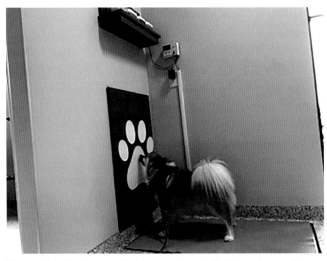

Figure 16.8 Placing a treat holder near the scale facilitates the use of treats for luring and treat trails on the scale. This dog is licking food off of the wall while getting weighed. *(Attribution: Colleen Koch, DVM, DACVB.)*

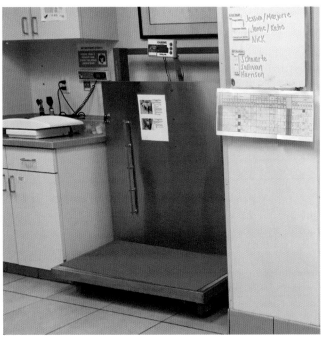

Figure 16.9 Incorrect floor scale location. This scale is elevated and positioned between the cabinet and the wall, making it difficult to get dogs on and off easily. *(Attribution: Lisa Radosta.)*

side table (see Figure 16.8). Ideally, floor scales should be located such that dogs can walk on and off directly (see Figures 16.9 and 16.10). When designing or renovating hospitals, scales can be inset to be flush with the floor or built into exam tabletops.

Moving the patient

When moving a pet from the reception area to the exam room, use nonretractable leashes to keep the patient close and walking in the same direction as the pet parent. If the

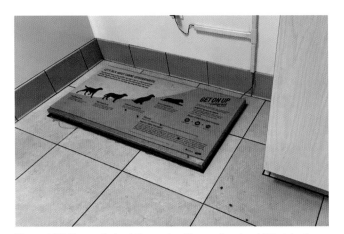

Figure 16.7 Treat trails should be made with treats less than 1/4 inch in diameter, spaced only a few inches apart. *(Attribution: Lisa Radosta.)*

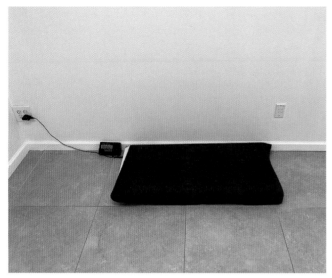

Figure 16.10 Correct scale location. Position floor scales so that dogs can easily walk on and off. *(Attribution: Lisa Radosta.)*

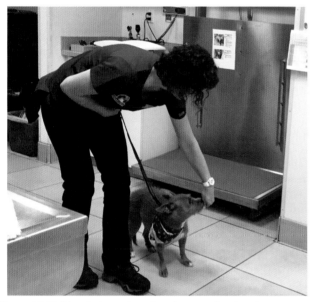

Figure 16.11 When luring patients, face the same direction that you want them to go. Do not stand in front of them. *(Attribution: Lisa Radosta.)*

approach to get the food. The veterinary healthcare team member should have already reviewed the emotional record of the pet, knowing which treats the pet prefers at the veterinarian's office. A good exam room is one that is easy to clean and also comfortable for the pet. By rearranging a few things, we can transform the room into a place where patients and pet parents feel safe and comfortable, and that the veterinary team can properly disinfect. Slippery surfaces such as the floor and the exam table should be covered with readily cleanable mats (e.g., yoga mats, comfort mats) so that they are nonskid. Nonskid surfaces can be covered with towels or washable soft bedding for comfort (see Figures 16.12 and 16.13).

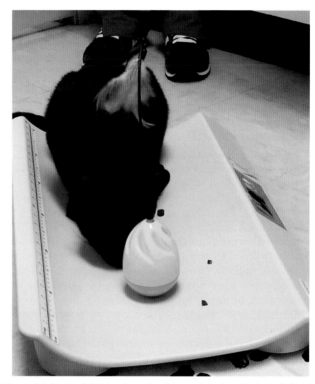

Figure 16.12 Small dogs and cats should be weighed on a baby scale. Treats and toys can entice pets to weigh themselves. *(Attribution: Lisa Radosta.)*

pet does not want to walk with the pet parent and/or the technician/nurse, food can be used as a lure or in a treat trail as above. Do not drag pets into the exam room. When luring or moving with treats, do not stand in front of the pet. Instead, face the way that you would like the pet to go and stand off to the side (see Figure 16.11). If the pet is in a carrier assist, instruct the pet parent so that the pet is carried in a secure way, supported from underneath.

The exam room

While the history is taken, the pet should be observed for signs of stress. If the pet is not presenting for gastrointestinal upset or is not food restricted, toss small food rewards just behind or to the side of the pet so that they do not have to

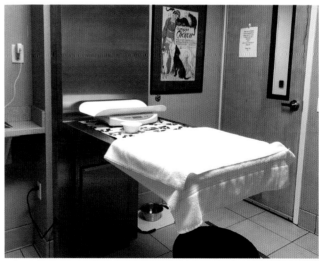

Figure 16.13 This exam room has a nonskid mat on the floor and on the table, a towel on the exam table, and a baby scale. *(Attribution: Lisa Radosta.)*

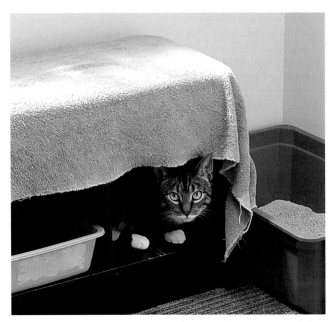

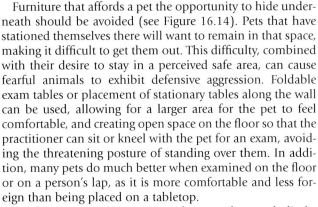

Figure 16.14 Avoid benches and other furniture where patients can hide underneath. *(Attribution: Amy Learn, VMD.)*

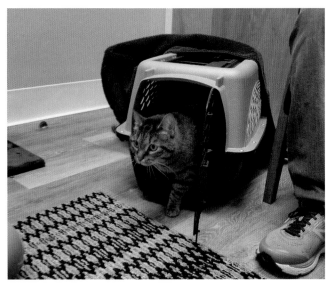

Figure 16.15 Letting cats exit the carrier on their own eases stress. *(Attribution: Amy Learn, VMD.)*

Furniture that affords a pet the opportunity to hide underneath should be avoided (see Figure 16.14). Pets that have stationed themselves there will want to remain in that space, making it difficult to get them out. This difficulty, combined with their desire to stay in a perceived safe area, can cause fearful animals to exhibit defensive aggression. Foldable exam tables or placement of stationary tables along the wall can be used, allowing for a larger area for the pet to feel comfortable, and creating open space on the floor so that the practitioner can sit or kneel with the pet for an exam, avoiding the threatening posture of standing over them. In addition, many pets do much better when examined on the floor or on a person's lap, as it is more comfortable and less foreign than being placed on a tabletop.

Food toys, treats, interesting odors, perches, and climbs should be provided for cats to encourage positive exploration. Food toys can be provided for dogs. When greeting, keep the torso upright, bend at the knees, and do not make direct eye contact if possible. For most pets, ignoring the pet except for tossing food is the most effective way to help the pet calm down. Pet parents should be encouraged to interact with their pet by petting them if it is safe, offering a food toy which can be prepared by the veterinary team and handed to the pet parent, or talking calmly to them. If a cat will not come out of the carrier voluntarily, food and toys can be placed near the carrier opening to encourage leaving the carrier. Alternately, the top of the carrier can be removed to allow the cat to exit, or the cat may be allowed to remain in the bottom of the carrier for examination or lifted out gently with the aid of a towel if necessary. In one study, over 90% of carrier-trained cats chose to stay in the bottom half of the carrier as a retreat for most of the examination.[39] Allow dogs and cats time to explore the room whenever possible before interacting with them. Consider the pet's sensory experience and acuity (e.g., visual, tactile, olfactory, auditory) to make the social and physical environment positive (pheromones, music, tone of voice, surface coverings), and prevent or eliminate what is negative (emotional state, fear odors) (see Figure 16.15).

Many patients are food motivated if they are not too stressed and the food is desirable.

Rightly so, veterinarians may be concerned that the use of food may send the wrong message to pet parents about treats and weight gain, potential gastrointestinal upset, or causing lipemia which could affect lab work results. For each of these concerns, there is a solution which addresses patient stress without negatively affecting pet parent or patient care.

Technicians/nurses can educate pet parents as to why the food is being used and how veterinary visits are different than what should happen at home. Trips to the veterinarian can be stressful, making this a unique, rare occasion where more, potentially higher calorie treats are given. It is unlikely that this one incident will cause significant weight gain, especially if pet parents follow the guideline of reducing the pet's next meal if the use of food during the appointment was excessive. Using low-fat, higher-value treats such as Zuke's, freeze-dried chicken breast, freeze-dried fish, Churu (loved by many cats), meat-flavored baby food, limited-ingredient treats, and canned food, and keeping the individual rewards to no larger than 1/4 inch or 1/16 teaspoon (about the size of a pea) gastrointestinal distress can be avoided in most cases. When using spreadable foods, use a spoon, spatula, pretzel stick, or oral-dosing syringe. Avoid using tongue depressors because some pets may try to ingest them. It is unlikely that feeding during the time of an outpatient appointment would cause significant lipemia or alter laboratory blood test results because postprandial blood triglycerides typically peak 2–6 hours after a meal, so treats given during an exam visit should not likely be problematic, as blood is being drawn at the time of feeding. Always check the chart for pet and human adverse food reactions, medical conditions, or cultural preferences that would prohibit certain treats from being offered in an acceptable manner. In that

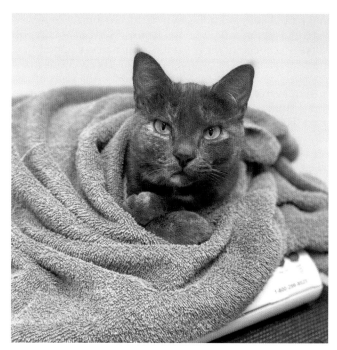

Figure 16.16 Towels are essential tools for low-stress restraint, and they protect team members from bites. *(Attribution: Amy Learn, VMD.)*

case, other types of distraction can be used, including tennis balls, rubber squeaky toys, or catnip mice and crinkly balls. If your hospital is set up for comfort and calm, most dogs and cats will accept or at least sniff a treat. If the appointment is scheduled near the pet's mealtime, half the meal can be fed at the normal time and half given after the veterinary visit to entice the pet to eat during the visit. Skipping entire meals can have ramifications including changes in mood, aggression, and cognition, and should generally be avoided. See Chapters 10 and 13. Cats have specific needs. Whenever possible, rooms should be set up with that in mind. Cat rooms should have two to three plush towels which have been sprayed with pheromone analogs 15–30 minutes prior to the appointment time. Towels can be used to provide a soft surface to lie on, serve as a cover to hide under while remaining in the bottom of their carrier for an examination, or to create a snuggly wrap to safely restrain a cat that is fearful and otherwise untreatable. Towels can also be used in the same ways for small dogs (see Figure 16.16).

Treatment, ICU, and pet care

Treatment areas, intensive care units (ICUs), and kennels are often congested, high-traffic areas with a plethora of sights and sounds. These may be the most challenging areas, as some of the sights and sounds are inescapable: beeping fluid pumps, animals recovering from surgery, critical patients that need handling and frequent treatments, opening and closing of metal cage doors, barking dogs erupting as people walk past, vacuums, clippers, oxygen cages, emergencies, and team members calling to one another over the din to get help with a patient as soon as possible. Hospitalized pets are kept in cages which trap them, restrict their movement, and house them in close proximity to veterinary staff, unfamiliar animals, noises,

odors, and sights, with no opportunity to escape or retreat. How can we possibly prevent or minimize stress in these areas?

The hospital environment can be managed to decrease patient's FASCP, decreasing the negative impact on immune health and recovery and pain and fear conditioning. Management and treatment of the pet's medical or surgical needs and preventing or alleviating pain or discomfort must be a priority. For those pets that are boarding or require extended hospital care, it may take two to three days for reduction of stress levels.[41,42]

The biggest challenges in these areas of the hospital are a result of patient placement and management of the environment. Pets that are stressed should be placed in areas which are quiet and safe. While glass-sided runs allow veterinary healthcare team members to easily see patients, they also allow patients to easily see each other. Stressed and aggressive pets should be in areas where visual access to other pets is blocked. Hanging a sheet with suction cup clips or using temporary window vinyl can serve as visual barriers. Placing these pets so that they are not directly across from another patient is best. A quiet environment (away from dogs) is especially important for cats because they tend to be less well socialized and adaptable to unfamiliar environments than dogs. In addition to the basic needs of the feline patient (e.g., litterbox, food, water) hide boxes, their cat carrier, cardboard boxes, polyester fleece bedding or towels in the bottom of the cage, and a cage cover for sight and sound abatement can reduce stress[41,43] (see Figure 16.17). Pheromone analogs can help to alleviate stress in dogs and cats when hospitalized.[44,45] See Chapter 12 for more information on pheromone analogs.

There are some dogs that respond positively to the sights and sounds of other animals, with this serving as enrichment. Those dogs can be placed in more high-traffic areas along with dogs that are calm in this environment and those that benefit from seeing the veterinary team, such as dogs with confinement distress, isolation distress, or separation-related disorders. Veterinary healthcare team members should be well versed in the body language of dogs and cats to ensure recognition of the difference between a relaxed pet and one that is in the freeze stage of the stress response. For confinement-related frustration, cage-enrichment

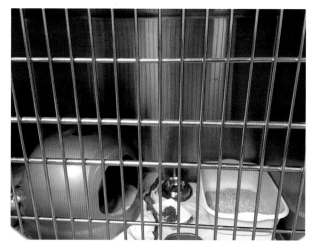

Figure 16.17 Cats should have hiding spaces and soft bedding in addition to food, water, and a litterbox. *(Attribution: Lisa Radosta.)*

opportunities can be provided, such as food toys or safe chew toys (see Chapters 5 and 13).

For treatment areas, consideration must be made about how to control anxiety-provoking sounds in these areas such as clanging of metal cage doors, clippers, ultrasonic dental scalers, Doppler blood pressure measurement, patients recovering from anesthesia, and the vacuum. Several studies have documented increased patient stress with increased hospital noise.[46,47] In fact, noise levels in ICU have been shown to spike at over 80 decibels, a level that can disrupt sleep and compound stress.[48]

Ambient sound can be used to mute the sounds of the ICU, treatment, or kennel. White or brown noise, classical music, and/or species-specific music for cats should be used.[49–51] Certain types of music and even audiobooks have been shown to increase the amount of time that shelter dogs spent resting and decrease vocalization.[52–55] In addition, classical music may not only be calming to pets but also pet parents and the members of the veterinary healthcare team.[50,51,56] The cost of using music in these areas is relatively modest and the potential benefits are many. Placement of speakers should be near the space where the patient is housed and between the source of the noise and the patient.

Cages can be purchased with sound-dampening designs so that they open and close more quietly. If the hospital is not equipped with these types of cages, staff must take extra care to quietly open and close the doors. Barking dogs should be kept in locations where they can be more relaxed and thus quieter. Vocalization in such a setting can be contagious, setting off a cacophony of yips, barks, and growls. Some dogs will not quiet, even with all of the strategies outlined here. These pets may need medications to ease their stress enough so that they can relax. In order for this step to take place, nurses and technicians must be able to recognize stress and must feel comfortable going to the doctor with their observations, and the doctor must understand medications well enough to prescribe wisely.

The behavior of the veterinary healthcare team affects the patient's behavior as well. Emotional contagion is discussed in more detail in Chapter 14. Something as simple as dropping treats into a kennel as one walks by can help to create a quiet and calm environment.[57] Most veterinary healthcare team members have experienced the situation of a team member yelling at or kicking at the cage door of a barking dog. This is counterproductive, unprofessional, and unkind. What would you consider to be the appropriate response to a child who is crying or trembling in fear and calling out for her mother? Is the appropriate response to yell at her or throw something at her? Of course not! We can all agree that will scare her more and keep her from being able to calm down. Dogs and cats are no different. When a dog or cat is scared, yelling or the expression of any negative emotional state is contraindicated and will make the pet more scared. In addition, the other members of the team working in that area are subjected to the toxicity of that behavior.

You never get a second chance to make a first impression. This is especially true for fearful dogs and cats. Most pets are stressed at the hospital. For some, the message is clearer, conveyed via barking, low growls, lunging, snapping, hissing, swatting, or biting. For others, the signs are less obvious, such as refusal to move, attempts to flee, cowering, or freezing. Some patients are resilient and will tolerate inappropriate

interactions such as leaning over, direct eye contact, and over-restraint without serious consequences. However, many will not. The sequelae of the veterinary team's lack of appropriate interactions may not be apparent immediately. It may take several appointments for a pet to exhibit overt signs of distress or aggression. If you have ever experienced a situation where a previously "fine" patient is suddenly aggressive, you most likely have experienced this phenomenon.

A proper greeting is deliberate, not fast. It is respectful of the dog or cat's personal space, considering the body language exhibited and responding appropriately. As much as possible, species-appropriate body language should be used by the team members interacting with the patient. For example, avoid sudden movements, direct eye contact, staring, direct approach, or reaching toward the face or neck/collar. These are all considered threats by dogs and cats. Move gradually, slowly, steadily, calmly, and softly. Many pets will be too stressed to greet the veterinary team. In these cases, it is better not to try to make friends but instead to refrain from interacting with the pet outside of using food as described above, tossed behind the pet. For pets that are not showing aggression, team members can turn sideways, kneel down to the pet's level if safe to do so, use small food rewards to make a treat trail, and allow the pet to approach. Allow the pet to investigate, explore, and initiate or solicit interaction. Contact should begin where the pet solicits or is most likely to accept touch. Pair the interaction with food reinforcement and proceed gently and gradually, provided the pet is calm, to potentially more stressful or painful touch or procedures. Many dogs and cats are not reinforced or rewarded nor soothed from petting. This is especially true of petting from strangers. Generally, this should be avoided unless the patient is clearly soliciting petting. Soliciting petting is not the same as the pet approaching. When you approach another person at work, do you expect them to stroke your hair? Of course not! It is just as undesirable to dogs and cats. If there is doubt about the pet's intention and what they are soliciting, it is better to refrain from petting. Veterinary team members should avoid bending over the pet and putting their faces near the pet's face. These are direct threats and can lead to serious bites to team members.

Some pet parents and staff respond by reprimanding or punishing the dog when it reacts. In this situation, it is unlikely that the punishment will have a positive long-lasting effect on the target behavior, which is aggression at the veterinarian's office. The stress response interferes with rational learning but facilitates emotional learning in this situation. See Chapter 14 for more information on the stress response. In this situation, the dog is unlikely to learn that growling is not an appropriate strategy at the veterinarian's office, but it is likely to learn that trips to the veterinarian's office not only include negative interactions with the veterinary team but also with the pet parent. This type of inadvertent but common learning at the veterinarian's office contributes directly to FASCP and aggression. One unfortunate but prevalent consequence of punishing warning signals such as growling is the reduction in the frequency of exhibition of those signals and escalation of more intense signals such as biting. Because the warning signal has been punished and is no longer exhibited, biting appears to come suddenly and without warning. See Chapter 10 for more information on punishment and reinforcement of behaviors including aggression. See Chapter 2, the recommended reading at the end of this chapter, and Appendix A for more information on cat and dog body language and how to properly greet a pet.

Separation from pet parents coupled with examination location can result in increased stress in cats and dogs, with FASCP also demonstrated to be higher in the treatment area than in the examination room with the pet parent.[58,59] Therefore, wherever possible, all procedures should take place in the same location with equipment and supplies brought to the pet, rather than the pet brought to the procedures. Studies show that dogs are less stressed, more secure, calmer, and easier to handle when the pet parent is in the room and talking to the pet than with the veterinarian, a stranger, or left alone.[14] Pet parent contact with dogs has been shown to reduce fear and reduce escape attempts (jumping off the table).[60] In cats, pet parent proximity and familiarity is also reassuring.[2,58] However, some pets may be more fearful or defensive in the pet parent's presence, particularly if the pet parent is distressed, anxious, fearful, or nervous.[7] Therefore, work to engage pet parents to be safely involved to reduce their pet's stress with positive contact and handling; giving treats; engaging with a toy; or with hands-off verbal and emotional support. If it is best to separate pet parent and pet for procedures, consider having the pet parent leave the room and perform procedures in the exam room to which the pet has already acclimated. However, separating the pet parent and the pet should be the exception rather than the rule.

If there is a need to move the pet for treatment, plan, prepare, and scout the route. Avoid visual and auditory stimuli that might evoke fear along the way. Cats should be moved in covered carriers while dogs might be carried or encouraged to walk on loose leash (not force) by luring or tossing treats.

The animal centric approach

Our behavior affects the patient's behavior

As professionals who love animals and work tirelessly to help and heal them, it might feel strange that a dog or cat would be afraid of veterinary team members. Unfortunately, most of our patients are at minimum stressed by us if not overtly fearful of us. The intention of the veterinary team is to show love by helping heal patients, but that intention is not necessarily clear to animals from our actions. It is critical that the point of view be pivoted to the way that a pet might interpret the experience. If you are afraid of heights and your friend wanted to help you by dragging you to the top of a skyscraper to enjoy the view, you might lose trust in her and assume that she does not really know you or care about you. If you do not know how to swim, but somebody thinks the best way for you to learn is to be thrown into the deep end of the pool, you likely won't embrace the concept. This is similar to the experience of our patients. When we approach inappropriately (by dog and cat standards), overrestrain, or ignore their sometimes desperate attempts to communicate with us, we lose their trust and scare them, resulting in increased physiologic stress, FASCP, and aggression. Simple alterations to our behavior and approach restraint can turn

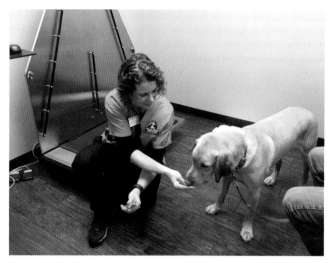

Figure 16.18 If you stand or kneel with your side to the dog and avert your gaze, you will look less threatening. Let the dog approach at its own rate. You can also toss treats or let the dog take the treats out of your hand while still averting your gaze. *(Attribution: Lisa Radosta.)*

the situation around, improve our medical care, and increase the accuracy of our diagnostic tests (see Figure 16.18).

Even if the initial meet and greet goes smoothly, it is important to recognize that most pets remain wary of the veterinary environment and any quick movement may startle them. Moving slowly, deliberately, and smoothly throughout the visit will help that pet remain calm.

Moving patients out of carriers and cages

When the pet is in a carrier or a cage, they are likely to feel trapped. Use the same skills when removing a pet from a cage. If you approach head on and reach for them, there is nowhere for the patient to hide or flee, often resulting in a defense response. Instead, position your body to the side and approach sideways or indirectly and allow the pet to approach you. You can hold the leash loop loosely for the dog to walk into or use a towel to scoop the patient up. For dogs that are fearful, but have shown no aggression, a food lure can be used in front of their mouth like a magnet drawing them forward to get them into position and keep them occupied while they are moved.

The animal-centric approach to handling

Once a good first impression has been made, the next hurdle is restraint. Think of restraint as animal-centric instead of veterinary team member or procedure-centric, and as a form of positioning or gentle handling. Instead of thinking of it as a way to hold the pet still, think of it as a way to get the pet into a comfortable position where it feels safe while still allowing the physical examination and procedures to occur. Where is the pet comfortable? Can the procedure be brought to the pet? Can the cat be examined in the carrier? Can the dog be examined on the ground? Patients do not know what to expect or worse yet, have negative experiences, which causes them to expect the worst. Handling can be tolerable and potentially a positive experience for many patients. Animal-centric restraint starts with understanding the patient's body language and communication (see Chapter 2 and Appendix A). Another essential step is to give the patient choices. For example, if a dog is more comfortable on the floor, consider examining it there. Letting patients come out of the carrier, explore the room and settle where they feel comfortable before an exam, and moving the exam to that location starts the relationship off on a positive note (see Figures 16.19–16.22).

Food is a primary reinforcer and is very powerful. Start with food as the pet is picked up and continue throughout the procedure. Many clinics use food for exams and handling, but the food is used incorrectly. Food should follow the pet. If their head goes down, so does the food. It should be used to move the pet. If the pet needs to move forward, the food moves in the direction that is desired to move the pet without physical force. In addition, if food immediately follows the stimulus, a positive emotional response can be

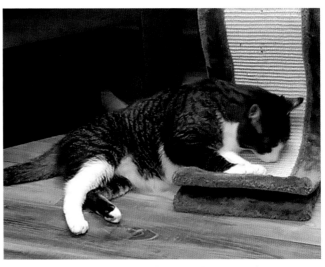

Figure 16.21 Scratching posts like this one with catnip or silver vine may help the pet relax in the clinic. *(Attribution: Amy Learn, VMD.)*

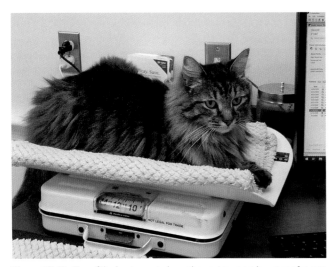

Figure 16.19 One of the best ways to keep the environment low stress for cats is to let them choose where they would like to rest. With a cozy towel and some treats on the scale, this cat made herself at home. *(Attribution: Amy Learn, VMD.)*

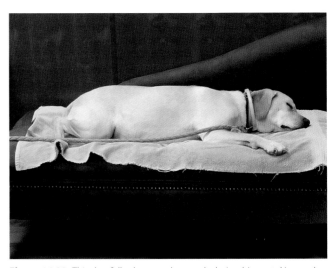

Figure 16.22 This dog fell asleep on the couch during history taking and enjoyed some treats for examination. *(Attribution: Amy Learn, VMD.)*

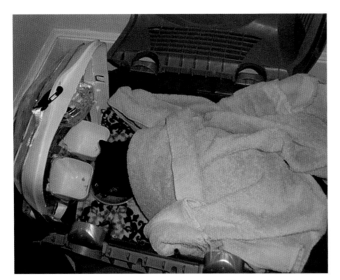

Figure 16.20 This cat chose to stay in the carrier with a towel covering her while eating some canned food. *(Attribution: Amy Learn, VMD.)*

conditioned. This looks and sounds easy; however, using food properly as a handling tool is an art and a science. Team members will need to practice on biddable, relaxed patients before they are ready for patients that are more fearful or stressed. Use the highest-value foods if needed in order to motivate patients to eat.

When the veterinary healthcare team has addressed any underlying pain, fear, anxiety, stress, conflict, and panic; type and location of handling preference; food preference; and if the procedure can be brought to the pet, handling can begin. Approach handling with consideration of the different directions that the pet might move: up/down, side to side, and back to front. Then, assess how a box can be built around that patient with the team member's bodies, the pet parent if it is safe, a food bowl, towels, the wall, or a piece of furniture. For example, a large dog might fare better lined up against a wall (side to side movement), standing on a mat with a technician holding the leash (side to side movement and forward/backward movement), the pet parent feeding in the front (forward movement), and the veterinarian examining from back to front (backward movement). This type of handling is more comfortable for many dogs and allows physical examinations and blood draws to be completed with minimal handling. Cats should be offered food as well during physical examinations and procedures. Cats will often eat in the hospital for the "right" food and in the right conditions (in the carrier, covered by a towel).

It is important to control movement in a humane way that is safe for all and prevent the pet from pacing or squirming because doing so may increase its arousal level or anxiety, causing it to become more reactive. There is a fine balance between minimal handling to keep the pet calm and handling it safely enough that no staff members are scratched or bitten. Watching the patient's body language and assessing appetite is the best way to moderate that balance. For small dogs and cats, a towel or blanket can be used to wrap or swaddle the pet or cover its head to help it feel more secure. Some cats will be more comfortable remaining in the bottom of their carrier. Allow them to gradually habituate and investigate, use food, and gradually increase intensity.

The veterinary healthcare team should be able to read and recognize body postures, facial expressions and vocalizations that indicate a relaxed state, a desire to positively interact, emerging signs of fear and anxiety, and any signs of pain or discomfort. It would seem obvious that veterinary healthcare team members have inherent knowledge of animal behavior because of their experience in the veterinary hospital. However, one study found that for cats in particular, veterinary professionals often had the same level of knowledge as pet parents when asked about the behavioral needs of cats.[61] In a recent veterinary study of Chilean veterinary practitioners, less than 20% were able to identify canine anxiety from videos and photographs, and less than 60% were able to interpret signs of aggression without error. Veterinarians with greater experience excelled at recognizing canine behavior, while those with mild to moderate experience did poorly.[62] What would you do if 60% of the members of your team could not assess the plane of anesthesia in animals during procedures? Would you go for it, given this lack of knowledge and hope for the best? Would you let your team learn as they go even if it compromised patient care? Of course not! Then, why would we ignore the skill set needed to alleviate a problem which affects up to 80% of your patients? Training in the recognition and interpretation of canine and feline body language for every person on the team who interacts with animals is essential.

Use appetite together with body language as a barometer of fear. If the pet stops taking treats or no longer responds to cues for rewards (e.g., sit or down for dogs), this likely indicates the onset or escalation of anxiety. When this is noted, the team should pause to assess what might be causing increased threat or discomfort, give the pet time to return to baseline, and resume when the pet will resume taking treats. A pause in handling means that the team stops the procedure and lets the pet regroup without changing the handling dramatically. For example, if a physical examination is being conducted and the pet stops eating, the veterinary technician should inform the doctor. The doctor who may be palpating the abdomen, for example, would move her hands away

from that spot or leave them hovering there and reduce the pressure significantly. If the signs of fear do not sufficiently decrease or the pet will not resume taking treats, determine whether some or all of the remaining procedures might be rescheduled with a new plan of action for a later day, including positive conditioning and previsit medication; or whether to medicate immediately to complete the necessary procedures on the same day. Otherwise, the pet should be immediately sedated or anesthetized with appropriate analgesia before proceeding. If the pet resumes eating and the stress level goes down, the procedure can continue. Often veterinary healthcare team members regard the pause as a moment to completely stop restraining the pet. The challenge with this strategy is that the pet will then have to be restrained again, which is likely to be even more stressful. It is better to communicate, pause, assess, and weigh if the procedure is necessary on that day. By postponing, revisions could be made to prevent or avoid the negative outcomes, through scheduling, modifying the location (where the pet might prefer), modifying the environment (accentuate the positive and eliminate the negative), altering restraint and handling (what the pet prefers), maximizing reward value (fasting, favored treats or toys), using desensitization and classical counterconditioning to handling, travel, hospital, and equipment, cueing reward training to teach alternative desirable behaviors (operant counterconditioning), giving previsit medications, and selecting and using positive conditioning or management products that might help to calm or improve safety. Rescheduling can also provide the opportunity to prepare the pet for injectable sedation to minimize fear. Previsit nutraceuticals and pharmaceuticals (PVP) should be dispensed where needed and trialed in advance (see Tables 16.3a and b).

When adjusting positioning, do so gently and deliberately. How would you want your 2-year-old child handled by the nurse at the pediatrician's office? That is how we want to handle pets, with great care and respect. With any indication of pain or prior to any procedure that will cause pain, analgesia in the form of topical, local, regional, or systemic medication should be administered.

For small dogs and cats, a towel or blanket can be used to wrap or swaddle the pet or cover its head. Eliminate visual threats by directing the pet's focus away from the stimuli (e.g., needles), hiding them from sight, or using visual barriers such as an Elizabethan collar, ThunderCap, cat muzzle, or blanket. Injections can be prepared in advance, hidden, given with new, small gauge needles, warmed to room temperature, and injected with the pet distracted with treats, toys, or stroking. Use pain management in advance of any pain-evoking stimulus, including a topical lidocaine/prilocaine mixture (20–30 minutes in advance),[29,30] local and regional blocks, and systemic medications (previsit oral or injectable).

As discussed above, the more gentle and passive the handling of feline patients, the less the fear and the more positive (cat friendly) the outcome, while full-body restraint increases negative responses. Unfortunately, the traditional method for handling, scruffing, is still widely used. Often this is the case, not because it is more effective, but because the technician may not know another way to safely handle cats, demonstrating another deficit in the training of many veterinary healthcare teams.

The American Association of Feline Practitioners' feline-friendly handling guidelines recommend against scruffing.[63] Scruffing increases stress, can increase aggression, and is more forceful than is necessary. In two recent studies comparing full-body restraint (cat in lateral recumbency with the technician holding the legs and their arm resting on the cat's neck) with passive control, where the cat is held with the least amount of restraint possible, either sitting, standing, or lying (chosen by the cat), full-body restraint took more time, cats demonstrated more negative behavioral (lip licking, ear position, vocalization) and physiological (pupil dilation, respiratory rate) responses, and were more likely to jump off the table immediately following release compared to the cats that were passively restrained.[64] In fact, the cats that were most unfriendly had the greatest changes in pupillary dilation, demonstrating that the most fearful cats will have the most extreme changes in emotional and physiological states when restrained traditionally and with force. Comparing full-body restraint to clipping, scruffing, and passive restraint, full-body restraint and clipping, followed by scruffing resulted in the most negative responses, with the least associated with passive restraint.[65] Cats should be handled and positioned gently and calmly by first choosing the place where the cat feels most comfortable for examination. This can be in the carrier with the top removed, on the owner's or veterinarian's lap, on a fuzzy bed on the scale, or wrapped in a comforting towel so that the cat does not need to struggle. If the cat cannot be examined and fear kept to a minimum with gentle handling and/or a towel wrap, anxiolytic or sedative medications should be considered.

In addition to the varying of touch and intensity, a gradation should also be made of procedural priority from most important (needs) to least important (wants). Then the plan should be followed, starting at the least aversive and highest importance and working along a gradient to end with or postpone those that are of highest aversiveness and lowest importance (e.g., rectal temperature for routine healthcare visits).[66]

Cooperative care for the fearful pet

When the techniques outlined above have been adopted, pet parents should notice a dramatic difference in the way their pet behaves at the veterinary hospital.[5,35,39,60,64–67] Even so, there are some pets that need more. These pets may have had a traumatic experience or be predisposed to FASCP. They may need more time to acclimate, or different reinforcement or specialized behavior modification. Patients can be conditioned to wear a muzzle, cooperate with examinations, injections, venipuncture, and certain medical procedures so that they have a sense of agency, lowering stress for the patient, pet parent, and the veterinary team.

Cooperative care is a process which conditions the pet to accept calmly and participate willingly in the handling and procedures that facilitate veterinary care, and specifically the handling and procedures that trigger FASCP. The intent of cooperative care training is to communicate, reorient, and guide the pet into alternative desirable behaviors that can be rewarded, as well as to assess choice and consent in situations that might evoke fear. Cues for veterinary, medical, and maintenance care that could serve as a foundation for calming, reorienting, and maintaining focus and for operant conditioning include touch (targeting), chin rest (with focus), check (investigating objects), and stationing to relax on a "place" or "mat."

Cooperative care also includes classical counterconditioning (changing a negative association with a stimulus into one that is positive) or systematic desensitization (exposure to the frightening stimulus in small increments below the threshold for fear and increasing in intensity over many sessions while keeping the pet calm). Cooperative care can be straightforward such as teaching the pet to offer a paw for claw (nail) trims or complicated and lengthy, such as teaching the pet all of the steps necessary to have blood drawn in the veterinary hospital without fear.

Cooperative care should be guided and taught by skilled professionals to achieve the most positive outcome. Like using food as a part of handling, cooperative care plans look simple to implement, especially when demonstrated by a skilled professional. However, there is always the risk that the nurse/technician or trainer will move too quickly or read body language incorrectly, causing the pet to be fearful. Setbacks like these are expected to some extent and will slow the time to achieve the goals set forth in the plan.

To create a plan, each stimulus that evokes fear is determined, and the intensity of each stimulus that is tolerated by the pet without fear is noted. These could include the carrier, travel, the veterinary facility, personnel, products (e.g., muzzles or head halters), instruments, and the specific body parts (handling) and procedures (ears, eyes, injections). The pet parent's goals and the veterinary team's goals should be in the plan to keep the process on track with the goals set initially. Pet parent goals may be very different than veterinary team goals, so this is an important step. Before cooperative care plans are made, an honest conversation should be had with the pet parent about the time and financial commitments required to complete the plan for their pet. They might be completely satisfied with a plan focused on getting the pet to accept an intramuscular injection for sedation instead of teaching the pet to accept the procedure awake. Partnering with the pet parent is essential for a positive outcome.

DS/CC may be a part of a cooperative care plan. In one study, a standardized four-week DS/CC program was mildly effective at reducing signs of veterinary fear; however, over 40% of pet parents were not compliant.[68] The behavior plan should therefore be tailored to the individual pet by identifying, desensitizing, and counterconditioning to the specific stimuli (social, physical, sensory, environments) that trigger the fear. The greater the skills of the person creating and implementing the plan, the quicker and more successful the process can go. In addition, explanation of the commitment and time required to complete the procedure is essential. Often pet parents will "go for it" in the exam room, feeling like they can accomplish anything suggested. Then, when they get home and move into their daily routine, they realize that their commitment was not realistic for their family. It is better to realize this in the exam room, facilitating an honest and realistic revamp of the plan, than for the pet parent to feel failure, disappointment, and potentially embarrassment when they cannot complete the plan, causing them to avoid communicating with the veterinary team for fear of judgment. DS/CC are described in more detail in Chapter 10.

Scheduling technician/nurse sessions as a value-added service

Veterinary healthcare team members are accustomed to assessing the health of pets and recommending treatment even if the patient was presented for a different problem. For example, if a dog presents for diarrhea and during the exam, fleas were noticed, the pet parent would be informed so that treatment for both could be instituted. This rule should apply to both physical and behavioral problems. In other words, if a patient is showing signs of fear, treatment should be offered, potentially including medications for future visits, resources, or cooperative care treatment.

Cooperative care appointments can be conducted outside of the hospital by skilled dog-training professionals; however, at some point in the procedure, the pet must be transitioned to the hospital setting, as that is where the procedures will occur. In addition, veterinary healthcare team members know the nuances of how a pet will have to stand, sit, lie down, offer its paw, or hold its head for procedures. Simple changes that occur in the hospital such as the placement of the hand when holding off the cephalic vein during a blood draw must be conditioned. If the pet is conditioned to accept the hand in the incorrect position because the practitioner has never themselves done this procedure, the treatment will be ineffective. Whenever possible, veterinary team members should spearhead these appointments.

Pricing of cooperative care appointments can be based on the labor, material, and overhead costs to schedule, check in, conduct, and check out the appointment as well as any base costs and premium which is typical for the hospital. Appointments can last 15–60 minutes, although shorter sessions of 20 minutes are usually recommended to start. During the appointment, the technician/nurse will explain the procedure, the timing of reinforcers or motivators, judgment of body language, and how to use the resources which will be sent home. Technicians/nurses should start with procedures they feel comfortable performing and then add on other DS/CC procedures as they gain more skill.

Similar to when a treatment plan is presented to pet parents for physical disorders, a treatment plan should be presented to the pet parent for emotional disorders. Pet parents should receive options such as a medication-only plan, a plan with a target goal of sedating the pet with injectable medications, and a cooperative care plan. Then the pet parents can decide what is best for their pet with full knowledge of the financial and time commitments associated as well as the consequences of declining care. If the pet parents decline and request more aversive techniques, the hospital is under no obligation to use any techniques which do not line up with the hospital's standard of care. In other words, aversive techniques, even when requested by the pet parent, are not recommended and, in many cases, may not be acceptable.

Managing fearful and aggressive pets

Pets that display aggression in the veterinary clinic are suffering from FASCP or frustration. How a pet responds to a fear-evoking event varies with the situation, type, and intensity of stimulus, previous experience, personality of the individual, circumstances (e.g., presence or absence of the pet parents, type and level of handling), and the control to avoid, hide, or seek comfort. Fear-evoking stimuli can be environmental (auditory, visual, olfactory, tactile/discomfort) or social (responses of pet parents, veterinary staff, or other pets) and can be related to visual, auditory, tactile, odor, or procedures and handling. Social stimuli (people, other animals) and uncontrollable stressors (physical handling, leash restraint, restricting avoidance) may increase aggression. Pets that freeze or flee may become aggressive if approached or further threatened (reaching, grabbing, pulling), especially if the pet is hiding (e.g., under a chair), confined (e.g., hospital cage), has retreated to a secure base or safe haven (carrier, pet parent), or unable to retreat further (e.g., back of cage, wall). If the pet learns that aggression is successful at removing the threat, the behavior is negatively reinforced. Even if the pet can be subdued to allow completion of the procedure, the process increases fear and the potential for aggression. See Chapter 10 for more detail on negative reinforcement.

Pharmacologic management of fearful and aggressive pets

Whenever a fear, anxiety, or pain-evoking veterinary visit or procedure is predictable or inevitable, and whenever fear, anxiety, or stress cannot be prevented, alleviated, or sufficiently abated with considerate and pet-centric veterinary care, medications should be dispensed, either preventively and proactively before travel and/or administered immediately and without hesitation at the visit should fear begin to escalate. Increased restraint, increased fear or anxiety by the pet parent or veterinary personnel, unfamiliar management tools, and procedural fear and pain will only serve to further increase FASCP. As fear escalates, response to drug therapy becomes more variable and less predictable, onset of effect is delayed, and drug protocols and doses may need to be increased, with increased potential for risks and adverse effects.[67,69]

Medications do not change the pet's relationship or alter the pet's conditioned fear response to a stimulus. What they can do is help to alleviate the underlying fear, anxiety, stress, conflict, panic, arousal, and impulsivity to help normalize the pet's mental state, improve the pet's emotional health and welfare, and create an environment in which the pet can learn, and behavior can be modified. Use of previsit and in-clinic anxiolytics, sedatives, antiemetics, and analgesics enables the veterinary team to prevent or alleviate pain and suffering, optimize safety, practice better medicine with more complete physical examination findings, more accurate assessment of vital signs and laboratory findings, prevent stress-induced immunosuppression, delayed wound healing and gastrointestinal upset, speed recovery, and prevent further fear conditioning and sensitization.

Previsit oral medications

For behavioral medications to be effective, they must be administered in advance of the onset of the fearful event and associated physiologic and behavioral response. Regarding previsit pharmaceuticals, medications should be administered 1–3 hours preemptively before the onset of any signs of FASCP. Alprazolam in dogs and cats, and diazepam and lorazepam in dogs, may be an exception and can be administered 30–60 minutes prior to visits, and dexmedetomidine oromucosal gel administered to dogs 20–60 minutes in advance.[70–72] However, medications intended for reducing FASCP prior to veterinary visits should be administered so that their effect takes place prior to triggering events. They should be administered when the pet is relaxed prior to exposure to the fearful stimulus or immediately upon showing initial signs. Often practitioners recommend that medications be administered 1 hour prior to the visit. However, FASCP can be associated with stimuli related to preparation and travel for many pets. For example, if a pet parent brings out the cat carrier the night before the veterinary visit, medications should be administered the night before and then again before the appointment. In this way, cumulative stress can be avoided. Any stimulus can be linked with an event, even if unnoticed by the pet parent. For example, if the pet parent carries a file or notebook or a certain tote bag when the dog is taken to veterinary appointments, those stimuli could very well be paired with a negative CER. Patients that have a negative CER to stimuli should receive their medications so that they have taken effect prior to the onset of the emotional response. As there can be marked individual variability, a trial in advance of the visit is recommended to assess effect, side effects, dose, duration, and onset so that the medication can be administered far in advance to achieve peak effect and sufficient duration. When that is not possible, for example, with next-day appointments, 3-hour dosing is recommended, with the exception of the medications listed above, such as dexmedetomidine and quick-acting benzodiazepines. Some medications such as acepromazine may be more effective when administered 4 hours prior to the visit. It should be noted that a sedated response in the home environment often does not translate to a sedated or calm response in the veterinary hospital. For this reason, pet parents should be informed that they may have to make several visits to the hospital before the right medication combination or dosage is established (see Tables 16.3a and b).

While it has been recommended that once an effective dose is determined, an additional dose might be considered 12 hours in advance or dosing started 24–48 hours in advance, this often is not necessary because of the short half-lives of most of these medications. For the most part, they are eliminated within 8–12 hours. For medications with short half-lives such as alprazolam and dexmedetomidine oromucosal gel, this generally is not advantageous. If the pet has significant ramp-up the day before the visit because of pet parent preparations or other conditioned stimuli associated with the veterinary visit (e.g., cat carrier, travel accessories, pet medical record notebook or files), predosing can reduce ramp-up. Natural supplements (see Chapter 12) may also be administered prior to the visit for preventing and reducing mild fear and anxiety if started and dosed sufficiently prior to the visit.

For FASCP in dogs, the use of trazodone, benzodiazepines (e.g., alprazolam, diazepam, or lorazepam), gabapentin, clonidine, dexmedetomidine oromucosal gel or tasipimidine can be effective prior to travel and veterinary visits.[71–77] Trazodone may be more rapidly absorbed in dogs if food is withheld, although it can be effective when administered with food. Its peak effect in dogs can be over 2.5 hours, which makes trial dosing particularly important to determine peak effect and duration of action.[78] Before administering dexmedetomidine (Sileo), pets should be positively conditioned to dosing with the syringe. In addition, because the mechanism used in syringe dosing is one with which most pet parents are not familiar, potentially contributing to inaccurate dosing, all pet parents should be given an explanation of the mechanism, hold the syringe in their hand, and demonstrate proficiency in dosing before they take the product home. In cats, gabapentin, trazodone, and benzodiazepines such as lorazepam or alprazolam can be effective as previsit pharmaceuticals if given sufficiently in advance (2–3 hours) of the veterinary appointment.[79–82] Another option for cats is pregabalin which is now approved in Europe for anxiety and fear associated with transportation and veterinary visits in cats at a dose of 5mg/kg PO 90 minutes prior to travel.[83] Dexmedetomidine oromucosal gel is not licensed or labeled for use in cats. Several studies have shown variable effect on reducing FASCP during travel and veterinary visits, with salivation as the primary adverse event.[84,85] Previsit medications should include pain relief and nausea/motion sickness relief as well as stress-reducing medications. Benzodiazepines, Entyce, or mirtazapine can be added prior to the visit to stimulate appetite for counterconditioning and restraint.[86] For some pets, anxiolytics such as benzodiazepines might disinhibit their behavior, resulting in an increase in aggression.

Table 16.3a Doses for single-dose oral preveterinary visit medication in dogs for relief of fear, anxiety, stress, conflict, and panic (FASCP)

Drug	Dose	Administration
Alprazolam	0.02–0.1 mg/kg	30–60 minutes prior to onset of FASCP
Clonidine	0.01–0.05 mg/kg	1.5–2 hours prior to onset of FASCP
Dexmedetomidine oromucosal gel	125 µg/m²	20–60 minutes prior to onset of FASCP
Diazepam	0.5–2.2 mg/kg	45–90 minutes prior to onset of FASCP
Gabapentin	10–50 mg/kg	1.5–3 hours prior to onset of FASCP
Imepitoin	20–30 mg/kg	2 hours prior to onset of FASCP – begin 30 mg bid two days prior to event
Lorazepam	0.02–0.5 mg/kg	30–60 minutes prior to onset of FASCP
Pregabalin	2–5 mg/kg	1.5–3 hours prior to onset of FASCP
Tasipimidine	10–30µg/kg	1 hr in advance of onset of FASCP
Trazodone	3–19.5 mg/kg	2–3 hours prior to onset of FASCP – onset is delayed by feeding
Add-on sedation		
Acepromazine	0.5–2.0 mg/kg	1–4 hours prior to onset of FASCP

References: 69, 70–78, 88 and Behavioral Drug Resources.
Note: Administration prior to the onset of FASCP is essential for optimal outcomes. Some animals mount a stress response hours prior to the veterinary visit and may need medications 3–4 hours prior to the visit or the night before and the day of the visit.

Table 16.3b Doses for single-dose oral preveterinary visit medication in cats for relief of fear, anxiety, stress, conflict, and panic (FASCP)

Drug	Dose	Administration
Alprazolam	0.125 mg–0.25 mg/cat (up to 1 mg/cat)	30–60 minutes prior to onset of FASCP
Clonidine	5–10 mcg/kg	1.5 hours prior to onset of FASCP
Gabapentin	10–40 mg/kg 50–200 mg/cat	1.5–2 hours prior to onset of FASCP
Lorazepam*	0.03–0.08 mg/kg 0.25–0.5 mg/cat	1.5 hours prior to onset of FASCP
Pregabalin	5–10 mg/kg	1.5 hours prior to onset of FASCP
Trazodone	25–100 mg/cat	1–2 hours prior to onset of FASCP
Add-on sedation		
Acepromazine	0.5–2.0 mg/kg	1–2 hours prior to onset of FASCP

References: 69, 80–83, 88, 89 and Behavioral Drug Resources.
Note: Administration prior to the onset of FASCP is essential for optimal outcomes. Some animals mount a stress response hours prior to the veterinary visit and may need medications 3–4 hours prior to the visit or the night before and the day of the visit.
*Time to peak efficacy has not been established in cats.

If after dose assessment and titration single products have not been sufficiently effective, combination use with drugs or natural products might be considered. For example, while trazodone and gabapentin might be calming as sole agents, they might also be used in combination, alprazolam or dexmedetomidine oromucosal gel (dogs) might be administered 30–60 minutes prior to the onset of FASCP, or acepromazine combined where greater sedation is indicated (see Tables 16.3a and b). More information can be found on previsit oral medications in Chapters 9 and 11.

Transmucosal administration (OTM)

For greater sedation in healthy, highly fearful, fractious pets, transmucosal medications might be administered 20–60 minutes in advance. The dose can be administered by syringe into the buccal pouch or mixed with a palatable viscous food or liquid such as honey, molasses, maple syrup, or peanut butter to enhance buccal contact and slow absorption. Sufficient additional sedation might be achieved with transmucosal use of injectable acepromazine or dexmedetomidine in dogs and cats or with buprenorphine in cats.[70,87–93] Satisfactory sedation was achieved in four aggressive dogs with 32.6 µg/kg of dexmedetomidine OTM, while 20 µg/kg provided equivalent but longer duration and slower onset (73 ± 33 minutes) than IV administration of 5 µg/kg.[87,91] Detomidine gel (Dormosedan) has also demonstrated effect in dogs.[94] For more intense fear and anxiety or where sole agents are insufficient, greater sedation can be achieved with a combination of a sedative (acepromazine or dexmedetomidine) plus a narcotic such as buprenorphine, butorphanol, or methadone in dogs and cats.[90,95–98] When further sedation is required, oral or transmucosal ketamine might

be added.[89,99] Alternately, buccal tiletamine-midazolam has been demonstrated to be effective for chemical restraint in cats from 15 to 120 minutes after dosing.[100] The Chill protocol, developed at the Tufts Cummings School of Veterinary Medicine, combines both oral and transmucosal medication for the management of fearful and aggressive dogs, with oral gabapentin dosed the evening before the appointment, gabapentin and melatonin administered 1–2 hours before the appointment, and transmucosal acepromazine given 30 minutes in advance[101] (see Table 16.4).

It is also important for the staff to realize that a pet sedated with oral medications may appear sedated, but caution should be exercised as some pets will be suddenly aroused such as by loud noises. As a result, pets on oral sedatives must be cautiously monitored for the possibility that they may unexpectedly lunge or bite.

Injectable sedation

When oral sedation is not sufficient, and for procedures in which anesthesia will be required intramuscular sedation is

Table 16.4 Doses for transmucosal administration

Drug	Dogs	Cats
Dexmedetomidine	0.01–0.04 mg/kg	0.02–0.04 mg/kg
Acepromazine	0.025–0.05 mg/kg	0.02–0.05 mg/kg
Buprenorphine	0.02–0.05 mg/kg (small dogs)	0.02–0.05 mg/kg
Dexmedetomidine + morphine	0.01–0.04 mg/kg + 1.0 mg/kg	
Dexmedetomidine + butorphanol	0.01–0.04 mg/kg + 0.2 mg/kg	
Dexmedetomidine + buprenorphine	0.01–0.04 mg/kg + 0.02–0.05 mg/kg	0.02–0.04 mg/kg + 0.02–0.05 mg/kg
Dexmedetomidine + methadone	0.01–0.04 mg/kg + 0.4–0.75 mg/kg	0.02–0.04 mg/kg + 0.3–0.75 mg/kg
Detomidine gel	0.5–2.0 mg/m² OR 0.1 mL (0.76 mg)/11 kg	
Ketamine (additional if needed)		10 mg/kg
Tiletamine-zolazepam		1–2 mg/kg buccally
Chill Protocol: transmucosal acepromazine + oral gabapentin and melatonin)	• Evening before: 20–25 mg gabapentin evening before • 1–2 hours before appointment: 20–25 mg gabapentin PO+ melatonin PO (small dogs, 0.5–1 mg; medium dogs, 1–3 mg; large dogs 5 mg • 30 minutes before appointment: acepromazine transmucosal 0.025–0.05 mg/kg	

References: 69, 87–101 and Behavioral Drug Resources.

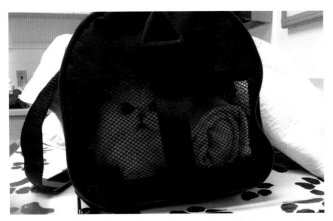

Figure 16.23 Soft carriers can be used to restrain pets for intramuscular injection. *(Attribution: Susan Barrett, DVM and Traci Shreyer, MA.)*

usually the safest and most effective means of restraint. Training dogs to wear a basket muzzle prior to the visit provides a quick and safe method of administering intramuscular injections. More information on basket muzzle training can be found at www.muzzleupproject.com and Appendix A. The ThunderCap (see Chapter 12) might also help by reducing visual stimuli. Training dogs to wear an Elizabeth an collar may also aid in more safely and efficiently administering medication. Muzzles that cover a cat's mouth and eyes are available; however, most cats can be injected while remaining in a carrier with the top removed, with the gentle use of a thick towel wrapped over them, or in a soft carrier with a rolled towel next to them (Figure 16.23).

While oral and transmucosal medications might provide sufficient calming or sedation to proceed with procedures when the pet is admitted to the veterinary hospital, they can also serve to facilitate the use of intramuscular sedation. If the pet is fearful or aroused and cannot be sufficiently calmed during the visit, injectable sedatives should be considered. In fact, sedatives should be used before the pet has a chance to become highly aroused or reactive, since they have a more consistent effect when used before the stress response ramps up. Sedatives may be necessary, not only for the safety of the pet parents and staff but also for the health and welfare of the pet. By preventing further fear, arousal, discomfort, and psychological trauma, we can avoid a highly negative experience for all. When using injectable sedation, consider that the greater the level of fear, anxiety, or arousal at the time of administration, the more variable the sedative response may be and the higher the dose and greater the risks of induction and anesthesia.[67,69] Therefore, prompt and calm injections when the pet is minimally stressed are safest and most effective. Also consider what previsit medications the pet has received when selecting and dosing intramuscular drugs to avoid overdoses or harmful interactions.

Not only is injectable sedation beneficial to the health, welfare, and safety of the pet, pet parent, and veterinary team, the cost is less than manual restraint in cases where pets are stressed. It is a misnomer that manual restraint takes less time, is less risky, and less costly. In one study, manual restraint was shown to require the most personnel (2.4) and the longest contact time (18 minutes) when compared to sedation. This was decreased with low-dose dexmedetomidine (125 μg/m²),

but high-dose dexmedetomidine (375 μg/m²) or the combination of dexmedetomidine and butorphanol (0.4 mg/kg) required still less restraint, lower mean contact time, and had the best behavioral and cooperative scores.[102] This is consistent with human studies in which patient tractability, procedural costs, and drug costs were lowered, hospital stays were shortened, and ICU stays and the need for ventilator-assisted respiration were reduced in patients receiving sedation with dexmedetomidine.[103,104]

Remember that up to 85% of pets are stressed at the veterinarian's office. With that in mind, many of your patients may require some sort of medication to accept handling without stress.

Drug selection should be based on the patient's level of FASCP and pain, planned procedure, and ASA (American Association of Anesthetists) risk (https://www.ncbi.nlm.nih.gov/books/NBK441940/) See table 16.5.

Dexmedetomidine is an alpha-2 agonist which provides fairly rapid analgesia and sedation (e.g., 20 minutes) and can be reversed with intramuscular injection of atipamezole if a more rapid recovery is desired. The use of an alpha-2 agonist decreases sympathetic outflow by inhibiting release of catecholamines and can lower stress associated with anesthesia and surgery.[105] Dexmedetomidine and medetomidine should be avoided in pets with cardiovascular compromise as it causes vasoconstriction and hypertension, leading to increased cardiac work. A newer alternative is medetomidine/vatinoxan (Zenalpha), which is labeled for intramuscular injection at a dose of 1 mg medetomidine/m² and has a more rapid onset (5–15 minutes) with a short duration (45 minutes) and can also be reversed with atipamezole. Vatinoxan is an alpha-2-antagonist that can counteract some of the cardiovascular side effects seen in traditional alpha-2-agonists (see https://dailymed.nlm.nih.gov/dailymed/drugInfo.cfm?setid5623f44bf-07c7-4704-8114-5e42e1316fb1). The level of sedation with dexmedetomidine and medetomidine will vary between individuals, and pets that appear sedated may be suddenly responsive to stimuli, including pain. These drugs require lower doses in combination with an opioid.

Optimal and balanced sedation in dogs and cats may be achieved with intramuscular injections of low-dose dexmedetomidine combined with a narcotic such as butorphanol. In one study of hospitalized dogs, salivary cortisol was lower in dogs that had been given butorphanol and dexmedetomidine 6 hours previously compared to unsedated dogs.[106] In place of butorphanol, buprenorphine might provide more analgesia but less sedation; and mu agonists such as hydromorphone, oxymorphone, morphine, or methadone offer greater pain control and greater sedation, and are reversible[69,88–90,95,96,98,107] (see Table 16.6). The addition of midazolam may provide anxiolytic and muscle relaxant effects and greater sedation, reduce the necessary dose of alpha-2 agonist required, reduce dose requirements for anesthetic induction, act as an appetite stimulant for a faster return to eating, provide short-term amnesia of the handling and procedure and fear it might have otherwise induced, and reduce the likelihood of postreversal excitation with atipamezole.[67,69,89,108] However, it may contribute to a paradoxical excitement in some pets.[69] Opioids may cause emesis, but administration of maropitant prior to the visit may reduce this risk as well as hasten return to eating.[31,32]

Acepromazine may be combined with an anxiolytic or opioid in lieu of dexmedetomidine. Acepromazine has a longer

Table 16.5 Injectable drugs for intramuscular sedation (used in combination)

Sedation	Butorphanol (minimal analgesia)[1]	0.2 mg/kg dog or cat
	+dexmedetomidine[2,3]	0.003–0.01 mg/kg dog
		0.005–0.015 mg/kg cat
	±midazolam[4]	0.1–0.2 mg/kg dog or cat
Greater fear/deeper sedation	Butorphanol (minimal analgesia)[1]	0.2–0.4 mg/kg dog or cat
	+dexmedetomidine[2,3]	0.008–0.028 mg/kg dog
		0.02–0.04 mg/kg cat
	±midazolam[4]	0.1–0.2 mg/kg dog or cat
Additional sedation	Ketamine	1–2 mg/kg (cat/small dog)
	or alfaxalone	0.5–2.0 mg/kg (10 mg IM limit to small dog or cat)
	or tiletamine/zolazepam	1–2 mg/kg dog or cat
Geriatric/ill (ASA III or IV)	Butorphanol[1]	0.2 mg/kg dog or cat
	+midazolam	0.1–0.2 mg/kg dog or cat
	and/or alfaxalone	0.5–1 mg/kg dog or cat

[1]The need for analgesia should determine the type of opioid to be administered. Select and substitute opioid for level of pain, procedure, and patient health (ASA level). For geriatric and ill pets, use opioids at low end of dose range and titrate to effect. **See Table 16.6 for selection, dosing, and use of opioids.**

[2]Could substitute acepromazine at 0.01–0.05 mg/kg dogs and 0.03–0.05 mg/kg cats (up to 0.1 mg/kg). Not anxiolytic so may add benzodiazepine.

[3]The dosage of medetomidine is double the dexmedetomidine in mg/kg.

[4]May provide anxiolytic, muscle relaxation, and amnesic effect but may cause paradoxical excitation. Reversible with flumazenil at 0.01–0.03 mg/kg IV to effect.

References: 69, 88–91, 95, 96, 98, 105, 107, 108, 110–112 and Behavioral Drug Resources.

Table 16.6 Selecting opioids (IM dosing)

Butorphanol	0.2–0.4 mg/kg (dog or cat)	Minimal pain – enhanced sedation
Buprenorphine	0.02–0.03 mg/kg (dog) 0.02–0.04 mg/kg cat	Mild to moderate pain
Morphine	0.2–1 mg/kg (dog)	Moderate to severe pain
Oxymorphone	0.05–0.2 mg/kg (dog) 0.02–0.1 mg/kg (cat)	Moderate to severe pain
Hydromorphone	0.05–0.2 mg/kg (dog) 0.05–0.1 mg/kg (cat)	Moderate to severe pain
Methadone	0.2–0.5 (dog or cat)	Moderate to severe pain

References: 69, 88–90, 95, 96, 98, 107, 108, 110–112 and Behavioral Drug Resources.

duration of action, but it may provide less reliable and less profound sedation; has no anxiolytic or analgesic effect; and is not reversible.[69,109] Therefore, the addition of midazolam would provide an anxiolytic effect. In cats, alfaxalone might be added to the opioid (e.g., butorphanol, hydromorphone, methadone) in place of dexmedetomidine.[108,110,111] Adding midazalom to the combination may provide greater sedation and less resistance to procedures such as catheter placement than hydromorphone and alfaxalone alone.[108]

To better manage more fractious patients, the dosage of dexmedetomidine can be increased, and ketamine might be added to the dexmedetomidine and narcotic combination.[69,88,89] While doses of ketamine of 1–3 mg/kg might be sufficient in many patients for additional sedation, a dose of 5–10 mg/kg could provide anesthesia in cats, although the volume is too high to be used in medium to large dogs.[69,88,89,112] As another alternative, alfaxalone or Telazol (tiletamine/zolazepam) might be added to the narcotic and dexmedetomidine combination for small dogs and cats.[69,88,89,111] However, recovery may be prolonged and associated with greater excitement, reactivity, and ataxia with the addition of alfaxalone. As ketamine, Telazol, and alfaxalone are anesthetic agents, patients given these drugs require anesthesia monitoring.

Reversal agents for midazolam (flumazenil at 0.01–0.02 mg/kg IV),[69] dexmedetomidine (atipamezole given IM equal to the same volume of dexmedetomidine [0.5 mg/kg] given IM or 5000 mcg/m² dog [Antisedan prescribing information]),[89,113,114] and mu agonists (naloxone or partial reversal with butorphanol) are also available to counteract adverse effects or if faster recovery is required.[69,89] However, recovery may be smoother and less stressful if the patient is not reversed.[69] In fact, reversing the sedative and sympatholytic effects of dexmedetomidine (or too rapid a reversal) could result in increased vigilance, excitability, sympathoactivation, self-trauma, and an increase in norepinephrine levels.[69,115] The use of naloxone should be reserved for patients with adverse effects (e.g., significant hypotension, respiratory depression, bradycardia) and titrated slowly until side effects abate, as full reversal will antagonize analgesic effects and may result in hyperexcitability and cardiac arrhythmias.[69] Therefore, the decision to reverse any of these drugs should be decided on an individual basis.

Home care instructions

After the in-hospital steps for nervous or fearful pets are completed, discharge instructions and billing might best be managed in the examination room or before bringing the pet to the pet parent. If the reception area needs to be utilized for discharge, the same considerations should be taken as upon arrival of the patient. Focused medical or postprocedural instructions should be calmly provided along with behavioral guidance for travel and returning the pet to the home, taking into consideration the pet, the procedures, and the home environment. Some degree of limited or gradual introduction may be warranted, especially for those pets returning to homes in which there are other pets present or that might be fearful or stressed for extended periods after the visit. Consider pheromones in the home, positive social interactions (treats, play, affection) while avoiding those that might be negative or evoke fear; and possibly even dispensing of medications for fear, anxiety, nausea, intestinal upset, or pain.

Conclusion

Fear and anxiety are common during an animal's visit to the veterinary hospital. However, most of the techniques described in this chapter should lessen the potential for this fear and improve the experience of the pet and pet parent, as well as the veterinary staff. These techniques do not take more time; they just require that staff interact with pets in a more skilled or refined manner, and that the hospital be set up with the patient's best interest in mind. Truly, by focusing your hospital's practices around keeping the patient both comfortable and feeling safe, you can get back to the roots of veterinary practice. It is about helping pets to be healthier and happier while forging a great, mutually respectful relationship with both patients and pet parents.

References

1. *Partners for Healthy Pets.* Reversing the decline in veterinary care utilization; progress made, challenges remain. AAHA/AVMA White Paper. https://cdn.ymaws.com/www.movma.org/resource/resmgr/Docs/VetCareUsageStudy_WhitePaper.pdf
2. Mariti C, Pierantoni L, Sighieri C, et al. Guardians' perceptions of dogs' welfare and behaviors related to visiting the veterinary clinic. *J Appl Welf Sci.* 2017; 20:24–33.
3. Mariti C, Bowen J, Campa S, et al. Guardians' perception of cats' welfare and behavior regarding veterinary visits. *J Appl Anim Welf Sci.* 2016;19:375–384.
4. Stanford TL. Behavior of dogs entering a veterinary clinic. *Appl Anim Ethol.* 1981;7:271–279.
5. Doring D, Roscher A, Scheipl F, et al. Fear related behavior of dogs in veterinary practice. *Vet J.* 2009;182:38–43.
6. Edwards PT, Smith BP, McArthur ML, et al. Fearful Fido: investigating dog experience in the veterinary context in an effort to reduce distress. *Appl Anim Behav Sci.* 2019;213:14–25.
7. Stellato AC, Flint HE, Dewey CE, et al. Risk-factors associated with veterinary-related fear and aggression in owned domestic dogs. *Appl Anim Behav Sci.* 2021;241:105374.
8. Volk JO, Felsted KE, Thomas JG, et al. Executive summary of the Bayer veterinary care usage study. *J Am Vet Med Assoc.* 2011;238:1275–1282.
9. Tateo A, Zappaterra M, Covella A, et al. Factors influencing stress and fear-related behaviour of cats during veterinary examinations. *Ital J Anim Sci.* 2021; 20:46–58.
10. Nibblett BM, Ketzis JK, Grigg EK. Comparison of stress exhibited by cats examined in a clinic versus a home setting. *Appl Anim Behav Sci.* 2015;173:68–75.
11. Bragg RF, Bennett JS, Cummings A, et al. Evaluation of the effects of hospital visit stress on physiologic variables in dogs. *J Am Vet Med Assoc.* 2015;246:212–215.
12. Marino CL, Cober RE, Iazbik MC, et al. White-coat effect on systemic blood pressure in retired racing greyhounds. *J Vet Int Med.* 2011;25:861–865.
13. Belew AM, Barlett T, Brown SA. Evaluation of the white-coat effect in cats. *J Vet Intern Med.* 1999;13:134–142.
14. Hoglund K, Hanas S., Carnabuci C, et al. Blood pressure, heart rate, and urinary catecholamines in healthy dogs subjected to different clinical settings. *J Vet Intern Med.* 2012;26:1300–1308.
15. Vaisanen MA-M, Valros AE, Hakoja EH, et al. Pre-operative stress in dogs – a preliminary investigation of behavior and heart rate variability in healthy hospitalized dogs. *Vet Anaesth Analg.* 2005;32:158–167.
16. Mills D, Karagiannis C, Zulch H. Stress—its effects on health and behavior: a guide for practitioners. *Vet Clin North Am Small Anim.* 2014;44:525–541.
17. Hekman J, Karas AZ, Sharp CR. Psychogenic stress in hospitalized dogs; cross species comparisons, implications for health care, and the challenges of evaluation. *Animals.* 2014;4:331–347.
18. Dhabbar FS. Enhancing versus suppressive effects of stress on immune function: implications for immunoprotection and immunopathology. *Neuroimmunomodulation.* 2009;16:300–317.
19. Walburn J, Vedhara K, Hankins M, et al. Psychological stress and wound healing in humans: a systematic review and meta-analysis. *J Psychosom Res.* 2009;67(3): 253–271.
20. Van Vonderen IK, Kooistra HS, Rijnberk A. Influence of veterinary care on the urine corticoid: creatine ration in dogs. *J Vet Int Med.* 1998;12:431–435.
21. Siracusa C, Manteca X, Cuenca R, et al. Effect of a synthetic appeasing pheromone on behavioral, neuroendocrine, immune, and acute-phase perioperative stress responses in dogs. *J Am Vet Med Assoc.* 2010;237:673–681.
22. Dreschel NA. Anxiety, fear, disease and lifespan in domestic dogs. *J Vet Behav.* 2009;4:249–250.
23. Lopes F, Hewison AL, McPeake L, et al. Noise sensitivities in dogs: an exploration of signs in dogs with and without musculoskeletal pain using qualitative content analysis. *Front Vet Sci.* 2018;5:17.
24. Mills DS, Demontigny-Bédard I, Gruen M, et al. Pain and problem behavior in cats and dogs. *Animals.* 2020;10:318.
25. Merola I, Prato-Previde E, Marshall-Pescini S. Social referencing in dog-owner dyads? *Anim Cogn.* 2012;15:175–185.
26. Huber A, Barber ALA, Faragó T, et al. Investigating emotional contagion in dogs (*Canis familiaris*) to emotional sounds of humans and conspecifics. *Anim Cogn.* 2017;20:703–715.
27. D'Aniello B, Semin GR, Alterisio A, et al. Interspecies transmission of emotional information via chemosignals; from humans to dogs (Canis lupus familiaris). *Anim Cogn.* 2018;21:67–68.
28. Bayrak A, Sagiroglu G, Copuroglu E. Effects of preoperative anxiety on intraoperative hemodynamics and postoperative pain. *J Coll Physicians Surg Pak.* 2019;29:868–873.
29. Leask E. Efficacy of EMLA™ cream for reducing pain associated with venepuncture in felines. *Vet Evid.* 6(3). doi:10.18849/ve.v6i3.456.

30. Chávez C, Ubilla MJ, Goich M, et al. Decrease in behaviors associated with pain during catheter placement using a topical anesthetic formulation in cats. *J Vet Behav.* 2021;46:15–17.

31. Kraus BLH. Efficacy of orally administered maropitant citrate in preventing vomiting associated with hydromorphone administration in dogs. *J Am Vet Med Assoc.* 2014;244:1164–1169.

32. Ramsey D, Fleck T, Berg T, et al. Cerenia prevents perioperative nausea and vomiting and improves recovery in dogs undergoing routine surgery. *Int J Appl Res Vet Med.* 2014;12:228–237.

33. Quimby JM, Brock WT, Moses K, et al. Chronic use of maropitant for the management of vomiting and inappetence in cats with chronic kidney disease: a blinded placebo controlled clinical trial. *J Feline Med Surg.* 2015;17:692–697.

34. Stella JL, Lord LK, Buffington CT. Sickness behaviors in response to unusual external events in healthy cats and cats with feline interstitial cystitis. *J Am Vet Med Assoc.* 2011;238:67–73.

35. Dunn LS. Positive impact of Fear Free Certification in Veterinary Practices. https://cdn-ffpets2.pressidium.com/wp-content/uploads/2019/10/The-Positive-Impact-of-Fear-Free-Certification.pdf; 2019.

36. Lloyd, J.K.F. Minimising stress for patients in the veterinary hospital: why it is important and what can be done about it. *Vet Sci.* 2017;4:22.

37. Riemer S, Heritier C, Windschnurer I, et al. A review on mitigating fear and aggression in dogs and cats in a veterinary setting. *Animals.* 2021;11:158.

38. McBroom CF, Caron M. Reducing fear in canine veterinary appointments through fear free tactics. https://keep.lib.asu.edu/items/133962; 2018 [Bachelor of Science, Honors, Student Thesis, Arizona State University].

39. Pratsch L, Mohr N, Palme R, et al. Carrier training cats reduces stress on transport to a veterinary practice. *Appl Anim Behav Sci.* 2018;206:64–74.

40. Hernander, L. Factors influencing dogs' stress level in the waiting room at a veterinary clinic. Available online: http://ex-epsilon.slu.se/3006/1/huvudversion_klar_lollo.pdf; 2008 (accessed on 11 October 2021) [Student Report. Swedish University of Agricultural Sciences, Department of Animal Environment and Health, Ethology and Animal Welfare Programme].

41. Moore AM, Bain MJ. Evaluation of the addition of in-cage hiding structures and toys and timing of administration of behavioral assessments with newly relinquished shelter cats. *J Vet Behav.* 2013;8:450–457.

42. Zeiler GE, Fosgate GT, van Vollenhollen E, et al. Assessment of behavioural changes in domestic cats during short term hospitalization. *J Feline Med Surg.* 2014;16:499–503.

43. Stoneburner RM, Naughton B, Sherman B, et al. Evaluation of a stimulus attenuation strategy to reduce stress in hospitalized cats. *J Vet Behav.* 2021;41:33–38.

44. Cerissa A, Griffith CA, Steigerwald ES, et al. Effects of a synthetic facial pheromone on behavior of cats. *J Am Vet Med Assoc.* 2000;217:1154–1156.

45. Siracusa C, Manteca X, Cuenca R, et al. Effect of a synthetic appeasing pheromone on behavioral, neuroendocrine, immune and acute-phase perioperative stress responses in dogs. *J Am Vet Med Assoc.* 2010;6:673–681.

46. Gilbert C, Mikaelsson A, Gilbert S. Enhancing dogs' welfare during a veterinary consultation; impact of environmental factors and positive interactions before the consultation. In: *Proceedings of the first annual meeting of the European Congress of Behavioral Medicine and Animal Welfare.* Berlin; 2018: 254–255.

47. Stellato AC, et al. Effect of high levels of background noise on dog responses to a routine physical examination in a veterinary setting. *App Anim Behav Sci.* 2019;214:64–71.

48. Fullagar B, Boysen S, Toy M, et al. Sound pressure levels in 2 veterinary intensive care units. *J Vet Intern Med.* 2015;29:1013–1021.

49. Snowdon CT, Teie D, Savage M. Cats prefer species-appropriate music. *Appl Anim Behav Sci.* 2015;166:106–111.

50. Hampton A, Ford A, Kox RE. Effects of music on behavior and physiological stress response of domestic cats in a veterinary clinic. *J Feline Med Surg.* 2020;22(2):122–128.

51. McDonald C, Zaki, S. A role for classical music in veterinary practice: does exposure to classical music reduce stress in hospitalized dogs? *Aus Vet J.* 2020;98(1-2):31–36.

52. Brayley C, Montrose VT. The effects of audiobooks on the behaviour of dogs at a rehoming kennel. *Appl Animal Behav Sci.* 2016;174:111–115.

53. Wells DL, Graham L, Hepper, PG. The influence of auditory stimulation on the behaviour of dogs housed in a rescue shelter. *Anim Welf.* 2002;11:385–393.

54. Kogan LR, Schoenfeld-Tacher R, Simon AA. Behavioral effects of auditory stimulation on kenneled dogs. *J Vet Behav.* 2012;7:268–275.

55. Amaya V, Paterson M, Descovich K, et al. Effects of olfactory and auditory enrichment on heart rate variability in shelter dogs. *Animals.* 2020;10(8):1385.

56. Engler W, Bain M. Effect of different types of classical music played at a veterinary hospital on dog behavior and owner satisfaction. *J Am Vet Med Assoc.* 2017;251:195–200.

57. Protopopova A, Wynne CD. Improving in-kennel presentation of shelter dogs through response-dependent and response-independent treat delivery. *J Appl Behav Anal.* 2015;48:590–601.

58. Griffin FC, Mandese WW, Reynolds PS, et al. Evaluation of clinical examination location on stress in cats: a randomized crossover trial. *J Feline Med Surg.* 2021;23:364–369.

59. Mandese WW, Griffin FC, Reynolds PS, et al. Stress in client-owned dogs related to clinical exam location: a randomized crossover trial. *J Small Anim Pract.* 2021;62:82–88.

60. Csoltova E, Martineau M, Boissy A, et al. Behavioral and physiological reactions in dogs to a veterinary examination: *Physiol Behav.* 2017;177:270–281.

61. Pereira GDG, Fragosos S, Morais, D. Comparison of interpretation of cat's behavioral needs between veterinarians, veterinary nurses, and cat owners. *J Vet Behav.* 2014;9:324–328.

62. Catalán AI, Rojas CA, Chávez GA. Recognition of aggressive and anxious behaviors in canines by a group of Chilean veterinarians. *J Vet Behav.* 2020;38:8–13.

63. American Association of Feline Practitioners and International of Society of Feline Medicine. Feline-friendly handling guidelines. *J Feline Med Surg.* 2011;13:364–375.

64. Moody CM, Picketts VA, Mason GJ, et al. Can you handle it. Validating negative responses to restraint in cats. *Appl Anim Behav Sci.* 2018;204:94–100.

65. Moody CM, Mason GJ, Dewey CE, et al. Getting a grip: cats respond negatively to scruffing and clips. *Vet Rec.* 2020;186:385. doi:10.1136/vr.1052616.

66. Bigras-Fontaine C, Bazin I, Desmarchelier M. Clinical relevance of rectal temperature measurement in cats showing marked signs of stress during routine veterinary visits: pilot study on 101 cats. In: Proc Veterinary Behavior Symposium. Austin, Tx; 2022: 11.

67. Argüelles J, Echaniz M, Bowen J, et al. The impact of a stress-reducing protocol on the quality of pre-anesthesia in cats. *Vet Rec.* 2021;188:e138. doi:10.1002/vetr.138.

68. Stellato A, Jajou S, Dewey CE, et al. Effect of a standardized four-week desensitization and counter-conditioning training program on pre-existing veterinary fear in companion dogs. *Animals.* 2019;9:767.

69. Steele A, Grubb T. Managing the aggressive patient. In: Mathews C, Sinclair M, Steele AM, et al., eds. *Analgesia and anesthesia for the Ill and injured dog and cat.* Hoboken, NJ: Wiley-Blackwell; 2018:270–278.

70. Korpivaara M, Huhtinen M, Aspegrén J, et al. Dexmedetomidine oromucosal gel reduces fear and anxiety in dogs during veterinary visits: a randomised, double-blind, placebo-controlled clinical pilot study. *Vet Rec.* 2021;e832. doi:10.1002/vetr.832.

71. Hauser H, Campbell S, Korpivaara M, et al. In-hospital administration of dexmedetomidine oromucosal gel for stress reduction in dogs during veterinary visits: a randomized, double-blinded, placebo-controlled study. *J Vet Behav.* 2020;39:77–85.

72. Landsberg G, Mougeot I, Kosziwka W, et al. Development and validation of a dog

travel anxiety model. In: *Proceedings of the 12th International Veterinary Behaviour Meeting.* Washington, D.C. IVBM, Upton, UK: 2019:21–23.

73. Gruen ME, Roe RC, Griffith E, et al. Use of trazodone to facilitate postsurgical confinement in dogs. *J Am Vet Med Assoc.* 2014;245:296–301.

74. Herron M, Shofer FS, Reisner IR. Restrospective evaluation of the effects of diazepam in dogs with anxiety-related behavior problems. *J Am Vet Med Assoc.* 2008;233:1420–1424.

75. Ogata N, et al. The use of clonidine in the treatment of fear-based behavior problems in dogs: An open trial. *J Vet Behav.* 2011;6:130–137.

76. Stollar O, Moore GE, Mukhopadhyay A, et al. Effects of a single dose of oral gabapentin in dogs during a veterinary visit: a double-blinded, placebo-controlled study. *J Am Vet Med Assoc.* 2022;260:2031–1040.

77. Kim S, Borchardt MR, Lee K, et al. Effects of trazodone on behavioral and physiological signs of stress in dogs during veterinary visits: a randomized double-blind placebo-controlled crossover clinical trial. *J Am Vet Med Assoc.* 2022;260:876–883.

78. Jay AR, Krotscheck U, Parsley E, et al. Pharmacokinetics, bioavailability, and hemodynamic effects of trazodone after intravenous and oral administration of a single dose to dogs. *Am J Vet Res.* 2013;74:1450–1456.

79. Pankratz KE, Ferris KK, Griffith EH, et al. Use of single dose oral gabapentin to attenuate fear response in cage-trap confined community cats: a double-blind, placebo-controlled field trial. *J Feline Med Surg.* 2018;20:535–543.

80. Stevens BJ, Frantz EM, Orlando JM, et al. Efficacy of a single dose of trazodone hydrochloride given to cats prior to veterinary visits to reduce signs of transport- and examination-related anxiety. *J Am Vet Med Assoc.* 2016;249:202–207.

81. van Haaften KA, Eichstadt Forseith LR, Stelow EA, et al. Effects of a single pre-appointment dose of gabapentin on signs of stress in cats during transportation and veterinary examination. *J Am Vet Med Assoc.* 2017;251:1175–1181.

82. Kruszka M, Graff E, Medam T, et al. Clinical evaluation of the effects of a single oral dose of gabapentin on fear-based aggressive behaviors in cats during veterinary examinations. *J Am Vet Med Assoc.* 2021;259:1285–1291.

83. Lamminen Terttu, Korpivaara M, Suokko M, et al. Efficacy of a single dose of pregabalin on signs of anxiety in cats during transportation-a pilot study. *Front Vet Sci.* 2021. doi:10.3389/fvets.2021.711816.

84. Landsberg G, Dunn D, Keys D, et al. Anxiolytic effect of dexmedetomidine oromucosal gel (Sileo) and gabapentin in a feline travel anxiety model. In: *Proceedings of the European Veterinary Animal Behaviour and Welfare Congress.* Berlin; 2018b:127–128.

85. Carson MA, Pankratz KE, Messenger KM, et al. Efficacy of dexmedetomidine oromucosal gel to attenuate anxiety in client owned cats presented for routine veterinary care. *Proc Vet Behav Symposium.* 2020:5.

86. Arguelles J, Enriquez J, Bowen J, et al. Mirtazapine as a potential drug to treat social fears in dogs: five case examples. In: Denenberg S, ed. *Proceedings of the 11th International Veterinary Behaviour Meeting.* CABI Oxfordshire UK; 2018:84–85.

87. Cohen A, Bennett SL. Oral transmucosal administration of dexmedetomidine for sedation in 4 dogs. *Can Vet J.* 2015;56: 1144–1148.

88. Herron ME, Shreyer TA. Fear and Aggression in Veterinary Visits – Dogs and Cats. In: Tilley LP, Smith Jr. FWK, Sleeper MM, et al., eds. *Blackwell's five minute veterinary consult: canine and feline.* 7th ed. Wiley-Blackwell; 2021:490–493.

89. Simon BT, Steagall PV. Feline procedural sedation and analgesia. When, why and how. *J Feline Med Surg.* 2020;22:1029–1045.

90. Santos LCP, Ludders JW, Erb HN, et al. Sedative and cardiorespiratory effects of dexmedetomidine and buprenorphine administered to cats via transmucosal and intramuscular routes. *Vet Anaesth Analg.* 2010;37:417–424.

91. Dent BT, Aarnes TK, Wavreille VA, et al. Pharmacokinetics and pharmacodynamic effects of oral transmucosal and intravenous administration of dexmedetomidine in dogs. *Am J Vet Res.* 2019;80:969–975.

92. Robertson SA, Lascelles BD, Taylor PM, et al. PK-PD modeling of buprenorphine in cats: intravenous and oral transmucosal administration. *J Vet Pharmacol Ther.* 2005;28:453–460.

93. Catbagan DL, Quimby JM, Mama KR, et al. Comparison of the efficacy and adverse effects of sustained-release buprenorphine hydrochloride following subcutaneous administration and buprenorphine hydrochloride following oral transmucosal administration in cats undergoing ovariohysterectomy. *Am J Vet Res.* 2011;72:461–466.

94. Messenger KM, Hopfensperger M, Knych HK, et al. Pharmacokinetics of detomidine following intravenous or oro-transmucosal administration and sedative effects of the oro-transmucosal treatment in dogs. *Am J Vet Res.* 2016;77:413–420.

95. Porters N, Bosmans T, Debille M, et al. Sedative and antinociceptive effects of dexmedetomidine and buprenorphine after oral transmucosal or intramuscular administration in cats. *Vet Anaesth Analg.* 2014;41:90–96.

96. Gioeni D, Brioschi FA, Di Cesare F, et al. Oral transmucosal or intramuscular administration of dexmedetomidine–methadone combination in dogs: sedative and physiological effects. *Animals.* 2020; 10(11):2057. doi:10.3390/ani10112057.

97. Ferreira TH, Rezende ML, Mama KR, et al. Plasma concentrations and behavioral, antinociceptive, and physiologic effects of methadone after intravenous and oral transmucosal administration in cats. *Am J Vet Res.* 2011;72:764–771.

98. Di Cesare F, Cagnardi P, Gioeni D, et al. Pharmacokinetics of dexmedetomidine combined with methadone following oral-transmucosal and intramuscular administration in dogs. *Int J Health Anim Sci Food Saf.* 2017;4(1). doi:10.13130/2283-3927/8416.

99. Grove DM, Ramsay EC. Sedative and physiologic effects of orally administered α2-adrenoceptor agonists and ketamine in cats. *J Am Vet Med Assoc.* 2000;216: 1929–1932.

100. Nejamkin P, Cavilla V, Clausse M, et al. Sedative and physiologic effects of tiletamine–zolazepam following buccal administration in cats. *J Feline Med Surg.* 2020;22:108–113.

101. Costa RS, Karas AZ, Borns-Weil S. Chill protocol to manage aggressive and fearful dogs. https://www.cliniciansbrief.com/article/chill-protocol-manage-aggressive-fearful-dogs; [Clinicians Brief, May 2019, 63–65].

102. Barletta M, Rafee M. Behavioral response and cost of comparison of manual versus pharmacologic restraint protocols in healthy dogs. *Can Vet.* 2016;57:258–264.

103. Dasta JF, Kane-Gill SL, Pencina M, et al. A cost-minimization analysis of dexmedetomidine compared with midazolam for long-term sedation in the intensive care unit. *Crit Care Med.* 2010;38:497–503.

104. Lachaine J, Beauchemin C. Economic evaluation of dexmedetomidine relative to midazolam for sedation in the intensive care unit. *Can J Hosp Pharm.* 2012;65:103–110.

105. Benson GJ, Grubb TL, Neff-Davis C, et al. Perioperative stress response in the dog; effect of pre-emptive administration of medetomidine. *Vet Surg.* 2000;29:85–91.

106. Hekman J, Karas A, Dreschel NA. Salivary cortisol concentrations and behaviours in a population of healthy dogs hospitalized for elective procedures. *Appl Anim Behav Sci.* 2012;141(3–4):149–157.

107. Moser KL, Hasiuk MM, Armstrong T, Gunn M, Pang DS. A randomized clinical trial comparing butorphanol and buprenorphine within a multimodal analgesic protocol in cats undergoing orchiectomy. *J Feline Med Surg.* 2020;22:760–767.

108. Wheeler EP, Abelson AL, Lindsey JC, et al. Sedative effects of alfaxalone and hydromorphone with or without midazolam in cats: a pilot study. *J Feline Med Surg.* 2021;23(12):1109–1116.

109. Verstegen J, Deleforge J, Dernblon D, et al. Non-linear relationship between bioavailability and dose after oral administration of four single doses of acepromazine in dogs and cats. *J Vet Anaes.* 1996;23:47–51.

110. Reader RC, Barton BA, Abelson AL. Comparison of two intramuscular sedation protocols on sedation, recovery

and ease of venipuncture for cats undergoing blood donation. *J Feline Med Surg.* 2019;21:95–102.

111. Bufalari A, Moretti G, Pepe A, et al. The use of alfaxalone in combination with opioids for cat sedation: preliminary results. *AgroLife Sci J.* 2020;9:48–53.

112. Ko JC, Austin BR, Barletta M, et al. Evaluation of dexmedetomidine and ketamine in combination with various opioids as injectable anesthetic combinations for cats. *J Am Vet Med Assoc.* 2011;239:1452–1462.

113. Mathews K, Grubb T. Pharmacologic and clinical principles of adjunct analgesia. In: Mathews C, Sinclair M, Steele AM, et al., eds. *Analgesia and anesthesia for the Ill and injured dog and cat.* Wiley-Blackwell; 2018:144–164.

114. Papich M. *Handbook of veterinary drugs.* 5th ed. St. Louis: Elsevier; 2021.

115. Scheinin H, Aantaa R, Hakola P, et al. Reversal of the sedative and sympatholytic effects of dexmedetomidine with a specific alpha2-adrenoceptor antagonist atipamezole: a pharmacodynamic and kinetic study in healthy volunteers. *Anesthesiology,* 1998;89:574–584.

Resources and recommended reading

AAFP Cat friendly handling videos for cat owners - AAFP Cat friendly handling videos for cat owners - https://catvets.com/education/online/videos.

Becker M, Radosta L, Sung W, Becker M. From fearful to fear free. Irvine: Limina Media; 2017.

Cat friendly homes – https://catvets.com/cfp/veterinary-professionals.

Cattledog Publishing. https://cattledog publishing.com/

Caney SM, Robinson NJ, Gunn-Moore DA, et al. Happy cats: stress in cats and their carers associated with outpatient visits to the clinic. *J Fel Med Surg.* 2022. doi:10.1177/10986 12X221121907.

Ellis SLH. Recognizing and assessing feline emotions during the consultation. *J Feline Med Surg.* 2018;20:445–456.

Fear Free Happy Homes (Pet Parents): https://www.fearfreehappyhomes.com/kit/fear-free-vet-visits/.

Fear Free Shelter Personnel: fearfreeshelters.com.

Happy visits and victory visits - https://todaysveterinarynurse.com/behavior/fear-free-happy-visits-and-victory-visits/.

Howell A, Feyrecilde M. Cooperative Veterinary Care, Wiley-Blackwell; 2018.

International Care - cat friendly handling videos https://icatcare.org/veterinary/resources.

Karn-Buehler J, Kuhne F. Perception of stress in cats by German cat owners and influencing factors regarding veterinary care. *J Feline Med Surg.* 2022;24(8):700-708.

Rodan I, Dowgray N, Carney HC, et al. 2022 AAFP/ISFM Cat Friendly Veterinary Interaction Guidelines: Approach and Handling Techniques. *J Fel Med Surg.* 2022;24(11):1093–1132.

Wess L, Böhm A, Schützinger M, et al. Effect of cooperative care training on physiological parameters and compliance in dogs undergoing a veterinary examination – A pilot study. *Appl Anim Behav Sci.* 2022;250:105615.

Behavioral drug resources and recommended reading

Crowell-Davis SL, Murray, TF, de Souza Dantas LM. *Veterinary psychopharmacology.* 2nd ed. John Wiley and Sons, Inc.; 2019.

Erickson A, Harbin K, MacPherson J, et al. A review of pre-appointment medications to reduce fear and anxiety in dogs and cats at veterinary visits. *Can Vet J.* 2021;62:952–960.

Fear free Toolbox - fearfreepets.com/toolbox/fear_free_drug_charts/ (requires registration)

Grubb T, Sager J, Gaynor JS, et al. 2020 AAHA Anesthesia and Monitoring Guidelines for Dogs and Cats. https://www.aaha.org/aaha-guidelines/2020-aaha-anesthesia-and-monitoring-guidelines-for-dogs-and-cats/anesthesia-and-monitoring-home/.

Herron ME, Shreyer TA. Fear and aggression in veterinary visits. In: Tilley LP, Smith FWK, Sleeper MM, et al., eds. *Blackwell's 5 minute veterinary consult: canine and feline.* 7th ed., John Wiley and Sons; 2021:490–493.

Korpivaara M, Huhtinen M, Pohjanjousi P, et al. Tasipimidine, a noveral orally active alpha-2 adrenoceptor agonist, alleviates signs of anxiety shown during veterinary examination- a pilot study. *Proc European Veterinary Congress of Behavioural Medicine and Animal Welfare,* 2021:96–97.

Korpivaara M, Pohjanjousi P, Huhtinen M, et al. Tasipimidine, a novel orally dosed alpha 2 adrenoceptor agonist, alleviates canine acute anxiety and fear associated with travel – a pilot study. *Proc 3rd European Veterinary Congress of Behavioural Medicine and Animal Welfare.* 2021: 149–150.

Mathews C, Sinclair M, Steele AM, et al. *Analgesia and anesthesia for the Ill and injured dog and cat.* Wiley-Blackwell; 2018.

National Library of Medicine – Daily Meds (FDA regulated products) - https://dailymed.nlm.nih.gov/dailymed/index.cfm.

Overall KL. Pharmacotherapeutics in clinical ethology: treatment efficacy, clinical pathology and outcome. 2021;158:1355–1419.

Papich M. *Handbook of veterinary drugs.* 5th ed. St. Louis: Elsevier; 2021.

Plumbs Veterinary Formulary – plumbs.com (requires registration)

Pregabalin (Bonqat – Orion Corporation) – European Medicines Agency. https://www.ema.europa.eu/en/medicines/veterinary/EPAR/bonqat

Veterinary Anesthesia and Support Group – vasg.org

Zenalpha -vatinoxan hydrochloride and medetomidine hydrochloride injection www.ema.europa.eu/en/medicines/veterinary/EPAR/zenalpha https://animaldrugsatfda.fda.gov/adafda/app/search/public/document/downloadFoi/12187

Continuing education and certification courses for veterinarians and pet care professionals

AAFP Educational Videos for Veterinary Teams – https://catvets.com/education/online/videos

Cat friendly Practice Program – https://catvets.com/cfp/veterinary-professionals

Fear Free (Pet Professionals): fearfreepets.com

Feline friendly handling webinar – https://catvets.com/education/online/webinars/feline-friendly-handling-interactions

International Cat Care – https://icatcare.org/veterinary/resources/

Karen Pryor Academy – Better Veterinary Visits https://karenpryoracademy.com/courses/better-vet/

Low stress handling – cattledogpublishing.com/

Ready, set for groomer, and Vet – https://www.lauramonacotorelli.com/ready-set-groomer-vet

CHAPTER 17

Separation-related disorders

Ariel Fagen, DVM, DACVB

Chapter contents

Introduction

Previously diagnosed as separation anxiety, separation-related anxiety syndrome, separation distress, or separation-related distress,[1-7] nomenclature is shifting in the literature to recognize a cluster of disorders related to separation and isolation from attachment figures (e.g., social group members, family members, human, or animal), termed separation-related problems[8-10] or separation-related disorders.[11,12] Separation-related disorders (SRDs) are distressing behavior problems for the pet parent and the pet that can deteriorate the relationship, negatively impact the bond, and affect the quality of life of the pet and the pet parent.[2,4-6,13-15] Dogs with SRD exhibit signs of anxiety, fear, frustration, phobia, or panic when they do not have access to attachment figures.[2,4,5,16] The clinical signs of SRD usually occur when the attachment figure is away from home but may occur when they are home, but the pet does not have access to them (i.e., virtual absence).[1,4,17] Distress displayed during attachment figure departures can range from a mild response to severe panic attacks. Treatment involves assessment of overall wellness, management of the environment to prevent or minimize distress, behavioral therapies to teach independence, and new associations with departures and neurochemical modulation (i.e., supplements, medications) to aid in the learning process and relieve suffering.

Prevalence

SRDs are common with as many as 36% of dogs referred to veterinary behaviorists,[14,17,18] and 6–33%[19–23] of all dogs showing signs of SRD; yet in one study, only 13% of pet parents seek help.[21] In senior dogs, up to 50% of referred cases may be due to SRD.[24] Evidence supports that older dogs (>7 years) with SRD may handle separations from their attachment figures differently and cope with stress less efficiently than younger dogs, displaying more passive and inhibited anxiety responses, decreasing activity, less escape behavior, more whining at the door, and elevated stress levels (higher salivary cortisol levels) than in younger dogs with SRD.[9,25] The more passive stress responses may originate from the dogs, motivational or behavioral state, rather than physical motor problems; however, anxiety may also be heightened and behavior responses altered by concomitant physical problems, age-related cognitive decline, or decrease in sensory capacity with the lowered capacity to sense and respond to the environment.

SRDs are grossly understudied and likely underdiagnosed and undertreated in cats. In surveys of cat pet parents, between 13.5% and 19% of cats had at least one of the criteria necessary to diagnose SRD.[3,10] Cats are more likely to purr, rub against the pet parents, and stretch, while pet parents are more likely to have verbal contract with their cats after a 4-hour departure when compared to a 30-minute departure.[26] In the aforementioned study, the amount of attention paid to the cat was not associated with the cat's likelihood of purring or rubbing against the pet parent. This information demonstrates that cats, at least to some extent, are aware of the length of pet parent departures. Like dogs, some clinicians describe signs of hyperattachment like persistent shadowing or contact-seeking and attention-seeking behaviors. Consistent with anxiety disorders, some cats start to display signs of distress with predeparture cues.

SRDs are more common in dogs adopted from shelters, rescues, and veterinary hospitals, or that lived as strays prior to adoption (see Box 17.1).[21,27–29] It is estimated that up to 30% of dogs in shelters were relinquished for SRD,[27,30] leading to the increased likelihood of those dogs showing SRD in their new homes.[7,27,31,32] Of dogs rehomed by an RSPCA rescue center in the UK, after three months, 38% of dogs receiving no treatment advice at the time of rehoming were diagnosed with separation anxiety.[27] There also could be something about abandonment and the rehoming process which may contribute to SRD development, with abandoned dogs adopted from rescues or shelters being more anxious and perhaps less securely bonded to the pet parent than dogs reared from puppyhood in the same family home.[33,34] Dogs purchased from pet stores (and thus likely sourced from commercial breeders) were more anxious and more likely to exhibit signs of SRD than those obtained from noncommercial breeders.[14,35] SRD is most commonly reported in males,[5,7,17,36–39] though this difference was not found consistently,[2,28] with one study finding females presented with more anxiety disorders.[14] While studies support that neutered males might be predisposed,[40] others support that both intact and neutered males are more likely to show signs,[39] and that female neutered dogs were less likely to exhibit destructive behaviors compared to intact males and females and neutered males.[27]

As with many behavioral disorders, there is most likely a genetic component to SRD (see Box 17.2). Certain breeds may exhibit different clinical signs of SRD as well as have a hereditary predisposition.[4,12,17,23,41] The following breeds have been suggested in different studies to have higher frequencies, although differences may be attributable to geographic demographics, breed distribution, recruitment populations, and the years in which the study were conducted: Golden Retrievers, English Springer Spaniels, Cocker Spaniels, Schnauzers, Dachshunds, Wheaten Terriers,[2,17,23,40] and mixed-breed dogs.[17,23,29,37] However, mixed breeds represent a large proportion of shelter dogs and adoption from a shelter is a risk factor for SRD.[4,11,21] Younger dogs may be predisposed to SRD development, with more than 50% of dogs reported to present with signs of SRD before 18 months of age, although there may be a further increase in prevalence in older dogs.[2,5,21,24] Dogs that were ill as puppies have also been shown to develop more separation-related barking.[4,42] Dogs that had more daily exercise[43] and dogs that engaged in game playing with their pet parents[39] were less likely to be reported by their pet parents to have SRD, but other studies have shown no correlation.[27] Dogs that have had obedience training and those trained through positive reinforcement appear to have less separation anxiety and other behavior problems, according to some studies,[15,44–46] while the use of aversive training has been associated with increased SRD.[47] Other studies show that general obedience and purpose of pet parentship (working dog versus companion dog) are unrelated to the presence of SRD.[48,49] Length of typical departures, frequency of typical departures, living with other dogs (in puppyhood or otherwise), and whether or not a dog is crated were not found to be predisposing factors in most studies.[7,27,50] Predisposing factors in cats include the number of female humans living in the home, little or no access to toys, and no other animal residing in the house (see Box 17.2).

Box 17.1 Risk factors for separation-related disorder

- Acquisition method: shelter, rescue, veterinary hospital, commercial breeder, pet store, stray
- M > F
- Breed: mixed breed, Golden Retrievers, English Springer Spaniels, Cocker Spaniels, Schnauzers, Dachshunds, Wheaten Terriers
- Younger dogs
- Smaller dogs
- Puppyhood illness

Box 17.2 Potential etiologies of separation-related disorder

- Frustration
- Attachment style of dog
- Attachment style of pet parent
- Cognitive processes and emotional regulation
- Genetic predisposition
- Early environment

Multiple etiologies for SRDs are examined in the literature; however, no definitive cause has been elucidated. If due to the rearing environment puppies are unable to explore independently by 14 weeks old, they may have a much harder time learning independence. After adoption, puppies that come to expect excessive social interactions, particularly in the first month after adoption, may be unable to psychologically cope with subsequent decreases in social interaction as schedule or lifestyle changes occur in the family, while dogs provided with a variety of social experiences between 5 and 10 months were at reduced risk.[21] Loss of attachment figure, history of abandonment, premature separation from the mother, poor maternal care, lack of early socialization, lack of habituation to short departures, and traumatic experiences occurring while alone have all been shown to potentially contribute to the development of SRD.[1,4,40-43,50,51] Recently, an early socialization program tailored to the behavioral and physiological needs of puppies during the first six weeks of life has been shown to contribute to a reduction in separation anxiety behaviors.[52]

While early life and learning experiences may influence the development of SRD, it is likely that genetic predisposition to fear, anxiety, stress, conflict, and panic also plays a role in the disorder.[2,11,23,53] Studies have started to explore specific genetic sequences as being risk or protective haplotypes, with a few found to be related to clinical signs of SRD in Golden Retrievers.[1,12] In addition, IGF1 and HMGA2 loci variants, small body size,[54] and genes that code for certain oxytocin, vasopressin, and dopamine receptors have been associated with SRD.[1]

Earlier literature suggested that SRDs are a result of hyperattachment or overattachment to a person or animal, as demonstrated by clingy and persistent shadowing or contact-seeking behaviors.[2,4,21,40,55] Highly social species, such as dogs, exhibit attachment behaviors that serve to maintain social contact and bonds between adult individuals as well as between parents and offspring. When an individual loses contact with the group, the resultant anxiety can trigger behaviors that will attract other members (vocalizations), help remove barriers (digging, chewing), or facilitate the restoration of contact (increased activity). In dogs, domestication and selective breeding (genetics) along with early socialization have further contributed to increasingly affectionate, socially dependent, and infantilized dogs, which might be predisposed to excessive pet parent attachment and intolerance to being left alone.[11,42,34] It is this underlying drive to be with members of the established social group that may provide the foundation for the development of attachment problems.

However, more recent data suggest that dogs with SRD are not necessarily *hyperattached* but rather have a problematic, insecure, or pathologic attachment style rather than the quantity of the attachment.[11,56] Consistent with this supposition is that dogs with SRD were not shown to exhibit more contact or proximity-seeking behaviors upon greeting after an absence,[11,56] nor were they assessed by pet parents as being more attached than non-SRD dogs.[27] Persistent shadowing and distress behaviors with separation within the home were not more likely in SRD dogs than non-SRD dogs.[27] Furthermore, genetic research points to proximity seeking and reaction to separation as being phenotypic features with different underlying genetic polymorphisms,[57] though significantly more

research is needed on the topic. Hyperattachment behaviors can occur in dogs with and without separation anxiety and is not a requirement for diagnosis.[4,5,56]

To further explore the idea that SRD may be rooted in disordered or pathologic attachment, many recent studies examine the application of attachment theory as described in the human literature[58,59] to dogs.[11,25,32,34,36,49,56,60-63] Attachment style is assessed by Ainsworth's Adapted Strange Situation Test (ASST), which has been modified to apply to dogs as an in-clinic test that assesses the dog's reaction to being in a novel environment, with and without the pet parent present, and being faced with a novel or threatening person, with and without the pet parent present. As with infants, securely attached dogs should be more willing to explore with their parent present, exhibit some level of distress and searching when separated from their parent in a strange situation, and exhibit contact-seeking behaviors upon return of the parent after a period of separation.

Evidence supports that healthy dogs have this "safe haven" or "secure base" attachment with their pet parents.[60-63,64] For example, dogs exhibited more social play with a stranger when their pet parent was present than when their pet parent was not present.[34,49] Dogs exhibited a variety of distress, protest, and searching behaviors when their pet parents were absent, most intensely during social isolation.[34,49] Upon return, the dogs exhibited proximity and contact-seeking behaviors that differed from the greeting behaviors exhibited toward a stranger.[34,49] Dogs' heart rates were higher when faced with a threatening stranger when their pet parents were not present compared to when they were. Among dogs that exhibited stress vocalizations with separation, heart rates were relatively higher when they faced the stranger for the first time without the pet parent present, compared to those that faced the stranger for the first time with the pet parent present. The pet parent's presence during initial introduction seemed to be an emotional buffer for the dogs. Heart rate variability decreased significantly, which is an indicator of high sympathetic tone, when dogs experienced the threatening stranger without their pet parent present.[62] All of these measures are consistent with the idea that the pet parent's presence is somewhat of a buffer against stressors.

The ASST has also been used to evaluate attachment in cats. In one study using the ASST, significant differences were found in the frequency of play and environmental exploration when cats were with the pet parent, as opposed to when they were alone or with a stranger, indicating a secure base attachment as described above.[65] Cats were also found to be more alert when left with the stranger and more inactive when left alone.[65] In contrast, Mills and Potter found that while cats were more likely to vocalize when the pet parent left the room as opposed to when a stranger left the room, there were no other differences in their behaviors when evaluated using the ASST.[66] The temporal patterns in behavior of cats are influenced by the personality and behavior of their pet parents, implying that there is a bond formed between the two.[67] Cats apparently do form bonds with their social group members. More investigation is needed to determine the extent and type of those bonds.

Alterations to the secure base pattern reflect three different insecure, disordered attachment styles (see Box 17.3). The first is the insecure-avoidant pattern, in which the dog does

Box 17.3 Aberrant attachment styles and resultant behavioral signs

Aberrant attachment styles	Relation to caregiver	Behavioral effect
Insecure-avoidant	Dog does not utilize caregiver as safety base	Minimal outward behaviors, avoids contact seeking, repression
Insecure-anxious	Caregiver is safety base	Hyperactivation of attachment behaviors, distress behaviors with separation, proximity seeking
Insecure-disorganized/disoriented	Conflicted about caregiver as safety base	Approach-avoidance behaviors, freezing behaviors, fear on reunion

not utilize the caregiver as a safety base, avoids contact seeking, and while it may experience distress in the strange situation, does so with minimal outward behaviors. These dogs may repress attachment behaviors.[11,23] The second is the insecure-anxious pattern (a.k.a. insecure-ambivalent or insecure-resistant), in which the dog hyperactivates their attachment behaviors; they resist parent departure, express distress to separation, are intensely proximity seeking, and are unable to explore a novel environment without their attachment figure present.[11,23,61] The third is the insecure-disorganized/disoriented pattern, in which the dog shows approach-avoidance behaviors, indicating conflict, fear on reunion, or dissociated/freezing behaviors.[60,61,68] The vast majority of pet dogs exhibit a secure attachment style in the studies that have been performed.[11,60,61]

Alterations from secure attachment has been postulated as an etiology for SRD. The literature shows that dogs with SRDs overall (1) do not use their pet parents as a secure base for exploring the environment, (2) are more likely to remain near their pet parent in a strange situation, and (3) do not show rapid decrease in stress behaviors immediately upon return.[11,36,69] Salivary cortisol changes over the course of ASST varied based on attachment style, with securely attached dogs showing lower cortisol reactivity than insecure-disorganized dogs, demonstrating less physiologic stress.[61] The attachment style proposed to be most similar to the behavioral repertoire of SRD dogs is the insecure-anxious attachment style.[11,36]

Based on the human literature, researchers have explored whether the attachment style of the dog is dictated by parenting style. The primary determinant of attachment style in people has been shown to be caregiver sensitivity and response to attachment signals of the infant. Studies support that caregiver responsiveness to the dog during a threatening situation is correlated with attachment style.[60,61] Konok et al. established clusters of dog–pet parent dyads that they considered comparable to the four attachment styles described above. Pet parents who often ignore their dogs' attention-seeking behaviors and score high on avoidance questionnaires are more likely to have a dog with clinical signs of SRD, which is consistent with adult–children data supporting that pet parents with insecure-avoidant attachment styles have children with insecure-anxious attachment.[21] One study showed that pet parents who self-report as having a permis-

sive and inconsistent dog-parenting style have dogs that bark, rather than whine, during departures.[41] Dogs that exhibit food-begging behaviors also tend to bark and not whine during departures.[41] Pet parents who exhibited an insecure-ambivalent attachment to their dog or considered their dog to be a social support to them also had dogs with increased cortisol reactivity, suggesting that caregiver interaction style influences how the dog handles these stressful situations.[61] Calmer canine temperament was associated with a secure attachment style, though this does not indicate whether the dogs were calmer because of their caregiver responsiveness, their caregiver responsiveness was because of their calm demeanor, or if both were related to a third factor not evaluated.[60] Perhaps the lack of appropriate pet parent responsiveness as well as inconsistency and unpredictability in interactions contribute to SRD or frustration intolerance.

Frustration has been postulated as the core originator in some SRD cases. Frustration occurs when an animal is prohibited from accessing a resource or when expectation of reinforcement based off learning history is not satisfied and has been associated with fear and autonomic signs when prolonged.[2,41,70] Pet parents may be the missing resource as well as the missing source of reinforcement. Inconsistent pet parent interaction style may lead to a dog that has a lower frustration tolerance and thus be more likely to exhibit frustration behavior, primarily barking, when the dog does not have access to their pet parent.[41] Frustration can lead to hyperresponsive reactions to environmental stimuli, as well as general activity levels and vocalization.[70] Disinhibition of displacement behaviors associated with frustration-like object play and exploratory behavior can lead to destructive behaviors.[70]

While frustration may be the originator for some, for others, a pure fear response seems a more appropriate explanation. Consistent with this is some evidence that the phenotypic presentation of SRD in some patients consists primarily of autonomic signs (e.g., urination in the home) without the classic contact seeking (barking, escape attempts) or destructive behaviors one might expect of a frustrated pet.[11,41] These dogs do not necessarily exhibit intense greeting behavior that may be a helpful tip-off to their pet parents that they have been distressed.[11] Pet parents are less likely to be concerned about their pet as suffering from SRD in this autonomic-only group.[11] This population may be the "silent sufferers" that go largely underdiagnosed and undertreated. Consistent with this is the finding that whining may be a more accurate correlator with SRD than barking,[71] which may be expected from an attention-seeking or frustrated pet.[41] Perhaps this shutdown, fearful group of dogs represents the insecure-avoidant cluster of attachment styles.[11]

Cognitive processes and lack of emotional self-regulation may play a role as well. Dogs with SRD may have a decreased adaptability[36] and are reliant on social contact to maintain a certain emotional homeostasis,[55] and are thus seeking contact to return to homeostasis. Overdependence on the pet parent for emotional regulation may inadvertently be fostered or reinforced by pet parents, and pet parent permissiveness may be associated with frustration-related, separation-related problem signs.[4,41] Some dogs may have been reliant on a conspecific for emotional feedback on how to respond to potential stressors in their world, and with the loss of other household dogs, their ability to regulate to the environmental trigger of the separation falters.[72] Additionally, dogs with SRDs have been shown to have negative cognitive biases[73] postulated as representing a more pessimistic view of the world, though this is just correlational data, not causational, and may actually be secondary to SRD.

Precipitating factors

Regardless of the etiology, multiple precipitating factors have been noted to be associated with the acute onset of clinical signs (see Box 17.4). SRD may arise or a relapse can occur in a stable dog with SRD when the dog is suddenly separated from its pet parents following a period of constant contact or after a sudden change in routine; any change in the household group or changes to the pet's environment; the death of a pet or family member or rehoming of a companion; systemic illness and other traumatizing separation-related events.[2,4,5,21,41,50,72]

Prevention

Elements of the early rearing environment have shown to be correlated with the likelihood of exhibiting separation-related behaviors at 12 months old. The findings of one study suggest that caregivers of litters should allow as much play as possible with other dogs,[54,69] though further research is needed to fully understand the effects of these efforts over the lifetime of the dog. Because illness in puppyhood has been associated with increased separation barking,[42] ensuring standard puppy health protocols, including hygiene, veterinary care, vaccination, diet, and appropriate conspecific contact is advised. Screening and assessment of shelter dogs and provision of appropriate advice to those who adopt these pets can effectively reduce separation-related behaviors in some cases.[7,27] While a short preadoption counseling session had minimal effect, provision of written recommendations was shown to correlate with lower rates (38–22%) of separation-related behaviors 12 weeks post adoption.[27,31] Advising pet parents with newly adopted dogs to always provide a food puzzle upon departure was shown to be a simple method that pet parents were able to comply with.[7,27] Advising pet parents to be calm at departure time may be helpful[27] as well. Pet parents should be advised to introduce puppies and new adoptees to separation gradually and enforce time away from the pet parents to help them cope better with spending time alone.[7,32,42] One to two

Box 17.4 Precipitating factors for separation-related disorder emergence

- Change in the pet parent's routine
- Pet parent returning to school or work
- Move to a new home
- Visit to a new environment
- Following a stay in a kennel
- Altered social relationships (new baby, new pet, new partner)
- Other fears, phobias, and anxiety disorders
- Medical, cognitive disorders

Box 17.5 Prevention of separation-related disorder

- Short departures starting in puppyhood
- Potentially play with other dogs in puppyhood
- Socialization, reinforcement-based training – no aversive training
- Postadoption counseling
- Written instructions for preventing SRD
- Slow changes to the schedule, environment, or lifestyle

hours of unattended time on weekends, in comparison to 0–1 hours of unattended time in puppies, has been shown to be correlated with a lower amount of separation-related behaviors at 1 year old.[69] Similarly, when the pet parent anticipates a significant alteration in schedule or in the amount of time spent with the dog, the changeover should be made as slowly as possible (see Box 17.5).

Diagnosis and potential outcomes

General health assessment

The initial step is the general health assessment. Each patient should receive a thorough physical examination, including orthopedic, neurologic, dermatologic, and baseline health screening, including a complete blood count, chemistry panel, urinalysis, fecal antigen test + Giardia, and thyroid profile, as well as additional assessment as indicated by age, health, examination, and clinical signs. For more on the link between systemic diseases and behavioral clinical signs, see Chapter 6. Additional testing would depend on clinical presentation. On physical exam, special attention should be paid to nail beds, foot pads, forelimbs, chin hair, skin around the muzzle, teeth, and gums for evidence of excessive wear, and injury associated with escape and destructive behavior, or saliva staining from hypersalivation (see Figures 17.1 and 17.2).[1,6,72]

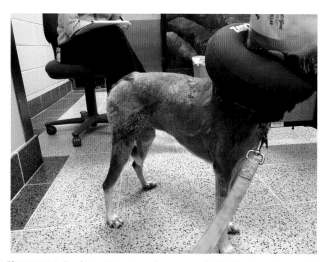

Figure 17.1 Degloving injury to a dog as a result of trying to escape a crate. (*Attribution: Julie Albright.*)

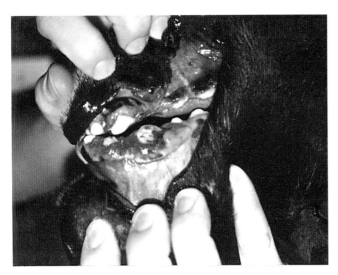

Figure 17.2 Dogs may wear down their teeth trying to escape the house or crates. *(Courtesy Kelly Moffat.)*

Diagnosis

The diagnosis of SRD involves collecting historical information about the pet that should reveal at least one of the following: abnormal attachment to one or more family/social group members, distress at the time of the attachment figure's departure, and attachment figure-absent behavioral clinical signs for which other physical and behavioral causes have been ruled out (see Box 17.6).[29] Pet parent report has been significantly correlated with video evidence,[1,36] making it a valuable modality for evaluation.

Many dogs exhibit mild distress when separated from their pet parents, and this may not be a psychopathological condition.[11] Unaffected dogs may show similar signs of distress when alone in an unfamiliar location, but the behavior signs quickly subside as the dog adapts to the environment.[36] Thus, mild signs of distress, especially in a novel environment, that resolve quickly would not constitute a diagnosable condition. Relevant clinical information that can shed light on possible diagnoses as well as steer treatment plans includes:

1) Clinical signs - The most common clinical signs of SRDs are vocalization, destructiveness, visual scanning, excessive motor activity, and house soiling during the pet parent's absence (see Box 17.7).[1,17,27,70,74] House soiling may be an involuntary physiologic and autonomic response or may be a goal-directed behavior of marking in situations of stress.[3,4,6] Vocalization may be an expression of distress, frustration, or contact-seeking calls.[3,6,41] Destructive behaviors may be attempts at escape or displaced frustration behaviors.[3–5,70] Other signs related to the pet's anxiety might include anorexia during departure (which disappears when the pet parent is home), hypersalivation, tachypnea, tachycardia, vomiting, diarrhea, increased motor activity, decreased motor activity (hiding, withdrawal, freezing), excessive licking or grooming, restlessness, shivering and shaking, orienting toward the environment, rearing to the wall or door, stereotypic behaviors such as ritualized circling and pacing, and self-injurious behaviors.[4,5,75] Occasionally, cases exhibit

aggression as the pet parents prepare to depart or place the animal in their containment area, perhaps in an attempt to prevent the departure.[2,11,14,17,38] In comparison, dogs without SRD have been shown to engage in passive behaviors during departures, such as resting or sleeping, and exploratory behavior was minimal unless a new stimulus was present.[76,77]

Upon the pet parent's return, dogs affected with SRDs have been shown to exhibit excited greeting behaviors for longer than a 2-minute duration and reduced ability to calm down.[11,17,36,40] These greeting behaviors were shown to involve more running and less proximity seeking compared to non-SRD dogs. In fact, levels of affection and proximity seeking upon reunion did not differ between SRD and non-SRD dogs.[36,56] Duration of pet parent absence may affect greeting behavior in those without SRD, but greeting behaviors remain consistently intense in those with SRD, no matter the length of departure.[36,77] This suggests that dogs with SRD experience the departure as stressful, no matter how long the duration of departure, whereas unaffected dogs have a graduated level of excitement, depending on how long a time has passed since they have seen their pet parent.

Clinical signs may be behavioral, emotional, and physiological responses to stress, which may include vocalization, destruction, agitation-anxiety, gastrointestinal signs (diarrhea, vomiting), inappetence, hypersalivation, withdrawal, inactivity, depression-apathy, house soiling, repetitive motor activity, escape behavior, and self-trauma when actually or virtually separated from preferred people.[2,4,5,32,40] The most commonly reported separation-related behaviors in cats are destruction (66.67%), vocalization (63.33%), urination outside of the litterbox (60%), depression (53.33%) aggressiveness (36.67%), agitation/anxiety (36.67%), defecation outside of the litterbox (23.33%),[10] and over grooming (6%).[3]

2) Duration of clinical signs – How long the problem behaviors have been going on is important in establishing the diagnosis, as well if there were any inciting events or lifestyle changes associated with the onset. While some puppies show stress reactions when first left home alone, most of these behaviors do not persist after 1–2 months.[78] Separation-distress reactions that persist beyond the puppy stage are maladaptive and may be indicative of either dysfunctional attachment or perhaps even a pathological state.[43,56] If the clinical signs have only been going on for a few days, there is an insufficient pattern for which a firm diagnosis could be established, especially if a significant life change just occurred. Studies examining SRDs use a variety of durations of clinical signs as criteria for the diagnosis for the purposes of their studies, from one month[79] to six months.[1] There is insufficient literature in cats to draw conclusions about length of clinical signs in cats.

3) Latency – The latency to arousal is the moment of onset of grossly observable signs of distress. Most signs arise prior to or within the first 10–30 minutes of departure in dogs.[27,70,74,80] Many dogs learn predeparture cues or environmental stimuli that predict that a separation is impending, such as the pet parent picking up their purse or putting on certain shoes. Identification of these

Box 17.6 Differential diagnosis of separation-related disorder

Problem	Differentials
Destructive behavior	Exploration – object play • May be related to scent/texture/odor/taste/novelty • Signs when pet parents are at home but may be suppressed by supervision Activity – energy • Inadequate exercise, mental stimulation Scavenging – usually garbage or food • Signs when pet parents are at home but may be suppressed by supervision Territorial – targets may be windows/doors • Signs when pet parents are at home Other fears and phobias, e.g., noise, storms • Signs when pet parents are at home, may be worsened when pet parents are absent Predation • Digging, scratching at drapes, window molding, walls and floor boards • Signs may occur when pet parents are at home; look for circadian pattern Confinement distress – escape attempts from confinement area • May be seen if confined during pet parent's presence Separation-related disorders – doors, windows, confinement areas, pet parent possessions • Predeparture anxiety may be present – may increase immediately following departure
Vocalization	Alarm/outside stimuli – territorial barking • Signs when pet parents are at home but may be suppressed by supervision Social facilitation Play Other fears and phobias, e.g., noise, storms • Signs when pet parents are at home Confinement distress • May be seen when pet parents are at home

Problem	Differentials
	Frustration - bark Physical – sensory loss, cognitive dysfunction syndrome, pain/discomfort Separation-related disorders – distressed, whine, high-pitched, howl • May be predeparture signs or immediately following departure
House soiling	Inadequate house training • Signs when pet parents are at home but may be suppressed by supervision Lack of sufficient opportunities to eliminate for age, needs, health • Duration of departure, scheduling Physical – monitor for other clinical and behavioral signs • Increased frequency, volume, urge, decreased control, cognitive dysfunction syndrome Excitement, conflict, or anxiety-related urination • Generally on pet parent homecoming, greeting Marking – vertical surfaces, often intact male – selected prominent surfaces • Signs when pet parents are at home but may be suppressed by supervision Other fears and phobias, e.g., noise, storms • Signs when pet parents are at home, may be worsened when pet parents are absent Separation-related disorders – other concurrent signs – seldom only sign • Occurs during virtually every departure, even if short and the pet has eliminated outdoors prior to the departure
Aggression	Other aggression diagnoses such as fear-induced aggression, anxiety-induced aggression, etc. See Chapter 23. Aggression occurs primarily when pet parents try to depart and is directed at the pet parent or redirected to another pet, another social group member, or an object.

Note: Concurrent signs, predeparture signs, and timing of signs supportive: video can confirm.

Box 17.7 Clinical signs consistent with separation-related disorder (not all clinical signs need to be present for diagnosis)

• Vocalization, destructiveness, visual scanning, excessive motor activity, and house soiling during the pet parent's absence
• Attempts to escape confinement and from the home
• Anorexia during departures but not when the pet parent is home
• Hypersalivation, tachypnea, tachycardia, vomiting, diarrhea, increased motor activity, decreased motor activity (hiding, withdrawal, freezing), depression/apathy, excessive licking or grooming, restlessness, shivering and shaking, orienting toward the environment, rearing to the wall or door, stereotypic behaviors such as ritualized circling and pacing, and self-injurious behaviors
• Excited greeting behaviors for longer than a 2-minute duration and reduced ability to calm down
• Anxious behaviors occur consistently with certain types of absences
• The pet shows signs of anxiety as the family member leaves
• Problem behaviors usually only occur when family members are absent or when the pets cannot gain access to family members when they are at home
• The anxious behaviors begin very shortly after the family member leaves and often occur even during very short absences
• The pet shows excited and long greeting behavior regardless of the duration of the departure

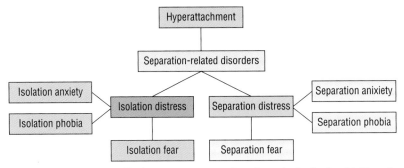

Figure 17.3 A new way of looking at separation anxiety diagnosis. *(Attribution: Ariel Fagen.)*

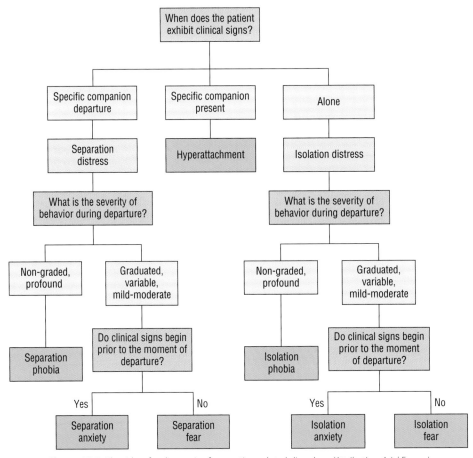

Figure 17.4 Algorithm for diagnosis of separation related disorders. *(Attribution: Ariel Fagen.)*

predeparture cues is suggestive of SRD, though must be differentiated from excitement about the possibility of the dog going with the pet parents on a walk or drive. The latency can have important implications about how to diagnose and implement treatment – see below. While there is no published literature in latency in cats suffering from SRD, this is still a measurable piece of the history which can be obtained and assessed in reexaminations to track progress.

4) Frequency – Dogs and cats must exhibit the behaviors nearly every time a triggering situation occurs, though not necessarily every separation. For example, some patients are able to remain calm for "regular" departures, as in departures that occur at approximately the same

time and for the same duration each week (e.g., working 9 am–5 pm Monday through Friday), while exhibiting signs of distress for "irregular" departures.[27,81] Or, some patients may trigger differently, depending on the order of departure of the people in the home. Look for consistency in a given environmental context. If there is no consistency in the same environmental context, then that is an indicator to look for other differentials that may be responsible.

5) Recovery time – This value represents how long it takes the dog or cat to recover from their clinical distress. Evidence supports that for many patients, the behavioral signs are most intense shortly after departure.[2,50,70,74] Signs often decrease over time in dogs but

may remain static for the duration of the departure, increase over time, or have a cyclical nature ranging from 25 to 60 minutes.[1,2,11,36,37,70,74] External stimuli can also lead to rearousal.[2,70] Dogs without SRD are more likely to show progressively less activity over the first 5 minutes of a separation[36] and when looking at the departure overall, tend to have even patterns of behavior with no peak or cyclicity noted.[77] Dogs with SRD show a tendency toward persistently elevated activity levels within the first 5 minutes of a departure.[36]

6) Intensity – Categorizing clinical signs at initial presentation as worsening, static, improving, or waxing and waning can be helpful for tracking response to treatment. For example, if a patient has been progressively worsening for three months prior to presentation and at the first recheck, the intensity has plateaued, this may indicate a response to treatment and that the treatment plan is headed in the right direction. Furthermore, a general understanding of intensity can inform quality of life and urgency in treatment decisions.

7) The pet parent's response to behavior and treatments that have already been tried – While this information does not help you diagnose the problem, it can direct treatment going forward. Medications that have been appropriately trialed in the past may not be worth repeating, and behavioral therapies that have been inappropriately applied may require some significant coaching to straighten out. Similarly, you may identify some attempts at correcting the behavior that may be making the problem worse that you can put a stop to.

Diagnostic tools

Pet parent accuracy in reporting of clinical signs is variable and while important, must be understood to have its limitations. When questioning pet parents, one must ask about specific behavioral descriptors and not just whether a pet is "afraid." Studies support that pet parents are able to identify certain behavioral descriptors in their pet but may not necessarily interpret the emotional state as fearful or anxious. Reports on relative amounts of destruction, howling, and whining have been shown to be decently correlated with video evidence, while restlessness, agitation, and pacing are easy to miss.[1] Because many of the clinical signs of SRD leave no "evidence" upon return home, pet monitoring and video recordings of departures are considered a standard and critical diagnostic tool in clinical practice. For example, one of the most frequent clinical signs observed in SRD patients is visual scanning,[1,74] a "silent" clinical sign, and some dogs, especially older dogs, may show more passive, withdrawn, or subtle signs. Video is essential for tracking response to treatment as well. With modern technology, video is becoming an easier tool to implement. Many home security cameras, baby monitors, computers, tablets, or phones with recording features and streaming applications can be used to this end.

Other diagnostic tools employed include activity monitors, some specifically designed for pet motion detection when pet parents are not available to monitor. These are of specific utility, and reliability and accuracy of each device need to be assessed carefully but may provide a means to track how *much* pacing is occurring during a departure, for

example. Likewise, decibel monitors may be helpful in certain cases to assess barking.

A new model for diagnosis

While many clinicians continue to use the terms separation anxiety or SRD, a new model for diagnosis is proposed here that further emphasizes that SRDs are really a cluster of related conditions (Figure 17.3). This new model differentiates between a fear response, anxiety, frustration, and panic disorder, as well as separation from preferred social beings versus total isolation (see Figure 17.4). To determine whether or not a patient has anxiety, we look at the interdeparture period, especially just prior to a departure, for clinical signs of distress related to the departure. To determine whether or not a patient has a fear versus a phobia, we look at the patient's response in the interdeparture period, at the moment of departure, and severity of signs through the duration of the departure. To determine whether the patient has concerns about separation versus isolation, we look at who and under what conditions the clinical signs emerge.

Fear, anxiety, stress, panic, phobias, and the physiologic stress response are discussed in Chapters 7, 14, and 15. For that reason, the discussion here will primarily focus on the differences between the emotional states. Evidence supports that the brain processes fear differently than anxiety and that they are generally distinct, though not unrelated, affective states.[82,83] In a fear response, the inciting stimulus is present, resulting in a rapid response in the amygdala. The response is involuntary, brief, instantaneous, associated with autonomic arousal and specific behaviors, and is precipitated by an antecedent event.[83,84,64]

Whereas in anxiety, a slower onset of distress activated by less predictable, more ambiguous, distant, or potential antecedent events can lead to chronic hypervigilance, arousal, and worry regarding a future or possible threat.[83,85] Anxiety can be anticipatory in nature and is not time bound in the way fear is, with longer recovery times.[64,83,84,86] Patients with anxiety exhibit heightened contextual anxiety,[83] meaning they pick up on the environmental cues that are associated with the fear-evoking stimulus (e.g., the blinds have been shut and all the lights turned off). The anticipatory feature of anxiety can be demonstrated in dogs as behavioral and physiologic signs of distress in *anticipation* of people leaving, not only at the moment of departure or once left. This anticipatory and chronic distress may present as generalized signs of anxiety, such as hypervigilance about their companion potentially leaving, and raises significant chronic quality of life concerns.[87] In one study, about 75% of dogs showed signs of distress when the pet parents prepared for a departure.[17]

A phobic response is an elevated, out of context, fear response, evoked by a stimulus which is present and can be associated with anticipatory anxiety.[83] Thus, here, if a patient is diagnosed with a phobia, then their disorder is characterized by both intensive phobic episodes associated with departures and potentially interepisode anticipatory anxiety as well. These diagnoses represent essentially a combination of intensive fear plus anxiety and therefore represent the most severe of the SRD cases. These cases raise particular quality of life and human–animal bond concerns and demand an aggressive and comprehensive treatment approach, necessitating emergency medications if the pet parent is unable to avoid departures.

The separation versus isolation specification speaks to whether the pet exhibits clinical signs of distress when separated from their preferred social companions (people or animals) versus when totally alone. This distinction is relevant, as it impacts treatment approaches. Research supports that some dogs have different responses to separation from their pet parent when a stranger is present or with a companion dog compared to social isolation.[34,88] For example, some dogs were less stressed in the presence of the cohabitant dog or utilized the stranger for social support when their pet parents were absent, similar to the use of dog sitters to relieve the signs of separation-related distress.[34,89] On the other hand, dogs with a specific attachment to one person that do not receive comfort from other human or animal social group members pose a huge emotional strain on the preferred person, whereby they feel "trapped" or "held hostage" by their pet, invoking feelings of desperation, frustration, anger, and stress, and thus risking the human–animal bond (see Box 17.8).

Patients can exhibit more than one of these conditions. If insufficient information is available to differentiate, then a diagnosis of *Separation Distress (unspecified)*, *Isolation Distress (unspecified)*, or *Separation-Related Disorder (unspecified)* could be made. If multiple diagnoses would be appropriate, the veterinarian could list each diagnosis separately or diagnose the patient with *Separation-Related Disorder (complicated)*. For example, the dog that exhibits panting, whining, and visual scanning for the first 5 minutes after the husband leaves the home when the wife is still home, but escalates to chewing at the door, urinating, howling, and salivating with elevated heart rate that starts when he sees the whole family putting their jackets on to leave the home and persists for 1–2 hours post departure, qualifies for the individual diagnoses of: Separation Fear and Isolation Phobia. Alternatively, this patient could be diagnosed with the more generic term *Separation-Related Disorder (complicated)*.

Patient mental state is dynamic and as such, diagnoses can change with time as learning experiences accumulate. For this reason, diagnoses should be reevaluated periodically, as treatment progresses and may need to be reclassified.

Hyperattachment

Clinical signs for diagnosing a patient with *hyperattachment* include contact seeking and persistent shadowing behaviors when the pet parent is home, increasing distress with increased distance from their preferred person, distress with preparation to leave the home, and excitement behaviors upon return to the home.[90] Proximity-seeking behavior alone is not sufficient evidence for a diagnosis of *hyperattachment*. Some level of distress associated with prohibition of contact and efforts on the dog's part to avoid the distress of being away from the person should be demonstrated. Proximity-seeking behaviors may result from reinforcement for proximity and not necessarily secondary to pathological anxiety disorder. Life may just be more fun when you hang near mom and dad!

Hyperattachment may be diagnosed along with other SRDs, may be a feature of generalized anxiety disorder,[21] or may be a standalone diagnosis.[11,91] Improvement of SRDs may not show concurrent improvement with signs of hyperattachment.[90] In fact, patients with hyperattachment may not show distress signs once the pet parent is out of the home. There is conflicting evidence as to whether or not patients diagnosed within the framework outlined here would be more or less likely to exhibit signs of hyperattachment.[17,40,56] Reexaminination of hyperattachment with respect to the different SRD diagnoses are warranted to further understand the interplay (see Figure 17.3).

Differential diagnosis

Although the presence of destruction, vocalization, and, to a lesser extent, elimination when the pet parent departs may be due to SRD, other possible causes for these signs must be ruled out (see Box 17.6). Two reasons to consider etiologies other than SRD would be: (1) the behavior also occurs when the family is home; and (2) the problem behavior occurs only randomly instead of consistently whenever the pet parent is gone. Should the problem behavior occur inconsistently, question the pet parents about characteristics of the departures when the problem behavior does occur and does not occur, as an important pattern may be revealed that may in fact be consistent with a context-dependent SRD. In addition, if signs arise with increasing duration of absence (rather than arising prior to, during, or immediately

---

Box 17.8 Six distinct diagnoses within separation-related disorders

	Fear	Anxiety	Phobia
Separation distress	Separation fear Physiological, physical, and/or behavioral signs of distress associated with separation from preferred social companions, such as specific family members	Separation anxiety Physiological, physical, and/or behavioral signs of distress in anticipation of and with separation from preferred social companions	Separation phobia Profound, nongraded, physiological, physical, and behavioral signs of panic with separation from preferred social companions along with physiological, physical, and/or behavioral signs of distress in anticipation of separation from preferred social companions
Isolation distress	Isolation fear Physiological, physical, and/or behavioral signs of distress associated with being alone	Isolation anxiety Physiological, physical, and/or behavioral signs of distress in anticipation of and with being alone	Isolation phobia Profound, nongraded, physiological, physical, and behavioral signs of panic associated with being alone along with physiological, physical, and/or behavioral signs of distress in anticipation of being alone

following departure), SRD should be questioned; however, this alone does not rule out SRD.

Major behavioral differentials to consider are confinement distress, territorial behaviors, cognitive dysfunction, noise aversions, thunderstorm phobia, other panic disorders, boredom, play, exploration, food-seeking behaviors, incomplete house training, urine marking, and more.[2,38,72] SRDs are commonly associated with fearfulness and other anxiety disorders, such as noise and storm phobias.[17,20,28,38,40,43] In one study, 83% of SRD dogs had a comorbid behavioral diagnosis, 43.7% with noise sensitivity.[17]

Among Finnish dogs, SRD patients were more likely to be characterized as hyperactive, impulsive, inattentive, fearful, and compulsive.[23] Noise aversions, thunderstorm phobias, and SRDs have been shown to have up to 50% comorbidity with separation anxiety.[14,17,40,43] In a Finnish study, almost 60% of dogs with separation anxiety were reported to be generally fearful and significantly more aggressive to other dogs, unfamiliar people, and pet parents.[17] One study analyzing frequencies of storm phobia, separation anxiety, and noise phobia in a veterinary behavior caseload found a probability that 85% of dogs with noise or storm phobia had separation anxiety, while 63% of dogs with separation anxiety had noise phobia.[38] However, in general population surveys of pet parents, there was low co-occurrence of separation anxiety with fear of noises,[27] and only 23% of noise-sensitive dogs with signs of separation anxiety.[43] Pet parents may see signs of noise aversions or thunderstorm fears when they are with the pet, but these may intensify when the pet parent is not present.[5,6]

Pets that are crated or otherwise confined may be distressed about the confinement itself and may react with anxiety, destructive behavior, escape attempts, and vocalization without having actual SRD. Therefore, dogs should be evaluated while crated or confined when the pet parents are with them (see Figure 17.5 and 17.6).[92] If they only show clinical signs when in the crate, for example, but not when separated from the pet parent in other contexts, then confinement distress would be a more appropriate diagnosis. To complicate matters further, patients with confinement anxiety can show anticipatory signs of distress prior to departures *only* when being crated and still struggle with departures when not crated but significantly less so and without any anticipatory signs. Thus, these patients may actually have Confinement Anxiety and Separation Fear but could easily be mistaken for an SRD case.

Additionally, dogs that react when viewing or hearing things outside of a window may show signs of destruction toward the exits and entrances to the home or the window where they watch their pet parent depart and people pass by. This destruction, vocalization, and other high-arousal behaviors can be mistaken for SRD. Video with a view to the outside may be revealing, though certainly SRD and territorial behaviors can co-occur and the clinical signs compound on each other at triggering moments (Figure 17.7).

Other differentials to consider are based on the individual clinical signs reported. For example, what may appear to be destruction and evidence of hypersalivation may be the result of seizures. What may appear to be stress-related urination in the home may be a clinical sign of polyuria or a lower urinary tract disease. Self-trauma may actually represent a dermatologic or neurologic condition. Veterinarians should consider

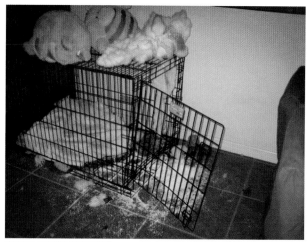

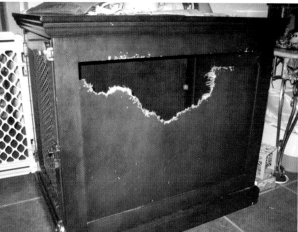

Figures 17.5 and 6 Confinement during departures can result in destruction and injury to the pet. *(Attribution: Lisa Radosta.)*

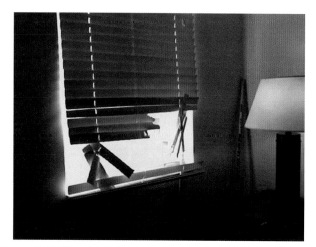

Figure 17.7 When destruction is primarily at windows other diagnoses should be ruled out. *(Attribution: Lisa Radosta.)*

intracranial and extracranial CNS disease, cognitive dysfunction, sensory decline, metabolic disorders, endocrinopathies, gastrointestinal disease, and medical factors contributing to house soiling. Any medical condition that causes pain or discomfort can exacerbate behavior problems and potentially cause behavioral clinical signs. Hence the importance of our complete physical exam, history taking, basic screening tests, thorough workups, and video evidence.

It is important to rule out that the behavior might be behaviorally appropriate given the life circumstances and the pet's history. For example, lack of sufficient opportunity to reach a potty area or history of adequate house training may result in accidents in the home. The drive to roam, especially in intact male dogs, may motivate escape behaviors. Normal social facilitation among housemate dogs can promote barking, exploratory, and play behaviors.[4,5,72] Lack of stimulation can appear as destructive behaviors. Dogs that show intensification of signs with duration of departure may be getting progressively more bored.[70] This may be of particular consideration when destructive behaviors are focused around food (e.g., the garbage or pantry) or items that might be particularly fun to chew or destroy (e.g., toothbrushes, underwear, or cardboard boxes). If all destructive behavior is oriented toward internal items and not at doorways, windows, and other external perimeters, have boredom higher on your rule-out list than you otherwise might.

Prognosis

The prognosis depends on the severity and chronicity of the disorder; the stress level of the pet parents; family schedule; the ability of the family to follow through on medication, management- and behavior-modification recommendations; the general wellness of the pet; and the pet's response to psychotropic medications. There is no magic formula for prognosis. Like much of medicine, it is individual and may change as treatment progresses. One study found that if treated within one year of onset of clinical signs, 80% of dogs showed improvement or were cured, compared to 67.9% of all the SRD dogs in the study.[37] Combining behavior modification with pheromones, SSRIs (fluoxetine, paroxetine, sertraline), or TCAs (clomipramine) given daily, combined with a benzodiazepine (alprazolam, diazepam) or clonidine given 1 hour prior to departures, improves the prognosis above using behavior modification alone.[89,93,94] Some dogs require long-term treatment.[93] Dogs with SRDs have been shown to have a "pessimistic" cognitive bias, representing an underlying negative affective state. Treatment has been shown to bring about a more "optimistic" cognitive bias, indicating an improvement in welfare and well-being.[94]

Treatment

As is the case with all behavior disorders, four modalities are employed in the treatment of SRDs: evaluation of general wellness, neurochemical modulation, management, and behavioral treatments. One size does not fit all. Giving pet parents options will help them to choose what works for them. It is possible to have a positive outcome in the treatment of SRDs with medication and management alone. While that is not ideal, it is the only option for some pet parents. Pet parents who choose this option should understand that the likelihood that they will ever be able to change the management of their dog, loosening the routine, for example, or lowering the pet's medications without behavioral therapies is very low. For SRDs in particular, treatment adherence is poorest when more than five instructions are given to the pet parent at one time.[37] In fact, while a treatment plan specifically tailored to the pet parent, pet, and household would have the greatest success and compliance, 56% of pet parents receiving a standardized, generic behavior modification plan reported a significant improvement after 12 weeks, and 25% reported slight improvement, while most untreated dogs were not improved.[89] Comparatively, a simple standardized treatment plan combined with fluoxetine therapy resulted in 73% overall improvement over eight weeks.[95] Therefore, the program should focus on a few simple steps, including: (1) avoiding panic responses and continued learning experiences while working toward a sustainable plan, (2) ameliorating distress for needed departures while a longer-term treatment plan is under way, (3) teaching the pet how to relax in the pet parent's absence or when alone, (4) and teaching the pet that good things can be associated with departures and if needed, predeparture cues. For most cases, drug therapy will also be needed to address the pet's intense distress. See Chapter 11 for more information on medications. As treatment proceeds, coach the pet parents to keep a log or journal of changes made and results for tracking purposes.[71] For most dogs, if you can get them through the first 30–90 minutes of the departure without recurrence of clinical signs, then the departure should go well, though there is likely a population of dogs for which this does not hold true.[49] While there are no studies examining the efficacy of different treatment protocols in cats, there is a good probability that at least some of the strategies outlined here will be effective for cats. See Box 17.9 for a summary of treatments for Separation Related Disorders.

Box 17.9 Treatment Recommendations for Separation Related Disorders	
Step	**Description**
Social/exercise	• Provide interactive times regularly throughout the day to ensure sufficient aerobic exercise, social time, play, and additional positive reinforcement-based training. • Maintain structure and predictability in interactions with the pet and in setting up the pet's routine and lifestyle. • Learn to read dog body language so you may more readily respond to subtle communications from your dog.
Confinement	• Confining your pet may result in increased anxiety unless the pet is accustomed to confinement while you are at home (crate, child gate, room, pen, tied down). Acclimating the pet to confinement should be done gradually using food and chew toys. Allowing your pet to choose its own desirable resting site and then rewarding its use can improve compliance. • Trial alternative confinement options like baby gating a room, an exercise pen, or part of the home. • Trial not confining your pet after dog proofing.

Box 17.9 Treatment Recommendations for Separation Related Disorders—cont'd

Step	Description
Protect the home	• When confinement is not an option or not the best option, take measures to protect the home as best you can. • Put up baby gates and close doors to block off any particularly destructive or sensitive areas. • Stack cardboard boxes, foam, newspapers, or other destructible, affordable padding on areas that the pet has focused destructive tendencies before. Alternatively, putting up metal scratch plates or plexiglass protective barriers may be helpful for certain cases – note that extreme destroyers may cause self-injury on these as they would on wood, etc.

Safe zone	• Set up a safe zone – every day, place your dog in the safe zone with a meal in a food puzzle, a recording of your voice playing, white noise or music in the background, and clothing scented like you on their dog bed. Then, either:
	  • Wait until you are ready to start a desensitization and counterconditioning to departures program, and do it within the safe zone with an extra-delicious food puzzle. This approach necessitates you having another safe location for the pet to be in the meantime for departures.
	  • Or place your pet in the safe zone for all departures with an extra-delicious food puzzle immediately. When you start the desensitization and counterconditioning to departures, ensure that either the relaxation mat or another safety signal is included.

Relaxation	• Teach your dog to relax on a mat by following the 5 Ds Relaxation Protocol. Only bring the mat out for practice and real use sessions; otherwise keep it stored away. Use low-moderate value treats when first teaching the protocol and practice in a quiet environment.
	  1. The Drive – put the mat down. The moment the pet steps on the mat, drop a treat on the mat every 1 second for 10 seconds as long as the pet stays on the mat. Call the dog off, or if the dog gets off on their own, pick the mat up and put it down somewhere different, and repeat until the dog does not want to get off the mat and/or immediately runs to the mat when it is put down.
	  2. The Doublecheck – put the mat down and turn your body 45 degrees from the mat. If the dog gets on the mat, reward as before and repeat. Practice at 90-degree turns, then 90-degree turns + 1 step away from the mat, then 90-degree turns + 2 steps away from the mat in all different orientations. If your dog lines up in front of you instead of getting on the mat, then back up to an earlier step or make it easier for your dog by orienting closer to the mat on your next repetition.
	  3. The Default Down – the moment your dog steps on the mat, cue the down. Reward as you have been with the dog in the down position, dropping treats in between his front paws so he has to move minimally to retrieve them. If the dog gets up, stop rewarding and reset. If your dog is unable to down on cue, then work with a trainer to either teach the down or lure the dog into a down.
	  4. The Duration – the moment your dog steps on the mat and lies down, count 1 second in your head, deliver the first treat, count another second, deliver the second treat, count another second, deliver the third treat. Note: you do your first count before you deliver your first treat. If your dog stays lying down this whole time, increase the interval to 2 seconds, and repeat for a total of three treats. Continue in this fashion, building up to a treat every 60 seconds three times in a row. A general guide for how to increase the time increments in seconds: 1, 2, 3, 5, 7, 10, 15, 20, 30, 45, 60. Practice at least some if not all of these sessions with the mat put down next to you while you relax in a chair or couch. Try to keep this boring and do not engage your dog aside from dropping the treats.
	  5. The Disengage and Destress – switch from rewarding for time intervals to body language signs that the dog is disengaging from "training mode" and is physically relaxing. Body language signs to reward for include: looking away from you, lowering the head, tail dropping to flatten on the ground, shifting a hip into lateral, settling in, deep breath, lying in lateral, closing the eyes, any observable muscular tension relaxation. Importantly, you must reward for a variety of body language signs so as to effectively reward for an inner state of relaxation and not just a specific body position like lying down in lateral. Initially, you may be able to capture more signs of disengagement, and over time, this should progress to true relaxation.
	The protocol is complete when the dog immediately gets on the mat when it is presented and lies down into a relaxed and comfortable position. At this point, the mat can start to be used for DS/CC protocols and in real-life contexts where we need the pet to self-regulate.

For hyperattachment: reward independence	• Teach independence by having your dog rest on a bed or mat with no physical contact. Give treats or toys to keep your dog occupied and gradually increase the length of time, and then move further away (ideally into a different room). • Reward independent, calm, and relaxed behavior frequently. • Set up a sanctuary space as directed above. Sit with them to start and slowly work yourself out of the room over many sessions: If the dog is able to eat comfortably, completely ignoring you for three days in a row, on the next day, move 1 foot closer to the door. If the dog looks up and then resumes eating, do not move closer to the door until you get three sessions with your dog completely comfortable. If your dog leaves his food, follows you, barks, whines, or shows any other sign of distress, return to your pet, help them resume eating, and then on your next session, practice a few feet closer to your pet than where you had been when they got distressed. Resume the protocol from there. • Play Find It games with increasing distance to promote independence and confidence building.
Never punish	• Punishment can increase fear and anxiety.
Departure cues	• Until departures are significantly improved, do not worry about addressing any predeparture cues. • Do not try to hide predeparture cues or practice them when you are not actually leaving – this can decrease predictability, which can increase anxiety over time. • Once departures themselves are much improved, manage cues that are still triggering so the pet is not exposed to them when possible. • If the predeparture cues remain triggering after departures themselves are much improved, there are three approaches to decreasing stress associated with departure cues:

continued

Box 17.9 Treatment Recommendations for Separation Related Disorders—cont'd

Step	Description
Departure training	• Either after relaxation conditioning has been solidified or right away, start a desensitization and counterconditioning plan for departures.
	• Set your pet up in their sanctuary space +/− on their relaxation mat. If no relaxation mat is being utilized, ensure that a different environmental stimulus is being used to help your dog understand that this is a "safe" departure, e.g., lavender-scented diffuser. Give them an extra-delicious food puzzle – multiple food puzzles are even better.
	• Rough plan: Slowly work up the duration of the departures while the pet is focused on their food puzzles in small increments. Video stream them during the process so you can observe for body language signs that indicate concern. Do not increase to longer durations until you have had two to three successful departures in a row with no signs of concern from your dog. Try to return BEFORE any signs of concern are noticed. If you do notice signs of concern, immediately return and at the next practice session, shorten your departure duration.
	• Tailored plan: With your dog on the relaxation mat, do reps of moving away from your dog and returning, gradually making the reps harder and longer, progressing from going through the door, to starting the car and driving away, and then gradually longer departures. If using a remote treat dispensing device, deliver a reinforcer at the hardest moment in that repetition. Monitor on live stream video to ensure no signs of concern are noted.
Pheromones/ medications	• Fluoxetine, a selective serotonin reuptake inhibitor (SSRI), or clomipramine, a tricyclic antidepressant, are licensed products for dogs that have demonstrated efficacy in conjunction with a behavior program of 2–4 months. Other SSRIs or TCAs might be an alternative.
	• Dog pheromone analogues Adaptil (formerly DAP) and Zenidog might be beneficial alone or together with drugs.
	• Benzodiazepines such as alprazolam and diazepam, dexmedetomidine oromucosal gel, gabapentin, clonidine, tasipimidine or trazodone, might be used concurrently with SSRIs on an as-needed basis prior to departures.
	• Selegiline might be considered for chronic anxiety disorders and in senior pets where cognitive dysfunction might be contributing to anxiety but not concurrently with SSRIs, TCAs, or trazodone.
Monitoring	• To assess the pet's behavior when out of sight or away from home, monitor with a video monitor, nanny cam, security camera, or live stream app or device.

Help the pet parent understand

Most pet parents do not understand why their pet is destroying the house or barking all day. The family needs to understand that the dog is distressed because it cannot cope with separation from them, not because it is "mad" at them. Some pet parents are convinced that the pet is "retaliating" about being left alone or confined. Having the pet parents record or monitor their pet's behavior during departure will help to convince them that the underlying motivation is fear and anxiety. These can be truly heartbreaking to watch. The "guilty look" that the pet parent sometimes sees on arrival when items have been damaged or the house has been soiled is a fear or conflict response, relieved to see their pet parents but fearful of their response. The dog's "guilty" look is simply a response to pet parent cues and an attempt to avoid conflict.[96] Once the pet parent understands the motivation behind the behavior, this can buy a lot of sympathy, partnership, and patience that otherwise would be absent.

Management

Stop punishment

Once the pet parent understands the motivation, having the discussion about discontinuing punishment becomes easier. Many pet parents, even when coached not to, verbally chastise their pet, show their pet the "evidence," or even physically reprimand their pet when they return home to find a mess.[27] They do so in an effort to help teach the dog not to perform the behavior in the future, but in reality, they may be increasing their pet's fear or anxiety levels. Because the punishment comes so long after the actual behavior occurred, the dogs are extremely unlikely to make the connection and learn the lesson the pet parent wants to teach. See Chapter 10 for a detailed discussion of punishment and reinforcement. Coach the pet parent to stop all punishment behaviors, just clean up their house, and then change the setup next time to minimize risk of destruction/elimination in the future. This is something the veterinarian or veterinary technician can help troubleshoot with them. Written instruction has been shown to help adjust pet parent's punishment behaviors upon return home.[27]

Avoidance

While working on a full treatment plan, pet parents should do what they can to avoid separations so the dog does not continue to have negative learning experiences and distressed moments. Day boarding, doggie day care, hiring a pet sitter or a dog walker, taking the dog to work, or having a neighbor, family member, or friend watch the dog are options for some. When avoidance is not possible and moderate to significant distress is occurring, fast-acting anxiolytic medications are necessary. Avoid stimuli or situations which contribute to stress. For example, if the dog panics in the crate in response to departures, recommend discontinuation of the crate. Some dogs do worse if pet parents come home mid-departure to check on the patient.[6] For these dogs, recommend whenever possible that the pet parent make one or as few as possible departures for the day (e.g., going straight from work to the grocery store or gym before returning home).

Set them up for success

Diet, systemic disease, and environment affect behavioral clinical signs. To that end, ensure that the pet's basic psychological and physical needs are served will set the pet parent and the dog up for success. Ensure the patient is getting a nutritious, well-balanced diet of appropriate amounts, adequate and healthy social experiences, and appropriate mental and physical stimulation.

One study found that there was correlation between the amount of exercise and the development of separation-related behaviors and noise sensitivity.[43] Dogs that received fewer daily walks were also found to spend more time alone and engage in fewer activities with the pet parents, thus the correlation may indicate that poorer overall quality of care or interaction with pet parents is related to SRD.[43] For patients that are receiving adequate exercise, switching up exercise routines so that they occur before departures instead of after departures could be helpful for some. A pilot study incorporating 15 minutes a day of exercise as part of a comprehensive behavioral therapy plan showed overall improvement in clinical signs; however, when compliance for exercise was assessed, the amount of exercise the dog received was not correlated with treatment success, implying that there was some benefit to the pet parent–dog relationship from exercise, but it was not a linear relationship, meaning that the number of minutes exercising was not correlated with a certain percentage improvement in behavioral clinical signs.[50] Given the paucity of evidence on exercise and the aforementioned need to keep recommendations to less than 5 for maximum compliance, this may be considered a low-priority endeavor, especially given pet parent time restrictions.

As suggested by the effect of parenting style on attachment disorders outlined earlier in this chapter, consistency and predictability may help contribute to a healthy attachment style. Educate pet parents on reading dog body language and how to respond appropriately so that they can assess and respond to their dog's emotional state appropriately, fostering predictability, anxiety relief, and a healthier attachment. This can be as simple as responding to calm, polite behaviors instead of nudgy ones with attention and other reinforcers. Furthermore, introducing structure and routine to the dog's day can go a long way in increasing predictability.

While no specific studies have looked at the effect of diet on SRD, ensuring appropriate quantity, quality, and appropriateness of diet helps to set the patient up for the least likelihood of physical problems (e.g., GI upset) or food-seeking problems contributing to any behavioral presentation. Veterinary calming-formulated diets might also be considered (see Chapters 12 and 13). Additionally, timing meals so that the pet is more motivated to participate in feeding as part of the treatment plan can be helpful. Many dogs with SRD are too anxious to eat during departures initially; therefore, increased appetite can be an indicator of improvement.[72]

Confinement

Confining the pet to a crate or small room in the home will prevent house soiling and destructive behavior in other areas of the home; however, many dogs with SRD have associated the crate with departures or have confinement distress/fear/ phobia. Therefore, confinement is generally contraindicated unless there is evidence that the dog does not panic and is comfortable and secure in the crate. Ideally, a safe place would be created in a place where the dog already feels comfortable. If a pet parent has not attempted letting the dog have free access to the home or part of the home and is willing to, then this can be trialed with video monitoring to assess results. Medications are often needed to facilitate giving the dog more freedom. Tethering should not be used and collars should be removed for any dog that has a history of destruction or escape attempts, as these can pose a strangulation risk.[72]

If confinement is absolutely needed but causes the pet stress, one approach is to continue to use the current confinement arrangement and trying to soften the experience as much as possible by providing treats, chews, puzzle toys, and favored toys in the area, then, at the same time, conditioning a sanctuary space (see below) within the home to use once the pet is comfortable in that location. The new conditioned sanctuary space is utilized in the context of teaching the pet to tolerate departures at the pace the dog can handle and thus avoid "spoiling" the safe location with needed departures in the old confinement arrangement. In addition, a specific desensitization and counterconditioning to crating plan may be needed, best administered under the guidance of a board-certified veterinary behaviorist, veterinary behavior technician, or skilled positive reinforcement trainer.

Protect the home

Nothing threatens the human–animal bond more in some of these cases than repeated and costly destruction of the pet parent's home and property (see Figures 17.8 and 17.9). If the dog is not confined during departures, prophylactic measures should be taken to prevent access to items that might be chewed or soiled. A goal of these protective measures is to buy time to institute the treatment plan for the desperate pet parent. If your pet parent elects to rehome or euthanize before you can find an effective medication protocol or condition the pet to tolerate departures, then the opportunity to help the pet is lost.

Protective measures are temporary for the families who opt for behavioral treatments as well as medications and management. For those who opt for medication and management alone, they will be permanent recommendations. For dogs that are destructive, blocking off areas, cabinets, and garbage cans with baby gates, exercise pens, and locks can be helpful. If there is a certain focal point of destruction, such as the front door, pet parents can put up purposefully destructible barriers to help protect their home, such as a stack of cardboard boxes, taped-up newspaper, foam, or easel paper pads for the dog to fixate on. Assess carefully with each pet parent what the relative foreign body risk is for the individual dog. Many of these dogs are swallowing drywall or wood anyway, so the relative increase risk in using a destructible is minimal. Other pet parents choose to install tougher barriers to protect their home, such as plexiglass or metal "scratch plates." Pull up blinds or remove them entirely, or block access to those areas. Place wood boards on couches if needed. Relative stress levels may need to be considered if confinement is the only option. As discussed

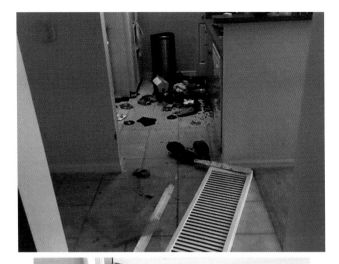

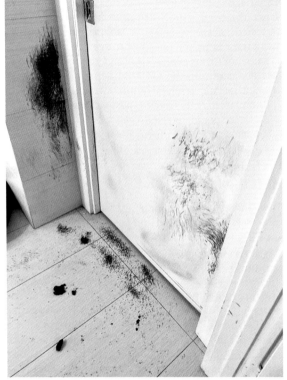

Figures 17.8 and 9 Damage to the home is distressing to pet parents and can cause serious injury to the pet. *(Attribution: Lisa Radosta, DVM, DACVB.)*

can be successful without a sanctuary space, ideally sanctuary space conditioning would be attempted in each patient. Once the pet has been conditioned to the sanctuary space and has a calm and relaxed physiologic response when exposed to that space, desensitization and counterconditioning to departures can begin. In this way, all practice departures will start from a place of relaxation, calm, and predictability, and the pet only has to contend with the auditory stimuli associated with departure, not additional visual stimuli.

For this to be successful, it must be completely conditioned before using it for departures or any other stressful event. To condition a sanctuary space, the dog should get daily exposure with positive consequences. The sanctuary space should be comfortable, with a bed, water bowl, food puzzle toys, other toys enjoyed by the pet, music (classical or whatever calms the pet), white noise (if the pet also has noise aversion), and calming scents such as lavender.[6,97] Sanctuary spaces can be fashioned for dogs and cats (see Figures 17.10 and 17.11).

An audio recording of the pet parent calmly speaking could be played, and a well-worn, unlaundered clothing item with the pet parent's scent on it should be placed on the dog's resting area. Both have been shown to decrease salivary cortisol levels in the first 5 minutes of a departure and potentially calm the dog.[34,98] If the dog is reactive to visual triggers out the windows, then blinds should be closed or window film put up to obscure the view. The goal is for the dog to calmly spend at least 10–15 minutes in that space on a daily basis without the pet parent's presence.

Variations can be made depending on the dog and pet parents' needs. If the plan is to have the dog confined to this space for real departures, then the practice sessions should include confinement in the space. If the dog does not

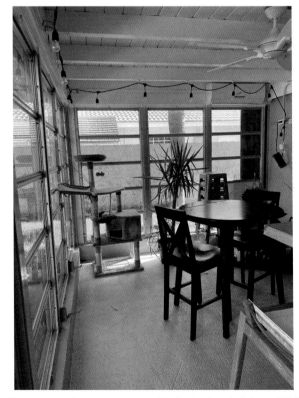

Figure 17.10 Cat sanctuary space. *(Attribution: Pamela Colareta, DVM.)*

above, dogs can cause serious self-injury attempting to escape the crate.

For dogs that house soil, sometimes enclosing them in a cleanable location is the easiest approach – such as a master bathroom or kitchen if they do not have distress with the confinement. Clean areas thoroughly. Place pee pads, indoor potty patches, or other waterproof barriers (e.g., tarps, shower curtains) over areas which have been soiled. Diapers or belly bands can be instituted for some pets; however, the pet parent should be careful to avoid urine scalding.

Sanctuary space

The sanctuary space is the foundation of creating a positive emotional response to departures. While treatment of SRD

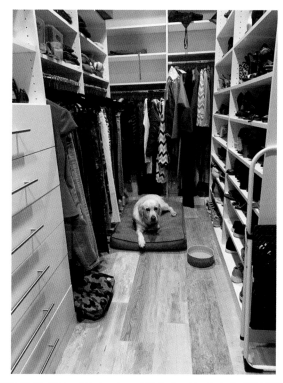

Figure 17.11 Dog sanctuary space. *(Attribution: Lisa Radosta, DVM, DACVB.)*

can use canned dog food, kibble mixed with water, chicken broth, low-fat yogurt, or other high-water content nontoxic foods. To make it last longer, the toy with the food in it can be frozen. Well packed and frozen, these can last 30–60 minutes.

When using the sanctuary space for real departures, the setup should look exactly the same as it does for the practice sessions, with the exception that the value of the food inside the food puzzle should be high and hard to resist. The dog should be placed in the space before the first signs of anxiety start, which may be prior to any identified predeparture cues. Ideally, the dog should be eating out of the food toy as the pet parent departs and immediately after the departure to get them through the hardest part of the departure for most dogs, which is the initial stages.

There are two options as to the *timing* of when to start using the sanctuary space for real departures. The first option, which is most ideal, is to only use this space in the context of desensitization and counterconditioning (DS/CC) to departures protocol and continue to have the dog elsewhere for real departures in the meantime. This is ideal because the sanctuary space becomes part of the strong "safety signal" to the pet for departures and is separate from the location where ongoing anxiety and fear is experienced. When fear is experienced in certain environments, the environment itself can be a trigger for anxiety in the future, known as contextual fear.[87] In an ideal world, we would eliminate risk of creating any contextual fear in the sanctuary space by waiting until the pet is truly ready to use it without distress. The down side of this strategy is that it can take weeks to months before the sanctuary space can be of help, and typically pet parents and dogs need some help right away.

For this reason, in many cases, we can successfully use the sanctuary space relatively quickly for real departures (in combination with anxiolytic medications) to try and combat the fear and anxiety with the positive conditioned emotional response which has been created. The pharmaceuticals plus the many pleasant practice sessions decrease the risk of creating a contextual fear in this space. Then, when the other therapies like relaxation and DS/CC to departures are ready, they can be worked within the sanctuary space. For severe cases or those with insufficient medication support, however, this may not be appropriate, and the sanctuary space should be combined with relaxation therapy and DS/CC to departures before being employed in real-life departures, otherwise the panic may override the positive conditioned emotional response to the space the pet parent has been working to obtain. Some pet parents elect to condition two sanctuary spaces, one for immediate use and one reserved for the DS/CC to departures plan. Others start using their sanctuary space right away but create a specific contextual safety signal when they are working the DS/CC plan (e.g., different music or scent).

experience distress when separated from the pet parents while everyone is still home, then the dog can be enclosed alone for the time that it takes him to finish his meal. If the dog would get distressed by being left alone in the space while the pet parent is home, then the pet parent should sit in the sanctuary space with the pet until they are able to be left alone. See below for more detailed descriptions of how to get the pet parent out of the room.

If containment is not needed, then doors can be left open. If the dog tends to pick up the food puzzle and move it out of the space, then the toy can be fixed in place to prevent this (e.g., use a leash passed through the Kong toy and then stuff with food) (Figure 17.12). Food toys are helpful because they are stuffed with food that motivates the dog. Pet parents

Vocalization

Products that suppress or punish barking, such as bark-activated shock and citronella collars or ultrasonic frequency bark, activated devices are contraindicated. These may stop the barking in some dogs but do not address the dog's underlying anxiety and fear. Furthermore, they can result in increased anxiety and over the long term, actually worsen

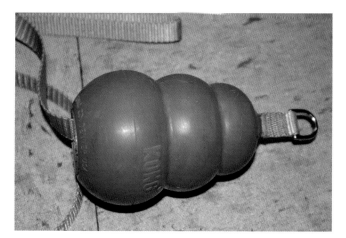

Figure 17.12 If the pet leaves the sanctuary space with the food toy during conditioning the food toy (not the pet) can be tied to something fixed. *(Attribution: Lisa Radosta.)*

signs of anxiety during departures and in other contexts. Many dogs with fear or anxiety bark through these anyway as they habituate to the punishment. Convincing pet parents whose residency is at risk in apartment complexes due to their dogs, barking behavior to NOT use these devices can be challenging. The best approach is to encourage the pet parent to use alternatives like day boarding, day care, and pet sitting for the pet, and to use short-acting medications immediately. Playing soothing music or white noise and keeping the pet away from doors and windows may reduce exposure to environmental stimuli that might trigger barking. Remote treat-dispensing devices may be creatively used to help reinforce quiet behavior by pet parents manually delivering treats through their phones or computers. Some even have settings that automatically deliver treats when the pet is not barking.

Adding another pet

In rare situations where the dog clearly enjoys the company of other dogs and is calmer with a dog present, providing another pet may alleviate signs of SRDs.[1,49] However, presence of a conspecific was not protective against the development of separation anxiety[7] and did not reduce time spent in anxiety during pet parent departure,[1] nor has occurrence of separation anxiety been correlated with another dog in the home.[40,74]

Pet parent departure and greeting behavior

Historically, it was thought to keep departures and homecomings low key or even ignore the dog to decrease the "emotional rollercoaster" associated with departures. Research is inconclusive as to whether pet parent greeting behavior affects greeting behavior of dogs.[77] In a laboratory test, talking and petting upon return of a familiar person resulted in elevated oxytocin levels and a more pronounced curve decrease in cortisol.[77] Petting and calm affection prior to departure was shown to decrease heart rate and extend calm behaviors after brief departures in dogs without SRDs in an unfamiliar environment but had no effect on salivary cortisol levels or distress behaviors.[99] Some pet parents may find it especially difficult to stay calm upon return home.[27] A more recent study has also shown that excitement and play during greetings and departures did not increase the development of SRDs.[100] This suggests that asking pet parents to not be affectionate upon return with their desperately seeking attention dogs may be a waste of time. Konok et al. postulated after analyzing attachment styles of pet parents of dogs with SRD that rejection of attachment behaviors by the dog might actually contribute to dog's stress and be related to their anxious attachment behaviors.[32] While providing attention at the time of departures and greeting does not contribute to the development of SRDs, attending to the dog with petting and verbal greeting without amping them up may be the best approach to the treatment for dogs with SRDs.[100]

Behavior modification

Relaxation therapy

Relaxation therapy is a cornerstone of treatment that can be used to give the dog a way to emotionally self-regulate (see online handout and list of handouts in Appendix C.). There are a variety of ways to perform relaxation therapies with multiple protocols proposed, to varying effect. Here we describe a goal-directed method of achieving a conditioned emotional response of relaxation to the presence of a mat when no distractions are around that can then be used in multiple anxiety or fear-provoking environments, departures among them. See Box 17.9.

To start, the pet parent should select a mat that the dog has no prior exposure to that is large enough for the dog to stretch out on comfortably and contains a nonslip backing. The mat should ideally be transportable and stored away out of sight between sessions. Yoga mats, bath mats, some crate pads, and small rugs work great. Lavender or pheromone analogues could be sprayed onto the mat before sessions to help ease anxiety and stress.

Pet parents should have low- to moderate-value treats – the dog's kibble might be a perfect choice so part of their regular ration can be used for sessions. Each treat can be no larger than the size of a pea. The dog just needs a taste for it to be an effective reinforcer. Treats should be kept out of sight of the dog during the sessions, either in a treat pouch or container on a counter. The pet parent should not reach to retrieve the treat until indicated in the protocol. Having a treat chronically in their hand can lead to a dog that gets very attentive to what that hand is doing, which can make relaxation very difficult. Avoid the use of clickers in this protocol as for many dogs, clickers are quite activating. Pet parents should practice in a quiet area of the home at a quiet time of the day when no other pets or distractions are around. Only once the protocol has been completed should it be used in stressful situations. The protocol described here assumes that the dog already knows a lie down cue reliably. If not, then the protocol will need to be modified under the guidance of a board-certified veterinary behaviorist, veterinary behavior technician, or skilled behavior modification trainer to help lure or capture a down.

Once relaxation is complete, the moment you place the mat down, the dog will trot onto the mat, lie down, and settle into a relaxation response within 1–3 minutes. Once this happens, the relaxation mat is ready for use with desensitization and counterconditioning to departures and other therapies as described below.

Independence therapies

For dogs that exhibit hyperattachment, independence therapies are important to help the dog "stand on its own 4 feet," so to speak. If these dogs cannot handle being in a separate room from the pet parents, then it may be too much to expect them to handle a full pet parent absence. We have multiple ways of teaching dogs to tolerate independence. Listed below are a few therapies, but no doubt many other creative options could be useful. Note that these treatments may not be indicated if a dog does not exhibit hyperattachment.

Demonstrations of independence. One simple way to foster independence is for the pet parent to reinforce calm independence and reward it. The reward may be anything the dog values, such as a piece of kibble or small treat tossed its way, a toy, a chew, a game, attention, pets, praise, walks, etc. The reinforcer does not need to be the same each time, just as long as the dog finds it motivating in the moment. Attention from their preferred person may be especially rewarding for some. Help your pet parent set a specific daily goal for how many times a day they will reinforce a demonstration of independence, say 30, 50, or 100. Counting out a fixed number of treats or pieces of kibble each morning and making sure the stash is used by the end of the day is one simple method to stick with the daily goal. Help your pet parent list out what will be considered demonstrations of independence for that dog. It may be as small as being willing to rest 4 feet away from the pet parent, or each step it takes away from the pet parent, to resting in a separate room or going into the yard alone. The criteria may change over time as the dog makes progress.

Shifting out of the sanctuary space. For those pet parents who have been staying with the pet during the practice sanctuary space sessions, once the pet is into the new routine, we can use this as an excellent base to work on independence. On day 1 of starting the shift out of the sanctuary space, the pet parent should sit one foot closer to the door than they typically have been for the duration of the sanctuary space session. If the dog is able to calmly continue eating like it has been and does not visually track the pet parent, stop eating, or move closer to the pet parent, then the next day, the pet parent should sit in the same location again. Once two to three successful sessions have been completed where the dog exhibits no sign of concern about the location of the pet parent, then on the next session, the pet parent should move one foot closer to the door. If at any point the dog appears to be monitoring the pet parents' whereabouts or demonstrates mild discomfort, the pet parent should stay where they are, not moving or talking to the pet. Some pets will work through this and settle back down. If the dog settles back down, the pet parent should reinforce that behavior by going back to their seat in the room. Then, the next repetition should be slightly less difficult. If the pet remains uncomfortable or experiences significant distress, end the session early, and then the pet parent should move back to the last position and repeat a few sessions with the patient comfortable there, before continuing forward with the protocol. Once the pet parent gets to the door, they should sit in the doorway with the door open, then in the doorway with the door half closed, then in the doorway with the door almost closed, then just on the other side of the door with the door almost closed, then on the other side of the door with the door fully closed, following the same progression described. Once out of the room, the pet parent can work farther away from the door as makes sense with their house arrangement. While in the room, the pet parent should largely ignore the dog and sit down and read, work on the computer, or otherwise engage in a stationary activity.

Independence games. Independence games are those which foster independent work or play. Examples include find it, tracking, and nosework. Information on these games can be found easily online.

Counterconditioning to being alone. This simple strategy can be used for food-motivated dogs that exhibit relatively mild concern about being without their pet parent and are willing to be away without stress when otherwise engaged. All it entails is providing the dog with food, a favored long-lasting chew, or other highly engaging item that the dog can enjoy by itself, which is given when the pet parent is not present.

If a pet parent is practicing sanctuary space, then this practice is inherently folded into that and need not be a separate exercise. If the dog experiences distress with the pet parent gone, picks up the item, and follows the pet parent, or stops engaging with the item, then either the item is not engaging enough or this dog needs a more graduated approach and this is not an appropriate therapy.

Desensitization and counterconditioning to the pet parent leaving the room. Any desensitization counterconditioning protocol should be performed under the guidance of a board-certified veterinary behaviorist, veterinary behavior technician, or skilled positive reinforcement-based trainer. As with all DS/CC therapies, if the dog is pushed too far too fast, then the plan could backfire and actually sensitize the patient to their pet parent leaving. See Chapter 10 for more detail on DS/CC. This exercise starts with a stationary behavior such as lying or sitting on a mat. A relaxation that is a useful tool for this purpose. The pet parent exposes the dog to longer and longer periods alone starting with 1 second. Remote treat dispensing devices can be very useful because they allow food rewards to be delivered without the pet parent being present, reinforcing at exactly the correct moment.

Desensitization and counterconditioning to departures. Desensitization and counterconditioning to full departures is the heart of treating SRD. The protocol proposed here is essentially an extension of the DS/CC plan for pet parent's leaving the room. In this protocol, the process extends to approaching the door, touching the door, exiting the door, potentially starting up a car and driving away and then the duration the pet parent is absent. Using the relaxation protocol described above as the base for this helps the patient not just tolerate but actually relax through the process. Video live streaming can be very helpful for a protocol like this so the pet parent can monitor the patient's body language through out a session.[6] Remote treat dispensing machines, some with cameras and the ability for pet parents to talk to their pet, can be valuable with these protocols. If not possible to use a remote treat dispensing device, then a treat can be delivered upon returning home if the pet is still relaxing on their mat.

A stepwise plan might look like this:
Setup:
Set up the relaxation mat in the pet's sanctuary space. The pet parent (monitoring the dog on live stream camera) walks out of the room, releases a treat from the remote treat dispenser, and returns. Repeat at the same level until there are three consecutive repetitions with the dog maintaining the relaxed body posture that is typical of the relaxation mat when not working on DS/CC. Take frequent breaks to facilitate learning.

1) Repeat with the pet parent walking up to the door.
2) Repeat with the pet parent walking up to the door and touching the doorknob.
3) Repeat with the pet parent opening the door.
4) Repeat with the pet parent going through the threshold of the door.
5) Repeat with the pet parent going through the door and almost closing the door.
6) Repeat with the pet parent going through the door and closing the door behind them.
7) Repeat with the pet parent going through the door and walking to the car.

8) Repeat with the pet parent exiting and getting in the car, closing the door behind them.

9) Repeat with the pet parent exiting, getting in, and starting the car.

10) Repeat with the pet parent driving down the driveway and returning.

11) Repeat with the pet parent driving down the street and returning.

12) Repeat with the pet parent driving around the block and returning.

13) Repeat with the pet parent absent for 5 minutes.

14) From there, slowly increase the time interval until a functional time is reached.

If at any point in the practice sessions the dog does not appear relaxed, the pet parent should stop and assess the situation. If the stress is mild, they should wait for the dog to calm down and then return to the dog. If the dog exhibits signs of outright distress, then the session should be stopped and at the next session, the pet parent should drop back to an easier step and continue moving forward.

This is just a sample plan, and what may work best for an individual varies. Some pets may need smaller steps or bigger ones. Others will need longer sessions or shorter ones. This is where having the skilled guidance of a practiced coach in the area can help ensure the plan moves along efficiently but not beyond what the patient can handle. This type of treatment is easily done incorrectly, which can cause the dog to be sensitized, not desensitized, to departures, making the clinical signs worsen. The value of an experienced practitioner cannot be overemphasized.

An alteration to this plan may look similar, but instead of distinctive repetitions with a remote treat dispensing device in practice sessions, the pet parent may elect to leave their dog with a long-lasting food puzzle and proceed with incrementally gradually longer departures, being sure to return before the food puzzle is finished and the pet gets distressed. Additionally, the presence of a food puzzle may provide some level of distraction and focus for the dog, which for some may be helpful. For other dogs, this distraction may work against our goals because they may be too distracted to learn or process that their person is leaving, then panic when the food puzzle is gone and they realize they are alone. Both a food puzzle and remote treat dispenser with even higher-value treats in it could be combined into one protocol as well.

Treatment plans with DS/CC protocols have established efficacy for treating SRD with decreased intensity of signs, longer duration of departures, and persistent improvement demonstrated three months after the completion of the treatment program.[50] Among these studies, there was variability in how quickly they reached treatment efficacy, what was considered treatment efficacy, duration of departures, and the use of counterconditioning and reinforcers. Despite this inconsistency, treatment can be quite successful.[50]

Predeparture cues

For many dogs, once desensitization and counterconditioning to departures is completed, the dog is comfortable with the whole process, and no work needs to be done on conditioning to predeparture cues. Thus, waiting to make it through the above protocols and reassessing the need for predeparture cue work can save the pet parent time, effort, and money. Additionally, working on predeparture cues too early in the process or only working on predeparture cues before the dog has become comfortable with departures themselves poses some risk. Some dogs become triggered by the predeparture cues because they are reliable predictors of the pet parent leaving. Unpredictability can contribute to the development of anxiety and frustration.[41,83] Take away this reliable predictor for them and you make departures more unpredictable and thus potentially more stressful! These anxious dogs are extremely perceptive to the environment, especially around the time of departure, because this information is very relevant to what feels like an imminent threat. The dog very well may learn to discern an alternative predeparture cue so as to relieve the chronic stress of the unpredictability. This results in a dog that just keeps accumulating new predeparture cues. Therefore, hiding the predeparture cue or mixing up how you do departures each time may intensify anxiety. Really, what we would like to be teaching these dogs is that "when we do departures this specific way, they are safe." Then the safety can be generalized and flexibly applied to more and more departures. When we practice sanctuary space and relaxation therapies and only use them in the context of "safe" departures, we are essentially giving them a new predeparture cue that indicates safety.[87] For all of these reasons, decoupling, desensitization, and counterconditioning are no longer widely recommended treatments for SRDs and instead are reserved for those dogs that do not completely respond to the treatments above.

Some dogs, however, really hone in on those predeparture cues, and even once they are much more tolerant of being alone, the predeparture cues still send them into a spiral of stress. These dogs likely have such a strong conditioned emotional response of distress to the cue that a sympathetic nervous system response is triggered by the cue itself. It has taken on its own meaning. For these dogs, we do really need to address the predeparture cues themselves and there are a few approaches on how to deal with this.

1) Management of predeparture cues. This essentially means changing up the pet parent's departure routine so that the dog is not exposed to the predeparture cue at all. For example, if a dog is set off by the pet parent picking up their purse, the purse can be left in the garage or the car. The dog does not see the purse and so is able to stay calm through the moment of departure.

2) Habituation to predeparture cues. This approach has been talked about a lot and historically has been advised; however, it is no longer generally recommended. With this approach, pet parents randomly engage in the predeparture cue but then do not leave. The goal is to decouple the predeparture cue with leaving so the activity is no longer predictive of a departure. For pets with moderate to significant anxiety, you risk increasing their anxiety because now, all of a sudden, departures have become more unpredictable (unless you have given them a very specific safety cue they can rely on).

3) Counterconditioning predeparture cues. This is one step up from habituation in that when the pet parent engages in the predeparture cue, they immediately follow up with returning to the pet and/or delivering a treat or other reinforcer. The goal is to outweigh the number of times the

predeparture cue is associated with something negative (a departure) to something positive (attention and a treat). For example, randomly throughout the day, the pet parent might pick up their keys and jingle them, then walk over to the dog wherever it is and drop a small piece of hot dog. This approach may be sufficient for many patients if they are not sent into a full-blown panic when the predeparture stimulus is shown.

4) DS/CC to predeparture cues. For those dogs with significant fear or phobia of the predeparture cue, a carefully constructed DS/CC plan may need to be followed to effectively calm this response.[91] This can be rolled into the DS/CC plan with departures, along with sanctuary space and relaxation work as well. This can take months and should be recommended only in the cases where it is necessary.

Medication

Medications are an important and powerful tool to immediately and chronically alleviate stress and treat SRD. See Chapters 11 and 12 for information on medications and supplements. Many pet parents cannot avoid departures completely while the behavioral therapies are still under way and thus, pet parents and dogs are left with sometimes intense, unavoidable distress. These dogs need your help and they need it now. There are two different general types of medications that can be used for the treatment of SRD; long-term medications and short-term or as-needed medications. Long-term medications are generally antidepressants such as, selective serotonin/norepinephrine reuptake inhibitors, and tricyclic antidepressants. Short-term, situational medications include benzodiazepines, alpha-2 agonists, phenothiazines, and gabapentin analogues. See Chapters 9 and 11 for information on indications for prescribing medications.

Fast-acting or as-needed medication

Fast-acting anxiolytic medications have an effect relatively quickly (30 minutes–2 hours) and may wear off relatively quickly (2–8 hours later). Fast-acting medications should be administered situationally so that the medication is causing an effect on the animal's emotional state prior to the time at which the anxiety about the pet parents' departure would usually begin. Anxiety, stress, and phobia can ramp up, so to speak. It is important to get ahead of the ramp-up by making sure that the medication is taking effect prior to the onset of fear, anxiety, stress, conflict, and panic. Therefore, situational use of medications in advance of departures may reduce anxiety and stress levels associated with the triggering events, prevent the ramping up of anxiety and arousal, and help to maintain a calmer emotional state throughout the departure.

Most patients will need a fast-acting medication in order to alleviate suffering immediately. Longer-acting medication will often be used with a faster-acting medication; however, longer-acting medications often take 4–8 weeks to be efficacious and that is too long for many patients to wait. While the goal is always for patients to be on as few medications at as low a dose as possible, the reality for many of these patients is that they will stay on a short-term and a long-term

medication for the duration of treatment. For some families, departures are infrequent enough and predictable enough, and the distress mild enough, that a long term is not needed and only a fast-acting anxiolytic is needed. And for others, just a daily or a combination of a daily and one or more fast-acting anxiolytics may be needed for the long haul to maintain a decent quality of life for the pet. Decisions about which medication and what type of medication to use are heavily influenced by a good history and discussing frankly the family's needs.

Benzodiazepines such as alprazolam, diazepam, or lorazepam may be useful for immediate control of clinical signs on a short-term or as-needed basis, approximately 1 hour prior to departure although for some medications, 1.5-2 hours is required. Duration of action can be anywhere from 3 to 8 hours, with alprazolam tending to be on the shorter side and diazepam and clonazepam on the longer side. They can be given alone but are more commonly used concurrently with the daily SSRI, SNRi or TCA. Clonidine, tasipimidine gabapentin, pregabalin, and trazodone may be beneficial prior to departures and are used commonly by veterinary behaviorists. Tasipimidine is approved for use in many European countries for short term alleviation of sitautional anxiety and fear in dogs triggered by owner departure. See Recommended Reading. These generally are given at least 1.5–2 hours prior to the onset of stressors and can last in the system for up to 8 hours. Oral transmucosal dexmedetomidine gel (Sileo, Zoetis) may be another good option and is on label for noise aversions, thus has a substantial body of data supporting its safety and efficacy for situational anxieties in dogs. This should be given approximately 30 minutes prior to the first sign of departure and may only last 2 hours. Choice of fast-acting anxiolytic depends on clinical signs the pet exhibits, duration of departures the medication is needed for, how long in advance the pet parent is able to predose, duration of action of the particular medication in the particular dog, and effects and side effects of the medication in the particular dog. Choice is certainly influenced by concurrent medications, underlying medical conditions, and comfort level with prescribing controlled substances. Sometimes polypharmacy is needed.

Phenothiazines block dopamine receptors in the brain, causing a nonspecific depression of the central nervous system, resulting in a reduction of motor function and reduced awareness of external stimuli. They do not reduce anxiety. For those reasons, they are considered adjunctive treatments, and their use should be limited to those cases where additional sedation might be needed, such as when significant self-injury or significant property damage is occurring, in conjunction with medications which do affect anxiety. For further details on the selection, use, timing (and references) for the situational or as-needed use of drugs, see Chapters 9 and 11.

Daily medications

Indications for prescribing long-term medications would include unpredictability of pet parent schedule, if the pet is at risk of harming itself or at risk of euthanasia or relinquishment, inability to premedicate prior to departures, chronicity of the disorder, comorbidities with other behavior disorders which will complicate treatment, and an environment which is not conducive to a positive outcome. As noted above, assessment of systemic disease prior to starting treatment is critical. With that said, animals with SRDs are suffering and they are at high risk of relinquishment. Treatment should not be delayed unless there is a medical reason to do so. For example, a short-term medication can be started while the veterinarian waits for the results of the lab work to come back. When lab work results come in, a long-term medication can be started.

The medications presently approved for separation anxiety in dogs in combination with behavior modification include the SSRI fluoxetine (Reconcile, PRN Pharmaceuticals) and the TCA clomipramine (Clomicalm).[95,101] In one study, fluoxetine was compared to placebo with no concurrent behavior modification and, while a significant drug effect was demonstrated, greater and more significant improvement was achieved using a combination of behavior modification and fluoxetine, emphasizing the importance of behavior modification and management in positive outcomes.[101] Other SSRIs, such as paroxetine and sertraline, may also be effective but have not been tested in clinical trials. Amitriptyline is generally not used as it appears to be less effective than fluoxetine or clomipramine at treating SRD (56% success rate in the former versus 75% in the latter) and has a wider scope of side effects than most SSRIs.[37,90]

While improvement may begin to be seen in 1–2 weeks, generally 4–8 weeks are required to achieve optimal clinical effects and, in most cases, drugs may need to be maintained for several months or longer. In one follow-up study, some dogs remained on clomipramine for over a year with no adverse effects and 10 of 12 dogs improved further over that time.[90]

Effective medications should be continued in dogs until the pet has stabilized and remains stable for at least six months. At that point, a slow wean can be considered. Weaning protocols vary but depending on duration of medication use, dose, and individual drug, generally a dose drop of ~25% every 1–4 weeks is reasonable. Video monitor as the wean is underway to ensure no relapse. If relapse occurs, keep the pet on the minimum effective dose. These medications can be used long term (years) as long as the pet does not develop a contraindication and lab work is routinely performed every 6–12 months or more often as medically indicated.

Natural supplements and pheromone analogues

Natural supplements, aromatherapy, and music therapy that might aid in calming or alleviating stress (see Chapter 12 for administration details) can also be used adjunctively prior to departures or on a daily basis; however, these supplements alone most likely will not provide sufficient anxiolysis for pets with SRDs.

Conflicting evidence exists as to whether dog-appeasing pheromone (Adaptil) could be helpful for ameliorating separation-related distress (see Chapter 12). Adaptil has been demonstrated to improve signs of separation anxiety in conjunction with behavior modification at a level similar to clomipramine in one study. However, it showed little effect on behavior, heart rate, and temperature with pet parent separation in another.[102] Given that Adaptil is essentially a risk-free intervention, if finances are not a concern and the pet parent wants to implement everything possible, Adaptil can be utilized. If the pet parent has financial concerns or is overwhelmed by the treatment process already, dog-appeasing pheromone may not be a priority treatment.

CASE EXAMPLE

Presentation

Melvina, a 3-year-old, 20 kg, spayed female mixed-breed dog was presented for destructive behavior and excessive vocalization when Caroline, the pet parent, departed the home.

History

Melvina's clinical signs started soon after her pet parent, Caroline, went back to work following summer break from her job as a teacher at a school. Melvina was constantly at Caroline's side whenever she was home and frequently nudged, pawed, or whined to get attention from her. Caroline could not even take a shower without Melvina whining at the door to be let in. If Caroline got up to get a snack or check on something in another room, even out of a deep sleep, Melvina would startle up into a stand and walk with Caroline. When Melvina observed the pet parent put on a specific pair of shoes and pick up her purse, she would pace, pant, whine, and body block her pet parent from exiting the front door. While the pet parent was at work, she would bark, pace, scratch, and chew at the front door and occasionally chew holes in pillows and stuffed furniture. Upon the pet parent's arrival, Melvina became extremely excited, running in big loops around the room, jumping over the coffee table. The panic behaviors occurred every time Caroline left Melvina and at no other times when Caroline was home.

Caroline had tried a few things to help the situation, but all had failed. She had tried crating Melvina but that just resulted in her chewing at the bars of the crate, eventually fracturing two teeth and vocalizing louder when she was alone. She tried leaving an ultrasonic noise maker that activated when Melvina barked. Melvina barked less with this on but continued to whine, pace, and destroy the home, so that was discontinued. Caroline had tried to drop her off at her sister's house to spend the day with her and her dog, but the pacing, whining, and trembling occurred, nonetheless.

At presentation Caroline had run out of ideas and was in a desperate state. She could not even go to the grocery store without fear of something else in her home being ruined or Melvina hurting herself. She needed help and she needed help immediately. She was doing what she could to avoid extra departures, but she could not stay home with Melvina during the workday. She had collected video of one workday and Melvina exhibited all the described behaviors, plus excessive panting and visual scanning. She was not observed to lie down until 5 hours into the departure, at which point she fell asleep, exhausted.

Workup

Melvina's physical examination, fecal antigen, and lab work were within normal limits.

Differential diagnosis

The differential diagnoses include: noise aversion, separation anxiety, separation fear, separation phobia, hyperattachment, generalized anxiety, frustration, attention-seeking behavior, confinement distress, and

CASE EXAMPLE—cont'd

territorial behavior. Melvina was diagnosed with separation phobia and hyperattachment.

Treatment

Caroline was instructed to start working on the sanctuary space therapy right away and test out what Melvina's favorite foods were so they could be stuffed into puzzle toys for real departures. The relaxation protocol and independence building were recommended. The pet parent was coached on clear, effective, simple communication with Melvina, how to read dog body language, and clicker training. Caroline and Melvina were referred to a positive reinforcement trainer who was experienced with separation anxiety to help them implement the plan.

Clonidine was initiated at 0.01 mg/kg PO 2 hours prior to Caroline leaving for work, with instructions that she could titrate up to 0.03 mg/kg if needed and no side effects. Reconcile (1 mg/kg PO SID) was started three days later, once Caroline was able to determine there were no side effects and the most efficacious dose of the clonidine. Caroline stacked boxes of cardboard up against the front door in an attempt to refocus Melvina's destructive behavior. Caroline was to continue video monitoring departures to watch for response to treatment.

Follow-up

The veterinary technician called Caroline later that week. Within four days of initiating treatment, Melvina was improved. She still exhibited the same stress behaviors as Caroline was preparing to leave, but her behavior during the departures was improved. Immediately after Caroline left, she was knocking the boxes down and spent 5–10 minutes tearing them up. Then, after standing and staring at the front door and whining for another few minutes, she was able to go into her sanctuary space and engage with her food puzzle for 30 minutes. After the food puzzle was empty, she paced for 10–15 minutes and then settled down for a nap on her bed in her sanctuary space. Occasionally, through the rest of the departure, she would get up to pace around and then settle back down. Melvina was assessed as improved but still experiencing distress. Caroline was then instructed to increase the clonidine dose to 0.04-0.05 mg/kg PO 2 hours prior to departures.

In five weeks, Melvina came in for a reevaluation. By this time, Caroline could tell the Reconcile was having an effect, and the relaxation mat was ready to be used as a base for a desensitization and counterconditioning program to departures. Under careful guidance of the dog training professional to whom she was referred, Caroline progressed from putting on her shoes and exiting the home to departures of 20-30 minutes, duration while Melvina remained relaxed in her sanctuary space working on her food puzzles. Occasionally, she would look up and alert as if she was listening for a few moments, but then would return to her food puzzle or lie back down and drowse. Caroline successfully weaned Melvina off the predeparture clonidine at this time, and she was maintained on her Reconcile long-term.

Conclusion

Separation anxiety is most likely more complex than we had assumed in years past. By separating out diagnosis into more specific categories, treatment can be personalized for the pet. Cats can be affected by SRDs, although at this time, not to the extent that we appreciate it in dogs. More research is needed in cats. Medications, management, and behavior modification are necessary for the best outcome.

References

1. van Rooy D, Arnott ER, Thomson PC, et al. Using a pet parent-based questionnaire to phenotype dogs with separation-related distress: do pet parents know what their dogs do when they are absent? *J Vet Behav*. 2018;23:58–65.

2. Ogata N. Review: separation anxiety in dogs: what progress has been made in our understanding of the most common behavioral problems in dogs? *J Vet Behav*. 2016;16:28–35.

3. Schwartz S. Separation anxiety syndrome in cats: 136 cases (1991–2000). *J Am Vet Med Assoc*. 2002;220(7):1028–1033.

4. Sherman BL, Mills DS. Canine anxieties and phobias: an update on separation anxiety and noise aversions. *Vet Clin North Am Small Anim Pract*. 2008;38:1081–1107.

5. Horwitz D. Separation anxiety syndrome. In: Tilley LP, Smith FWK, Sleeper MM, et al. eds. *Blackwell's 5 Minute Veterinary Consult: Canine and Feline*. 7th ed. New Jersey: John Wiley and Sons; 2021: 1231–1234.

6. Ballantyne KC. Separation, confinement, or noises: what is scaring that dog? *Vet Clin North Am Small Anim Pract*. 2018;48: 367–386.

7. Herron ME, Lord LK, Husseini SE. Effects of preadoption counseling on the prevention of separation anxiety in newly adopted shelter dogs. *J Vet Behav*. 2014;9:13–21.

8. de Assis LS, Matos R, Pike TW, et al. Developing diagnostic frameworks in veterinary behavioral medicine: disambiguating separation related problems in dogs. *Front Vet Sci*. 2020; 6(January):499. doi:10.3389/fvets.2019.00499.

9. Marx A, Lenkei R, Pérez Fraga P, et al. Age-dependent changes in dogs' (Canis familiaris) separation-related behaviours in a longitudinal study. *Appl Anim Behav Sci*. 2021;242:105422.

10. de Souza Machado D, Oliveira PMB, Machado JC, et al. Identification of separation-related problems in domestic cats: a questionnaire survey. *PLoS One*. 2020;15(4):e0230999. doi: 10.1371/journal.pone.0230999.

11. Konok V, Marx A, Faragó T. Attachment styles in dogs and their relationship with separation-related disorder–a questionnaire based clustering. *Appl Anim Behav Sci*. 2019;213:81–90.

12. Pongrácz P, Gómez SA, Lenkei R. Separation-related behaviour indicates the effect of functional breed selection in dogs (Canis familiaris). *Appl Anim Behav Sci*. 2020;222:104884.

13. Buller K, Ballantyne KC. Living with and loving a pet with behavioral problems: pet owners' experiences. *J Vet Behav*. 2020;37:41–47.

14. Cannas S, Talamonti Z, Mazzola S, et al. Factors associated with dog behavioral problems referred to a behavior clinic. *J Vet Behav*. 2018;24:42–47.

15. Doane M, Sarenbo S. A modified combined C-BARQ and QoL for both the companion dog and its owner. An embryo to a companion dog welfare assessment? *Appl Anim Behav Sci*. 2019; 213:91–106.

16. van Rooy D, Haase B, McGreevy PD, et al. Evaluating candidate genes oprm1, drd2, avpr1a, and oxtr in golden retrievers with separation-related behaviors. *J Vet Behav*. 2016;16:22–27.

17. Storengen LM, Boge SCK, Strøm SJ, et al. A descriptive study of 215 dogs diagnosed with separation anxiety. *Appl Anim Behav Sci*. 2014;159:82–89.

18. Denenberg S, Landsberg GM, Horwitz D. A comparison of cases referred to behaviorists in three different countries. In: Mills D, Levine E, Landsberg GM, et al. eds. *Current Issues and Research in Veterinary Behavioral Medicine.* West Lafayette, Ind: Purdue University Press; 2005:56–62.

19. Tiira K, Sulkama S, Lohi H. Prevalence, comorbidity, and behavioral variation in canine anxiety. *J Vet Behav.* 2016;16:36–44.

20. Dinwoodie IR, Dwyer B, Zottola V, et al. Demographics and comorbidity of behavior problems in dogs. *J Vet Behav.* 2019;32:62–71.

21. Bradshaw JWS, McPherson JA, Casey RA, et al. Aetiology of separation-related behaviour problems in domestic dogs. *Vet Rec.* 2002;151:43–46.

22. Konok V, Kosztolányi A, Rainer W, et al. Influence of owners' attachment style and personality on their dogs' (*Canis familiaris*) separation-related disorder. *PLoS One.* 2015;10:e0118375.

23. Salonen M, Sulkama S, Mikkola S, et al. Prevalence, comorbidity, and breed differences in canine anxiety in 13,700 Finnish pet dogs. *Sci Rep.* 2020;10:2962. doi:10.1038/s41598-020-59837-z.

24. Landsberg G. The most common behavior problems in older dogs. *Vet Med.* 1995;90(suppl):16–24.

25. Mongillo P, Pitteri E, Carnier P, et al. Does the attachment system toward owners change in aged dogs? *Physiol Behav.* 2013;120:64–69.

26. Eriksson M, Keeling L, Tehn T. Cats and owners interact more with each other after a longer duration of separation. *PLoS One.* 2017;12(10):e0185599. doi: 10.1371/journal.pone.0185599.

27. Blackwell EJ, Casey RA, Bradshaw JW. Efficacy of written behavioral advice for separation-related behavior problems in dogs newly adopted from a rehoming center. *J Vet Behav.* 2016;12:13–19.

28. Kurachi T, Irimajiri M, Mizuta Y, et al. Dogs predisposed to anxiety disorders and related factors in Japan. *Appl Anim Behav Sci.* 2017;196:69–75.

29. McCrave EA. Diagnostic criteria for separation anxiety in the dog. *Vet Clin North Am Small Anim Pract.* 1991;21:247–255.

30. Diesel G, Brodbelt D, Pfeiffer DU. Characteristics of relinquished dogs and their owners at 14 rehoming centers in the United Kingdom. *J Appl Anin Welf Sci.* 2010;13:15–30.

31. Segurson SA, Serpell JA, Hart BJ. Evaluation of a behavioral assessment questionnaire for use in the characterization of behavioral problems of dogs relinquished to animal shelters. *J Am Vet Med Assoc.* 2005;227:1755–1761.

32. Marder AR, VanDriel M, Engel J. A comparison of canine behavior in pre-adoptive and post-adoptive homes. In: Mills D, Levine E, eds. *Current Issues and Research in Veterinary Behavioral Medicine.* West Lafayette, Indiana: Purdue University Press; 2005:262–263.

33. Prato-Previde EP, Valsechhi P. Effect of abandonment on attachment behaviour of pet dogs. In: Landsberg G, et al. eds. *Proc 6th IVBM-CA, Brescia, Italy: Fondazione Iniziative Zooprofilattiche e Zootechniche.* 2007:31–32.

34. Prato-Previde E, Spiezio C, Sabatini F, et al. Is the dog-human relationship an attachment bond? An observational study using Ainsworth's strange situation. *Behaviour.* 2003;140:225–254.

35. McMillan FD, Serpell JA, Duffy DL, et al. Differences in behavioral characteristics between dogs obtained as puppies from pet stores and those obtained from noncommercial breeders. *J Am Vet Med Assoc.* 2013;242:1359–1363.

36. Konok V, Dóka A, Miklósi Á. The behavior of the domestic dog (*Canis familiaris*) during separation from and reunion with the owner: a questionnaire and an experimental study. *Appl Anim Behav Sci.* 2011;135:300–308.

37. Takeuchi Y, Ogata N, Houpt KA, et al. Differences in background and outcome of three behavior problems of dogs. *Appl Anim Behav Sci.* 2001;70:297–308.

38. Overall KL, Dunham AE, Frank D. Frequency of nonspecific clinical signs in dogs with separation anxiety, thunderstorm phobia, and noise phobia, alone or in combination. *J Am Vet Med Assoc.* 2001;219:467–473.

39. McGreevy PD, Masters AM. Risk factors for separation-related distress and feed-related aggression in dogs: additional findings from a survey of Australian dog owners. *Appl Anim Behav Sci.* 2008;109:320–328.

40. Flannigan G, Dodman NH. Risk factors and behaviors associated with separation anxiety in dogs. *J Am Vet Med Assoc.* 2001;219:4604–4606.

41. Dietz L, Arnold A-MK, Goerlich-Jansson VC, et al. The importance of early life experiences for the development of behavioural disorders in domestic dogs. *Behaviour.* 2018;155:83–114.

42. Serpell JA, Jagoe JA. Early experience and the development of behaviour. In: Serpell JA, ed. *The Domestic Dog; Its Evolution, Behaviour and Interactions with People.* Cambridge: Cambridge University Press; 1995:131–138.

43. Tiira K, Lohi H. Early life experiences and exercise associate with canine anxieties. *PLoS One.* 2015;10:e0141907.

44. Clark GI, Boyer WN. The effects of dog obedience training and behavioural counseling upon the human–canine relationship. *Appl Anim Behav Sci.* 1993;37:147–159.

45. Blackwell EJ, Twells C, Seawright A, et al. The relationship between training methods and the occurrence of behaviour problems as reported by owners, in a population of domestic dogs. *J Vet Behav.* 2008;3:207–217.

46. Jagoe A, Serpell J. Owner characteristics and interactions and the prevalence of canine behavior problems. *Appl Anim Behav Sci.* 1996;47:31–42.

47. Dodman NH, Brown DC, Serpell JA. Associations between owner personality and psychological status and the prevalence of canine behavior problems. *PLoS One.* 2018;13(2):e0192846. doi:10.1371/journal. pone.0192846.

48. Lenkei R, Alvarez Gomez S, Pongrácz P. Fear vs. frustration – possible factors behind canine separation related behaviour. *Behav Process.* 2018;157:115–124.

49. Mariti C, Ricci E, Carlone B, et al. Dog attachment to man: a comparison between pet and working dogs. *J Vet Behav.* 2013;8:135–145.

50. Butler R, Sargisson RJ, Elliffe D. The efficacy of systematic desensitization for treating the separation-related problem behaviour of domestic dogs. *Appl Anim Behav Sci.* 2011;129:136–145.

51. Overall KL, Hamilton SP, Change ML. Understanding the genetic basis of canine anxiety: phenotyping dogs for behavioral, neurochemical, and genetic assessment. *J Vet Behav.* 2006;1:124–141.

52. Vaterlaws-Whiteside H, Hartmann A. Improving puppy behavior using a new standardized socialization program. *Appl Anim Behav Sci.* 2017;197:55–61.

53. Blackwell EJ, Bradshaw JWS, Casey RA. Fear responses to noises in domestic dogs: prevalence, risk factors and cooccurrence with other fear related behaviour. *Appl Anim Behav Sci.* 2013;145:15–25.

54. Zapata I, Serpell JA, Alvarez CE. Genetic mapping of canine fear and aggression. *BMC genomics.* 2016;17:572. doi:10.1186/s12864-016-2936-3.

55. Appleby D, Plujimakers J. Separation anxiety in dogs. The function of homeostasis in its development and treatment. *Vet Clin North Am Small Anim Pract.* 2003;33:321–344.

56. Parthasarathy V, Crowell-Davis S. Relationship between attachment to owners and separation anxiety in pet dogs (Canis lupus familiaris). *J Vet Behav.* 2006;1:109–120.

57. Kis A, Bence M, Lakatos G, et al. Oxytocin receptor gene polymorphisms are associated with human directed social behavior in dogs (Canis familiaris). *PLoS One.* 2014;9(1):e83993. doi: 10.1371/journal.pone.0083993.

58. Ainsworth MDS. Object relations, dependency, and attachment: a theoretical review of the infant-mother relationship. *Child Dev.* 1969;969–1025.

59. Ainsworth MDS, Bell SM. Attachment, exploration, and separation: illustrated by the behavior of one-year-olds in a strange situation. *Child Dev.* 1970;49–67.

60. Solomon J, Beetz A, Schöberl I, et al. Attachment security in companion dogs: adaptation of Ainsworth's strange situation and classification procedures to dogs and their human caregivers. *Attach Hum Dev.* 2019;21:389–417.

61. Schöberl I, Beetz A, Solomon J, et al. Social factors influencing cortisol modulation in dogs during a strange situation procedure. *J Vet Behav.* 2016;11:77–85.

62. Gácsi M, Maros K, Sernkvist S, et al. Human analogue safe haven effect of the owner: behavioral and heart rate response to stressful social stimuli in dogs. *PLoS One.* 2013;8(3):e58475. doi: 10.1371/journal.pone.0058475.

63. Mariti C, Ricci E, Zilocchi M, et al. Owners as a secure base for their dogs. *Behaviour.* 2013;150:1275–1294.

64. Hofmann SG, Ellard KK, Siegle GJ. Neurobiological correlates of cognitions in fear and anxiety: a cognitive–neurobiological information-processing model. *Cogn Emot.* 2012;26:282–299.

65. Edwards C, Heiblum M, Tejeda A. Experimental evaluation of attachment behaviors in owned cats. *J Vet Behav.* 2007;2:119–125.

66. Potter A, Mills DS. Domestic cats (Felis silvestris catus) do not show signs of secure attachment to their owners. *PLoS One.* 2015. doi:10.1371/journal.pone.0135109.

67. Wedl M, Bauer B, Gracey D. Factors influencing the temporal patterns of dyadic behaviours and interactions between domestic cats and their owners. *Behav Process.* 2011;86:58–67.

68. Main M, Soloman J. Procedures for identifying infants as disorganized/disoriented during the Ainsworth Strange Situation. In: Cicchetti D, Cummings EM, Greenberg MT, eds. *Theory, Research and Intervention.* Chicago: University of Chicago Press; 1993.

69. Harvey ND, Craigon PJ, Blythe SA, England GC, et al. Social rearing environment influences dog behavioral development. *J Vet Behav.* 2016;16:13–21.

70. Lund DJ, Jorgensen MC. Behavior patterns and time course of activity in dogs with separation problems. *Appl Anim Behav Sci.* 1999;63:219–236.

71. Pongrácz P, Lenkei R, Andras M, et al. Should I whine or should I bark? Qualitative and quantitative differences between the vocalizations of dogs with and without separation related symptoms. *Appl Anim Behav Sci.* 2017;196:61–68.

72. Overall K. *Manual of Clinical Behavioral Medicine for Dogs and Cats-e book.* Elsevier Health Sciences; 2013.

73. Mendl M, Brooks J, Basse C, et al. Dogs showing separation-related behaviour exhibit a 'pessimistic' cognitive bias. *Curr Biol.* 2010;20:R839-R840.

74. Palestrini C, Minero M, Cannas S, et al. Video analysis of dogs with separation related behaviors. *Appl Anim Behav Sci.* 2010:124:61–67.

75. Cannas S, Frank D, Minero M. Video analysis of dogs suffering from anxiety when left home alone and treated with clomipramine. *J Vet Behav.* 2014:9:50–57.

76. Scaglia E, Cannas S, Minero M, et al. Video analysis of adult dogs when left home alone. *J Vet Behav.* 2013;8:412–417.

77. Rehn T, Handlin L, Uvnäs-Moberg K, et al. Dogs' endocrine and behavioural responses at reunion are affected by how the human initiates contact. *Physiol Behav.* 2014;124:45–53.

78. Cannas S, Frank D, Minero M, et al. Puppy behavior when left alone: changes during the first few months after adoption. *J Vet Behav.* 2010;5:94–100.

79. Moesta A, Kim G, Wilson-Frank CR, et al. Comparison of serum brain-derived neurotrophic factor in dogs with and without separation anxiety. *J Vet Behav.* 2020;35:14–18.

80. Takeuchi Y, Houpt KA, Scarlett JM. Evaluation of treatments for separation anxiety in dogs. *J Am Vet Med Assoc.* 2000;217:342–345.

81. Seksel K. Separation anxiety in dogs and cats with reference to homeostasis. Veterinary Behavior Chapter Proceedings, *Science Week.* 2013;22.

82. Sylvers P, Lilienfeld SO, LaPrairie JL. Differences between trait fear and trait anxiety: Implications for psychopathology. *Clin Psychol Rev.* 2011;31:122–137.

83. Davis M, Walker DL, Miles L, et al. Phasic vs sustained fear in rats and humans: role of the extended amygdala in fear vs anxiety. *Neuropsychopharmacology.* 2010;35: 105–135.

84. Ekman, P. An argument for basic emotions. *Cogn Emot.* 1992:6:169–200.

85. Blackford JU, Pine DS. Neural substrates of childhood anxiety disorders: a review of neuroimaging findings. *Child Adolesc Psychiatr Clin N Am.* 2012;21:501–525.

86. Chua P, Krams M, Toni I, et al. A functional anatomy of anticipatory anxiety. *Neuroimage.* 1999;9:563–571.

87. Amat M, Camps T, Brech SL, et al. Separation anxiety in dogs: the implications of predictability and contextual fear for behavioural treatment. *Anim Welf.* 2014;23:263–266.

88. Mariti C, Carlone B, Ricci E, et al. Intraspecific attachment in adult domestic dogs (Canis familiaris): preliminary results. *Appl Anim Behav Sci.* 2014;152:64–72.

89. Blackwell E, Casey RA, Bradshaw JW. Controlled trial of behavioural therapy for separation-related disorders in dogs. *Vet Rec.* 2006;158:551–554.

90. King JN, Simpson BS, Overall KL, et al. Treatment of separation anxiety in dogs with clomipramine: results from a prospective, randomised, double-blind, placebo-controlled, parallel-group multicenter clinical trial. *Appl Anim Behav Sci.* 2000;67:255–275.

91. Mundell P, Liu S, Guérin NA, et al. An automated behavior shaping intervention reduces signs of separation anxiety-related distress in a mixed-breed dog. *J Vet Behav.* 2020;37:71–75.

92. Irimajiri M, Crowell-Davis SL. Animal behavior case of the month. Separation anxiety. *J Am Vet Med Assoc.* 2014;245:1007–1009.

93. King JN, Overall KL, Appleby BS, et al. Results of a follow-up investigation to a clinical trial testing the efficacy of clomipramine in the treatment of separation anxiety. *Appl Anim Behav Sci.* 2004;89:233–242.

94. Karagiannis CI, Burman OH, Mills DS. Dogs with separation-related problems show a "less pessimistic" cognitive bias during treatment with fluoxetine (Reconcile™) and a behaviour modification plan. *BMC Vet Res.* 2015;11:80. doi:10.1186/s12917-015-0373-1.

95. Landsberg GM, Melese P, Sherman BL. Effectiveness of fluoxetine chewable tablets in the treatment of canine separation anxiety. *J Vet Behav.* 2008;3:12–19.

96. Horowitz A. Disambiguating guilty looks; salient prompts to a familiar dog behavior. *Behav Process.* 2009;8: 447–452.

97. Komiya M, Sugiyama A, Tanabe K, Uchino T, Takeuchi T. Evaluation of the effect of topical application of lavender oil on autonomic nerve activity in dogs. *Am J Vet Res.* 2009;70(6): 764–769.

98. Shin YJ, Shin NS. Evaluation of effects of olfactory and auditory stimulation on separation anxiety by salivary cortisol measurement in dogs. *J Vet Sci.* 2016;17: 153–158.

99. Mariti C, Carlone B, Protti M, et al. Effects of petting before a brief separation from the owner on dog behavior and physiology: a pilot study. *J Vet Behav.* 2018;27:41–46.

100. Texeira AR, Hall NJ. Effect of greeting and departure interactions on the development of increased separation-related behaviors in newly adopted adult dogs. *J Vet Behav.* 2021;41:22–32.

101. Podberscek AL, Hsu Y, Serpell JA. Evaluation of clomipramine as an adjunct to behavioural therapy in the treatment of separation related problems in dogs. *Vet Rec.* 1999;145: 365–369.

102. Taylor S, Webb L, Montrose VT, et al. the behavioral and physiological effects of dog appeasing pheromone upon canine behavior during separation from owner. *J Vet Behav.* 2020;40:36–42.

Resources and recommended reading

European Medicines Agency. Tessie (tasipimidine). https://www.ema.europa.eu/en/medicines/veterinary/EPAR/tessie.

Korpivaara M, Huhtinen M, Pohjanjousi P, et al. Tasipimidine, a novel orally dosed alpha-2 Adrenoceptor agonist, alleviates separation anxiety in dogs - a 5-week study. *Proc 3rd European Veterinary Congress of Behavioural Medicine and Animal Welfare* [Online]. October 7-9, 2021:151–152.

Linsetedt J, Kirjavainen M, Korpivaara M. Concurrent use of tasipimidine and clomipramine - an interaction study. *Proc 4th Annual Meeting of the European Veterinary Congress of Behavioural Medicine and Animal Welfare,* Palma, Mallorca: October 28th-31st 2022:123.

Meneses T, Robinson J, Rose J, et al. Review of epidemiological, pathological, genetic, and epigenetic factors that may contribute to the development of separation anxiety in dogs. *J Am Vet Med Assoc.* 2021;259(10):1118–1128.

Meneses T, Robinson J, Rose J, et al. Development of and pharmacological treatment option and future research opportunities for separation anxiety in dogs. *J Am Vet Med Assoc.* 2021;259(10):1130–1139.

CHAPTER 18

Abnormal repetitive behaviors: stereotypies and compulsive disorders

Valarie V. Tynes, DVM, DACVB, DACAW

Chapter contents

Introduction

The terms stereotypy and compulsive disorder (CD) refer to a group of heterogenous behaviors that have both been described as repetitive, invariant, occurring out of context, and appearing to be purposeless or functionless. The actual definitions of stereotypies and CDs in the veterinary literature often overlap creating confusion. In many cases, the words are used interchangeably. The result is a lack of clear diagnostic criteria that differentiates stereotypies from CD in animals. At times, the definitions have led to the suggestion that stereotypies and CDs may lie on a spectrum of behavior, but more current information suggests that these different conditions arise from pathology in different areas of the

brain.[1] Since the diagnosis of stereotypies and CDs is phenotypic (based on observable signs) and so little is known regarding the actual neurobiology or pathophysiology of the conditions, the term "abnormal repetitive behaviors" has been suggested and will be used throughout this chapter.[2,3]

Traditionally, our understanding, categorization, and descriptions of many abnormal animal behaviors have been based on our knowledge of similar conditions in human mental disorders. Many of the conditions appear analogous (performing a similar function but having a different evolutionary origin) and many appear homologous (similar in evolutionary origin but not necessarily in function) to human mental disorders. Structural and functional elements of neural systems are highly conserved across vertebrate species, so it is logical that some mammals and birds might exhibit similar neuropsychiatric conditions to humans.[4] Animal models for some human psychiatric diseases have been validated and can aid in our understanding of these conditions. However, when faced with a pet performing unusual or atypical behaviors for which no physical cause can be found, trying too quickly to assign a "behavioral" diagnosis can result in a failure to recognize underlying pain or discomfort, leading to further unnecessary suffering for the animal.

Generally speaking, in human medicine, abnormal repetitive behaviors are divided into stereotypies and impulsive/CDs, but even in humans many of these problems have been categorized and labeled in a somewhat inconsistent manner. Many human repetitive behaviors are also further described and categorized on the basis of patient reports, something that cannot be relied on in veterinary medicine. These are a complex set of behavior problems and it is still unclear if behaviors such as tail chasing, fly snapping, overgrooming, pica or flank sucking share any underlying neurobiological or pathophysiological similarities, even though much of the veterinary research continues to lump them together under the heading of compulsive disorders. Thus, one should avoid trying to "force" any particular animal repetitive behavior into these categories because the label does not really inform us as to the cause of the clinical signs, the function of the behavior, or its treatment. In addition, many of the unusual or strange behaviors that have typically been categorized as compulsive have recently been shown to be indicative of underlying physical conditions affecting a variety of body systems.

Problem overview

Stereotypies

A stereotypy can be defined as the invariant repetition of a motor pattern that serves no apparent goal or function. These behaviors have been commonly reported in farm, zoo, and laboratory animal species, and initially arise in situations of conflict or frustration related to a variety of different aspects of the captive environment. Maternal deprivation has also been shown to contribute to the development of stereotypic behaviors[2] and a genetic predisposition to stereotypical behaviors has been noted in some species.[5-7] However, the one feature noted to be shared by all nonhuman animals with stereotypies is the presence of frustration.[8]

In humans, stereotypies are usually associated with autism and other severe developmental disorders. They also can occur as secondary signs in a variety of other mental health disorders such as schizophrenia or Tourette's syndrome. Stereotypies can also be triggered by certain drugs such as amphetamines.

Stereotypical behaviors are typically derived from normal motor patterns and may begin in response to a variety of different environmental factors that lead to frustration. In the beginning, there is variability in the appearance of the repeated behavior, but with time and repetition, the behavior becomes more fixed or rigid and eventually continues, even in the absence of the initial triggering stimuli. At which point, they can be referred to as "emancipated." While it has been suggested that the performance of stereotypies may help animals cope with a poor environment, there is no sound evidence that all stereotypies serve as coping mechanisms.[8]

Obsessive/compulsive disorders

Obsessive/compulsive disorders in humans (OCDs) are characterized by obsessions; recurrent, persistent, and intrusive thoughts, urges, or images that cause them distress. The compulsions are the repetitive mental acts or behaviors that they feel driven to perform in order to relieve anxiety. A diagnosis of OCD requires the presence of obsessions and/or compulsions that are time consuming (more than 1 hour a day), cause significant distress, and impair work or social functioning. The exact cause of OCD in humans is not fully understood, but it is likely that the tendency to develop OCD is inherited and certain environmental factors or stressful life experiences trigger the development of the problem. In people, OCDs will usually develop prior to or around adolescence.

The rationale for labeling these disorders in pets as compulsive is based in part on the use of the dog as a model for human OCD. Abnormal serotonin transmission has been identified as a primary mechanism by which CDs are induced and in humans, the condition preferentially responds to drugs that inhibit serotonin reuptake.[9,10] Using dogs with acral lick dermatitis (ALD) as a model for the human disorder, drugs that inhibit serotonin reuptake, such as clomipramine, fluoxetine, and citalopram, were found to improve clinical signs, while drugs that had more effect on norepinephrine reuptake, such as desipramine, were not effective.[11-14] This is evidence of predictive validity (response to the same therapeutic agents), but construct validity (evidence of shared biological basis) is still lacking. Since we cannot know if animals are experiencing obsessions, the term compulsive disorder (CD) has been suggested for use in animals.

Pathogenesis of repetitive disorders

It has been suggested that CDs in animals are most commonly seen in genetically predisposed individuals that are subjected to chronic or recurrent conflict or frustration, or whose behavioral needs are not adequately met. In a study in Brazil of 20 dogs with ALD that could not be attributed to underlying physical causes, all dogs were described as having an anxious personality. None of the pet parents played with their dogs routinely and 70% of the dogs were never walked.[15] In another study, dogs with abnormal repetitive and stereotypical behavior were more resistant than control dogs to extinction trials for a previously conditioned behavior.[16] This may be used to predict an individual dog's predisposition toward developing compulsive and stereotypical behaviors are less plastic or able to adapt to changes in their social or physical environment.

In predisposed breeds such as Doberman Pinschers, abnormal repetitive behaviors and CDs have been linked to structural brain differences (see Table 18.1).[17] Flank sucking, which is primarily seen in Doberman Pinschers, might have a physical component, but could also be a behavioral disorder (related to blanket sucking) for which a genetic component (gene cadherin 2, CDH2) has been identified.[5,6,18] Other inherited susceptibilities include tail chasing and spinning in German Shepherd Dogs, Bull Terriers, Staffordshire Bull Terriers, Anatolian Sheepdogs, and Australian

Table 18.1 Manifestations of abnormal repetitive behaviors (ARB) in dogs and cats

ARBs in dogs	ARBs in cats
Self-trauma, injurious, or self-directed	
Tail mutilation/chewing	Tail mutilation/attacking
Face and neck scratching	Face and neck scratching
Acral lick dermatitis	Symmetrical alopecia (overgrooming)
Compulsive licking or chewing	Hair plucking/pulling
Claw (nail) biting	Claw (nail) biting
Self-nursing	Self-nursing
Flank sucking	
Locomotor, predatory	
Tail chasing, spinning	Tail chasing
Pacing, circling	Chasing, predatory sequences
Chasing lights/shadows	Freezing, staring
Rhythmic barking	Excessive vocalization
Freezing, staring	
Fence running	
Neurologic, hallucinatory	
Snapping at air	Fixed stare
Checking rear	Hyperesthesia
Head shaking	
Oral/ingestive	
Pica	Pica
Sucking, for example, blankets, pet parent	Sucking wool/pet parent
Licking – environment/pet parent	Licking – environment/pet parent
Polyphagia – voracious eating	
Glugging[a]	
Psychogenic polydipsia	
Social, sexual	
Masturbation	Mounting, humping
Mounting, humping	Penis licking
Penis sucking	

[a]Dodman NH, Cottman N. Animal behavior case of the month. *J Am Vet Med Assoc.* 2004;225:1339–1341.

Cattle Dogs, and pica and wool sucking in Burmese and Siamese cats.[19–23] And in at least one breed, the Bull Terrier, tail chasing may occur with aggression and fear or may resemble partial seizures with normal electroencephalogram (EEG) results which are responsive to phenobarbital.[24] Tail chasing may be associated with structural brain abnormalities, as have been other stereotypical locomotor behaviors and compulsive disorders.[25]

In animals, repetitive behaviors typically arise in situations of conflict or frustration where it is assumed that the pet does not have any other strategy for effectively dealing with the situation. Conflict and frustration often result in displacement behaviors or redirected behaviors. Displacement behaviors are behaviors that appear inappropriate or out of context for the circumstances (e.g., circling, tail chasing, excessive grooming). Redirected behaviors are those exhibited toward a target other than the one that prompted the behavior (e.g., redirected aggression or light and shadow chasing). Conflict occurs when an individual is motivated to perform two opposing behaviors at the same time. This might occur when a pet is uncertain about the outcome or when the pet parent's responses to the pet's behavior have been inconsistent in the past. Inconsistent or unpredictable consequences and punishment, especially if inappropriately timed or particularly aversive, often result in conflict or frustration. For example, if a pet parent arrives home to find that their pet has destroyed something, eliminated in the home, or torn open the trash, and responds by punishing the dog, the dog may develop anxiety related to the pet parent's return to the home. At the same time, the dog may be eager to greet the pet parent, experiencing conflicting desires; rush to greet (excitement, affiliative behavior) or stay back (fear). Internal emotional conflict is stressful and can result in displacement behaviors and other unwanted behavioral responses.

Frustration refers to a situation in which an individual is motivated to perform a behavior but is not able to do so. This might occur when a pet is aroused by other animals, people, or prey outside the window. Pets placed in a yard or confined to crates or runs for long periods may begin repetitive pacing, circling, or barking if unable to exercise or to access potential playmates, territorial intruders, or prey. Pets may also be mentally frustrated if they are inhibited from playing, chasing, jumping up, or barking, especially if punishment has been used in an attempt to stop the behavior (see Table 18.2).

Conflict and frustration can also arise from housing in unnatural, restrictive, or suboptimal environments for the pet's needs. Illness, injury, and inadequate attention to welfare issues such as food, water, temperature control, and freedom from pain or discomfort might also contribute to emotional conflict or frustration. These situations can lead to the displacement or redirected behaviors becoming repetitive.

Maternal deprivation has also been shown to predispose individuals to stereotypic behavior in some species due to frustrated motivations to suckle or insufficient social contact. While some of these behaviors may be transient, some may persist into adulthood.[2] In a study of hand-reared kittens, being orphaned, bottle fed, and separated earlier from the mother, were all found to be risk factors for cross-sucking behavior. This behavior, where kittens repetitively suckle on the body parts of litter mates, can be so persistent as to cause injury to suckled kittens.[26] Maternal deprivation has also been shown to lead to heightened fearfulness, anxiety, and alterations in how the individual responds to stress, which may contribute to a greater potential for the development of stereotypic behaviors as well as fears when exposed to stressors later in life.[2]

Conflict and frustration-induced displacement behaviors are usually seen in response to a specific stimulus (e.g., visual,

Table 18.2 Glossary of terms

Conflict-induced behaviors	Conflict occurs when the pet is motivated to perform two opposing behaviors (e.g., approach and withdrawal). Because the pet is unable to display the two behaviors simultaneously, a displacement behavior may be exhibited.
Frustration-induced behaviors	Frustration refers to a situation in which the pet is motivated to perform a behavior but is not able to do so. The barrier may be physical (as when access to the stimulus is blocked, such as when fenced in the yard) or behavioral (the pet suppresses its response because of possible consequences, such as punishment). The resultant behavior could be a displacement behavior or a redirected behavior.
Displacement behavior	A displacement behavior is a normal behavior shown at an inappropriate time, appearing out of context for the situation, often as a result of frustration or conflict. Displacement behaviors may also be observed in situations of arousal when there is no appropriate outlet for dearousal. Examples of displacement behaviors include yawning, eating, vocalizing, lip licking, grooming, circling, spinning, and tail chasing.
Redirected behavior	When an animal is motivated to perform an activity (e.g., territorial protection, fear aggression, marking) but is unable (frustrated) to gain access to the principal target, the behavior may be directed at an alternative target (e.g., a nearby person, another animal, or an object).
Vacuum activity	The performance of a behavior in the absence of the normal substrate required for the performance of the behavior. Typically, when an animal is highly motivated to perform an instinctive behavior but there is no available appropriate substrate, a vacuum activity may be exhibited (flank sucking, wool or fabric sucking, licking).
Stereotypies	A stereotypy is an abnormal, invariant, repetition of a motor pattern that serves no apparent function. Stereotypies may be induced by conflict, frustration, deprivation, or central nervous system dysfunction.
Compulsive disorders	Compulsive behaviors are abnormal and repetitive but unlike stereotypies, appear to be goal directed. The animal lacks complete control over the initiation and cessation of the behavior and it interferes with normal behavior, such as eating and social interaction, and/or is self-injurious.

auditory, odor, tactile) or event and are likely to resolve when the inciting factors are removed. However, pet parent responses may further aggravate the problem by inadvertently reinforcing the behavior or increasing fear and conflict through the use of punishment.

Physical factors may also aggravate repetitive behaviors, especially if the consequences of the behavior (e.g., tail chasing, excessive licking) lead to pain, injury, or infection. After all, it is completely normal for most animals to lick a wound or painful area. Alternatively, the presence of chronic pain can also result in anxiety, which can be the stimulus for a displacement or redirected behavior. Deep infections can also result in additional pain and prevent a lesion from healing, which will promote continued licking. In these cases, attention must be paid to holistic treatment of the animal. Every affected body system will need to be treated concurrently in order to change the behavior and solve the problem.[27]

Providing optimal housing with adequate social and environmental enrichment has been shown to decrease stereotypies in many species but does not always stop them completely. The age at which the problems developed and how long they exist prior to attempting to change them may all affect the likelihood of resolution. In many cases, it may be difficult to identify the original stimulus or event that led to the behavior, making it even more difficult to resolve.

Pet parent inadvertent reinforcement or unintentional environmental reinforcement of the behavior has been shown to be a significant factor, at least in some cases, of canine repetitive behaviors and CDs, with 43% of pet parents overtly reinforcing their dogs (some inadvertently with laughter or attention) for the behavior.[28] Most respond by either punishing the dog with a verbal cue; ignoring the dog; preventing the behavior; giving something desirable such as attention, a toy, or a treat; or attempting to distract

the dog, remove the item, or cue the dog to do something else.[28] In situations where the behavior is not directly controlled by the pet parent but instead affected mostly by the environment such as is the case with light chasing, the presence of light in the environment can serve to reinforce the behavior. For the best outcomes, all reinforcement should be controlled and/or eliminated.

Pathophysiology of repetitive disorders

There may be a common pathophysiology for all of the disorders labeled as compulsive, but it is equally likely that the neurotransmitters involved vary between presenting complaints and that there may be changing involvement as the problem progresses. Locomotor repetitive disorders, such as tail chasing, that tend to develop after repeated conflict are displayed most commonly in situations of high arousal and are often so intense that it may be difficult to calm the pet or interrupt the behavior. By contrast, oral repetitive behaviors (such as flank sucking and ALD) may develop more acutely, are most likely to be displayed in situations of minimal or insufficient stimulation, and may appear to help the pet to cope or settle. Animals exhibiting these behaviors are often described as being "zoned out" or in a trancelike state. It is unknown if these different mental states are a result of different pathophysiology, however it has been suggested that locomotor stereotypies might involve the mesolimbic dopaminergic system, while oral stereotypies may involve activation of the nigrostriatal dopaminergic system.[29] Hallucinatory-type behaviors such as fly snapping and pouncing may involve different pathophysiologic mechanisms. There also may be differing levels of cognition ranging from spontaneous, seemingly uncontrollable reactions to pets that search for or fixate on specific targets.

One investigation into the differences and similarities between stereotypies and OCDs, using a systems approach to the problem, has led to the hypothesis that all stereotypies arise from disruption of basal ganglia systems. OCDs and related impulse control disorders arise from disruptions in the prefrontal cortex and the numerous pathways between the prefrontal cortex and the rest of the brain.[1] These suggestions are based on research in humans with brain damage or dysfunction which found evidence that different neurologic signs exist, depending on which part of the brain is affected. These problems each represent failure in different behavioral control systems. Mechanisms which would normally inhibit a behavior are not functioning normally, so the individual is unable to stop repeating a motor pattern or readily switch goal-directed behaviors.[1]

Beta-endorphins, dopamine, glutamate, and serotonin have all been implicated in repetitive disorders, primarily based on response to therapy. Altered glutaminergic neurotransmission may also be a factor, since blocking glutamate-sensitive N-methyl-D-aspartic acid (NMDA) with drugs such as memantine or dextromethorphan has been shown to be effective in some cases.[30,31] However, it has been suggested that the role of gamma-aminobutyric acid, neuroactive peptides such as cholecystokinin, corticotrophin-releasing factor, neuropeptide Y, and tachykinins such as substance P should also be considered.[32]

It has long been believed that some repetitive disorders are mediated through opioid receptors, since opioid antagonists such as naltrexone have been successful at reducing stereotypies in dogs, sows, and horses.[33–35] In addition, medications that supply an exogenous source of opiates, such as hydrocodone, have been reported to be effective for ALD.[36] It has been theorized that endorphins act as an internal mechanism for reinforcement and that they might play a role in the early development of stereotypies. This suggests that when performing these repetitive behaviors, animals may be self-narcotizing and this helps them to cope with the distressing environment. However, an increase in blood endorphin levels has not been identified and there is no consistent evidence that repetitive behaviors result in the animal feeling better or less stressed. It has been shown, however, that animals experiencing high levels of stress release high levels of endogenous opioids that modulate dopaminergic pathways. Thus, rather than simply having an effect due to their rewarding properties, these opioids may be sensitizing the dopaminergic pathways in the basal ganglia.[37]

Dopaminergic drugs such as amphetamines may induce stereotypies and dopamine antagonists such as haloperidol may result in suppression of stereotypies.[33,38,39] In one study, higher prolactin levels were found in dogs with chronic stress, stereotypic behaviors, fear, aggression, and autonomic signs, while lower levels of prolactin were associated with acute fearful and phobic events.[40] Thus, drugs that enhance dopamine transmission such as selegiline might be indicated in stereotypies associated with chronic stress.

Abnormal serotonin transmission has been suggested to be the primary mechanism by which some repetitive disorders are induced. As in human models of OCDs, drugs that inhibit serotonin reuptake (e.g., clomipramine, fluoxetine, fluvoxamine, citalopram) have been shown to be most effective in the treatment of canine and feline repetitive disorders.[11–15,19,41–43] Animal studies have also identified direct evidence of serotonin involvement.[9] In some animal studies, the serotonin reuptake inhibitor citalopram and not the neuroleptic clozapine was effective in reducing stereotypic behavior in female voles.[44] Abnormalities in serotonergic and dopaminergic pathways have been found in dogs that exhibit compulsive behaviors when compared to dogs that do not.[45] Changes in serum levels of neurotensin and corticotropin-releasing hormone have been found in Bull Terriers that exhibit signs of CDs when compared to Bull Terriers that are unaffected, as has been described in humans with CDs.[46]

In time, it is probable that different neuropathological mechanisms may be identified for different presentations. In fact, the French (Pageat) approach espouses that abnormal repetitive behaviors arise as a result of a number of different behavioral disorders, including permanent anxiety disorder, where the dog is constantly in a state of inhibition and prone to displacement behaviors [which may respond to selegiline, a TCA (clomipramine) or an selective serotonin reuptake inhibitor (SSRI)]; unipolar disorder, where the dog may be hypervigilant, overexcitable, and unable to stop behavioral sequences (which may respond to selegiline); hyperactivity disorder or attention deficit disorder with hyperactivity (which might respond to methylphenidate, fluvoxamine, fluoxetine, imipramine, or amitriptyline); deritualization anxiety, where there has been a change in the social group and the dog becomes withdrawn and overly defensive (which may respond to selegiline); and dissociate disorders, where the dog becomes increasingly less receptive and may have hallucinatory events (which may respond to risperidone)[47] (see Chapters 9 and 25).

The effect of diet and certain vitamins on abnormal repetitive behaviors is unclear; however, one study demonstrated that in dogs that displayed repetitive tail chasing those regularly taking a multivitamin were less likely to develop tail chasing.[48]

Prevention

We do not fully understand why some animals in similarly barren or inappropriate environments do or do show repetitive behaviors. The causes and contributing factors are complex and not completely consistent between different ARBs. Breed, individual differences, maternal effects, early development, and socialization all play a role in how pets manage stress (see Box 18.1). Therefore, one cannot confidently describe what can be done to prevent the problems from developing. However, providing appropriate and sufficient enrichment in the form of social interactions and play, a predictable and comfortable environment that meets the individuals' behavioral needs, and predictable consequences that focus on rewarding desirable behavior can reduce stress for most pets. Abnormal repetitive behaviors, specifically tail chasing, can begin as early as three months of age.[48] Puppies or kittens that present with stereotypical behaviors should be treated immediately and aggressively to prevent the progression of the disorder.[48] Neutered males may be at greater risk than females for tail chasing. Informing parents of these risks and offering preventative care, especially to at-risk breeds, should be the standard of care.[48] At least one study has found significant differences in hematologic parameters between dogs that were diagnosed with CD and those that did not display CD. In the aforementioned study, dogs with CDs were statistically more likely to have polycythemia.[49]

The following suggestions include many which could simply be described as good practices when raising or training any animal, and they may serve to prevent the further development of many problem behaviors.

1. Provide consistent and predictable family–pet interactions using a positive approach to training and communication. Predictability in rewards means that the pet learns what behaviors get rewarded and what behaviors do not. This can only be achieved if the family is consistent in each response (e.g., you will get affection only if you sit calmly or lie down you will be greeted only if you are quiet and sitting, we will continue to walk forward only if you keep the leash slack, you will get this chew toy only when you lie on the mat, etc.).

2. Avoid positive punishment as it can cause fear and damage the bond with the pet. Positive punishment can be especially problematic if it is harsh or used inconsistently. This can cause internal conflict and anxiety and can worsen repetitive behaviors. The need for punishment can be avoided by proper supervision, confinement, or pet proofing to prevent undesirable behaviors, and rewarding alternate desirable behaviors.

3. Provide an environment that is secure, comfortable, and stimulating and meets the pet's needs. This should include comfortable bedding or resting areas, enrichment toys, opportunities for climbing and exploration (paper bags, boxes, perches), and scratching areas (cats). Catnip, chew products (dogs), food and puzzle toys, and scavenger hunts for treats can provide mental stimulation and contribute to an enriched environment.

4. Provide sufficient social enrichment at times that are most suitable to family and pet. This should include quality time together such as positive training, play, and exercise. Weekly explorations of new or variable environments provide enjoyable shared activity. Social play with

other pets and people can also be encouraged (e.g., play dates). Avoid these shared outings if they result in undesirable responses from the dog (e.g., barking, lunging, or hyperarousal of any kind). Adequate play, training, and exercise can be achieved in the yard or home if necessary and is preferable to forcing the dog into situations that may make it uncomfortable.

5. Some degree of structure in the pet's schedule and routine can increase predictability and decrease conflict.

6. Genetics, healthy maternal behavior, gentle handling, socialization, and exposure to environmental stimuli during early development and through the sensitive socialization period can have a strong influence on future behavior. Therefore, these should be considered when first obtaining a pet and in particular through the first few critical months with the pet when it learns about its new home and family (see Chapters 2, 4 and 5).

7. Be proactive and screen every patient for early signs of problem behaviors. This can be easily accomplished with a brief questionnaire given to every pet parent at each appointment (see Chapter 1, Appendix C and online forms). Encourage pet parents to report not only any signs of physical illness but also any new, or unusual behaviors, or changes in behavior, as soon as they arise. In most cases, the longer a repetitive behavior exists, the more difficult it is to treat.

Diagnosis and potential outcomes

Diagnosing a repetitive behavior as a neuropsychiatric disorder must be done with caution. It is essentially a diagnosis of exclusion because all other organ system conditions must first be ruled out. For example, neurological signs may be due to partial (focal) seizures; self-traumatic disorders may be due to adverse food reactions; and oral and ingestive behaviors may be caused by gastrointestinal (GI) diseases (see Chapter 6 and below). Feline hyperesthesia is a clinical sign or group of signs that can have dermatologic, neuromuscular, or behavioral causes. Unusual behavior can too often be an animal's response to a disease process such as pain, neuropathy, pruritus, or other form of altered sensation. Since the animal cannot verbalize what it is experiencing, it is often wise to err on the side of caution and presumptively treat an animal for pain or other physiological condition before determining that its behavior is a result of a learned or pathologic condition such as a ARB.

In addition, one must never ignore the role that stress can play in initiating and/or perpetuating any behavioral disorder. Unmitigated, chronic stress can ultimately lead to impairment of the immune system and gastrointestinal and dermatologic conditions. For example, the skin and the central nervous system share many of the same hormones, neuropeptides, and receptors. Many of these substances are involved in neurogenic inflammation, pruritus, and pain sensation, and stress can alter their release. This stress can cause pathophysiologic responses that can perpetuate the itch-scratch cycle, contributing to repetitive licking or overgrooming (see Chapters 6 and 7).

To further confuse the subject, a variety of therapeutic options have been reported to be effective for the same phenotypic presentation. Therefore, in addition to diagnostic tests, therapeutic response trials with medications that target a specific body system (e.g., food trial, parasite control, seizure medication, gastrointestinal medication) may be invaluable in both diagnosis and treatment. However, the diagnosis may be further complicated by the fact that many medications (e.g., memantine, doxepin, clonazepam, carbamazepine, gabapentin, pregabalin) have multiple effects (e.g., pain, seizure, anxiety, compulsion, pruritus). For example, tail chasing and self-trauma, pawing or scratching of the face, and hyperesthesia in cats may potentially have dermatologic, neurologic, pain (including neuropathic pain), or mental causes. Tail chasing in dogs has been described by different authors as resulting from pain, an opioid-mediated stereotypy,[35] a CD responsive to tricyclic antidepressant (TCA) and SSRI therapy,[41,42] a seizure-related neurological disorder,[50] or perhaps a disorder similar to human autism.[21] Therefore, caution should be used when basing a diagnosis purely on the response to a particular therapeutic approach.

Differentiating a stereotypy from a CD can be challenging, but the systems-level research suggests that the difference between stereotypies and impulsive/compulsive disorders lies in *what* is repeated. In impulsive/compulsive disorders, an inappropriate goal is repeated (such as the plucking of hair by a person with trichotillomania or the chasing of lights by a dog), and in stereotypies, a particular motor pattern is repeated.[1] This may not seem helpful to some who might ask is tail chasing simply a repeated motor pattern or is it goal oriented? Is a dog with ALD simply repeating the motor pattern of licking or is the behavior an attempt to achieve a goal? One thing to keep in mind when considering the difference: just because the motor patterns are not extremely fixed or rigid (e.g., the dog that spins to the right and spins to the left) does not mean that it may not be a *developing stereotypy* since part of the definition is that the behavior patterns are more flexible in the beginning and become fixed with repetition.

More important than classifying the behavior as a stereotypy or CD and ruling out disease in other body systems is to try to identify the antecedents or triggers that lead to the behavior, although most pet parents cannot identify these when asked.[51] Even if the behaviors have already become emancipated from their original cause, identifying any antecedents (triggers) will aid in developing a treatment plan.

History taking must therefore include information regarding:

- The pet, including the signalment, developmental history, adoption, early socialization, and training, and any other concurrent behavior or physical health conditions.
- The pet's personality, how the pet responds to different stimuli (e.g., people, animals, locations, situations, noises), and whether there are issues of fear, anxiety, stress, conflict, or panic.
- What methods the pet parents use for training, including reinforcement (when, where, what, and how), punishment (when, where, what, how, and why), and control products or devices, including collar and type, body harness, head halter, or remote training devices.
- The family, including other pets and their relationships, the pet's daily schedule, and the environment, including specific questions on social enrichment and object/toy play.

- The problem, how and when it started; how it has progressed or changed; when, where, and how often the problem occurs; triggers, antecedents, or events that precede the problem; the pet parent's response and how the dog responds; and a detailed description (including video if available) of the problem, including the sequence of events and the dog's body language; frequency, duration, intensity, situations in which the problems arise, and whether the pet parent can prevent or interrupt it.
- Concurrent behavioral problems and somatic signs that might indicate whether the stereotypy is a component of another problem (e.g., cognitive dysfunction syndrome, attention deficit hyperactivity disorder).

If all conditions of other body systems have been ruled out, managed, or resolved and the behavior problem persists, then a behavioral diagnosis of a repetitive disorder can be made. The repetitive behavior might then be further classified as a stereotypy, displacement or redirected behavior, reinforced or conditioned behavior, or even a CD. Even if a physical condition is identified, the initiating cause may have been due to the behavior. For example, a dog that presents with an ALD may have initiated the lesion by licking due to stress or conflict but may have developed a deep infection that must now be treated along with the anxiety-related issues in order for the ALD to be cured. Conversely, the lesion may have come first (due to atopy, injury, or infection) and persists due to the dog's continual licking of the lesion. This example demonstrates how intimately physical and mental health can be linked and why an holistic approach is always important. One-health approach to health is always important.

When abnormal behaviors are exhibited only in the pet parent's presence, it is possible that the pet parent's responses to the behavior are a primary factor in development and maintenance of the problem (conditioned or reinforced). Other possible differentials are the repetitive, hallucinatory, fixated, or stereotypic behaviors that are seen in the Pageat (French) diagnoses (see Chapters 9 and 25).

It is clear, however, that repetition of a behavior further strengthens the neuronal pathways involved, so some action should be taken immediately upon a report of a behavior being demonstrated in a repetitive fashion.

Management

By evaluating the pet's household, daily routine, and the undesirable behavior itself, including when and where it occurs and the consequences that arise from engaging in the behavior, a specific program can be designed to reduce stress and conflict and direct the pet into acceptable and desirable alternative behaviors. For some problems, such as flank sucking in Doberman Pinschers or the Golden Retriever that carries towels in its mouth, the problem may be sufficiently benign that treatment may not be necessary or may be more disruptive than the problem itself. If the behavior appears to be a successful coping mechanism for reducing stress or resolving underlying conflict and the family is addressing the pet's needs effectively, additional treatment may not be warranted. However, if the pet's welfare is affected (e.g., the pet continues to live with chronic conflict, frustration, or anxiety) or if the problem is unacceptable for the family, appropriate environmental management will be crucial. In addition, if the behavior significantly reduces the amount of time that the pet engages in normal behaviors, negatively impacts relationships with other pets or people in the home, or leads to secondary physical problems such as pain, inflammation, or infection, then treatment using pharmaceutical agents may also be important.

A management plan for reduction of repetitive behaviors should include most aspects of the prevention strategies described earlier in addition to the following:

1. Consistent and predictable environment and daily routine over which the pet has control to engage in desirable activities (e.g., resting, perching, object play) and undesirable behaviors are prevented (set the pet up to succeed; see Chapter 5).
2. Consistent and predictable consequences using rewards to encourage desirable behavior rather than punishment to discourage undesirable behavior (see Chapter 10).
3. Providing sufficient enrichment and outlets to meet the pet's behavioral needs (see Chapters 5 and 10).
4. Ensuring pet parent responses do not further reinforce or aggravate the undesirable behavior (e.g., anger, punishment, agitation, inconsistent responses to the pet's behavior).
5. Identification and removal or reduction of stressors that lead to fear, anxiety, stress, conflict, panic, or frustration.
6. Identification and prevention or avoidance of triggers that precede displacement or redirected behaviors.
7. Teaching pet parents to identify triggers and read facial and body language to be able to preempt the behavior and direct the pet to an acceptable behavior.
8. Developing techniques and tools for pet parent interruption of the behavior on the occasion where it is displayed in spite of the other interventions being used.

Predictability and control: environment, routine, and consequences

Pets that develop repetitive behaviors may be particularly sensitive to inconsistency or lack of predictability in their daily schedule and in their interactions with the family. The pet's regular routine should include social interaction with people in the form of reward-based training, play, and exercise, and opportunities for social interactions with other pets (if these are not a source of conflict). Pet parents might be encouraged to focus on play that simulates the normal activities of the species or breed (e.g., pulling carts, herding or retrieving for dogs, hunting games for cats). Feeding times could be scheduled throughout the day, utilizing feeding toys and foraging stations so that the pet can work (or play) and expend energy to obtain food. Following social sessions with the pet parent, the pet must learn to settle or play with its own toys (rest or object play) without the need for attention (i.e., learning to accept inattention). Cats can be encouraged to use an elevated area for perching or a cat play center. Dogs can be encouraged to use a resting or bedding area and, if not inclined to nap or sleep, offered enrichment toys (feeding, chew, and manipulation toys) that provide novelty and complexity to keep the pet motivated and challenged.

Minimizing access to conflict- and frustration-inducing stimuli

Music, radio, TV, or white noise can help reduce anxiety and minimize audible stimuli that might contribute to stress or anxiety. Other products that might help reduce anxiety in some pets include ThunderShirt, anxiety wraps or pheromones, ThunderCaps, and goggles that reduce visual stimuli, Rex Specs, Mutt Muffs or sound baffling that reduces audible stimuli (see Chapter 15).

Treatment

As is the case with most behavior problems, the likelihood of success will increase if the plan includes appropriate environmental management, behavior modification, and when appropriate, pharmacological therapy. Pharmacological therapy may be necessary to decrease anxiety in order to keep the pet in a state where it can learn the new responses being taught, relieve pain and distress, and improve welfare.

Complete plans for behavioral clinical signs include:

1. Avoidance of triggers.
2. Modulation of fear, anxiety, stress, conflict, panic, pain, and discomfort through environmental management, medications, diet, and supplements as needed.
3. Management of the environment to provide adequate outlets necessary to address breed-typical needs, increase enrichment, keep the pet and the family safe, and remove reinforcement for undesirable behaviors.
4. Pathways to teach desirable behaviors with positive reinforcement.
5. Education on proper interactions with the pet, species-specific body language, and proper training.
6. Discontinuation of all positive punishment techniques.
7. Discussion of quality of life of the patient.

Training – predictable consequences

Training or behavior modification should focus on encouraging behaviors that are desirable rather than punishing behaviors that are undesirable. Casual and inconsistent pet parent interactions should be replaced by a program of predictable rewards where the pet parents ensure that all rewards, including affection, toys, and food, are given for behaviors that are incompatible with the CD (e.g., resting on a mat instead of chasing their tail, playing with a favored toy rather than chasing lights) (see Chapter 10). Encouraging desirable outcomes helps reduce stress and can be achieved by several means: encouraging settled behaviors; maintaining a calm household; calm and consistent pet parent responses; and the appropriate use of rewards. Clicker training can help immediately reinforce desirable behaviors. Keeping the dog or cat on leash may help to inhibit, disrupt, or prevent undesirable behavior. Remote treat dispensers are also a useful for training dogs to settle on a mat or bed for progressively longer and more relaxed responses. All positive punishment must be avoided. Positive punishment is very difficult to use effectively, although most people feel that they effectively punish their pet. The literature supports the pitfalls of positive punishment. It increases fear, anxiety, stress, conflict, and panic, is less effective than positive reinforcement techniques, is difficult to implement effectively, and it increases aggression (see Chapter 10).

Differential reinforcement of other or alternate behaviors (DRO, DRA)

Pets with repetitive behaviors should be taught an appropriate desirable behavior to replace the undesirable one (DRO, DRA) using positive reinforcement-based techniques. Ideally the pet parents should be aware of when and where the behaviors are about to arise so that they can proactively or preemptively focus on achieving the desirable behavior. If compulsive behaviors arise in the pet parent's presence, the pet should be interrupted immediately and calmly with a novel, nonfrightening sound such as the shake of a treat jar or verbal cue and then cued to engage in an appropriate alternative behavior (e.g., lie down, go to your mat, play with your toy) which can then be reinforced. Pets that cannot be easily distracted and redirected are candidates for medication as a part of the treatment plan. Pet parents should not give the reward until the alternative desired behavior is achieved. When the family cannot be present to interrupt the behavior, some other means of prevention may be needed. Crate confinement or Elizabethan collars may be useful, but these products can further aggravate the pet's anxiety and should be avoided if the pet is not completely comfortable with them.

Pharmacological therapy

Based on human models for the treatment of OCD, drugs that inhibit serotonin reuptake, including SSRIs (e.g., fluoxetine) and TCAs (e.g., clomipramine) have been shown to be most effective in the treatment of disorders described as compulsive in the cat and dog.[11,12,14,19,42,43,52,53] In fact, in a retrospective study examining the treatment of 24 dogs with fly snapping, more dogs responded and had better outcomes when treated with fluoxetine compared with phenobarbital.[54]

Clinical studies and case studies on the treatment of CDs in dogs and cats have confirmed the use of a TCA, such as clomipramine, or an SSRI, such as fluoxetine, as the most effective primary form of drug therapy for dogs and cats, with a decrease in behaviors reported of at least 50–75% within four weeks.[19,41,43]

Clomipramine is the most selective inhibitor of serotonin reuptake of all the TCAs and has been reported to be effective in the treatment of ALD, spinning, and tail chasing.[11,12,19,41,43] It has also been utilized successfully in repetitive disorders in cats, including psychogenic alopecia.[51,52,55] TCAs other than clomipramine have not been found to be as effective since they have less effect on serotonin reuptake inhibition. However, in addition to effects on mood and anxiety, other TCAs such as doxepin and amitriptyline have strong antihistaminic effects or may reduce neuropathic pain associated with self-traumatic disorders, while a combination of nortriptyline and gabapentin has been shown to achieve good pain relief in humans.[56]

SSRIs such as paroxetine, fluoxetine, sertraline, fluvoxamine, or citalopram may often be effective. In a study of 13 cases of ALD, improvement was seen with clomipramine (43%), fluoxetine (39%), and sertraline (21%) in comparison to placebo, desipramine, and fenfluramine (a serotonin-releasing agent).[12] In other studies, significant improvement in ALD in dogs was demonstrated with fluoxetine and citalopram.[13,14] One study found clomipramine and fluoxetine to be equally effective in reducing tail chasing behavior in dogs.[23] See Table 18.3. Doses can be increased through the dosing range after four to six weeks if there is insufficient response, and every two weeks thereafter until there is an adequate response as long as there are no adverse effects. See Chapter 9 for more information on the approach to prescribing. If the problem improves, the medication should be continued for at least six months past complete remission of the problem and then decreased slowly. Slowly decreasing the dose of most of these medications allows the family to watch for signs of the undesirable behavior returning so that further reduction in the drug dosage can be stopped. Many patients may need to be maintained on some level of medication throughout their lives.

Altered glutaminergic neurotransmission may also be a factor in the pathogenesis of some repetitive disorders. Therefore, using an NMDA receptor antagonist to block glutamate-sensitive NMDA may be an effective treatment option. In one case series, memantine, an NMDA receptor antagonist, reduced the severity of CDs in 64% of 11 treated dogs within two weeks of treatment.[30] Memantine may be effective alone or may have a synergistic effect when combined with fluoxetine.[57] Dextromethorphan may also be useful because of its NMDA-antagonist properties.[44] However, due to its short half-life, rapid clearance, and variable absorption in dogs, it may not be a reliable form of therapy.[58] See Table 18.3.

Opiate antagonists such as naltrexone and naloxone have also been reported to be effective in some cases, perhaps due to differing pathology with perhaps greater effect in the early stages of the disorder or by blocking the release of endorphins released during stereotypic behaviors such as self-trauma. In one case of compulsive tail chasing, an injection of naloxone 0.01 mg/kg was reported to be effective within 20 minutes and clinical improvement was maintained for 3 hours.[35] In another study, injections of nalmefene or naltrexone reduced chewing, licking, and scratching in dogs with ALD, atopy, and other causes of pruritus for up to 3 hours after injection. In a study using oral naltrexone for ALD at 2.2 mg/kg once or twice daily, improvement was seen in 7 of 11 dogs, but all dogs relapsed after treatment was stopped.[59] On the other hand, it has been suggested that there is low oral bioavailability and inconsistent therapeutic value, and that the active metabolite 6-beta naltrexol is not formed in dogs.[34,60]

A monoamine oxidase inhibitor, such as selegiline, may be another consideration for pets with stereotypic behaviors since chronic stress has been associated with elevated prolactin.[40] Selegiline is licensed in Europe for emotional disorders which are often associated with states of chronic anxiety and concurrent physical signs, including alterations in eating, drinking, sleep, or elimination. It has also been reported to be effective in cats with emotional disorders, including repetitive self-licking.[61] See Table 18.3.

Since dopamine agonists such as apomorphine and amphetamines can induce stereotypic behavior and antipsychotics have been effective in treating stereotypies in other species, it is perhaps surprising that antipsychotics such as haloperidol have not proven to be effective for stereotypic behaviors in pets.[33,38,62]

Medications which might be effective in combination with an SSRI or clomipramine (see Table 18.3) include:

- Buspirone or tryptophan; however, caution should be taken to monitor for signs of serotonin toxicity.
- Gabapentin, pregabalin, or carbamazepine, which also might act on partial seizures, neuropathic pain, or anxiety.
- Clonazepam (or other benzodiazepines such as lorazepam or diazepam), which might have effects on anxiety or as adjunct therapy for partial seizures.
- Tramadol (caution should be taken to monitor for signs of serotonin toxicity), opioids, or meloxicam for concurrent pain.
- Phenobarbital, potassium bromide, or levetiracetam for temporal lobe epilepsy or partial seizures.

Pheromones, L-theanine, alpha-casozepine, melatonin, aromatherapy, valerian, and other natural supplements might also be used concurrently to further reduce any underlying anxiety, but compelling evidence for efficacy in the treatment of repetitive disorders is lacking (see Chapter 12).

Specific repetitive behaviors

Repetitive behaviors in pets are typically categorized as locomotor, oral, hallucinatory, and those that result in self-trauma. However, another, more useful way to categorize them may be by body systems affected (e.g., neurologic, gastrointestinal, or dermatologic). Regardless of the classification applied, many of these conditions appear to overlap. Although general approaches to diagnosing and treating repetitive disorders apply to each presentation, there may be additional considerations based on the body system affected.

Repetitive disorders with neurological and locomotor signs

Some of the most difficult and frustrating repetitive behaviors to treat are those that include signs that could be of neurologic origin, such as fly snapping, tail chasing, pouncing, fixed staring, star gazing, head shaking, spinning, checking, and the tremors of Boxers, Bulldogs, Doberman Pinschers, and Great Danes. Similar feline conditions include staring, and pouncing, chasing, and hunting behaviors toward "imaginary prey." Any of these behaviors could occur as a result of a neurologic problem; however, as is the case with many compulsive or stereotypical repetitive behaviors, a gastrointestinal component was found in at least one case of stargazing behavior in a dog.[63] In some cases, a tentative diagnosis may need to be made and presumptive treatment begun. Pets with primary neurological diseases may present with no other physical signs or neurologic deficits. Some of these repetitive behaviors can be a presentation of a focal seizure. Focal seizures are involuntary movements that may be localized to a single limb or part of the face.

The animal experiencing a focal seizure may be somewhat responsive to other stimuli and may or may not demonstrate an aura and preictal and postictal phases, as is common with generalized seizures. Focal seizures can be divided into motor and sensory -type seizures. While motor seizures involve involuntary movement of one part of

Table 18.3 Drug therapy for compulsive disorders and abnormal repetitive behaviors

Drug	Dog	Cat
Clonazepam	0.1–1.0 mg/kg q8–12 hours	0.02–0.2 mg/kg q12–24 hours
Other benzodiazepines	See Appendix B	See Appendix B
Clomipramine	1–3 mg/kg q12 hours*	0.3–0.5 mg/kg q24 hours
Doxepin	2–5 mg/kg q12–24 hours	0.5–1 mg/kg q12–24 hours
Fluoxetine	1.0–2.0 mg/kg q24 hours*	0.5–1.5 mg/kg q24 hours
Sertraline	1–3 mg/kg q12-24 hours*	0.5–1.5 mg/kg q24 hours
Fluvoxamine	1–2 mg/kg q24 hours*	0.25–1.0 mg/kg q24 hours
Citalopram	1 mg/kg q24 hours*	0.5–1 mg/kg q24 hours
Paroxetine	0.5–2.0 mg/kg q12-24 hours*	0.5–1 mg/kg q24 hours
Naltrexone	1–2.2 mg/kg q12 hours	25–50 mg/cat q24 hours
Carbamazepine	4–8 mg/kg q8–12 hours	2–6 mg/kg q12–24 hours
Phenobarbital	2–5 mg/kg q12 hours	1–3 mg/kg q12 hours
Gabapentin	10–30 mg/kg q8–12 hours	3–10 mg/kg q12 hours
Pregabalin	2–4 mg/kg q8 hours	1–2 mg/kg q12 hours
Potassium bromide	20–40 mg/kg daily or divided q12 hours	Not recommended
Levetiracetam	5–30 mg/kg q8–12 hours	10–20 mg/kg q8 hours
Selegiline	0.5–1 mg/kg q24 hours in morning	0.5–1 mg/kg q24 hours in morning
Memantine	0.3–1 mg/kg q24 hours	
Dextromethorphan	2 mg/kg q6–12 hours	0.5–2 mg/kg up to q8 hours

*Higher doses may be required for treatment of compulsive disorders with cautious oversight for any signs of serotonin syndrome (especially if combining with other drugs that might enhance serotonin transmission).

the body, sensory focal seizures may result in abnormal sensations such as tingling, pain, or visual hallucinations. Fly-biting or fly-snapping behaviors may occur as a result of focal seizures with visual hallucinations. However, evidence linking these and similar behaviors to gastrointestinal distress confirms the possibility of multiple etiologies that can be associated with this nonspecific behavioral sign.[64,65] In a study retrospectively examining the records of 24 dogs with fly biting or fly snapping, abnormalities found included EEG spike activity, bilateral deafness (BAER), Chiari malformation (25%), syringohydromyelia, and falx cerebri.[54]

Complex focal seizures (formerly known as psychomotor seizures) are focal seizures with alterations in awareness. Affected dogs may exhibit repetitive motor activities such as head pressing, vocalizing, aimless walking, running, or circling.[66]

Circling and spinning behaviors could also be a result of complex focal seizures, but pain or altered sensation from peripheral neuropathies must be ruled out. Pain in the tail and back has been determined to be the cause of some cases of tail-chasing behaviors in dogs. In at least two cases, MRI and computed tomographic scans have documented lumbosacral disease in tail-chasing dogs (Marsha Reich, DVM, DACVB, personal communication). These patients responded well to treatment with varying combinations of surgery and antiinflammatories.

Although hydrocephalus has been suggested as a contributing factor in spinning Bull Terriers, a causative relationship has not been established.[22,24,67] One study comparing 145 tail-chasing Bull Terriers to 188 unaffected dogs found that males had an increased susceptibility for tail chasing and that associations were made with anxious behavior, episodic aggression, and trancelike staring. While these signs are most likely associated with a CD or partial complex seizure, some similarity between the condition in Bull Terriers and human autism has been speculated.[21] Although it has been investigated preliminarily, no association has been determined between tail chasing and a specific gene (CDH2) in Bull Terriers, Staffordshire Bull Terriers, and German Shepherd Dogs.[48] Treatment with anticonvulsants, serotonin reuptake inhibitors (SSRIs, TCAs), or both might be used; however, many cases have proven refractory, especially when there are other concurrent problems and risks such as aggression.

Cavalier King Charles Spaniels with syringomyelia accompanied by a Chiari-like malformation (where there is a mismatch between a brain that is too big and a skull that is too small, with the cerebellum and medulla pushed into the foramen magnum) can experience spinal pain as well as neuropathic pain affecting the head, shoulders, neck, and face. Diagnosis can be confirmed by computed tomography scan or magnetic resonance imaging. Signs might include face and neck scratching, paw licking, and unusual positioning of the head and neck. However, circling and fly biting have also been reported in Cavalier King Charles Spaniels and this may be a result of the malformation[68,69] or even GI disturbance.[62] Humans with syringomyelia report a wide range of uncomfortable symptoms including headaches, suboccipital or neck pain, back pain, and trigeminal pain, but the most debilitating is dysesthesia, which is variously described as a burning pain, hyperesthesia (pins and needles), and stretching or pressure of the skin over the shoulders.[70] Treatment options for clinical signs of Chiari malformation include corticosteroids or nonsteroidal antiinflammatory drugs, drugs for neuropathic pain including gabapentin, drugs to reduce cerebrospinal fluid such as furosemide, cimetidine, and omeprazole, and possibly surgery.[69]

When diagnostic testing is unable to yield a definitive diagnosis, the veterinarian may need to take into account all presenting signs, breed, signalment, history, and the extent to which other differential diagnoses have been ruled out to determine how best to treat the problem. Monitoring response to therapy may be the next best option for the patient, the family and the veterinarian to be able to control the signs and make a presumptive diagnosis.

Therapeutic trials

1. When the behavior is associated with a loss of consciousness or motor signs, then a seizure should be considered and a clinical trial with seizure medication performed. Pets that appear to have an aura, an ictal stage in which the behavior appears, and a postictal stage, or when the signs persist into the interictal interval, may also improve with seizure medication. However, when there are no psychomotor signs and no loss of consciousness, a partial (focal) seizure might still be a possible cause; therefore, a trial with levetiracetam might be an option, while clonazepam, gabapentin, pregabalin, or carbamazepine alone or in combination with other seizure medications might be added for refractory cases.[71]

2. When pain is suspected, analgesics or antiinflammatories are warranted. If neuropathic pain is a consideration, a trial with gabapentin, carbamazepine, or amitriptyline should be considered as well.

3. If the repetitive behavior is believed to be a result of conflict, frustration, anxiety, or compulsion, a trial with clomipramine or fluoxetine can be considered. However, if a neurologic cause has not been ruled out there is the potential that TCAs, and to a lesser extent SSRIs, could potentiate seizure conditions.

4. For tail chasing, efficacy has been reported using fluoxetine, clomipramine, naloxone, memantine (alone or in combination with fluoxetine), and dextromethorphan.[19,23,30,35,41,53]

Repetitive disorders with oral or ingestive signs

Licking, chewing, sucking, pica, and polyphagia

Unusual oral behaviors, including licking, sucking, smacking lips, or gulping, have a high likelihood of being associated with underlying gastrointestinal conditions. Other physical differentials would include partial complex seizure, pet parent-conditioned behaviors, stereotypies, and CDs. In a recent study of dogs with excessive licking of surfaces, gastrointestinal disorders, including eosinophilic and lymphoplasmacytic infiltration, delayed gastric emptying, irritable bowel syndrome, giardiasis, pancreatitis, and gastric foreign bodies, were identified and the problems in 9/18 dogs were completely resolved after treatment.[72] The presence of other concurrent gastrointestinal or neurological signs might also help to differentiate other potential causes. Dogs that have a history of chronic eructation, flatulence, borborygmi, vomiting, or frequent soft stools in combination with any of the oral repetitive behaviors should be closely examined for underlying GI problems. Keep in mind that chronic anxiety can lead to GI upset and the discomfort associated with chronic GI issues could increase anxiety. In these cases, if finances or other limitations preclude an ideal diagnostic workup, a trial of medications such as gastrointestinal protectants, H2 antagonists, proton pump inhibitors, or dietary management such as with a limited antigen, hydrolyzed protein, or low-residue diet should be considered to rule out a potential gastrointestinal cause for oral behaviors.

Problems associated with pica, sucking, and chewing are less well understood and the tendency of researchers to lump sucking, chewing, and ingestion into a single behavioral category when collecting data further confuses the subject. Pica is defined as the consumption of nonnutritive items and is likely to have a different pathophysiology from the conditions associated with just sucking or chewing. Dogs and cats might suck and chew on themselves (flank sucking in Dobermans), each other (as with intersucking in kittens), and fabrics such as wool or cotton. Sucking and chewing behaviors have been described as infantile behaviors and may represent redirected suckling behaviors due to early weaning or a variety of other possible environmental stressors. The behavior may be reinforced because the pet finds it self-soothing. In these cases, sucking and chewing may be more appropriately diagnosed as stereotypies.

Pica can occur in dogs and cats and has been found to include consumption of a variety of different items commonly found in the household such as rubber bands, electrical cords and cables, wallpaper, wood, items from the garbage, leather shoes and gloves, fabrics, children's toys, baby bottle nipples, and plants. Cats also seem to be attracted to string and thread. While these behaviors might appear obsessive and pose danger to the pet (resulting from foreign body obstruction or injury), they are likely a variant of normal exploration, scavenging, and predation. Cats in particular evolved to hunt and given the choice, have been shown to eat about 13 meals in a 24-hour period.[73] Thus, the chewing and ingestion of nonfood items may reflect a redirected appetitive behavior that cats are otherwise unable to express due to the manner in which they are fed commercial diets. Even when dry food is available throughout the day, these cats may be seeking items that have a different "mouth feel" or require more chewing and manipulation and serve as a partial outlet for their predatory drive. Self-reinforcement due to the taste or texture will further increase the repetition of these behaviors. Pet parents who chase the cat or yell at it may inadvertently reinforce the behavior by giving the cat attention that it finds rewarding but are more likely to cause fear, anxiety, stress, and conflict, worsening the behavior.

Target preferences of cats with oral repetitive behaviors in one study were found to include 93% wool, 64% cotton, 53% synthetic fabrics, 22% rubber and plastic, and 8% paper and cardboard.[20] Pica in cats was most commonly observed either within two months of rehoming or between 6 and 18 months of age (i.e., at the time of sexual or territorial maturity), suggesting that stress might also play a role in predispose cats to pica.[20] In a recent survey of wool-sucking Siamese and Birman cats, all of the cats were found to have an abnormally intense appetite.[74] Early weaning and a smaller litter size were found to be associated with a higher risk of wool sucking in Birmans, but physical conditions such as dental disease, gastrointestinal upset, conjunctivitis, ruptured anal glands, and urinary crystals were associated with a risk of wool sucking in Siamese cats.[74] In another study of eight cats with pica, every cat demonstrated some form of gastrointestinal disease, including delayed gastric emptying, gastric reflux, and eosinophilic inflammation of the GI tract.[75] Mild hypercholesterolemia was found in seven of the eight cats. It is impossible to say exactly how these conditions are associated with pica because GI disease could be a result of the cat consuming nonfood items that lead to GI upset, but hyperlipidemia has been documented to result in waxing and waning vomiting, diarrhea, and abdominal discomfort. Primary hypercholesterolemia is rare in cats so its association with pica deserves further investigation. As is the case with dogs, underlying physical causes for pica should always be investigated and ruled out through appropriate diagnostics. Presumptive treatment of gastrointestinal disease may be necessary when a full physical workup cannot be completed.

In a recent survey study of 42 dogs requiring surgery due to the ingestion of foreign items and 42 control dogs, 88% of dogs that required foreign body surgery had behavioral clinical signs. These disorders were identified as hyperactivity, impulsivity, and anxiety based on pet parent-completed questionnaires.[76] Twelve percent of the dogs were identified as having gastrointestinal pain, but the presence of other gastrointestinal disorders was ruled out. However, in a recent case report, a 5.5-year-old dog with a 4.5-year history of pica (eating rocks) resolved when diagnosed and treated for mild hip dysplasia.[63] These different reports underscore the importance of considering all of the possible conditions that can contribute to pica before making a diagnosis and limiting treatment to behavioral management and psychotropic drugs.

Numerous physical conditions have been identified in association with pica. These include portacaval shunts, iron deficiency anemia, pyruvate kinase deficiency, ehrlichiosis, gastrointestinal disorders, neurologic damage, feline infectious peritonitis (FIP), and other physical conditions.[75,77–83] Conditions such as metabolic diseases or medications that result in an increased appetite (e.g., corticosteroids and some benzodiazepines) can also lead to pica. Pets that are underfed and those placed on calorie-restrictive diets may begin to seek out new items to eat. Anxiety disorders and phobias may cause destruction of household objects, but ingestion is less common. Pet parents will need to be instructed to be observant to determine when destruction of items may also include consumption (see Chapters 17 and 19).

Management and treatment

For a treatment overview, see the section on management and treatment of repetitive disorders above. The family needs to focus on reducing sources of anxiety and conflict; increasing predictability and enrichment; reinforcing alternate, other; or incompatible behaviors; and identifying stimuli or situations that might incite the problem and avoiding them.

Specific recommendations for problematic licking, sucking, chewing, or picas include:
- Supervision to keep the pet engaged in desirable exploration and play and to prevent or interrupt undesirable behavior.
- Ensuring that the area is pet proofed or the pet is confined away from possible targets when the family cannot supervise or the use of a muzzle in dogs. Prolonged avoidance may decrease interest provided other outlets are provided.
- Increasing oral stimulation by stuffing or freezing dog toys with food, increasing dietary bulk (fiber, roughage), increasing oral stimulation with dental food and treats, or bones with meat or gristle (provided they are large

enough that the dog does not swallow them and not too dense to fracture teeth). Food toys that require manipulation to obtain each piece of food and games of food hide and seek can greatly slow eating for pets that ingest their food too quickly. Placing toys among the dry food inside the food bowl can slow eating.

- For cats that suck or chew on fabric but do not ingest it, the primary concern may be the damage that the cat does to fabrics. In these cases, providing a sheepskin, blanket, or other objects made of wool for the cat to focus its behavior on can be helpful. Other nonacceptable objects will need to be kept away from the cat, but many cats appear to be satisfied with having some outlet for the behavior.
- In cases where the cat is actually ingesting nonfood items, a variety of different items have been suggested for providing the cat the oral stimulation it needs without the risk of blockage or other GI problems. These include increased fiber in the diet, offering potted cat grass for the cat to chew on, and even providing canine dental chews such as rawhides. Feeding cats their ration in food-dispensing toys should also be considered as an option that allows the cat to express some of its predatory behavior in an acceptable fashion.
- There is a single documented case study that successfully utilized behavior modification (desensitization and counter conditioning) to diminish the occurrence of pica in a cat.[84] Although there is only one published study demonstrating the effectiveness of behavior modification in cats, it is very likely that a behavior modification treatment plan is effective in modifying this behavior as it is in other species.

Psychogenic polydipsia

Increased drinking and urinating are most often due to physical causes. Water intake measurement and urine concentration should first confirm that there is indeed an excess in drinking and urination. Differentials include diabetes mellitus, chronic kidney disease, pyometra, hypercalcemia, hepatic insufficiency, pyelonephritis, Cushing's disease, hypokalemia, hypoadrenocorticism, hyperthyroidism, gastrointestinal disease, and iatrogenic causes. While both central diabetes insipidus and primary polydipsia (psychogenic) are rare, a positive response to desmopressin acetate (DDAVP) would be very suggestive of a physical cause, most likely diabetes insipidus, although Cushing's syndrome could still be a possibility.[85] Polydipsia can be due to gastrointestinal disease a some patients. Patients that may suffer from nausea, gastrointestinal discomfort, or inappetence due to primary gastrointestinal disease may drink more to alleviate the discomfort or feel satiated. True psychogenic polydipsia is rare. Always investigate fully all other body systems.

Management and treatment of behavioral polydipsia

If disease or disorder in all other body systems can be ruled out, then excessive drinking may be determined to be psychogenic. The first step will be to try to identify an antecedent or trigger for the behavior and to determine if some stressor or anxiety exists that is contributing to the behavior. A behavior modification plan would need to be aimed at changing the pet's response to the antecedent, stressor, or anxiety-provoking stimulus. Medication might be used for decreasing anxiety. Some psychotropic medications also increase thirst and so may be contraindicated.

Pet parents should keep a diary to determine when the pet is likely to seek water and engage the pet in other productive activities at these times (social times, play and exercise, training, object play). Food, treats, and chews that are low in sodium should be selected. Excessive drinking can be prevented by restricting water access to measured amounts at scheduled times throughout the day, teaching the dog to leave its water bowl to engage in other activities (and to ensure drinking behaviors are not inadvertently reinforced), and with the use of ice cubes, frozen food treats, drinking bottles, self-watering devices, and drinking bowls (e.g., DrinkBetter) that can slow and limit drinking.

Repetitive disorders involving excessive grooming and/or self-trauma

Self-trauma is often secondary to repetitive behaviors such as spinning and tail chasing, attacking some other body part, or excessive self-grooming behavior. Stressors such as relocation have also been known to lead to self-injurious behavior (SIB) in some species.[86] One syndrome that might be mistaken for a primary behavioral problem is excessive scratching, especially in the area of the head, face, and mouth. In cats and possibly dogs, a neuropathy may cause head, muzzle, or neck scratching. Feline orofacial pain syndrome may also present with signs of oral discomfort and tongue mutilation. A breed disposition in Burmese cats has been reported.[87] Dental disease, dermatologic disease, trigeminal neuropathy, genetic disorders, and behavioral factors such as stress or anxiety should all be considered; however, in most cases, treatment will need to focus on reducing the neuropathic pain with medications such as gabapentin along with concurrent antiinflammatory, pain, and behavioral medications for anxiety and stress. Differentials include any disease process that leads to pain, dysesthesia, paresthesia or pruritus (e.g., hypersensitivity reactions, neuropathies), infections (e.g., bacterial, fungal, parasitic), endocrinopathies, genetic disorders, tumors, or skin disorders associated with systemic diseases (e.g., hepatocutaneous syndrome). While behavioral disorders should be on the differential list for animals that lick, bite scratch or chew, they should be considered a diagnosis of exclusion or a contributing cause.

Up to 40% of companion animals suffer from itchiness (pruritus), needing examination by a veterinarian.[88] Pruritus or any dermatologic discomfort can cause an increase in fear, anxiety, and stress. Pets may lick, bite, or chew incessantly. When pet parents attempt to stop the pet, the dog or cat may become aggressive. The licking may also be reinforced by the pet parent, resulting in an increase in the behavior, or the pet may simply move away to lick, bite, or chew. Pain including pruritus (itch) can lead to and/or compound existing emotional stress directly through a physiologic response or by leading to fear or anxiety. In addition, clinical signs associated with pain (e.g., trembling) and pruritus (e.g., licking, biting, chewing) can be difficult to distinguish from signs of emotional stress.

In humans, primary dermatologic disorders such as eczema and psoriasis are regarded as psychophysiologic because emotional stress can cause worsening of clinical signs.[89] In fact, in humans, atopic dermatitis has been associated with reduced coping tools, anxiety, irritability, and aggression.[90] Dogs with atopic dermatitis are more likely to show fear, anxiety and stress, and more likely to display aggression to strangers, owners and familiar dogs, as well as nonsocial fear, touch sensitivity, excitability, attention-seeking, decreased trainability, hyperactivity, chewing, mounting, coprophagia, begging for food, stealing food and excessive grooming, when compared with their nonitchy counterparts.[91,92] While the clinical presentations of atopic syndrome in cats are often quite different from those seen in dogs, it is likely that they could likewise be exacerbated by fear, anxiety, and stress responses.

Suspected psychodermatologic disorders (e.g., psychogenic alopecia, ALD) should always include a thorough dermatologic evaluation. In these cases, treatment of emotional stress should accompany treatment of underlying dermatologic disorders. Supplements and medications which alter emotional stress may also sedate patients and may appear to abate clinical signs associated with pruritus and pain. For this reason, a workup of other body systems is paramount.

In one case of a 30-month-old Labrador Retriever that presented with acute onset tail mutilation,[93] radiographs of the tail revealed soft tissue swelling and a mineralized ossicle in one intervertebral space that may have caused discomfort. Administration of analgesics led to complete resolution of the behavior. Self-mutilation has been documented in several other species secondary to nerve injury, pain, and altered sensation, so self-mutilation behaviors should always lead to a thorough physical exam and imaging, if possible, to rule out underlying physical causes. In the case of long standing problems, the pet parent may not remember if the lesion or the behavior came first. This can make diagnosis challenging, and empirical treatment with analgesics or antiinflammatories may be warranted in some patients before beginning behavior modification or treatment with psychotropic medications.

Dogs

Acral lick dermatitis, claw (nail) biting, head and face scratching, tail mutilation

For ALD or other self-traumatic disorders in dogs, a physical examination, CBC, serum chemistry, thyroid screening, fecal antigen, urinalysis, and a dermatologic workup, including a skin scraping, fungal culture, cytology, radiographs, and biopsy, may all be indicated. When diagnostic tests do not reveal the underlying cause, therapeutic trials with antibiotics, pain medication, antiinflammatory drugs, parasiticides, and/or food trials may be necessary. Referral to a board-certified dermatologist may be required to fully rule out dermatologic disease.

ALD occurs as a result of a primary dermatological condition that results in repeated self-trauma to a focal area, often on the leg. Dogs can initiate the development of a lesion due to the fact that their normal response is to lick a lesion or any area that is causing pain, pruritus, or discomfort. The constant licking behavior maintains and worsens the lesion. In one published account, six dogs presumed to have ALD were diagnosed with other issues, including lymphoblastic lymphoma, irritation from a Kirschner pin, furunculosis, a mast cell tumor, leishmaniasis, and sporotrichosis.[94] In another study in

which biopsies were obtained from 29 ALD lesions, bacteria were isolated from 30 of 31 cases. In only 8 of 22 cases (36%) were superficial cultures consistent with deep cultures and 48% of deep cultures were multidrug resistant, with 20% methicillin resistant.[27] Therefore long-term bactericidal antibiotic therapy (often for 4–12 weeks and sometimes longer) based on the results of culture and sensitivity from deep tissue is almost always required. Treatment may also include ancillary medications to break the itch-scratch cycle (e.g., glucocorticoids, antihistamines). Pet parent supervision to physically prevent the dog from licking the lesion may be necessary to ensure resolution and/or protection of the lesion with the use of Elizabethan collars, bandages, socks, body suits, or leggings, depending on what the individual patient tolerates.

Even when the primary dermatological or pain-causing disorder is treated, the behavioral clinical signs may persist, although to a lesser degree than upon initial presentation. Contributing behavioral causes include stress, anxiety, phobias, attention seeking and inadequate exercise, mental stimulation, or social interaction have all been suggested as a cause for excessive licking, biting, and chewing.

Grooming is a common displacement behavior so animals may persist in grooming to the point of causing hair loss and open lesions secondary to anxiety and stress from many possible causes. For claw (nail) biting, any disease of the claw or claw beds (immune, inflammatory, or infectious, including in particular Malassezia) must first be ruled out (Figure 18.1).

Flank sucking appears as follows: the dog may grab a section of flank skin in its mouth and hold the position, resulting in changes as simple as a dampened, ruffled haircoat to more severe changes including raw, open sores, necessitating treatment with antibiotics and preventive measures such as Elizabethan collars in some cases in conjunction with behavior therapy and drugs. As with any abnormal repetitive behavior, every stone must be overturned to search for underlying physical causes. Even disorders as counterintuitive as hypoadrenocorticism have been linked with flank sucking in Doberman Pinschers. It may in fact simply be a coping mechanism

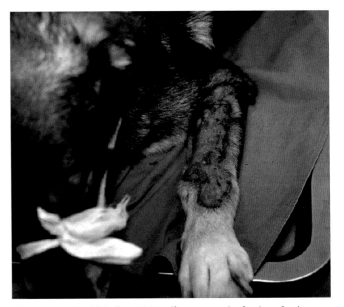

Figure 18.1 Acral lick dermatitis: self-trauma to the foreleg of a dog. *(Reproduced with permission from Ackerman L. Practical Canine Dermatology. Goleta, CA: American Veterinary Publications; 1989.)*

that Dobermans are predisposed to whenever they feel stress, fear, anxiety, conflict, panic, pain, or discomfort.

Management and treatment

Treatment of canine self-trauma requires the same approach as other repetitive disorders discussed above. The behavior history should identify when the problem began and what might have been the inciting factors. Pet parent responses and attempts to correct the factors that are contributing to the problem must be identified and removed. When there are identifiable problems in other body systems, their involvement as an initiating factor or as a secondary complication will need to be determined; regardless, any pain, inflammation, infection, or other physical issues will need to be treated. Specific stressors or anxiety-provoking stimuli in the home should be identified so that these can be resolved. Enrichment should be scheduled to provide alternative acceptable outlets for the behavior, especially at times when the self-trauma might be displayed. Alternate acceptable behaviors such as resting with head down, picking up toys and holding them, or chewing on appropriate toys, should be reinforced. Clicker training can help to mark, reinforce, and shape progressively more desirable behaviors. If the pet begins to engage in the undesirable behavior, it should be given no social feedback at all, including scolding, consoling, obedience cues, or eye contact. The pet should be calmly interrupted with a cue to perform an alternate behavior for which it can be rewarded. SSRIs (e.g., fluoxetine, paroxetine, or citalopram) or TCAs (e.g., clomipramine) are generally the medications of choice (see Chapter 11). The addition of other medications and natural products to reduce anxiety further or adjunctive therapy with NMDA antagonists, such as memantine or dextromethorphan, might be considered. Medications such as doxepin have also been reported previously to be useful in treating ALD, but it is likely that while there may be some behavioral effect, the strong antihistaminic effects may be most beneficial effect from this medication when treating ALD.

Cats

Self-trauma and psychogenic alopecia

Cats spend between 30% and 50% of their awake time grooming. It is an important maintenance and social behavior.[95] Grooming is also common displacement behavior in cats and may be seen during situations of conflict, frustration, or stress.[55] In some cases, cats overgroom themselves to the point where alopecia and even skin lesions develop. However, physical problems are often the primary or sole reason for hair loss. When presented with a cat that has hair loss, licking, or scratching, the diagnostic workup should begin with an examination, skin scrapings, cytology, parasite assessment, trichogram, fungal culture, anal sac expression, CBC, serum chemistry, thyroid evaluation, urinalysis, proBNP, fecal antigen testing, and a viral profile may also be needed, as well as biopsies for histopathologic assessment. Unlike the situation in dogs in which atopic dermatitis is primarily a skin disease, asthma may play a significant role in feline atopic syndrome and must be considered, in addition to dermatologic manifestations that are often quite different from those seen in dogs (including papulocrustous eruptions, inflammatory plaques, and even granulomatous reactions). So, unlike the typical diagnostic approach often adequate for canine atopic dermatitis, the dermatologic evaluation for feline atopic dermatitis would typically continue with a trichogram, fungal culture, skin scraping, and possible biopsy. Assuming no abnormal findings, this does not yet confirm a behavioral cause since parasitic hypersensitivity, adverse food reactions, and other hypersensitivity reactions may have similar presentations with hair loss and no primary skin lesions. Therefore, a therapeutic response trial with novel or hydrolyzed protein diets for at least eight weeks, a parasite control trial, and trials with appropriate anti-inflammatory agents might be used sequentially or together to rule out pruritic causes. Using this protocol in 21 cases presented for psychogenic alopecia to a referral practice, 76.2% had a physical etiology, 9.5% were deemed compulsive, and 14.3% were combined physical and behavioral. A combination of adverse food reaction and atopic dermatitis (six cases) was the most common diagnosis. Some cats had atopic dermatitis, parasitic hypersensitivity, or an adverse food reaction alone (see Figures 18.2 and 18.3). Although biopsies indicated an inflammatory response for most physical cases, some cats with histologically normal skin still had an underlying physical cause.[96] Even when there is an underlying cause which is not behavioral, fear, anxiety, stress, and distress need to be treated to improve patient quality of life. A response to medication that alters behavior does not denote a lack of underlying physical cause.

Tail attacking and mutilation in cats may have a behavioral cause, but numerous other differentials must first be ruled out. Tail mutilation may begin as a play behavior or a conflict-induced behavior in which the cat circles and chases its tail. However, should the cat bite into its tail, the resultant pain, infection, and possible neuropathy could incite further chewing and attacking. Skin disease, trauma, spinal pain, and other neuropathies could initiate the behavior or be a secondary contributing factor.

Management and treatment

Treatment should focus on identifying the underlying cause, often with the aid of a therapeutic response trial. Repetitive disorders will require a program of predictability, enrichment, and identification and elimination of stressors that might cause or contribute to the problem (discussed previously). Temporary use of Elizabethan collars or bandaging might also be required to prevent further self-trauma, however, these might further contribute to the pet's stress. The family should keep a journal to determine when the problem is most likely to arise, so they can provide entertaining distractions and alternative activities in a timely manner. While clomipramine and fluoxetine are likely to be effective if the diagnosis is a compulsive or conflict-induced behavior, concurrent medications might be needed if there are also elements of pain, neuropathic pain, or other physical conditions.[19,52,55]

Hyperesthesia in dogs and cats

Feline hyperesthesia syndrome

This is a poorly understood condition that possibly has neurological, dermatological, pain, and behavioral components.[97] It is also known as rippling, rolling, or twitching skin disease. The clinical picture varies between cats such that individuals may exhibit all or a select few of the described signs. Clinical signs include: pacing, agitation, licking at the tail or back legs, hissing, growling, and biting at the tail or sides, exaggerated tail wagging or thumping, and jumping up as if startled.[98] Some cats will bite and scratch at their front legs or paws. They may vocalize, suddenly run and hide, and defecate while running. The hallmark sign of this condition is rippling or twitching of the thoracolumbar skin and spasm of the epaxial muscles. The cat may appear agitated during the episode, pupils may dilate, and there may be episodes of self-directed aggression or redirected aggression. The behavior is often difficult or impossible to interrupt and can be induced simply by rubbing the cat's back, although episodes most commonly begin without any apparent environmental stimulation. Some cats exhibit skin rolling and vacuum licking when the dorsal lumbar area is touched. In a recent case series, most cats that presented for signs of feline hyperesthesia were less than a year of age, had access to outdoors, and were male.[98] In the same study, extensive diagnostic workups did not reveal any physical causes; however, hypersensitive dermatitis was suspected in two cases. Medication used in this case series included gabapentin, meloxicam, antibiotics, phenobarbital, prednisone, topiramate, clomipramine, fluoxetine, amitriptyline, and tramadol. Of the six cases treated, all improved and five cats showed complete remission. Based on this limited case series, gabapentin may be a very important part of improvement in these cases.

The first step is to rule out physical conditions. Dermatologic conditions such as parasites (e.g., fleas, cheyletiellosis, *Demodex gatoi*), yeast infections, allergies, adverse food reactions, and immune-mediated disease can cause pain, cutaneous sensitivity, and irritation in the area. Neurologic diseases such as neuritis, cranial disease, partial seizures, spinal diseases including myelitis, disk protrusion and trauma, genetic disorders, and neuropathic pain can induce clinical signs.[99] Musculoskeletal diseases, including a myelopathy induced by feline leukemia virus and a vacuolar myopathy similar to inclusion-body myositis in humans, have also been identified in some cats.[100,101] Pain might also arise from the gastrointestinal tract or anal sacs. It has also been suggested that in some cats, pain pathways may be overly sensitive to relatively innocuous touch sensations.[102] Any form of arousal could potentially induce hyperesthesia, as can conflict, frustration, and CDs.

Management and treatment

Therapeutic response trials should only be attempted if they will not interfere with diagnosis and treatment of the underlying problem, the pet's welfare will not be negatively affected, they are appropriate for safely relieving clinical signs, and a diagnostic workup is under way. For example, if a patient is suffering and/or the pet parent is considering euthanasia of the pet, treatment with fluoxetine and clonidine may be started to alleviate suffering. In this case, medications such as clomipramine would be avoided during the dermatologic workup because of their potent antihistaminic effects. In another example, gabapentin may be prescribed for pain; however, it also has anticonvulsant and antianxiety effects. Therefore, if the pet responds with less frequent behavioral signs, it does not confirm a specific underlying cause. That is not to say that medications should not be prescribed which will help the patient. Delay causing an increase in fear, anxiety, stress, or pain is not ethical or in the pet's best interest. However, the limitations of the medications used should be considered. Pet parents should be counseled that response to psychotropic medications does not lead to a behavioral diagnosis. In most cases, this behavior is the result of the cat experiencing some sensation and not a CD. Just because the underlying condition cannot be identified does not mean that the cat is not experiencing a real physical sensation, so presumptive therapy for dermatologic or neurologic conditions should be the first approach.

Other treatments will vary with underlying cause. If arousal, conflict, frustration, or anxiety contributes to the problem, the environment should be modified to avoid triggers that might incite the behavior and the cat provided with a predictable environment that provides for all of its behavioral needs. Increased enrichment by increasing predatory chase sessions, providing feeding toys, and increasing exploration with boxes or three-dimensional space and perching areas might be beneficial, provided they do not increase the cat's arousal to a level that might incite the behavior.

Canine hyperesthesia

Hyperesthesia, with twitching of the skin and epaxial muscles, which might be associated with circling or self-trauma such as licking or biting, is also recognized in the canine. Possible causes might include arousal and conflict, cranial and spinal diseases including intervertebral disk disease, dermatologic conditions, neuropathic pain, or as a component of anxiety, arousal or CDs, especially when accompanied by other signs such as tail chasing in German Shepherd Dogs. This is rarely seen and should be addressed similarly to feline hyperesthesia. See above.

CASE EXAMPLES

Case 1

Presentation

Twilight, a 2-year-old, 37-kg spayed female Labrador Retriever, was presented for a 2-cm thickened ulcerated lesion on the left foreleg.

History

The pet parent had a baby two months prior to the onset of the problem, but the initial licking had started intermittently approximately four months previously. During the past month, the licking had been constant. Yelling at the dog was only successful in distracting her temporarily. Prior to the pregnancy, the female pet parent and the dog often jogged together and spent a lot of time in the park. The dog had minimal training and was not consistently responsive to any verbal cues. Since the baby was born, the dog could not be successfully settled and the pet parent frequently found herself scolding the dog.

CASE EXAMPLES—cont'd

Workup

A thorough physical workup, including CBC, serum chemistry, thyroid screening, urinalysis, fecal antigen, skin scrapings, cytology, and fungal culture, uncovered no other problems. The skin appeared indurated and superficially eroded with evidence of suspected deep infection; an aspirate from the lesion was submitted for culture and sensitivity.

Treatment

Since Twilight also had evidence of folliculitis and mild cheilitis, both behavioral and dermatologic therapy was suggested. Twilight was already on a monthly topical flea and heartworm medication and was placed on an eight-week course of bactericidal antibiotic on the basis of culture and sensitivity, as well as a commercial novel protein diet. The pet parents were instructed that they were to give at least 50% of the food out of feeding toys or as training treats. The pet parents filled food toys with a mixture of oatmeal and dog food, and occasionally purchased some rabbit meat and pumpkin to use as fresh treats.

Behaviorally, the pet parents were instructed to focus on reducing the conflict and anxiety associated with the dog's change in routine, which had unintentionally decreased the quality of daily life and altered the relationship with the pet parent. The pet parents were encouraged to alternate in taking the pet on at least one long walk each day, and to hire a dog-walking service to provide a second daily walk with a group of dogs. The pet parents were shown how to train sit, lie down, and stay on command using food lures and a head halter. Toys filled with food were provided during times when Twilight was likely to lick and when the baby was present. When not supervising, the pet parents were to use an Elizabethan collar to allow the lesion to heal and attempt to break the cycle. Close supervision and preemptive measures were to be used and all punishment was to cease. The family was told that if Twilight began to lick, they were to redirect her to her bed and when she settled, reinforce her. If the pet stopped for 10 seconds or more, they were to provide a toy filled with food for her to lick instead of her leg, play with her, or take her for a walk. After walks, training, and play, the pet parents were advised to develop a consistent routine where they could provide Twilight with toys filled with food or rabbit meat on her mat while they attended to the baby.

Followup

After eight weeks, all skin problems were resolved except the lesion on the foreleg, which was mildly improved. Whenever the pet parents were unable to supervise and Twilight was not actively engaged with toys or food, she would begin to lick at the site. When they were present, they could interrupt the behavior. Antibiotics and diet were extended for an additional four weeks and fluoxetine was prescribed at a dose of 0.5 mg/kg PO q24 for 14 days, then 1 mg/kg PO q24. A positive reinforcement dog trainer was recommended to assist with training relaxation and an alternate behavior that Twilight could perform instead of licking, such as carrying a toy.

Twelve weeks after the initial appointment, the pet parents noted that the licking had virtually ceased at any time the dog was supervised and verbal cues were sufficient to keep her attention. She was able to settle on her bed with a food toy and not lick her leg when they were taking care of the baby and unable to attend to her. She had learned to hold a specific toy, which she could also lick when she was stressed. The dog training professional was working with them to send her to that toy when they saw her licking. The Elizabethan collar was only used at night.

Sixteen weeks after the original appointment, the skin remained well controlled, the lesion had virtually healed, and the Elizabethan collar was only left applied at nights or when the pet parents were away from home. Over the long term, attempts at reduction in dose of fluoxetine led to recurrence and it was still in use at 2-year followup. Recurrence of skin lesions could be controlled with antibacterial shampoos and conditioner.

Case 2

Presentation

Tyson, a 7-year-old neutered male domestic short-haired cat, had a two-year history of hair loss along the belly and the posterior surfaces of all four legs.

History

Tyson previously had a dermatologic diagnostic workup but with minimal response to treatment trials with oral corticosteroid trials and flea treatments. The behavior had persisted. The pet parents could not recall an inciting incident or any changes when the behavior first started. They felt confident that they had "done everything" and that this behavior was a result of their cat's personality.

Workup

A CBC, serum chemistry, thyroid screening, urinalysis, proBNP, and fecal antigen test were within normal limits. There were no abnormalities seen on physical examination, and the trichogram revealed that the hairs were predominantly in anagen (growth phase) but had been broken by licking. A skin biopsy showed no evidence of any underlying cause (mild perivascular inflammation presumed due to licking), and the dermatophyte culture and skin scrapings were negative.

Treatment and followup

A parasiticide response trial and an eight-week trial with a hydrolyzed protein diet trial achieved an improvement of over 50%. The food was continued and a corticosteroid-response trial was initiated. After three weeks, all licking had ceased and hair regrowth was occurring at all sites of previous hair loss. At this point, treatment was continued and Tyson was challenged with his original diet. Within two weeks, licking and hair loss had resumed. Over time and through challenge feeding, it was determined that Tyson could not tolerate beef or pork, but could be completely controlled with a single antigen diet of chicken and rice, chicken, or pieces of game meats as treats, and low-dose oral cyclosporine therapy ranging from daily to twice weekly depending on season. Although there had been no skin lesions, Tyson's diagnosis was a combination of adverse food reactions and feline atopic dermatitis (see Figure 18.2).

Case 3

Presentation

Sassy, a 6-kg, 4-year-old female spayed Burmese cat, was referred for psychogenic alopecia.

History

Although Sassy was occasionally allowed outdoors, she preferred to stay indoors, resting on the top of the couch, looking out the window. She occasionally played with the other cat in the home and there were few, if any, reported conflicts. Both cats were fed free choice, had kitty grass to chew, and were given play sessions with chase toys and catnip every few days. Approximately 1.5 years earlier, Sassy began pulling out her hair on her belly, midback, and both hind legs, and fleas were identified. However, after treatment of both cats, the hair loss and licking in Sassy continued and her skin could be seen rippling along the back as often as once daily, after which she would lick

continued

herself incessantly. After reviewing the behavior history with the pet parents, the only apparent stressor was that the husband did not want Sassy on the couch and would punish her by yelling or block her access by placing an upside-down plastic carpet runner (nubs up) on the couch.

Workup

After the full dermatologic workup, food trial, parasite control, and corticosteroid therapy (as detailed in Case 2), there was no improvement in the hair loss or hyperesthesia.

Treatment and follow-up

Feeding toys, daily play sessions with chase toys, a new perching area, and avoiding further punishment were discussed and Sassy was placed on 5 mg clomipramine daily. After two weeks, the pet parents reported that hyperesthesia had ceased. At a followup visit at three months, there was good hair regrowth, no further hair loss or hyperesthesia, and the pet parents had ceased all punishment but had initiated only minimal additional play. Attempts to reduce the clomipramine to every other day therapy and an attempt at transdermal clomipramine therapy both led to recurrence, and an oral dose of 5 mg daily PO was still being used at 18-month followup. Sassy was diagnosed as having psychogenic alopecia (see Figure 18.3).

Case 4

Presentation

Rocky was a 3-year-old male neutered Lhasa Apso that barked incessantly and chased his tail whenever the pet parent entered the home.

History

The problem began about one year earlier during a time when Rocky had a lapse in house training and for several weeks in a row, the pet parent frequently punished Rocky upon arriving home and finding a mess in the house. Rocky would start to approach the pet parent,

then back away and run in circles while barking. The pet parents admitted that at the start they had found the tail chasing "funny" and "cute" and had encouraged the behavior. When the behavior became incessant, the pet parent then attempted to calm Rocky down by patting or lifting him, but recently had resorted to interrupting the behavior by feeding Rocky as soon as the behavior started.

Workup

A CBC, serum chemistry, thyroid screening, and urinalysis were within normal limits. However, the fecal antigen test revealed Giardia infection. There were no abnormalities seen on physical examination.

Treatment and followup

Treatment for the Giardia infection was initiated. In addition, the pet parents were instructed to stop punishing him with any form of physical or verbal punishment. They were also instructed to work with a positive reinforcement trainer to help them have more consistent interactions with him because the barking and tail chasing had initially developed as a result of conflict at the time of pet parent arrival, since he was motivated to greet the pet parent but fearful of being punished.

In two weeks, the pet parents had seen a decrease in tail chasing by 50%. A review of reward-based training and sessions with a reinforcement-based trainer were recommended to help Rocky learn desirable behaviors, including down–stay, sit and focus, and mat training, that might then be used each time a problem might arise. Each time Rocky approached for anything of value (food, play, or attention), the pet parents were advised to use one of the behaviors predictably and consistently (sit or down–stay) to reduce Rocky's arousal and to teach him proper greeting behaviors that would earn rewards. The pet parents were advised as to how to distract and redirect him with treats in cases where he was not yet able to respond to cues adequately. In addition, the pet parents were advised to keep departures and returns low key. Within six weeks, the behavior had ceased.

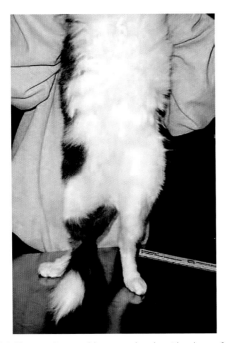

Figure 18.2 Tyson: a 7 year old neutered male with adverse food reaction and atopic dermatitis.

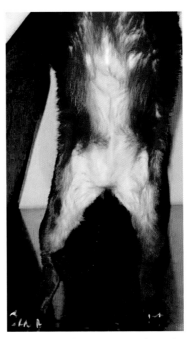

Figure 18.3 Sassy: a 4 year old Burmese cat with psychogenic alopecia.

Prognosis

The prognosis for any repetitive disorder will be dependent upon the underlying cause being identified and appropriately treated, especially in cases where pain, pruritus, neuropathy, or seizures may be present. When physical conditions can be identified and successfully treated, the prognosis may be good. When pet parent responses and a poor environment have contributed to the problem, the prognosis can be good if the family is able to change their behavior and commit to modifying the environment. If no underlying physical cause can be identified and the problem is determined to be a repetitive disorder due to displacement, redirection, conflict, or anxiety, then again, success will be dependent upon the ability of the pet parent to modify the environment appropriately to meet the pet's behavioral needs and implement behavior modification. However, the pet parent should be warned that stereotypical behavior is notoriously difficult to stop completely. There are many documented cases where behavioral modification, environmental management, and psychotropic medications decrease the behaviors but never completely stop it. These disorders may take some time and effort to find the best combination of behavior therapy and medications to be able to control the problem effectively, and long-term ongoing treatment is likely to be required. Ultimately, the most important criteria to evaluate are that the animal's behavioral needs are being met and their welfare remains good, even if they continue to perform the behavior occasionally.

Conclusion

Abnormal repetitive behaviors are not common in dogs and cats and are most commonly associated with physical disorders. In many cases, the underlying disorder may not be obvious and may involve significant workup. Medications which alter behavioral state should be used immediately to relieve fear, anxiety, stress, and pain. However, pet parents and the veterinarian should be aware of the limitations of these medications on some diagnostic tests and that they should not be considered therapeutic trials. Finally, behavior modification and environmental enrichment should be considered in all cases.

References

1. Garner JP. Perseveration and stereotypy – systems-level insights from clinical psychology. In: Mason G, Rushen J, eds. *Stereotypic Animal Behaviour: Fundamentals and Applications to Welfare*. 2nd ed. Wallingford: CABI; 2006:121–152.

2. Latham NR, Mason GJ. Maternal deprivation and the development of stereotypic behaviour. *Appl Anim Behav Sci*. 2008;110:84–108.

3. Kaulfuss P, Wuerbel H, Failing K. Studies on classifying abnormal-repetitive behaviours in dogs. In: *Proceedings of the 2010 European Veterinary Behavior Meeting*. Hamburg: 2010:92–96.

4. Devinsky O, Boesch JM, Cerda-Gonzalez S, et al. A cross-species approach to disorders affecting brain and behaviour. *Nat Rev Neurol*. 2018;14(11). doi:10.1038/s41582-018-0074 z.

5. Dodman NH, Karlsson EK, Moon-Fanelli A, et al. A canine chromosomes 7 locus confers compulsive disorders susceptibility. *Mol Psychiatry*. 2009;15:8–10.

6. Dodman NH, Ginns EI, Schuster L, et al. Compulsive disorder, a dog model of human OCD. *Int J Appl Res Vet Med*. 2016;14(1):1–18.

7. Schoenecker B, Heller KE. Indication of a genetic basis of stereotypies in laboratory-bred bank voles (Clethrionomys glareolus) *Appl Anim Behav Sci*. 2000;68:339–347.

8. Rushen J, Mason G. A decade-or-more's progress in understanding stereotypic behavior. In: Mason G, Rushen J, eds. *Stereotypic Animal Behaviour: Fundamentals and Applications to Welfare*. 2nd ed. Wallingford: CABI; 2006:1–18.

9. Vanderbroek I, Odberg FO, Caemaert J. Microdialysis study of the caudate nucleus of stereotyping and non-stereotyping bank voles. In: *Proceedings of the International Society of Applied Ethology*. Potters Bar: Universities Federation for Animal Welfare; 1995:245.

10. Math SB, Janardhan Reddy YC. Issues in the pharmacological treatment of obsessive-compulsive disorder. *Int J Clin Pract*. 2008;61:1170–1180.

11. Goldberger E, Rapaport JL. Canine acral lick dermatitis: response to the antiobsessional drug clomipramine. *J Am Anim Hosp Assoc*. 1990;27:179–182.

12. Rapaport JL, Ryland DH, Kriete M. Drug treatment of canine acral lick; an animal model of obsessive-compulsive disorder. *Arch Gen Psychiatry*. 1992;49,517–521.

13. Stein DJ, Mendelsohn I, Potocnik F, et al. Use of the selective serotonin reuptake inhibitor citalopram in a possible animal analogue of obsessive-compulsive disorder. *Depress Anxiety*. 1998;8:39–42.

14. Wynchank D, Berk M. Fluoxetine treatment of acral lick dermatitis in dogs: a placebo-controlled randomized double-blind trial. *Depress Anxiety*. 1998;8:21–23.

15. Pereira JT, Larsson CE, Ramos D. Environmental, individual, and triggering aspects of dogs presenting with acral lick dermatitis. Abstract. In: Heath S, ed. *Proceedings of the 7th International Meeting of Veterinary Behaviour Medicine*. ESVCE Belgium; 2009:278–279.

16. Protopopova A, Hall NJ, Wynne CD. Association between increased behavioral persistence and stereotypy in the pet dog. *Behav Proc*. 2014;106:77–81.

17. Ogata N, Gillis TE, Liu X, Cunningham SM, et al. Brain structure abnormalities in Doberman Pinschers with canine compulsive disorder. *Prog Neuropsychopharmacol Biol Psychiatry*. 2013;45:1–6.

18. Moon-Fanelli AA, Dodman NH, Cottam N. Blanket and flank sucking in Doberman Pinschers. *J Am Vet Med Assoc*. 2007;231:907–912.

19. Overall KL, Dunham AE. Clinical features and outcome in dogs and cats with obsessive-compulsive disorder: 126 cases (1989–2000). *J Am Vet Med Assoc*. 2002;221:1445–1452.

20. Bradshaw JWS, Neville PF, Sawyer D. Factors affecting pica in the domestic cat. *Appl Anim Behav Sci*. 1997;52:373–379.

21. Moon-Fanelli AA, Dodman NH, Famula TR. Characteristics of compulsive tail chasing and associated risk factors in Bull Terriers. *J Am Vet Med Assoc*. 2011;238:883–889.

22. Blackshaw JK. Tail chasing and circling in dogs. *Can Pract*. 1994;19:7–11.

23. Yalcin E. Comparison of clomipramine and fluoxetine treatment of dogs with tail chasing. *Tierarzt Prax*. 2010;28:295–299.

24. Dodman NH, Knowles K, Shuster L, MoonFanelli A, Tidwell A, et al. Behavioral changes associated with suspected complex partial seizures in Bull Terriers. *J Am Vet Med Assoc*. 1996;208:688–691.

25. Ucchedu S, Gallucci A, Briguglio P, et al. Tail chasing a dog with brain atrophy: a case report. *J Vet Behav*. 2018;25:52–55.

26. Delgado MM, Walcher I, Buffington CAT. A survey-based assessment of risk factors

for cross-sucking behaviors in neonatal kittens, Felis catus. *Appl Anim Behav Sci.* 2020;230:105069.

27. Schumaker AK, Angus JC, Coyner KS, et al. Microbiological and histopathological features of canine acral lick dermatitis. *Vet Dermatol.* 2008;19:288–298.

28. Burn CC. A vicious cycle: a cross-sectional study of canine tail-chasing and human responses to it, using a free video-sharing website. *PLoS One.* 2011;6:e26553.

29. Cabib S. Neurobiological basis of stereotypies. In: Lawrence AB, Rushen J, eds. *Stereotypic Animal Behavior; Fundamentals and Applications to Welfare.* Wallingford: CABI; 1993:119–145.

30. Schneider B, Dodman NH, Maranda L. Use of memantine in treatment of canine compulsive disorders. *J Vet Behav.* 2009; 4:118–126.

31. Dodman NH, Shuster L, Nesbitt G, et al. The use of dextromethorphan to treat repetitive self-directed, scratching, biting or chewing in dogs with allergic dermatitis. *J Vet Pharmacol Ther.* 2004;27:99–104.

32. Korff S, Harvey BH. Animal models of obsessive-compulsive disorder: rationale to understanding psychobiology and pharmacology. *Psychiatr Clin North Am.* 2006;29:371–390.

33. Kennes D, Odberg FO, Bouquet Y, et al. Changes in naloxone and haloperidol effects during the development of captivity induced jumping stereotypy in bank voles. *J Pharmacol.* 1988;153: 19–24.

34. Dodman NH, Shuster L, White SD, et al. Use of narcotic antagonists to modify stereotypic self-licking, self-chewing and scratching behavior. *J Am Vet Med Assoc.* 1988;193:815–819.

35. Brown SA, Crowell-Davis S, Malcolm T, et al. Naloxone-responsive compulsive tail chasing in a dog. *J Am Vet Med Assoc.* 1987;190:884–886.

36. Brignac MM. Hydrocodone treatment of acral lick dermatitis. In: *Proceedings of the 2nd Annual World Congress of Veterinary Dermatology.* Montreal; 1992:50.

37. Longoni R, Spina L, Mulas A, et al. (D-Ala2) deltrophin II: D1-dependent stereotypies and stimulation of dopamine release in the nucleus accumbens. *J Neurosci.* 1991;11:1565–1576.

38. Hartgraves SL, Randall PK. Dopamine agonist-induced stereotypic grooming and self-mutilation following striatal dopamine depletion. *Psychopharmacology.* 1986;90:358–363.

39. Iglauer F, Rasim R. Treatment of psychogenic feather picking in birds with a dopamine antagonist. *J Small Anim Pract.* 1993;34:564–566.

40. Pageat P, Lafont C, Falewee C, et al. An evaluation of serum prolactin in anxious dogs and response to treatment with selegiline or fluoxetine. *Appl Anim Behav Sci.* 2007;105:342–350.

41. Moon-Fanelli AA, Dodman NH. Description and development of compulsive tail chasing in terriers and

42. Irimajiri M, Luescher AU, Douglass G, et al. Randomized, controlled clinical trial of the efficacy of fluoxetine for treatment of compulsive disorders in dogs. *J Am Vet Med Assoc.* 2009;235:707–709.

43. Hewson CJ, Luescher UA, Parent JM, et al. Efficacy of clomipramine in the treatment of canine compulsive disorder. *J Am Vet Med Assoc.* 1998;213:1760–1765.

44. Schoenecker B, Heller KE. Stimulation of serotonin (5-HT) activity reduces spontaneous stereotypies in female but not in male bank voles (Clethrionomys glareolus). Stereotyping female voles as a new animal model for human anxiety and mood disorders? *Appl Anim Behav Sci.* 2003;80:161–170.

45. Vermeire S, Audenaert K, De Meester RD, et al. Serotonin 2A receptor, serotonin transporter and dopamine transporter alterations in dogs with compulsive behaviour as a promising model for human obsessive-compulsive disorder. *Psychiatry Res Neuroimag.* 2012:201:78–87.

46. Tsilioni I, Dodman N, Petra AI, et al. Elevated serum neurotensin and see our age levels and children with autistic spectrum disorders and tail chasing Bull Terriers with a phenotype similar to autism. *Transl Psychiatry.* 2014;4:e466. doi:10.1038/tp.2014.106.

47. Dehasse J. Clinical management of stereotypies in dogs. In: *Presented to the AVSAB Annual Conference.* AVMA; 1998.

48. Tiira K, Hakosalo O, Kareinen L, et al. Environmental effects on compulsive tail-chasing in dogs. *PLoS One.* 2012;7:e41684.

49. Irimajiri M, Jay EE, Glickman LT. Mild polycythemia associated with compulsive disorder in dogs. *J Vet Behav.* 2006;1: 23–28.

50. Dodman NH, Knowles KE, Shuster L, et al. Behavioral changes associated with suspected complex partial seizures in bull terriers. *J Am Vet Med Assoc.* 1996;208: 688–691.

51. Hall NJ, Protopopova A, Wynn CDL. The role of environmental and owner-provided consequences in canine stereotypy and compulsive behavior. *J Vet Behav.* 2015:10:24–35.

52. Seksel K, Lindeman MJ. Use of clomipramine in the treatment of anxiety-related and obsessive-compulsive disorders in cats. *Aust Vet J.* 1998;76: 317–321.

53. Irimajiri M, Luescher UA. Effect of fluoxetine hydrochloride in treating canine compulsive disorder. In: Mills D, Levine E, eds. *Current Issues and Research in Veterinary Behavioral Medicine.* West Lafayette, Indiana: Purdue University Press; 2005:198–200.

54. Wrzosek M, Plonek M, Nicpon J, et al. Retrospective multicenter evaluation of the "fly-catching syndrome" in 24 dogs: EEG, BAER, MRI, CSF findings and response to antiepileptic and antidepressant treatment. *Epilepsy Behav.* 2015;53:184–189.

55. Sawyer LS, Moon-Fanelli AA, Dodman NH. Psychogenic alopecia in cats: 11 cases (1993–1996). *J Am Vet Med Assoc.* 1999;214:71–74.

56. Gilron I, Bailey JM, Tu D. Nortriptyline and gabapentin, alone or in combination for neuropathic pain: a double-blind randomized controlled crossover trial. *Lancet.* 2009;374:252–262.

57. Wald R, Dodman N, Shuster L. The combined effects of memantine and fluoxetine on an animal model of obsessive-compulsive disorder. *Exp Clin Psychopharmacol.* 2009:17;191–197.

58. Kukanich B, Papich MG. Plasma profile and pharmokinetics of dextromethorphan after intravenous and oral administration in dogs. *J Vet Pharmacol Ther.* 2004;27: 337–341.

59. White SD. Naltrexone for treatment of acral lick dermatitis in dogs. *J Am Vet Med Assoc.* 1990;196:1073–1076.

60. Beaver BV. *Canine Behavior Insights and Answers.* 2nd ed. St. Louis: Saunders Elsevier; 2009:83.

61. Dehasse J. Retrospective study on the use of Selgian (selegiline) in cats. In: *Proceedings of the American Veterinary Society of Animal Behavior.* 1999.

62. Willemse T, Spruijt BM. Preliminary evidence for dopaminergic involvement in stress-induced excessive grooming in cats. *Neurosci Res Commun.* 1995;17:203–208.

63. Poirer-Guay MP, Belanger MC, Frank D. Stargazing in a dog: atypical manifestation of upper gastrointestinal disease. *Can Vet J.* 2014;55:1079–1082.

64. Frank D, Bélanger M, Bécuwe-Bonnet V, et al. Prospective physical evaluation of 7 dogs presented with fly biting. *Can Vet J.* 2012;1253(12):1279.

65. Mills DS, Demontigny-Bedard I, Gruen M, et al. Pain and problem behavior in cats and dogs. *Animals.* 2020;10(2):318. doi:10.3390/ani10020318.

66. Berendt M, Gram L. Epilepsy and seizure classification in 63 dogs: a reappraisal of veterinary epilepsy terminology. *J Vet Int Med.* 1999;13:14–20.

67. Dodman NH, Bronson R, Gliatto J. Tail chasing in a bull terrier. *J Am Vet Med Assoc.* 1993;202:758–760.

68. Rusbridge C. Neurological diseases of the Cavalier King Charles spaniel. *J Small Anim Pract.* 2005;46:265–272.

69. Rusbridge C. *Chiari-Like Malformation and Syringomyelia in Cavalier King Charles Spaniels.* Doctoral Thesis. Utrecht: Utrecht University; 2007.

70. Todor D R, Harrison TM, Milhorat TH. Pain and syringomyelia: a review. *Neurosurg Focus.* 2000;8:1–6.

71. Dewey CW, Cerda-Gonzalez S, Levine JM. Pregabalin as an adjunct to phenobarbital, potassium bromide, or a combination of phenobarbital and potassium bromide for treatment of dogs with suspected idiopathic epilepsy. *J Am Vet Med Assoc.* 2009;235:1442–1449.

72. Bécuwe-Bonnet V, Bélanger M, Frank D, et al. Gastrointestinal disorders in dogs

with excessive licking of surfaces. *J Vet Behav.* 2012;7:194–204.

73. Mugford RA. External influences on the feeding of carnivores. In: Kare MR, Maller O, eds. *The Chemical Senses and Nutrition.* New York: Academic Press Inc.; 1977.

74. Bornes-Weil S, Emmanuel C, Longo J, et al. A case-control study of compulsive wool-sucking in Siamese and Birman cats (n = 204). *J Vet Behav.* 2015;10:543–548.

75. Demontigny-Bédard I, Bélanger M, Hélie P, et al. Physical and behavioral evaluation of 8 cats presenting with fabric ingestion: An exploratory pilot study. *Can Vet J.* 2019;60:1081–1088.

76. Masson S, Guitaut N, Medam T, et al. Link between foreign body ingestion and behavioural disorder in dogs. *J Vet Behav.* 2021;45:25–32.

77. Thomas CW, Rising JL, Moore JK. Blood lead concentrations of children and dogs from 83 Illinois families. *J Am Vet Med Assoc.* 1976;169:1237–1240.

78. Black AM. The pathophysiology and laboratory diagnosis of congenital portosystemic shunts in dogs. *N Z Vet J.* 1994;42:75.

79. Goldman EE, Breitschwerdt EB, Grindem CB, et al. Granulocytic ehrlichiosis in dogs from North Carolina and Virginia. *J Vet Intern Med.* 1998;12(2):61–70.

80. Kohn B, Weingart C, Eckmann V, et al. Primary immune-mediated hemolytic anemia in 19 cats: diagnosis, therapy, and outcome (1998–2004). *J Vet Intern Med.* 2006;20:159–166.

81. Kohn B, Fumi C. Clinical course of pyruvate kinase deficiency in Abyssinian and Somali cats. *J Feline Med Surg.* 2008; 10:145–153.

82. Berset-Istratescu CM, Glardon OJ, Magouras I, et al. Follow-up of 100 dogs with acute diarrhea in a primary care practice. *Vet J.* 2014;199:188–190.

83. Demontigny-Bédard I, Beauchamp G, Bélanger M, et al. Characterization of pica and chewing behaviors in privately owned cats: a case-control study. *J Feline Med Surg.* 2016;18(8):652–657.

84. Mongillo P, Adamelli S, Bernardini M, et al. Successful treatment of abnormal feeding behavior in a cat. *J Vet Behav.* 2012;7:390–393.

85. Feldman EC. Diagnosis and treatment of pd/pu. In: *Proceedings of the Western Veterinary Conference.* 2005.

86. Davenport MD, Lutz CK, Tiefenbacher S, et al. A rhesus monkey model of self-injury: effects of relocation stress on behavior and neuroendocrine function. *Biol Psychiatry.* 2008;63:990–996.

87. Rusbridge C, Heath S, Gunn-Moore DA, et al. Feline orofacial pain syndrome (FOPS); a retrospective study of 113 cases. *J Feline Med Surg.* 2010;12,498–508.

88. Hill PB, et al. Survey of the prevalence, diagnosis and treatment of dermatologic conditions in the small animals in general practice. *Vet Rec.* 2006;158:533–539.

89. Panconesi E, Hautman G. Psychophysiology of stress in dermatology. *Dermatol Clinic.* 1996;14:399–422.

90. Scheich G, Florin I, Rudolph R, et al. Personality characteristics and serum IgE level in patients with atopic dermatitis. *J Psychosom Res.* 1993;37:637–642.

91. McAuliffe LR, Koch CS, Serpell J, et al. Associations between atopic dermatitis and anxiety aggression, and fear-based behaviors in dogs. *J Am Anim Hosp Assoc.* 2022;58(4):161–167.

92. Harvey N, Craigon P, Shaw S, Blott S, England G. Behavioral differences in dogs with atopic dermatitis suggest stress could be a significant problem associated with pruritus. *Animals.* 2019:813.

93. Zulch HE, Mills DS, Lambert R. et al. The use of tramadol in a Labrador retriever presenting with self-mutilation of the tail. *J Vet Behav.* 2012;7(4):252–258.

94. Denerolle P, White SD, Taylor TS, et al. Organic diseases mimicking acral lick dermatitis in six dogs. *J Am Anim Hosp Assoc.* 2007;243:215–220.

95. Houpt KA. *Domestic Animal Behavior.* 4th ed. Ames, IA: Blackwell Publishing; 2005.

96. Waisglass SE, Landsberg GM, Yager JA, et al. Underlying physical conditions in cats with presumptive psychogenic alopecia. *J Am Vet Med Assoc.* 2006:228;1705–1709.

97. Shell LG. Feline hyperesthesia syndrome. *Feline Pract.* 1994;6:10.

98. Batle PA, Rusbridge C, Nuttal T, et al. Feline hyperaesthesia syndrome with self-trauma to the tail: retrospective study of seven cases and proposal for integrated multidisciplinary diagnostic approach. *J Feline Med Surg.* 2019;21(2):178–185.

99. Croates JR, Dewey CW. Cervical spinal hyperesthesia as a clinical sign of cranial disease. *Compend Contin Educ Pract Vet.* 1998;20:1025–1027.

100. March P, Fischer JR, Potthoff A, et al. Electromyographic and histological abnormalities in epaxial muscles of cats with feline hyperesthesia syndrome. *J Vet Int Med.* 1999;13:238.

101. Carmichael KP, Bienzle D, McDonnell JJ. Feline leukemia virus-associated myelopathy in cats. *Vet Pathol.* 2002;39: 536–545.

102. Drew LJ, MacDermott AB. Neuroscience: unbearable lightness of touch. *Nature.* 2009;462:580–581.

Resources and recommended reading

Bennett SL, Zahn MZ. Managing compulsive disorders in cats. *Today's Veterinary Practice.* September/October 2021; 11(5):99–102.

Kinsman R, Casey R, Murray J. Owner-reported pica in domestic cats enrolled onto a Birth Cohort Study. *Animals.* 2021;11(4):1101. doi:10.3390/ani11041101.

Mason G, Rushen J, eds. *Stereotypic Animal Behavior Fundamentals and Applications to Welfare.* 2nd ed. Oxfordshire, UK: CAB International; 2006.

Older CE, Diesel AB, Heseltine JC, et al. Cytokine expression in feline allergic dermatitis and feline asthma. *Vet Dermatol.* 2021;32(6):613-e163. doi:10.1111/vde 13022,Epub2021.

Santoro D, Pucheu-Haston CM, Prost C, et al. Clinical signs and diagnosis of feline atopic syndrome: detailed guidelines for a correct diagnosis. *Vet Dermatol.* 2021;32(1):26-e6. doi:10.1111. vde.12935.

Schnedeker AH, Cole LK, Diaz SF, et al. Is low-level laser therapy useful as an adjunctive treatment for canine acral lick dermatitis? A randomized, double-blind, sham-controlled study. *Vet Dermatol.* 2021;32(2):148-e35. doi:10.1111/vde.12921.

Sulkama S, Salonen M, Mikkola S, et al. Aggressiveness, ADHD like behaviour, and environment influence repetitive behaviour in dogs. *Sci Rep.* 2022;12(1):3520. doi:10.1038/s41598-022-07443-6.

Walsh BR. A critical review of the evidence for the equivalence of canine and human compulsions. *Appl Anim Behav Sci.* 2021;234:105166.

CHAPTER 19

Unruly and destructive behaviors – canine

**Wailani Sung, MS, PhD, DVM, DACVB and
Lisa Radosta, DVM, DACVB**

Contents

Introduction

Among the most frequently reported behavior problems and causes of relinquishment to shelters include unruly behaviors such as excessive barking, jumping, general disobedience, excessive energy, and destructive behaviors,[1-4] with 12–21% of pet dogs exhibiting problematic unruly or destructive behavior.[5-7] The behavioral issues discussed in this chapter are most often normal canine behaviors that are undesirable to the pet parents, although fear, anxiety, stress, conflict, panic (FASCP), or frustration may be a contributing factor in the development or perpetuation of the problem (e.g., if pet parent responses include punishment or are inconsistent). Unruly behaviors represent about 5%

or more of cases at behavior practices indicating they can be sufficiently problematic or abnormal to require specialist referral.[8] When not sleeping or resting, a dog's day would normally be spent in social play, and exploration with an emphasis on food acquisition (e.g., scavenging, hunting). Problems arise if the family does not provide the dog with an enriched environment, sufficient and appropriate outlets to meet its behavioral needs, and the direction needed to behave in a way that is desirable to the pet parents. Many, if not most of these behaviors which are referred to as unruly for the purposes of this chapter, are normal behavioral responses to the environment and consequences (reinforcement, punishment), that also are undesirable to the pet parents. Helping pet parents understand that the behavior is undesirable, but expected given the environment will aid in a complete understanding of their dog, which will in turn facilitate altering the dog's behavior.

Factors contributing to the development of any behavior include genetics, epigenetics (effect of environment and external factors on the expression of genes), the animal's coping style, environmental experience, and learning. Maintenance of behaviors occurs through positive and negative consequences to those behaviors. Behaviors that are reinforced will occur more frequently in the future. For example, if the pet obtained food by chewing into a cabinet, the behavior will be more likely to occur in the future. Regarding chewing, if the dog has an object it should not have and the pet parent chases the dog to retrieve it, the "stealing" behavior may be reinforced, as chase may be perceived as play by the dog. Even if the dog is verbally scolded when the pet parent finally retrieves the object, the behavior of running with the object was reinforced. The behavior of giving the object back (when the pet parent takes it and yells) is punished. The dog in this case will steal and run more because the behaviors have been reinforced, and be less likely to give the item back to the pet parent because that behavior has been punished. In this way, pet parents reinforce and punish behaviors incorrectly, actually increasing the undesirable behavior.

Even if the pet parent is implementing training procedures correctly, if the pet still continues to be reinforced, the undesirable behavior will continue. For this reason, removal of all reinforcement for the undesirable behavior is vital for improvement. On the other hand, unless the pet is provided with appropriate and sufficient outlets for its energy and reinforced for desirable behaviors, this will cause or contribute to FASCP and frustration. See Chapter 10 for more information on reinforcement and maintenance of behaviors.

It is imperative that families receive counseling and resources and enroll puppies in socialization classes before the window for socialization closes (see Recommended Reading, Chapter 2, and Appendix A). Preventive counseling and screening at each veterinary visit can provide the family with the advice and resources they need to understand normal behavior, meet the behavioral requirements of the pet, and set the pet up for success (see Chapters 1 and 5). Research consistently shows that proper education of pet parents can be protective against relinquishment.[3,4,9] In addition, a recent study found that relinquished dogs had significantly more behavior issues than dogs not relinquished, including excitability, training difficulty, and excessive energy, yet these were less likely to be recognized as problems by relinquishing pet parents, indicating a lack of understanding of dog behavior and how to manage these problems.[10] Dogs under the age of two years, dogs that are overly active, and dogs that did not attend obedience classes were more likely to be relinquished to shelters, and behavioral advice by the veterinarian is associated with a lower risk of relinquishment.[9,11] In fact, a single behavior counseling session for puppy parents at the first veterinary visit significantly reduced mounting or mouthing at pet parents, disturbing pet parents while eating, and persistent play, as well as soiling and aggression toward unfamiliar people and dogs.[12] Puppies that are not adequately socialized are more likely to develop behavioral problems (see Chapters 2 and 5). Pet parents should also be encouraged to continue to take their dogs to formal obedience classes well after the socialization period

and potentially through social maturity, which ends at three years of age. This will provide a mental and physical outlet for the dog, setting the foundation of positive interactions with the family and the dog so that pet parents can teach and communicate with their dogs, strengthening the human–animal bond. Puppies that attended properly conducted puppy classes had reduced risk of social fear and aggression, nonsocial fears, fear of crates, touch sensitivity, behavior problems later in life, the use of punishment-based techniques in the home, higher retention rates in the home, and improved trainability.[13–16] In addition, puppies and dogs that were enrolled in obedience classes were more responsive to the cues of pet parents.[17] Families are often misinformed or misguided into using punishment or physical dominance to suppress undesirable behaviors. Punishment is counterproductive, as it does not train the pet how to behave acceptably in the situation and can cause FASCP and frustration. There may also be the misconception that using positive punishment techniques is more effective in addressing problematic behavior. The use of positive punishment techniques is no more effective than the use of positive reinforcement techniques and in many cases, compromise the dogs' welfare,[18] and at least one study indicated that positive reinforcement techniques were more effective in addressing problematic behaviors when compared to dogs trained using positive punishment.[19] In addition, the risk of injury from choke, shock, or prong collars is significant (see Figure 19.1 and 19.2). Also see on line client handout: Why not to use shock. While all pet parents cannot use positive reinforcement effectively and may need instruction, there is very little chance that they will do physical harm and injure their dog with a food reward. See Appendix A and Chapter 10 for further information on reinforcement training. See Box 19.1 for causes of unruly behavior.

Approach to diagnosis and treatment in general practice

The approach to the diagnosis and treatment of unruly behaviors is not unlike the approach to other behavioral

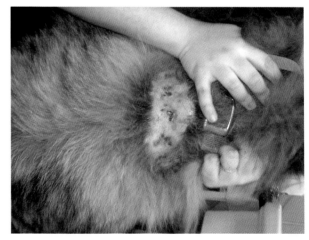

Figure 19.1 Physical injury from training with a prong collar. (*Attribution: Gary Landsberg, DVM, DACVB.*)

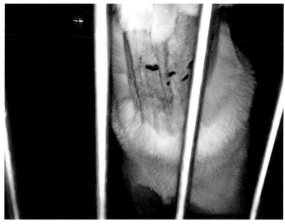

Figure 19.2 Injury due to shock collar use. *(Attribution: Jeannine Berger, DVM, DACVB, DACAW, CAWA.)*

problems and disorders except that it may be less complex. Ideally, a veterinary nurse or technician would be a part of the team to participate in education, training, and follow-up. One of the primary objectives in history taking for unruly behaviors is to determine if the behavior is species or breed typical (normal and expected) or if there is behavioral pathology. Always consider the potential for inputs to the behavior from FASCP and especially frustration. Behaviors which are expected for the species or breed but cannot be expressed and for which no alternative opportunity for expression exists can often lead to frustration and conflict. Once these elements are present, they fuel the behavior, potentially leading to conditioned arousal, overarousal, and behavioral pathology.

Variables to assess include:
- Signalment, including age and breed.
- Appetite, hunger, and diet.
- Recent changes in health or behavior.
- How the pet responds to family absences.
- How and where the pet is confined and acceptance of confinement.
- Whether the behavior includes licking, sucking, or ingestion.
- What is chewed.
- When, where, and in what situations the behavior occurs.
- Whether the chewing occurs when pet parents are home, absent, or both.
- How the pet responds to prey.
- Response to loud noises.
- The response to territorial stimuli.
- What the pet parent has done to try to stop the behavior.
- The pet's daily activities.

Treatment for unruly behaviors is fairly straightforward. The same six steps can be applied to most unruly behaviors (see Box 19.2).
1. Assess for underlying fear, anxiety, stress, conflict, and panic.
2. Provide adequate outlets necessary to address breed-typical needs.
3. Teach desirable behaviors with positive reinforcement.
4. Manage the environment to remove reinforcement for and prevent undesirable behaviors.
5. Reinforce desirable behaviors.
6. Stop positive punishment techniques.

Jumping on people

This is a common, annoying problem, especially for pet parents of young, friendly dogs, representing over 25% of reported behavior problems.[20] Dogs jump up on people as a greeting and to solicit play or attention or interaction.[21] Even if the intent is to greet happily, jumping up can be dangerous if there is a large size differential between the dog and the person (e.g., large dog, small child), if the person is immunocompromised and/or weak, or has poor balance (e.g., elderly, young).[22]

Families often find it difficult to stop the behavior because:
- They have not taught the pet a desirable way to interact in social situations.
- They have no effective, humane way to interrupt the undesirable behavior.
- The family is inconsistent in their response to the pet, including intermittent reinforcement and/or punishment of the behavior.

- The pet requires more environmental enrichment than is being provided.
- The family only trains the dog when it is overly aroused, distracted, or stressed.

Prevention

Jumping up can be prevented by encouraging pet parents to use reward-based training to teach desired greeting behaviors as early as eight weeks of age and ensuring that attention is not given until the puppy greets in a calm way.

Pet parents should follow these guidelines:

- Attend training classes starting one week after the first vaccination and deworming. See Appendix A for Guidelines for Humane Training.
- Teach the puppy or newly adopted dog to perform a greeting behavior (e.g., sit, down, hand touch) to greet and ask for attention.
- Instruct people who interact with the dog to wait for the pet parent's OK and be prepared to break off the greeting if the pet starts to jump.
- Never reinforce the dog when it jumps. Avoid lifting, giving food, play, touch, or eye contact if the pet starts to jump.
- Reward the dog each time it approaches and does not jump.
- Have a toy or treat handy to lure the dog into position before jumping begins.
- Use the same greeting behavior for all greetings, family and strangers alike.

- Limit petting to one to two strokes under the chin and chest if the pet has difficulty maintaining the greeting behavior for long periods of time.
- Keep the dog on leash attached to a no-pull harness or head halter or keep the dog behind a physical barrier to prevent jumping up until it is fluent at the greeting behavior.
- Make sure all family members and visitors abide by the same rules.

Diagnosis and prognosis

Patients that have underlying FASCP fueling the jumping should be treated for those disorders in order to achieve full resolution. It is best to not assume that the behavior is unruly and without a component of FASCP without a complete history and physical examination. In addition, certain medications and supplements can cause agitation and increased energy. If family and visitors are consistent, there is an excellent prognosis for resolution of the problem if the dog has not been consistently or intermittently reinforced for the behavior previously and if FASCP or frustration are not underlying drivers of the behavior.

Management and treatment

In order to manage this jumping, all family members should interact consistently with the dog using positive reinforcement to reward desirable greeting behavior and removing reinforcement for any undesirable jumping behavior. See Online handout Jumping up and Table 19.1 for complete management and treatment guidelines.

Table 19.1 Management and treatment for the dog that jumps up (Also see online handout Jumping up)

Methods	Comments
Assess for underlying fear, anxiety, stress, conflict, and panic, systemic disease, and behavioral pathology	• Rule out systemic disease and medications which may cause agitation and increased energy; disorders of fear, anxiety, stress, conflict or panic, attention-seeking behavior, and displacement behavior.
Teach desirable behaviors with positive reinforcement	• Teach a greeting behavior (e.g., sit, down, touch, go to mat) using reward-based training to be used for all interactions with people. Also See online handouts sit and relax and tips for effective training. • A remote treat dispenser (See Figures 19.3 and 19.4) is useful for immediately and remotely rewarding the dog for going to a mat. Use any reward that the dog values, including food, petting, praise, and toys.
Provide adequate outlets necessary to address breed- and species-typical needs	Regularly scheduled exercise, play, and training provide for the pet's physical and social needs.
Manage the environment to remove reinforcement for and prevent undesirable behaviors	• Keep greetings low-key. • Never encourage jumping up. • Be consistent, even with visitors. • Do not look at pet or acknowledge the dog until they are performing the desired behavior instead of jumping. • Confine the dog behind a door, baby gate, outside in a fenced yard, or in a crate until visitors are settled in the house, then bring the dog out on leash for greetings. • Scatter treats on the floor, toss toys, or use treats to lure the dog into a sit position. • Remove all attention and any other reinforcement immediately if the dog begins to jump. This is the most powerful way to correct this behavior if it is driven by attention.
Stop positive punishment techniques	• Techniques such as hitting, pushing the dog off, grabbing the dog, using a loud noise, or yelling are not recommended. • If punishment is the only treatment used, there is an increased chance of fear, anxiety, stress, conflict, panic, and frustration. Fear and pain via physical punishment is never the correct choice and leads to serious behavior problems.
Surgery	• Neutering has no effect on this behavior except to reduce male sexual mounting.
Medications and supplements	• There are no indications for using a medication or supplement with this behavior problem.

Provide adequate outlets necessary to address breed- and species-typical needs

Well-exercised and enriched dogs that understand how to engage in independent activities such as nosework or puzzle solving may be less likely to intensely seek attention when greeting. While it is not always possible to exercise a dog prior to the entry of visitors into the home, daily exercise within the dog's physical limits cannot hurt. A daily regimen that includes structured, consistent interactions, play, exercise, and multiple short training sessions is important for reducing arousal.

Teach desirable behaviors with positive reinforcement

Rather than trying to train the pet what not to do (i.e., jump), the focus should be on training desirable greeting behaviors – standing (four on the floor), sitting, lying down, performing touch, or having the dog wait on its bed or mat. The touch cue directs the dog's attention to the person's hand positioned neutrally at the person's side. When the dog touches the hand with its nose, it receives a treat.

To be successful, the family will need to train these behaviors until the dog can reliably perform them in most situations 9 out of 10 times when asked the first time. Then they are ready to use them for real greetings. If the dog does not know the cue for the desired behavior, the dog should not be greeting people at the door. It is better for the dog to be behind a barrier when visitors come into the house, then come out on a leash and work on obedience cues with the pet parent than for the dog to learn incorrect behavior from mishandled greetings. Timing is a crucial element of any training. For the dog to pair the reinforcement with the behavior, the reinforcer should be given while the dog is engaged in the desired behavior or immediately after. Of course, once the dog has learned to stand, sit, or lie down on cue, this will speed the process, as the pet parent can ask the dog for the behavior and immediately reward the dog's correct response. Clicker or marker-based training ensures immediate timing of rewards to quicken the learning process (see Chapter 10).

Even in training situations, someone may inadvertently reinforce the undesirable behavior. If the dog knows what is expected and which behaviors will be reinforced and that reinforcement is more likely than the inadvertent reinforcement from people, there is a good chance that the dog will perform the desirable behavior, even in less than perfect conditions.

When the dog is fluent at the new greeting behavior, it is time for practice greetings with familiar people. This can be accomplished by having familiar people enter and depart several times in the same training session. At first, they should be kept low key with little to no eye contact or petting except when the dog is calm. The person should be told not to give any attention to the dog until the dog is in the desired position. Attention includes eye contact, touching (even to push the dog away), or talking to the pet. A leash attached to a flat collar, head halter, or no-pull harness (once the dog has been positively accustomed to wearing one) can be used to prevent the dog from jumping up. When the desirable behavior is offered, the dog can then be reinforced. If the pet starts to jump, the person should stand up straight and turn sideways, keeping the pet in peripheral vision, but removing all attention and cueing the pet into a desirable behavior. Alternatively, the person can walk away. As mentioned above, if the dog does not calm down when ignored, consider underlying causes associated with FASCP or frustration. These dogs may simply have been intermittently reinforced for arousal or jumping and thus are continuing to offer this behavior in an extinction burst.

All treats should be offered at the pet's nose level directly in front of the mouth or tossed to the floor. If treats are offered above the pet's nose level or out of reach, this will encourage jumping or moving to get the treat, which is contrary to the purpose of the training. The pet parent should continually give small treats as long as the pet maintains the desired behavior. After a few moments of success, the pet parent and dog should walk away from the person. Then the exercise is repeated. When the pet can stay calm as people enter the house, the criteria can be raised to include calm petting under the chin. Once the dog can reliably perform this behavior with family members, practice can begin with visitors. With persistently jumping dogs, the visitors may need to walk out and close the door behind them. This behavior effectively indicates to the dog when it jumps, the visitor leaves. After 15–60 seconds, the person reappears and the dog is immediately instructed to perform the desired behavior. When the dog complies, the person enters the room and proceeds with the greeting behavior.

Dogs can also be taught to go to a mat, bed, or crate when visitors arrive. While this may sound simple, it is challenging for many dogs. Remote-activated treat dispensers such as the Manners Minder, Treat&Train, Furbo, and Pet Tutor can aid in teaching a dog to lie on a mat or stay in one place away from the door[20] (see Figures 19.3 and 19.4). Significant improvement was observed in the reduction of jumping and barking when the pet parents followed a written protocol that incorporated the use of the remote-controlled reward dispenser to reinforce alternate behavior.[20] Proper greeting behavior must also be taught when releasing the dog from

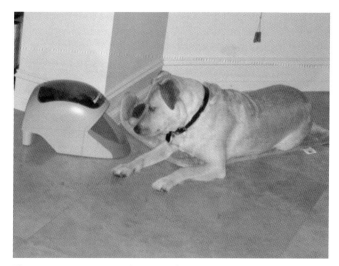

Figure 19.3 Remote treat dispensing devices are excellent ways to remotely reinforce desirable behaviors. Manners Minder. *(Attribution: Lisa Radosta.)*

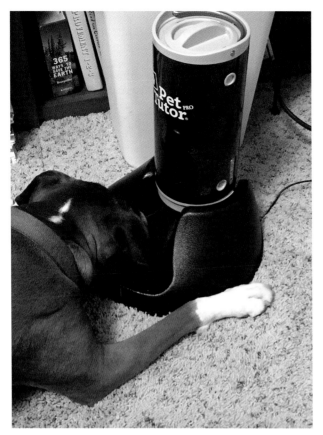

Figure 19.4 Remote treat dispensing devices are excellent ways to remotely reinforce desirable behaviors. Pet Tutor. *(Attribution: Ashley Elzerman, DVM, DACVB.)*

its crate or confinement area. Make sure the dog performs a behavior, mark the behavior, and offer the reinforcer before release. If necessary, use a leash and humane collar so that the dog leaves the confinement area calmly and under control.

Manage the environment to remove reinforcement for and prevent undesirable behaviors

Attention in the form of petting, eye contact, verbal interaction, tossing of toys, and other types of play will perpetuate jumping in that situation. For the best outcome, people who interact with the dog should not respond to jumping with any attention at all. All reinforcement for jumping should be identified and removed. Some dogs that have been intermittently reinforced will jump more when attention is removed. Dogs that do not have underlying FASCP will usually decrease the rate of jumping in three to five days. However, some dogs have an emotional component to the behavior. In these cases, it is less likely to respond to removal of attention

because attention is not the only motivator for the behavior. Outside of training sessions, under no circumstances should family members or visitors give the pet any attention for jumping up, including games that involve jumping up. Techniques for avoiding reinforcement are listed above.

Sometimes avoiding and turning away may not be practical, especially when the pet is overly excited or the visitor is unsteady on their feet. In those cases, pet parents can keep a basket of balls or toys at the door for tossing. As the dog goes to get the toy, the visitors can enter the house. Then, they can toss the next ball as the pet is coming back toward them. Another strategy involves scattering small treats on the floor away from the door. While the dog cleans them up, the visitors can enter. Treats can also be scattered in a nearby room. Then, when the visitors have entered or are settled, the dog can be let out of the room. If the dog understands the basic behaviors but has a difficult time performing them when distracted by visitors, a leash attached to a flat collar, no-pull harness- or head halter can help to keep the dog near the pet parent so that they can direct their behavior. With that said, the pet parent should not pull on the dog, as the dog will not learn to make correct choices, thus the importance of teaching appropriate behaviors which can be rewarded. Ideally, the pet would be behind a pet gate or in an exercise pen until it can comply with the pet parent's cues.

Reinforce desirable behaviors

In some situations, dogs can respond to the reinforcement of other desirable behaviors which are not necessarily taught in a formal way. For example, if before jumping, a dog pauses to stand calmly and look at the visitor or runs into a room to look out the window calmly in order to see the visitor coming up to the house, those behaviors can be reinforced using a clicker and treats or a remote treat dispensing device. If the pet is reinforced for those behaviors, jumping will become less likely. Instructing pet parents to reinforce any behavior in which the pet is not jumping (e.g., standing, sitting, lying down) frees them from formal training, which may overwhelm them, and achieves the goal of decreasing jumping.

Stop positive punishment techniques

Punitive or painful corrections such as hitting, a knee to the chest, stepping on feet, pinch collars, or pinning are not appropriate and are contraindicated. These types of behaviors cause conflict, fear, and deterioration of the human–animal bond. The dogs may not be deterred and may learn to escalate the strength and intensity of their behavior.

Once the pet has learned that a specific greeting behavior or calm behavior in general earns rewards and that jumping results in no rewards, the jumping behavior will stop.

CASE EXAMPLE

Presentation

Lucy, an 8-month-old spayed female Irish Setter, was presented for jumping on the pet parents and visitors when they came into the home.

History

Lucy enjoyed greeting people and as a young puppy, people generally petted her and talked to her when she greeted enthusiastically, including jumping up on them and pawing at them. As Lucy grew bigger and stronger, some people were pushed back and scratched by her nails when she jumped. The pet parents had tried yelling, telling her "no," pulling on the leash, grabbing her by her neck, kneeing her the chest, pushing her off of them, grabbing the collar, and holding her down. But as the corrections escalated, the jumping just got worse. Now, when people came to the door and the pet parents tried to reach for her, she put her head down and ran away.

Differential diagnoses

The differential diagnoses included attention-seeking behavior, displacement behavior, lack of enrichment and exercise, lack of training, and specific/situational fear of the pet parents. She was found to have lack of training, lack of exercise and enrichment, and a specific/situational fear of the pet parents when reached for during arousing situations at the door.

Workup

Lucy's physical examination and laboratory results were within normal limits.

Treatment

Due to Lucy's fear of the pet parents, medication and supplements were discussed but not recommended because there was a good likelihood that a change to entirely positive reinforcement-based training techniques would decrease her fear. The pet parents were instructed to stop all physical and verbal punishment immediately. In addition, they were referred to a qualified positive reinforcement dog trainer in order to teach the following behaviors: sit, lie down, go to mat/place, and accept confinement behind a baby gate. Once Lucy could perform these behaviors with fluency, the sit - stay and down - stay were to be introduced. Since Lucy enjoyed playing with her ball, it was used along with food for training. They were given resources for enrichment and exercise ideas. Until Lucy was fluent at the recommended behaviors, she was to be put behind a pet gate when the pet parents were not home. They were instructed on how to make the space comfortable and how to use food-stuffed toys to help her accept confinement. When one pet parent was home, she could be loose in the house and placed behind the pet gate before the other parent

was expected to arrive. Finally, they were taught how to countercondition her to their hands moving toward her neck. They were to reach and toss a treat at her feet, then walk away and let her eat the treat.

Follow-up

In one month, the veterinary technician followed up by phone with Lucy's pet parents. They reported that when they entered the home, if Lucy did not immediately respond to a sit or down cue, they ignored her completely and kept walking forward. If she persistently jumped on them, the pet parents walked out of the door again or into another room and closed the door. After a 15- to 30-second break, the pet parents would open the door and immediately direct Lucy to perform a sit-stay. If she did, they handed her a treat and petted her, or they tossed the ball to the back of the room. This was working and they had seen a significant decrease in the jumping. They reported that she was a high- energy dog and that tossing the ball seemed to be more effective than handing her a food reward. The dog training professional had taught them how to teach her to drop the ball. As a result, they used this strategy when anyone entered the house. If Lucy sat, they tossed the ball. She ran to get the ball, came back to them, dropped the ball, and sat again for another toss. The pet parents had stopped yelling at her and reported that they were enjoying her personality more as well. They had stopped formally counterconditioning her to hands reaching with treats because they reached for her so frequently when tossing the ball that the fearful body language had disappeared due to inadvertent counterconditioning her.

Discussion

There were several factors in Lucy's case contributing to her behavior. The pet parents had not taught her which behaviors were desirable; she did not have a base of positive reinforcement training with which to communicate with the pet parents; she was underexercised and underenriched; and she was reinforced by much of the pushing and handling that the pet parents viewed as punishment. That and her habituation to the punishment contributed to the escalation of the physicality of the strategies leading to fear. If left unchecked, this type of situation often leads to conflict, increased fear, and aggression.

Stealing and trash raiding

Food stealing and garbage raiding are normal investigative, exploratory, and scavenging behavior which can occur in up to 40% of pet dogs and 53% of trained assistance dogs.[23,24] These are self-reinforcing behaviors of opportunity and chance which even with the pet parent's best efforts may end up being intermittently reinforced. For these reasons, stealing food can be a persistent behavior, even in dogs that are rehomed.[25] Dogs may raid trash bins and food cupboards if attracted by odor, taste, or texture. Some of these items can be dangerous if swallowed (i.e., plastic, cooked bones, corn cobs, peach pits) or may have bacterial contamination. Long-skulled dogs may be more likely to engage in food stealing when compared to short-skulled dogs.[26] Dogs are more likely to steal food in the dark as compared to a well-lit room[27] and prevalence increases with the presence of children in the household.[28] Attempts at correction often fail because instead of focusing on providing alternative outlets that are appealing to the pet, many pet parents resort to punishing undesirable behavior, sometimes long after the behavior is finished.

Pet parents are often certain that their pets know they have misbehaved because they report that their dog looks guilty and because they often believe that their dog inherently understands how much a certain behavior annoys or irritates the pet parent. When a pet appears to look guilty, it is merely using species-specific body language intended to defuse the situation and avoid conflict. If this is effective at causing the pet parent to avoid using punishment, they may continue to exhibit this body language when they see the pet parent. Some pets also learn in which situations they get punished, such as when the pet parent arrives home and trash is on the ground. Instead of learning not to get into the garbage, the dog learns that the pet parent's arrival home ends in punishment for the dog, regardless of what he was doing just before (e.g., resting, staring out the window), and that there are no unpleasant consequences if the pet parents are not watching. This leads to confusion and conflict, not learning.

Diagnosis and prognosis

Dogs that raid the garbage may have underlying physical problems, including any condition that increases or alters appetite such as endocrine disorders (e.g., diabetes, hyperadrenocorticism), iatrogenic appetite (e.g., glucocorticoids, phenobarbital, benzodiazepines), or gastrointestinal disease; may be underenriched or underexercised; may not have a nutritionally balanced diet; may have been recently placed on reduced calories; or may have simply learned that a certain behavior is reinforcing. Dogs that lick, chew, or suck on objects in the environment and those with picas should be assessed for gastrointestinal disease.[29] Switching to a calorie-restricted diet, feeding a puppy insufficient amounts (e.g., feeding according to recommendations on the food bag rather than the pup's actual needs), and drugs that increase appetite such as corticosteroids may increase scavenging, food stealing, garbage raiding, and even picas. They may even contribute to food guarding and possessive aggression. While a basic body system workup would include a complete blood count, serum chemistry, urinalysis, thyroid profile, and fecal PCR antigen, assessment for endocrine function (adrenal, thyroid), gastrointestinal disease, and exocrine pancreatic insufficiency tests may also be warranted.

As with all behavior disorders, what seems straightforward often is not. Do not skip the physical examination and systemic wellness workup in these dogs because their behavior appears unruly in nature (see Chapter 6).

Dogs may also perform these behaviors if they are effective in gaining attention. If these behaviors occur only during pet parent departures or during noise events, separation-related disorders and noise aversion should be ruled out, respectively (see Chapters 15 and 17). Finally, dogs with possessive aggression frequently steal items and then act aggressively when the pet parent tries to remove them. Prognosis depends on the family's ability to manage the pet, train alternate behaviors, and manage the environment. Dogs that have underlying fear, anxiety, stress, conflict, and panic will need more detailed treatment which may include medications, behavior modification, and environmental management (see Chapter 23).

Prevention

These problems can be prevented by providing dogs with the necessary amounts of physical and mental stimulation, and supervising to encourage desirable behaviors and prevent or interrupt undesirable behaviors. In addition, one study found that dogs prefer fresh odors as opposed to those that are aged and meat odors to nonmeat odors.[30] Pet parents may consider throwing meat away in a garbage that is inaccessible to the dog. The family must focus on training the pet as to which objects are acceptable to chew and play with and where to sleep rather than punishing unacceptable behaviors. When the family cannot supervise, the pet must be prevented from gaining access to areas where problems might arise. While confinement training young dogs generally works best, blocking entry to problem areas or using child locks, baby gates, or tie-downs are alternative ways of preventing undesirable behaviors.

Management and treatment

Provide adequate outlets necessary to address breed- and species-typical needs

Encouraging the pet to chew on items that are acceptable to the pet parent and appealing to the pet is the first course of action and should start from the first day that the pet is in the home regardless of age (see Table 19.2). Provide the pet with a variety of interesting toys. Finding toys that appeal to the pet, rotating through toys to maintain novelty, and adding food stuffing or

Table 19.2 Management and treatment of stealing and trash raiding (Also see online handout Stealing)

Steps	Comments
Assess for underlying fear, anxiety, stress, conflict, and panic, systemic disease, and behavioral pathology	• Rule out systemic disease and medications which may cause agitation and increased energy; disorders of fear, anxiety, stress, conflict or panic, attention-seeking behavior, and displacement behavior.
Provide adequate outlets necessary to address breed- and species-typical needs	• Regularly scheduled exercise, play, and training provide for the pet's physical and social needs.
Manage the environment to remove reinforcement for and prevent undesirable behaviors	• Prevent access by closing off areas or confining away from where the dog might steal, picking up items easily stolen, and securing trash and cabinets. • Do not look at pet or acknowledge the dog when they have stolen something that is not valuable and that will not injure them. Trade up with a higher value reinforcer when the dog has stolen something that he cannot keep.
Teach desirable behaviors with positive reinforcement	• Reward-based training to teach leave it and drop it.
Reinforce desirable behaviors	• Use any reward that the dog values, including food, petting, praise, and toys to trade up for items that he has stolen and have to be retrieved.
Stop positive punishment techniques	• Techniques such as hitting, pushing, grabbing the dog, using a loud noise, or yelling are not recommended. Many dogs steal when the pet parent is not watching. If punishment is used, they will very likely continue to perform the behavior when they are unsupervised, worsening the problem. Increasing fear and pain via physical punishment is never the correct choice and leads to FASCP. Stop all punishment.
Surgery	• Neutering has no effect on this behavior, except that dogs are calmer after gonadectomy. • There is no evidence that calmer dogs are less likely to steal or raid the garbage.
Medications and supplements	• There are no indications for using a medication or supplement with this behavior problem.

coatings can help to encourage and maintain interest in chew and feeding toys (see Chapters 5, 10, and 13). The family should provide regular sessions of play, exercise, training, and attention to provide predictability to the pet's daily routine and ensure that its needs are being met. Provide appropriate supervision to keep the pet engaged in acceptable activities and prevent them by closing doors or keeping the dog on leash to keep the pet from sneaking off to explore and scavenge.

Pet parents should use food-dispensing and food-filled toys instead of feeding from a food bowl. For dogs that are used to eating out of a bowl, slow introduction to the use of food toys may be necessary (see Chapter 13). Higher-bulk diets may help to satiate the pet better, while dental chews and dental diets and pet-safe chew toys can provide additional outlets for chewing. Before the behavior is likely to occur during the day whether the pet parents are home or will be departing, meals can be provided in several food-dispensing toys. This provides the dog with an opportunity to "scavenge" for his meals and prolongs the time spent in feeding while the pet parent is not able to supervise.

Teach desirable behaviors with positive reinforcement

Teach appropriate behaviors for which the pet can earn reinforcement such as the "leave it" and/or "drop" cues, so the dog learns to give up items on cue. The pet parent should start with lower-value items first and reinforce a reliable response. Then subsequently work on items of greater value and variety so the dog consistently is rewarded for leaving the items alone. Once the pet is fluent in leave it and/or drop it, they can leave out two to three appropriate items and one unacceptable item. When the dog approaches or sniffs the unacceptable item, the pet parent calmly tells the dog to "leave it," then calls the dog over to engage in another toy and offers effusive praise and treats. Repeat several times. Every time the dog leaves the unacceptable item alone, it receives praise and treats. From here, the pet parents can use the "leave it" cue when the pet approaches items and does not pick them up, then reinforcing this behavior instead of stealing.

Manage the environment to remove reinforcement for and prevent undesirable behaviors

Because stealing and garbage raiding can be reinforced in various ways, determination of the factors reinforcing the behavior can be helpful. Dogs that are reinforced by attention can be ignored when they steal if it is safe to do so. Often dogs that are solely motivated by attention from the pet parent will walk away from the item if they are not chased by the pet parent. Then, they can be reinforced for walking away from the item. If the dog is stealing food because the food is reinforcing, use the management strategies above to prevent the dog from accessing the items or keep the items securely away from the dog.

Pet parents should not use their things (e.g., old shoes) as playthings, as this makes it difficult for the pet to distinguish between household items and chew toys. All items likely to be stolen should be picked up. Pets should be confined in a room, hallway, exercise pen, or crate when they cannot be supervised (see Chapters 5, 14, and 17 for more information

on how to create a sanctuary space.). Use locks, baby gates, closed doors, or other physical barriers to prevent garbage raiding by either blocking access to rooms or confining the pet to areas of the home away from potential targets. Use secure containers for food placement and place the trash in a location the pet cannot access.

If a pet does steal something, the pet parent's behavior will directly affect the likelihood of the dog stealing in the future. Pet parents should follow the guideline that if the pet steals something, they should give the pet something even higher in value in trade or give the pet something higher in value in trade and give the item back (if it is safe to do so). This strategy teaches the pet that it is in their best interest to give the item up to the pet parent. If the dog is found chewing on a household item, the pet parent should refrain from trying to wrestle the forbidden item from the dog (which could become a game for the pet or increase FASCP) and instead trade the item the dog has for one it values more. The dog can then be directed to suitable toys and chews. Pet parents are often concerned that they are reinforcing their dog for stealing if they trade up with a higher-value reward. In some cases, the dog may learn to steal items and then wait for the pet parent to come and trade up for them. Even if this is the case, it is much easier to manage than a dog that runs away, hides, or acts aggressively. When this happens, the dog usually picks up the item, waits for the pet parent to approach, drops the item, and then gets their reward. The interaction has been repurposed into a positive one, which is much easier to change.

Reinforce desirable behaviors

The pet parents should provide a large variety of appropriate objects the dog can chew on, and provide plenty of positive reinforcement when the dog chews on appropriate items and ignores unacceptable items.

Stop positive punishment techniques

Harsh correction, prolonged scolding, delayed punishment, and physical punishment are not appropriate. They do not teach the pet what is correct to do, increasing the likelihood of conflict and aggression in that situation in the future. Pet parents may be attracted to the use of aversive methods to teach the pet to avoid a particular area, such as the use of a remote-controlled spray or shock collar, motion-activated alarm, or a variety of bitter/hot sprays on the contraband items. Keep in mind the use of any aversive method such as these may inhibit behavior but can also increase FASCP in the dog. These emotional states are not conducive to the resolution of behavior problems. The pet parent should use the alternate methods listed above and provide the dog a way to fulfill its needs.

Getting on furniture

There is a myth which is still circulating on the internet and in other places that dogs will become aggressive, develop serious behavior problems, or will consider themselves dominant if they have access to furniture. Studies have shown that this is untrue. Dogs that are "spoiled" resting with the pet parents or sleeping on furniture are no more likely to have serious behavior problems than those that are not allowed to do so.[31]

With that said, in one study, dogs that were permitted to sleep on the bed within the first two months of adoption were more likely to be at risk of developing aggression compared to those that were not.[32] In addition, some dogs prefer or require a sleeping area where they will not be disturbed while resting. There is no law of behavior that states that dogs cannot be on the bed or the couch, and it is not necessary to prevent or stop the practice if it does not lead to any associated problems for the pet parent. If the pet parent does not want the dog on the furniture or if aggression occurs on the furniture, relegation to dog-only furniture is necessary. Potentially for new pets to the home, the dog should use dog-only furniture, for the first two to three months after adoption and then be taught to ask politely to get on furniture shared by the pet parent. The most important thing is consistency and training. If the family decides that the pet should not be allowed on furniture, then no exceptions can be made.

Management and treatment

Provide adequate outlets necessary to address breed- and species-typical needs

Just like us, dogs need comfortable places to rest. The family should choose suitable resting locations (dog bed, crate, carpet remnant, alternate piece of furniture not used by people) that appeal to the dog. The dog should have at least one resting space in each room where it frequently settles or sleeps to reduce drive to get on the furniture. If there is a sofa or comfy ottoman on which to lie in that room and the room does not have a bed for the dog, the dog is more likely to get on the furniture. To feel safe, dogs may need elevated resting spaces.

Teach desirable behaviors with positive reinforcement

Encourage the dog to approach the desired resting area by placing favored toys and chews in the area and rewarding with treats or attention when using the area. The dog should be consistently reinforced for lying down on the mat or bed.

Whenever the dog is given a puzzle toy or long-lasting chew to work on, it should be directed to go to the mat and lie down and encouraged to stay there while working on the toy/treat by the pet parent periodically dropping high values treats on he mat the longer the stays on in that location. Whenever the dog lies in the desirable location without pet parent prompting, plenty of verbal praise and high-value treats should be given to the dog.

Manage the environment to remove reinforcement for and prevent undesirable behaviors

If a family member wants to have the pet in their lap, the person should get on the floor with the pet. They should teach the dog a cue to be invited into the person's lap using positive reinforcement. Keeping the pet off of the furniture when the pet parent is not around requires a preventive strategy. If the family had previously allowed the dog on the furniture, it is difficult to prevent the dog from jumping on furniture when family members are not present. Easy solutions to this include closing doors; confining the dog to an area where it cannot access the furniture; placing a less-comfortable or undesirable surface covering on the furniture such as plastic furniture covers or upside-down plastic carpet runners or bristle door mats; and placing items on the furniture which make it impossible for the dog to get up on the furniture at all, such as dining room chairs and baby gates. The pet should constantly be supervised by the family to prevent use of the furniture. Block access to the furniture when the family is not present. Monitors and motion detectors can aid in supervision should the pet move out of direct sight.

Stop positive punishment techniques

Grabbing dogs, pulling them off of the couch, or pushing them off will only increase fear and eventually in some dogs increase aggression. Instruct pet parents not to do this.

CASE EXAMPLE

Presentation

Gilligan, a 2-year-old male Standard Poodle, was presented for food stealing, trash raiding, climbing on furniture, and destroying furniture when he was unsupervised or alone.

History

Gilligan exhibited exploratory, playful, and destructive behaviors that persisted into adulthood. Whenever he was left alone or unsupervised, he went into rooms where he would steal food off tables, raid trash cans, climb onto furniture, and chew on the upholstery. Gilligan enjoyed playing with family members and other dogs. The pet parents attempted to confine Gilligan to a crate but this resulted in extreme howling, salivating, and chewing at the bars, so confinement proved to be impractical. Many of the potential problem areas could be closed off, but a few of the rooms had no physical way of blocking entry.

Differential diagnoses

The differential diagnoses for Gilligan's behavior include lack of enrichment, lack of exercise, separation-related disorder, confinement distress, noise aversion, and attention-seeking behavior. Because these behaviors occurred outside of any sounds and he had shown no evidence of fear of sounds, noise aversion was ruled out. His behaviors occurred when he had access to the pet parents as well as when they were not home, so separation-related disorders were ruled out. He performed the behaviors when the pet parents were not home or were not supervising him, so attention-seeking behaviors were ruled out. It was determined that Gilligan had a lack of enrichment and lack of exercise and was exhibiting normal opportunistic behaviors. He was also diagnosed with confinement distress.

Workup

Gilligan's physical exam was within normal limits. Laboratory tests, including a fecal antigen, were performed in order to assess for any underlying disorders which might be fueling the food stealing and trash raiding. All were within normal limits.

Treatment

The pet parents were given resources to educate them on providing additional enrichment, including regular play and exercise sessions at least twice a day, feeding out of food toys, rotating toys, and enrolling him in an obedience tricks class and doggie day care. They were referred to a positive reinforcement trainer in order to teach the following exercises: leave it, drop it, and settle. Although obtaining a second compatible, playful dog for the household may have helped, the family was concerned another dog might add to their problems. When the pet parents departed, all except for the dining room and kitchen were closed off. Child locks were placed on the kitchen cupboards and trash was placed in the garage before the family departed. They were told to avoid the crate, but with the help of the dog training professional, condition him to a secure and enriched confinement area with a tall baby gate secured to the wall.

Follow-up

The veterinary technician checked in on Gilligan's progress after two weeks. He was no longer stealing, but his explorations into the dining room occasionally led to destruction. The pet parents agreed to block off the dining room. Whenever he approached the pet gate, the pet parents redirected him to lie down on his mat placed several feet away. He was praised and rewarded for lying down on the mat. During dinner time, Gilligan was instructed to lie down on the mat. Before the family started their meal, he was given a treat-filled puzzle toy or long-lasting chew to work on. Gilligan learned to stay away from the dining room and lie down on the mat.

Pulling/forging ahead on lead

Many dogs lunge ahead on their leash and pull their pet parents during a walk. This is most often a normal behavior. Nonetheless, it is not enjoyable or safe for the pet parents. While this is a normal behavior, there are some predispositions or trends which can be found in the literature. Male dogs are more likely to pull on leash and with greater force than female dogs.[33] Leash tension, either applied by the pet parent and intended to control the dog or a result of the dog pulling, affects learning and gait. Dogs are intermittently reinforced for pulling in many cases because they are permitted to pull to investigate an object of interest, for example, and habituate to the punishment of the tension on the leash. Tension on the leash is more likely to be applied when the pet parent and dog need to navigate precarious situations such as when the dog is trying to get to an item or when they have to move past a distraction.[34] If the dog is not trained to respond to a tight leash by slowing down or turning back to engage with the pet parent, it is more likely to learn to habituate to the tension on the leash and will often be reinforced for that behavior as it explores the environment.

Prevention

Pulling on the leash can be prevented by teaching dogs when they are young that the walk will only progress forward if the leash remains loose. Rewards such as food and toys can be used to encourage, motivate, and reinforce walking by the pet parent's side (heeling). Front-attach (chest-led) harnesses and head halters can be useful training tools for managing dogs that pull and lunge and for training loose leash walks. The use of shock, choke, and pinch collars are unnecessary and detrimental. They cause physical pain and emotional distress and are never recommended. See Chapter 10 for more detail on these types of training tools.

Diagnosis and prognosis

As discussed above, this is typically a normal behavior which has been reinforced; however, in some dogs, pulling on the leash can be a result of fear of a particular stimulus in the environment, displacement behavior, generalized anxiety, and noise aversion as well as other fears and phobias not listed here. The assumption that a behavior is normal cannot be made unless the pet is first evaluated for FASCP. Dogs that lunge almost always have an underlying FASCP and need further evaluation. Lunging on the leash is discussed in more detail in Chapters 10 and 23.

Management and treatment

Provide adequate outlets necessary to address breed- and species-typical needs

Some dogs need more exercise than others. Pet parents should be advised that a leisurely walk may not be enough for their pet. Pets that are well exercised are less likely to forge ahead and pull on the pet parent. Exercise options include but are not limited to swimming, training classes, or tossing a ball, or a flying disc in the yard.

Teach desirable behaviors with positive reinforcement

Pulling on the leash is much easier to prevent than to treat but can be improved effectively with training and proper equipment. The guidance of a good positive reinforcement trainer is invaluable. Training consists of using a humane tool to control forward movement, avoiding reinforcement for pulling, reinforcing calm behavior on the leash, checking in with the pet parent, and proximity to the pet parent on leash. This is a common problem in dogs and there is a wealth of good information available on how to teach loose leash walking (see Chapter 10 and Appendix A).

Manage the environment to remove reinforcement for and prevent undesirable behaviors

In situations where the dog has already learned to pull, use a head halter or no-pull harness. Dogs habituate to harnesses fairly quickly; however, individual dogs will need training to fit and accept harnesses or head collars (see Figures 19.5–19.7). Traditional harnesses where the leash attaches at the top and back of the harness are a good option

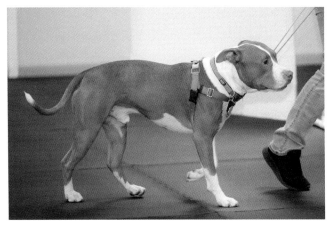

Figure 19.5 No pull harnesses can be helpful in preventing undesirable be-haviors. *(Attribution: Lisa Radosta.)*

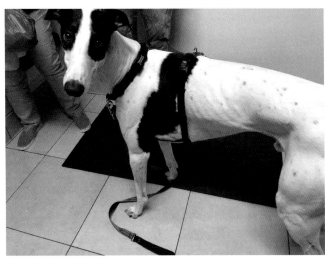

Figure 19.7 No pull harnesses can be helpful in preventing undesirable be-haviors. Blue-9 Balance Harness. *(Attribution: Lisa Radosta.)*

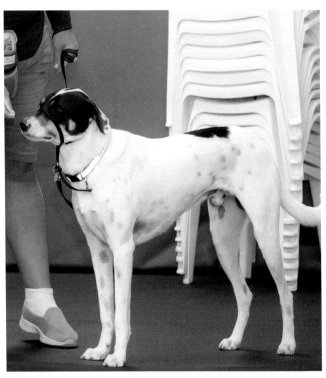

Figure 19.6 Head collars can be helpful in preventing undesirable behaviors. *(Attribution: Lisa Radosta.)*

for dogs that do not pull since they avoid pressure on the neck or trachea. However, they encourage pulling and should not be used in dogs that already have this behavior or in young dogs that do not know yet how to walk calmly on a leash.

The use of a double-ended leash, in which one end clips to the ring on head halter or the front of the harness and the second end clips to the back of the harness, provides the pet parent with more control and leverage when the dog pulls. Instead of being off centered, pulled to one side, the pet parent can grab each end of the leash and have more leverage by bracing heir arms against the pressure the dog applies.

Reinforce desirable behaviors

Pet parents should be encouraged to reinforce their pet by either letting them investigate something interesting, play-ing with them, or using small treats each time that their pet is walking calmly next to them.

Stop positive punishment techniques

There is no place for chill choke, shock, or pinch collars in when training dogs to walk politely on the leash. There are humane, more effective ways to teach controlled walking (see Chapter 10 and Appendix A).

CASE EXAMPLE

Presentation

Fester, a 4-year-old, 50-kg intact male Rottweiler, was presented for pulling on the leash.

History

The male pet parent had taken Fester to obedience classes as a puppy, where a pinch collar was used to teach loose leash walking. As Fester

grew, the collar was less and less effective. Fester, a regular at day care, was very friendly toward other dogs and pulled toward dogs in the neighborhood with loose mouth, soft ears, and a wagging tail. Nonetheless, his breed and size were scaring the neighbors and the homeowner's association had gotten involved. At the time of presenta-tion, the female pet parent, who was small in stature, could not walk Fester at all because it was too dangerous. The male pet parent had purchased a shock collar recently for walks. When Fester pulled on the leash, they activated the shock collar on the level 1 setting. They had slowly increased the intensity because he was not responding. They had also noticed that now, when he saw other dogs, he sometimes growled. This was a new behavior.

Workup

Fester's physical examination and laboratory tests were within normal limits.

Differential diagnoses

Lack of training, learned behavior due to inappropriate training, and fear-induced aggression were determined to be contributing to Fester's behavior.

Treatment

The pet parents were informed of the risk that the aggression would get worse with use of the shock collar or any form of punishment. They were given resources to help them understand that the shock collar was contraindicated. While the damage had been done to some extent by using the shock collar, there was still time to change the course of the aggression. They were referred to a positive reinforcement dog trainer,

who fit Fester with head collar, helped the pet parents to condition him to wear it, and taught them how to reinforce him when he looked at them on walks and every time that he was not pulling. They began working on loose leash walking in the yard so that the female pet parent would gain confidence without feeling unsafe. Until both parents and Fester were successful in the back yard, they were not to walk him outside of the yard. His behavior had not changed at day care (he was not shocked there), so he continued to attend twice weekly.

In one month, the veterinary technician checked on Fester via phone. The pet parents had just started walking him outside of the yard. They were doing well but only taking short walks so far. They had stopped using the shock collar. At this time, the dog training professional had recommended that they treat the fear-induced aggression, so high-value treats were given for counterconditioning every time he saw another dog. Counterconditioning was used to reinforce a different emotional response and behavior incompatible with the initial reaction. Within two months, Fester was able to walk outside with the pet parents in the neighborhood. He was not growling at other dogs but would instead look at the pet parents when he saw another dog. The dog training professional had recommended that they continue to reinforce him when he did this so that this behavior would be maintained.

Excessive barking

Barking is a normal means of canine communication. Barking may be seen in conjunction with hunting, herding, territorial defense, threat displays, fear, distress, attention seeking, care seeking, and play. Repetitive, aimless barking may be a part of canine cognitive dysfunction syndrome. Barking exhibited for attention will increase in frequency when the dog is reinforced, which often happens when pet parents try to quiet the dog with food, play, or attention. Barking is reinforced when the perceived threat (e.g., a stranger approaching) is successfully removed (stranger retreats). Attempts at punishment, especially light scolding, may also serve to reinforce the behavior, while a more intense punishment and bark-suppressing collars may contribute to or aggravate underlying FASCP and do not address the underlying motivation for the behavior or teach the desirable response. Excessive barking can be due to FASCP. In some circumstances, barking may start as a normal behavior and worsen over time as the pet gets frustrated. The prevalence of barking problems in a survey of 4144 dogs was 18%, while over 5% of relinquished dogs were reported as displaying problematic barking.[3,6]

Prevention

Prevention includes teaching a quiet cue so that barking can be controlled and never reinforcing undesirable barking (e.g., by giving attention, food, or play) at any point in the dog's life. Young dogs should be socialized and habituated to sounds, situations, and people that otherwise might initiate barking. Immediately and consistently distract to interrupt any undesirable barking at its commencement and immediately reinforce quiet behavior.

Diagnosis and prognosis

In order to make a proper diagnosis, the veterinarian should obtain an accurate history, including the triggers and situations in which the barking occurs; environmental factors (visitors, sounds outside); who is present; if the pet parent is home, absent, or both; the pet parent's response to the barking; the dog's response to the pet parent's efforts; the location of the barking (e.g., at the windows, doors); and if there are any other animals present that may be contributing to the barking. By the time the case is presented to the practitioner, the barking may have multiple contributing factors and there may be more than one type of barking occurring. Differential diagnoses include separation-related disorders, noise aversion, attention-seeking behavior, territorial aggression or barking, confinement distress or anxiety, situational or specific fears or phobias, lack of enrichment and exercise, and learned behavior. As with all behavioral clinical signs, an assessment for underlying FASCP and physical illness should always be completed.

Barking categories include greeting, play initiation, self-defense, territorial barking, distance increasing, attention getting, care seeking, food soliciting, pain, loneliness, group-facilitated behavior, learned or conditioned behavior, physical causes (e.g., pain, cognitive dysfunction), fear, anxiety, stress, and panic.[35]

Management and treatment

Provide adequate outlets necessary to address breed- and species-typical needs

Provide adequate outlets necessary to address species- and breed-typical needs (see Table 19.3). Dogs that bark because they are understimulated or bored may benefit from exercise before the times when they would typically bark and the use of food puzzle toys.

Table 19.3 Management and treatment of barking

Steps	Comments
Assess for underlying fear, anxiety, stress, conflict, and panic, systemic disease, and behavioral pathology	• Rule out systemic disease and medications which may cause agitation and increased energy; disorders of fear, anxiety, stress, conflict, or panic, attention-seeking behavior, and displacement behavior.
Manage the environment to remove reinforcement for and prevent undesirable behaviors	• Determine all stimuli that lead to barking so that exposure can be prevented or the pet's response to the stimulus altered. Prevent access to the stimuli by closing drapes, confining, installing privacy fence, denying access to rooms where passersby can be seen, etc. Use of white noise or classical music to help muffle outside sounds.
Stop positive punishment techniques	• Yelling or physically punishing the dog after the fact will only make the dog afraid of the pet parent. Don't recommend this. Handheld or ultrasonic devices rarely work in the long term. Shock collars are contraindicated. Some efficacy has been shown with citronella collars; however, without positive reinforcement of alternate behaviors, they were ineffective in the long term.
Teach desirable behaviors with positive reinforcement	• Train and reward acceptable alternative behaviors such as get a toy, quiet, go to your spot, and settle. • Consider desensitization and counterconditioning. • Identify all stimuli that lead to vocalization and develop a gradient for presentation, either by starting at a distance or in a different room, or by muting the stimulus so that it is less intense. Use favored rewards to ensure a calm, positive response during exposure to the stimulus.
Reinforce desirable behaviors	• The pet parent should look for quiet behavior and use high-value rewards to reinforce. Avoid reinforcing barking with praise or petting.
Surgery	• Debarking surgery may reduce the volume of the bark, but some level of vocalization may continue since it does not address the underlying cause. • Regrowth and resumption of louder barking may occur. Debarking is considered inhumane and may be illegal in some countries. This is not a recommended treatment.
Medications and supplements	• There are no indications for using a medication or supplement with this behavior problem unless an underlying behavioral pathology is present.

Teach desirable behaviors with positive reinforcement

Teach a quiet cue so that the pet parent can control the barking. There are many ways to train quiet. In general, the dog is stimulated to bark with a very low-level stimulus (e.g., one knock on the door). The pet parent can capture the dog being quiet, mark, and reward. They can also offer a treat when the dog is barking and when the dog is quiet, say quiet and reinforce the dog. These are just a few ways to teach this behavior. Regardless of how it is taught initially, the pet parent will need to put this behavior under stimulus control (give it a name/cue) and then use it in different situations to make sure that the pet is fluent. It can also be chained with go to your spot/settle to move the dog away from the stimulus.

For some dogs, executing a quiet or settle cue may be difficult. These dogs may respond better to more active engagement, such as redirecting the dog to grab a ball or toy or coming to the pet parent to perform a touch cue. Most dogs will close their mouths when they perform a touch cue, thereby effectively interrupting the barking behavior. If more treatment is necessary, the pet parent can pursue desensitization and counterconditioning to change the response to stimuli. In cases where this is indicated, recommend a skilled dog training professional or board-certified veterinary behaviorist.

Manage the environment to remove reinforcement for and prevent undesirable behaviors

Before the dog knows how to perform the required cues, the pet parents can distract the dog with the sound of a treat bag or squeaky toy, then immediately redirect the dog to perform alternate behaviors. Then the pet parent needs to reinforce the dog and remove it from the situation, continue to keep the dog occupied in performing a series of behaviors, or provide the dog with a task that requires more engagement such as playing with a puzzle toy or working on a long-lasting chewy.

Identify and eliminate the cause by controlling or avoiding stimuli that elicit barking. Use brown or white noise, the television, radio, or calming music to help mask or muffle sound stimuli that elicit barking. Use Thunder-Caps, Doggles, Happy Hoodies, and Mutt Muffs to reduce exposure to stimuli. Remove reinforcement for undesirable behaviors by limiting exposure to triggers that elicit barking, such as using window blinds or curtains to limit the view out the window if the dog barks at people, dogs, and other stimuli passing by the house. Removing all reinforcement means constant supervision in the situations where the dog may bark or entirely preventing access (sight, sound) to the stimuli. This can be challenging for some pet parents. For example, if the dog barks in the yard, the pet parents need to supervise the dog in the yard and block the dog's access to those things that cause barking.

Reinforce desirable behaviors

Reward quiet behavior with praise and attention. Often dogs get the most attention when they act up. When the dog is quiet and calm, pet parents should acknowledge this and calmly praise or toss a treat.

Stop positive punishment techniques

Pet parents might be attracted to positive punishment techniques for a quick fix, but a long-lasting positive outcome with these methods is unlikely; thus they are not recommended. While the punishment may inhibit the barking in the presence of the pet parent, it will continue in the pet parent's absence because the motivation to bark has not been altered and the punisher (the pet parent) is not present. In addition, yelling at a dog may very well incite it to bark more due to the effects of social facilitation and emotional contagion.

Regarding barking in particular, several studies have looked at the use of positive punishment. Use of a water hose reduced fence barking, but by 90 days, the effect was negligible, as 86% of dogs had resumed. In another study where a bark-activated citronella collar was used to disrupt barking and play was used as a reward as soon as the dog quieted, 4% of fence barking recurred over 90 days. Because this study used positive reinforcement immediately after disruption, a conclusion about the effectiveness of either alone is not possible.[36] In another study investigating the efficacy of a bark-activated citronella spray collar, while barking was reduced in the short term, it increased when the use of the collar was discontinued and was no longer effective after 30 days regardless of whether it was used daily or intermittently, demonstrating that dogs will habituate to punishment and that mode of changing behavior almost never leads to a long-lasting positive outcome.[37]

Devices intended to interrupt barking may act as a punisher, may act to interrupt the behavior (allowing for a window of opportunity for retraining), or may have no effect on some dogs but may be aversive and could cause or increase FASCP in some dogs. Interruption with a squeak toy, shaking a treat box, tossing a toy or a few treats, calling the dog's name, or giving effectively trained cues (recall, touch/target, mat) can be used to engage the pet in an alternative desirable behavior for rewards without any FASCP. In one study, barking decreased in 88.9% of cases with the citronella spray collar, but in only 50% of cases with a bark-activated shock collar,[38] demonstrating that the shock collar is not as effective as other methods, contrary to what pet parents may believe. The risks of shock are high (see Chapter 10) and it has not been shown to be the most efficacious treatment for barking. For those reasons, it is never recommended. In a study of 41 barking dogs at two veterinary hospitals, 77% of dogs wearing a citronella spray collar and about 59% of dogs wearing a scentless spray collar had a significant reduction in barking in a veterinary hospital setting.[39] However, the long-term outcome regarding barking and psychological effects were not investigated. In short, aversives, confrontation, and positive punishment are not appropriate and are contraindicated for the prevention or treatment of undesirable behavior. In addition to causing fear and discomfort, even if punishment successfully suppresses what is undesirable in the short term, it does not address the underlying cause, does not train desirable responses, and has high likelihood of relapse in the long term. For more on shock collars, see Chapter 10. As discussed above, the best outcomes are achieved when the dog knows what to do and that behavior is reinforced.

CASE EXAMPLE

Presentation

Mr. Ed, a 2-year-old, neutered male Shetland Sheepdog, was presented for barking at people or pets that approached the property.

History

The pet parents lived in a townhouse and the neighbors had lodged a complaint. Mr. Ed barked when the pet parents were home and when they were not home. The barking would continue until the person or pet was out of sight or until they came inside and Mr. Ed had a chance to greet them. The only way that the pet parents could stop Mr. Ed from barking was to get his tug toy and initiate play. He was not exhibiting any aggression and seemed more interested in meeting the visitor than in chasing the person away. Barking ceased when Mr. Ed was rewarded by giving him attention or when the stimulus was removed (the visitor or animal moved out of sight).

Differential diagnoses

It was determined that Mr. Ed had excitement-induced barking, which had been reinforced many times over the course of his lifetime.

Treatment

The pet parents were instructed to block all the windows so that Mr. Ed could not see outside; use white or brown noise to drown out the sound of people in neighboring townhouses and those walking on the street; and to interrupt all barking with a shake of a treat bag followed by calling his name. When Mr. Ed came to them after being interrupted with the shake of the treat bag, they were to reinforce him with a small food treat or toss his ball for him.

In addition, it was recommended that they work with a positive reinforcement dog training professional to teach quiet, and then chain that behavior with go to your spot and settle.

Follow-up

The veterinary technician checked in with the family two weeks after the initial appointment. The pet parents were very pleased because now Mr. Ed would, most of the time, bark once and then immediately run to them to get a treat. While he was still barking, the barking had significantly decreased. They also reported that they were not having to shake the treat bag nearly as often. They had not called the dog training professional yet. The technician reminded them of the importance of working with a dog training professional for a positive long-term outcome. If they wanted to be able to open their blinds and see outside, they needed to call the dog trainer.

The veterinary technician checked in on the family in another two weeks. The pet parents had declined to call the dog trainer but reported that they were very pleased with Mr. Ed's behavior. They did not mind keeping their blinds closed on the first floor of the townhouse and the neighbors had not complained since they started interrupting his behavior. They also noticed that he was more attentive to them in general and more responsive when they called his name after they had started following through with the recommendations made at the initial appointment.

Unruliness

Unruliness tends to be a catch-all phrase for dogs that the family cannot get under control, respond poorly to verbal cues, and engage in behaviors the family finds obnoxious. Most unruly dogs are understimulated, genetically predisposed to high levels of energy and activity (working dogs), or their unruly behaviors have been inadvertently reinforced (or all three). Problem situations are likely to occur when the need for exercise, proper social interaction, and control is neglected, and treatment requires a more structured program of predictability, mental and physical enrichment, and reinforcement-based learning, focused on foundation training to calm/relax on cue and remain settled for increasing longer durations.

While many pet parents will say that their dog is hyperactive or has attention deficit hyperactivity disorder (ADHD), true hyperactivity disorders, also referred to as hyperkinesis or ADHD, are rare in dogs. The prevalence of reported (not diagnosed) hyperactivity in a survey of 4144 dogs was 12%, while approximately 7% of relinquished dogs were reported as hyperactive.[3,6] If intensity, frequency, or behavioral signs are excessive, abnormal, repetitive, or accompanied by signs of FASCP, altered appetite, or altered sleep, then the problem may be abnormal or pathologic, such as an impulsive, anxiety, compulsive, or hyperactivity disorder. Diagnosis and treatment of hyperactivity behavior are discussed in Chapter 6. Dogs with compulsive disorders (spinning, shadow chasing, tail chasing) may present for being overly active and out of control. Diagnosis and treatment of stereotypic behaviors are discussed in Chapter 18. Increased outlets for expending energy, obedience training, leash control, and other techniques designed to give pet parents more control over their dogs' behaviors are required to correct these problems. However, training techniques need to be adjusted to suit the individual dog, family, and household.

Prevention

Dogs, especially puppies and adolescent dogs, should be provided with a regular daily routine of play, exercise, mental stimulation, and social interaction to meet their individual needs (see Table 19.4 and see Chapter 5). Positive reinforcement training from adoption can help dogs to understand how to interact with people and the environment.

Diagnosis and prognosis

Unruly dogs can easily be confused with hyperactive dogs and dogs with impulse control disorders. Before deeming a dog disobedient or unruly, care should be taken to differentiate other behavior disorders. Those cases where the behaviors have been inadvertently rewarded by the pet parents can usually be improved with behavioral modification techniques, while those with an innately high energy level and insufficient outlets may be difficult or impractical to resolve. Some dogs may go through a phase during their adolescence in which they do not consistently listen to the pet parents; however, this disobedient phase does not last long if handled correctly.[40] Pet parents need to be aware that this may be a passing phase in dogs which should be met with structure, positive reinforcement training, and adequate outlets for stimulation. Young dogs that are playful and active may improve with maturity. Puppy classes and provision of resources and counseling at first puppy visits and early in the onset of the problem have been demonstrated to be preventive for behavior problems including excessive play and reduced use of punishment-based discipline.[5,12,15]

Management and treatment

Treatment of unruly behavior must be tailored to the individual pet. Important considerations include the breed, the family's response to the dog's behavior, the environment,

Table 19.4 Management of the overactive dog

Methods	Comments
Assess for underlying fear, anxiety, stress, conflict, and panic, systemic disease, and behavioral pathology	• Rule out systemic disease and medications which increase agitation or energy level, underenriched, underexercised, attention-seeking behavior, generalized anxiety, specific or situational fear or phobia, displacement behavior.
Provide adequate outlets necessary to address breed- and species-typical needs	• Provide a regular routine of play and exercise designed to suit the dog's individual needs (e.g., retrieve, swimming, flyball, agility), encourage independent play.
Manage the environment to remove reinforcement for and prevent undesirable behaviors	• Do not look at or acknowledge the dog when they are performing undesirable behaviors which are reinforced by attention.
Reinforce desirable behaviors	• Use any reward that the dog values, including food, petting, praise, and toys to reinforce calm behavior. Look for the absence of the negative behavior and reinforce that.
Teach desirable behaviors with positive reinforcement	• Enroll the pet in puppy classes at eight weeks of age, and adult classes at 9–12 months of age. Excitable pets may do better in low-distraction, quiet environments or with private lessons.
Stop positive punishment techniques	• Positive punishment of increased energy is ineffective and is not recommended, as it does not address the underlying cause and can increase FASCP and frustration.
Medications and supplements	• There are no indications for using a medication or supplement with this behavior problem unless an underlying behavioral pathology is present.

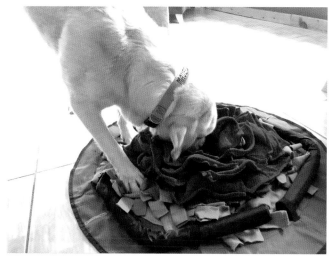

Figure 19.8 Snuffle mat. *(Attribution: Cheryl Van Voorhies, M.ed..)*

family social dynamics, and the amount of successful previous training. To design an effective treatment program, it is first necessary to identify and address the motivation or underlying cause for the behavior. Situations that cause the pet to become exceptionally excited, like greetings or putting on a leash, should be kept low key. If the pet has not learned foundation behaviors, obedience training is important. Once the pet learns basic cues, sits and downs should be requested before the pet gets anything from any person with whom it interacts. Provide an alternative activity to reward the dog and keep it engaged and occupied such as a food toy or stuffed or frozen-food toys, puzzle toys, or food hidden in snuffle mats (see Figure 19.8). Attention-seeking behavior must be ignored.

Provide adequate outlets necessary to address breed- and species-typical needs

Dogs of all ages need enrichment and exercise. If the desire or innate need is present, the dog will find a way to fulfill that need. It is always better to provide the pet with adequate outlets for its energy in the way of physical exercise (e.g., play, training sessions, swimming, dog sports), mental exercise (e.g., puzzle toys, food toys, find it games, training classes), and positive reinforcement training than to try to treat a behavior problem. Some dogs have energy levels so high that long walks or runs will not be enough. Pet parents need education as to their pet's individual needs.

Teach desirable behaviors with positive reinforcement

The simplest way to teach desirable behaviors is with the help of a positive reinforcement dog training professional. Classes are excellent ways to wear a dog out physically and mentally while teaching impulse control and proper behaviors. Pet parents often opt for in-home private lessons. While those may be helpful, classes provide stimulation and can be just as helpful if not better for the dog and pet parent. Even after vigorous exercise and play, some dogs remain unsettled. For those dogs, play sessions can end with a short training session focusing on settle.

Manage the environment to remove reinforcement for and prevent undesirable behaviors

If the behavior is fueled by attention, pet parents must completely ignore the dog when it is performing the behavior. Ignoring, walking away, shutting the door, or "time out" is preferable to providing attention. If the unruly behavior begins, cue the dog to perform a behavior and reinforce the dog. Then, exercise or play can be provided. Some behaviors are self-reinforcing. In those cases, the behavior is best prevented in the first place.

Reinforce desirable behaviors

Rewards (e.g., play, food, attention) should only be given for desirable behaviors. Since immediately providing a play period or exercise when the pet is unruly may reward the behavior, it is best to initiate play and exercise when the dog is calm or playing with its toys and before attention-seeking behaviors begin. Alternatively, the pet parent can ask for an interrupting behavior that is easy for the pet, such as sit or down, and then begin play. Finally, the pet parent can move away from the pet, stepping behind a baby gate, for example. When the pet is calm, they can ask for a behavior such as sit or down and then reinforce.

Stop positive punishment techniques

Unruly dogs usually get an overwhelming amount of negative and conflicting information from the family. The family may yell, scold, grab, or hold the dog down. These types of behaviors on the pet parent's part will make the dog more conflicted, potentially fearful, and increase the likelihood of negative behaviors such as aggression in the future. They are counterproductive. The dog is seeking information about how to get what it needs. Yelling or physical information only informs it that the pet parents are not able to understand the way that it is communicating and that they themselves are unpredictable.

Destructive behaviors

Destructive behaviors, such as chewing, scratching, and digging, can cause household damage, injure the pet, and weaken the family–pet bond. Destructive behaviors severe enough to be considered problematic in dogs occur in up to 21% of the pet dog population, are not affected by gonadectomy, get better with age, and are more common in pets adopted at older ages.[5] Dogs may be destructive because they are engaging in normal, exploratory, predatory, or play behaviors; digging into furniture to retrieve a toy or to settle or rest; chewing at doors or windows due to territorial arousal; chewing on clothing or carpeting because of an interesting or appealing odor or taste; or as a result of separation-related disorders, compulsive behavior, confinement distress, pica, and escape behavior arising from fears and phobias. To determine whether destructive behavior is a normal but undesirable behavior versus an abnormal behavior and to implement an appropriate treatment plan, it is necessary to make an accurate diagnosis. The behavioral history should consider the age and breed of the pet, the targets of the destructive behavior, the family's response, and if there are specific stimuli, situations, or times in which problems arise. Video clips can often help make the diagnosis.

Pets that are frustrated from exhibiting their normal repertoire of behaviors may engage in less-desirable behaviors to help fill the void, such as chewing, barking, or displacement behaviors (circling, excessive grooming) which may progress to compulsive disorders in genetically predisposed individuals, such as acral lick dermatitis (see Chapter 18). For pets with FASCP disorders, behavior modification and medication may be necessary (see Chapters 10–12). Dogs that chew because of FASCP or frustration when confined need positive, systematic exposure to their confinement area (see Chapter 17). Diagnosis and treatment of destructive behaviors related to fears and phobias, separation-related disorders, and compulsive disorders are discussed in other chapters within this text.

Prevention

Dogs should be provided with an environment that is predictable, comfortable, interesting, complex, and stimulating, and that provides both physical and psychological choices. Many pets are understimulated because sufficient outlets are not available or the opportunities offered do not address their needs. Young dogs also need ample exercise as an outlet for some of their boundless energy. Social interaction and play with the family (e.g., tug games, fetch, hide and seek), play with other dogs, physical exercise, and reward training should be provided frequently. More challenging activities such as agility, flyball, herding trials, disc dog competition, hunting, treibball (herding large balls), and pulling carts all provide outlets to help meet the social, physical, and mental needs of the breed or the individual. The best way to prevent destructive behaviors is to provide newly adopted dogs of any age with appropriate chew and food-filled toys and which are not. Until the dog is clearly choosing his own toys for chewing consistently, it should be under constant supervision or confined to a safe dog-proofed area.

Oral exploration can be encouraged by placing food in appealing and durable toys that require chewing and/or physical manipulation to release the food, by playing feeding games of hide and seek, using snuffle mats, or scattering food over a safe area (scatter feeding). Placing food in toys instead of bowl feeding can extend feeding time and provide increased enrichment (see Figures 19.9 and 19.10 and Chapters 5 and 13).

However, even with a good repertoire of appealing toys, regular sessions of social play, physical exercise, and reward-based training, many dogs still find time to explore, chew, scavenge, or dig. Therefore, to ensure safety and prevent damage to pet parent possessions, preventive measures will also need to be implemented. The focus should be on setting the pet up to succeed by providing, encouraging, and reinforcing behaviors that are desirable while preventing behaviors that are undesirable. Pet parents should not play tug games with towels or socks or give items like old shoes to chew. Advise pet parents to find toys that are appealing because of their texture or can be filled, stuffed, or coated. Destructive behavior can be prevented by dog-proofing areas, preventing access to areas where the dog might do damage, and supervising to distract, interrupt the behavior, and direct the dog to an alternative acceptable outlet.

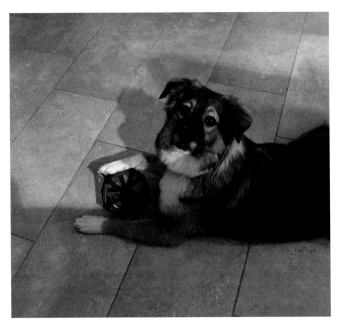

Figure 19.9 Food toys provide mental enrichment and occupy the dog during times when undesirable behaviors would otherwise be occurring. *(Courtesy Lisa Radosta.)*

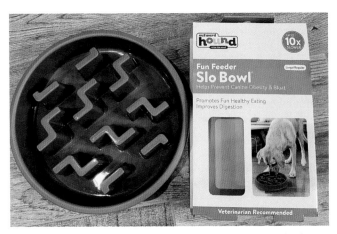

Figure 19.10 Food toys provide mental enrichment and occupy the dog during times when undesirable behaviors would otherwise be occurring. *(Attribution: Lisa Radosta.)*

Diagnosis and prognosis

Most destructive behaviors by young dogs are normal but unacceptable behaviors. Pet parents should be questioned about the dog's daily schedule, including the amount of exercise and training the pet receives; the amount and types of food, toys, and chews that are offered; how the pet is housed when the pet parent cannot supervise; and what steps have been implemented to correct the problem to date. The cause of destructive chewing in adult dogs can be more of a challenge to diagnose and manage successfully. Some dogs, especially those that retain juvenile characteristics and dogs with the energy and stamina required in working breeds, may continue to chew and scavenge as adults. Destructive behaviors that persist into adulthood may be due to reinforcement by the pet parent or by the behavior (i.e., the activity itself is enjoyable). Additional underlying causes in adult dogs include predation, hunger, separation-related disorders, noise phobias, confinement distress, compulsive disorders, and territorial behavior. Problems of other body systems may contribute to any behavioral clinical sign, even if it seems unlikely. For that reason, a physical examination and appropriate baseline workup is always necessary. Animals are voiceless. Any deviation from what is considered normal or clinical signs which might appear excessive should trigger a physical evaluation.

The prognosis varies with the age, breed, and temperament of the pet, the pet's environment, family dynamics, and, especially, the underlying cause of the chewing. With proper diagnosis, training, and adequate supervision, the prognosis for complete control of most normal chewing problems by young pets is good to excellent. Destructive behaviors may take time to improve or resolve and in some situations, may get worse before getting better. In one study, 25.5% of adopted dogs displayed destructive behavior one week after adoption, which increased to 41% of dogs one month after adoption.[41] In a recent survey with over 4000 dogs, prevalence of destructive behavior was 12%, while 7% of relinquished dogs were reported as destructive, indicating that some destructive behaviors are sufficiently problematic to require referral[3,6] (see Table 19.5).

Management and treatment

Provide adequate outlets necessary to address species-and breed-typical needs

While destruction is more likely in young dogs, dogs of any age can exhibit this behavior. The goal is to ensure that a regular daily routine with sufficient enrichment in the form of exercise, training, and play is provided. Provide appealing, durable, and time-consuming items with which to play and chew. Begin with a variety of toys to determine which the dog prefers. Good choices are those designed for food to be stuffed into the openings. This will increase the dog's level of interest in the toys and extend the length of time it spends licking and chewing. Other toys that might maintain a dog's interest include those that must be manipulated to release small pieces of food or kibble. If most of the dog's food is fed from these toys, feeding time can be longer, more challenging, and more enriching than eating from a food bowl. Toys should be rotated in and out every few days to keep them interesting.

Teach desirable behaviors with positive reinforcement

Pet parents can teach cues to decrease the likelihood of destructive chewing which occurs when they are home such as find it, leave it, and drop it.

Manage the environment to remove reinforcement for and prevent undesirable behaviors

Supervise closely until the dog is reliably choosing its own things. When supervision is not possible, the dog should be placed in a safe, destruction-proofed area with its bedding, toys, and chews. All dogs do not innately feel comfortable in small, enclosed areas. Time should be taken to introduce the

Table 19.5 Management of destructive behavior in dogs

Course of action	Comments
Assess for underlying fear, anxiety, stress, conflict, and panic, systemic disease, and behavioral pathology	• Rule out systemic disease and medications which increase agitation or energy level, underenriched, underexercised, attention seeking behavior, generalized anxiety, specific or situational fear or phobia, displacement behavior.
Provide adequate outlets necessary to address breed-and species-typical needs	• Provide opportunities for the pet to chew appropriately. • Offer a wide selection until preferred toys are determined. • Provide toys that are durable (e.g., plastic, rubber), that can be filled with biscuits, dog food, rawhide, or pieces of meat or cheese. Spread cheese, yogurt, or peanut butter on toys. Freeze food-filled toys to lengthen their desirability. • Pet parents should provide a regular schedule of physical activity ranging from long walks or runs to opportunities to sniff and explore. • Additional activities might also be needed for high-energy individuals and working breeds, such as playing ball or flying disc, tug games, retrieving, herding trials, flyball, and agility. • Hiding toys and treats around house or yard for pet to seek and find. • Provide a variety of toys. Keep interest by rotating, providing novel toys, or adding new food and treats.
Manage the environment to remove reinforcement for and prevent undesirable behaviors	• Do not use possessions to chew or encourage play with them. • Whenever the pet parent cannot supervise, the dog should be confined to a crate, exercise pen, or dog-proofed room so that it does not have the opportunity to engage in unacceptable chewing until the pet can reliably be left alone. • Sprays or ointments which taste hot or bitter can be applied to household objects; however, this is rarely effective.
Reinforce desirable behaviors	• When the pet chews or plays with one of its toys, that behavior should be reinforced with praise, play, or food treats to reinforce the behavior.
Teach desirable behaviors with positive reinforcement	• Obedience training to teach calm and focused behaviors.
Stop positive punishment techniques	• In general, physical punishment should be avoided as it can cause fear, avoidance, and aggression. It only stops the behavior in the pet parent's presence and may inadvertently reinforce the behavior.

pet slowly to the idea of confinement in a positive manner. See Chapters 15 and 17 for information on how to introduce a dog to confinement or condition a sanctuary space.

The pet may have a preference for certain off-limits items. The easiest and safest thing to do is to make sure that the pet does not have access to those items. While pet parents may want to have a dog that gets to roam the house freely without supervision, it may not be safe or advisable for some dogs. As discussed above, avoidance techniques are only likely to succeed if more desirable outlets for feeding and chewing (from the dog's perspective) are also available.

Additional management may include increasing the amount fed, switching to a higher-bulk diet, or changing the feeding schedule to match the times the dog might chew. Trap and remove prey if this is the reason for scratching or chewing on walls or floors. Chewing at windows and drapes during territorial displays can be prevented by keeping the dog away from these areas and providing appropriate supervision during times where stimuli are present outside.

If the dog does engage in chewing inappropriate things and it knows an attention behavior such as watch, come, or leave it, it is best to use that cue. When it returns to the pet parent, it can be reinforced. If the dog is not fluent in any particular behavior in that circumstance, any sound which distracts but does not scare it can be used to interrupt the behavior (e.g., squeaky toy, treat bag, calling the dog's name, hand clap). Then, when the pet parent has the dog's attention, they should immediately engage the dog in a desirable outlet for play or chewing and reinforce. The pet parent may ask you if they are in fact reinforcing their pet for the undesirable behavior by distracting their dog with the shake of a treat bag, for example. Should not their dog be punished when they are doing the wrong thing? The pet parent is not reinforcing the negative behavior when they distract with a sound such as the shake of a treat jar or a treat bag. They are getting the dog's attention. Then, they will ask the dog to perform a behavior such as sit or direct the dog to an appropriate behavior such as chewing on a dog toy, which is then reinforced. The behavior that is reinforced is the one that immediately precedes the reinforcement. In this case, that would be chewing on a dog toy or sitting.

Reinforce desirable behaviors

When the dog chooses its own items on which to chew, the pet parent should reinforce that behavior. A clicker or marker word can be helpful when capturing behaviors which may be offered throughout the day.

Stop positive punishment techniques

Pet parents who use punishment to suppress undesirable behaviors rather than encouraging and reinforcing desirable behavior may cause FASCP, which can lead to further destructive behavior. If it is mild and not sufficiently aversive, it can serve as social reinforcement. See Chapter 10 for more information on punishment and reinforcement. Punishment can teach some pets to avoid the behavior only in the family's presence. At worst, punishment can cause fear of family members or a confused and conflicted pet.

CASE EXAMPLE

Presentation

Barney, a 9-month-old neutered male Labrador Retriever, was presented for destroying items around the house when the pet parents were home.

History

Barney was loose in the house when the pet parents were home and confined to a large crate when they were not. He went into the crate easily for a food-filled toy. They watched him on their home cameras when they were at work and he spent most of the time sleeping. The pet parents rarely had time to exercise Barney. He had not been to puppy classes nor obedience training classes. He loved playing with other dogs and played with the neighbor's dog on the weekends. The pet parents noted that he was less likely to destroy on the weekends. Since his adoption at two months of age, he had eaten holes in the carpet, chewed large holes in expensive pieces of furniture, destroyed books, and dug up or chewed every plant in the home.

Workup

Barney's physical examination and the results of laboratory tests were within normal limits.

Differential diagnoses

Potential causes of Barney's behavior include lack of enrichment, lack of exercise, lack of training, separation-related disorders, noise aversion, compulsive behavior, and normal behavior. It was determined that he had normal behavior and was underenriched, underexercised, and undertrained. Because he did not show any signs of fear of sounds and his behavior occurred when the pet parents were home and he had access to them, noise aversion and separation-related disorders were ruled out.

Treatment

The veterinarian discussed with the pet parents that Labrador Retrievers very commonly present for foreign body surgery and that this problem had to be treated immediately. Because he loved playing with other dogs, and the pet parents did not have time to exercise him, doggie day care and increased playdates with the neighbor's dog were recommended. A professional dog walker was recommended to help out with an extra midday walk.

The pet parents were to find a small room or a hallway in which to confine him which had no carpeting and could easily be dog proofed. Ideally, this would be a room where he could see the family. Barney was only allowed out of this space if and when he could be kept in sight. The family was instructed to provide physical, mental, and social enrichment, including retrieving games, physical exercise, and reward-based training each day. When the pet parents were at home, they provided Barney with durable, rubber food-stuffed toys and toys with beef hide attached to direct and maintain desirable chewing. Whenever he initiated chewing on any of his toys, the pet parents were to praise him and occasionally throw him a small treat. Household items that Barney had chewed were coated with a commercial antichew spray. Small plants were placed out of reach. A second group of food-dispensing manipulation toys was also purchased to be left with Barney in his crate when the pet parent left for the day. After the midday walk, the dog walker refilled the toys and again provided them in the crate. A positive reinforcement training class was recommended. Barney's training was focused on sit and watch, relaxed down-stays, and come.

Follow-up

The veterinary technician followed up in two weeks with a phone call. Barney was enjoying day care and his food toys. They did not have time for more play dates and they could not afford both a dog walker and day care, so they had opted for day care. They had not enrolled in a training class yet. They felt guilty about putting him in the hallway, even though he did not cry or scratch to get out and he had toys to play with there. They admitted that they let him out frequently and did not supervise him. During that time, Barney would find household items to chew, although at decreased frequency than before they started treating him. The pet parents were upset but resisted the temptation to punish Barney. The veterinary technician advised them to rotate food toys and other toys so that Barney had three new toys each day. In addition, they were to feed all of his food out of food toys. While meals were not to be delayed

significantly, most of the food should come at times when the pet parents were home so that he would be occupied during the time when he would usually be destructive. It was also recommended that they block off other areas of the house, effectively confining him in the room where they were. Finally, they were told to carry 20 small treats and a clicker with them. They were to click him any time that he was in the room with an item that he might chew and he did not choose that item. The technician gave them online resources for training go to your spot, stay, and settle. She also recommended a self-guided training program online.

The veterinary technician followed up in two weeks by phone. Barney's parents had signed up for the online course and were working at their own pace on the weekends. They were rotating toys and feeding as recommended. He was still going to day care. They had used the clicker as directed. Barney was rarely chewing on the pet parent's things anymore, but he was following them around frequently, waiting for a click and treat. They were instructed to slowly, over a month or so, decrease supervision.

Digging

Digging may be a nuisance but is an innate trait for many dogs. The behavior often arises in many of the same situations as other destructive behaviors, often due to a lack of sufficient alternative forms of stimulation. Breeds that are bred to flush out prey such as terriers, which may dig as part of the hunt, may be stimulated to dig wherever there are odors of food or prey in the ground. Dogs will also dig to bury and retrieve bones. Some dogs dig to escape confinement. In addition, some dogs are motivated to dig cooling and nesting sites.

Prevention

Dogs should be closely supervised when outdoors for a few months after adoption to keep them engaged in desirable activities, to prevent undesirable digging, and to redirect undesirable digging into alternate desirable activities. Immediately after adoption, for dogs that desire to dig, the pet parent should provide a designated place to dig outside (e.g., digging pit, digging box). They can bury toys or chews in that area to entice the dog to dig. When the dog digs there, the pet parent should reinforce with food or play which occurs at the dig site. When the dog goes to another site and starts to dig, the pet parent can interrupt with a nonfrightening sound such as the shake of a treat bag, a treat jar, calling the dog's name, or a hand clap. They then call the dog to them, reinforce (the dog came when called and must be reinforced for this behavior) and direct the dog to the acceptable site. The drive to dig after prey is very strong and may be stronger than the reinforcement provided by the pet parent. When leaving the dog outdoors unsupervised, block access to the areas where it is undesirable for the dog to dig, and provide a secure confinement area (with motivating outlets for enrichment) to prevent digging access to the undesirable sites or to limit digging to that area.

Diagnosis and prognosis

Since dogs dig for a number of reasons, it is important to determine the underlying cause to be able to formulate an effective program for management and treatment. Carefully interview the pet parent as to the circumstances surrounding the digging. If the digging is along the fence or near a gate, the dog may be digging to escape. Escape attempts could be due to separation-related disorders, noise phobias, or sights, sounds, and odors outside the yard, including potential playmates, threats, prey, or an intact female (if the dog is an intact male). Digging for prey might be at single or multiple sites in the yard; however, depending on the prey species (e.g., voles), it may be difficult to identify these as the cause of digging. The prognosis varies considerably with the underlying cause. Even with additional stimulation, neutering of intact males, and minimizing access to the stimuli that might incite escape, some dogs require either supervision whenever outdoors or a suitable confinement area to prevent undesirable digging.

Management and treatment

Provide adequate outlets necessary to address breed- and species-typical needs

Dogs that engage in digging are seeking something, whether that is to cool off or expend excess energy. Determination of the motivation will allow the pet parent to provide adequate stimulation. For example, if the pet is digging to cool off, the pet parent may provide cool mats, only let the dog outside when it is not too hot, provide cover, install ceiling fans on an outside porch, or provide a baby pool with a couple of inches of water for splashing.

Teach desirable behaviors with positive reinforcement

The pet parents can teach or capture the digging behavior and elicit the cue when the dog is provided an appropriate substrate to dig in. The dog should be offered plenty of praise and treats for digging on cue in the appropriate substrate or area.

Manage the environment to remove reinforcement for and prevent undesirable behaviors

Supervise dogs that dig inappropriately when outdoors. Do not allow the dog outside unsupervised until trained. Block off areas that are undesirable. Limit access to the yard at times when prey is likely to be out if that contributes to the behavior. Create a digging pit or safe and desirable (to the pet parent) place for the dog to dig. Educate the pet parent that the dog has an underlying motivation for digging. If the designated digging area differs significantly from the dog's preference, it will be challenging to entice the dog to dig there as part of a long-term solution. For dogs that are digging to escape, the motivation for the behavior should be determined. Barriers to visual stimuli, neutering intact males, increased opportunities for play and enrichment in the yard, and secure confinement might be needed. If the motivation is to escape and the dog has already escaped via digging out of the yard, it has already been reinforced for that behavior. In all cases, dogs should only be let out into yards that are secured. That may mean putting locks on the gates so they are not accidentally left open or digging a trench into the ground where additional fencing or rebar can be installed. Holes dug in undesirable places can be filled with rocks, gravel, or water, or covered with chicken wire or fencing, but the pet may just choose another site to dig. Supervising will help deter undesirable behavior, but digging will likely resume when the pet parent is not present.

Reinforce desirable behaviors

Pet parents should always reinforce digging in appropriate areas. This can be done remotely by burying desirable things such as bones in those areas. That way, when the dog digs there, it will find a prize, enticing digging in that area in the future.

Stop positive punishment techniques

Motion-activated sprinklers can deter the dog from digging in a particular place. However, the desire to dig will still be present. For that reason, the strategies above must be implemented for a positive long-term outcome.

CASE EXAMPLE

Presentation

Sonic, an intact male Border Collie, was presented for digging under the gate and roaming the neighborhood when the pet parent was at work during the day.

History

Upon arriving home, the pet parent would see Sonic wandering around the neighborhood, call him, grab him by the collar, and punish him for escaping.

Workup

Sonic's physical examination and lab work were within normal limits.

Differential diagnoses

Potential causes of Sonic's digging included seeking out females in heat, lack of enrichment, lack of exercise, lack of appropriate places to dig, reinforced behavior (neighbors feeding and playing with him, play with other dogs), lack of adequate fencing, and specific fear or phobia. On presentation and by pet parent report, he was not fearful of sounds or situations, to their knowledge. The most likely differentials were that he was seeking out females in heat, was underenriched, underexercised, and was being reinforced by the neighbors.

Treatment

The pet parent was told that punishing the dog after he had escaped was counterproductive. In fact, Sonic was starting to avoid the pet parent when he came home and was more hesitant to come when called. Neutering was recommended to decrease sexually motivated escape and roaming behavior. Increased exercise, including jogging and games of fetch, was suggested each afternoon when arriving home. They were told to walk the fence line and block off any areas of potential escape and provide a safe and desirable digging area.

The veterinary technician followed up by phone in two weeks. Sonic was doing well and had not escaped the yard. The pet parent purchased several inexpensive soccer balls and encouraged Sonic to play with them by throwing and kicking them around the yard. The pet parent covered the space below the gate with chicken wire where Sonic had escaped and installed a motion-activated sprinkler near the gate. They agreed to keep Sonic in the house when they were not home. Each morning before departing, Sonic was provided with a frozen food-filled rubber dog toy and his morning diet.

Sonic would occupy himself with his toys and food when the pet parents departed and was excited when the pet parents returned home. However, he did have relapses any time that he was let outside. He did not dig by the gate, but he was digging in other areas around the fence. The pet parents made it clear that they had a yard so that they would not have to watch their dog when outside and did not intend to stay out with him.

At this time, neutering was recommended again, as roaming is one of the few behavior problems which responds to gonadectomy with a decrease in frequency. In addition, the pet parents were told to contact the fencing company and ask them to dig a trench into the yard and lay wire into the trench so that it would be very difficult for Sonic to dig out. In this way, they could eliminate all reinforcement for this behavior. The neuter was scheduled for a time when the fence would be constructed and Sonic boarded at the veterinary hospital until the fence had been completed.

One month after Sonic went home, the veterinary technician followed up by phone. Sonic was calmer and was not digging to get out. When he did try to dig at the fence, he was unable to dig deep enough to get out. The pet parents were happy with the results.

Nocturnal activity

Most pets that do not sleep through the night have a physical or behavioral condition which underlies their behavior and are not exhibiting unruly behavior. If a pet cannot sleep through the night, all other behavioral disorders such as generalized anxiety, specific or situational phobia, noise phobia, cognitive dysfunction, sleep disorders, and separation-related disorders should be considered. It is possible that dogs may need more exercise mental and physical activities than they are getting causing them to continue to be active at night. In cases such as those, it should be recommended that more exercise and environmental enrichment should be provided for the pet during the day. Also see chapter 8 Restlessness, wakign at night.

Conclusion

Most often unruly and destructive behaviors are the result of inadequate attention to the needs of the dog. These are generally easily prevented and treated. However, behavioral clinical signs are vague and behavioral pathology as well as physical illness must always be ruled out before an assumption of "normal behavior" is made. In some cases, normal behaviors which are met with punishment as the primary training tool can grow into frustration-related, displacement, conflict-related, or compulsive behaviors. Just because these types of behaviors are considered normal, they should not be ignored.

References

1. Fatjo J. The epidemiology of behavioural problems in dogs and cats: a survey of veterinary practitioners. *Anim Welf.* 2006;15:2.
2. Salman MD, Hutchinson J, Ruch-Gallie R. Behavioral reasons for relinquishment of dogs and cats to 12 shelters. *J Appl Anim Wel Sci.* 2000;3:93–106.
3. Diesel G, Brodbelt D, Pfeiffer DU. Characteristics of relinquished dogs and their owners at 14 rehoming centers in the United Kingdom. *J Appl Anim Welf Sci.* 2010;13:15–30.
4. Coe JB, Young I, Lambert K, et al. A scoping review of published research on the relinquishment of companion animals. *J Appl Anim Welf Sci.* 2014;17(3):253–273.
5. Martinez AG, Pernas GS, Casalta FJD, et al. Risk factors associated with behavioral problems in dogs. *J Vet Behav.* 2011;6:225–231.
6. Dinwoodie IR, Dwyer B, Zottola V, et al. Demographics and comorbidity of behavior problems in dogs. *J Vet Behav.* 2019;32:62–71.
7. Bamberger M, Houpt KA. Signalment factors, comorbidity, and trends in behavior diagnoses in dogs: 1644 cases (1991–2001). *J Am Vet Med Assoc.* 2006; 229:1591–1601.
8. Denenberg S, Landsberg GM, Horwitz D. A comparison of cases referred to behaviorists in three different countries. In: Mills D, Levine E, Landsberg GM, et al., eds. In: *Current Issues and Research in Veterinary Behavioral Medicine.* West Lafayette, IN: Purdue University Press; 2005: 56–62.
9. Patronek GJ, Glickman LT, Beck AM, McCabe GP, Ecker C. Risk factors for relinquishment of dogs to an animal shelter. *J Am Vet Med Assoc.* 1996;209:572–581.
10. Powell L, Duffy DL, Kruger KA, et al. Relinquishing owners underestimate their dog's behavioral problems: deception or lack of knowledge? *Front Vet Sci.* 2021; 8:734973. doi:10.3389/fvets.2021.734973.
11. New JC, Salman MD, King M, et al. Characteristics of shelter-relinquished animals and their pet parents compared with animals and their pet parents in U.S. pet-owning households. *J Appl Anim Welf Sci.* 2000;3:179–201. doi:10.1207/ S15327604JAWS0303_1.
12. Gazzano A, Mariti C, Alvares S, et al. The prevention of undesirable behaviors in dogs: effectiveness of veterinary behaviorists' advice given to puppy owners. *J Vet Behav.* 2008;3:125–133.
13. González-Martínez Á, Martínez MF, Rosado B, et al. Association between puppy classes and adulthood behavior of the dog. *J Vet Behav.* 2019;32:36–41.
14. Blackwell EJ, Twells C, Seawright A, et al. The relationship between training methods and the occurrence of behaviour problems as reported by owners, in a population of domestic dogs. *J Vet Behav.* 2008;3:207–217.
15. Cutler JH, Coe JB, Niel L. Puppy socialization practices of a sample of dog owners from across Canada and the United States. *J Am Vet Med Assoc.* 2017;251:1415–1423.
16. Duxbury MM, Jackson JA, Line SW, et al. Evaluation of association between retention in the home and attendance at puppy socialization classes. *J Am Vet Med Assoc.* 2003;223(1):61–66.
17. Kutsumi A, Nagasawa M, Ohta M, et al. Importance of puppy training for future behavior of the dog. *J Vet Med Sci.* 2013;75(2):141–149.
18. Cooper JJ, Cracknell N, Hardiman J, et al. The welfare consequences and efficacy of training pet dogs with remote electronic training collars in comparison to reward based training. *PLoS One.* 2014;9(9): e102722. doi:10.1371/journal.pone. 0102722.
19. China L, Mills DS, Cooper JJ. Efficacy of dog training with and without remote electronic collars vs. a focus on positive reinforcement. *Front Vet Sci.* 2020;7:508. doi:10.3389/fvets.2020.00508.
20. Yin S, Fernandez EJ, Pagan S, et al. Efficacy of a remote-controlled, positive-reinforcement, dog-training system for modifying problem behaviors exhibited when people arrive at the door. *Appl Anim Behav Sci.* 2008;113:123–138.
21. Rezac P, Koru E, Havlicek Z, et al. Factors affecting dog jumping on people. *Appl Anim Behav Sci.* 2017;197:40–44.
22. Dorey NR, Tobias JS, Udell MAR, et al. Decreasing dog problem behavior with functional analysis: linking diagnoses to treatment. *J Vet Behav.* 2012;7:276 282.
23. Hubbard K, Skelly BJ, McKelvi J, et al. Risk of vomiting and diarrhoea in dogs. *Vet Rec.* 2007;161:755–757.
24. Davis BW, Nattrass S, O'Brien G, et al. Assistance dog placement in the pediatric population: benefits, risks, and recommendations for future application. *Anthrozoos.* 2004;17:130–145.
25. Stephen J, Ledger R. Relinquishing dog pet parents' ability to predict behavioral problems in shelter dogs post adoption. *Appl Anim Behav Sci.* 2007;107:88–99.
26. McGreevy PD, Georgevsky D, Carrasco J, et al. Dog behavior co-varies with height, bodyweight and skull shape 2013. *PLoS One.* 2013;8(12):e80529. doi:10.1371/ journal.pone.0080529.
27. Kaminski J, Pitsch A, Tomasello M. Dogs steal in the dark. *Anim Cogn.* 2013;16: 385–394.
28. Blackwell EJ, Twells C, Seawright W, et al. The relationship between training methods and the occurrence of behavior problems, as reported by pet parents, in a population of domestic dogs. *J Vet Behav.* 2008;3:207–217.

29. Becuwe-Bonnet V, Belanger MC, Frank D, et al. Gastrointestinal disorders in dogs with excessive licking of surfaces. *J Vet Behav.* 2012;7:194–204.

30. Beaver B, Fishcer M, Atkinson C. Determination of favorite components of garbage by dogs. *Appl Anim Behav Sci.* 1992;34:29–136.

31. Voith V, Wright JC, Danneman PJ. Is there a relationship between canine behavior problems and spoiling activities, anthromorphism and obedience training? *Appl Anim Behav Sci.* 1992;32:263–271.

32. Guy NC, Luescher UA, Dohoo SE, et al. Risk factors for dog bites to pet parents in a general veterinary caseload. *Appl Anim Behav Sci.* 2001;74:29–42.

33. Hao-Yu S, Paterson MBA, Georgiou F, et al. Who is pulling the leash? Effects of human gender and dog sex on human–dog dyads when walking on-leash. *Animals.* 2020;10:1894. doi:10.3390/ani10101894.

34. van Herwijnen IR, van der Borg J, Naguib, et al. Rein sensor leash tension measurements in pet parent-dog dyads navigating a course with distractions. *J Vet Behav.* 2020;35:45–46.

35. Pongracz P, Molnar C, Miklosi A. Barking in family dogs: an ethological approach. *Vet J.* 2010;10:141–147.

36. Pageat P, Tessier Y. Disruptive stimulus: definition and application in behavior therapy. In: *Proceedings of the First International Conference of Veterinary Behavioral Medicine.* UK: Universities Federation for Animal Welfare, Potter's Bar; 1997:187.

37. Wells D. The effectiveness of a citronella spray collar in reducing certain forms of barking in dogs. *Appl Anim Behav Sci.* 2001;73:299–309.

38. Juarbe-Diaz SV, Houpt KA. Comparison of two antibarking collars for treatment of nuisance barking. *J Am Anim Hosp Assoc.* 1996;5:231–235.

39. Moffat KM, Landsberg GM, Beaudet R. Effectiveness and comparison of both a citronella and scentless spray bark collar for the control of barking in a veterinary hospital setting. *J Am Anim Hosp Assoc.* 2003;39:343–348.

40. Asher L, Englad GCW, Sommerville R, et al. Teenage dogs? Evidence for adolescent-phase conflict behaviour and an association between attachment to humans and pubertal timing in the domestic dog. *Biol Lett.* 2020;16: 20200097. doi:10.1098/rsbl.2020.0097.

41. Lord LK, Reider L, Herron ME, et al. Health and behavior problems in dogs and cats one week and one month after adoption from animal shelters. *J Am Vet Med Assoc.* 2008;233:1715–1722.

Resources and recommended reading

Fear Free Happy Homes – www.fearfreehappyhomes.com.

Ohio State Indoor Pet Initiative. https://indoorpet.osu.edu.

American College of Veterinary Behaviorists et al. *Decoding Your Dog: The Ultimate Experts Explain Common Dog Behaviors and Reveal How to Prevent or Change Unwanted Ones.* New York, NY; Houghton Mifflin Harcourt; 2014.

Today's Veterinary Practice - Puppy training https://todaysveterinarypractice.com/pet-owner-resources/puppy-training-handout/

CHAPTER 20

Unruly and destructive behaviors – feline

Ellen Lindell, DVM, DACVB and Lisa Radosta, DVM, DACVB

Chapter contents

Introduction

Domestic cats exhibit many normal, species-typical behaviors that are poorly tolerated yet inadvertently reinforced by their pet parents. Indoor cats live underenriched lives, which may lead to increased expression of normal, destructive, and unruly behaviors. These behaviors can range from destruction of property to vocalization that interferes with a person's ability to relax or sleep.

When a pet parent expresses a concern about their cat's undesirable behavior, it should be considered serious. The pet parent's perception of a problematic behavior, regardless of whether the behavior might be within normal limits for a cat, determines whether the cat will be able to remain in the home. Accurate assessment requires a behavioral history, physical examination, and screening lab work.

Educating pet parents about normal behavior and screening for behavioral concerns should be a part of all well-visit appointments. Encourage conversation by initiating a dialog. Prevention and early intervention can create and sustain a lasting bond among the pet parent, their cat, and your veterinary team.

General behavior modification principles

Cats are willing and able to learn many behaviors. When an undesirable behavior is exhibited, it is common for a pet parent to ask, "How can I stop this behavior?" The better question would be, "How can I find a suitable replacement for this behavior?" When interventions focus on *stopping* behaviors, fear, anxiety, and conflict ensue. Frustration occurs when a cat's needs are not met. Emotional conflict can progress to fear of the pet parent when interventions include the use of positive or physical punishment, whether delivered through a remotely activated device or directly from the pet parent.

Help pet parents shift their focus to teaching rather than correcting. Reward-based methods of training work very well with all species, including cats. At a minimum, training should be used to encourage and reward the cat for engaging in behaviors that satisfy the cat's motivation and serve as acceptable substitutes for unwanted or "unruly" behaviors.

In addition to teaching skills that can be used to modify specific problematic behaviors, pet parents can teach behaviors that are fun to watch, fun to perform, and even practical. Trick training provides social and cognitive enrichment for cats (and people) and strengthens the bond between the family and the cat. All cats are not receptive to food-based training. Some may be motivated by freedom to go outside in a catio, play with a remote toy, or play with the pet parent. Finding the right motivation and reinforcement is essential to quick and effective training. Training improves communication and predictability, increases the frequency of exhibiting acceptable behaviors, and when properly done, can improve a cat's tolerance for frustration.

Destructive behavior

Problem overview

Cats can damage homes and property with their teeth or claws. Curtains, carpet, and soft furniture are common targets. Scratching in particular is one of the most common complaints from cat pet parents.[1,2] It is estimated that as many as 50% to over 80% of cat pet parents report this behavior, and is the second most common behavioral complaint after house soiling, although most were not appreciably bothered.[2–6] However, fewer than half of pet parents were aware of how to encourage scratching on appropriately designated surfaces and only about 10% had received advice from their veterinarian.[4] Scratching behavior is a normal feline maintenance behavior that can be part of environmental exploration, play, claw maintenance, communication (visual, olfactory), attention seeking, and territorial marking.[7–11] The motivation to engage in this behavior is so strong that declawed cats continue to engage in it.[12] Cats tend to use the same spot repeatedly (up to six times a day), enhancing the strength of the olfactory and visual signals.[9,13,14] Cats typically choose to scratch on surfaces located in the main living areas, the places where they spend most of their time.[9,15] Most common targets of inappropriate scratching were furniture, including chairs, sofas, and tables, followed by carpet, with the highest frequency on vertical surfaces of furniture-covered fabric.[4] Scratching can be triggered by an emotion; cats experiencing anxiety, fear, excitement or stress may scratch to communicate a message, presumably with the intention of affecting the behavior of the recipient.[8,16] Expression may be a sign of excitement, anxiety, fear, or stress. As such, positive punishment of this behavior by the pet parents can lead to increased conflict and worsening of the behavior. Cats have been observed scratching more in the presence of other cats, which may lead to the conclusion that the behavior is influenced by social facilitation or that it acts as a displacement behavior performed when cats are stressed.[9,11]

Scratching decreases with age. There is no difference etween males and females in their tendency to scratch.

Damage through chewing is less common than scratching and pet parents are often unprepared. Cats may chew houseplants, wood, or cloth. Cats may initiate play with stringlike items such as shoelaces and yarn; these strings may be swallowed in the course of play. Destructive chewing may be part of normal exploration and play but can also reflect underlying disease. For more discussion of ingestion of nonfood items, see Chapters 6 and 13.

Prevention

Educate and provide resources to new cat pet parents about normal cat behavior and cat behavioral needs. Providing cat pet parents with educational material was associated with a reduced risk of relinquishment. A single counseling session for new kitten parents aimed at preventing behavioral problems was effective in reducing undesirable behavior including climbing on curtains and furniture, disturbing pet parents when lying down, excess vocalization, and resistance to body handling.[17,18] All cats, regardless of age, should be supervised until they consistently use appropriate surfaces for scratching and suitable toys for chewing. When a cat has access to a scratching post in their living area, they use it![10] Until appropriate behavior patterns are established, when supervision is not available, gates or closed doors may be used to block the cat's access to valuable property. If cats are to be confined, they should be provided with an assortment of toys and scratching posts along with the basic essentials (food, water, litterbox, and comfortable resting spots).

Opportunities and outlets for scratching are a basic environmental need.[11] Cats are self-motivated to scratch surfaces; however, each cat will have its own preferences for textures, locations, and orientations of scratching surfaces. New cats and kittens should be offered a wide selection of scratching posts in order to find their preference, with scratching posts reported to be preferred over scratch pads.[4] However, placing cats near designated scratching items in an attempt to encourage scratching has been shown to significantly lower the use of those items.[4] While pet parents often prefer or at least offer carpet, most likely because that is what is widely available, in one study, younger cats preferred rope and older cats preferred carpet.[6] Additional findings from that study include that cats are more likely to scratch a post with a <3 feet (1 m) base when compared with those with a >5 feet (1.5 m) base, upright posts and posts with several levels, further demonstrating that finding the cat's preference is the foundation to solving this behavior problem. In another study, when presented with chenille, suede, synthetic leather, and waterproof grosgrain, the cats preferred chenille and liked synthetic leather the least.[19] To find the cat's preference, provide different textures including cardboard, ropes, and loosely woven rugs or fabrics, and different orientations (vertical, angled, and horizontal). Place posts in prominent, well-traveled areas and near favored resting places to mimic the sequence which would occur in nonpet cats and because cats often scratch when they wake up from sleeping. Cats that have scratching posts available in their core areas and to whom a variety of scratching posts are available are unlikely to use undesirable (to the pet parent) places to scratch.[6,10] Find what the cat likes, and provide that substrate and others (diversity) in the areas where the cat rests and plays (Figures 20.1–20.3).

Several posts may be needed in order to be sure that there is a post available in any area that the cat has demonstrated a preference for scratching. Catnip and silver vine might further encourage and stimulate scratching post use.[20] In addition, areas where the pet parent doesn't want the cat to scratch can be made less appealing by covering them with plastic sheeting, double-sided tape, or carpet runner pointy side up.

Teach pet parents how to trim their cat's nails safely and without stress. Condition the cat to accept nail trims as soon as they are adopted using positive reinforcement and cooperative care techniques. If nail caps are to be used, condition the cat to accept them.

A common mistake is to offer the cat the substrates, styles and location of scratching post preferred by the family and not necessarily preferred by the cat. The best thing that the family can do is provide the cat with their preferred items where they want to scratch. There is almost always a way to marry the pet parent's and the cat's preferences so that all can be happy.

Similarly, a wide range of safe toys, including food-dispensing toys, should be provided in many locations until play preferences have been determined. Once the pet parent has

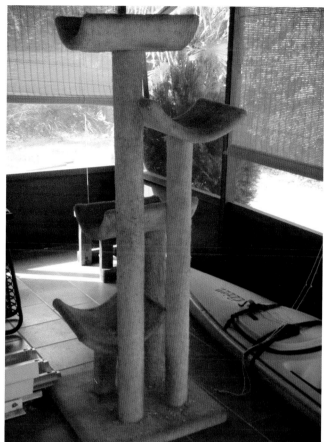

Figure 20.2 Scratching posts with bases less than 3 feet in width and upright columns may be preferred over scratching posts with larger bases and horizontal scratching areas. *(Attribution: Lisa Radosta.)*

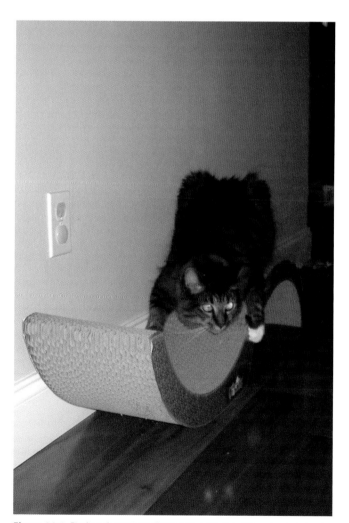

Figure 20.1 Finding the cat's preferences by offering different substrates is the best way to curb destructive scratching. *(Attribution: Lisa Radosta.)*

determined the types of toys preferred by the cat, they should purchase enough of those types of toys so that they can rotate the toys daily, giving the cat three different toys per day.

The veterinarian plays a crucial role in counseling pet parents that destructive scratching can be prevented and treated. Declawing (onychectomy) should not be considered an appropriate preventive or intervention strategy for destructive scratching (Box 20.1). See treatment below for more information on declawing.

Diagnosis and potential outcomes

A diagnosis of normal destructive behavior can be made based on observation of the cat's posture and the timing of the behavior. During normal exploratory and play-based scratching and chewing, cats assume a relaxed or playful posture; bouts of chewing or scratching are typically short. These normal behaviors will be demonstrated at various times of day, whether or not the pet parent is nearby. Cats may vocalize using the same vocalization pattern used in other play contexts. Normal destructive behavior can be easily modified with a good outcome. Cats that ingest objects, particularly stringlike items, may require surgical intervention.

Destructive behavior may occur secondary to frustration when a desired reward or interaction is not immediately available. This behavior generally occurs when the pet parent

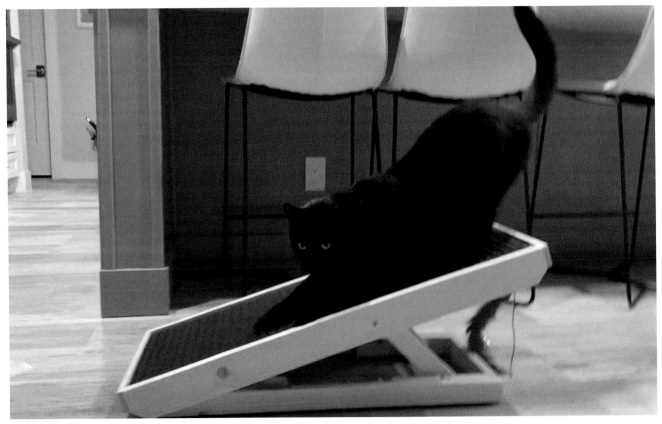

Figure 20.3 Sturdy scratching ramps may be preferred by larger cats. *(Attribution: Lisa Radosta.)*

Box 20.1 Onychectomy-Factors and Outcomes

- Short- and long-term physical complications can occur in up to 40% of patients.
- Short- and long-term complications include pain, bleeding, limping (abscesses, decreased energy, claw regrowth, draining tracts, radial nerve paralysis, swelling, infection, wound dehiscence, incomplete healing, protrusion or loss of the second phalanx, tissue necrosis from incorrect bandaging, changes in stance and gait, aversion to having the feet touched, sudden vocalizing for no reason, running around as if stung by a bee, and chronic lameness.
- Declawed cats are more likely to jump on counters and tables, exhibit reduced activity and playfulness, develop back pain and may be at increased risk for behavior problems including biting, aggression, excess barbering and periuria/perichezia.
- Up to 86% of declawed cats showed radiographic evidence of retained P3 fragments.
- Declawing bans have not been linked to increased relinquishment.

is nearby and is inadvertently reinforced by the family's response. The intensity of the behavior may increase during a bout; bouts may continue for extended periods and cats may appear distressed; vocalization is common. The behavior generally resolves with appropriate intervention and the outcome is positive.

Further assessment is needed when the level of destructive behavior suddenly changes in a mature cat. If the behavior occurs only when pet parents are not available, differentials include separation-related disorders and fear or frustration related to an external trigger. Scratch marking is a communication-based scratching that can develop in response to social conflict or a change in the relationships among cats within the home.[16] The prognosis will be based on the diagnosis and ability to identify and treat the primary condition.

Sudden onset of destructive chewing may occur secondary to pain, GI disease, change in appetite, or change in diet. When cats consistently pursue nonfood items to suckle, chew, or ingest, further diagnostics are needed to rule out compulsive behavior. Oriental breeds may be at increased risk (see Chapters 6, 13, and 18).

Management

Keeping cats' claws trimmed will reduce damage to objects and may reduce the frequency of destructive scratching. Offer the cat several different, family approved, scratching posts in the locations which have been selected by the cat for scratching. If a particular object, such as a chair or carpet, has been a consistent target for the cat, place the scratching post as close as reasonable to that object. Use catnip treats, or silver vine to entice and reward the cat for interacting with the scratching post.[20] Cats that were rewarded were more likely to use the preferred post while punishment did not reduce the frequency of undesirable scratching behavior.[4,6] A less appealing material or covering such as a drop cloth, double-sided sticky tape, or carpet runner pointy side up can be used on or around the target object until the cat has been conditioned to use the preferred post or location.

Box 20.2 Managing and treating destructive behavior

- Educate the family about normal cat behavior.
- Supervise newly adopted cats and kittens.
- Block the cat's access to valuable property.
- Find the cat's preference for substrate, location, and orientation.
- Place scratching areas in prominent, well-traveled areas and near favored resting places.
- Provide several scratching places with diversity of texture within the cat's preferences but close to the areas that the cat prefers.
- Reduce appeal or attraction to scratching of undesirable surfaces with contact paper sticky side up, citrus rinds, double-sided tape, a loosely draped drop sheet or carpet runner pointy side up.
- Enrich the environment by providing a wide range of safe toys.
- Use food dispensing toys.
- Keep cats' claws trimmed.
- Use catnip, treats, or silver vine to entice the cat to interact with the scratching post.
- Reinforce with praise, treats, and potentially petting if the cat views that interaction as reinforcing.
- Cats that like to chew should be provided with objects that they can safely carry and gnaw.
- Use SoftPaws to reduce damage.

Provide cats with an assortment of activities in many locations. Environmental enrichment can be designed to create attractive activity pods that enable the cat to safely climb, scratch, manipulate, and pursue objects. Provide comfortable perches with engaging but nonthreatening views. Cat TV, iPad games for cats, and wildlife outside can be used to keep cats focused for extended periods. Time for social enrichment should be arranged at least twice daily. The type of social interactions should be designed with consideration of the cat's personality and can include petting, brushing, training, and interactive games (see Appendix A and Recommended reading below).

Cats that like to chew should be provided with objects that they can safely carry and gnaw. Food toys, cat grass, and in some cases, bones designed for dogs may be provided. Wires may need to be covered with PVC wraps for the cat's safety and some irresistible items may need to be removed (see Box 20.2).

Treatment

Treatment should focus on addressing the cat's needs rather than on trying to stop the cat from engaging in the behavior completely. There is an underlying motivation for the behavior, which is normal and necessary. Prevention without redirection to an appropriate surface will increase the frustration of the cat and the pet parent. Simply blocking areas or making them less appealing or uncomfortable without providing a suitable scratching surface will increase the frustration of the cat and the pet parent. Blocking does not serve as an effective treatment strategy as cats with a strong innate motivation to scratch will seek another scratchable surface. While access to undesirable and problem areas and objects should be blocked for safety and protection, giving the cat a choice of more appealing, desirable, and appropriate alternative outlets should be the first and primary focus.

Consider the diagnosis and the cat's motivation when designing an intervention. Pet parents who are risk averse can be offered claw covers such as SoftPaws until appropriate scratching behavior is established.

Declawing is not an acceptable treatment for cats that engage in scratching behavior. In years past, declawing was offered when cats were gonadectomized. Since that time, much has been published and learned about declawing. Now, it is clear that this is not a benign surgery and even when done "right", causes long-term pain and poor quality of life. At the time of this writing elective onychectomy is illegal in many provices, cities, states and countries with many more pending legislation approval.

Short- and long-term physical complications can occur in up to 40% of patients and include pain, bleeding, limping (for up to 96 months after surgery), abscess, decreased energy, claw regrowth, draining tracts, radial nerve paralysis, swelling, infection, wound dehiscence, incomplete healing, protrusion or loss of the second phalanx, tissue necrosis from incorrect bandaging, changes in stance and gait, aversion to having the feet touched, sudden vocalizing for no reason, running around as if stung by a bee, and chronic lameness.[21-26] When blade and laser techniques were compared, cats that underwent blade onychectomies had increased blood and urine cortisol concentrations 24 hours postop were less willing to play or use their paws 48 hours postop were more likely to have pain after being discharged, and were more likely to eliminate outside of the litterbox.[18,27-30] Regardless of the surgical technique, onychectomy has serious short- and long-term complications which compromise the quality of life of the patient.

The literature varies on the incidence of behavior problems in cats that have been declawed. Some studies show no difference between declawed cats and those that are not declawed regarding aggression to family members or house soiling and exhibit less destructive and predatory behavior.[5,21,25,31-33] However, other studies show that when compared to clawed cats, declawed cats are more likely to jump on counters and tables,[3] exhibit reduced activity and playfulness,[34] develop back pain and may exhibit increased behavior problems including biting, aggression, excess barbering and periuria/perichezia.[5,35,36] In one study, 86% of cats showed radiographic evidence of retained P3 fragments and of those cats, the likelihood of back pain and periuria/perichezia was even more likely than cats that did not have retained P3 fragments.[36] Veterinarians may be concerned that if they do not conduct declaw surgeries, more cats will be relinquished to shelters in their area. However, a recent study has demonstrated that there was no difference in the number of cats surrendered for destructive scratching after a ban on declawing in that province.[37] Declawing has been linked to a multitude of behavior problems regardless of surgical technique and has not been shown to increase relinquishments when made illegal. (see Box 20.1).

Scratching secondary to frustration can be addressed by anticipating the cat's needs and providing access to suitable rewards. Food toys and motorized toys which move independently help can be used when the cat is likely to be active and before undesirable scratching begins. Cats that scratch to gain access to specific areas can be provided with alternative areas to explore. Closet doors and bureau drawers can be left open randomly; food and toys can be hidden in tunnels or boxes. Offer interactive social time when cats are quiet to avoid rewarding demanding behaviors. See Chapters 5 and 13 for enrichment ideas.

A treatment plan for destructive behavior should not include punishment. Punishment can permanently damage the relationship between the cat and family. Emotional consequences include increased conflict and distress that can affect the cat's well-being and have significant health consequences for all body systems.

Jumping on counters and climbing

Problem overview

Cats are attracted to high surfaces. In the course of playing and exploring their environment, cats frequently climb onto counters. Pet parents become frustrated and often try assorted correction-based techniques to stop this normal behavior.

Prevention

Prevention, as with scratching, involves finding the underlying motivation for the behavior, providing the cat with alternate ways to fulfill that need, and ensuring that all of the cat's behavioral needs are being met. Supervise young kittens and newly adopted adult cats until it is clear that they are unlikely to jump on the counter. Offer resting places in the same room which are as high or higher. Many cats get excited and jump up when food is being prepared. Prepare food in the area where the cat is fed or teach the cat to sit and wait for food in the feeding area. This can easily be taught using clicker training. See Appendix A. Reduce reinforcement of the behavior by keeping counters spare, free of food and resting spaces such as towels or dish-drying mats when the cat is unsupervised. Provide opportunities for exploring and perching on alternative surfaces at assorted levels. Confinement can be used when supervision is not available.

Diagnosis and prognosis

Climbing onto counters is normal behavior that is typically highly rewarded by the discovery of food, interesting objects to investigate, or attention from the pet parent. Frequently, cats jump on counters or tables to get closer to the family. For example, if a cat jumps on the counter as soon as the pet parents arrive home, the cat may be seeking attention or he may have a separation-related disorder and be anxious about greeting. If a cat rests on the counter, it may be because there are soft towels on the counter and the cat doesn't have similar soft, high spaces to rest. Cats of any age with the physical ability to jump are likely to engage in this behavior. A sudden onset of jumping onto kitchen counters may reflect an increase in hunger. Consider all causes for increased appetite (see Chapters 6 and 13). The prognosis for improvement with management and treatment is very good.

Management

Once the underlying cause has been determined, focus on changing the environment to fulfill the cat's needs in other ways and avoid reinforcement. Reduce reinforcement associated with accessing food by removing unattended food items or any other items to which the cat is attracted such as plants or objects to explore or for play from counters and table tops. Remove dish towels or other soft resting substrates by hanging them instead of folding them on the counter. Bend down to greet cats immediately or pick them up if they prefer in order to prevent jumping on the counter to get closer to the pet parent. Provide ample opportunities for exploration, climbing, perching, and resting in other locations with appealing treats, catnip, or toys, or with windows for outdoor viewing, to entice and reinforce locations. Food and toys may be hidden in assorted areas of the house and on several levels by using cat trees and walkways. Caches can be placed in tunnels, boxes, dresser drawers, or any location that is not objectionable from the pet parent's standpoint. When possible, establish multiple feeding stations and offer meals in toys instead of dishes. Be sure to check these stations regularly to be sure that the cat is eating an appropriate daily ration.

Treatment

Cats can be taught to wait patiently at a specific location such as a chair or stool while pet parents prepare or consume food. Training is accomplished by delivering highly desirable treats to the cat as it waits at the designated location. For the cats that want to greet the family and jump up to be close, they can be taught to station on a cat tree or sit and wait on another piece of furniture. Sometimes other pets block the offending cat from getting to the pet parent. In that case, the other pets would need to be trained as well. For example, larger pets such as dogs can learn to sit and wait for greeting so that the cat can be petted on the floor. Teach the cat an off cue so that the pet parent can get the cat off of the counter without conflict. This can be taught using a toy or treats. Use food to entice the cat onto the cat tree or work with him when he has chosen to be there. Then, toss a treat or toy to the floor. When the cat gets the treat or toy, mark the behavior with a clicker or another conditioned reinforcer and reinforce with a small treat or play. Repeat this sequence, keeping in mind that cats learn best with very short sessions (3–5 repetitions). Also, asking a cat to jump repeatedly for five minutes may not be healthy or comfortable for him. That will cause a negative conditioned emotional response, which is the opposite of what we are trying to achieve. When the cat reliably is moving off of the cat tree, the pet parent can add the off cue before they toss the toy. When that has been repeated over many short sessions, eliminate the lure and use only the cue. Continue to reward the correct response, jumping off the counter, by delivering a food or toy reward. Always reinforce when the cat is correct. While variable reinforcement is very powerful at maintaining behaviors, many pets cats work best with continuous reinforcement — they are undermotivated to follow trained cues since food and attention are freely available. In these cases, continuous reinforcement for behaviors is often best. See Recommended Reading, Chapter 10, and Appendix A for information and resources on how to train cats.

Make the counters or tables less appealing or uncomfortable by adding citrus rinds, carpet runner pointy side up, shallow pans with water, or double-sided tape. Identify the cat's motivation for climbing in a specific location, and provide alternative, acceptable locations that meet these needs. For example, provide a surface that is physically comfortable and, provides the cat with a similar view. Make the other spaces more desirable for resting by using catnip silver vine, pheromone analogues, and treats. Reinforce cats when they are lying in desirable resting spaces.

If the cat is caught on the counter and does not immediately jump down, the pet parent can cue the cat into an alternative desirable behavior (e.g., off, station) or quietly pick the cat up and place it on an acceptable resting space nearby. For cats that don't appreciate being picked up, they can easily be lured from counters and other surfaces using play, a toy, or a treat. Pet parents may feel that luring the cat off of the counter will reward the behavior. This is unlikely to happen as the cat's motivation to jump up will not be affected by the lure to jump down. Rather, the cat may be more likely to jump off and find an acceptable resting place more quickly. Instead, this moves the cat off of the undesirable location and onto a more desirable location.

Pet parents should not shout or chase their cat. Punishment can trigger fear or aggression and seriously damage the cat's relationship with the person (see Box 20.3).

Excessive nocturnal activity in cats

Problem overview

Cats are generally regarded as having crepuscular patterns, being most active at dawn and dusk, presumably because those are the patterns of their prey; however, each cat may have its own patterns.[16] It is reasonable to assume that many cats can and have adapted their patterns to those of their humans. Bothersome nocturnal behaviors are more common in kittens and often decrease with maturity. While most cats are socially mature by about two years of age, some cats remain playful, active, and interactive. Nocturnal wakefulness in cats negatively impacts the well-being of the family and tolerance of this behavior may be limited. Cats with excessive nocturnal activity should be treated immediately

> **Box 20.3** Management and treatment of cats getting on the furniture or counters, or into rooms where they are not allowed
>
> 1. Set clear boundaries defining where the cat is allowed to go. The entire family should cooperate.
> 2. Provide enrichment in the way of toys, scents, surfaces, food and puzzle toys, and safe access to outdoors.
> 3. Provide acceptable (to the pet parent and the cat) resting spaces of the same height or higher and similar texture or surface to the unacceptable area or surface.
> 4. Reinforce the cat for being in alternate resting spaces.
> 5. Lure the cat from areas where he should not be. Reinforce him for voluntarily getting off of those areas.
> 6. Make certain that there is nothing that might attract the cat to off-limits areas, such as food or toys.
> 7. Prevent access when the cat cannot be supervised.
> 8. Use upside-down vinyl carpet runners, citrus rinds, shallow pans with water, contact paper sticky side up, and double-sided tape to reduce the appeal and attraction to areas which are unacceptable.
> 9. Train the cat to get off on cue using positive reinforcement.

to address the welfare of the cat and the family and prevent potential relinquishment.

Prevention

If soon after adoption, a cat or kitten shows signs of having excessive nocturnal activity or even a pattern of sleep that is different from the family, they can use strategies to set up a different nocturnal pattern. It is always better to introduce management strategies in anticipation of concerns. Pet parents who are light sleepers should plan ahead and introduce their new cat to a private sleeping area which can also be used as a sanctuary space (see Chapters 5 and 17). An adult cat may be given free run of the house if there are no other behavioral concerns requiring supervision; a kitten should be confined to a kitten-safe area. A confined cat should have a comfortable, elevated resting spot, water, a litterbox, toys, and several food toys/feeders. Keeping the cat exercised during the day and increasing environmental enrichment can also help to keep the pattern from developing. Automatic feeders may be generally helpful to avoid inadvertent reinforcement of food-seeking behavior. Many owners are tempted to wake up during the night to feed a vocalizing cat and this response can contribute to sustained nighttime vocalization. This way, if an automatic feeder is used, the cat will not be in advertently reinforced for waking the pet parents who may then give the cat food to entice him to go back to sleep.

Diagnosis and potential outcomes

Nocturnal wakefulness can be a variation of a normal feline behavior pattern and should be suspected in young, healthy cats that engage in play-related or foraging behaviors at various times during the night. The prognosis for cases such as these is generally good.

Nocturnal activity in cats may be linked to other behavioral disorders and clinical signs such as aggression and fabric chewing, and negative correlations were found between nocturnal activity and overgrooming and cat-directed sociability.[38] Based on these findings, it is possible that nocturnal activity in some cats is tied to anxiety or stress. Other potential causes include inadvertent reinforcement from the pet parent (e.g., letting the cat outside, feeding the cat); fear, anxiety, stress, conflict, or panic about interactions with other animals or people in the home; change in the feeding or elimination behavior of the cat; lack of enrichment and stimulation during the day; and activities of the other pets or prey influencing the activity of the cat.[16] Older cats can suffer from cognitive dysfunction, causing changes in the sleep – wake cycle.[39] When there is a sudden increase in nocturnal activity, especially in a middle-aged or older cat, a complete physical and behavioral workup is needed, as there may be underlying disease contributing to this change. Differentials include hyperthyroidism, diseases that can increase appetite, and cognitive dysfunction. Increased nocturnal activity can also be due to physical causes such as pain, hyperthyroidism, Cushing's disease, dermatologic disease, gastrointestinal pain, lower urinary tract disease, seizure activity, polyuria/polydipsia due to renal disease or other systemic disease, hyperesthesia, and changes in appetite.[16] Treatment of the primary disease can cure or improve the behavior. Age-related cognitive decline is progressive (see Chapters 6 and 8).

When a pet is presented for increased nocturnal activity, it is important to remember that the pet parent may not be aware of whether or not there was a triggering stimulus such as a noise or a cat outside. In other words, the cat may be responding to a noise or become startled by a cat outside and then become more active. In cases like this, the family experiences this situation as increased activity directed toward them but was not present for the experience with the cat outside. If the inciting stimulus isn't addressed, the behavior is unlikely to resolve. In addition, most pet parents wake up when a cat jumps on them or sits on their chest while they are sleeping. That can be reinforcing. Like most pets, cats are creatures of habit and often wake up at the same time each night. During the behavioral assessment, learn the timing of the onset of the cat's excessive evening activity. Is it at the start of bedtime, during the middle of the sleep period, or early in the morning just before the alarm is set to go off? If it occurs at the same time each night, finding the inciting cause will be more straightforward. Ask about the interactions between the cat and other animals in the household. Overt conflicts between cats are often more frequent at night—perhaps the cats are inhibited by the family's presence during the day.

Frustration-related nocturnal activity or play-induced aggression/behavior may occur around the pet parent's bedtime routine (see Chapter 24).

Cats that are fed shortly after their pet parent's alarm sounds may learn to anticipate the alarm and become active earlier and earlier even as their person tries to sleep. Risk factors include being fed immediately upon the pet parent's wakening or a recent diet change (type of food or quantity provided). In the absence of a disease related to hunger, gastrointestinal disturbances, or metabolism, the prognosis for resolution is excellent.

Management

Pet parents need immediate relief. Most kittens tolerate being confined and some adult cats tolerate being closed out of the bedroom for the short term until treatment can be completed. Cats should be provided with food, water, a litterbox and toys as described under prevention. For cats that cannot tolerate being without the pet parent at night, a dog crate or indoor fenced area may be provided in the pet parent's bedroom. Since treatment can take a few weeks, in some urgent situations, situational use of medications that will help the cat sleep such as trazodone, gabapentin, or perhaps a benzodiazepine such as clonazepam (depending on signs, health, age, and therapeutic response) can be used.

Meanwhile, if the cat does wake the pet parent up, they should be as neutral as possible. If safe, it is best to avoid responding to the cat. With no reinforcement, the behavior may extinguish over 5–7 nights although for some cats, it will take more time. If ignoring is not an option, the cat can quietly be removed from the room and if needed, put into the enriched confinement area. Explain to pet parents that ignoring the cat entails no interaction at all, including looking at, petting, feeding, or talking to the cat. It is important to avoid reinforcement of attention-seeking behaviors during waking hours. Be sure the cat receives adequate social play that ends at least one hour before bedtime.

Pet parents may be tempted to throw pillows at the cat, spray it with water, yell at it, or otherwise punish it. These responses may appear to be effective as the behavior could stop abruptly for the moment, but long term, punishment carries many risks, including the risk of fear which could ultimately exacerbate the underlying behavior as well as permanently damage the relationship between the cat and person. The alternative may be and often is much worse than the initial presentation. Recommend addressing the underlying cause. Punishment generates fear and can permanently damage the relationship between the cat and the pet parent, which is never a desired outcome.

Treatment

A treatment plan for a cat diagnosed with normal nocturnal activity should incorporate the pet parent's long-term management goals. Long-term maintenance of separate sleeping locations for the pet parent and cat is sustainable as long as the cat does not exhibit signs of distress. Enrichment, including automatic feeders and preferred self-operated toys, may be sufficient for resolution of the behavior. Treatment should focus on increasing the cat's ability to rest and play independently and, when possible, coordinating the cat's schedule with that of the pet parents. Cats should be provided with ample play outlets when family members are present. End play at least an hour before bedtime to give the cat some time to unwind before the pet parent retires.

Cats that are distressed when confined away from their pet parents can be desensitized systematically. Introduce the cat to the enriched confinement room or area for gradually increasing periods of time when the pet parent is at home. Between lessons, be sure that pet parents provide ample social and interactive play time. See Chapters 5 and 17 for more information on independence training and creation of a sanctuary space.

If the family is home during the day, when they sit down to relax, they can encourage their cat to also relax by providing a soft blanket that has been sprayed with a pheromone analogue. Social cats that are alone much of the day may benefit from a visit from a pet sitter who can provide activity and refresh any food toys. Giving the cat structure throughout the day may be helpful. This includes scheduled play, petting, brushing, or cuddle times. Ideally, the cat's drive for affection would be met during the day and lessened at night. In addition, pet parents can teach the cat how to ask politely for attention (e.g., sit, touch, high five) and reinforce that behavior during the day.

If there are underlying fear, anxiety, stress, conflict or panic (FASCP) or behavioral comorbidities, medications or supplements may be needed to effectively treat the disorder (see Chapters 11 and 12).

When nocturnal wakefulness relates to food seeking, the nature of food delivery should be explored. Be sure the cat receives sufficient calories. Choose foods that are satisfying – explore diets that are designed to increase satiety. When introducing a weight reduction diet, consider the cat's body score and the health risk to the cat if the body score were to increase slightly versus the risk that the pet parent will not keep the cat in the home. A balanced approach to weight loss should consider diet, exercise, and emotional well-being.

Delay the morning feeding by a couple of minutes so that the cat does not expect food as soon as the pet parent is awake. Use food puzzles and create multiple hidden feeding stations to encourage the cat to hunt, explore, and find food

Box 20.4 Management and treatment of increased nocturnal activity

- Assess for all underlying physical disorders.
- Create a private sleeping area or sanctuary space. Condition the cat to accept that space.
- Avoid reinforcement by using automated feeders.
- Provide enrichment in the way of toys, scents, surfaces, food and puzzle toys, and safe access to outdoors.
- Medications may be needed to help the cat sleep or treat concurrent behavior disorders.
- Teach the cat to rest and play independently.
- Coordinate the cat's schedule by playing with and exercising the cat during the day.
- Use pheromone analogs to decrease stress.
- Avoid intermittent reinforcement of the behavior.
- Consider changing the diet or how the cat acquires the food.
- Assess the diet and the caloric intake of the cat.
- Do not feed the cat as soon as the pet parent wakes up. Use automatic feeders overnight and delay feeding by 15–30 minutes after the pet parent gets up.
- Schedule play, petting, and cuddle time during the day.
- Teach the cat a cue which can be offered for attention and reinforce during the day.

without assistance. Avoid delivering food when the cat is demanding. Cats can be taught to exhibit specific behaviors on cue such as stationing on a mat or a calm sit in order to receive food (see Box 20.4).

Excessive vocalization

Problem overview

Vocalizations convey general information regarding the underlying emotional or motivational state of the cat within four main contexts: (1) social interactions with other animals (conflict or affiliative); (2) sexual behavior; (3) parental behavior; and (4) interactions with people. Cats may vocalize at night for attention, because they are fearful or distressed, or to receive food. In addition, physical causes contribute to vocalizations as does cognitive dysfunction.

Cats have developed and use vocalizations in good part to communicate with humans. Like any behavior, vocalizations can be reinforced or punished, increasing or decreasing the likelihood of occurrence in the future. In addition, selective breeding has produced breeds that are more likely to be vocal, such as the Siamese. Lack of socialization to the stimuli likely to be encountered in the environment can influence vocalization with less socialized cats using higher-pitched calls for longer periods of time.[40] See Chapter 2 for more information on cat vocalizations. Pet parents mainly complain when the behavior occurs during the night. As described in the previous section, this nocturnal behavior is frequently inadvertently reinforced.

Prevention

Vocalization as a normal communication is routinely reinforced. It can be fun to talk back to a vocalizing cat but less fun when the cat starts the conversation at night. Prevention of normal but excessive vocalization is best accomplished by refraining from engaging in interactions when the cat is vocalizing. Anticipate the cat's needs and provide play, attention, and meals when the cat is quiet and calm. As is the case with virtually all cat behavioral disorders, enrichment of the environment will improve this behavior, as will independence training.

Diagnosis and potential outcomes

The key to finding the underlying cause is assessment of the pet's body language in the situations in which the vocalization occurs. With that said, with inadvertent reinforcement, situations in which the behavior is displayed will change. Often these cats are presented when the behavior is chronic, making it challenging to find the underlying cause. Excessive vocalization as a normal communicative behavior typically occurs in presence of family members and the cat's body language is consistent with affiliative behavior. There is usually a history of reinforcement – the cat learns to expect a specific response for vocalizing and increases the intensity of its behavior until the pet parent finally responds. When the cat has been previously reinforced for vocalization and reinforcement is suddenly discontinued or is delivered inconsistently, the cat can become frustrated. Signs of frustration can include an increased intensity or volume of vocalization and increased duration of bouts. There may be increased activity or displacement behaviors, such as knocking objects off furniture, during or between bouts. This may also be a response to the family ignoring the behavior. If safe and humane, the family may be advised to completely ignore the behavior until it is extinguished (see Chapter 10). Fear-based vocalization may occur in a specific area of the home, is exhibited with body language consistent with FASCP and may be associated with rapid aimless movement or hiding.

When there is a sudden onset of vocalization, an external trigger or illness, including behavioral illness, should be considered. Cats may excessively vocalize due to FASCP, physical disease (e.g., hyperthyroidism, renal disease, pain, FLUTD, constipation, endocrine disorders causing polyuria/polydipsia), stressful interactions with other animals and household, storm or noise fear or phobia, and separation-related disorders. Hyperthyroidism and feline cognitive decline should be ruled out in age-appropriate cats. Treatment of the primary disease may be curative. Intact cats vocalize normally – female cats when in estrus and male cats when near estrous queens. Desexing (neutering) is usually curative.

Management

The management of excessive vocalization is similar to the management of nocturnal activity. Reduce human-generated reinforcement for vocalization, enrich the environment identify triggers for vocalization, and reduce the cat's exposure to the triggers as much as possible while treatment is under way. External triggers for fear or frustration may be managed by keeping the cat away from specific locations or by using window coverings. Management for attention-seeking and food-seeking behaviors is discussed in the previous section.

Treatment

Vocalization secondary to reinforcement is treated by removing the reward for the behavior. Pet parents can train their cat to engage in alternative behaviors to change the nature of the communication. For example, cats seeking social interaction can be trained to sit or lie quietly before receiving verbal or physical attention. The expectation is that over time, the cat will begin to offer reinforced quiet behaviors in lieu of vocalizing and will develop an increased tolerance of a delay in reward delivery. See Chapter 10 for information on how to train this behavior. Fear-based vocalization is treated by reducing the emotional component. Medications or supplements may be necessary to treat underlying FASCP (see Chapters 11 and 12). In addition, a complete plan potentially including avoidance of triggers and eventual desensitization and counterconditioning to specific triggers can be implemented. See Box 20.5.

Box 20.5 Management and treatment of excessive vocalization

- Assess for all underlying physical disorders.
- Create a private sleeping area or sanctuary space. Condition the cat to accept that space if the behavior occurs overnight.
- Avoid misplaced reinforcement by using automated feeders.
- Provide enrichment in the way of toys, scents, surfaces, food and puzzle toys, and safe access to outdoors.
- If the cat has underlying FASCP, consider medications or supplements to treat the underlying disorder.
- Teach the cat to rest and play independently.
- Play and exercise the cat during the day.
- Use pheromone analogs to decrease stress.
- Avoid intermittent reinforcement of the behavior.
- Schedule play, petting, and cuddle time during the day.
- Teach the cat a cue which can be offered for attention and reinforce during the day.
- Assess environment for stressful or frightening situations.

CASE EXAMPLE

Presentation

Howie, a 14-month-old, 5-kg DSH, was presented for climbing on counters and stealing food.

History

Howie climbs onto the counters and steals food as well as nonfood items. He consumes the food items for the most part. He moves the nonfood items to a hiding spot in his cat tree. Howie had lived indoors since he was adopted at two months of age and was fed a good-quality commercial cat food. He is fed two meals daily. The pet parents assumed he would outgrow the climbing and stealing behavior. When Howie was a small kitten and made his first successful leaps, the pet parents would gently remove him for fear he might be injured. When the behavior persisted, interventions were applied to thwart the behavior. If they caught him on the counter, they sprayed him with water. If the bottle was not handy, they clapped their hands loudly. Howie always ran away in response to these punishers, and sometimes remained in hiding for more than an hour. Howie quickly stopped going onto the counters in the presence of the pet parents, but stealing continued when they were not in the room. The next intervention tried was to set booby traps – noise-generating motion detectors. Howie could carefully navigate around some of the traps. As such, the frequency of counter jumping was reduced, but not eliminated. A new behavior developed: climbing onto high shelves and dressers. There Howie would find small, often valuable items to remove and carry about. The pet parents were frustrated. They felt that they had done a good job kitten-proofing, but Howie was no longer a kitten. Besides, he had plenty of toys.

Workup

Howie's physical examination was within normal limits. Because he was consuming food items, a CBC, serum chemistry, fecal float and antigen test, and urinalysis was completed and within normal limits. His body score was 4/9. His coat was healthy. The option to do further diagnostics, including a digestion/absorption panel, was offered. The pet parents declined further diagnostics until after initial treatments were applied and their efficacy was assessed.

Differentials

Differential diagnoses included reinforced behavior, attention-seeking behavior, pica, gastrointestinal disease (e.g., IBD, food intolerance), increased hunger, normal exploratory behavior, and lack of enrichment/stimulation. The risk of a physiologic abnormality was considered low given Howie's age, appropriate growth pattern, normal laboratory testing results normal body score, normal stool volume, and the gradual progression of a behavior that including stealing both food and nonfood items. It was determined that Howie had normal exploratory activity and lack of enrichment. In addition, there may have been a component of lack of satiety from the diet he was being fed. Finally, the consistent use of punishment had caused a specific fear of the water bottle and certain loud noises (e.g., hand clapping).

Treatment

The pet parents were educated on and given additional resources regarding normal cat behavior, the need for enrichment beyond the toys that they had already provided, and the pitfalls of punishment. Instead of trying to stop Howie's exploratory behavior, they were advised to create an environment in which his needs could be satisfied without disrupting their personal property.

To start, two cat trees were added – one in the corner of the large kitchen, and another beside Howie's favorite dresser. In addition, a cat "highway" was created using a series of tunnels and boxes that could be baited with snacks and toys that Howie was known to prefer. Howie could now prowl through the house and discover new and interesting objects.

Howie was to continue to receive his meals twice daily, but in between, food toys would be selectively placed in areas that the pet parents agreed Howie could safely explore. Exploring the desired areas would yield rewards. Furthermore, while Howie was establishing new patterns, the family was asked to keep the counters clear of food, to remove appealing items from Howie's favorite shelves and dresser, and use carpet runner with the pointy side up on all surfaces that they didn't want him to use. These items could gradually be replaced after several weeks of progress.

The family was counseled on the danger and consequences of using punishment. Howie became very frightened when he was scolded. Fortunately, he did recover, but it is important to remember that the cat–human bond can be fragile. To build Howie's trust and confidence, the pet parents were asked to schedule interactive play with Howie every day and to start a routine of training for food rewards so that Howie would know that it is safe to take food that is handed to him.

CASE EXAMPLE—cont'd

Follow-up

The veterinary technician followed up with weekly phone calls were for one month. The pet parents reported steady and rapid improvement. Howie participated in appropriate activities and was rarely found in possession of his pet parent's valuables or food items.

An eight-week progress appointment was done with the veterinary technician. At this time, Howie had relapsed slightly and was sometimes jumping on the counters. The pet parents expressed that they were tired of having the carpet runner on their kitchen island. When questioned, it was also reported that they had stopped rotating toys and setting up mazes for him to explore. The veterinary technician reminded them that these management techniques would need to be in place for months to years and potentially for Howie's entire life. The drive to explore is innate and Howie has a strong drive. The pet parents inquired about medications and supplements. The technician reminded them that medications were not indicated for Howie at this time and that medicating their cat for his entire lifetime was going to be a challenge. The pet parents agreed to continue management but not the use of aversives on the surfaces where they didn't want him to go. The technician recommended a positive reinforcement trainer who worked with

cats and resources online and in print to teach the pet parents how to train him to get off of the counter.

The veterinary technician followed up in two weeks by phone. The pet parents were doing well and had accepted who Howie was. They had a routine and switched responsibility for Howie between family members every couple of days. Finally, they were in the process of working with a positive reinforcement trainer via video conference to teach Howie to go to his cat tree and get off of the counters. At this time, the veterinary technician asked Howie's family to check in every three months until Howie was at least two years old.

Discussion

We share our home with cats and often overlook the fact that cats are predators and maintain a genetic predisposition to engage in exploratory behavior. Howie's motivation to engage with his environment had not been satisfied. When punishers were applied to try to eliminate this innate behavior, Howie adapted by seeking alternative locations to explore. In addition, punishment had altered the relationship between a behaviorally normal cat and his family in a negative way.

Conclusion

Many of the behaviors that humans dislike are normal cat behaviors. Indoor cats are wholly underenriched, causing frustration and boredom. If these behaviors are then punished, causing

FASCP, the relationship between the cat and pet parent begins to deteriorate. This leads to all kinds of negative sequelae, including relinquishment. For the welfare of cats and their families, no matter the behavior problem, early intervention and enrichment are always the right things to do.

References

1. Heidenberger E. Housing conditions and behavioral problems of indoor cats as assessed by their owners. *Appl Anim Behav Sci.* 1997;52:345–364.
2. Fatjó J, Ruiz-de-la-Torre JL, Manteca X. The epidemiology of behavioural problems in dogs and cats: a survey of veterinary practitioners. *Anim Welf.* 2006; 15:179–185.
3. Morgan M, Houpt KA. Feline behaviour problems: the influence of declawing. *Anthrozoös.* 1990;3:50–53.
4. Moesta A, Keys D, Crowell-Davis S. Survey of cat owners on features of, and preventative measures for, feline scratching of inappropriate objects: a pilot study. *J Feline Med Surg.* 2018; 20(10):891–899.
5. Grigg WK, Kogan LR. Owners' attitudes, knowledge, and care practices: exploring the implications for domestic cat behavior and welfare in the home. *Animals.* 2019;9:978. doi:10.3390/ani9110978.
6. Wilson C, Bain M, DePorter T, et al. Owner observations regarding cat scratching behavior: an internet based survey. *J Feline Med Surg.* 2016;18:791–797.
7. Lindell E. Destructive and scratching behavior cats. In: Tilley LP, Smith FWK, Sleeper MM et al., eds. *Blackwell's 5 Minute Veterinary Consult: Canine and Feline.* 7th ed. Hoboken, NJ: John Wiley and Sons; 2021:388.
8. Heath S. Behaviour problems and welfare. In: Rochlitz I, ed. *The Welfare of Cats.* Dordrecht: Springer; 2007: 91–118.
9. Bradshaw JWS, Casey RA, Brown SL. *The Behaviour in the Domestic Cat.* 2nd ed. Wallingford: CAB International; 2012.
10. Mengoli M, Mariti C, Cozzi A, et al. Scratching behavior and its features: questionnaire based study in an Italian sample of domestic cats. *J Feline Med Surg.* 2013;15:886–892.
11. Ellis SL, Rodan I, Carney HC, et al. AAFP and ISFM feline environmental needs guidelines. *J Feline Med Surg.* 2013;15(3): 219–230.
12. Landsberg GM. Cat owners attitudes to declawing. *Anthrozoos.* 1991;4:192–197.
13. Pageat P, Gaultier E. Current research in canine and feline pheromones. *Vet Clin North Am Smal Anim Pract.* 2003;33: 187–211.
14. Panaman R. Behavior and ecology of free-ranging female farm cats (Felis catus L.). *Z Tierpsychol.* 1981;56:59–73.
15. Feldman H. Methods of scent marking in the domestic cat. *Can J Zool.* 1994;72: 1093–1099.
16. Casey R. Management problem in cats. In: Horwitz DF, Mills DS, eds. *BSAVA Manual of Canine and Feline Behavioural Medicine.* 2nd ed. Gloucester: BSAVA; 2009: 98–110.
17. Gazzano A, Bianchi L, Campa S, et al. The prevention of undesirable behavior in cats: effectiveness of a veterinary behaviorists' advice given to kitten owners. *J Vet Behav.* 2015;10:535–542.
18. Patronek GJ, McCabe, GP, Ecker C. Risk factors for relinquishment of cats to an animal shelter. *J Am Vet Med Assoc.* 1996; 209:582–588.
19. Rossi AP, dos Santos CRC, Maia CM, et al. Rescued cats prefer to scratch fabrics commonly used to cover upholstered furniture. *J Appl Anim Welf Sci.* 2021. doi: 10.1080/10888705.2021.1949595.
20. Zhang, L, John JM. Scratcher preferences of adult in-home cats and effects of olfactory supplements on cat scratching. *Appl Anim Behav Sci.* 2020;227:104997.
21. Patronek GJ. Assessment of claims of short and long-term complications associated with onychectomy in cats. *J Am Vet Med Assoc.* 2001;219:932–937.
22. Martinez SA, Hauptmann J, Walshaw R. Comparing two techniques for onychectomy in cats and two adhesives for wound closure. *Vet Med.* 1993;88: 516–525.
23. Tobias KS. Feline onychectomy at a teaching institution: a retrospective study of 163 cases. *Vet Surg.* 1994;23: 274–280.
24. Jankowski AJ, Brown DC, Duval J, et al. Comparison of effects of elective

tenectomy or onychectomy in cats. *J Am Vet Med Assoc.* 1998;213:370–373.

25. Landsberg GM. Feline scratching and destruction and the effects of declawing. *Vet Clin North Am Small Anim Pract.* 1991; 21:265–279.

26. Robertson S, Lascelles D. Long-term pain in cats. How much do we know about this important welfare issue? *J Feline Med Surg.* 2010;12:188–199.

27. Pollari FL, Bonnett BN. Evaluation of postoperative complications following elective surgeries of dogs and cats at private practices using computer records. *Can Vet J.* 1996;37:672–678.

28. Pollari FL, Bonnett BN, Bamsey SC, et al. Postoperative complications of elective surgeries in dogs and cats determined by examining electronic and paper medical records. *J Am Vet Med Assoc.* 1996;208: 1882–1886.

29. Tobias KS. Feline onychectomy at a teaching institution: a retrospective study of 163 cases. *Vet Surg.* 1994;23:274–280.

30. Gerard AF, Larson M, Baldwin CJ, et al. Telephone survey to investigate relationships between onychectomy or onychectomy technique and house soiling in cats. *J Am Vet Med Assoc.* 2016;249:638–643.

31. Borchelt PL, Voith VL. Aggressive behavior in cats. *Compend Contin Educ Pract Vet.* 1987;9:49–57.

32. Fritscher SJ, Ha J. Declawing has no effect on biting behavior but does affect adoption outcomes for domestic cats in an animal shelter. *Appl Anim Behav Sci.* 2016;180:107–113.

33. Sung W, Crowell-Davis SL. Elimination behavior patterns of domestic cats (Felis catus) with and without elimination behavior problems. *Am J Vet Res.* 2006;67:1500–1504.

34. Duffy DL, Dinez de Moura RT, Serpell JA. Development and evaluation of the Fe-BARQ: A new survery instrument for measuring behavior in domestic cats (Felis s. catus). *Behav Process.* 2017;141:329–341.

35. Yeon SC, Flanders JA, Scarlett JM, et al. Attitudes of owners regarding tendonectomy and onychectomy in cats. *J Am Vet Med Assoc.* 2001;218:43–47.

36. Martell-Moran NK, Solano M, Townsend HGG. Pain and adverse behavior in declawed cats. *J Feline Med Surg.* 2018;20: 280–288.

37. Ellis A, van Haaften K, Protopopova, et al. Effect of a provincial feline onychectomy ban on cat intake and euthanasia in a British Columbia animal shelter system. *J Feline Med Surg.* 2022; 24(8):739–744.

38. Kendall K, Ley J. Owner observations can provide data for constructive behavior analysis in normal pet cats in Australia. *J Vet Behav.* 2008;3:244–247.

39. Sordo L, Gunn-Moore DA. Cognitive dysfunction in cats: update on neuropathological and behavioural changes plus clinical management. *Vet Rec.* 2021;188. doi:10.1002/vetr.3.

40. Yeon SC, Kim YK, Park SJ, et al. Differences between vocalization evoked by social stimuli in feral cats and house cats. *Behav Process.* 2011;87: 183–189.

Recommended reading and resources

AAFP and ISFM Feline Environmental Needs Guidelines. *J Feline Med Surg.* 2013;(15): 219–230.

AAFP Cat Parent Resources. Available at: https://catvets.com/guidelines/client-brochures

AAFP – How to feed a cat. Available at: https://catvets.com/guidelines/practice-guidelines/how-to-feed

AAFP Cat Scratching Resources. https://catvets.com/claw-friendly-toolkit/scratching-resources

American College of Veterinary Behaviorists. *Decoding your Cat.* Mariner Books; 2020.

Bradshaw, J; Ellis, S. *The Trainable Cat*; Basic Books; 2017.

Dantas LM, Delgado MM, Johnson I et al. Food puzzles for cats. Feeding for physical and emotional wellbeing. *J Feline Med Surg.* 2016;18:723–732.

Fear Free Happy Homes - Cats need to scratch. Here's how to help them do it right. https://www.fearfreehappyhomes.com/cats-scratch/

Ohio State University. Available at: https://indoorpet.osu.edu/cats .

Schroll S. Kitten Kindergarten; 2017. Books on Demand.

CHAPTER 21

House Soiling – Canine

Valarie V. Tynes, DVM, DACVB, DACAW

Introduction

The primary purpose of micturition and defecation is to rid the body of wastes but in the adult dog, elimination behavior can serve a number of additional functions, including communicating information about sexual status, individual identity, and territory. It may also occur in a variety of situations as a component of fear, anxiety, and excitement.

House soiling can begin due to a urogenital condition or any other physical condition leading to polyuria, polydipsia, constipation, or diarrhea, to name a few. Even after successful treatment of the physical condition, the problem may continue due to the experience in which the dog has learned that the new location is an acceptable, additional place for elimination. Therefore, every dog presented with a complaint of house soiling should have a workup including physical examination, complete blood count (CBC), serum chemistry, urinalysis, thyroid profile, and fecal antigen + Giardia, and any additional diagnostics such as imaging or scoping indicated by clinical signs, examination, and laboratory findings. In addition, a determination should be made as to whether or not the dog was ever completely house trained prior to presentation. Any dog that has been previously well house trained and begins house soiling should have physical causes strongly considered (see Chapter 6).

If the dog has never been well house trained, then the history may need to focus on what prompted the pet parent to present for the problem at this time. Some pet parents, especially of smaller dogs, will tolerate house soiling for some period of time before becoming frustrated with the problem and seeking help. The factors that lead to this eventual change in tolerance of a behavior can be varied and numerous and include such things as moving to a new home, replacing carpeting, or adding a roommate who is less tolerant of the behavior. But changes in the nature of the elimination can also result in a change in tolerance for the behavior (e.g., development of diarrhea making feces harder to clean or increased frequency of urination requiring increased cleaning efforts). In the cases where house training has never been complete, any change in frequency or quantity of urine or feces and any change in consistency of feces should also lead to a thorough physical evaluation before progressing with the house training discussion.

House soiling is a common problem faced by dog pet parents and is a major risk factor for canine relinquishment.[1–3] In fact, dogs that urinate in the house weekly are two to four times more likely to be relinquished to a shelter.[3] In two extensive internet-based surveys of pet parents, between 15% and 30% of dogs were reported to house soil, while in a Spanish study of veterinary practitioners, destructiveness, aggression, and house soiling were the three most common behavior complaints of pet parents.[4–6] The most prevalent form of house soiling involved both feces and urine (65%), followed by urine only (29%) and feces only at 6%.[5] Therefore, screening for behavioral problems such as house soiling should be a part of every routine visit due to the fact that many pet parents will tolerate a problem for varying lengths of time before seeking help. In many cases, by the time they seek help from their veterinarian, the bond between the pet and pet parent may be so damaged that the pet parent is past the point of being willing to invest much time, energy, or money in correcting the problem. If the problem had been discovered earlier and appropriate interventions initiated, successful treatment may have been easier and the likelihood of success probably greater.

The importance of preventive counseling

Veterinarians must never assume that pet parents have an understanding of normal canine behaviors or knowledge of appropriate approaches to behavior problems. Undeniably, appropriate veterinary intervention can make the difference between relinquishment and a dog staying in its forever home. One study showed that dogs with periuria and perichezia had a seven times lower risk of relinquishment if they had two veterinary visits in a year compared to less than once a year.[7] In addition, when advice is given at the first puppy appointment regarding house training, dogs are less likely to house soil a year later when compared with dogs whose pet parents did not receive that advice.[8] However, only 25% of dog pet parents report receiving veterinary behavioral advice,[7] so veterinarians must make a point of giving clear behavioral advice with the same belief and determination that they do physical recommendations such as heartworm prevention if they expect pet parents to remember it and follow their instructions. If the veterinarian does not make their commitment

to behavioral health clear as well as their ability to offer sound solutions, the pet parent will assume that they have neither and may search elsewhere for solutions, with potentially dire consequences.

Problem overview

House training dogs should not be difficult but will need to be at least briefly explained to some pet parents since many myths and misconceptions abound. One study of dog pet parents who were relinquishing their pets showed that almost 50% believed that rubbing a dog's nose in a mess when it soiled was helpful or were unsure if this was appropriate.[9] Since this type of response and in fact, any form of confrontation or punishment has the potential to do great harm, proper counseling of pet parents of newly adopted puppy or adult dogs is critical.[10]

There is also a commonly held belief that small dogs are more difficult to house train than larger dogs. One recent study supported this idea and confirmed that in fact, in the population surveyed, small dogs (66.8%) were significantly less likely to be house trained than larger dogs (95.0%).[11] A second study found small dogs to be 3.21 times more likely to have soiling problems than medium-sized dogs.[12] The reasons behind this remain unclear, but one hypothesis is that people are generally more forgiving of a smaller dog's accidents than they would be of a larger dog, so less effort may be put into the house training. Other hypotheses to consider are that smaller dogs have smaller bladders and may need to eliminate more frequently. This knowledge could be used to increase pet parent awareness and educate them regarding relative frequencies of outings for different-sized dogs. Sex (males 2.1 times more frequent) and age (decreasing with age) have also been identified as risk factors for house soiling.[12]

Prevention

Preadoption counseling, when available, can be beneficial in the prevention of elimination behavior problems. An important ally in this regard is the animal shelter, adoption service, or breeder. Although house soiling was the primary problem reported in 35% of dogs one week following adoption, most dogs were house trained within one month.[7] However, significantly more of the pet parents who had preadoption counseling considered their dogs house trained (86.4–98.1%), and pet parents who received counseling used less verbal punishment and were more likely to clean soiled areas with enzymatic cleaners.[13]

Once the pet is seen by the veterinarian, printed or emailed handouts or the provision of appropriate web resources should be used to be certain that pet parents are given the correct information and that they take it home to share with the remainder of the family. See Appendix A and Recommended Reading below.

At about three weeks of age, most puppies begin eliminating away from the nesting area on their own. By five weeks of age, locations and substrates for elimination are chosen and by eight to nine weeks of age, puppies are attracted by the odors of urine and feces to specific areas for elimination and begin to avoid soiling their den (sleeping quarters)[14] (see Figure 21.1). Good house training strategies will take advantage of the dog's innate proclivity to avoid eliminating in its den and combine

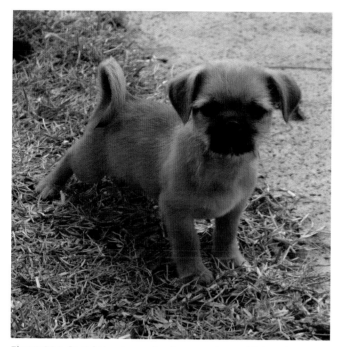

Figure 21.1 By eight to nine weeks of age, puppies establish a substrate preference for elimination. *(Attribution: Lisa Radosta.)*

- Manage the environment to prevent accidents.
- Supervise closely and proactively until house training is complete.
- Use confinement in a crate or room to prevent accidents when not well supervised.
- Consider keeping the dog close to the pet parent and supervised using a harness or collar and leash.
- Feed on a schedule with the last feeding well before bedtime.
- Take the dog or puppy out frequently, every 1 to 2 hours in the beginning.
- Praise immediately after elimination in the elimination area and follow with reinforcement (food or play), not when the pup leaves that area or goes back to the house.
- Keep adult dogs on leash in the elimination area even if the area is fenced.
- Avoid punishment such as yelling, pushing the dog's face into the urine or feces, or spanking.

Manage the environment and schedule

Management for house training requires that elimination in undesirable areas be prevented by providing close supervision or confinement at all times until the dog is fully trained to eliminate in its appropriate area and no longer eliminates in inappropriate areas. One means of accomplishing this is to use a wire or plastic crate to provide a safe confinement area where the pet can be placed at times when it cannot be closely observed. Another alternative is to use a harness or collar and leash to keep the dog or puppy near the pet parent. This provides an effective means of keeping the puppy in sight, and gently and effectively interrupting indoor elimination and guiding the pet to the desirable area without the need for verbal reprimands or any form of punishment. When leaving a leash attached, the puppy must be constantly supervised and the leash should not be left attached to a collar that might choke when tightened. Maintaining a feeding schedule will influence the pet's elimination schedule. Food should be offered at consistent times each day for 20–30 minutes. The pet should be taken to its elimination area within 15–20 minutes of eating. The last meal should be finished 3–5 hours prior to bedtime. For adult dogs for which the feeding schedule is already set, the pet parents may have to feed a bit earlier in order to be able to give the dog adequate time to eliminate before they leave the house. Adult dogs that are soiling might be fed a lower fiber diet to reduce the amount of stool produced. Water should be available all day and taken up just prior to bedtime unless there are physical reasons for which restriction of nocturnal water intake would be inappropriate. The pet parent must regularly accompany the dog to the desired location for elimination. This location must be easily accessible to the puppy as well as desirable for the pet parent. Use of the same location repeatedly allows residual smells to accumulate that should serve to increase the dog's interest in the location and the likelihood that it will eliminate when taken there. At eight weeks of age, the puppy should probably be taken out on average about once every hour as well as immediately after napping, playing, drinking, and after meals as described above before being returned to confinement and immediately before bed at night. As a general rule of thumb, puppies should not be expected to wait for

this inclination with the puppies' acquired substrate preferences and operant and classical conditioning.

This tendency to keep the den area clean of wastes can be overcome by a number of factors. For instance, a dog that is confined for long periods will soil its living areas if not given the opportunity to relieve itself in a more appropriate area. Dogs that are anxious or distressed about being crated or confined may eliminate in their confinement area. Dogs that learn to eliminate in their crate (e.g., from pet store or puppy mills) before they are adopted may be refractory to having this behavior altered because they become habituated to living in a soiled area or in some cases, the hard surface of their crate floor actually becomes their preferred substrate.

As environments and lifestyles change, some pet parents, such as those with small dogs living in high-rise urban dwellings, may prefer to train their pets to an indoor elimination site (i.e., doggy litter, potty pads). Training to eliminate on a new surface can be achieved with most dogs. Patience and consistency are necessary, as well as an understanding that one is attempting to overcome the substrate preference already developed by the dog at a young age and that this can be challenging but rarely impossible, as long as one takes the appropriate, science-based approach.

As is the case with most behaviors we wish to change, house training will be most successfully accomplished by following these basic principles: manage the environment so that the appropriate behavior is easy to achieve; reinforce the desired behavior at every possible opportunity; and avoid using punishment if the unwanted behavior occurs. By consistently following these basic principles, within a few months, most pet parents will be able to train a dog of any age to eliminate in the area that the pet parent desires and to cease eliminating in areas the pet parent deems inappropriate (see Box 21.1).

elimination for approximately more than 1 hour or less for each month of life. For example, a 12-week-old puppy should be taken outside every 2 to 3 hours and a 16-week-old puppy every 3 to 4 hours. This decreases the opportunity for the puppy to eliminate in an undesirable location. If the pet parent is still struggling to house train a puppy at 16–24 weeks of age, they may need to continue taking the puppy to the desired spot for elimination every 1 to 2 hours. Every puppy is an individual and their physical size, activity level, and metabolism, as well as their age, may affect how often they need to eliminate.

Some 10- to 14-week-old puppies will begin sleeping through the night and be able to go without eliminating for 8 hours at night but not be able to do the same during the day. Pet parents of young puppies should consider setting an alarm to wake themselves up once in the middle of the night for the first few nights to weeks after bringing the new puppy home so that they can take the puppy outside for elimination. By being proactive in this way, the puppy is prevented from having to learn to whine and cry to be let out of the crate. The pet parent can slowly discontinue doing this as they note the puppy sleeping more soundly through the night and developing more control of its elimination.

Even if the desired location is in an enclosed yard, having the dog on leash allows the pet parent to take the dog to the area for elimination and keep them from wandering or beginning to play. The pet parent should stand quietly and allow the dog time to sniff and explore the immediate area. The dog will learn that this is different from play time or walking time, based on the pet parent's behavior and the specific location. If the dog does not show signs of interest in eliminating within 5–10 minutes, return to the house, monitor closely or confine, and return to the outdoors to try again frequently. Depending on how long since the last elimination, the pet parent may want to try again in 15–20 minutes. With time and experience, the pet parent will begin to recognize the cues that the puppy is preparing to eliminate; abruptly stopping one activity, walking slowly, looking around, sniffing, circling, etc.

Each dog is an individual and the pet parent is responsible for being observant and determining how long their dog can retain urine and stool, and when and how often they should take it to its elimination site in order to ensure that the opportunity for elimination in the appropriate site is always provided before elimination in an unacceptable location can occur.

Reinforce elimination in desired locations

The dog should then be praised lavishly and given a small treat as soon as it completes its elimination in the appropriate place. A clicker or marker word can be used to mark the appropriate behavior and then food reinforcement can follow. The pet parent should not wait until the pet is back indoors to give the reward since this actually reinforces returning to the home, not elimination. If the puppy wants to play, this can also be used as a reward immediately following elimination. When time allows, spending some time playing with the puppy after eliminating also teaches the puppy that eliminating promptly is not punished by having to immediately return inside (i.e., the fun does not end just because they have eliminated). Some puppies will learn to postpone elimination as they mature once they have discovered that

elimination always results in less time outdoors. This can make house training more difficult if the pet parent becomes impatient and returns the puppy indoors before it has eliminated, increasing the chance that the puppy will have an accident in the house.

Avoid punishment

Physical punishment, scolding, and rubbing the pet's nose in urine or feces are ineffective and inhumane methods for attempting to house train dogs, yet most pet parents rely more on punishing unwanted behaviors than reinforcing desired behaviors. For the pet, it is far simpler to learn in which areas elimination is regularly and consistently rewarded than to learn all of the potentially thousands of indoor locations where it might get punished for eliminating.

Attempting to teach desirable elimination habits with punishment is further complicated by the fact that elimination is always inherently rewarding. The act of elimination relieves pressure and results in feelings of increased comfort, thus providing immediate reinforcement. Unless the animal is discovered as it prepares to eliminate (sniffing, circling, squatting), punishment is simply unlikely to be very effective in the face of this reinforcement. If caught at that moment, the most valuable thing a pet parent can do is to rush the pet outside to the desired location for elimination and hope that the animal completes the act there so it can also be praised and rewarded.

Punishment comes with many dangers, especially when used for elimination; it can result in a dog that simply fears eliminating in the presence of people, making it even more difficult to house train, especially if the pet parent has no fenced yard and must walk the dog for outdoor elimination. Dogs punished for eliminating in the house may learn that they must simply avoid the pet parent in order to eliminate. In these cases, the dogs often try to get as far from the pet parent as possible for elimination, often appearing to sneak away to another room in order to eliminate so they will not be caught. This behavior also makes house training very difficult but cannot happen if the dog is properly supervised, another reason why supervision is critical to effective and humane house training.

Punishment may teach the dog not to eliminate in one particular place. It may also teach the dog to not eliminate in that place in the presence of the pet parent, but it cannot teach the dog where exactly the pet parent wishes the dog to eliminate. In addition, punishment has been shown to potentially result in fear-related aggression directed toward the pet parent.

Teaching a verbal cue for elimination

Teaching a verbal cue for elimination can be a helpful tool for assisting with house training and come in handy in the future if any circumstances require that the dog eliminate in an unfamiliar environment or on an unfamiliar substrate (see Box 21.2). To teach a verbal cue for elimination, the pet parent must first decide on a word that all family members can and will use consistently. In the beginning, every time the puppy or newly adopted dog is taken outside for the purpose of elimination, the word must be spoken immediately after they begin eliminating. The pet is then praised

- Decide on a word that all family members will use.
- Say the cue word as the puppy or newly adopted dog begins to eliminate.
- Repeat, repeat, repeat.
- When the pet parent can recognize the pet's cues that they are about to eliminate (as opposed to when they are actually eliminating), they are ready to change how they use the cue word. Instead of saying it when the pet is in the act of eliminating, they should say the cue word when the pet is showing signs that they will eliminate soon.
- When the pet has been hearing the cue word consistently for two weeks when they are about to eliminate, the pet parent can move to the next step.

- If the puppy is caught in the act of eliminating in the house, it should be scooped up quickly and moved to the appropriate elimination area. Reinforce if it completes elimination there.
- Do not punish the dog for elimination in the house. If the puppy eliminates in the house, the responsible party is the human who was charged with watching the puppy or newly adopted dog, not the dog! The delivery of punishment will serve to make the dog scared of the pet parent and potentially teach them to urinate in private, which will deter house training.
- Thoroughly clean all soiled areas.

and rewarded as described above. Within a relatively short period of time (days to weeks, depending on the puppy and the pet parent), the pet parent will begin recognizing the signs that elimination is imminent (circling or sniffing, squatting or leg lifting) and can begin to say the verbal cue when they know the pet is going to eliminate within the next couple of seconds. It is critical that the pet parent not repeat the word multiple times while waiting for the dog to eliminate. If they find they are saying the verbal cue prematurely, then they should go back to saying it only after the pet begins eliminating and continue observing and learning the reliable cues that predict that the dog is going to eliminate. After a few weeks of using the verbal cue immediately before the pet begins to eliminate, the pet should learn to associate the verbal cue with the act of eliminating and the cue can then be used to encourage elimination. Pet parents must be cautioned to not use the cue unless they know the pet has some need to eliminate. Frequent repetition of the word without subsequent elimination will cause the verbal cue to become meaningless to the pet.

Troubleshooting house training

If the pet parent sees the puppy in the act of eliminating in an undesirable place, the first thing they must do is to try to get his attention without frightening him (see Box 21.3). Calling the puppies name or giving it the cue for come (assuming that it has learned that cue) may be effective but yelling "No," stomping feet, or clapping hands should be avoided. Depending on the size of the puppy, they can calmly but quickly scoop it up and take it directly to the desired location for elimination or try to quickly lead it there. If the puppy completes the act in the desired location once moved, they should be praised and reinforced with a treat or play. If the dog or puppy has had an accident in the house, the person responsible is the family member, not the dog. It is perfectly natural to eliminate in the house, from the dog's point of view. Pet parents should examine who made the mistake and alter the procedure for supervising the puppy. A properly supervised puppy rarely has an accident in the house. For example, was the puppy not being supervised closely enough? Had it been allowed to wander too far away from the pet parent? Had it been allowed outside unsupervised and

someone assumed the puppy had eliminated outdoors when in fact it had not? Whatever the problem, it usually lies in the management of the puppy, so the pet parent must correct the problem and prevent the situation from occurring again in the future. Any location in the home that is soiled by the pet must be thoroughly cleaned and treated with an effective odor neutralizer.[15] Carpeting should be soaked with the product since spraying the surface does not get to all parts of the odor. In some cases, a pet might also be deterred from eliminating in the area by changing the substrate to one that is less appealing (e.g., plastic drop sheets, nubs-up plastic carpet runner, or double-sided sticky tape) or by physically blocking access to the soiled areas. Whenever recommending the use of sticky tape, consideration should always be taken for the welfare of the pet. For example, long-haired pets can get caught in the tape if it is sticky enough, causing pain and distress.

Using the method described above, dogs of any age can be house trained or taught to use indoor toileting systems or potty pads. Successful completion of house training may take anywhere from several weeks to many months depending on the age of the dog, the duration of soiling in the home, the consistency of family members, and how often mistakes occur. In general, a dog should not be considered house trained until it has gone for at least four to eight consecutive weeks without soiling in the home. Adult dogs that have been house soiling for many years may take six months or more before they are dependably trained. When several weeks have passed without any accidents, pet parents should gradually begin giving the dog more unsupervised access to more areas of the home.

Signaling

Pet parents often indicate that their dogs do not give any sign or ask them to go outdoors. Signaling may be learned by repeated high-level reinforcement of outdoor elimination. These dogs may then engage in behaviors to get the pet parents to notice that it is time to go outdoors (e.g., going to the exit door and scratching or vocalizing, or just sitting in front of the pet parent and staring at them). However, when the dog cannot move away because it is leashed next to the person or confined to a crate or kennel, it may begin to show signs of conflict and anxiety (whining, circling, barking, pacing). If the pet parent consistently takes the pet out to eliminate each time these behaviors are noted, the pet will eventually learn to perform them actively to be taken to the elimination area. Pet parents who claim their dog is not signaling are often simply not observing the dog closely enough to recognize the more subtle signs that the dog needs to eliminate. The key to training the dog to signal is to identify these signs and take the dog immediately to its elimination site, where it is immediately rewarded for elimination. Over time, most dogs will learn to signal in some manner (whining, pacing, barking, or even going to the exit door and waiting) when they feel the urge to eliminate.

Challenging circumstances

If pet parents cannot be home to let the dog out as often as necessary based on the guidelines above, they may need to:
- Hire a dog walker.
- Provide for indoor elimination alternatives. These can include newspapers, potty pads, or commercial litterbox systems for dogs. If using one of these methods, the puppy's confinement area should be a larger enclosure such as a bathroom, laundry room, an exercise pen (ex-pen), or gated area of the home. The dog's crate can be placed inside the larger enclosure and the door left open for all but the shortest departures. The entire floor of the enclosure (excluding the crate and bedding and in the case of an adult dog, feeding and watering area) should be covered with the paper or potty pads. The papered area can be made smaller as the dog begins limiting elimination to one specific area. Pet parents desiring to paper train their puppies should be cautioned that dogs may generalize what they learn and attempt to use any other paper found on the floor later in life, so it will be the pet parent's responsibility to keep these items picked up. However, if the potty pad or elimination area is designated by using a commercial indoor house training system or a plastic frame around the potty pad, the pet may be able to better distinguish between what is the appropriate elimination area (see Figure 21.2).
- On the other hand, puppies cannot be left confined, alone, or unattended with no social contact for hours on end. Puppies require social interaction, socialization,

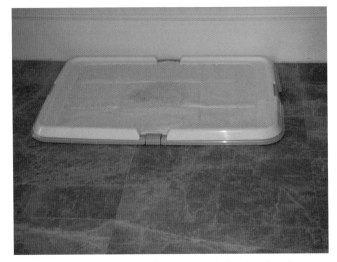

Figure 21.2 Making the indoor elimination area look unique by using a plastic frame around the potty pad can help the dog to distinguish between acceptable indoor elimination locations and unacceptable ones. *(Attribution: Lisa Radosta.)*

and training. Confinement is for the purpose of independence training and house training. It is not to be used as punishment for house soiling or as a hours-long method of confinement.
- If a pet door is available, a pen or other indoor confinement area can be arranged around the flap so that the dog has access to the yard for elimination, but the indoor area is only large enough for bedding, toys, and in the case of an adult dog, food and water. Dogs that have access to a yard or elimination area via a pet door may be more difficult to adequately house train because they always have access to preferred substrates. Pet parents should be cautioned to use pet doors once their dog or puppy has completed the house training process.

Some adult dogs and an occasional young puppy will be resistant to crating or confinement.
- Dogs of any age should be introduced to the crate gradually and in a positive manner. Feeding in the crate, tossing toys in the crate, and hiding treats for them to find in the crate should all help the pet adjust to confinement. The dog should be praised when it explores the crate willingly and chooses to rest there. Comfortable bedding and toys should always be present in the crate to help the pup make a positive association with the crate. Begin by closing the door for very short periods of time initially, always giving the dog a special treat when the door is closed and allowing the dog out before it begins acting distressed about being confined. It is helpful to avoid letting the dog out of the crate in response to its whining or crying since this can teach the dog that vocalizing is what is required in order to get released. However, dogs should also not be left in confinement if they are vocalizing and/or distressed since experiencing stress while being confined will worsen their feelings of anxiety and distress regarding being confined.
- It is common for puppies to vocalize when left alone the first few times they are in a new home and separated from their dam and siblings, but this should last for no more than a few minutes each night and within a few nights, the vocalizing should have stopped.
- Some puppies will vocalize less if their crate can be placed in the bedroom where pet parents are sleeping. Some dogs might even be allowed to have freedom in the bedroom during the night as long as the bedroom door is closed, and may learn to scratch at the door or vocalize at night when they need to eliminate. Pheromone analogs may be helpful to accustom puppies to crate confinement by decreasing stress.
- A crate should never be used to punish a pet for unwanted behaviors. The crate cannot continue to be viewed as a pleasant, positive place for the pet while at the same time being used as a place to isolate the pet when it has performed an unwanted behavior.
- Dogs that are distressed by crating may be able to be confined to a small room such as a laundry room, kitchen, bathroom, or a gated portion of the home. However, if they eliminate in the room, then it may be too large to serve as a confinement area for the purpose of house training.
- No dog or puppy should ever be forced into a crate or confinement if it is unwilling to enter on its own, if it must be lured to get it inside, or if it shows any distress after being confined.

Crate soiling

Puppies or adult dogs that soil their crates present a challenge that should be addressed immediately. If allowed to continue, crate soiling can make house training difficult because the dog can become accustomed to being in a dirty crate and lose its innate tendency to avoid soiling its den area. The first time that crate soiling happens, the pet parent should attempt to determine what circumstances likely led to the incident. Assuming the dog or puppy did not come from a facility (i.e., shelter, puppy mill, or other environment where the habit of crate soiling had already developed), then some of the more common causes for crate soiling to be considered include:

- The dog was put away without first having the opportunity to empty its bladder or bowels.
- The dog was left confined too long without a timely opportunity to empty its bladder or bowels.
- The dog is experiencing a physical condition leading to increased frequency and/or urgency of elimination.
- The dog was fed just prior to confinement.
- A recent diet change (high-fiber diet, diet that causes polyuria/polydipsia).
- Anxiety (separation-related disorder or confinement anxiety or distress, noise aversion, fear or phobia).

House soiling related to physical conditions

Problem overview

A variety of different physiological conditions can result in canine house soiling in even the best trained of dogs, regardless of age (see Table 21.1). A puppy that is difficult to house train in spite of the pet parent following all of the appropriate recommendations could have a congenital problem such as ectopic ureters or a urinary tract infection (UTI) leading to house soiling. Any condition leading to polyuria, polydipsia, diarrhea or constipation, increased urgency or frequency of defecation, pain or discomfort associated with accessing the usual elimination site, or incontinence can all result in house soiling. Aging pets can experience a decline in cognitive function that results in confusion, disorientation, and a loss of previously learned skills such as house training.

Prevention

In addition to offering good preventive care and regular physical exams at all stages of the dog's life, veterinarians can proactively educate pet parents about the behavior changes they can expect with certain physical conditions and medications. If, for example, corticosteroids have just been prescribed, part of the discharge instructions should include a reminder that the dog may need access to more water than usual. It will also need to urinate more often so asking the pet parent if the dog has access to a dog door, or inquiring as to the pet parent's schedule and availability for increased frequency of outings could all be part of the discussion at discharge. If pet parents can prepare for the changes in behavior known to be associated with particular physical conditions or medications, they can possibly prevent the first

Table 21.1 Physical causes of house soiling

Physical causes of fecal house soiling	Physical causes of urinary house soiling
• Increased volume of feces	• Increased volume of urine – polyuria
• Maldigestion/malabsorption	• Renal, hepatic, hypercalcemia, pyometra
• High-fiber diets	• Hyperadrenocorticism, diabetes
• Increased frequency of voiding	• Increased frequency of voiding
• Colitis, diarrhea, and underlying diseases	• Urinary tract infection – calculi – bladder tumors
• Reduced control – incontinence	• Reduced control – incontinence

• Compromised neurologic function
  • Peripheral nerve impairment
  • Spinal impairment
  • Sphincter impairment
	• Compromised neurologic function
	  • Peripheral nerve impairment
	  • Spinal impairment
	  • Sphincter impairment/ incompetence

• Painful defecation
  • Arthritis/anal sacculitis/colitis
	• Painful urination – pollakiuria
	  • Arthritis, urinary tract infection, calculi, prostatitis

• Cranial disease/central control (tumors, encephalitis, infection)	• Cranial/central control (tumors, encephalitis, infection)
• Sensory decline	• Sensory decline
• Cognitive dysfunction syndrome	• Cognitive dysfunction syndrome
• Altered mobility – arthritis/ neuromuscular	• Altered mobility – arthritis/ neuromuscular
• Medications altering stool consistency	• Medications altering urination frequency or volume

	• Marking
	  • Increased anxiety, for example, endocrinopathy
	  • Hormonal (e.g., androgen-producing tumors, such as interstitial cell tumor)

accident that so often leads to additional accidents. Olfactory cues as well as learned substrate preferences and the internal reinforcement associated with the act of elimination all act together to increase the chance that a dog may return to a location in the house they have soiled. Prevention by limiting access, using confinement and/or increased close supervision, plus increased frequency of outings can be highly effective when expecting a condition involving increased frequency or urgency.

Increased access to the outdoors can be achieved in numerous possible ways: if the pet parent cannot come home from work more often and does not have a dog door installed, they could add one. They could hire a dog walker to walk the dog during the day or ask a friend or neighbor to let the dog out once or twice during the day, depending on the pet parent's schedule and the presence or absence of a yard. They can send the dog to doggie day care or day board at the veterinarian's office. If none of these are possible, the pet parent may wish to confine the dog to one room and provide a crate pan with artificial grass or sod for elimination. Even the most well house-trained dog will use these when needing to eliminate if they are provided and if access to other areas is limited. Ex-pens or baby gates may both be helpful for containing the dog in this manner. The space must be large enough to provide the dog with a place for sleeping, food, and water at some distance from the elimination area. Initially, the paper or pads may need to cover most of the space but as the dog begins using them, the amount of space they cover can be decreased each day until the paper is limited to one area that the dog has chosen for elimination.

Diagnosis and potential outcomes

Diagnosis of house soiling secondary to a physical condition will first require collection of history and signalment. If the dog is an adult that has always been well house trained, then this raises the index of suspicion for a problem associated with the urinary or gastrointestinal tract or possibly a metabolic condition. If the dog has never been well house trained, ruling out a contributing physical condition will still be necessary, so even more attention must be paid to the history. As mentioned above, pet parents may regard their pet as house trained and when asked, they may answer that their dog is house trained when upon further questioning, the dog may have had accidents throughout its life. The details are critical. Is the dog urinating, defecating, or both? Has there been an overall increase in frequency and if so, when did it start? Are there other behavioral changes consistent with systemic illness, such as anorexia or lethargy? Have there been changes in the pet's management or lifestyle, such as a new diet, changes to the schedule, or new pets in the home? Before this recent bout of accidents, how often did your dog have accidents in the house of urine or feces? When the dog eliminates, is there a change in posture, straining, apparent discomfort during or following elimination, or has urine or fecal appearance or fecal consistency changed?

Mental or emotional health issues should be ruled out as well. Does the dog have a history of any anxiety or fear-related behaviors (e.g., noise fear or phobias, fear of strangers)? If a dog does not have a history of a shy or fearful temperament and it develops a house-soiling problem as an adult, then this should raise the index of suspicion for a physical condition. With that said, pet parents often do not remember or would not have been able to recognize if their pet was anxious or fearful prior to presentation or as a puppy. Similar to the historical questions above, how the question is asked is critical to acquisition of quality information. Instead of asking if the dog was anxious as a puppy or historically, ask specific questions about body language and behavior (see Box 21.4).

Once a dog is of an advanced age and is considered a senior or geriatric patient, then anxiety-related causes should be considered at the same time as one is investigating the possible physical conditions. Certain anxiety-related conditions become more common in aging patients, and both mental and physical health problems could be contributing to house soiling in the aged animal.

Several different physical conditions can lead to urinary incontinence, so it will be important to determine if the pet

> **Box 21.4** Accurate history taking for dogs presented for house soiling
>
> - Urination, defecation, or both?
> - Where are the accidents occurring?
> - When are the accidents occurring? Is the pet parent home, not home, or both?
>   - If the accidents occur when the pet parent is not home:
>   - What does the dog look like and what does he do before and during pet parent departures and when left alone?
>   - Do the pet parents have cameras in their house? If so, what does the pet do when they are left alone?
> - How does the pet react to storms or loud noises?
>   - If the pet has any reaction to storms or loud noises, ask about reaction, not only the pet parent's assessment of the pet's fear, anxiety, stress, conflict and panic.
>   - What does he do when he is exposed to storms and loud noises?
> - When did this start?
> - Was your dog previously house trained before this problem started? House trained means that your dog rarely if ever had accidents in the house.
> - Has your dog recently begun drinking more, eating more, panting more or had any changes in activity, mobility, personality, or behavior?
> - Are there any changes to urine or fecal appearance (e.g., color, soft or mucus-filled stools) or frequency of elimination (urine or feces)?
> - Are you giving any medications or supplements?
> - Did you recently change your dog's diet?
> - Overall, how is your dog feeling?
> - Do you find puddles in the house or tiny drops?
> - Are the surfaces vertical or horizontal?
> - If the dog is male, does he lift his leg when he urinates outside?
> - Do you find your dog lying in a puddle of urine or is his fur wet?
> - Have you witnessed your dog urinating in the house? If so, what is his posture?

has voluntary control over urination some of the time, all of the time, or none of the time. Incontinence can range in appearance from constant dribbling, leaking during activities with abdominal push (getting up from lying down, jumping up, stretching, changing positions), leaking only when sleeping, intermittent dribbling while maintaining the ability to signal and void, and/or sometimes appearing to be under conscious control. Some animals can experience urinary incontinence some of the time and still have voluntary control of urination at other times. This usually occurs with nonneurogenic disorders. The most common nonneurogenic disorder of micturition seen in dogs is hormone-responsive incontinence. This form of incontinence is further defined as that which occurs secondary to urethral sphincter mechanism incompetence (UMSI) in gonadectomized female dogs and results in incontinence most often when the animal is relaxed or asleep. Other conditions which can lead to USMI and occasional dribbling of urine are UTI, inflammation, prostatic disease, or a history of prostate surgery. Urinary bladder storage dysfunction can also result in frequent leakage of small amounts of urine. Continuous dribbling of urine with the ability to urinate voluntarily can also occur in cases of ectopic ureters. The presence of uroliths can result in continuous dribbling of urine without the ability to voluntarily control urination but in some cases of urolithiasis, the dog will occasionally leak urine while appearing to have control at other times. Some dogs with urolithiasis may never demonstrate apparent incontinence, making this an easily overlooked cause of urinary house soiling in dogs. See Chapter 6 for a full discussion of the physical causes of behavioral clinical signs.

After collecting the history and determining the presence or absence of conscious control, the posture associated with elimination should be documented. Posture (e.g., lowered ears and body, tail lowered and/or wagging rapidly) can help to identify if there is an excitement or fear or anxiety-related component to the behavior.

A comprehensive physical examination, including palpation of the distended and empty urinary bladder, a digital rectal examination, and an orthopedic and neurologic examination are all recommended. Radiography and/or ultrasonography may be necessary to confirm the presence or absence of uroliths. Cystoscopy, ultrasonography, contrast urography, or cystourethrovaginoscopy may be required to diagnose ectopic ureters. A complete blood count, serum chemistry analysis, urinalysis, fT4 (ed) and fecal antigen including Giardia are the baseline needed for all behavior cases. It is easy to label something as behavioral and not go any further. However, up to 82% of dogs that were referred to board-certified veterinary behaviorists for behavior problems have pain and up to 45% have undiagnosed systemic illness.[16] The likelihood of systemic illness and/or pain is high and all patients should be thoroughly evaluated.

Fecal incontinence can occur due to reservoir incontinence, nonneurogenic sphincter incontinence, or neurogenic sphincter incontinence. If a pet parent presents a dog with a complaint of fecal house soiling where the dog appears to have no control over its bowels, reservoir incontinence will be the most likely cause. Neurogenic and nonneurogenic fecal incontinence will most likely develop due to trauma, anorectal disease and surgery, central nervous system disease, or peripheral neuropathy, in which case the history will likely point to one of these other problems. Multiple other clinical signs will also likely be present, suggestive of these other disease processes.

Reservoir incontinence is usually secondary to colorectal disease such as colitis, irritable bowel syndrome, neoplasia, or any condition causing diarrhea. In addition to the diagnostics already discussed, fecal antigen including Giardia is recommended to rule out parasitism.

Once the presence of voluntary control is confirmed, the dog should also be carefully examined for signs of osteoarthritis or neuromuscular conditions that might make accessing the desired elimination site difficult or even painful for them. History must include determining where the dog has typically eliminated and if there have been changes in where the pet parent expects the dog to eliminate. Many pet parents underestimate the challenge that an additional step or two may pose for an aging dog with worsening osteoarthritis.

Some of the possible conditions may be surgically correctable or curable, resulting in a good prognosis for successful resolution of the house-soiling problem. Other conditions may be lifelong and some may continue to worsen with age, requiring that the pet parent be taught new ways to manage the dog's elimination to prevent house soiling (see Table 21.1).

Management

When managing a case of house soiling secondary to a physical condition caused by another organ system, the initial conversation with the pet parent should include a discussion of how long it may realistically take to treat the condition or bring it under control. Regardless of how long this time may be, the pet parent may need to be prepared for how to mitigate household damage in the meantime. It is important that they not expect to go home with a medication that will correct the dog's problem immediately since even if that is likely, the issue of learning, including new substrate and location habits and preferences, intrinsically reinforced by elimination must also be addressed. Conversely, if there is discomfort on elimination, the pet may develop an avoidance of a site or choose more easily accessible sites.

Initial recommendations should include:
- House the animal in a location where any accidents will cause minimal damage to the home (e.g., on an easily cleanable surface such as tile or linoleum). Restrict the dog's access to other areas of the home.
- Clean all previously soiled areas in the home using a cleanser specifically for animal odors (i.e., chemical modification, enzymes, bacterial odor removal).
- Return to basic house training procedures as described previously; closely supervise or confine the pet and take it to the appropriate toileting location as frequently as necessary to avoid house soiling. Praise immediately after completion of elimination in the appropriate location. If the dog cannot be taken to the appropriate location as often as necessary, then confinement with an alternative surface such as potty pads, newspapers, or other indoor canine toileting systems will be necessary.
- Provide education on the ability of the pet to avoid accidents, considering the physical limitations now in place by the systemic disease or pain and the medical prognosis for resolution or control.

Treatment

If the house soiling is due to a physical condition that can be treated and cured, then successful treatment of the condition combined with the management described above should lead to ultimate successful resolution of house soiling. If the physical condition is likely to be chronic and/or progressive, then the long-term management of the dog may have to change and the prognosis for complete resolution of the house soiling may be guarded. The pet parent will need to be counseled as to what is realistically possible for the dog. For example, the dog may not ever be able to roam the home unsupervised again. Some degree of confinement may always be required.

Retraining the dog to using an indoor elimination system may be necessary, as not all dogs will readily begin eliminating indoors in the desired location without some training. With some effort, retraining the dog to use a specific indoor substrate is not that difficult. If the dog has been using grass for most of its life, then squares of sod can be acquired from a local garden store during all except the coldest part of the year. If sod is not available, then artificial grass or an indoor commercial potty device may suffice in some cases. A piece of sod or artificial grass can be laid on the surface that the pet parent wishes the dog to use for elimination. Feces can be manually removed as necessary and urine may be rinsed off outside. The sod will have to be replaced regularly until the dog is using it reliably, then the sod or artificial grass can be cut away in small pieces (a small amount every few days) until all that remains is the surface that the pet parent desires the dog to use. Most dogs retrain to a new substrate in a few days to weeks. Commercial self-cleaning indoor elimination areas with realistic artificial turf are readily available as well.

House soiling secondary to fear or anxiety

Problem overview

House soiling due to anxiety or fear can occur in a variety of different circumstances. Dogs may eliminate in the home due to separation-related disorders, aversion, fear, or phobia of noises or thunderstorms. Where house soiling was associated with fear and anxiety, the majority (53%) were reported to be marking in specific locations, with the remainder house soiling in random locations.[5] Some dogs urinate when greeted because they are excited or conflicted, anxious, stressed, or afraid. House soiling in dogs with separation-related disorders or confinement problems may be just one sign in a spectrum of clinical signs or it may be the primary sign. Some dogs with severe noise aversions will house soil. This may occur in the presence or absence of the pet parent and if occurring only in the absence of the pet parent should be differentiated from house soiling due to separation-related disorders. But for some dogs with noise aversions, fears, or phobias, the presence of the pet parent provides social support and may result in some mitigation of clinical signs. Thus, clinical signs may be mild in the pet parent's presence and more severe in their absence, resulting in some behaviors, such as house soiling, that only occur when a storm or other frightening noise occurs in the pet parent's absence.

Some dogs are unable to voluntarily control their urination in social situations that lead to fear, anxiety, or high levels of excitement. This problem is seen more often in young dogs, especially young females that have not yet developed good sphincter control.

In some cases, dogs may experience conflict (approach avoidance) because they are uncertain as to how to greet or interact in certain situations.

All of these behaviors have one thing in common: they occur when the dog is sympathetically aroused so that the dog does not have complete control over their elimination. These are examples of behaviors that occur as a result of an emotional state, so attempting to treat the behavior without first attending to the emotional state will often result in failure.

Prevention

Prevention of urination secondary to fear, anxiety, stress, conflict, panic, or excitement is most straightforward when dealing with a young dog that urinates when being greeted. The problem is worsened by the bladder being full so plans should always be made to give the puppy opportunities to empty its bladder prior to greetings. When greeting puppies or dogs with a tendency to urinate when excited or anxious,

it is often helpful to avoid making eye contact with the dog, bending over it or reaching to pet the dog. Pet parents may need to remind all visitors to the home to avoid immediately greeting the puppy in an excited manner as well. High-pitched voices should also be avoided when greeting the dog. Instead, everyone should wait until the initial excitement associated with arrival and greeting is over and allow the dog to approach them if it desires. Then the dog should be greeted calmly using low, soothing tones while squatting or sitting, turned sideways to the dog and avoiding direct eye contact. New puppy pet parents should be reminded to avoid using punishment when training young puppies or dogs with shy or anxious personalities, especially when dealing with periuria and perichezia. Punishment only increases fear, anxiety, and conflict, and will subsequently worsen many problem behaviors. Even using a stern voice or facial expression can be enough to cause urination due to fear, anxiety, or conflict in some dogs.

Diagnosis and potential outcomes

Good history taking will usually allow the clinician to identify house soiling due to separation-related disorders. The house soiling in this case should only occur in the absence or the perceived absence of the pet parent or when completely isolated. It may not occur every single time the dog is alone, but unless there are compounding causes for house soiling, should never occur when the dog can have access to the pet parent. The clinician may have to question the pet parent carefully to differentiate the house soiling that occurs in the absence of the pet parent from that which occurs when the dog leaves the presence of the pet parent and goes to another room or area to eliminate. This can be a feature of incomplete house training that occurs when the dog has learned that eliminating in the presence of the pet parent can result in punishment of some kind. See Chapter 17 for more information on separation-related disorders.

House soiling due to aversion, fear, or phobia associated with noises can be more challenging to diagnose because the pet parents will not always know whether a storm or other frightening event occurred in their absence. Pet parents should be questioned regarding the dog's behavior during fireworks, storms, or other frightening events when the pet parent is present. If the dog demonstrates any signs of fear or anxiety associated with loud noises, then the possibility must be considered that house soiling in the pet parent's absence could be occurring due to one of these noises. Dogs that have a noise phobia have 88% chance and those with thunderstorm phobia have an 86% chance of developing separation-related disorders.[17] The fact that the incidence of aversion, fear, and phobia of noises and storms in dogs that also experience separation-related disorders is high can make differentiating the two difficult in some cases. Ultimately, however, the best, if not the only way, to accurately diagnose this condition is for a trained professional such as a veterinarian or veterinary technician to watch or ask the pet parent to watch and describe video of the dog while alone. Many families have webcams and can watch or record their pets when they are not home. A few minutes of video can be enough to confirm that a dog is experiencing distress during separation or isolation. Once that is known, determining that house soiling is also or only associated with fear of noises can require a period of extra attention by the pet parents to weather patterns or other events that may be occurring in their absence. If possible, installing cameras that can allow them to monitor their dog's behavior for the entire time that the pet parent is away, will allow them to confirm the diagnosis more quickly, including *when* during the absence the dog is eliminating and whether there are stimuli or events associated with the elimination.

Elimination due to excitement, anxiety, or conflict associated with greetings can be diagnosed in part because the elimination should only occur in these contexts and is limited to urination. These dogs typically urinate and defecate in the appropriate places at all other times, unless they are also incompletely house trained. They will also assume a posture typical of fear, anxiety, or conflict when urinating; their entire body may be curved or hunched over, their head bowed with their ears lowered or pressed flat against their head, their rear end lowered to the ground, and their tail tucked under their body. Their tail may wag stiffly while tucked between their rear legs. Many dogs will roll over soon after greeting with this posture. See Chapter 2 and Appendix A for information on body language (see Box 21.5).

Management

Both diapers and wraps or belly bands are available for dogs. These may be used in some situations to prevent damage to the home while treatment options are initiated. However, where in some cases these may prevent dogs from eliminating because it finds the experience of eliminating into the devices uncomfortable or unpleasant, in the case of fear, anxiety, stress, conflict, or panic-associated elimination, the dog is most likely not making a choice to eliminate. The elimination is out of the dog's control because it is associated with sympathetic arousal. Therefore, pet parents can try these devices but if they do not appear to help decrease the frequency of the elimination, they should be avoided so as not to cause irritation and further discomfort to the dog due to the presence of urine or even feces against their skin for prolonged periods.

Other forms of management may include simply housing the dog in areas where their soiling will be less problematic

---

Box 21.5 Differential diagnoses for house soiling

- Inadequate house training
- Excitement-induced urination
- Conflict-induced urination
- Anxiety-induced urination
- Fear-induced urination
- Stress-induced urination
- Social or environmental stress marking
- Territorial marking
- Noise aversion, fear, or phobia
- Separation-related disorders
- Physical problems
- Management-related problems
- Location or surface preferences
- Learned preference for an unacceptable location or surface

---

for the pet parent, for example, confining the dog to a room with a linoleum or tile floor rather than a room with carpet or possibly even a kennel, crate or ex-pen. However, in cases of separation-related disorders, this must be done with great caution as confinement may worsen feelings of distress in some dogs, ultimately making the problem worse and successful treatment more difficult.

Treatment

House soiling due to fear, anxiety, stress, conflict, or panic is a clinical sign of an emotional problem such as separation-related disorders, noise aversion, fear, or phobias. Treatment must therefore be aimed at correction of the emotional disorder. Once that condition is diagnosed and treated, with a treatment plan for management, behavioral modification, and medication when indicated, then the unwanted behavioral signs of house soiling should stop. See Chapters 14, 15, and 17 for treatment of separation-related disorders, and fears of noises.

Marking

Problem overview

Urine marking behavior is a normal means of olfactory communication in dogs. It is likely that dogs are able to identify individuals based on the information in the scent of the urine.[18] Although urination is considered sexually dimorphic in dogs, urination postures vary significantly, with the possibility of up to 12 postures being displayed by males and females.[8,19,20] In most cases, urine marking involves an intact male dog standing, raising a leg, and directing a stream of urine at an upright object.[14,20] However, dogs of both sexes, even if neutered or spayed, may urine mark, although intact male dogs are more likely to urine mark than neutered males or females.[14] It makes sense then that castration reduces scent marking in intact male dogs,[21] although if there is an emotional component to the marking, it will most likely not be reduced and may be increased with neutering. Female dogs often mark while assuming their normal squatting posture. Dogs mark their territory with urine, most likely indicating to future passing dogs that another dog has passed this way. Dogs will also mark in response to other olfactory cues, with some dogs actually overmarking other dog's urine. Female dogs will mark more frequently when in estrus.[19] Urine marking in the home, by a neutered dog that has been previously well house trained, is usually a result of fear, anxiety, stress, conflict, or panic. Marking with feces is quite rare in dogs.

Prevention

Marking can be reduced 70–80% by castration in male dogs[12] and castration, as well as spaying of females, is the recommended way to prevent marking behavior in most cases. However, even a well house-trained neutered dog may urine mark when exposed to certain olfactory cues. If moving into a new home where dogs previously house soiled, the odors left by prior canine occupants can result in urine marking. When possible, determining if dogs lived in a home prior to purchase or renting can be helpful. The new pet parent may need to consider professional cleaning prior to moving to avoid urine marking by the new canine occupant.

Many dogs will mark anything that provides a novel olfactory stimulus such as dirty laundry or new furniture. When aware that a dog has a penchant for marking novel items in the home, pet parents should be instructed to avoid placing these items where the dog can have access to them. Since urine marking in the home is often a result of anxiety, preventing anxiety-provoking stimuli, to the extent possible will be the best approach.

Diagnosis and potential outcomes

Since both male and female dogs may urine mark, it can be challenging to determine when a dog is urine marking (for the purpose of communication) versus simply eliminating due to a full bladder. The posture alone i.e. standing versus squatting will not be the most reliable indicator. The behavioral history should include a description of the posture that the dog normally assumes when eliminating outdoors (assuming it has been house trained prior to the development of this problem) and whether or not it normally marks numerous items when outdoors. Urine marking typically involves producing small quantities of urine in multiple places as opposed to a complete emptying of the bladder, and explaining this to the pet parent will usually allow them to better understand and describe what their dog normally does when urinating. A video recording can aid the veterinarian in diagnosing whether the elimination behavior is marking. Questions regarding when, on what, and where the urine marking is occurring will be necessary in order to determine underlying causes. For example, marking might occur secondary to conflict between two family dogs or a change in the family dynamic, resulting in anxiety. If a dog is marking near windows or doors on or a visitor's possessions, this can suggest territorial marking, possibly due to anxiety.

A retained testicle may begin to produce testosterone as the dog passes sexual maturity. Interstitial cell tumors in a retained testicle or testicular remnant could be involved in testosterone production.[22] Retained testicles can be found on ultrasound[23] and via serum testosterone. Although baseline testosterone may be high, a gonadotropin-releasing hormone (GnRH) response test comparing baseline testosterone to a sample drawn 2–3 hours after 50 µg IM GnRH administration may be more sensitive.[24] Physical conditions that contribute to anxiety and those that might lead to an increased frequency of urination should also be ruled out; therefore, a minimum baseline should be completed as discussed above.

If a neutered dog has previously been well house trained, does not have any physical conditions leading to polyuria or pain upon elimination, and there has been no change in the pet parent's schedule resulting in the dog not being taken to its place of elimination frequently enough, then a diagnosis of urine marking as a result of anxiety or stress should be considered. When the cause of the dog's anxiety can be identified and either removed or decreased to some extent, the prognosis for resolution is good.

Management

Management should initially include attempts to remove or decrease anxiety-causing stimuli wherever possible. For example, simply eliminating access to objects that the dogs have been marking by confining the dog away from those items may be all that is necessary. Another option might include habituating the dog to a belly band or a diaper. Most dogs would rather not soil themselves and if they can avoid it, they will, so simply wearing the device can lead to a decrease in marking. However, if the stimulus leading to the marking behavior is not eliminated, then the behavior is likely to return every time the dog is not wearing the band or diaper.

Confinement can work similarly for managing a urine marking problem as it does for any other house-soiling problem. Limiting a dog to the confines of a crate or pen decreases the chance that it will willingly soil in the limited area.

Treatment

If the pet parent is willing, castration or spaying should be considered in the urine-marking animal. If already neutered and urine marking is due to anxiety, then appropriate treatment of the anxiety problem will be necessary. Dog-appeasing pheromone (spray, collar, or diffuser), medications (selective serotonin reuptake inhibitors, tricyclic antidepressants), (Chapter 11) and natural supplements (Chapter 12) may be helpful for decreasing anxiety of marking dogs. At the same time that efforts are being made to ameliorate the anxiety, the dog will still need to be prevented from marking. This can be accomplished using confinement when the dog cannot be completely supervised or tethering if the pet parent prefers. Dogs can be tethered to their pet parents using an approximately 4–6-foot (1.5–2-m) leash. The pet parent must then be observant and if the dog is seen to begin investigating an area as if to mark it, the pet parent can gently redirect the dog, take it outside, and encourage marking or elimination there. The dog should at least be reinforced with treats or play.

The geriatric patient

Problem overview

The geriatric dog is susceptible to many physical conditions that can increase the frequency of elimination as well as limit its ability to locate and/or access its previously learned elimination locations. House training requires voluntary control of the detrusor reflex at a cortical level. As the dog ages, physical and physiologic changes occur in the central nervous system that result in a general decrease in cerebral function.[25] Impaired cerebral function can affect the geriatric pet's house training by reducing voluntary control of the emptying reflex and by reducing awareness. Loss of voluntary control can result in urge incontinence (the dog has a warning that micturition is about to occur but cannot stop it) or unconscious urination (there is no awareness or control). Reduced awareness may also result in the pet being less cognizant of its external environment, making it less likely to signal to the pet parent when it has to eliminate. For further discussion of cognitive dysfunction, see Chapter 8.

Prevention

As a result of organ function decline (renal, hepatic), endocrinopathies (e.g., Cushing's, diabetes), and an increase in cystitis, pyelonephritis, and prostatitis with declining immune function, many geriatric dogs require more frequent access to elimination areas. Problems such as arthritis, muscle atrophy, and weakness can make rising and/or navigating stairs challenging. Sensory decline may impact the pet's awareness, communication, signaling, and navigating of the environment. Educating pet parents regarding these changes and encouraging them to be proactive in recognizing them in their dog will allow them to prepare. These preparations could include access to doggie doors, having a friend, neighbor, or dog walker give the dog extra outings, or even providing an indoor potty system. Adding ramps or carpeting (or other nonslip surfaces) to stairs or walkways can aid the geriatric dog in accessing the outdoors. Senior dogs may be less willing to go outside in inclement weather to eliminate so they may need to be supervised more closely and possibly provided with indoor options.

Diagnosis and potential outcomes

When presented with a house-soiling geriatric dog, the clinician will first need to determine if the dog has conscious control of urination (see the section "House soiling related to physical conditions"). If the dog does not, then whatever underlying physiological conditions are resulting in the lack of control will need to be treated or managed. If the dog has physical control but is determined to have other physiological conditions that are resulting in pain, discomfort, or increased urgency or frequency of elimination, then these will need to be managed as well. The dog should be screened for cognitive decline or dysfunction since house soiling is one of the common signs of this problem.[25,26]

Many of these conditions that can contribute to house soiling in the geriatric dog are not conditions that will be cured. The clinician should help pet parents understand that the dog may never again have the complete control that it had as a young dog (assuming it was previously house trained). Many pet parents do not recognize their dog's pain or failing health since the changes can occur very gradually and most dogs are very good at masking signs of pain or discomfort. They may thus believe that the dog is acting out of "spite" for some reason or being "lazy" or "stubborn." Increased awareness of the dog's challenges may help pet parents to be more patient and tolerant regarding the occasional accident that may occur with a geriatric dog.

Management

Management of underlying health conditions will be paramount but recognizing the need to change the environment to make it easier for the dog to access the elimination site that the pet parent wishes them to use is also critical. Closer observation and supervision when the pet parents are home will be important as well. Taking the dog to the desired site for elimination and observing the dog, just as one would a puppy being house trained, may be necessary. Confining the dog (when no one can supervise it) in a crate, pen, or small room with an indoor potty system of some type may be the easiest thing for many pet parents to do. Senior pets may be less able to adapt to change, so attempts should be made to give them some degree of routine and avoid sudden changes in schedules or household status. Steps should be taken to gradually prepare the dog for any expected changes when at all possible.

Treatment

If a geriatric dog begins house soiling, he may quickly develop a preference for this more convenient or accessible location, assuming that the cause is not cognitive decline and the dog's memory is relatively intact. In this case, the chosen location will need to be made unavailable to him, supervision increased, and confinement or tethering used as described above to prevent repeats of the behavior. If the dog is experiencing arthritis, medications and supplements to reduce pain and stiffness should be considered even if the dog does not appear to be uncomfortable to the pet parents (see Box 21.6).

Box 21.6 Summary of treatment for canine house soiling

- Diagnose and treat or rule out physical problems
- Treat underlying emotional issues (e.g., separation-related disorders, noise aversion, fear or phobia)
- Choose a location and substrate for elimination that is desirable for the pet and pet parent
    - Take regularly to location
    - Immediately reinforce (praise, treats, play) the pet when it eliminates in an appropriate area
- Control the feeding schedule to control elimination schedule
- Supervision
    - To train/reinforce desirable behavior
    - To prevent/interrupt (e.g., auditory, leash) undesirable behavior
- Prevent resoiling at previously soiled areas
    - Prevent access/confinement
    - Change substrate
    - Odor elimination
- Focus on rewarding desirable behavior, not punishment of undesirable behaviors

---

CASE EXAMPLES

Case 1

Presentation

Herman, a 4-month-old, 5 kg Dachshund puppy, was presented for urination in his crate and throughout the house but never in the presence of the pet parent.

History

Herman would eliminate outdoors in the yard and the pet parent would give appropriate rewards. He would regularly defecate outdoors morning and night and the pet parents reported no perichezia. He would not eliminate indoors if a family member was closely

Continued

supervising but would occasionally sneak away and urinate in another room. When the pet parents found the soiled area, they would immediately take him to the spot, put his nose in the urine, and verbally reprimand him. Herman slept in the bedroom with the pet parents during the night. On occasion, he would go downstairs to urinate while they slept. On weekdays, Herman was left in a crate in the laundry room from about 8.30 a.m. to 4.00 p.m. and on most days, the pet parent would find urine in the crate. Whenever the pet parents found urine in the crate, they would yell at him and send him outdoors in the yard, where he was ignored for 30 minutes. The pet parents were convinced that Herman knew that he was misbehaving because he would act "guilty" whenever they found urine in an inappropriate location.

Workup

Herman's physical examination and baseline workup was within normal limits.

Differential diagnoses

Separation-related disorders, noise aversion, fear and phobia, learned behavior, inadequate house training, and specific fears were considered as differential diagnoses for Herman's elimination behavior in the house. It was determined that Herman was eliminating in his crate because he could not hold his urine for the amount of time expected. He did not show any signs of distress when the pet parents were not home and he showed no fear of sounds.

Treatment

To provide the puppy with an opportunity to eliminate within 4 to 5 hours, the pet parents arranged for a dog walker to provide Herman with an additional walk during the lunch hour. Since the family wished to continue confining Herman when they were out, a crate training guide was provided to encourage positive association with crate confinement. The crate was relocated to the corner of the bedroom where the puppy normally slept, and the door was kept closed so that he could not wander downstairs at night. The pet parents continued to reward the puppy for outdoor elimination and were instructed to keep him in sight when indoors so that he could not sneak away. Since Herman would seldom eliminate in the first 2 hours after eliminating outdoors, the pet parents could be somewhat lax about supervision for the first hour after the walk, but would keep him in sight or put him in his crate with a chew toy if an hour had passed. With the noontime walk, Herman ceased urinating in his crate within a week and would sleep through the night in his crate. With increased supervision and withdrawal of punishment, all soiling was resolved by seven months of age, but noon walks were continued since they provided Herman with a needed opportunity to eliminate.

Discussion

Since Herman was being left alone for 7.5 hours daily, he could not control his urine until the pet parents arrived home. He had learned to avoid the pet parents when eliminating, which is why he would sneak away when he felt the urge to urinate. He would act fearful (which the pet parents assumed to be guilt) whenever the pet parents found urine because he had learned that he would get punished and berated. It was explained to the pet parents that unless he was deterred in the act, he could not understand the consequences of his actions. However, even with effectively timed punishment, he would merely avoid urinating indoors when the pet parents were supervising, which he had already learned.

Case 2

Presentation

Lily, a 11-month-old spayed female Bichon Frise, was presented for eliminating indoors whenever the pet parent was not supervising her.

History

Lily urinated in the house even if she had been outdoors recently. She sometimes sneaked away to eliminate. When the pet parents were away from home, Lily was left in the kitchen, where she eliminated on paper. While the pet parents were outdoors with the dog, she would not eliminate. During the first two months after adoption, each time that Lily eliminated indoors, they would yell or hit her. They would then put her outdoors unsupervised in the yard. At times, Lily had managed to sneak away from the pet parents and eliminate in other rooms.

Differential diagnoses

Lily could be urinating in the house due to lack of house training, incorrect house training, fear, anxiety, stress, learned behavior, or noise fear or phobia. Lily did not display any fear of sounds. It was determined that she had a lack of house training because of incorrect and inconsistent techniques used by the pet parents and had learned to prefer areas in which the pet parents were absent due to punishment-based techniques.

Workup

Lily's physical examination and laboratory tests were within normal limits.

Treatment

The first step was to teach Lily that she would receive valuable rewards (food treats, play toys) whenever she eliminated outdoors. This proved to be extremely difficult because she was fearful of eliminating in the pet parents' presence. Therefore, the pet parents were instructed to accompany the dog outdoors, stay at least 8 feet away, and ignore her until she eliminated (regardless of how long it took). When she eliminated, they were to click (mark the behavior with a clicker) and toss a toy or treat.

They were educated and given resources on proper house training, training in general, and relationship building. They were to stop yelling and positive punishment techniques. They were referred to a positive reinforcement trainer for basic training and relationship building.

As soon as Lily eliminated and expected rewards when the pet parents were present, they were instructed to add a "go pee" cue as urination ended and then follow with reinforcement. The pet parents were to supervise her at all times in the house. Lily was fitted with a comfortable harness. The pet parents kept her on a leash when they were home so that they could monitor her.

Follow-up

The veterinary technician followed up in three months and Lily was successfully house trained and had not had any accidents in the house in the past month. She had been given more freedom in the house and was not on leash anymore.

Discussion

Lily had learned to eliminate indoors on paper and had never learned to eliminate outdoors. In fact, because of the way punishment had been used, she was fearful of eliminating in the pet parents' presence, regardless of whether she was indoors or out. When this type of interaction frames the relationship between dog and pet parent, the relationship first has to be rebuilt on positive and structured interactions before the pet can successfully learn new behaviors.

Conclusion

Physical reasons for a break in house training should always be considered when working up the dog that is house soiling.

Unresolved physical problems will cause any attempts to correct the behavior problem to fail. However, even if physical problems can be resolved, new surface preferences, locations, and schedules that lead to house soiling may persist. The basic approach to treatment involves correcting the factors that initiated the problem, using supervision and rewards to retrain desired behavior, and preventing the undesirable behavior from occurring for a long enough period of time to reestablish regular elimination in the desired location.

References

1. Salman MD, Hutchinson J, Ruch-Gallie R, et al. Behavioral reasons for relinquishment dogs and cats to 12 shelters. *J Appl Anim Welf Sci.* 2000;3:93–106.
2. New JG, Salman MD, Scarlett JM, et al. Shelter relinquishment: characteristics of shelter-relinquished animals and their owners compared with animals and their owners in U.S. pet-owning households. *J Appl Anim Welf Sci.* 2000;3:179–201.
3. Patronek GJ, Glickman LT, Beck AM, et al. Risk factors for relinquishment of dogs to an animal shelter. *J Am Vet Med Assoc.* 1996;209:572–581.
4. Corridan CL. *The Role of Owner Expectation in Development of a Successful Human*: Dog Bond. Doctorate Thesis. Lincoln, UK: University of Lincoln; 2010.
5. Dinwoodie IR, Dwyer B, Zottola V, et al. Demographics and comorbidity of behavior problems in dogs. *J Vet Behav.* 2019;32:62–71.
6. Fatjó J, Ruiz-de-la-Torre JL, Manteca X. The epidemiology of behavioural problems in dogs and cats: a survey of veterinary practitioners. *Anim Welf.* 2006;15:179–185.
7. Lord LK, Reider L, Herron ME, et al. Health and behaviour problems in dogs and cats one week and one month after adoption from animal shelters. *J Am Vet Med Assoc.* 2008;233:1715–1722.
8. Gazzano A, Mraiti C, Alvares S, et al. The prevention of undesirable behaviors in dogs: effectiveness of veterinary behaviorists' advice given to puppy owners. *J Vet Behav.* 2006;3:125–133.
9. Kass PH, New JC Jr, Scarlet JM, et al. Understanding animal companion surplus in the United States: relinquishment of nonadoptables to animal shelters for euthanasia. *J Appl Anim Welf Sci.* 2001;4:237–248.
10. Herron ME, Shofer FS, Reisner IR. Survey of the use and outcome of confrontational and non-confrontational training methods in client-owned dogs showing undesired behaviors. *App Anim Behav Sci.* 2009;117: 47–54.
11. Learn A, Radosta L, Pike A. Preliminary Assessment of differences in completeness of housetraining between dogs based on size. *J Vet Behav.* 2020;35; 19 26.
12. Gonzalez Martinez A, Pernas GS, Casalta FJD, et al. Risk factors associated with behavioral problems in dogs. *J Vet Behav.* 2011;6:225–231.
13. Herron ME, Lord LK, Hill LN, et al. Effects of preadoption counselling for owners on house-training success among dogs acquired from shelters. *J Am Vet Med Assoc.* 2007;231:558–592.
14. Houpt KA. *Domestic Animal Behavior for Veterinarians and Animal Scientists.* 6th ed. Ithaca, NY: Cornell University; 2018.
15. Melese-d'Hospital P. Eliminating urine odors in the home. In: Voith VL, Borchelt PL, eds. *Readings in Companion Animal Behavior.* Trenton, NJ: Veterinary Learning Systems; 1996;191–197.
16. Mills DS, Demontigny-Bedard I, Gruen M, et al. Pain and problem behavior in cats and dogs. *Animals.* 2020;10:318. doi:10.3390/ani10020318.
17. Overall KL, Dunham AE, Frank D. Frequency of nonspecific clinical signs in dogs with separation anxiety, thunderstorm phobia and noise phobia, alone or in combination. *J Am Vet Med Assoc.* 2001;219:467–473.
18. Dunbar IF. Olfactory preferences in dogs: the response of male and female beagles to conspecific odors. *Behav Biol.* 1977;20: 471–481.
19. Wirant SC, McGuire B. Urinary behavior of female domestic dogs (Canis familiaris): influence of reproductive status, location, and age. *Appl Anim Behav Sci.* 2004;85:335–348.
20. Sprague RH, Anisko JJ. Elimination patterns in the laboratory beagle. *Behaviour.* 1973;47(3–4):257–267.
21. Hart BL. Environmental and hormonal influences on urine marking behavior in the adult male dog. *Behav Biol.* 1974;11: 167–176.
22. Johnston SD, Kustritz MV, Olson PNS. Disorders of the feline testes and epididymides. In: Johnston SD, Kustritz MV, Olson PNS, eds. *Canine and Feline Theriogenology.* Philadelphia: Saunders; 2001:525–536.
23. Felumlee AE, Reichle JK, Hecht S, et al. Use of ultrasound to locate retained testes in dogs and cats. *Vet Radiol Ultrasound.* 2012;53: 581–585.
24. Brewer M, Jesudoss Chelladuri JRJ. Cryptorchidism. In: Tilley LP, Smith FWK, Sleeper MM, et al., eds. *Blackwell's 5 Minute Veterinary Consult: Canine and Feline.* 7th ed. Hoboken, NJ: John Wiley and Sons; 2021;346–347.
25. Landsberg GM, Malamed R. Clinical picture of canine and feline cognitive impairment. In: Landsberg G, Madari A, Zilka N, eds. *Canine and Feline Dementia. Molecular Basis, Diagnosis and Therapy.* Cham, Switzerland: Springer International Publishing; 2017:1–11.
26. Azkona G, García-Belenguer S, Chacón G, Rosado B, León M, Palacio J. Prevalence and risk factors of behavioural changes associated with age-related cognitive impairment in geriatric dogs. *J Small Anim Pract.* 2009;50(2):87–91.

Recommended reading

American College of Veterinary Behaviorists, et al. *Decoding Your Dog: The Ultimate Experts Explain Common Dog Behaviors and Reveal How to Prevent or Change Unwanted Ones.* New York: Houghton Mifflin Harcourt; 2014.
BCSPCA – https://spca.bc.ca/faqs/house-train-dog/.
Ballantyne K. Today's Veterinary Practice - https://todaysveterinarypractice.com/canine-house-soiling-back-basics/
Fear Free Happy Homes - https://www.fearfreehappyhomes.com/how-to-house-train-your-puppy-the-fear-free-way/
Fear Free Happy Homes - https://www.fearfreehappyhomes.com/9-tips-to-housetrain-your-puppy-or-adult-dog/
Lindell E. *Clinician's Brief.* https://www.cliniciansbrief.com/article/canine-house-soiling.

House soiling – feline

Alison Gerken, DVM

Introduction

House soiling is the deposition of urine and/or feces on horizontal and/or vertical surfaces, including on objects and in locations that are considered unacceptable by pet parents. In a recent internet survey of cat parents, over half reported house soiling.[1] House soiling can significantly disrupt the human–animal bond and is a leading reason that many cats are relinquished or euthanized.[2–4] One survey of about 1600 cat parents[2] and another survey of about 1700 cat parents[5] who presented their cats to shelters for relinquishment found that 28%[2] and 18%[5] of cats were relinquished due to behavior problems with house soiling being the most frequently cited behavioral complaint in 43%[2] and 38%[5] of those cats.

House soiling is a normal feline behavior which may arise secondary to a multitude of pathologies including physical disease and/or acute or chronic stress. Feline house soiling problems may be transient or may resolve quickly in response to simple environmental management, or they may be chronic and necessitate that the clinician identify the underlying etiology and create a tailored treatment plan which may include environmental modification; diet change; supplements, psychotropic medications and/or pheromonotherapy; and behavior modification. Because feline house soiling is often a distressing, frustrating, and embarrassing problem for pet parents, regular follow-up, support, and guidance is required for a successful outcome.

Terminology

House soiling can be divided into two broad categories – toileting (also referred to as latrining or elimination), which is physiological micturition or defecation, and marking (also referred to as spraying), which is the deposition of urine or feces outside of the litterbox for communicative purposes.[1,6,7] Historically, nonmarking house soiling was referred to as feline inappropriate elimination or inappropriate toileting.[8] However, this terminology is not accurate because it implies that the cat is doing something unnatural or is acting out of spite or anger toward the pet parent when eliminating in undesirable locations when in fact, the cat is doing something wholly natural in response to environmental, emotional, and/or physical stimuli.[8] Elimination is a normal communicative behavior for cats, and Cats may eliminate outside of their previously used elimination areas when they develop a physical disorder or experience FASCP (fear, anxiety, stress, conflict, panic), when something unpleasant or aversive causes them to avoid that area or substrate (medical, physical, sensory), and/or when their physical, environmental, and social needs are not met.[9] When basic needs are not met, it is normal and appropriate for animals to attempt to fulfill those needs. In this case, the cat may seek alternative locations in which to eliminate that better suit his needs. Many humans would make the same choice if only offered a cramped, dirty, smelly latrine. Problems arise when the cat's elimination location choice is undesirable to the pet parent. The current terminology of feline behavioral house soiling is discussed below.

Table 22.1 House soiling terminology

Term	Definition
House soiling	Deposition of urine or feces in locations unacceptable to the caregiver irrespective of the underlying cause
Elimination or toileting	Urination (micturition) and/or defecation
Urine marking, urine spraying	Deposition of urine, usually on vertical surfaces but also including on horizontal surfaces outside of the litterbox for the purpose of communication
Periuria	Deposition of urine in unacceptable locations irrespective of underlying cause
Perichezia	Deposition of stool in unacceptable locations irrespective of underlying cause
Middening	Deposition of feces outside of the litterbox for the purpose of communication

House soiling: deposition of urine or feces in locations that are considered unacceptable or undesirable to pet parents.[8]

Elimination, toileting, latrining: physiological micturition or defecation.[8,10]

Undesirable elimination, toileting, latrining: deposition of urine or feces in locations that are considered unacceptable or undesirable to pet parents, not due to marking.[8,10]

Periuria: deposition of urine outside of acceptable locations.[1,8,10,11]

Perichezia: deposition of feces outside of acceptable locations.[11]

Urine marking, spraying: deposition of urine, usually smaller amounts, on vertical (and rarely horizontal) surfaces for communicative purposes.[1,6,8]

Fecal marking, middening: deposition of feces outside of acceptable locations for communicative purposes[1,8] (see Table 22.1).

Normal feline elimination behavior and preferences

Normal elimination behavior

For kittens, the purpose of elimination is purely to satiate a physiologic need. Before three weeks of age, the dam stimulates the kitten to urinate and defecate.[12,13] Kittens can voluntarily eliminate at 5–6 weeks of age and start to explore litter substrates, and lie down in litterboxes at 3–5 weeks. By 5–7 weeks, cats begin to eliminate in a litterbox, displaying species-typical behavior associated with elimination including digging, sniffing, circling, and squatting.[9,14] Kittens usually begin covering their eliminations when presented with litterlike substrate by about seven weeks.[9,14] The physiologic relief experienced after eliminating in the litterbox reinforces use of the litterbox, thus making continued use of the litterbox likely.[7,15] Therefore most kittens readily accept a litterbox for toileting.

Cats voluntarily eliminate in three ways: squat urination, defecation, and urine spraying.[16,17] Cats most commonly

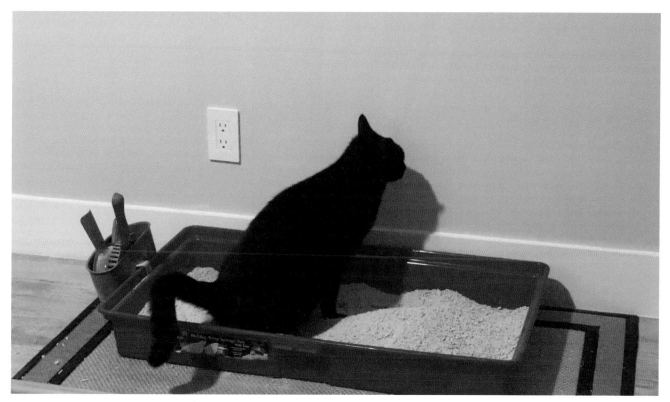

Figure 22.1 Normal posture for cat urination. *(Attribution: Lisa Radosta.)*

employ the method of squat urination for micturition, but they may start urinating in a squat position and finish in a standing position[16] (see Figure 22.1). A healthy cat urinates 2–5 times and defecates at least once daily.[15,16] One study found that the urination sequence consists of the cat digging a hole in the substrate for 12 seconds on average before urination, squatting over the hole to express urine, sniffing the area for 18 seconds on average, and covering the spot for an average of 16 seconds.[18] Cats may or may not sniff the voided urine and cover it.[7,16] The defecation sequence is similar, except the cat may not squat as deeply.[14,18] Cats with house soiling disorders spend less time digging before elimination.[18] In fact, digging for four seconds or less prior to elimination may be associated with the development of elimination problems.[16] Outdoor cats usually bury their feces when near their home (possibly to minimizing the spread of scent and endoparasitic disease) but may leave their feces exposed outside of their core territory.[17–21] Cats usually sniff the locations where they just buried feces but tend to not do this after leaving them exposed.[22]

Marking (spraying)

Urine marking or spraying is a normal felid behavior that is not intended to void the bladder[7,16,21,23]; is generally either sexual (to attract mates) or reactional (in response to environmental and social triggers);[9,24] is often accompanied by vocalization;[9] and serves as a form of communication among conspecifics with territorial, agonistic, and sexual connotations[11,14,23–26] (see Figure 22.2). The exact information obtained from urine marks is unclear.[24,25] Both males and females can mark, regardless of their reproductive status.[7,16,24] Scent communication is important within feline social groups and cats identify a collective "familiar" odor that is comprised of all the scents, including those expressed by the pets, humans, and inanimate objects, within the home.[9,20,27,28] Scent signals, including urine marks, are long-lasting, allowing cats that encounter the signals to receive the intended information long after the signaling cat has departed, making this type of scent signaling especially useful.[21]

All cats, especially male adult cats, investigate areas of deposition of the urine of other cats.[29,30] Urine from unfamiliar cats is sniffed longer than that of familiar cats,[31] particularly if produced by estrous females.[32] It may serve to advertise reproductive status and mate selection, identify individuals and their relatedness, provide information on individual health, establish a territory, coordinate movements, limit contact between individuals, and prevent agonistic encounters.[25] Cats are individuals and may respond to the urine of other cats in various ways such as avoidance, retreat, overmarking (marking with their own urine in that spot), or doing nothing at all outside of investigation (see Figure 22.2).[32] Cats often spend a longer time sniffing the feces of an unfamiliar cat when compared to their own or that of a familiar cat,[19] suggesting that fecal marks may convey important information.[16] Middening, or fecal marking, is the least common form of marking and is rare in domestic cats.[9,15,23]

Undesirable elimination

Undesirable elimination involves squatting to defecate or urinate on horizontal surfaces in locations that are undesirable and/or unacceptable to the pet parent.[7,10] It occurs with an

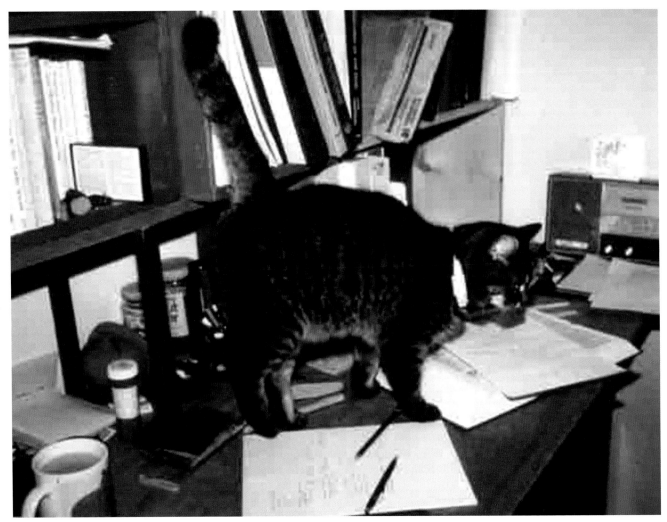

Figure 22.2 Normal posture for cat spraying or urine marking. *(Courtesy of Katherine Houpt, VMD, PhD, DACVB.)*

almost equal incidence in females and males,[17] and is generally accompanied by normal preelimination and postelimination behaviors[7] with the caveat that cats with house-soiling problems may spend less time digging before eliminating than cats without house-soiling problems[18,24] (see Table 22.2).

Elimination preferences

In general, cats prefer large boxes in safe and private places which have adequate amounts of litter and are pristinely clean.[7,8,23,33–36] If these needs are met, most cats will reliably use the provided litterboxes. The recommended minimum litterbox size is 86 cm × 39 cm or 1.5 times the length of the cat as an adult, whichever is larger.[7,33] In a study of box preferences, cats were found to prefer the biggest litterbox offered (86 × 39 × 14 cm) which exceeded the size of commercially available litterboxes, over a regular-sized litterbox (58 × 39 × 14 cm).[33] In general, the larger the box, the better. That way, the cat has the maximum likelihood of encountering a clean box which suits his needs (see Figure 22.3). High-sided boxes may be preferred by some cats because they provide better security.[9] While one study showed no relationship between elimination problems and the location of the litterbox,[18] generally cats prefer quiet and secluded locations where they will

Table 22.2 Differentiating marking from undesirable elimination

Marking	Undesirable elimination
Communicative function; not intended for voiding	Voiding behavior
Adults – postpubertal	Any age
Most common in intact males and females in estrus, followed by neutered males	Males or females, intact or neutered
Urine (in rare cases, feces)	Urine and/or feces
Usually small amounts	Usually larger amounts
Generally vertical surfaces; in rare cases, urine or feces on horizontal surfaces	Generally horizontal surfaces
Stands, tail erect, backs up, treads with rear legs, sprays urine	Squats
Prominent upright surfaces in the home: doors, windows, new objects, family member possessions, or frequently used furniture	May eliminate on specific surfaces or selected locations but may also have no obvious preference

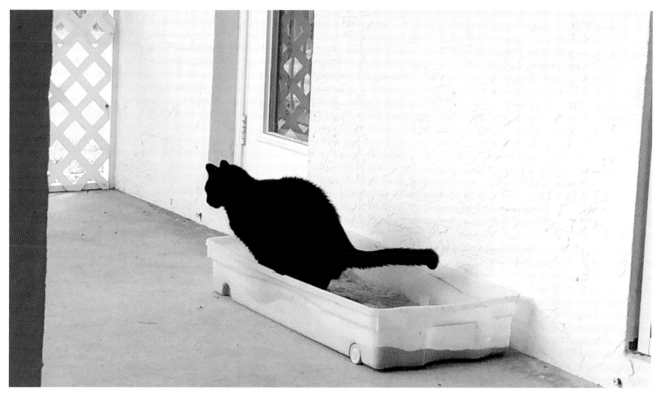

Figure 22.3 Appropriate litterbox size. *(Attribution: Lisa Radosta.)*

not be disturbed during elimination and sites away from feeding and resting areas.[7,9,17,22]

Cats, like us, have their own preferences. Litter preferences are no exception. Regarding scented versus unscented litter, studies to date have shown no general preference among cats[18,35]; however, cats do not like the odor of strong cleaning disinfectants.[37] In a number of studies, an activated carbon litter (i.e., Fresh Step) was preferred over similar clumping litters and those enhanced with baking soda,[38][10] but updated research on feline litter preference is needed.

The preferred substrate is usually absorbable, loose and soft, allowing the cat to dig and create an indentation in which to deposit urine or feces preelimination and allowing for the cat to perform a burying ritual post elimination.[7,8] Important substrate factors include texture, granularity, and coarseness. Although there may be wide individual variability between cats and households and although more recent studies are needed, prior studies have demonstrated that cats prefer fine-grained, clumping litter over coarse or pearl-like textures, clay, recycled paper, and a light-weight flushable litter with a pH indicator.[41-43] Some cats may prefer clay or silica substrates over wood pellets for urination, with cats preferring clay over silica for defecation specifically.[44] Other cats might be attracted to a mixture of potting soil or sand, especially if they also eliminate in these substrates outdoors.[9] In a study of 56 cats in a residential cattery, 93% of urine patches and 96% of deposited feces were covered when sufficient litter depth was provided.[45]

Whether the cat prefers a covered or uncovered litterbox depends on the individual. One study found no preference[46] while another study showed that most cats preferred uncovered litterboxes when offered appropriately sized boxes (86 × 39 × 14 cm).[37] Covered boxes of inadequate size compromise a larger cat's ability to posture normally and may trap unpleasant scent or odor, causing some cats to avoid covered litterboxes.[9]

Prevalence

House soiling is the most commonly reported behavior problem by general practitioners[47] and has historically been the most common behavior problem for which cat parents seek assistance at veterinary behavior specialty clinics, representing up to two-thirds of all cases; this frequency may be on the decline while aggression cases increase, possibly reflecting the changes in the skill set of the primary care practitioner.[17,48-52] The prevalence of house soiling disorders in cats has varied across studies. Of feline house-soiling cases presented to behavior specialty practices in four countries, 25–70% exhibited undesirable urination, 6–32% exhibited undesirable urination and defecation, 5.5–30% exhibited urine marking, and 9–20% exhibited unacceptable defecation only.[50-53] Male and female cats are equally as likely to house soil, but males are more likely to mark/spray.[14] In one study, 74% of cat parents sought help from their veterinarian for urine marking problems.[36] Persian cats are more frequently presented for elimination problems.[15,47,48,50-52]

Etiology and predisposing factors

Physical disease

Physical disease is often the primary cause of feline house soiling.[7] House soiling can be due to any condition that affects urinary tract health (e.g., feline lower urinary tract disease [FLUTD] including feline idiopathic cystitis [FIC], bacterial cystitis, urinary bladder tumor, cystolithiasis, urethrolithiasis; renal calculi);[8,10,17,53] causes changes in urine or fecal consistency (e.g., inflammatory bowel disease, infiltrative bowel disease, intestinal parasites, pancreatitis, endocrine disease, metabolic disease, or a space-occupying abdominal mass, food allergy, food sensitivity, constipation); volume or frequency (e.g., diabetes mellitus, kidney disease, hyperthyroidism) or control; causes increased pain, discomfort, or altered mobility during elimination (e.g., osteoarthritis, neuropathic pain, anal sacculitis, obesity, neuropathies); or affects cortical control of thirst and/or elimination.[1,7–9] Other physical health conditions affecting cognition and elimination behaviors include age-related cognitive decline, sensory impairment, neurological disease, and endocrine disease, including hyperthyroidism.[8,9]

FIC is an exclusionary diagnostic term for inflammatory changes in the urinary bladder than cannot be explained by identifiable physical causes. It is a complex disease that is not fully understood. It has also been termed Pandora's syndrome to describe a disorder that does not arise directly from the lower urinary tract and that is connected to underlying stress.[54] The condition bears some resemblance to interstitial cystitis in human females.[54] Like other forms of FLUTD, FIC can be associated with urinating in atypical locations, frequent urination, stranguria, hematuria or discolored urine, dysuria, and in emergency circumstances, an inability to void urine. When present, FIC may be self-limiting and only occur once, may occur intermittently throughout the cat's life at various frequencies, and may be chronic and persistent.[9] Having lower activity levels, living in a multicat household, and being indoor only may increase a cat's risk of FIC.[55,56] Research has found that comorbid disorders including problems with the nervous system[57,58] pet parent-observed gastrointestinal signs, self-scratching and fearful, nervous and aggressive behaviors commonly occur in cats with FIC.[57,59,60] It has also been suggested that feline interstitial cystitis may cause general anxiety in cats[61] and that behavioral changes including increased startle responses and excessive under- or over- attachment to pet parents may be present concomitantly with FIC.[62]

Periuria is the most common clinical sign reported by parents of cats with FLUTD,[63] and a history of lower urinary tract disease has been shown to increase the likelihood of periuria nearly threefold.[53] The most common causes of FLUTD in cats are FIC and uroliths, with neoplasia and bacterial cystitis more likely in older cats.[64–67] Approximately 20% of cats with feline lower urinary tract disease have cystic calculi.[68] Of cats with FLUTD, the majority (55–69%) of cases are idiopathic.[56,69,70] FIC may be difficult to distinguish from behavioral periuria since both conditions may be precipitated by stress.[71–73] Currently, no single specific diagnostic test or marker will confirm FIC. In one study, approximately half of cats with house soiling as the only reported sign were found to have idiopathic cystitis as diagnosed by uroendoscopy.[68]

While undesirable urination has been consistently associated with urinary tract abnormalities, the research on the association between FLUTD and urine marking is inconsistent. Some studies have found that urinary tract disease does not appear to be correlated with urine-marking behavior,[1,74] while other research has suggested that spraying behavior is associated with a higher level of urinary tract abnormalities.[10,75] Cats with FIC may urine mark.[10] Increases in testosterone may

result in urine marking and other tomcat behaviors in neutered cats.[76–78] In one study, physical conditions were more frequent (38.9%) in spraying cats than controls in the same household (5.5%). In that study, physical problems were diagnosed in 39.1% of cats with undesirable toileting compared to 26.1% of controls, indicating that households with undesirable toileting may have higher levels of concurrent physical disease than in spraying households.[10]

Any disease that causes decreased mobility or pain, especially related to passing urine or feces or accessing the litterbox, may lead to house soiling.[8,9,61,79] Cats with osteoarthritis or intervertebral disc disease may be unable or unwilling to access litterboxes that require them to walk up a flight of stairs, jump onto a raised surface, or step over high sides.[61,80] Declawed cats are at greater risk of developing chronic pain and house soiling. In a study comparing 137 declawed to 137 nondeclawed cats in which cats were assessed for pain and behavior problems, and were radiographed, declawed cats were more likely to experience back pain, barbering, have an altered gait, and exhibit periuria, perichezia, and aggression when compared to the nondeclawed cats.[81] In that study, the use of optimal surgical technique did not eliminate the risk of adverse behaviors developing subsequent to onychectomy.[81] However, another study did not find a greater incidence of house soiling in declawed cats when compared to nondeclawed cats; however, in this study, radiographs and pain assessment were not conducted.[18] The assessment of pain in animals is challenging, but it is central to veterinary practice and patient welfare, and should be a component of every physical examination.[80,82] Therefore, the veterinarian should be familiarized with pain recognition and assessment in cats (see Chapter 6).

Obesity can increase the risk of urinary tract disease in cats,[83] which can, in turn, increase the risk of house soiling. Age-related conditions such as cognitive dysfunction and any disorders that cause impairment of neurologic and sensory functions should also be considered potential causes of feline house soiling.[1,8,84] One study found that 36% of cats over the age of 11 years reported to suffer from cognitive dysfunction syndrome.[85]

If a physical disorder is found, it should not be assumed to be the cause of the house soiling,[1] as the cat may have multiple problems. All other potential physical, environmental, and social causes of house soiling should be considered for all cases. This is no different than a dog with hypoadrenocorticism that presents with vomiting needing a full workup to ensure that the dog did not develop a gastrointestinal obstruction or pancreatitis concomitant to their Addison's disease.

Furthermore, house soiling due to an organic disease may continue even after the physical problem is resolved. Pain or discomfort associated with elimination can lead to the development of learned negative associations between painful micturition with the litterbox and/or site of the litterbox,[8,61] leading to avoidance of the litterbox, substrate, or location, and the development of new location or substrate preferences, thereby not returning to litterbox use after the physical issue has been treated.[7,18] Therefore, finding and treating a physical disorder does not exclude the presence of a comorbid emotional disorder (and vice versa) and the need for environmental management and behavioral modification, even if the physical disorder is controlled or resolved.[8]

Urine marking

Urine marking is a sexually dimorphic behavior, occurring with a higher frequency in male cats.[50,52] In one study of 256 cats presented to a university behavior service for urine marking or spraying, 75% of the cats were male.[50] Intact male cat urine has a particularly powerful pungency, likely due in part to felinine levels.[86] The behavior appears to be facilitated by sexual hormones because the incidence of spraying is higher in intact animals and enhanced in the springtime by females in estrus.[87] Therefore, intact male and female cats may urine mark to communicate their availability for mating. However, urine marking is not completely dependent on hormones since 10% or more of males and 5% or less of females will continue to spray following gonadectomy.[88–90] In clinical trials for a urine-marking study, neutered males were significantly overrepresented at 85% of cases.[91] This is likely because the neural circuitry in the male is established prior to birth.[92]

In addition to intact status increasing the risk of urine marking, one study found that marking cats were more likely to be older (median of 9.5 years) and have free access to the outdoors or cat flaps, and were less likely to be described as "relaxed," which may indicate that in pet cats, urine marking has a stress or anxiety component.[1] Living in multicat households is also a risk factor for both urine-marking and toileting behaviors, although the influence appears to be greater with marking.[1,7,8,93]

Undesirable elimination – aversions and preferences

Undesirable elimination outside of a physical etiology is generally divided into two main categories – aversions and preferences. The cat may develop aversions to litterbox factors (i.e., size and cleanliness of the box), the litterbox substrate (e.g., type of litter) or the litterbox site (e.g., location, reduced access due to the presence of other pets or children). Preferences may develop for certain surfaces (e.g., soft, absorbent, unscented litter) and/or locations (e.g., quiet location, bed, rug).[93]

Litterbox aversion is a common diagnosis in house-soiling cats.[64] With litterbox aversion, cats may object to any aspect of the toileting experience including how clean the box is kept, its size, whether it is covered or uncovered, the presence of a liner and use by other cats. Poor litter hygiene is considered the leading cause of undesirable elimination.[9,11] The physical accumulation of waste or odors may create an aversion to the box. One study found that the visual presence of waste was more aversive than the odor of waste.[94] In that study, the presence of fake, odorless urine and/or feces caused cats to avoid using the litterbox in which the fake deposits were placed, suggesting that it wasn't the odor, or the identity of the user, but the visual and physical presence of the deposits that caused cats to avoid dirty litterboxes. In another study, cats shifted their preference for a larger litterbox to a cleaner litterbox as the larger box became more soiled.[37]

Because cats prefer larger boxes, smaller boxes may deter cats from using them. Litters fragranced with perfumes or baking soda to reduce the odors associated with elimination, while appealing to people, may be aversive to cats.[9,53] However, one study found no association between litterbox

factors – including size of the litterbox, absolute and relative number of the litterboxes, and type of litter – and periuria.[1] Yet another study found that a history of previous infection, the use of scented litter, and cats that did not cover their elimination were the only statistically significant risk factors for undesirable toileting.[53] Emphasizing that each cat will have his own preferences and that each household will differ in the challenges presented to the individual cat. See below for more information on diagnosis and treatment.

Aversions to the litterbox or litterbox location may also develop secondary to learning if a negative experience associated with the litterbox previously occurred,[9,61] including being medicated, disciplined, frightened by a sudden noise, or chased by another pet in the vicinity of the box.

Cats may develop a preference for a location that is quieter and more secure (e.g., further away from noisy appliances, protected from other animals or children)[7,9] or for a substrate which is more comfortable. Some cats may feel safest on the pet parent's bed, hence eliminating there instead of the litterbox.[9] Furthermore, the cat may have started eliminating in secluded areas in order to avoid family members, especially if they had been previously punished (e.g., scolded, squirted with a water bottle, yelled at, swatted, pushed away, hit) in or near the litterbox. Some cats may prefer a substrate that is softer, less coarse and more absorbent than litter, such as carpet, clothing, or bedding.[7,11,23,44] This is not surprising, considering that not only are these materials soft and absorbent, but they are often located in spacious areas that offer easy access and retreat, and are extremely well cleaned by the pet parent each time urine or feces is found. Some cats may prefer tubs, showers, and sinks, perhaps because the waste is immediately eliminated through the drain.

Indoor only

The availability of access to the outdoors has been associated with a lower incidence of undesirable elimination, which may be due to less frequent litterbox use leading to increased litterbox cleanliness or to an increased appeal of the outdoor substrates and locations.[1,95–96] Indoor-only cats rely only on what has been provided for them for mental, emotional, and physical enrichment. This may be problematic if solely indoor cats do not have the provisions to meet their needs,[97] which may lead to house-soiling problems. Granting outdoor access to indoor cats with undesirable elimination is not a recommended solution, as this poses significant health, safety, and welfare issues, but the importance of sufficient environmental enrichment that encourages natural feline behaviors in the household cannot be overstated.[98] With regard to urine marking, one study found that cats with free access to the outdoors (and cat flaps in the house) had a higher incidence of marking, possibly due to increased interactions with cats outside and increased exposure to novel scents.[1]

Role of fear, anxiety, stress, conflict, and panic (FASCP) in house soiling

Any physical, environmental or social change that causes FASCP or frustration, such as a new baby, adult, or animal household member, relocation to a new home, remodeling, change in the pet parent's daily schedule or routine, changes in pet parent interactions with the cat, and suboptimal litterbox management, as well as social tension and conflict with other pets, may contribute to the onset of house soiling.[1,7,11,93,95,99] A stressed cat may be less willing to tolerate substandard toilet facilities.[11]

Both environmental and social stressors are commonly implicated in the development of urine marking,[24,28,91] and cats described as "relaxed" being less likely to urine mark.[1] Because urine marking may develop secondary to sexually intact status, territoriality, and stress, both confident and anxious cats can mark.[7,9] In neutered cats, urine marking is largely caused by acute and chronic stress.[7] Spraying during situations of stress, anxiety, and conflict may be a form of displacement behavior, helping the pet to cope with stress. Potential stressors that may cause marking include intruders (usually in the form of nonresident cats outside of the home), novel sights, sounds, or odors, especially from other cats, insufficient mental stimulation, pet parent absences, fear-evoking interactions with family members, and tension between pets or with a family member.[9,24] Furthermore, urine-marking episodes may coincide with FIC relapses since they are both triggered by stress.[7,24]

Interspecies interactions

Despite their solitary ancestry, domestic cats are social animals.[100,101] Humans often act as integral social partners for cats, as many cats spend more time with humans than they do with conspecifics.[102–104] There is evidence that cats form attachment bonds to their pet parents.[100–101] and that how they perceive their daily interactions with people in the home affects their behavior.[97] There is evidence that pet parents who spent several hours throughout the day with their cats report fewer problem behaviors.[100] Affiliative behaviors that may indicate the cat has positive bonds to their pet parents include approaching with an erect tail curled like a question mark at the tip, purring during interactions, rubbing on their pet parent's legs or other body parts, lying on their pet parent's laps or against their pet parents, and greeting meowlike vocalizations.[21,100,105] See Chapters 2 and 24 for more information on body language and social behavior (see Figure 22.4).

Studies have shown that cats and dogs can live harmoniously with each other and develop amicable relationships including play, proximity, nose-to-nose greeting, sleeping together, and cats rubbing against dogs with which they are friendly.[106–108] In a survey of 1270 pet parents whose household consisted of at least one dog and one cat, more than half of the cats formed interspecific social bonds with familiar dogs, including friendly interactions, sleeping or playing together, while 18% did not and 1% had aggressive interactions.[109]

In a survey of 748 pet parents, 20.5% of the cats were reported as uncomfortable in the dog's presence once a week or more, approximately 50% rarely or never played together, and over 30% had an amicability rating of 5 or less (out of 10).[109] For these reasons, interactions between cats and dogs should be examined as a part of the history for any cat presenting for undesirable elimination.

Intraspecies interactions

While cats may cohabitate in the same household, this does not necessarily mean that they develop social cohesion. Cats

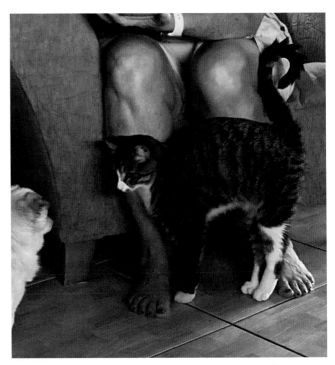

Figure 22.4 Question-mark tail is displayed before or during affiliative behavior. *(Attribution: Krista Sirois.)*

living with other animals occupy smaller ranges within a home,[110] which may limit access to space and resources in the home. Tension between housemate cats may arise in response to competition for resources, including food, space, and desirable elimination sites.[108] Certain cats may monopolize access to food, litterboxes, eating and perching spots, and attention,[9,16,108] which may cause other household cats to seek out undesirable places for elimination.[111,112] Aggression between housemate cats may occur secondary to social tension and is most likely to occur when a new cat is introduced to the household, when a resident cat has been absent and returns to the home (such as after a veterinary visit), and when there is competition for resources.[16] In a study of 2492 households with multiple cats, almost 17% of the households reported intercat aggression.[113]

Living in a multicat household has been shown to be a risk factor for house-soiling disorders,[1,7,17] with increased population density within the home appearing to have a greater influence on the incidence of marking in cats.[1,91,93] Cats are twice as likely to engage in undesirable elimination and six times more likely to engage in marking behavior if they live with one or more other cats,[1] with studies finding that 74–89% of marking cats lived in multicat households.[1,17,91] In one study, pet parents identified agonistic interactions with other cats in the household and outside of the household as common potential causes of their cat's urine spraying.[91] In multicat households, urine spraying may occur to delineate territory or may occur due to a lack of adequate resources or space, leading to increased stress.[7] Male cats that live with a female cat are more likely to spray than those living with another male.[89] Furthermore, cats with FIC are more likely to be in conflict with a housemate cat,[55] with more frequent flareups of FIC potentially leading to more frequent occurrences of house soiling. While one study did not find a significant association between living with at least one other cat, interactions with other cats outside, and living in conflict with other cats inside or outside of the home in cats with FIC compared to controls, living in conflict with another cat may have been underestimated as the signs of intercat conflict may be subtle and easily missed.[56] In situations where aggression between housemate cats exist, both the aggressor and the victim may develop undesirable elimination disorders or other undesirable behaviors.[16]

The role of learning

Behavior is always being reinforced or punished, even when pet parents are not involved. When a cat eliminates, the behavior is inherently reinforced because the pressure in the bladder subsides. The stimuli in the environment can become paired with the alleviation of urinary bladder pressure, causing the cat to repeat the behavior in the future. This can lead to the persistence of house-soiling behaviors, even if the physical or emotional ailment that caused it has been treated. See Chapter 10 for more information on reinforcement of behaviors. For example, a change in the type of litter may have caused the cat to initially avoid the litterbox; however, the cat may have acquired a new preference for carpet that persisted after the pet parent switched back to an acceptable brand of litter. In this example, the initiating factor was a litter change and the maintaining factor is the new preference for the softer material. As another example, a cat with FIC may have started urinating in a closet due to pain during micturition and developed a preference for the quiet location of the closet compared to the noisy location of the litterbox next to the washing machine. Even when the dysuria secondary to FIC diminishes, the cat may still prefer the quieter location and/or their aversion to the previous location or litter may persist. In these cases, identifying the factors maintaining the house soiling behavior is important to curtail the problem and to prevent the problem from recurring.

Stress

Being able to identify and assess FASCP in cats is essential to diagnosing and treating elimination problems. Cats communicate their emotional states through visual, tactile, olfactory, and auditory means. See to Chapter 2 for more discussion on how to interpret feline body language. More overt signs of FASCP including hissing, growling, spitting, swatting, and biting are often recognized by pet parents, but more subtle communication, including avoidance, withdrawal, decreased exploration and play behavior, hypervigilance, restlessness, decreased grooming, increased hiding, and changes in appetite (e.g., anorexia or overeating) may be overlooked.[16,111,114–117] Therefore, pet parents may not realize that social stress between cats can be related to the house-soiling problem, and they often assume that a lack of overt fighting is evidence that the cats are interacting comfortably.[7,117]

Specific body language changes that may be seen in cats with FASCP and frustration include holding the body close to the ground, tense musculature, flattening or rotation of the ears, tail wrapped closely or tucked under the body, gaze aversion, dilated pupils, piloerection, whiskers held back, and nose licking and wrinkling.[114] Avoidance is a preferred strategy for coping with stress in cats.[114,115] Avoidance behaviors range from gaze aversion to physically running away.[115]

The more commonly overlooked signs of social tension between cats include avoiding one another, walking around one another, blocking the movement of another cat, waiting for another cat to pass before moving into an area, retreating when another cat approaches, actively displacing another cat from a favorite resting location, avoiding eye contact, staring at another cat, pawing at another cat, or chasing another cat.[16,116,117] The lack of behaviors that indicate bonding between cats (such as play, allogrooming, sharing resources, and close proximity) may also be indicative of problems between cats.[7] One study found that conflict behavior between cats, from most to least frequently displayed, included staring, chasing, stalking, fleeing, twitching of the tail, hissing, and screaming.[113] A cat that is victim to aggression from another cat often becomes withdrawn.[16] If social tension exists between cats in the household, cats may seek seemingly more safe locations for elimination.[16]

If the cat is urinating on top of specific items, such as a family member's clothing, bed, favorite chair, or children's toys, this may suggest social tension with family and an anxiety-evoked problem should be considered.[7] On the other hand, for some cats, these surfaces may offer an appealing odor or texture for toileting (see Tables 22.3 and 22.4).

Table 22.3 Factors that may contribute to undesirable elimination

Litterbox aversion	• Aversive odor (deodorant, organic waste)
	• Box not cleaned frequently enough
	• Unacceptable litter (depth, texture, odor)
	• Unacceptable box (too small, covered, plastic liner)
	• Disciplined, medicated, or frightened in or near the box by humans, other pets
	• Discomfort during elimination
Location aversion	• Too much activity in the area
	• Traumatic/fearful experience in the area
Location preference	• Another area is more appealing to the cat
Surface preference	• Another surface is more appealing than the litter substrate
FASCP	• Pet parent absence • Multicat household • Environmental changes – moving, renovating, new people or pets in the household, new furniture • Punishment • Internal
Pathophysiological	• FLUTD • Pain (OA, IVDD, declawed, other) • Endocrine • Metabolic • Gastrointestinal • Neurological • Cognitive dysfunction • Sensory decline

Table 22.4 Factors that may contribute to marking

Sexual status	• Intact males • Estrus females
Territorial	• New cats in household or neighborhood • Scents from other cats on items entering the home
Social FASCP	• Multicat household • Punishment • Changes in pet parent schedule • Pet parent departures
Environmental FASCP	• Moving • Renovating • New people or pets in the household • Novel objects
Pathophysiological	• FLUTD • Pain (i.e., DJD, declawed, IVDD, other) • Endocrine • Metabolic • Gastrointestinal • Neurological • Cognitive dysfunction • Sensory decline

Prevention

Prevention of undesirable toileting centers on promptly addressing any physical issues that may cause pain or discomfort during elimination and providing an environment best suited to the cat's needs.

Optimizing the litterbox environment

Individual cat preferences should be determined and met as discussed above in the section Normal Feline Elimination Behavior and Preferences and the section Etiology and Predisposing Factors. With poor litter hygiene being the leading cause of elimination problems,[11] litterbox cleanliness and odor control should be primary considerations. Pet parents should scoop waste from the litterboxes at least once daily, with more frequent waste removal being even better.[9] The pet parents should also empty entire contents of the litterbox, wash the litterbox with dish soap and hot water, and refill the box with fresh litter once weekly, though every 2–4 weeks may be acceptable for some cats.[7,9] Though no research has evaluated how often litterboxes should be replaced, ideally used boxes should be replaced if they retain odor after being washed or if they are older than two years.[7]

A general rule of thumb is that the more boxes and the bigger the boxes, the better.[7–9,33,34] Pet parents should aim for at least one box per cat plus one additional box ($n + 1$).[7,9,112] While this is generally recommended for all households with cats, it may not be an absolute requirement, as socially affiliated cats may be willing to share litterboxes.[7,9] Litterboxes that are placed next to one another should be considered as one large box.[9] The opening of adjacent boxes should not face one another so that cats exiting the box can avoid an approaching cat.[9] Larger-sized boxes prevent an accumulation of waste from deterring cats from using them. Boxes should

be at least 1.5 times the length of the cat from nose to tail base or at least 91 cm in length, whichever is bigger.[9,33] Because many commercial litterboxes are often too small, pet parents should be encouraged to use under-the-bed storage bins, sweater boxes, and other large storage containers that can be purchased at a home improvement store or department store.

Whether to use open or closed litterboxes is decided by the cat's personal preference. Open boxes may be preferred by pet parents so that they can more easily monitor the hygiene of the litterbox and scoop eliminations from the litterbox,[9] while covered boxes may be preferred for cats that soil over the edge of the litterbox. Cats tend to dislike litterbox liners.[7] Automatic self-cleaning boxes may not be acceptable to some cats.

Scented litters, while appealing to people, may be aversive to cats, and they do not reduce or eliminate the need to regularly clean the litterbox and maintain its hygiene.[9] Therefore, it might be prudent to offer both scented and unscented litters in a preference test. Finer-textured, granular, sandlike litters should be used.[7,9,14,43] Most cats prefer clay clumping litter.[7,9,41] The litter depth should be at least 1.25 inches (3 cm);[7,9] greater litter depth may be preferred for feces.[45] If elimination frequency and/or volume are increased by disease, more frequent cleaning, more litterboxes, self-cleaning litterboxes, or a larger litterbox may be required.

Litterboxes should be placed in easy to access, low-traffic areas.[16] Litterboxes should be far from noisy appliances, including the washer and dryer, as well as from air vents and windows or doors that are adjacent to sidewalks or passersby. The litterboxes should also be placed in locations that are not too hot or too cold, such as in garages in the summer or winter or next to radiators. Litterboxes should be located away from the cat's other resources including food and water bowls as well as resting and hiding places,[9] though one study suggested that cats may prefer to have a litterbox closer to where they eat.[18] One exception to this is that geriatric or painful cats may need their litterboxes to be located closer to their resources with easy access and entry. Furthermore, litterboxes should be placed in multiple locations around the house so that the cat has options,[9] and on all floors of the home for geriatric cats and cats with mobility issues.[9,23] For cats that need privacy, the pet parent may offer a covered box or may place a baby gate in the doorway of the litter area to limit entry from other animals and people in the home. Children should be instructed not to approach litterboxes. All boxes should have more than one entry and exit point so that the cat can avoid or escape approaches from other pets or people while using the litterbox (see Figure 22.3).

Role of neutering in the prevention of urine marking

Neutering reduces urine marking and urine odor in intact male cats as well as the marking associated with estrus in female cats. It eliminates urine marking in 90% of adult male cats.[88,89] Age of gonadectomy does not appear to be a factor in the cat's tendency to spray as an adult.[78] One study that evaluated the effects of gonadectomy performed before 24 weeks and after 24 weeks of age also did not find an increased incidence of behavior problems in the early neutered cats three years after castration.[118] While neutering does prevent and decrease the frequency of spraying in most cats, it does not prevent the behavior in all cats. Of cats neutered between 6 and 10 months of age, about 10% of adult males and 5% of females become urine markers as adults.[89]

Preventing FASCP

Sufficient environmental enrichment is necessary to decrease environmental stress and social tension between cats and prevent elimination problems, particularly urine marking.[1,6,8,9,23,28,119,120] Ensuring that the cats can access a variety of resource-rich areas[23,28,97] permits them to disperse to different spaces in a restricted space,[10] thereby potentially reducing conflict between them. One study found that increased space improved play behavior, which is commonly accepted as an indicator of positive welfare.[121] Multiple feeding and water stations located at multiple levels and in quiet spots offer cats secure places to eat and drink apart from other household cats.[16] There should be plenty of vertical and horizontal space, vertical and horizontal scratching posts, hiding spaces, and toys such that each of these resources are accessible to all cats without the cats having to interact with one another. Large-sized enrichment items, such as cat trees, are recommended for multicat households.[97] Feeding stations, resting places, and hiding places should have more than one entry and exit point to minimize interactions between the cat and other pets or people in the household around these resources. Also see feline environmental needs, enrichment resources, and discussion of feline aggression in Appendix A, Chapters 5, and 24.

Pet parent interactions with the cat should be structured, predictable, and positive, and punishment in the form of yelling, startling, pushing, or hitting the cat should never occur, as this may cause FASCP, undermine the cat's relationship with the pet parent, and cause behavior problems or make existing behavior problems worse.[7,24] Changes in the environment, routine, or schedule should also be minimized or avoided. New scents, such as gym bags or furniture, and the scents of other cats, including clothing that may have picked up the scent of another cat, should not be brought into the home or should be washed before being brought into the home.[9,24]

Because urine marking may be due to territorial stress, if there are outdoor cats present, then the household cat's furniture, resting perches, food areas, and litterboxes should be placed away from locations where the cat might visualize the nonresident cats. This can be accomplished by using baby gates, window film, or closed doors. Outdoor cats should be deterred from remaining on the property by using pet repellants, sprays, or sprinklers. Nothing that might attract outdoor cats such as garbage, food, or bird feeders should be left out in the yard.

Introducing cats to multicat households

Properly introducing cats to a household with existing cats is key to preventing intercat aggression and feline elimination disorders.[8,28] The veterinary healthcare team is responsible for guiding pet parents through the process of successfully integrating new cats into the household, as pet parents often seek information from unreliable sources, including the internet and friends or family. Misinformation may lead to improper introductions, which may lead to increased FASCP of the cats in the household and the development of behavior problems. In a survey study completed by 128 people who introduced a new cat to a household with preexisting cats, half reported fighting between the new cat and existing cats when the new cat was introduced. Of these households, 35% of them reported that the fighting continued during the subsequent 12-month period.[122] To prevent aggression and conflict behaviors between cats, gradual introduction of the cat into the household is recommended.[123] See Chapter 2 for interpretation of feline body language and Chapter 24 for a complete discussion of how to introduce cats.

Litterbox training

Litterbox training newly acquired cats can help establish consistent elimination habits, preventing the onset of elimination problems. Litterbox training is often simple, as cats will naturally seek out the litterbox as long as it meets their needs. Litterbox training can begin around four weeks of age in kittens, which is the time that kittens start voluntarily eliminating and exploring new substrates,[14,112] or as soon as older kittens or adult cats are brought home. The household should contain one litterbox per cat plus an additional one, and the litterboxes should be of adequate size (see above). A combination of covered and uncovered litterboxes should be provided to help determine the cat's preferences. Initially, the litter which was used before adoption should continue to be used. Litter can be changed out based on the cat's preferences in the future, after the cat is fully litterbox trained. See sections above for a discussion on general feline litterbox preferences. Initially, the cat should be confined to a smaller room or area of the house, such as a large bathroom or a bedroom, so that the litterbox is more easily accessible. Remove other substrates including rugs, mats, clothing, and houseplants containing potted soil to reduce the likelihood that the cat develops an elimination preference for another substrate. The pet parent should show the cat the locations of each litterbox and allow the cat to sniff and investigate the boxes. Then the cat should be gently placed in the litterbox, as long as the cat is comfortable with being picked up. If the cat avoids, runs away or tries to get away, tenses, or becomes aggressive in response to being picked up, then the pet parent should lure them into the litterbox with a favored food or toy. Once inside of the litterbox, the cat may instinctively start digging in the litter. If they do not, then the pet parent may gently rub their fingers through the litter to stimulate the cat's natural digging action. The cat should be placed in the litterbox when they wake up, after they eat or drink, and after they play until they begin to use the box consistently on their own. When the cat eliminates in the litterbox, the pet parent should reinforce this behavior with a treat or by praising or petting, using whichever reinforcer is preferred by the cat. (See Chapter 10 for determining reinforcement preferences.) Clicker training is an efficient and effective way to immediately mark the desired behavior of elimination in the litterbox in order to facilitate quicker or more effective learning. (See Chapter 10 for more information on clicker training cats.) The box should initially be scooped after each elimination to reduce the risk that the cat develops an aversion to a dirty litterbox. Once the cat is consistently eliminating in the litterbox for at least two weeks, then the frequency of scooping may decrease to several times daily. At this time, the cat can be removed from the confined space, but the litterboxes should remain in their current locations. If the location of the current litterboxes is undesirable to the pet parents, then the parents may add litterboxes to more preferred locations without moving the original boxes. After four weeks of the cat consistently using the litterboxes in the preferred locations, the pet parents may remove the litterboxes from the unfavored locations one at a time, or they may begin to gradually move the litterboxes in the unfavored locations by several inches every 5–7 days to more preferred locations. After another 2-4 weeks of consistent litterbox use, the frequency of scooping may be reduced to once daily. The pet parents may consider using a pheromone diffuser in the area of the litterboxes to provide a calming effect. See Chapter 12 for more discussion on the use of pheromones. Note that some cats will immediately and readily accept a litterbox, so confinement and litterbox movement may not be necessary. In these cases, the cat should initially be reinforced for litterbox use, but this may be withdrawn after 2–4 weeks of regular and consistent litterbox use.

Diagnoses

Diagnoses are made based on a description of what the cat is doing (e.g., marking, undesirable toileting) and the cat's preferences or aversions (e.g., substrate preference, location aversion). In addition, there are qualifiers which may be applied to any diagnosis. They include: (1) social stress; (2) environmental stress; (3) pathophysiological; (4) territorial; (5) sexual; (6) FASCP (see Box 22.1).

Urine marking (spraying)

Urine marking (spraying) involves the deposition of small amounts of urine on vertical or horizontal surfaces.[1,6,8] The diagnosis of urine marking or spraying is based on body posture, amount of urine, locations where the urine is deposited, behavior before and after urination, and the orientation of the urine. As noted above in the section Etiology and Predisposing Factors, urine marking can be sexual in nature and may be due to physical disease but in pet cats, is more often due to fear, anxiety, stress, conflict, panic, or frustration. Qualifiers for urine marking include: (1) urine marking (social stress); (2) urine marking (environmental stress); (3) urine marking (physical disease, FLUTD, etc.); (4) urine marking (territorial); and (5) urine marking (sexual). The posture of urine marking is characterized by (1) the cat backing up to an object with his rear end held high; (2) tail erect and quivering; (3) direction of the urine backward onto a vertical surface; and (4) alternate treading of the ground with the rear paws.[7,9,16,17,36] It is uncommon for cats to dig before spraying or cover the area afterward.[16,21] Horizontal marking may occur with vertical marking or alone (as the sole type of marking) with similar characteristics to vertical marking such as quivering the tail and walking away without sniffing.[11,112,124] Marking on pet parent or dog possessions such as clothes or bedding may indicate that the cat is anxious or conflicted about these relationships and that the stressors triggering the marking originate from within the home.[9] There are no substrate preferences with marking unless the elimination disorder is multifactorial, meaning that cats that are marking and do not have periuria

Pathophysiological (urine)
- FLUTD (FIC, bacterial cystitis, urinary bladder tumor, cystolithiasis, urethrolithiasis)
- Conditions causing polyuria or polydipsia (e.g., diabetes, renal, hyperthyroidism, psychogenic polydipsia)

Pathophysiological (feces)
- Conditions causing increased frequency/urge (chronic enteropathy, colitis, diarrhea, infiltrative bowel disease, endo parasitic, pancreatitis)
- Conditions causing painful or difficult defecation (anal sacculitis, obstipation, constipation, neoplasia)

Pathophysiological (both)
- Conditions causing pain (e.g., osteoarthritis, neurologic, declawed, urinary bladder, abdominal)
- Conditions causing incontinence (e.g., central, neurogenic, neuropathy)
- Conditions affecting locomotion (e.g., osteoarthritis, disc disease, muscle atrophy, neurologic)
- Miscellaneous conditions (e.g., metabolic disorders such as hepatic, hyperthyroidism, cognitive dysfunction, sensory decline, obesity)

Fear, anxiety, stress, conflict, panic
- Internal
- Environmental (move, renovation, lack of sufficient enrichment)
- Social (multicat household, new pet or family member, social tension with existing pet or family member)

Communication (marking)
- Sexual status
- Identity
- Territory

Aversions and preferences (undesirable elimination)
- Litterbox aversion (i.e., presence of organic waste, insufficient number of litterboxes, litterbox too small)
- Substrate aversion (i.e., deodorized litter)
- Location aversion (i.e., litterbox near noisy appliances or in high-traffic area of house)
- Substrate preference (i.e., soft, absorbent material such as carpet or soil)
- Location preference (i.e., quiet and private or inaccessible to other animals or small children in the home)

Learned association
- Cat developed aversion to litterbox or location due to prior adverse experience (i.e., cat experienced pain during elimination due to organic disease, cat was punished or medicated in or near the litterbox) and developed subsequent preference for new location or substrate

will urinate on various surfaces.[7] Marking cats generally continue to use litter for micturition and defecation (although some cats will present with both toileting and marking), see Figure 22.2.[10,112]

Litterbox aversion

Litterbox aversion can be diagnosed when elimination in the box is decreased or absent entirely and the cause is not a substrate or location preference. Cats with litterbox aversion will urinate on any substrate and in any location, but they avoid the litterbox due to a characteristic of the box, such as the location, type of litterbox, litter, size, or cleanliness, to which the cat objects. If the characteristic to which the cat is averse is intermittent, such as cleanliness of the box or pain, they may use the box intermittently and still have a litterbox aversion. So, while generally cats that have a litterbox aversion do not use the box for urine or feces, they may occasionally or intermittently continue to use the box, especially early on before the learned association has been made or a preference for another substrate or location has developed.

Substrate aversion

Substrate aversions occur when cats develop an objection to the substrate provided in the litterbox.[9] This may be due to the texture, coarseness, scent, or depth of the litter. Cats may perch on the edge of the litterbox (this can also indicate that the box is too small), differing from litterbox aversion. The use of the box is usually not intermittent but instead does not occur at all because the substrate to which the cat is adverse is always present. Cats with substrate aversion may urinate or defecate on any substrate and in any location outside of the litterbox. In other words, they do not have a substrate preference but instead simply have an aversion to the substrate that they are being offered in the box.

Location aversion

Cats with location aversion will not urinate in the location to which they are averse, which is generally where the litterbox is located, will eliminate in various locations other than the litterbox, will use the litterbox if it is moved to a different location, and will urinate or defecate on a variety of substrates.

Substrate preference

Cats with substrate preferences always or almost always eliminate on the same type of substrates. For example, the cat may choose smooth surfaces such as countertops and floors, soft surfaces such as sheets and towels, or plush surfaces such as carpet and bath rugs. Cats that have a substrate preference will use that substrate when it is available to them. They are usually not averse to using the litterbox or other substrates and may continue to use the litterbox or other substrates when their preferred substrate is not available. However, cats can have preferences and aversions. For example, a cat may prefer rugs, urinating on those when available, but choosing his litter when they are not available. However, if he also has a location aversion or litterbox aversion, then he may not return to using his litterbox when rugs are made unavailable. In this case, even though the main diagnosis is a substrate preference, the additional diagnoses will influence the outcome if not treated.

Location preference

Cats with location preferences always or almost always eliminate in the same location. Cats that have a location preference will use that location or several locations when they are available to them. They are not averse to using the litterbox. As such, they often continue to use the litterbox when their preferred location isn't available (e.g., door to room is closed). As mentioned above, cats can have preferences and aversions. For example, a cat may use the corner of the bedroom for defecation when accessible. When not

available, he chooses the litterbox. However, if he also has a substrate aversion, even though the main diagnosis is location preference, the substrate aversion will also have to be treated to resolve the elimination problem.

Stress-induced urination

Many of the cats that will be presented for house soiling will have a component of fear, anxiety, stress, conflict, or frustration. As a matter of fact, this may be the primary cause of cats urinating in undesirable locations. Whether the stress is due to physical or emotional causes, it can drive house soiling. Often, the veterinarian will not be able to distinguish a preference from an aversion or the effects of a physical disease from the effects of environmental stressors. For cats that are under physiologic and/or physical stress for which a diagnosis cannot be made, or for which it is clear that FASCP are components of their behavior, a diagnosis of stress-induced urination can be made. Later, if a preference or aversion becomes apparent during follow-up and treatment, the diagnosis can be revised if needed.

Treatment

Treatment includes reducing stress through environmental and social changes, treating underlying or contributing physical diseases, finding the cat's preferences and aversions, and providing the substrate, litter, litterbox, and location that he desires. Individual treatments are outlined below.

Approach to diagnosis and treatment in general practice

As stated above, undesirable elimination regardless of the form it takes is a common problem in pet cats which can lead to relinquishment and euthanasia. In one study, 74% of pet parents sought help from the veterinarian for urine-marking problems;[36] however, 25% of pet parents whose cats were eliminating outside of the litterbox did not seek help because they did not feel that the veterinarian could help.[36] The most efficient way to screen for elimination problems is to do it at each visit using a short, general behavior questionnaire such as the one provided online and listed in Appendix C. If the pet parent answers yes, their cat is eliminating outside of the litterbox, then a conversation about the problem can be initiated with the pet parent and an appointment to address the house-soiling issue can be scheduled if necessary.

As is the case with any behavioral disorder, approaching feline house-soiling problems requires an assessment of overall wellness and a comprehensive behavioral history to identify the underlying cause(s) and design a treatment plan that is appropriate for the cat and household. The behavioral history should focus on three key factors that may cause or contribute to house soiling: social, physical, and environmental factors, keeping in mind that these causative factors may coexist.[1,9]

Historically, the recommended approach to feline house-soiling cases included the veterinarian spending an hour or more with the pet parent to review a detailed questionnaire, obtain a thorough history, view videos and images of the home environment, and devise a comprehensive treatment plan. While that is still the standard of care, achieving that in one 15–30-minute appointment in veterinary practice is unrealistic. Instead, the veterinarian can achieve the same result over 3–4 appointments every 1–2 weeks without delaying treatment.

When approaching feline house-soiling cases, the veterinarian should first determine how they would prefer to see these cases. Consider whether the practice allows for hour-long appointments and whether a dedicated technician is available for these cases. A technician should be able to obtain a comprehensive history, educate pet parents on typical feline communication, explain the doctor's treatment plan including environmental modification recommendations, describe the follow-up plan, and follow-up with the pet parent one week after the initial appointment. See Chapter 1 for more discussion on the role of support staff.

Utilizing a questionnaire specific to feline house soiling speeds up the history-taking process, but depending on the length of the appointments, it may not be possible to collect all information at once. If the veterinarian plans to see house-soiling cases in 20–30 appointments, then multiple short, one-page questionnaires can be used at the first 2–3 appointments to obtain all of the necessary information in a piecewise fashion. If the veterinarian plans to see house-soiling cases in 60 or more minutes, then a single, longer, more comprehensive, questionnaire can be used at the initial appointment. See Appendix C for long and short questionnaires to be used for feline house-soiling cases.

Ideally, the client care representative who schedules the appointment would send a link to the questionnaire online so that the veterinary healthcare team will have the information prior to the appointment and need only to ask clarifying questions during the appointment. This allows for more time to be spent during the appointment performing diagnostics and educating the pet parent on treatment recommendations. If the questionnaire is not completed beforehand, then request that the pet parent arrive 10 minutes prior to the appointment to complete the form. Some pet parents may not be able to complete an online form and the information may have to be collected in the examination room. The same questionnaire form can still be used and filled out by a veterinary healthcare team member; however, if fitted into a standard general practice appointment, most of the time will be taken up collecting history.

Initially, rechecks should be scheduled every 1–2 weeks. After that time, the frequency of rechecks will depend on the cat's response to treatment. Recheck the patient every 1–2 weeks if the house-soiling problem does not improve, every 4–8 weeks if the problem improves but does not resolve, and every 12–16 weeks if the problem resolves. If the veterinarian intends to see feline house-soiling cases in multiple 20–30-minute appointments, then the following appointment structure is recommended.

First visit:
- Abbreviated questionnaire to obtain the initial history
- General wellness assessment
- Relief of FASCP using medications, supplement, diet, pheromone analogues
- MEMO - multimodal environmental enrichment

See Figure 22.5 and Box 22.2.

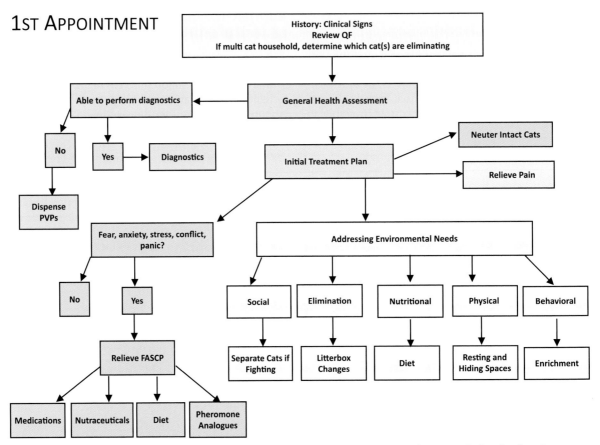

Figure 22.5 First appointment flow. *(Attribution: Alison Gerken.)* QF, Questionnaire Form (see Appendix C, online forms.)

Box 22.2 First appointment steps

1. Review initial questionnaire form. Ask clarifying questions.
2. If multicat household, determine which cats are eliminating
3. Perform general health assessment
   a. All house-soiling cats: physical, orthopedic, neurological exams; feline pain scale recommended
   b. Periuria: CBC, biochemisty, T4, UA, urinalysis, urine culture, whole-body radiographs ± abdominal ultrasound
   c. Perichezia: CBC, biochemistry, T4, fecal exam, whole-body radiographs ± abdominal ultrasound, rectal examination (under heavy sedation or anesthesia only)
   d. If unable to perform, start preveterinary visit pharmaceutical
4. Institute initial treatment plan
   a. Analgesic trial (NSAID, gabapentin)
   b. Anti-anxiety medications to reduce FASCP
   c. MEMO:
      i. Optimization of litterbox facilities:
         1. Increase number of boxes: $n + 1$
         2. Increase size of boxes: storage boxes
         3. Relocate boxes to quiet areas, all floors of the house
         4. Discontinue use of automatic litterbox
         5. Remove liners
         6. Use unscented, clay clumping litter
         7. Increase litter depth
         8. Try covered and uncovered litterboxes
         9. Scoop litterboxes at least once daily; more is better
         10. Empty box, clean with hot water and soap, and replace with fresh litter once weekly
      ii. Encourage litterbox reuse
         1. Clean elimination spots in the house with enzymatic cleaner
         2. Prevent access to undesirable elimination spots
      iii. Increase environmental enrichment
         1. Provide sufficient, multiple, and separated environmental resources including food and water stations, toileting areas, hiding, scratching, play and resting areas
         2. Provide safe space with places to hide
         3. Provide opportunities for play and predatory behavior
         4. Provide positive, consistent, predictable human–cat Interactions
         5. Discontinue all forms of punishment
   d. Separate fighting cats
   e. Neuter intact marking cats

Second visit (1–2 weeks later):

- Abbreviated questionnaire to obtain the history
- Evaluate pet parent treatment adherence and cat's response to treatment
- General wellness assessment
- Modifications to original plan
- MEMO - multimodal environmental enrichment
- Distinguishing between undesirable elimination and marking
- Specific recommendations to assess cat preferences and further lower stress in the household

See Figure 22.6 and Box 22.3.

If the veterinarian intends to see feline house-soiling cases in a one hour or longer initial assessment, then the first appointment would include a more detailed questionnaire to obtain a complete history, a diagnosis of the type of house soiling, a general wellness assessment, and a more tailored treatment plan. The first, second, and third appointments below could be combined into one or more longer appointments.

Ultimately, the treatment of feline house-soiling problems is dependent on regular followups to modify the treatment plan, guidance and support from the veterinary healthcare team to the pet parent, and pet parent adherence to recommendations. House soiling is an emotionally taxing problem for cat parents. Pet parents may remark that they are "at their wit's end" and considering relinquishment or euthanasia. When pet parents express hopelessness, it is important to show them empathy and provide them with realistic, tangible options. There are myriad environmental and social changes, as well as medications, that can be attempted to treat the house-soiling problem, so when pet parents express frustration or share that they are considering relinquishment or euthanasia, remind them of how many treatment options still exist and give them alternatives to what has proven unsuccessful. If a pet parent has expressed that they want to euthanize their cat for the house soiling problem, then the veterinarian may consider boarding the cat at their clinic to provide the pet parent with some immediate relief of the problem, allow more time for the pet parent to implement recommended changes to their environment, to observe the cat in a clinical setting for any signs that suggest that a physical condition may be underlying the house-soiling problem, and to initiate pharmaceutical therapy.[9] In addition, referral to a board-certified veterinary behaviorist should be considered for all cases where relinquishment or euthanasia is a potential outcome.

First appointment

At the first appointment, the team should focus on key factors to assess the environment and social interactions, perform a general health assessment, recommend changes to the environment which reflect the preferences of most cats, and reduce fear, anxiety, stress, conflict, and panic (see Figure 22.5 and Box 22.2).

First appointment history

As discussed above, the initial history for feline house-soiling cases that are being seen in a 20–30-minute general practice appointment is best obtained with a short questionnaire. While open-ended questions allow for the pet parent to express every observation, time in general practice is often limited. With this approach, closed-ended questions are utilized to get concise answers and guide treatment. Then, the pet parent can add additional information as needed.

Videos and pictures of the environment are valuable in that they allow the veterinarian to assess the environment entirely and to pick up on things that the pet parent may not have noticed. When the appointment is scheduled, the request should be made for pet parents to take short (no longer than one minute) videos and pictures including soiled areas, litterbox locations, feeding stations, drinking stations, sleeping and scratching locations, interactions with other animals and people inside and outside of the family, and enrichment opportunities. So that the videos can be viewed prior to the appointment, they can be sent by email, text, or file transfer link. Many pet parents will bring the videos on their smartphone, computer, or tablet to share. Some pet parents will not follow the recommendation to take images or videos. In that case, they can send them after the appointment, or the veterinarian can rely on history taking.

At the first appointment, the history should include:

Social factors

1. Is the cat indoor only or does it have access to the outdoors?
2. How many cats are in the household?
3. Which cat is house soiling?
4. Do the cats in the household sleep together and groom each other?
5. How often do the cats in the household avoid, hiss, growl, swat, or bite at each other?

Physical factors

1. What has been the duration of the house-soiling problem?
2. What are the frequencies of urination and defecation?
3. What is the frequency of house soiling?
4. How has the frequency of house soiling changed since the onset of the problem?
5. What is the appearance, volume, and consistency of feces and urine?
6. What is the cat's elimination posture? Does his posture remain consistent throughout the elimination sequence, or does he adjust his posture while eliminating?
7. Does the cat vocalize when eliminating?

Environmental factors

1. Where are urine and feces being deposited?
2. How many litterboxes does the cat have access to?
3. What sizes are the litterboxes?
4. Where are the litterboxes located?
5. Are there liners in the litterboxes?
6. Are the litterboxes covered or uncovered?
7. What type of litter is used in the litterboxes?
8. How often are the litterboxes cleaned?
9. What is used to clean the litterboxes and the eliminations outside of the litterbox?

Overall wellness

1. How is the cat's appetite?
2. Are there any changes in the cat's drinking habits?
3. Are there any changes to the frequency or volume of urine and/or stool?
4. How is the cat's activity level? Have there been any changes?
5. Does the cat run, jump, and play normally?
6. Have there been any changes to the cat's gait?

Previous treatments

1. What treatments have historically been implemented to address the house-soiling issue?
2. What was the cat's response to previous treatments?

Determine if any previous treatments, including changes to litterbox management, medications, pheromones, and behavior modification or training, have been instituted. Determine for how long each modality was applied and its efficacy. Keep in mind that previous treatments may not have been properly applied or used long enough. Inform pet parents that previous treatments may have to be repeated if they were tried incorrectly.

First appointment diagnosis

With the information collected in this initial appointment, the diagnosis may be apparent. On the other hand, only clinical signs may have been ascertained. A list of potential diagnoses is given in Box 22.1. At minimum, the veterinarian must be able to determine if there is fear, anxiety, stress, conflict, or panic in the household and any obvious deficits in the litterbox and social environments. A list of differentials or at minimum a description of the different manifestations of the cat's behavior should be made.

Social factors

Multicat households can pose a challenge in feline house-soiling cases since it may not be immediately evident which cat is soiling. Often, pet parents may feel very strongly that a certain cat is the culprit; however, the best practice is to assume that all cats are involved until proven otherwise. With urine marking, it is likely that more than one cat is marking.[7,17] In one recent study, fecal cortisol levels were significantly higher from all cats in households with urine spraying compared to households with toileting cats, suggesting that spraying cats are more aroused or stressed, as were their housemates that were not spraying. Therefore, appropriate management is required for all cats in the household and not just the spraying cat to alleviate stress.[6] Separation for a few days or weeks may seem adequate to find the perpetrator; however, separation changes the dynamics of the household and alters elimination habits. By separating the cats, one or all cats in the household may stop eliminating in undesirable areas, yielding no valuable insight as to which cat is the culprit. Another approach is to give fluorescein orally (0.5 mL of a 10% solution or the ends of six strips of 6-mg fluorescein into gel caps)[125] and assess any soiled areas with a Wood's lamp or black light for fluorescence, which will last up to 24 hours. However, one study found that fluorescein can stain carpet and does not fluoresce in acidic urine.[126] Bright-colored, nontoxic crayon shavings or nontoxic arts and crafts glitter can be added to canned food to identify which cat is fecal soiling. Often the best option is to monitor with a webcam or recording device to catch the culprit as well as view the soiling behavior, which will provide more information about its nature and potentially give clues as to its cause. Motion-activated webcams are readily available.

Furthermore, in multicat households, the nature of the cats' relationship needs to be considered, as social tension between cats may cause or contribute to house-soiling problems.[7] However, a thorough evaluation of these relationships is unlikely in a 20–30-minute appointment. Therefore, the initial assessment should focus on a few basic questions to assess for affiliative (sleeping together, allogrooming, allorubbing) or agonistic (avoidance, blocking, aggression) behaviors between the cats.

Physical factors

Evaluate the cat's elimination habits, including the duration of the house-soiling problem, the frequency of elimination, the appearance, consistency, and volume of urine and feces, the frequency of the house soiling, and changes to the frequency of house soiling over time (i.e., whether the frequency has increased, decreased, or maintained over time). Furthermore, the pet parent should describe the cat's posture when eliminating, including whether the cat is reluctant to crouch, crouches initially but then stands to complete the elimination, frequently adjusts their body posture when eliminating, hovers with some limbs inside of the litterbox and some limbs on the edge of the litterbox, and/or stumbles over the edge of the litterbox when entering or exiting the box.

Environmental factors

Obtain litterbox information, such as size, type of litterbox, number of litterboxes and locations, type of litter, whether the litterbox is covered or uncovered, the use of litterbox liners, whether there is a preferred litterbox, location, or litter and litterbox management, including frequency and type of cleaning. Also determine where the cat is depositing urine and feces outside of the litterbox and how those locations are being cleaned.

General health assessment

Identifying a physical health disorder early is essential for the treatment of the house-soiling problem as well as for the overall welfare of the cat. A general health assessment cannot be omitted and must be performed in all cats that present for house soiling, including a physical examination, orthopedic examination, and neurologic examination. At the initial appointment, the veterinarian should ask the pet parents about physical and behavior changes that may indicate pain in their cats. Using a validated pain assessment scale should be considered. See Appendix A resources Chapter 6 for a discussion on pain assessment tools. The cat's elimination posture may also provide a clue as to whether pain is contributing to the house-soiling problem. Cats that are reluctant to crouch, begin their elimination sequence crouched but finish standing (which may be a normal elimination pattern),[16] frequently shift their weight or reposition their body when postured, or stumble while entering the box may be painful. Furthermore, vocalization during elimination may also suggest pain[127] or distress and has been associated with periuria[128] and sexual marking.[9]

Reduced range of motion in joints, pain on palpation along the spine or on abdominal palpation, and/or hair loss on the caudoventrum may suggest orthopedic, musculoskeletal, neurological, abdominal, or urinary bladder pain.[9] Since animals, especially cats, have adaptive mechanisms which may mask signs of pain, the absence of overt signs of pain does not mean an absence of pain. For feline house-soiling cases, especially in older cats, pain should be a presumed possible cause of the soiling problem.

Baseline laboratory tests, including CBC, serum chemistry, T4, urinalysis, proBNP, fecal antigen + Giardia ELISA, urine culture, and radiographs to evaluate for cystic calculi and osteoarthritis, should also be performed on all cats with periuria.[7,9,10,129] If digital rectal examination is necessary, it should only be performed under sedation or anesthesia. Radiographs should be recommended in cats with house-soiling problems, especially in cats older than six years old, to evaluate for both calculi and osteoarthritis.[130] Other diagnostics should be recommended as indicated. Because some conditions such as FIC may occur intermittently and cause transient signs, repeat diagnostics may need to be performed. (See Chapter 6 on general wellness and physical influences of behavioral clinical signs.) The practitioner must bear in mind that a normal physical examination and normal laboratory results do not rule out some of the most common causes of feline house soiling, such as FIC and degenerative joint disease.[129]

In marking cats, determine if the cat has been gonadectomized. In male cats, examination of the penis for penile barbs or odorous urine might be indicative of the presence of male hormones arising from a retained testicle or testicle remnant.[131] In female cats, evidence of estrous behavior may exist. If these findings are present, hormonal assays should be performed. Standardized methods for evaluating testosterone levels in response to gonadotropin-releasing hormone have been developed.

First appointment treatment plan

See Tables 22.5 and 22.6, Box 22.2, and Figure 22.5.

Table 22.5 Treatment of urine marking

Goal	Approach
Rule out pathophysiological causes	• Perform diagnostic workup including CBC, biochemistry panel, T4, UA, urine culture and sensitivity, radiographs ± abdominal ultrasound.
Keep stimuli away from cat	• Eliminate outdoor stimuli. For example, if outdoor cats are the stimulus for spraying, discourage visits by humane removal or outdoor avoidance devices (e.g., motion detector sprinkler, cat repellents). • Move bird feeders and rubbish bins that attract cats. Remove stray cat urine from around windows and doors with odor eliminators. • Reduce the number of cats in the home. • Keep children, dogs, and visitors away from the cat.
Keep cat away from stimuli	• Keep the cat away from or block access to windows or other vantage points where he can view outdoor cats. • Use window coverings or close doors to prevent the cat from seeing stray cats. • White noise, TV, or music may reduce the sound of outdoor stimuli.
Surgery	• Castration reduces spraying in 90% of males and spaying in 95% of females.
Confinement	• When the cat cannot be supervised, confine away from areas where he sprays. • Relapses may be reduced by allowing the cat back into previously soiled areas gradually, with constant supervision and ensuring positive outcomes.

continued

Table 22.5 Treatment of urine marking—cont'd

Goal	Approach
Punishment	• Punishment should be avoided. If the pet parent views the cat as they are about to mark or is in the process of marking, they should interrupt the cat with a gentle noise such as a name-call or kiss, call them away, and then reward them. The pet parent should not use loud sounds (i.e., hand clap, shaking coins) or water spray as these may worsen fear and the problem.
Avoidance	• Avoidance devices might keep the cat away from areas where they mark. Place upside-down vinyl carpet runner (nubs up), double-sided tape, or aversive scents such as citrus, perfumes, or cat repellent in the area. However, this will only stop marking at the specific site. Do not use motion-activated sprays or alarms or mats that deliver a shock, as these may potentiate fear and worsen the problem.
Change function of sprayed area	• If a cat only marks one or two areas, consider placing their bedding, food bowls, scratching post, or toys in these areas.
Access to the outdoors	• Some cats will spray less indoors if they have some access to the outdoors, while others will do better if kept indoors all the time.
Provide alternate sites for marking	• If marking is limited to a specific area, provide litter box with higher sides, place box in tub or shower stall, or try covered box.
Environmental management	• Increasing the number of litterboxes, providing additional litter locations, increasing litterbox scooping to at least once a day, cleaning the box weekly, and using odor counteractants where the cat marks may address environmental factors that contribute to spraying. Also do preference testing to find the most appealing litter, box, and location.
Resolve social tension	• Inquire about body language when cat interacts with other cats, pets, or people in the home. • If social tension is present, separate cat from other cats or pets in the home. • Ensure resources, including enrichment items, are placed in multiple separate locations on all floors of the house and that there are different entry and exit points so that the cat can access resources without encountering another animal. • Do not permit small children to approach the cat during elimination.
Environmental enrichment to decrease FASCP	• Provide a calm, stable environment with sufficient enrichment, opportunities to engage in normal feline behaviors (e.g., climbing, perching, bedding, scratching, food, water, play, and exploration) and opportunities to avoid stressors/environmental control (perching, climbing, hiding).
Drug therapy to decrease FASCP	• Fluoxetine and clomipramine have been shown to be effective for eliminating or reducing marking, as may other drugs and supplements. • Pre-treatment lab tests should precede drug use to screen for underlying medical problems. • Transdermal application is unlikely to be effective for psychotropic drugs. • A drug response can be expected in one to four weeks, although eight weeks or longer may be required for maximal improvement. After two months or longer of effective control, the drug can be gradually reduced. Some cats may require long-term maintenance.
Pheromone therapy	• Feliway spray or diffuser may reduce spraying within one to four weeks. • Pheromone therapy can be combined with drug therapy.

Table 22.6 Treatment of undesirable elimination

Goal	Approach
Rule out pathophysiological causes	• Perform diagnostic workup including CBC, biochemistry panel, T4, UA, urine culture and sensitivity, radiographs ± abdominal ultrasound.
Litterbox optimization	• If the problem is due to litter or box aversion, then determine if the cause might be cleanliness, box size, litter liners, scent, covered box, or litter type through preference testing. • Increase number of boxes and size of boxes. • Determine favorite litter by providing additional boxes with a choice of substrates (e.g., clay clumping, recycled paper, etc.) • Determine favorite box by providing a choice of boxes (covered and uncovered, lower sides, larger, lined and unlined). • Scoop and refill litter at least once daily and clean boxes weekly. • Identify deterrents in the litter area (e.g., laundry equipment, temperature, lighting, flooring, furnace). Also determine if cat is being disturbed in the area by family members, other cats, or dogs. • If the problem is location aversion, move the box to the cat's preferred area and then gradually move it to a site preferable to the pet parents. • If the problem is substrate preference, offer the preferred substrate in the box, then gradually remove this substrate and replace with litter.

Table 22.6 Treatment of undesirable elimination—cont'd

Goal	Approach
Prevent access to soiled sites	• Move furniture over the soiled areas. • Block access or close doors to frequently soiled rooms.
Decrease desirability of inappropriate sites	• Reduce the appeal of previously soiled areas by removing carpet, placing a sheet of plastic, aluminum foil, vinyl carpet runner (nubs up), or double-sided tape in the area, or with aversive odors such as citrus or perfume. • Place food bowls, bedding, toys, scratching post, kitty condo, or a play center in the area. • Use chemical or enzymatic/bacterial odor eliminators. Be certain to use a sufficient amount of the product to saturate the entire area.
Confinement	• If soiling persists, confine the cat to a small area with litterbox where they do not soil and only allow them out when they can be supervised 100% of the time. Confinement should continue for long enough to reestablish reliable, consistent litterbox use. The cat can then be allowed out of confinement for gradually longer times each time the box has been successfully used as long as there is no recurrence of soiling.
Punishment	• Punishment should never be used. If the pet parent views the cat as they are about to mark or is in the process of marking, they should interrupt the cat with a gentle noise such as a name-call or tongue click, call them away, and then reward them. The pet parent should not use loud sounds (i.e., hand clap, shaking coins) or water spray, as these may worsen fear and the problem.
Reward desired behavior	• Give praise, food treats or play immediately following elimination in the box to reward litter use. Rewards can also be used to train the cat to go to his litter area. Clicker training can be particularly useful in timing of rewards for elimination.
Environmental enrichment to reduce FASCP	• Provide a calm, stable environment with sufficient enrichment, opportunities to engage in normal feline behaviors (e.g., climbing, perching, bedding, scratching, food, water, play, and exploration) and opportunities to avoid stressors (perching, climbing, hiding). • Make changes slowly and avoid punishment and any anxiety-evoking interactions.
Resolve social tension	• Inquire about body language when cat interacts with other cats, pets, or people in the home. • If social tension is present, separate cat from other cats or pets in the home. • Ensure resources, including enrichment items, are placed in multiple, separate locations on all floors of the house, and that there are different entry and exit points so that the cat can access resources without encountering another animal. • Do not permit small children to approach the cat during elimination.
Psychotropic medications and pheromonotherapy reduce FASCP	• Start anxiolytic and/or antidepressant medication to address acute or chronic FASCP. • Use Feliway diffuser for calming effect.

Communication with pet parents

Pet parents may be very distressed by their cat's house-soiling problem, and they may be considering relinquishment or euthanasia by the time that they seek help. A clinician with well-honed communication skills will be better able to manage strong emotions and establish a supportive alliance with pet parents. Allow the pet parent to speak without interruption but repeat key points and ask for clarification when needed. Acknowledge and empathize with pet parent emotions. Ask the pet parent to identify their goals and expectations of treatment outcome. Decide on the best therapeutic plan and recommend a strategy on how to proceed. Ask for the pet parent's response and collaborate on finalizing the plan. At the end of the meeting, summarize the discussion concisely and clearly, and check the pet parent's understanding. Clarify any questions and then make clear recommendations regarding follow-up.

House soiling diary

Recommend that the pet parents keep a diary of their cat's daily schedule of elimination, location of soiling, posture when eliminating, litterbox use, and whether there are any changes or stressors that can be correlated with house-soiling events. The diary is important to identify possible triggers of the house soiling and to assess the efficacy of treatments. See Appendix C for a sample diary available online.

Pharmaceuticals/pheromones/diet changes

At the first appointment, medications to treat pain should be dispensed if there is a suspicion of pain. In addition, first-line recommendations for all house-soiling cases could include pheromone analogues, calming probiotics, and changes in diet. FASCP should be identified and medications dispensed if necessary. Many cases can be resolved with environmental management and the first-line treatments mentioned above. Dispense psychotropic medications when needed but avoid overuse.

Medications are indicated to treat any physical disease that may be causing or contributing to house soiling. While that seems obvious, in some cases, it may be uncertain whether the cat is experiencing pain or discomfort, perhaps because the pet parent declined a full medical workup or because the cat was masking their pain on physical examination. Surveys have historically shown that veterinarians were less likely to treat pain in cats than in dogs due to difficulties recognizing pain, lack of knowledge regarding analgesia, and fear of drug side effects.[132,132a,132b] In feline house-soiling cases, a trial with an analgesic medication may be indicated even if a physical cause cannot be identified, especially if there is a change from normal behavior, development of new behaviors, or behavioral signs that might be associated with pain.[132] Withholding treatments such as analgesics can cause greater harm, as the pet's pain and suffering goes unaddressed and unnecessary treatments may be implemented instead. Therefore, suspected pain should be addressed first rather than after the cat does not respond to environmental and behavioral therapy.

To determine the duration of an analgesic trial and to evaluate the efficacy of the analgesic, the pet parent will need to have a good sense of the frequency of periuria or perichezia; the analgesic will need to be administered for at least 5–7 days longer than an occurrence of house soiling would be expected. In other words, if the cat regularly eliminates outside of the litterbox once daily, then the analgesic would need to be administered for 5–7 days to evaluate for response to treatment. On the other hand, if the cat eliminates outside of the litterbox on average once weekly or if the pet parent is unsure of the frequency, then the analgesic trial will need to be conducted for about 12–14 days.

Because osteoarthritis is one of the most common causes of chronic pain in cats,[133] the preferred analgesic trial would consist of a nonsteroidal antiinflammatory medication (NSAID), such as Onsior (robenacoxib), which has been approved for use up to three days in cats in the United States,[134] or meloxicam, a COX-2 preferential NSAID.[133,135–137] Several studies have shown that NSAIDs can increase activity in cats with DJD[138] and a recent study showed that cats with osteoarthritis that were treated with six weeks of robenacoxib showed improved temperament and happiness.[139]

Because of the potential NSAID effects on kidneys and liver (though idiosyncratic drug-induced hepatoxicity secondary to NSAIDs is rare in cats),[133,140] laboratory tests as mentioned above should be performed prior to starting an NSAID. Gabapentin is widely used to treat neuropathic and chronic pain and some acute pain situations.[141] One study of 20 cats with osteoarthritis receiving gabapentin 10 mg/kg PO every 12 hours for two weeks found improvements as identified by pet parents.[142] Another study evaluating long-term use of gabapentin for musculoskeletal pain or head trauma in three cats at an average dose of 6.5 mg/kg every 12 hours found that satisfactory pain management was achieved in all of the cats.[143] See Chapter 11 for more detail on medications.

If response to an analgesic trial is observed (i.e., the frequency of house soiling decreases, the cat's energy is increased, the cat is more socially engaged, the cat seems happier), then a medical workup to evaluate for sources of pain, if not already performed, ongoing analgesia, and modification of the environment to improve the painful cat's access to the litterbox facilities and other resources are indicated.

If FIC is suspected, common treatment modalities often include analgesics such as opioids including oral transmucosal buprenorphine, transdermal buprenorphine, alpha antagonists such as prazosin,[9] though further investigation is needed to determine how much benefit they provide, environmental enrichment, dietary alterations (which is beyond the scope of this chapter), and pheromone therapy.[63]

In addition to addressing any sources of pain or discomfort, reducing FASCP is an essential component of the initial treatment plan for feline house soiling. Reducing fear and anxiety has been shown to decrease urine-marking behavior and intercat aggression, and to improve quality of life for felines.[9,16,111] Improving environmental enrichment, including optimizing litterbox facilities, is an essential component of reducing stress in house-soiling cats.[9,23,24,28] Even if the soiling cat has been diagnosed with FLUTD, multimodal environmental modification (MEMO) alone has been shown to significantly decrease stress as well as the frequency of lower urinary tract signs.[144] In a study of 46 cats with FIC, 70–75% of the cats had no lower urinary tract signs after 10 months of MEMO.[144] In that study, the three most important modifications were shown to be optimal litterbox management, increased pet parent interaction, with the cat and pet parent education. Pheromones and probiotics can also be used to reduce stress. See below for specific recommendations.

While psychotropic medications are not necessary for all cases, there are circumstances that require that psychotropic medications must be considered. If the cat's FASCP during the assessment is too heightened for an examination and/or diagnostics to be performed, then pre-veterinary visit pharmaceuticals will be needed to complete the general wellness assessment (see Chapters 9, 11, and 16). If the initial history reveals moderate to severe FASCP at home and/or if the cat is in danger of being relinquished or euthanized, then short-term anxiolytics can be prescribed while initial recommendations are implemented.

Prevent resoiling

By providing a cat with their preferred litterbox, location, and litter, and by cleaning the litterbox regularly, regular litter use may be reestablished. However, some cats may also continue using sites where they have previously soiled. Access to soiled areas might be prevented by moving furniture, closing doors, or using gates. Removing urine and stool odor in soiled areas may reduce reuse of these sites. When urine or feces is found outside of the box, the pet parent should immediately remove the urine or feces and clean the area with an enzymatic cleaner according to the manufacturer's instructions, as enzymatic cleaners chemically break down the odor instead of masking it. Some cleaning products, such as citrus fragrances, may be aversive to cats. Therefore, the pet parent should carefully select the products to be used for cleaning soiled areas. The cleaning product should first be tested in a small area to check for discoloration, then ample amounts should be used to ensure penetration into deeper layers rather than just spraying the surface. Cats can likely detect odors for longer than humans, so keep in mind that evaluating the degree of cleanliness relying on human olfaction is limited. If elimination occurs on carpet, the carpet may need to be removed so that the underlying affected floor can be treated. If the cat eliminated on items that can be hand- or machine washed such as bedding, sofa cushions, clothes, rugs, or mats, the items should be immediately removed from the environment and washed.

Addressing environmental needs

MEMO is an acronym standing for multimodal environmental modification. As mentioned above, MEMO has shown usefulness in preventing recurrence in cats that have FIC.[144] When applied to house-soiling cases, it can be used to reduce stress without the use of pharmaceuticals. MEMO consists of five categories: social, physical, behavioral, nutritional, and elimination. Similarly, the American Association of Feline Practitioners (AAFP) and International Society of Feline Medicine (ISFM) Environmental Needs Guidelines describe five pillars of a healthy feline environment that support the cat's physical health, emotional well-being, and interaction with human companions and other animals.[9] These pillars include providing: a safe place; multiple and separated environmental resources including food, water, toileting areas, scratching areas, play areas, and resting or sleeping areas; opportunities for play and predatory behavior; positive, consistent, and predictable human–cat social interactions; and an environment that respects the importance of the cat's sense of smell. At each cat's house soiling appointment, these needs should be addressed.

Optimizing litterbox facilities

In order to avoid overwhelming the cat and increasing his stress, which may worsen the house soiling, changes to the litterbox should be made slowly, while always keeping the same choices available to the cat. In other words, an additional box which is different in style or has a different substrate may be offered initially; however, the existing box and substrate should still be available to the cat. Some cats will investigate new objects in the environment immediately and some take longer to habituate to them. Optimizing the litterbox entails addressing anything that may be aversive about the litterbox (liner, lid), litter (texture, scent, cleanliness), and location. Some cats are more flexible than others, and the preferred litterbox environment for one cat may not be the preferred environment for another; therefore, optimizing the litterbox environment requires that the pet parent identify the litterbox factors that best suit their individual cat. This is often done by offering the cat choices and making regular adjustments to the litterbox depending on the cat's preferences.

The boxes should be upgraded in size so that they are an appropriate size (see section above titled Normal feline elimination behavior and preferences). For some cats, even the jumbo or extra-large commercial sized litterboxes are not sufficient in size. Pet parents should be encouraged to use under-the-bed storage bins, sweater boxes, and other large storage containers that can be purchased at a home improvement store or department store.

The pet parents should provide a sufficient number of litterboxes and distribute them in appropriate places around the home. The general rule of thumb that has been historically recommended is that there should be one litterbox per cat in the household plus an additional litterbox ($n + 1$).[9,11] Some cats may need more boxes if they have a physical condition that causes an increased frequency of urination or defecation or volume of urine or stool. Any litterboxes that are placed side by side should be considered as one large litterbox.

Ensure that the cat can readily access the litterboxes. If the cat is geriatric, has mobility issues, has suspected chronic pain, and/or has impaired vision, then there should be at least one box on each floor of the home to prevent the cat from having to use stairs to access the litterbox.[7] Litterboxes that are flat or have very low sides should also be considered for these cats. All cats in the household should be able to obtain immediate access to the litterboxes without the risk of encountering another cat or animal.[9] Position the litterboxes so that they are away from food and water as well as resting places.[9] The exception to this is if the cat is geriatric or has mobility issues, in which case at least one litterbox may need to be nearby the cat's other resources, such as sleeping areas and feeding and water stations.[7] Night lights may aid cats with visual impairment to access their litterbox.[9] Additional litterboxes or litterboxes that are unused by the cat should be moved from noisy environments to low-traffic areas, away from appliances, air vents, entry and exit points, and windows, walls, or doors that are adjacent to outside traffic.[7,9] If the cat has only been offered an automatic self-cleaning litterbox, the pet parent should add non-automatic litterboxes, as the sudden noise and motion of these boxes can cause fear and create an aversion to the boxes.

The pet parent should provide a choice of hooded and open boxes. Cats that soil over the edge of a box should be provided with a covered box or one with higher sides in addition to the box that already is present. Do not make any changes to the litter or substrate at this time unless it is clear from the history that this is the appropriate thing to do. Simply switching from one type of litter, even if it is from clay litter to a different commercial clay litter, is not likely to successfully treat a litterbox aversion.[42] If pain is suspected, then offering a finer-textured litter in an additional box should be considered, as digging in gravel-type substrate may be uncomfortable for cats with pain, including pain secondary to declawing.[81] In one study, the frequency of elimination outside the box was reduced when Zero Odor was added to the litter.[145] In another study, cats were more likely to use a plant-based clumping litter with an added attractant (which was not specified in the study) over a control plant-based clumping litter.[146] The pet parent should provide an appropriate depth of litter of at least 1.25 inches (4 cm),[9] topping off the litter when necessary. Greater litter depth may be preferred for feces.[45] Liners should be removed from the boxes.[7]

The pet parent should be instructed to scoop waste from the boxes at least once daily, with more frequent waste removal being even better.[9] The entire contents of the litterbox should be emptied, the box should be washed with hot water and dish soap, dried, and refilled with fresh litter once weekly.[9] The pet parent should avoid cleaning the litterbox with scented detergents, bleach, ammonia-based products, and other scented cleaning products.[7,9] Even cats that are urine marking can improve with litterbox optimization. One study found that thoroughly cleaning the urine marks daily with enzymatic cleaner, scooping waste from the litterbox daily, and washing the litterbox and replacing the litterbox with fresh litter weekly resulted in up to a 50% decrease in urine-marking behavior.[91]

Making too many environmental changes at once may be overwhelming for cats and pet parents. At first, the pet parents might make simple changes to improve litter appeal by cleaning the box more frequently, changing the box location, or changing the type of box and/or litter. The practitioner can begin by suggesting changes that appear to be most appropriate based on the history of the house soiling problem. Leaving some options from the previous litterbox environment is necessary just in case the cat still prefers those options.

The cat's environment should give the cat an opportunity to engage in species-typical behavior (e.g., scratching, climbing, resting, perching, play) and to avoid stressors (e.g., climbing, perching, hiding). Hiding is an important coping mechanism for cats in stressful environments. Strategically placed crates, boxes, open closet doors, and climbing trees can all serve as retreats for cats.[16] Ensure that the cat has access to plenty of horizontal and vertical space and scratching posts. The cat should also be fed in a safe, quiet location; the use of food puzzles may provide greater mental stimulation than feeding from food bowls,[147,148] although a recent study showed that cats prefer freely available food.[149] A provision of toys to serve as outlets for play and to satiate the cat's natural predatory behavior should be provided. Although cats like predictability, small, regular changes in the environment, such as regularly rotating toys, provide novelty, renew the cat's motivation, and prevent boredom.[16] Natural hunting behavior can be encouraged by hiding food throughout the house and using food puzzles. Ensure that there are plenty of resources distributed throughout the home in multicat households.

Social interactions

A predictable routine can help decrease overall stress.[16] Cats should receive at least three structured, positive interactions with their pet parents daily. In a study on the effect of multimodal environmental modification on cats with FIC, increased pet parent interactions were one of the most significant modifications that led to a decrease in incidences of FIC.[144] The nature of these interactions depends on the cat's preferences; some cats prefer to be petted, some prefer to be groomed, and some prefer to play.

Pet parents should never punish (i.e., scold, push, swat, hit, smack, or startle-squirt water, clap their hands, or shake a jar of coins) their cat, including when they catch their cat in the act of house soiling. This can create or worsen FASCP in the cat, which may perpetuate the house soiling and damage the human–animal bond, which may already be fragile due to the elimination problem. If the pet parent catches the cat engaging in preelimination behaviors, such as scratching or posturing, or in the act of soiling outside of the litterbox, the pet parent should not respond by yelling, making a loud noise, spraying the cat with a water bottle, forcefully grabbing, pushing or physically disciplining the cat, or rubbing the cat's nose in the soiled area. This will only increase stress, and lead to the cat developing a negative association with the pet parent. Instead, the pet parent should use a more neutral or gentle sound, like a bell or crinkling of a treat bag, that may interrupt or stop the cat from eliminating without causing fear. The pet parent should reinforce the cat (i.e., praise) as soon as the cat stops engaging in the preelimination or undesirable elimination behavior, then gently pick up the cat and bring him to the litterbox, reinforcing him again once there. If the initial history reveals that the soiling cat is fighting with another pet in the household, then full-time separation from that animal should be implemented.[7] This can be achieved by having the pets live in separate bedrooms or in separate spaces in the home that are divided by tall gates.

Surgery

Castration eliminates urine marking in 78–90% of adult male cats and decreases the marking associated with estrus in female cats.[88,89] Should marking arise in adult male cats, the presence of male urine odor, secondary sexual characteristics, and penile barbs might indicate a retained testicle or residual extratesticular tissue, which might be confirmed by gonadotropin-releasing hormone response testing (see Chapter 6). Castration should be recommended for unaltered spraying cats; however, pet parents should be informed that it does not reduce marking behavior in all cats, as 10% or more of males and 5% or less of females will continue to spray following neutering.[88–90] In these cases, additional causes of marking need to be considered and treated.

Second appointment

The second appointment should begin with the clinician assessing the adherence to and efficacy of the initial treatment recommendations (see Box 22.3, Figure 22.6). If the house soiling has persisted, then the next goal of this visit is to determine the type of elimination disorder, the cat's preferences, and a clinical timeline. This will be used to identify specific stimuli and environmental changes that trigger the soiling behavior. Once this has been established, then the veterinarian will be better poised to tailor the treatment recommendations to the individual cat's needs and preferences, evaluate the need for medications or supplements, or make changes to the initial medical plan. See figure 22.6 and box 22.3.

Second appointment history

The history should include a list of changes made based on the recommendations from the first visit, changes in the frequency or pattern of the house soiling, previous treatment recommendations which were not instituted, and challenges faced since the first appointment. If the house soiling has improved or resolved, then the veterinarian should question the pet parent regarding the treatment timeline to determine if a particular change resulted in a return to the litterbox. For example, if the pet parent first changed the size of the litterbox and the cat continued house soiling, and then the pet parent removed the litterbox liners and the cat ceased house soiling, then the veterinarian may reasonably deduce that the liners were causing an aversion to the litterbox. With that said, cats are sometimes repelled by novelty and at other times, they are drawn to it. In many cases, it is best to leave changes for a minimum of two weeks to ensure that the change in the pet's behavior is lasting and consistent.

Similar to the first appointment, a short, one-page questionnaire can be utilized to obtain the additional history needed to differentiate the type of house soiling. The history will focus on three key factors that may cause or contribute to house soiling, including social, physical, and environmental factors. Because both the physical environment, including the litterbox and litterbox management, which were addressed in the first appointment, and the social environment, including the cat's interactions with

Box 22.3 Second appointment steps

1. Review second appointment questionnaire form; ask clarifying questions
2. Evaluate pet parent adherence to previous recommendations
3. Evaluate cat's response to changes and timeline of response in relation to any changes in house-soiling pattern
4. Evaluate pet parent's challenges with implementing first appointment recommendations
5. Use the history to distinguish marking versus toileting behavior
6. Establish temporal relationship between potential triggers and onset of house soiling
7. Determine if house soiling occurs only when pet parent departs the home; if it does, consider separation-related disorders
8. Tailor treatment plan to specific house-soiling diagnosis
   a. Marking
      i. Reduce exposure to inciting triggers
         1. Block access to windows, doors, cat flaps, perches, or rooms that have window view if outdoor cats present
         2. Deter neighborhood cats from accessing property – pet repellants; motion-activated sprays or sprinklers; remove garbage, food and birdseed; use microchip-activated cat flaps to prevent outdoor cats from entering the home
      ii. Prevent future spraying
         1. Avoid introducing new odors to the home
         2. Make sprayed areas undesirable
         3. Clean marked areas with enzymatic cleaner
      iii. Consider allowing marking station or stations in the home
         1. Use L-shaped litter station or litterboxes leaned upright against walls
   b. Undesirable elimination
      i. Reestablish litterbox use
         1. Increase number of boxes in the home
         2. Increase sizes of boxes
         3. Place boxes in quiet, low-traffic areas
         4. Provide option of covered and uncovered boxes
         5. Switch to unscented, clay clumping litter
         6. Remove liners
      ii. Change function of soiling location
      iii. Prevent access to preferred substrate – remove rugs and mats, close doors to prevent access to rooms with preferred substrate
      iv. Place preferred substrate in the boxes
   c. Resolve social tension with housemate cats
      i. Separate cats if indicated
      ii. Ensure items of enrichment are in multiple, separate locations and have more than one entry and exit point
      iii. Rehoming may be necessary
   d. Resolve tension with family members
      i. Provide predictable, consistent, and positive interactions
      ii. Eliminate all punishment
   e. Evaluate need for medications and supplements
      i. Cat has acute or chronic FASCP
      ii. Cat has relapses of FIC despite environmental changes
      iii. Cat is neutered and marking
      iv. Pet parent has made all recommended environmental modifications
      v. Pet parent is unable to eliminate stimuli that trigger marking
      vi. Cat at risk of relinquishment or euthanasia

2ND APPOINTMENT

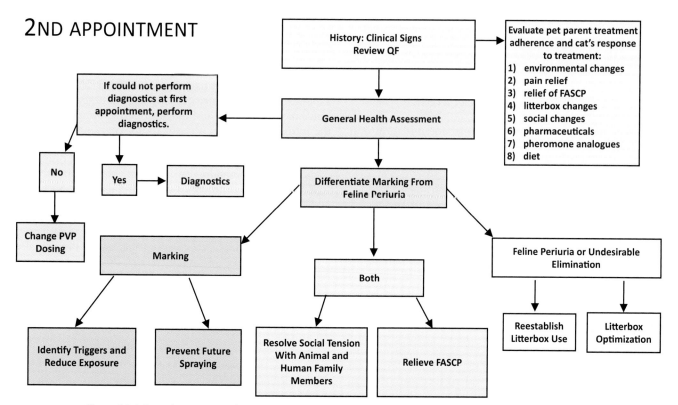

Figure 22.6 Second appointment flow. *(Atrribution: Alison Gerkin.)* QF, Questionnaire Form (see Appendix C, online forms.)

humans and other animals inside and outside of the home, may contribute equally to a house-soiling problem,[1,9] the history must focus on all aspects of the cat's physical and social environment.

At the second appointment, the minimum history should include:

Social factors

1. How many people live in the home? What are their ages?
2. How does the cat interact with family members? Strangers?
3. How often does the cat avoid, hide, run away from, and/or show aggression (growling, hissing, swatting, biting) toward familiar and/or unfamiliar people?
4. How often does the cat approach, sit next to or in the laps of, and/or rub on familiar and unfamiliar people?
5. How often do strangers visit the home?
6. How does the pet parent respond to the cat's house soiling?
7. What other animals are in the home? What are their species, ages, and breeds?
8. What was the order in which the pets were brought into the home?
9. How often does the cat avoid, hide, run away from, and/or show aggression toward (growling, hissing, swatting, biting) other pets in the home?
10. How often does the cat approach, rub on, groom, sleep with, and/or play with other pets in the home?
11. How do the pet parents believe the animals in the home get along?
12. Can the cat see other animals (i.e., other cats, squirrels, birds at a bird feeder etc.) from inside the home?

Physical factors

1. Does the cat eliminate on horizontal, vertical, or both surfaces?
2. What volume of urine and/or stool is being eliminated outside of the litterbox?
3. Describe the cat's preelimination and postelimination behaviors. Does the cat circle, dig, complete elimination in the box, or run away during or immediately after eliminating?
4. Does the cat try to cover the urine or feces?

Environmental factors

1. Which locations does the cat prefer for urination and defecation?
2. Does the cat only soil one type of surface (e.g., smooth, soft) or does it soil any surface?
3. Does the cat use the box for both urination and defecation?
4. How often does the cat use a litterbox for urination and defecation? Does the cat only use the box for one or the other?
5. Were there any changes to the environment indoors or outdoors prior to the onset of the elimination problem?
6. How many water and feeding stations are present and where are they located?
7. What enrichment does the cat have access to?

Social factors

Explore the daily social interactions between the human household members and the cat, and determine how the cat gets along with family members and visitors. Ask how the household members respond when they catch the cat in the act of house soiling and when they find soiled areas. The pet parents should be asked how often the soiling cat engages in affiliative and agonistic (aggressive, combative) behaviors with household cats. Because pet parents often overlook the more subtle signs of feline body language, the veterinarian should ask specific questions about the frequency that certain body language, such as avoidance, staring, blocking, allogrooming, and allorubbing, are demonstrated during interactions with housemate cats. If the pet parent is uncertain, they should be educated by the veterinary healthcare team on feline body language, provided with body language resources, and instructed to document instances of affiliative and agonistic behaviors in order to track the frequency in which the soiling cat engages in such interactions. The pet parent should be asked about any interactions between the soiling cat and other species in the home that may increase the cat's stress or decrease the cat's access to the litterbox. For example, dogs may lie in front of or next to the litterbox. Interactions with another animal in the house may also lead to cats perceiving their litterbox as unsafe. For example, dogs may bark, stick their noses into the litterbox, or chase the cat while the cat is using the litterbox. The veterinarian should also explore the daily social interactions between the human household members and the cat, and determine how the cat gets along with family members and visitors. Ask how the household members respond when they catch the cat in the act of house soiling and when they find soiled areas.

Physical factors

Questioning about physical features of the elimination behavior, including the cat's posture when urinating, whether the soiling is directed on horizontal, vertical; or both surfaces, the volume of urine being passed, how often the cat is eliminating outside of the litterbox, and the pre- and post-elimination behaviors is essential to differentiating marking behavior from toileting. Yet in one study, only 69% of veterinarians inquired about whether the soiling was on vertical or horizontal surfaces.[36]

Ways to accurately distinguish between urine marking and undesirable elimination are outlined above and in Table 22.2. The frequency of marking or undesirable elimination may vary greatly, and may not be temporally related to the introduction of the stressor to the environment. For example, if a stray cat is present daily, then the cat may mark daily. On the other hand, if the stray cat visits only once weekly, then the marking cat may mark that frequently. The marking cat may continue to void normal amounts of urine and feces in the litterbox.[9] While leaving urine and/or feces uncovered is not an indicator of a problem, a change from previously routine behavior (e.g., a cat used to cover their elimination but suddenly starts running out of the box after eliminating without covering their deposit) may be indicative of a problem.[7] Cats that balance on the edges of litterboxes with only one or two paws inside the box, investigate and then avoid entering a box, avoid digging and circling or covering waste while in the box, shake paws after stepping out of the litterbox, scratch the surrounding wall or sides of the litterbox rather than the litter, quickly run out of the box, and vocalize on the way to the box or while eliminating may have an aversion to a dirty litterbox or to the substrate.[7,9,23,42,145]

Less commonly, a cat may mark urine or stool on horizontal surfaces.[24] This type of marking can be more difficult to distinguish from toileting. In horizontal marking, the cat may squat, quiver the tail, and walk away without sniffing.[7,124]

Marking on horizontal surfaces is a consideration when the cat deposits small amounts of urine or feces on socially significant surfaces rather than specific substrates or locations and continues to use their litter for elimination of both urine and stools.[7] Most cats that mark on horizontal surfaces also mark on vertical surfaces.

A study that evaluated the sensitivity and specificity of the characteristics used to differentiate between elimination and marking found that while they were all significantly associated with their expected form of periuria, using any one of these features as a single criterion when differentiating between elimination and marking was unreliable.[1] Using urination on vertical surfaces as a criterion to diagnose marking was less likely to lead to a misdiagnosis than using volume of urine as a criterion to differentiate between periuria and marking, but urination on horizontal surfaces was less reliable, as a quarter of the cats urinating on horizontal surfaces were found to be marking.[1] The posture assumed while urinating and the presence or absence of attempts to cover the urine were more reliable indicators, but the study found that relying on either of these two criteria alone may lead to misdiagnosis.[1] Therefore, differentiating between elimination and marking behavior requires a thorough history so that multiple criteria can be considered when making the diagnosis.

Establishing the average number of urine or stool marks per day, week, or month is essential to determining the extent of the problem and to tracking response to treatment. Pet parents should continue using their house-soiling diary, and identify locations and the cats involved, as outlined above.

Environmental factors

Determining the house-soiling locations may provide clues as to what might be an inciting factor or motivation for the house soiling. Cats will frequently mark the same areas repeatedly, which are often socially significant places or objects.[7,9] Some cats will target new or novel objects, surfaces, or odors, such as purses, bags, and shoes, that have disrupted the scent in the environment after being brought into the home.[9] Cats that mark external walls, windows, and doorways may be responding to outdoor stimuli, such as outdoor cats, that they perceive as a threat.[7,9] Sometimes, the residual scent of another cat can cause the cat to spray. For example, if a visitor has cats at home, the cat may spray the visitor's coat when they he smells the odor of the nonresident cats. As another example, the cat may start spraying around the living-room fireplace if firewood that has been sprayed by neighborhood cats is brought inside the home. Cat doors or flaps may trigger urine marking due to the perceived or actual threat of other cats entering the home.[9]

With undesirable elimination, soiled areas typically have no social significance except perhaps in cases where the cat is avoiding the litterbox and choosing a new site due to interference or preventing access by other household pets or people.[7,9,23] Urine may be found in hidden areas such as under the bed or next to the litterbox. If the cat only eliminates on one type of surface (i.e., soft, absorbent surfaces such as carpets, bath mats and clothes), then he may have a substrate preference.[23] If the cat eliminates outside of the litterbox on multiple types of substrates (i.e., both soft surfaces and hard floors), then he does not have a substrate

preference and may have an aversion to the litterbox or litterbox location. If the cat eliminates outside of the box in a singular location or in a few locations that are similar (i.e., the showers in the house, behind furniture), then a location preference may be suspected. Cats with a location preference may also seek out previously soiled areas or locations where other cats have eliminated.[14,23] Cats that eliminate near the box and engage in preelimination and postelimination behavior (e.g., digging, covering) most likely have an aversion to the box itself.[7]

Cats that eliminate outside of their litterbox may or may not also regularly use their litterbox for urination and/or defecation.[7] Intermittent litterbox use might provide some clues as to when and why the box is used and when it is avoided. Cats that entirely avoid using the litterbox may have a preference for other surfaces or locations, or may have an aversion to returning to the box. If the cat consistently defecates in the box but urinates elsewhere, or vice versa, then the problem is unlikely to be due to the litterbox or substrate. Likely causes include physical problems such as pain, discomfort, or mobility issues, surface or location preferences for urine or feces, litter cleanliness, and intermittent situations (e.g., loud noises, presence of other pets) that might induce the cat to avoid the box. A litterbox that is too small in size might lead to litterbox avoidance, only when the box has not been adequately cleaned. In addition, cats that are sporadically confronted or have their access blocked by a pet or person during elimination may leave the box to eliminate elsewhere, leading to intermittent house soiling. Finally, some cats will not use the same box for urine and feces, so an insufficient number of boxes may lead to the cat urinating or defecating outside of the litterbox once a certain type of elimination has been deposited in the box.

Garner information about the cat's access to resources. Determine the number and location of feeding and water stations, feeding routine (i.e., what, when, and where the cat is fed), resources available to the cat (i.e., horizontal and vertical spaces, hiding places, scratching posts, toys), and access to windows, doors, lanais, porches, or transparent cat flaps. If the cat has access to the outdoors, ask if there have been any changes to the outdoor environment that may have reduced or eliminated the cat's access to elimination areas such as a structure being placed on previously vacant land, a garden being paved, or animals not previously present being spotted in the yard (see Tables 22.3 and 22.4).

Clinical timeline

Evaluate for a temporal relationship between any potential triggers of FASCP and the onset of house soiling by determining if there are specific events such as changes in the environment, changes in social interactions, changes in daily routine or schedule, and changes in physical health that preceded the house soiling (e.g., punishment, agonistic encounters with dogs or other cats, arrival of a new outdoor cat, addition of new pets or family members to the home, move or renovation of the house). Determine if the cat only house soils when separated from household members or a particular family member. If so, this may be suggestive of a separation-related disorder (see Chapter 17). In one study, 75% of cats with separation-related disorders urinated on the pet parent's bed.[150] Determine if the pet parent traveled prior to or after the onset of house soiling and if so, whether the cat was left home alone, left at home under the care of a familiar or unfamiliar person, or boarded at a cattery or veterinary clinic during the pet parent's travels.[7] Consider that some potential stressors, like seemingly small changes in the environment or lifestyle, may not have been recognized as problematic by the pet parent.

It is not uncommon for pet parents to report that a behavior is acute when in fact it is chronic or was intermittently displayed and is now more consistently exhibited. This can be avoided by using the questionnaire provided in Chapter 1 for all cat appointments. If the onset of house soiling is truly acute, it is more likely that a physical cause or contributing factor is present.

Second appointment diagnosis

With the information gleaned from the additional history collected in appointment two, the veterinarian should be able to reduce the length of the differential diagnosis list and tailor the treatment plan (see Box 22.1).

Second appointment treatment

Now that the type of elimination problem has been established, treatment can be better tailored. The principal approach to management of marking should focus on decreasing exposure to the inciting stimuli and target areas, preventing future spraying, optimizing litterbox facilities, addressing social tension, and initiating pheromone and/or pharmaceutical therapy if indicated. For undesirable elimination, continued modification of the cat's environment and social interactions to reduce social stress should be emphasized. Pheromone and pharmaceutical therapy may also be indicated for undesirable elimination disorders (see Tables 22.5 and 22.6).

Reduce exposure to the target areas and stimuli

The cat should be prevented from accessing stimuli that incite spraying by blocking access to windows or windowsills using baby gates (which may need to be stacked on top of one another to prevent the cat from jumping over them) or closing doors, moving furniture or cat perches away from the windows, or keeping the cat out of rooms that have an outdoor view. Window shades, drapes, blinds, window film, or other visual barriers might be used to block the sight of outdoor cats, and music and white noise might be used to reduce the sounds of outdoor stimuli. Potentially fear-evoking devices such as electronic pet mats or ultrasonic mats should be avoided as they increase stress, leading to worsening of the elimination problem or to development of other unwanted behaviors.[9]

If the stimulus for marking is the sight, sound, or odors of outdoor cats, then efforts should be made to stop these cats from coming onto the property. This may be possible by using pet repellents, motion-activated sprays, or sprinklers. Ultrasonic motion detectors are also available, but are seldom effective. Anything in the yard that might attract roaming cats should be removed or made inaccessible (e.g., bird feeders, garbage, food). Pet parents should be instructed to stop feeding any stray animals. If the pet parents cannot find a way to prevent stray cats from accessing their yard, they may need to consider having them humanely removed. The pet parents should remove or block cat doors or flaps that allow unwanted cats to enter the household, or use microchip-operated devices so that access is only granted to resident cats.[9]

Eliminating the factors that contribute to marking may not always be possible, especially when the problem is due to stray cats on the property or due to relationships between cats in the home. In these cases, behavior modification and/or pharmaceuticals are most likely indicated. However, by reducing exposure to the cat's spraying locations, damage to household possessions will be prevented and the urine-marking frequency will decrease in many cases. To prevent disruption of the cat's olfactory and chemical perception of their environment that they rely on to establish a sense of security and safety, pet parents should avoid introducing odors such as detergents, medications, cleaning products, new or unfamiliar clothing items, and other animal scents, and prevent access to items with a scent or texture that the cat might mark (e.g., new furniture, grocery bags, or visitors' shoes and boots).[9]

Make sprayed areas undesirable for future elimination. Deterrents such as double-sided tape, unpleasant odors (citrus, potpourri, cat repellents), or vinyl carpet runners with the nubs up, aluminum foil, or plastic sheeting could also be used to keep the cat away from areas where they might mark. In some cases where soiling is limited to one to a few sites, the function of the area might be changed by placing a food bowl, scratching post, kitty condo, bedding, or toys in the area. Cats that soil in a sink or bathtub might be deterred by leaving a small amount of water in the bottom. Always consider the possibility that repellents may cause the cat to become stressed. Even something as benign as aluminum foil can frighten a noise-phobic cat. The function of marking sites can be altered by placing food and water bowls, cat trees and beds, and toys at these sites.[9] However, while making soiled areas unpleasant may stop use of these site, if the stress of the cat isn't addressed, cats will often respond by simply moving to a new target, often a nearby spot. Therefore, simply making the urination spots undesirable is often not sufficient to resolve urine marking.

Marked areas should be cleaned frequently to deter a cat from refreshing their scent at a marking site.[9] Ammonia-based cleaning products should be avoided as they may smell like urine to a cat.[9]

Since urine marking is a normal feline behavior, for some cats, an acceptable compromise might be to allow one or two sites for indoor marking. Pet parents can create an L-shaped litter station arrangement with two litterboxes – one box positioned horizontally with litter inside and the other box positioned perpendicular to the other box with no litter inside. Furthermore, litterboxes can be leaned in an upright position against walls or other areas where the cat is marking. Some cats will limit their urine spraying to these locations.

Establish and offer the cat's preferences

Continued efforts to optimize the litterbox to suit the cat's individual preferences are essential to addressing periuria and perichezia. A possible aversion to the litterbox and the litterbox location was addressed in the first appointment by, if indicated, increasing the number of litterboxes in the home, increasing the size of the litterboxes, placing litterboxes in quiet, low-traffic areas, covering or uncovering the boxes, and removing liners from the litterboxes. If these changes have not been instituted, then they should be at this time.

Pet parents may best determine their cat's litterbox preferences by giving two boxes with one variable changed every 1–2 weeks (e.g., litter type, hooded versus uncovered box, lined or unlined) to determine the cat's preferred litter and box type. Care should be taken to make changes slowly. This will give the cat time to adjust to the change (some cats are neophobic, or fearful of new things) and give the pet parent time to evaluate efficacy. If the pet parent has sufficient space, three or four choices might be offered cafeteria style to give the cat more options. Litter additives have been developed to increase litter appeal, but no controlled data have been published as to their efficacy. One study showed that cats were more likely to use a plant-based clumping litter with an added attractant over a control plant-based clumping litter, but the attractant used was not specified.[146] If there are multiple cats present in the household, separating the cats may be the most practical way to evaluate litter preferences effectively. Another option is to place a monitor in the litter area to see which cat uses which litter.

If a location preference is suspected because the cat is eliminating in one or a few specific locations, a litterbox can be placed in the preferred location. If this is unacceptable to the pet parent, then once the litterbox is used consistently for at least two weeks in the cat's preferred location, it can be gradually relocated at a rate of several inches/centimeters a day to an area more desirable to the pet parent.[9]

For cats with a substrate preference, the appeal of the appropriate toileting facility should be optimized, while the cat's preferred substrate should be made less attractive or unavailable. Rugs or mats can be removed from the household and/or cats can be restricted from certain areas that contain the preferred substrate using gates and closed doors. The preferred substrate may be placed into litterboxes. For example, cats that prefer soil and seek out houseplants for their elimination may be attracted to the litterbox if a layer of soil is added on top of the litter. Then the amount of soil can be gradually reduced and the amount of litter in the box gradually increased. Similarly, for cats that prefer soft, absorbent materials like carpet or clothes, these materials could be placed alongside litter in a litterbox. Once the cat is consistently eliminating in the litterbox containing the preferred substrate, then the material could be gradually withdrawn. For example, if the cat appears to prefer hard flooring, then the cat may be offered an empty litterbox or a litterbox with only half covered with litter. As mentioned above, when making changes to any part of the environment, keep previous options available for approximately two weeks unless the cat is clearly averse to them. Making quick changes and eliminating old choices can cause increased stress and worsen house soiling.

Resolve social issues with family members and other pets

If the history is consistent with social tension between household cats, then separating the cats for some or all of the time to limit agonistic interactions may be necessary. These separate spaces should have food bowls, water bowls, litterboxes, and resting and hiding places. The cats can be rotated between the separate spaces. In some cases, rehoming a cat that is unhappy living with other cats may be beneficial[9] (see Chapter 24).

As discussed, in the initial treatment during the first appointment, the pet parent should ensure that resources in multicat households are plentiful and that the cat has secure access to resources. Food and water stations, resting places, perches, hiding places, and litterboxes should be provided throughout the environment. Access to these places should have more than one entry and exit point to prevent a cat from confronting another cat. If one of the cats in the household returns to the home after an absence, allow that cat to regain the group's scent before encountering the other cats. This cat should be placed in a separate room with clothing, bedding, or a cloth that has been in contact with an affiliate cat's cheek.[9]

Social interactions with pet parents must be predictable, consistent, and positive. The nature, frequency, and duration of interactions with family members depend on the cat's preferences. Some cats may prefer to be petted, some may prefer to be groomed, and some may prefer to play. Others may need less to no petting, and less social time. The most important factor is to avoid conflict, fear, anxiety, stress, and frustration. Training the cat may also offer a source of positive interactions with the family and will keep the cat mentally stimulated. Interactions should be stopped at the earliest signs of stress, and future interactions should be modified to meet the cat's preferences. Pet parents should never punish, yell at, or startle (by squirting water, clapping their hands, or shaking a jar of coins) their cat, including when they catch their cat in the act of house soiling. This can create fear and conflict in the cat, which will worsen the house-soiling problem and damage the human–animal bond.[7]

Pharmaceuticals/pheromones

While psychoactive medications are not a substitute for other treatment strategies, including addressing any physical disorders, optimization of the litterbox and environmental modification, psychoactive medications as well as pheromone analogue therapy can be extremely helpful in treating house-soiling problems which have stress, conflict or frustration as contributing or underlying factors. Psychotropic medications should be prescribed if the cat exhibits FASCP on a regular basis and the veterinarian has determined that those emotional states contribute to the behavioral clinical signs. Indications for initiating pharmaceutical therapy include:

1. The cat has signs of acute or chronic FASCP (see the section on FASCP in the first appointment and Chapter 2 [body language], Chapter 7 [effects of stress], Chapter 9 [approach to prescribing], and Chapters 11 and 12 [medications and supplements]).
2. The cat has relapses of FLUTD.[9]
3. The cat is neutered and marking.[151]
4. The house soiling has persisted despite the pet parent making all recommended litterbox and environmental modifications.

5. The pet parent is unable to eliminate stimuli that trigger marking (i.e., the presence of outdoor cats).
6. There is social tension between the soiling cat and other pets or family members in the household.
7. The cat is at risk of relinquishment, euthanasia, or poor quality of life (e.g., being placed outdoors indefinitely).

There is no need or use for psychoactive drugs if the house soiling is due to a management issue that must be addressed by the pet parents (i.e., poor litterbox hygiene).

See the section on medications in this chapter (see Tables 22.5 and 22.6).

Third appointment

If the veterinarian is seeing feline house soiling cases in multiple 20–30-minute appointments, then the foci of the third appointment include evaluating the efficacy of instituted treatments, modifying medications if indicated, and instituting behavior modification, including litterbox training. Similar to the second appointment, the third appointment should begin by evaluating the pet parent's adherence to prior treatment recommendations and the cat's response to implemented treatments.

If photos or videos of the cat's litterbox environment, enrichment, and interactions with housemate cats were requested at the previous visit, these videos can be reviewed at this appointment to ensure motivations for the elimination problem have been correctly identified and that the pet parent has implemented all prior recommendations. If medications started at the previous visit have been well tolerated but not sufficiently effective, then they may be modified at this visit. Keep in mind that some medications, including antidepressants, may take 4–6 weeks to have their effect. See the below section on medications and Chapters 9, 11, and 12 for modifying medication plans.

Since the litterbox should be optimized at this point, if all previous recommendations have been instituted, then behavior modification to reestablish litterbox use may be initiated.

Behavior modification to reestablish litterbox use

The ultimate goal of behavior modification for feline house-soiling problems is to reestablish positive associations with the litterbox, as well as its location and its substrate. To reestablish consistent use of the litterbox, the cat may need to be confined, at least when he cannot be effectively supervised.

When confined to a relatively small area, most cats will eliminate in the box if it is sufficiently appealing. However, confinement can increase stress and is not suitable for every cat.[119] If confinement to establish litterbox use is attempted, it should be a last resort when all other treatment recommendations have been followed and were ineffective. Ideally, the room should be big enough to perform preference testing using at least two litterboxes, with one variable in each box changed every five days (e.g., litter type, hooded versus uncovered box, lined or unlined). If the pet parent has sufficient space in the room where the cat will be confined, three or four choices might be offered, cafeteria style, to give the cat more options. For cats with a substrate preference, the cat's preferred substrate should be removed from the room, but the preferred substrate may be placed into litterboxes. For example, a layer of soil can be added on top of litter if the cat prefers soil for elimination; then the amount of soil can be gradually reduced and the amount of litter in the box gradually increased. Similarly, for cats that prefer soft, absorbent materials such as carpet or clothes, these materials could be placed alongside litter in a litterbox. Once the cat is consistently eliminating in the litterbox, then the material should be gradually withdrawn. If the cat appears to prefer hard flooring, then the cat may be offered an empty litterbox or a litterbox with only half covered with litter.

Because confinement can increase stress, which can worsen the house-soiling behavior, every attempt should be made to reduce anxiety associated with confinement by enriching the confinement area and providing consistent, structured, and positive interactions with the pet parent. The pet parent should reward the cat each time they enter the room, and provide perches, scratching posts, food and water stations, and toys in the room. The family should be advised to remove the cat from the confinement area as much as possible for socialization and play but never allow them out of sight. Keeping a journal of the cat's elimination, eating, and sleeping schedule (including frequency and times of day) can inform the pet parents on when to release the cat from confinement, aiming for release to occur at times when elimination is not expected. This is particularly useful for stool soiling; for example, if a cat has a bowel movement once daily, he can be released from confinement each day after the litterbox is used for defecation.

If the cat refuses to use the litterbox when confined to a separate room, the confinement area might need to be reduced in size to a large cage. A perch or shelf should be added inside the cage to provide a place for the cat to rest. The floor should be covered with litter to ensure it is used for elimination. When the litter is used regularly for one week, it should then be placed in a litterbox on the floor of the crate. When the cat is using this litterbox regularly for one week, he may be allowed access to the rest of the room with litterboxes arranged as described above. After two weeks without soiling in the room, the pet parent can begin to release the cat from the room for 60 minutes. Before each release, the pet parent should ensure that the litter has been used and the litterbox is thoroughly cleaned. The cat should be returned to his litter area when it might be time to eliminate if he does not voluntarily return on his own. The pet parent should supervise the cat the entire time that he is released from the room. If the cat uses the litter box, he should be immediately rewarded; if the cat does not eliminate, the pet parent should continue to supervise and return the cat to his litterbox every 60 minutes. If the pet parent is unable to supervise the cat, the cat should be confined to the room and released only after the litter is used again and the pet parent can supervise the cat. Once the cat is consistently using the litterbox for two weeks, then the amount of time that the cat is released from confinement with supervision can be gradually increased by 60 minutes until the cat is regularly using the litterbox without being confined for at least eight hours. At this point, the pet parents may elect to discontinue confining the cat altogether.

In addition, the pet parent should reward the cat for litterbox use to reinforce this desired behavior. Since timing of the reward delivery is critical for the cat to learn which behavior is being reinforced, clicker training might be the most effective way to immediately mark the cat's elimination inside of the litterbox and to signal to the cat that a reward will be delivered shortly. The sound of the clicker may evoke fear in some cats, so the pet parent should test the cat's response to the clicker prior to using it when the cat is in the litterbox. The pet parent should wrap the clicker in a thick towel to dampen its sound and stand at least 10 feet away from the cat when first discharging the click. Every time the clicker is discharged, a reward should immediately follow. Rewards may include food, praise, pets, or grooming, and should be selected based on the cat's individual preferences. If the cat tolerates the discharge of the click when the clicker is wrapped in a thick towel, then the pet parent should use a thinner fabric like a piece of clothing or paper towel to wrap the clicker. If the cat tolerates the sound of the click in this context, then the clicker may be used unwrapped. If at any point the cat shows signs of fear, including running away, startling, freezing, putting his ears back, lowering his tail, developing dilated pupils, or becoming piloerect, after the discharge of the clicker, then the sound is too intense and should continue to be muffled, or another conditioned reinforcer such as a unique word or softer sound could be used. Provided a click of the tongue is unique, this might be an alternative to a clicker. See Chapter 10. As soon as the cat eliminates in the litterbox, the pet parent should mark that behavior with the clicker or the marker word and the reward should then be delivered promptly to the cat once the cat has exited the litterbox.

The pet parent can also train the cat to go to the litterbox on cue. Once trained to go to the litter on cue, the pet parent might then be able to encourage the cat to return to their litter every couple of hours, or to call the cat to their litter if they begin to show any signs that they are about to eliminate.

Behavior modification for marking

Behavior modification utilizing desensitization and counterconditioning is generally not practical for marking except when a problem in a relationship might be addressed. If the house-soiling problem arises as a result of the cat's relationship with other cats, people, or dogs within the home, the long-term goal is to use desensitization and counterconditioning to improve these relationships (see Chapter 10). Furthermore, when the cat is observed moving away from a site previously utilized for marking without marking, the pet parent should mark this behavior with a clicker or marker word and then promptly provide the cat's preferred primary reinforcer (e.g., food, praise, play, pets).

Medications and supplements

Medications can be extremely helpful in treating housesoiling problems as they may decrease FASCP that underlie the problem. However, psychoactive drugs do not replace the need for other treatment strategies, including addressing any physical disorders, optimizing the litterbox and environment, and resolving social tension between the cat and other pets or family members.

If undesirable elimination is a result of litterbox aversions or substrate preferences, then medication is not indicated or helpful unless there is a component of anxiety or stress. If the avoidance of the box is caused by stress, anxiety, or pain, then cats are more likely to show a response to drug therapy once those underlying causes are addressed.

Medications are often necessary to control urine marking.[11,90,151,152] Because urine marking is a normal feline behavior, eliminating it can be challenging, especially when sources of stress cannot be reduced in the cat's environment. In such cases, pharmacologic therapy may significantly decrease or eliminate urine marking.[9] A meta-analysis that evaluated the use of pharmacotherapy (clomipramine or fluoxetine) and pheromone therapy in the treatment of feline urine marking showed a significant association between the use of any intervention and the number of cats that ceased or reduced urine spraying by at least 90%.[153]

Pharmaceutical options

Commonly used medications in the treatment of urine marking and undesirable elimination secondary to FASCP are selective serotonin reuptake inhibitors and tricyclic antidepressants. However, none of the currently used medications are approved for use in cats, except for clomipramine in Australia. Therefore, whenever medications are dispensed, pet parents should be informed of off-label or extra-label use when applicable. Pretreatment lab tests are important as a screening baseline as well as to identify cats that may have health problems, such as hepatic or renal disease that might be a contraindication for the use of drug therapy or that might contribute to the behavior problem itself. Pet parents should be instructed to monitor and report any side effects. Since individual responses may vary, pet parents should start medications when they are available to observe their cat's response for at least four hours. Similarly, pet parents should be advised as to how long it might take to achieve efficacy and at what point dose adjustments or a change in treatment regime may need to be implemented. While improvement may be seen within the first week after starting an antidepressant, eight weeks or longer might be needed to achieve maximal improvement.[90] Pet parent contact at least every two weeks to assess efficacy of and any side effects to drug therapy is necessary. For all pets on medication, every 6–12-month laboratory testing is recommended. This may be more frequent for cats with underlying medical disorders, such as hepatic or renal disease.

Studies on the use of psychoactive medication for the treatment of house soiling disorders, while limited, have shown that improvement in urine marking may be achieved with fluoxetine in combination with environmental management and increased litterbox hygiene. In one double-blind placebo-controlled study, fluoxetine was effective at a dose of 1 mg/kg when combined with cleaning urine marks, ensuring the household contained one litterbox per cat plus an additional litterbox, scooping the box daily, and washing and changing the litter once weekly.[152] While improvement may be seen within the first week, fluoxetine showed increased efficacy at reducing urine marking when administered eight weeks or longer; however, some cats needed to be treated for 32 weeks to reach more than 90% reduction in urine marking.[90]

Once there has been a cessation in spraying for at least two months, an attempt might then be made to slowly decrease the medication dosage. However, long-term therapy is often necessary and recurrence rates after drug withdrawal are likely to be high unless sufficient modifications can be made to the pet's behavior and/or environment. Therefore, gradual dose reduction over several months might be a more practical approach to determine if the drug can be successfully withdrawn. Some cats maintained on long-term therapy may ultimately show recurrence, perhaps associated with new or stronger environmental stressors or long-term tolerance.

Clomipramine has also been shown to be approximately as effective as fluoxetine for treating urine spraying and reducing FASCP in cats, but dose and effects may be somewhat more variable. Clomipramine has been shown to be effective for reducing or controlling urine marking in cats at a dose of 0.25–0.5 mg/kg per day.[26,90,154,155] In one study, 20 of 25 cats showed a greater than 75% reduction in spraying within four weeks.[154] In another study of 26 spraying cats, there was 75% reduction in urine spraying in 80% of the cats; in 35% of those cats, there was complete cessation of the urine spraying.[26] In a controlled multicenter center study of 67 neutered cats, compared with a placebo, clomipramine significantly reduced the frequency of urine spraying in cats. The effect appeared to be dose dependent, with number of urine spraying events per day during the third month of treatment decreased by 64%, 72%, and 85% among cats treated with clomipramine at a low (0.125 to 0.25 mg/kg PO q 24 hours), moderate (0.25 to 0.5 mg/kg PO q 24 hours), and high (0.5 to 1 mg/kg PO q 24 hours) dosage, respectively.[155] In one comparative study, the efficacy of clomipramine at 0.5 mg/kg per day and fluoxetine at 1 mg/kg per day was similar.[90] Furthermore, improvement in some cats with recurrent FLUTD treated with clomipramine has been anecdotally reported.[9]

A recent study evaluated the efficacy of venlafaxine 1 mg/kg PO q 24 hours administered for 60 days, combined with environmental changes and behavior modification, in cats presenting for a range of problem behaviors. The study found that venlafaxine was significantly more efficacious than placebo in reducing house soiling, aggression, and fear. In the six cats that received venlafaxine, improvement was seen at day 60 and none of the cats experienced side effects.[156] In another study, eight cats diagnosed with FLUTD (six of them had periuria) and seven cats with behavior-related periuria (five with undesirable elimination, two of which were secondary to intercat aggression, one which was related to cognitive dysfunction, and one cat with urine marking) were administered venlafaxine at 0.9–1.7 mg/kg PO q 24 hours.[157] Clinical resolution was achieved in 85% of cats with 62% of cats achieving resolution within one week.[157] However, duration of clinical resolution was variable, with four cats relapsing after 3, 5, and 12 months. Side effects reported in that study included sedation, increased social behavior, anxiety, and decreased appetite.[157]

Side effects of antidepressants may include physical effects such as gastrointestinal signs and anorexia and undesirable or paradoxical behavioral effects such as agitation (see Chapter 11).[158,159] Clomipramine may cause fecal and urinary retention.[154,160] Urinary retention has also been reported with fluoxetine administration.[158,161] Because of this potential risk, these medications should be used with caution in cats that may be urinary house soiling due to FLUTD to avoid increasing the risk of a urethral obstruction. Other selective serotonin reuptake inhibitors such as paroxetine and sertraline have also anecdotally been reported to be effective in the treatment of feline house soiling disorders.

Diazepam (at a dose of 0.25-0.5 mg/kg twice daily) has been reported to be effective at reducing spraying in up to 74% of cats, with greatest effect achieved in neutered males.[162,163] Rare reports of fatal hepatopathies have been reported with oral diazepam use.[164] For this reason, diazepam is not recommended. Other benzodiazepines such as alprazolam, lorazepam, clonazepam, and oxazepam might be used instead. More specifically, benzodiazepines without active metabolites, such as oxazepam and lorazepam, may be favored as they may reduce the potential for adverse hepatic effects.[165] Lorazepam may be particularly effective at reducing FASCP and frequency of periuria in cats while being very well tolerated. Benzodiazepines might cause ataxia, sedation, and increased appetite (desirable when using food for behavior modification).[165] Some cats may develop a paradoxical hyperactivity, which may resolve over a few days or may require dose adjustment or discontinuation.[165] Twice-daily treatment is generally required for most benzodiazepines; however, as-needed administration for stressful events can also be helpful. Gradual withdrawal is recommended to avoid rebound effects if benzodiazepines have been administered daily for more than two weeks.[165]

Buspirone has also been used with some success to treat spraying behavior. One study found a significant reduction in urine marking in cats that received oral buspirone at 1 mg/kg once daily and in cats that received transdermal buspirone at 4 mg/kg once daily for five weeks; however, it is unknown whether the transdermal formulation reached therapeutic levels.[166] In another study, buspirone reduced spraying in 55% of cats, with cessation in 33%.[163] After the drug was withdrawn in that study, buspirone had a lower relapse rate of 50% compared to diazepam (up to 90%), despite the two medications having about the same efficacy in the treatment of urine spraying.[163] Buspirone does not cause the sedation, ataxia, or increased appetite seen with most benzodiazepines, and it has not been associated with adverse hepatic events.[163,167] At a dose of 5 mg/kg PO, buspirone caused increased wakefulness and decreased REM sleep in cats, as did diazepam at 1 mg/kg PO.[168] Buspirone may also cause cats to become more friendly and social, assertive, agitated, and aggressive.[163] In one case report, a spraying cat not only stopped spraying, but also began venturing into other parts of the house when treated with buspirone 2.5 mg PO twice daily. The buspirone could not be withdrawn without recurrence of the spraying.[169] Improvement on buspirone may not be seen for 1–2 weeks.[163]

Cyproheptadine (at a dose of 2-4 mg per cat twice daily) may be useful of the control of urine marking in some neutered male cats.[170] However, in one comparative study, clomipramine was found to be more effective.[171] Selegiline has been used for elimination disorders related to cognitive decline and in some European literature, has been reported to be effective for urine marking.[172,173] Progestins were historically used to treat urine marking in cats, but appear to be less effective than other medications,[174] except perhaps in neutered males, where improvement reached 50% compared to 10% in spayed females.[174,175] However, due to their potential for side effects such as immunosuppression, mammary cancer, and diabetes mellitus, their use should only be considered in neutered males when other therapeutics are ineffective (see Table 22.7).[176]

Table 22.7 Psychopharmacologic options for treatment of house-soiling disorders

Drug	Dosage (see Appendix B)	Comments
Fluoxetine	0.5–1.5 mg/kg q 24 hours	Good data for efficacy
Paroxetine	0.25–1.5 mg/kg q 24 hours	Likely similar effect as fluoxetine but no data. May be more calming. Mild anticholinergic.
Sertraline	0.25–1.5 mg/kg q 24 hours	Likely similar to fluoxetine but no data
Clomipramine	0.5–1.3 mg/kg q 24 hours	Mild anticholinergic. Good data for efficacy.
Venlafaxine	0.5–2 mg/kg q 24 hours	Little data for efficacy. Possibly beneficial for treatment of FIC.
Amitriptyline	0.5–2.0 mg/kg q12–24	Anticholinergic. Highly bitter – no data.
Buspirone	0.5–1 mg/kg q 12–24 hours up to 7.5 mg per cat q 12 hours	Expensive. Minimal side effects. Twice-daily dosing. Moderate efficacy.
Alprazolam	0.125–0.25 mg per cat q 8–12 hours	No data for treatment of house soiling. May increase appetite and cause sedation, ataxia and paradoxical excitement.
Lorazepam	0.125–0.25 mg per cat q 12–24 hours	No data for treatment of house soiling. May increase appetite and cause sedation, ataxia and paradoxical excitement.
Oxazepam	0.2–0.5 mg/kg q 12–24 hours	No data. May be less potential for hepatotoxicity than diazepam.
Selegiline	0.25–1 mg/kg q 24 hours	Cognitive dysfunction or emotional disorders
Megestrol acetate	2.5–10 mg per cat q 24 hours for 1–2 weeks then reduce gradually to once to twice weekly	Poor efficacy except perhaps neutered males. Potential for adverse effects. Last resort.
Medroxyprogesterone acetate	5–20 mg/kg SC/IM q 3–4 months	Injectable. Potential for adverse effects. A possible last resort option for neutered males.

Note: All doses listed are for oral administration unless otherwise noted

Pharmaceutical withdrawal

Once there has been a cessation in spraying for at least 3-6 months, an attempt might then be made to decrease the medication dosage slowly by 25-50% or less per week while monitoring for recurrence and lowest effective dose. In most cases, and especially if the social and physical environment cannot be modified to suit the cat's needs and lower FASCP sufficiently, the discontinuation of medications will cause relapse. In one study, 25% of cats could be withdrawn from clomipramine without recurrence of spraying after six months.[154] After eight weeks of therapy, recurrence rates ranging from 53% to over 75% were reported after discontinuation of buspirone and diazepam, respectively.[163] In another study in which improvement with drug therapy was achieved after either 16 or 32 weeks of fluoxetine, most cats returned to marking after withdrawal of treatment; however, a second course of treatment was found to be as effective as the first.[90] Therefore, long-term therapy is often necessary and recurrence rates on drug withdrawal are likely to be high unless sufficient modifications can be made to the pet's behavior or environment. Cats with the greatest marking at baseline were most likely to recur after drug withdrawal.[152]

Gradual dose reduction over several months might be a more practical approach to determine if the drug can be successfully withdrawn to reduce the potential for adverse or rebound effects during withdrawal and to determine whether a lower maintenance dose might be effective.

Some cats maintained on long-term therapy may ultimately show recurrence, perhaps associated with new or stronger environmental stressors or perhaps related to long-term tolerance. It is not uncommon for medications which previously were effective to be less effective when instituted again after discontinuation. Veterinarians should inform the pet parents of this possibility when discussing the risks and benefits of weaning their cat off of an effective medication.

Route of administration

Medications such as clomipramine and fluoxetine come in a size and chewable format for dogs that might make dosing and administration impractical for some cats. However, attempts to use some of these medications as transdermal medication, including fluoxetine, amitriptyline, and buspirone, have found little or insufficient absorption compared to oral dosing although one study reported an effect of transdermal buspirone on urine marking at 4 mg/kg.[166,177–178] Therefore, compounding of medications into a size and formulation (e.g., tiny tab, liquid) more appropriate for cats may be necessary. However, relative potency and stability may be an issue with compounded products. Another useful option would be to hide the pill in a high-valued food that might mask the pill's flavor, or to crush the medication into a flavored paste (liver or fish spreads) or food (e.g., cream cheese, butter, wet cat food, ice cream).

Pheromones

Besides marking with urine, cats also use secretions from skin glands and paws for communication.[25] In fact, there may be an antagonistic relationship between urine marking and facial marking, as application of cheek gland secretions reduces both sexual and reactive urine marking.[9,153,179–182] Therefore, pheromone analogues have been used in spraying cats to encourage alternative forms of marking (i.e., facial rubbing). These are considered first-line recommendations for all house-soiling cases. Studies have found that pheromone analogues resulted in significant reduction of urine marking but had a lower probability of leading to cessation of the marking behavior compared to pharmaceuticals[75,153] and often do not eradicate urine marking.[179] Pheromone analogues do not require oral administration and are non-systemic.[9] The feline facial pheromone analogue spray Feliway Classic has been reported to reduce urine spraying in 57–97% of cats.[75,180,181] A Feliway diffuser has also been shown to reduce urine marking[182] and may make the litterbox more appealing for cats with undesirable elimination.[9] A meta-analysis found that use of Feliway Classic therapy reduced spraying by more than 90%.[153] This result can last even after four weeks of discontinuation of the pheromone product.[181] Another study saw a decrease in the number of urine marks with Feliway in 57% of households, but two-thirds of the cats continued to mark regularly after treatment.[180] Since these studies were generally four weeks or less and did not include any environmental management, greater improvement might be achieved with longer-term use and a concurrent behavioral management program.[153] When peruria is due to stress, Feliway has been shown to calm cats in unfamiliar or stressful environments or situations, including changes in the environment such as moving, the addition of new pets, etc.[9,183,184] One study did not find a statistical difference between cats with recurrent FIC treated with Feliway and a placebo group but did find a trend for the cats exposed to Feliway having less severe episodes and fewer recurrences of FIC.[185]

For cats that show agonistic interactions with other cats in or outside of the home or with family members, the feline-appeasing pheromone analogue Feliway Multicat (USA) or Feliway Friends (Europe) may diminish agonistic interactions and promote calmer behaviors.[186] However, pheromones may be less effective in multicat households or with marked intercat aggression. In a meta-analysis of studies that evaluated the efficacy of pheromonotherapy, there were no associations found between treatment success and either the duration of the problem or number of cats in the household.[153] It is uncertain whether this also applies to pharmacological intervention.[75,153,181] If sufficient improvement is not achieved with Feliway alone, concurrent drug therapy should be considered.

A variety of nutraceuticals, dietary supplements, and prescription diets might also reduce anxiety-induced urine marking, alone or in conjunction with drug therapy, but data are still lacking (see Chapters 12 and 13). These might include L-theanine and alpha-casozepine, or therapeutic diets supplemented with ingredients such as alpha-casozepine and L-tryptophan in an increased ratio to other large amino acids, such as Royal Canin Feline Calm and Feline Hill's Pet Nutrition Prescription Diet c/d Multicare Urinary Stress. In addition, these supplements might have indications for the treatment of underlying stress contributing to undesirable toileting and FIC.[187-189]

Prognosis

Successful treatment of feline house-soiling disorders depends on a number of factors, including whether initiating factors can be resolved; duration of the problem; the environment and the pet parent's ability to modify and manage the environment; number of areas and surfaces soiled; the temperament of the cat; and the patience, ability, and willingness of the family to commit to working with the cat. When physical issues have been addressed and a cat has access to an optimized litterbox in a location they prefer, undesirable elimination should improve. In one study, an overall improvement rate was achieved in 78.5% of 189 cats that were treated for undesirable elimination.[190] Improvement may be seen immediately once improved litterbox management is instituted, but in general, pet parents can expect improvement of the house-soiling behavior within 1–3 months with treatment. However, in one study, elimination disorders that had been present longer in duration were rated by pet parents as less improved or worse once treatment was implemented,[191] so pet parents must be informed that prognosis likely declines the longer the problem has been occurring.

For marking, prognosis is more variable. Because marking is a normal behavior, eliminating it can sometimes be impossible.[9] Medications and/or pheromone therapy are often necessary in the treatment of urine marking, but the marking behavior may persist to some degree or recur if medication is stopped, so long-term use of medication may be necessary. In some cases, despite aggressive management and pharmaceutical intervention, urine spraying may persist at levels that are considered unacceptable to the pet parents. Because urine marking most often persists in households with social tension among cats,[181] rehoming may ultimately be the most suitable option (see Boxes 22.4 and 22.5).

Box 22.4 Factors affecting the prognosis of urine-marking

- Cause of the problem
- Duration of the problem
- Frequency of marking incidents
- Number of areas and surfaces marked
- Number of cats in the home
- Ability to identify and control access to arousing stimuli
- Environmental control – practicality and limitations
- Temperament of the pet
- Pet parent commitment/expectations – human–animal bond
- Health of the pet
- Drug use – efficacy, compliance, and cost
- Veterinarian's ability to diagnose and develop a program that suits pet, pet parent, and household

---

Box 22.5 Factors affecting the prognosis of unacceptable toileting

- Cause of the problem
- Litterbox experience
- Substrate experience
- Duration of the problem
- Frequency of house-soiling incidents
- Number of areas and surfaces soiled
- Number of cats in the home
- Temperament of the pet
- Pet parent commitment to modifying behavior
- Environment/limitations
- Health of the pet
- Veterinarian's ability to diagnose and develop a program that suits pet, pet parent, and household

CASE EXAMPLES

Case 1

Presentation

Jenny, an 8-year-old spayed female Domestic Medium Hair cat, was presented for fecal soiling.

History

Jenny had always eliminated in the litterbox until about 1.5 years prior to presentation. Fecal matter was often found next to the litterbox. Jenny always used the litterbox for micturition and occasionally for defecation. There were two litterboxes in the home, both of which were located on a veranda that was surrounded by windows overlooking a lawn where dogs were frequently walked. The litterboxes contained unscented clumping litter, and they were both open and lined. Sometimes when the pet parent found feces on the floor, she yelled at Jenny and brought her over to the place of defecation, pushed her nose into this site, and then confined her to a room for up to a few hours.

Diagnosis

Physical examination was unremarkable. Jenny's pet parent declined laboratory testing. Several differential diagnoses for the fecal soiling were considered, including a litterbox aversion secondary to pain during defecation or a litterbox characteristic such as the presence of a liner, the size of the boxes, or suboptimal litterbox hygiene, as well as a location aversion due to the placement of the boxes in a location with frequent dog exposure.

Treatment

The pet parent added a third large litterbox to the home in a room separate from the veranda, and removed the liners in the litterboxes. She began scooping the litterboxes twice daily. Soiled areas were cleaned with enzymatic cleaner. Furthermore, the pet parent was instructed to eliminate all punishment, as this may worsen the problem. After one week of these changes being implemented, Jenny resumed using the litterboxes for all elimination.

Case 2

Presentation

Fiona, an 11-year-old spayed female Domestic Shorthair cat, was presented for urinating outside of the litterbox.

History

Fiona was diagnosed with a malunion right femoral fracture at the time of adoption at one year of age, and she always reacted to being touched on her right back limb and caudodorsal region. Fiona started urinating outside of the litterbox around the time that she was adopted, and the frequency of periuria had increased over time to occurring daily. She always defecated inside of the litterbox. When Fiona urinated outside and inside of the litterbox, she sometimes urinated while standing with her rear backed up to a vertical surface and her tail slightly raised but not quivering and she sometimes postured to urinate. She always urinated large volumes and she scratched the litter or the ground after urinating. When defecating inside of the litterbox, Fiona stood with three legs positioned on the rim of the litterbox and one limb in the litter. The home contained four litterboxes of variable sizes. They were scooped 2–3 times daily, they all contained unscented clumping litter, and they were dumped, cleaned, and replaced with fresh litter once weekly.

Diagnosis

Fiona was diagnosed with feline periuria. Marking behavior was considered since Jenny sometimes backed up to vertical surfaces when eliminating, but was ruled out because Fiona did not demonstrate the characteristic posture of spraying including an erect, quivering tail, always urinated large volumes and attempted to cover the elimination.

On physical examination, she repeatedly tensed, turned her head, and growled on palpation of her right hip and caudodorsum. Pain secondary to the historical right femoral fracture, neurologic disease such as intervertebral disc disease, or other orthopedic disease (i.e., osteoarthritis of the coxofemoral joint) was suspected. Any of these possible sources of pain may have led Fiona to develop a negative association with the litterbox, leading to a litterbox aversion.

Treatment

Lab work was recommended, but declined by the pet parent. Fiona was started on gabapentin 5 mg/kg PO q 8 hours to address pain. Fiona immediately began urinating in the litterbox more regularly, but the periuria persisted. The pet parents were unable to block Fiona's access to all of the sites where she soiled, so Fiona was confined to a separate bedroom with two litterboxes, a food and water station, boxes for hiding, a cat tree, a window perch, and toys. Fiona received 3–5 interactions with the pet parents daily. Fiona consistently used the litterboxes in this bedroom. After one week, the pet parents began to let Fiona out of the room after she urinated in the morning. They closely supervised her and placed her back into the room about two hours later. Whenever she was returned to the room, she was given a treat and praise. Fiona continued to eliminate in the litterboxes in the room, so she was allowed out of the room for gradually increasing amounts of time throughout the day. After six weeks, the pet parents began allowing Fiona out of the bedroom at all times and her soiling did not recur.

Case 3

Presentation

Jasmine, a 3-month-old female kitten that had been obtained at two months of age, was using the pet parent's indoor planter for elimination.

History

The kitten slept in the third-floor bedroom at night and the litterbox was located on the first floor in the laundry room. Jasmine had used her litterbox for the first few weeks but would no longer use it. The pet parent had tried a number of litter types and litterboxes for variable amounts of time, with no improvement.

Diagnosis

Physical examination revealed a healthy and very alert kitten. Urinalysis and fecal evaluation failed to show any physical cause for the elimination problem. Jasmine had apparently developed a preference for using the soil in the planter and had perhaps developed an aversion for the litterbox area. Since she exhibited fear of loud noises, it was suspected that the sounds of the washer and dryer could have caused her to avoid the laundry room.

Treatment

The pet parent was advised to prevent Jasmine from eliminating in the planter by covering the surface of the soil with chips of marble, providing an appropriate elimination area near the planter with a lightweight sand-like litter as closely as possible resembling soil, adding a box near her sleeping area and moving the box outside of the laundry room, making no more than one change every five days. The pet parent was to avoid yelling at her and scolding her but was to reinforce her with food whenever she used the appropriate box. Within two weeks, Jasmine was using the litter consistently. The pet parents were instructed that they could move the box up to 1–6 inches every day to a more acceptable location. They were further instructed to not change anything else about the litterbox environment.

Case 4

Presentation

Digger, a 2.5-year-old neutered male Burmese, was presented with fecal soiling which initially was found next to the litterbox in the laundry room but had progressed to a Persian rug in the dining room.

continued

CASE EXAMPLES—cont'd

History

The initial soiling was associated with signs of colitis with mucoid fecal matter and an increase in defection frequency to 2–3 times daily. After extensive workup, food intolerance was diagnosed, and the cat had been controlled for several months with a venison and green pea prescription diet. Although clinical signs of colitis were resolved, Digger continued to eliminate once daily, always on the Persian rug. All urine was in the litterbox.

Diagnosis

Digger was diagnosed with perichezia initiated by colitis. However, the soiling had persisted in the dining room due to either litterbox aversion and surface or location preferences.

Treatment

The pet parents were instructed to block off the dining room to prevent access to the Persian rug. If they could not do that, they were to provide a litterbox on top of the spot where Digger was defecating. The pet parents were unable to block off the dining room effectively, so they decided to provide a litterbox instead. Digger continued to defecate in the dining room about 12 inches from where the litterbox was placed. It was suspected at this time that Digger had a litterbox aversion for defecation only due to a negative conditioned emotional response when defecation was painful.

The pet parents were instructed to purchase a new litterbox which had completely different characteristics from the old box and was at least 1.5 times the length of Digger's body. Suggestions included different colors of boxes, cookie sheets, under-bed storage boxes, and cardboard commercial litterpans. They were to place the new box over the area where he was defecating.

Within days, Digger was eliminating in the new box. The pet parents were consulted as to which option they would like to employ next- they hey could either move the box to a more desirable location or they could try to condition him to appreciate a more typical box. The pet parents elected to move the box. After two weeks, the box was in the corner of the room, and he continued to defecate in that box.

Case 5

Presentation

Buddy, a 4-year-old neutered male Domestic Shorthair cat, was presented for urination outside of the litterbox.

History

Buddy was adopted as a kitten and began urinating outside of the litterbox after he had been living in the home for about 1.5 years. On numerous occasions, the pet parents had observed Buddy backing up to a vertical surface with his tail erect and quivering, and spraying urine onto a vertical surface or object. He did not attempt to cover his eliminations. The pet parents placed litterboxes in the locations where Buddy eliminated, and had a total of 10 litterboxes in the home. The boxes were scooped 2–3 times daily, and dumped, washed with soap and warm water, and replaced with fresh litter monthly. However, Buddy continued to urinate outside of the box. Buddy lived in a home with five other cats, and he hissed and growled when passing by or interacting with the other cats on a daily basis.

Diagnosis

Physical examination was unremarkable. Laboratory testing was within normal limits. Buddy was diagnosed with urine marking due to social tension with the other cats in the household.

Treatment

Standard litterbox changes were recommended including bigger boxes spread throughout the home so that no one cat had to pass another cat to get to the litterboxes. The boxes were to be scooped at least once daily and dumped and cleaned monthly. All soiled locations were to be treated with an odor-eliminating cleaner, and where possible, some furniture or other items that had been soiled were removed from the home. The pet parents were given resources on cat body language, enrichment, and intercat aggression. They were told to watch their cats for any of the most common but subtle, types of aggression such as body blocking and staring.

After one week, the spraying had decreased significantly but was still present. The veterinary technician encouraged the pet parent to use the cameras in the home to ensure that Buddy was not the only cat that was eliminating outside of the litterbox. Three weeks after the initial appointment, the pet parent called and reported that she had in fact seen another household cat urine marking. She had noticed staring down and body blocking from several of the cats throughout the day. It was recommended that the other cat in the household that was seen urine marking come in for an evaluation. All changes previously recommended should continue. Bebe, a spayed female 13-year-old cat from the same household, was presented for urine marking. Bebe was reportedly the "queen" of the house. She displaced other cats, and hissed at them and chased them.

Bebe's laboratory tests and physical examination were within normal limits. Both Buddy and Bebe were placed on fluoxetine 0.5 mg/kg PO q 24 hours. After two weeks, the pet parents reported a 50% decrease in elimination and that the cats were getting along better. The fluoxetine was then increased to 0.75 mg/kg PO q 24 hours in both cats. Eight weeks from the original appointment, the urine marking was reduced by 75% in Bebe and 100% in Buddy. The pet parents were satisfied with this progress and elected to continue the treatment plan.

Conclusions

House soiling is a common reason that cats present to veterinarians and compromises the human–animal bond, increasing the risk of relinquishment or euthanasia. For any cat presenting with periuria or perichezia, physical causes, including general urinary tract and/or gastrointestinal tract health and pain, must be ruled out. If the house soiling cannot be attributed to a physical problem, then the social environment, including relationships with other pets and family members in and outside the household, and the physical environment, including the litterbox environment and changes to environment, routine or structure must be evaluated for potential inciting house soiling triggers. The clinician must bear in mind that the cases of house soiling are often multifactorial.

Stress management and fulfillment of the cat's environmental and emotional needs are essential to the management of all cases, including those caused by physical diseases. Prognosis for feline house soiling disorders depends on the pet parent's adherence to treatment recommendations, the chronicity of the problem, and the cat's temperament. Most cats respond favorably to treatment, but some cats may continue to soil to some degree despite treatment. For some cats, long-term pharmaceutical treatment may be indicated.

References

1. Barcelos AM, McPeake K, Affenzellar N, et al. Common risk factors for urinary house soiling (periuria) in cats and its differentiation: the sensitivity and specificity of common diagnostic signs. *Front Vet Sci.* 2018;5:108.

2. Salman MD, Hutchison J, Ruch-Gallie R, et al. Behavioral reasons for relinquishment of dogs and cats to 12 shelters. *J Appl Anim Welf.* 2000;2:93–106.

3. Patronek GJ, Glickman LT, Beck AM, et al. Risk factors for relinquishment of cats to an animal shelter. *J Am Vet Med Assoc.* 1996:209(3):582–588.

4. Marder AR, Engel JM, Hekman JP. Feline behavior problems reported by owners after adoption from an animal shelter. In: *Proceedings of the 6th International Veterinary Behavior Meeting (IVBM)*, Riccione, Italy; 2007:138–139.

5. Kass PH, New JC, Scarlett JM, et al. Understanding animal companion surplus in the United States: relinquishment of nonadoptables to animal shelters for euthanasia. *J Appl Anim Welf Sci.* 2001;4: 237–248.

6. Ramos D, Reche-Junior A, Luzia Fragoso P, et al. A case-controlled comparison of behavioural arousal levels in urine spraying and latrining cats. *Animals.* 2020;10(1):117. doi:10.3390/ani10010117.

7. Dantas LMS. Vertical or horizontal? Diagnosing and treating cats who urinate outside the box. *Vet Clin North Am Small Anim.* 2018;48:403–417.

8. Heath S. Common feline problem behaviours: unacceptable indoor elimination. *J Feline Med Surg.* 2019; 21:199–208.

9. Carney HC, Sadek TP, Curtis TM, et al. AAFP and ISFM guidelines for diagnosis and solving house-soiling behavior in cats. *J Feline Med Surg.* 2014;16:579–598.

10. Ramos D, Reche-Junior A, Mills D, et al. A closer look at the health of cats showing urinary house-soiling (periuria): a case-control study. *J Feline Med Surg.* 2019,21.772–779.

11. Neilson J. Housesoiling in cats. In: Horwitz DF, Mills DS, eds. *BSAVA Manual of Canine and Feline Behavioural Medicine.* Gloucester, UK: British Small Animal Veterinary Association; 2009: 117–126.

12. Thor KB, Blais DP, de Groat WC. Behavioral analysis of the postnatal development of micturition in kittens. *Dev Brain Res.* 1989;46(1):137–144.

13. Bradshaw J. Behavior of cats. In: Jensen P, ed. *The Ethology of Domestic Animals: An Introductory Text.* 3rd ed. New York, NY: CABI; 2017 [Chapter 17].

14. Borchelt P, Voith V. Elimination behavior problems in cats. *Compend Contin Educ Pract Vet.* 1986;8:197–207.

15. Beaver BV. Feline eliminative behavior. In: *Feline Behavior: A Guide for Veterinarians.* 2nd ed. St. Louis, MO: Saunders; 2003.

16. Overall KL, Rodan I, Beaver B, et al. Feline behavior guidelines from the American Association of Feline Practitioners. *J Am Vet Med Assoc.* 2005;2007(1):70–84.

17. Olm DD, Houpt KA. Feline house-soiling problems. *J Appl Behav Sci.* 1988;20(3): 335–345.

18. Sung W, Crowell-Davis SL. Elimination behavior patterns of domestic cats (Felis catus) with and without elimination behavior problems. *Am J Vet Res.* 2006;67: 1500–1504.

19. Nakabayashi M, Yamaoka R, Nakashima Y. Do faecal odours enable domestic cats (Felis catus) to distinguish familiarity of the donors? *J Ethol.* 2012;30, 325–329.

20. Panaman R. Behaviour and ecology of free-ranging female farm cats (Felis catus L.). *Z Tierpsychol.* 1981;56:59–73.

21. Brown SL, Bradshaw JWS. Communication in the domestic cat: within-and between-species. In: Turner DC, Bateson P, eds. *The Domestic Cat: The Biology of Its Behaviour,* 3rd ed. Cambridge: Cambridge University Press; 2013 [Chapter 4].

22. MacDonald D, Apps PJ, Carr GM, et al. Social dynamics, nursing conditions and infanticide among farm cats, Felis catus. *Adv Ethol.* 1987;28:1–64.

23. Herron ME. Advances in understanding and treatment of feline inappropriate elimination. *Top Companion Anim Med.* 2010;25:195–202.

24. Horwitz D. Common feline problem behaviors: urine spraying. Clinical review. *J Feline Med Surg.* 2019;21: 209–219.

25. Mohorovic´ M, Krofel M. The scent world of cats: where to place a urine scent mark to increase signal persistence? *Anim Biol.* 2020;71(2):151–168.

26. Dehasse J. Feline urine spraying. *Appl Anim Beh Sci.* 1997;53:365–371.

27. Heath S. Feline housesoiling. In: *Proceedings World Small Animal Veterinary Association.* Sydney, Australia; 2007, August 19–23. www.ivis.org.

28. Ellis SLH, Rodan I, Carney HC, et al. AAFP and ISFM feline environmental needs guidelines. *J Feline Med Surg.* 2013; 15:219–230.

29. Natoli E. Behavioral responses of urban feral cats to different types of urine marks. *Behaviour.* 1985;94:234–243.

30. Passanisi WC, Macdonald DW. Group discrimination on the basis of urine in a farm cat colony. In: MacDonald DW, ed. *Chemical Signals in Vertebrates.* Oxford: Oxford University Press; 1990.

31. Hart BL, Hart LA, Bain MJ. Feline house soiling. In: *Canine and Feline Behavior Therapy.* 2nd ed. Ames, Iowa: Blackwell; 2006:265–286.

32. Verberne G, de Boer J. Chemocommunication among domestic cats, mediated by the olfactory and vomeronasal senses, I. Communication. *Z Tierpsycholog.* 1976;42:86–109.

33. Guy NC, Hopson M, Vanderstichel R. Litterbox size preference in domestic cats (Felis catus). *J Vet Behav.* 2014;9: 78–82.

34. Neilson J.C. Is bigger better? Litterbox size preference test. In: *Proceedings of the ACVB/AVSAB Annual Meeting.* New Orleans, LA, 2008:46–49.

35. Neilson JC. Litter preference in cats; scented vs. unscented. In: *Proceedings of the ACVB/AVSAB Scientific Session.* St. Louis, MO; 2011:8–10.

36. Bergman L, Hart BL, Bain M, et al. Evaluation of urine marking by cats as a model for understanding veterinary diagnostic and treatment approaches and client attitudes. *J Am Vet Med Assoc.* 2002; 221:1282–1286.

37. Neilson JC. Scent preferences in the domestic cat. In: *Proceedings of the 6th International Veterinary Behaviour Meeting.* 2007:171–172.

38. Neilson JC. Litter preference test; evaluating carbon enhanced litter. In: *Proceedings of the ACVB/AVSAB Annual Meeting.* Washington, DC; 2007:59–60.

39. Neilson JC. Litter odor control: carbon vs. bicarbonate of soda. In: *Proceedings of the ACVB/AVSAB Annual Meeting.* New Orleans, LA; 2008:31–34.

40. Neilson JC. Feline litter acceptance. A comparison of brands. In: *Proceedings of the ACVB/AVSAB Annual Meeting.* Seattle, WA; 2009:10.

41. Neilson JC. Pearl vs. clumping litter preference in a population of shelter cats. In: *Proceedings of the AVSAB Annual Meeting*; 2001:14.

42. Borchelt PL. Cat elimination behaviour problems. *Vet Clin North Am Small Anim.* 1991;21:257–264

43. Smith K, Dreschel NA. A comparison of cat preferences for litterbox substrates. *Newslett Am Vet Soc Anim Behav.* 2008; 30:6–7.

44. Villeneuve-Beugnet V, Beugnet F. Field assessment of cats' litter box substrate preferences. *J Vet Behav.* 2018;25:65–70.

45. Mills DS, Munster C. Litter depth preference in the domestic cat. In: *Proceedings of the 4th International Veterinary Behaviour Meeting.* Australia, Caloundra; 2003:201–202.

46. Grigg EK, Pick L, Nibblett B. litterbox preference in domestic cats: covered versus uncovered. *J Feline Med Surg.* 2013; 15(4):280–284.

47. Fatjó J, Ruiz-de-la-Torre JL, Manteca X. The epidemiology of behavioural problems in dogs and cats: a survey of veterinary practitioners. *Anim Welf.* 2006; 15:179–185.

48. Denenberg S, Landsberg GM, Horwitz D, et al. A comparison of cases referred to behaviourists in three different countries. In: Mills D, Levine E, eds. *Current Issues and Research in Veterinary Behavioral Medicine.* West Lafayette, Indiana: Purdue University Press; 2005:56–62.

49. Beaver BV. House soiling by cats: a retrospective study of 120 cases. *J Am Anim Hosp Assoc.* 1989;25:631–637.

50. Bamberger M, Houpt KA. Signalment factors, comorbidity, and trends in behaviour diagnosis in cats: 736 cases 1991–2001. *J Am Vet Med Assoc.* 2006; 229:1602–1606.

51. Amat M, de la Torre JLR, Fatjo J, et al. Potential risk factors associated with feline behavior problems. *Appl Anim Behav Sci.* 2009;121:134–139.

52. Wassink-van der Schot AA, Day C, Morton JM, et al. Risk factors for behavior problems in cats presented to an Australian companion animal behavior clinic. *J Vet Behav.* 2016;14:34–40.

53. Horwitz D. Behavioral and environmental factors associated with elimination behaviour problems in cats: a retrospective study. *Appl Anim Behav Sci.* 1997;52:129–137.

54. Buffington CAT, Westropp JL, Chew DJ. From FUS to Pandora syndrome: where are we, how did we get here, and where to now? *J Feline Med Surg.* 2014;16:385–394.

55. Cameron ME, Casey RA, Bradshaw JW, et al. A study of environmental and behavioural factors that may be associated with feline idiopathic cystitis. *J Small Anim Pract.* 2004;45:144–147.

56. Defauw PA, Van de Maele I, Duchateau L, et al. Risk factors and clinical presentation of cats with feline idiopathic cystitis. *J Feline Med Surg.* 2011;13:967–975.

57. Westropp JL, Kass PH, Buffington CA. Evaluation of the effects of stress in cats with idiopathic cystitis. *Am J Vet Res.* 2006;67:731–736.

58. Westropp JL, Welk K and Buffington CA. Small adrenal glands in cats with feline interstitial cystitis. *J Urol.* 2003;170: 2494–2497.

59. Buffington CA, Westropp JL, Chew DJ, et al. Risk factors associated with clinical signs of lower urinary tract disease in indoor housed cats. *J Am Vet Med Assoc.* 2006;228:722–725.

60. Stella JL, Lord LK, Buffington CA. Sickness behaviors in response to unusual external events in healthy cats and cats with feline interstitial cystitis. *J Am Vet Med Assoc.* 2011;238(1):67–73.

61. Mills DS, Demontigny-Bédard I, Gruen M, et al. Pain and problem behavior in cats and dogs. *Animals.* 2020;10(318). doi:10.3390/ani10020318.

62. Hague DW, Stella JL, Buffington CA. Effects of interstitial cystitis on the acoustic startle reflex in cats. *Am J Vet Res.* 2013;74:144–147.

63. Hostutler RA, Chew DJ, DiBartola SP. Recent concepts in feline lower urinary tract disease. *Vet Clin North Am Small Anim.* 2005;35:147–170.

64. Gerber B, Boretti S, Kley S, et al Evaluation of clinical signs and causes of lower urinary tract disease in European cats. *J. Small Anim. Pract.* 2005;46:571–577.

65. Walker D. Feline lower urinary tract disease: a clinical refresher. *Irish Vet JN.* 2009;62(4):272–277.

66. Dorsch R, Remer C, Sauter-Louis C, et al. Feline lower urinary tract disease in a German cat population A retrospective analysis of demographic data causes and clinical signs. *Tieraerztl. Prax. Ausg. K Kleintiere Heimtiere.* 2014;42(4):231–239.

67. Saevik BK, Trangerud C, Ottesen N, et al. Causes of lower urinary tract disease in Norwegian cats. *J Feline Med Surg.* 2011; 13(6):410–417.

68. Buffington CA, Chew DJ, Kendall MS, et al. Clinical evaluation of cats with nonobstructive urinary tract diseases. *J Am Vet Med Assoc.* 1997;210:46–50.

69. Lemberger SI, Deeg CA, Hauck SM, et al. Comparison of urine protein profiles in cats without urinary tract disease and cats with idiopathic cystitis, bacterial urinary tract infection, or urolithiasis. *Am J Vet Res.* 2011;72:1407–1415.

70. Dorsch R, Remer C, Sauter-Louis C, et al. Feline lower urinary tract disease in a German cat population. *Tierarztl Prax Ausg K Kleintiere Heimtiere.* 2014;4:1–9.

71. Buffington CAT. Idiopathic cystitis in domestic cats-beyond the lower urinary tract. *J Vet Intern Med.* 2011;25:784–796.

72. Buffington CA. Comorbidity of interstitial cystitis with other unexplained clinical conditions. *J Urol.* 2004;172:1242–1248.

73. Lund HS, Sævik BK, Finstad ØW, et al. Risk factors for idiopathic cystitis in Norwegian cats: a matched case-control study. *J Feline Med Surg.* 2016;18(6):483–491.

74. Tynes VV, Hart BL, Pryor PA, et al. Evaluation of the role of lower urinary tract disease in cats with urine marking behavior. *J Am Vet Med Assoc.* 2003;223: 457–461.

75. Frank DF, Erb HN, Houpt KA. Urine spraying in cats: presence of concurrent disease and effects of a pheromone treatment. *J Appl Anim Behav Sci.* 1999; 61:263–272.

76. Millard RP, Pickens EH, Wells KL. Excessive production of sex hormones in a cat with an adrenocortical tumor. *J Am Vet Med Assoc.* 2009;234(4):505–508.

77. Cafazzo S, Bonanni R, Natoli E. Neutering effects on social behavioiur of urban unowned free-roaming domestic cats. *Animals.* 2019;9(12):1105. doi:10.3390/ani9121105.

78. Hart BL, Eckstein RA. The role of gonadal hormones in the occurrence of objectionable behaviours in dogs and cats. *Appl Anim Behav Sci.* 1997;52:331–334.

79. Merola I, Mills DS. Behavioral signs of pain in cats: an expert consensus. *PLoS One.* 2016; 11(2):e0150040. doi:10.1371/journal.pone.0150040.

80. Steagall PV, Monteiro B. Acute pain in cats. Recent advances in clinical assessment. *J Feline Med Surg.* 2019a;21:25–34.

81. Martell-Moran N, Solano M, Townsend H. Pain and adverse behavior in declawed cats. *J Feline Med Surg.* 2017;20(4): 280–288.

82. Steagall PV, Monteiro B. Chronic pain in cats. Recent advances in clinical assessment. *J Feline Med Surg.* 2019b;21: 601–614.

83. German AJ, Ryan VH, German AC, et al. Obesity, its associated disorders and the role of inflammatory adipokines in companion animals. *Vet J.* 2010;185:4–9.

84. Sordo L, Gunn-Moore GA. Cognitive dysfunction in cats: Update on neuropathological and behavioural changes plus clinical management. *Vet Rec.* 2021;188(1). doi:10.1002/vetr.3.

85. Gunn-Moore DA. Cognitive dysfunction in cats: clinical assessment and management. *Top Companion Anim Med.* 2011;26(1):17–24.

86. Miyazaki M, Yamashita T, Suzuki Y, et al. A major urinary protein of the domestic cat regulates the production of felinine, a putative pheromone precursor. *Chem Biol.* 2006;13(10):1071–1079.

87. Bradshaw J, Cameron-Beaumont C. The signaling repertoire of the domestic cat and its unrelated relatives. In: Turner DC, Bateson P, eds. *The Domestic Cat: The Biology of its Behavior.* 2nd ed. Cambridge, UK; Cambridge University Press; 2000:67–93.

88. Hart BL, Barrett RE. Effects of castration on fighting, roaming, and urine spraying in adult male cats. *J Am Vet Med Assoc.* 1973;163:290–292.

89. Hart BL, Cooper L. Factors related to urine spraying and fighting in prepubertally gonadectomized cats. *J Am Vet Med Assoc.* 1984;184:1255–1258.

90. Hart BL, Cliff KD, Tynes VV, et al. Control of urine marking by use of long-term treatment with fluoxetine or clomipramine in cats. *J Am Vet Med Assoc.* 2005;226:378–382.

91. Pryor PA, Hart BL, Bain MJ, et al. Causes of urine marking in cats and effects of environmental management on frequency of marking. *J Am Vet Med Assoc.* 2001;219:1709–1713.

92. Hart BL. Gonadal androgen and social sexual behavior in male mammals. A comparative analysis. *Psychol Bull.* 1974;81:383–400.

93. Casey R, Murray J. Risk factors for inappropriate urination and urine spraying in domestic cats. In: *Proceedings of the 2010 European Veterinary Behaviour Meeting.* Belgium, Hamburg, Germany: ESVCE; 2010:82–84.

94. Ellis JJ, McGowan RTS, Martin F. Does previous use affect litterbox appeal in multicat households? *Behav Process.* 2017;141:284–290.

95. Sandøe P, Nørspang AP, Forkman B, et al. The burden of domestication: a representative study of welfare in privately owned cats in Demark. *Anim Welf.* 2017;26(1):1–10.

96. Schubnel E, Arpaillange C. Contribution to the study of indoor cats' behavioural problems. *Prat Med et Chir de l'Anim de Comp.* 2008;43(2):63–70.

97. Foreman-Worsley R, Farnworth MJ. A systematic review of social and environmental factors and their implications for indoor cat welfare. *Appl Anim Behav Sci.* 2019; 220. doi:10.1016/j.applanim.2019.104841.

98. Tan SML, Stellato AC, Niel L. Uncontrolled outdoor access for cats: an assessment of risks and benefits. *Animals*. 2020;10(2): 258. doi:10.3390/ani10020258.

99. Hart BL, Hart LA. Feline behavioural problems and solutions. In: Turner DC, Bateson P, editors. *The Domestic Cat: The Biology of its Behaviour*. Cambridge, UK: Cambridge University Press; 2014:201–212.

100. Heidenberger E. Housing conditions and behavioural problems of indoor cats as assessed by their owners. *Appl Anim Behav Sci*. 1997;52(3–4):345–364.

101. Merola I, Lazzaroni M, Marshall-Pescini S, et al. Social referencing and cat-human communication. *Anim Cogn*. 2015;18: 639–648.

102. Humphrey T, Proops L, Forman J, et al. The role of cat eye narrowing movements in cat–human communication. *Sci Rep*. 2020;10. doi:10.1038/s41598-020-73426-0.

103. Adamelli S, Marinelli L, Normando S, et al. Owner and cat features influence the quality of life of the cat. *Appl Anim Behav Sci*. 2005;94(1–2):89–98.

104. Ramos D, Arena MN, Reche-Junior A, et al. Factors affecting faecal glucocorticoid levels in domestic cats (Felis catus): a pilot study with single and large multi-cat households. *Anim Welf*. 2012;21(2):285–291.

105. Turner DC. A review of over three decades of research on cat-human and human-cat interactions and relationships. *Behav Processes*. 2017;141:297–304.

106. Menchetti L, Calipari S, Mariti C, et al. Cats and dogs: best friends or deadly enemies? What the owners of cats and dogs living in the same household think about their relationship with people and other pets. *PLoS One*. 2020;15(8): e0237822. doi:10.1371/journal. pone.0237822.

107. Feuerstein N, Terkel J. Interrelationships of dogs (Canis familiaris) and cats (Felis catus L.) living under the same roof. *Appl Anim Behav Sci*. 2008;113(1–3): 150–165.

108. Crowell-Davis SL, Curtis TM, Knowles RJ. Social organization in the cat: a modern understanding. *J Feline Med Surg*. 2004;6(1):19–28.

109. Thomson JE, Hall SS, Mills DS. Evaluation of the relationship between cats and dogs living in the same home. *J Vet Behav*. 2018;27:35–40.

110. Bernstein PL, Strack M. A game of cat and house: spatial patterns and behavior of 14 domestic cats (Felis catus) in the home). *Anthrozoos*. 1996;9(1):25–39.

111. Levine ED. Feline fear and anxiety. *Vet Clin North Am Small Anim*. 2008;38: 1065–1079.

112. Neilson J. Thinking outside the box: feline elimination. *J Feline Med Surg*. 2004;6:5–11.

113. Elzerman AL, DePorter TL, Beck A, et al. Conflict and affiliative behavior frequency between cats in multi-cat households: a survey-based study. *J Feline Med Surg*. 2019. doi:10.1177/1098612X19877988.

114. Ellis SLH. Recognising and assessing feline emotions during the consultation: history, body language and behaviour. *J Feline Med Surg*. 2018;20:445–456.

115. Heath S. Understanding feline emotions and their role in problem behaviours. *J Feline Med Surg*. 2018;20:437–444.

116. Clark C. Dealing with multi-cat households: understanding how problems develop. *Comp Ani*. 2016;21(1):8–14.

117. Pachel C. Multicat aggression: restoring harmony in the home: a guide for practitioners. *Vet Clin North Am Small Anim*. 2014;44(3):565–579.

118. Howe LM, Slater MR, Boothe HW, et al. Long-term outcome of gonadectomy performed at an early age or traditional age in cats. *J Am Vet Med Assoc*. 2000;217:1661–1665.

119. Rehnberg LK, Robert KA, Watson SJ, et al. The effects of social interaction and environmental enrichment on the space use, behaviour and stress of owned housecats facing a novel environment. *Appl Anim Behav Sci*. 2015;169:51–61.

120. Amat M, Camps T, Manteca X. Stress in owned cats: behavioural changes and welfare implications. *J Feline Med Surg*. 2016;18(8):577–586.

121. Loberg JM, Lundmark F. The effect of space on behaviour in large groups of domestic cats kept indoors. *Appl Anim Behav Sci*. 2016;182:23–29.

122. Levine E, Perry P, Scarlett J, et al. Intercat aggression in households following the introduction of a new cat. *Appl Anim Behav Sci*. 2005;90(3–4):325–336.

123. Ramos D. Common feline problem behaviors: Aggression in multi-cat households. *J Feline Med Surg*. 2019;21(3):221–233.

124. Bateson P, Turner DC. Questions about cats. In: Turner DC, Bateson P, eds. *The Domestic Cat: The Biology of its Behavior*. 2nd ed. Cambridge, UK: Cambridge University Press; 2000:231–232.

125. Hart BL, Leedy M. Identification of source of urine stains in multi-cat households. *J Am Vet Med Assoc*. 1982;180:77.

126. Neilson J. The use of fluorescein in cats to identify participants in housesoiling. In: *Proceedings of the ACVB Scientific Presentations*. Philadelphia, PA; 2004.

127. Kruger JM, Lulich JP, MacLeay J, et al. Comparison of foods with differing nutritional profiles for long-term management of acute nonobstructive idiopathic cystitis in cats. *J Am Vet Med Assoc*. 2015;247:508–517.

128. Dulaney DR, Hopfensperger M, Malinowski R, et al. Quantification of urine elimination behaviors in cats with a video recording system. *J Vet Intern Med*. 2017;31(2):486–491.

129. Scherk M. Urinary tract disorders. In: Little SE, ed. *The Cat Clinical Medicine and Management*. St. Louis, MO: Elsevier; 2012:935–1013.

130. Slingerland LI, Hazewinkel HA, Meij BP, et al. Cross-sectional study of the prevalence and clinical features of osteoarthritis in 100 cats. *Vet J*. 2011; 187:304–309. pmid:20083417.

131. Doxsee A, Yager JA, Best SJ, et al. Extratesticular interstitial and Sertoli cell tumors in previously neutered dogs and cats; a report of 17 cases. *Can Vet J*. 2006;47:763–766.

132. Monteiro BP, Lascelles BDX, Murrell J, et al. 2022 WSAVA guidelines for the recognition, assessment and treatment of pain. *J Small Anim Pract*. 2022. https://doi.org/10.1111/jsap.13566.

132a. Lascelles B, Capner C, Waterman-Pearson AE. Current British veterinary attitudes to perioperative analgesia for cats and small mammals. *Vet Rec*. 1999; 145:601–604.

132b. Hugonnard M, Leblond A, Keroack S. Attitudes and concerns of French veterinarians towards pain and analgesia in dogs and cats. *Vet Anaesth Analg*. 2004;31:154–163.

133. Sparkes AH, Heiene R, Lascelles DX. ISFM and AAFP consensus guidelines: long-term use of NSAIDs in cats. *J Feline Med Surg*. 2010;12:531–538.

134. *Onsior® (robenacoxib) Freedom of Information Summary*, NADA 141–320. 2011.

135. Guillot M, Moreau M, Heit M, et al. Characterization of osteoarthritis in cats and meloxicam efficacy using objective chronic pain evaluation tools. *Vet J*. 2013;196(3):360–367.

136. Robertson SA. Managing pain in feline patients. *Vet Clin North Am Small Anim*. 2008;38:1267–1290.

137. Bennett D, Zainal Ariffin SM, Johnston P. Osteoarthritis in the cat: 2. How should it be managed and treated? *J Feline Med Surg*. 2012;14(1):76–84.

138. Gruen ME, Griffith EH, Thomson AE, et al. Criterion validation testing of clinical metrology instruments for measuring degenerative joint disease associated mobility impairment in cats. *PLoS One*. 2015;10:e0131839. pmid:26162101.

139. Adrian D, King JN, Parrish RS, et al. Rodenacoxib shows efficacy for the treatment of chronic degenerative joint disease-associated pain in cats: a randomized and blinded pilot clinical trial. *Sci Rep*. 2021;7721. doi:10.1038/ s41598-021-87023-2.

140. Duncan B, Lascelles X, Court MH, et al. Nonsteroidal anti-inflammatory drugs in cats: a review. *Vet Anaesth Analges*. 2007; 34:228–250.

141. Mathews A. Physiologic and pharmacologic applications to manage neuropathic pain. In: Mathews KA, Sinclair M, Steele AS, et al. *Analgesia and Anesthesia for the Ill or Injured Dog and Cat*. Hoboken: John Wiley and Sons; 2018:17–50.

142. Guedes AG, Meadows JM, Pypendop BH, et al. Assessment of the effects of gabapentin on activity levels and owner-perceived mobility impairment and quality of life in osteoarthritic cats. *J Am Vet Med Assoc*. 2018;253(5):579–585.

143. Lorenz ND, Comerford EJ, Iff I. Long-term use of gabapentin for musculoskeletal disease and trauma in three cats. *J Feline Med Surg.* 2013;15(6):507–512.

144. Buffington CA, Westropp JL, Chew DJ, et al. Clinical evaluation of multimodal environmental modification (MEMO) in the management of cats with idiopathic cystitis. *J Feline Med Surg.* 2006;8: 261–268.

145. Cottam N, Dodman NH. Effect of an odor eliminator on feline litter behaviour. *J Feline Med Surg.* 2007;9:44–50.

146. Frayne J, MacDonald Murray S, Croney C, et al. The behavioural effects of innovative litter developed to attract cats. *Animals.* 2019;9(9):683. doi:10.3390/ani9090683.

147. Dantas LMS, Delgado MM, Johnson I, et al. Food puzzles for cats: feeding for physical and emotional wellbeing. *J Feline Med Surg.* 2016;18:723–732.

148. Delgado M, Bain MJ, Buffington CAT. A survey of feeding practices and use of food puzzles in owners of domestic cats. *J Feline Med Surg.* 2020; 22(2):193–198.

149. Delgado MM, Han BSG, Bain MJ. Domestic cats (Felis catus) prefer freely available food over food that requires effort. *Anim Cogn.* 2021;25(95-102). doi:10.1007/s10071-021-01530-3.

150. Schwartz S. Separation anxiety syndrome in cats: 136 cases (1991–2000). *J Am Vet Med Assoc.* 2002;220(7):1028–1033.

151. Eckstein RA, Hart BL. Pharmacologic approaches to urine-marking in cats. In: Dodman NH, Shuster L, eds. *Psychopharmacology of Animal Behavior Disorders.* Abingdon: Blackwell Science; 1998:264–276.

152. Pryor PA, Hart BL, Cliff KD, et al. Effects of a selective serotonin reuptake inhibitor on urine spraying behaviour in cats. *J Am Vet Med Assoc.* 2001;219: 1557–1561.

153. Mills DS, Redgate SE, Landsberg GM. A meta-analysis of studies of treatments for feline urine spraying. *PLoS One.* 2011;6(4):e18448.doi:10.1371/journal. pone.0018448.

154. Landsberg G, Wilson AL. Effects of clomipramine on cats presented for urine marking. *J Am Anim Hosp Assoc.* 2005;41:3–11.

155. King JN, Steffan J, Heath SE, et al. Determination of the dosage of clomipramine for the treatment of urine spraying in cats. *J Am Vet Med Assoc.* 2004;225:881–887.

156. Metz D, Medam T, Masson S. Double-blind, placebo-controlled trial of venlafaxine to treat behavioural disorders in cats: a pilot study. *J Feline Med Surg.* 2021;24(6):539–549.

157. Hopfensperger MJ. Use of oral venlafaxine in cats with feline idiopathic cystitis or behavioral causes of periuria. In: *Proceedings of the American College of Veterinary Behaviorists Annual Symposium.*, San Antonio, TX, USA; 2016 August 5: 13–17.

158. Ogata N, Mattos de Souza Dantas L, Crowell-Davis S. Selective serotonin reuptake inhibitors. In: Crowell-Davis S, Murray T, Mattos de Souza Dantas L, eds. *Veterinary Psychopharmacology.* 2nd ed. Ames, Iowa: Blackwell Publishing; 2019:103–128.

159. Crowell-Davis SL. Tricyclic Antidepressants. In: Crowell-Davis S, Murray T, Souza Dantas L, eds. In: *Veterinary Psychopharmacology.* 2nd ed. Ames, Iowa: Blackwell Publishing; 2019:231–256.

160. Pfeiffer E, Guy N, Cribb A. Clomipramine-induced urinary retention in a cat. *Can Vet J.* 1999;40(4):265–267.

161. Pflaum K, Bennett S. Investigation of the use of venlafaxine for treatment of refractory misdirected play and impulse-control aggression in a cat: a case report. *J Vet Behav.* 2021;42:22–25.

162. Marder A. Psychotropic drugs and behavioural therapy. *Vet Clin North Am Small Anim.* 1991;21:329–342.

163. Hart BL, Eckstein RA, Powell KL, et al. Effectiveness of buspirone on urine spraying and inappropriate urination in cats. *J Am Vet Med Assoc.* 1993;203:254–258.

164. Center SA, Elston TH, Rowland PH, et al. Fulminant hepatic failure associated with oral administration of diazepam in 11 cats. *J Am Vet Med Assoc.* 1996;209:618–625.

165. Mattos de Souza Dantas L, Crowell-Davis S. Benzodiazepines. In: Crowell-Davis S, Murray T, Mattos de Souza Dantas L, eds. *Veterinary Psychopharmacology.* 2nd ed. Ames, Iowa: Blackwell Publishing; 2019:67–102.

166. Chávez G, Pardoa P, Ubillab MJ, et al. Effects on behavioural variables of oral versus transdermal buspirone administration in cats displaying urine marking. *J Appl Anim Res.* 2015;44(1): 454–457.

167. Mattos de Souza Dantas L, Crowell-Davis SL. Miscellaneous serotonergic agents. In: Crowell-Davis S, Murray T, Mattos de Souza Dantas L, eds. *Veterinary Psychopharmacology.* 2nd ed. Ames, Iowa: Blackwell Publishing; 2019:129–146.

168. Hashimoto T, Hamada C, Wada T, et al. Comparative study on the behavioral and EEG changes induced by diazepam, buspirone and a novel anxioselective anxiolytic, DN-2327, in the cat. *Neuropsychobiology.* 1992;26:89–99.

169. Overall KL. Animal behavior case of the month. *J Am Vet Med Assoc.* 1994;205(5): 694–696.

170. Schwartz S. Use of cyproheptadine to control urine spraying in a castrated male domestic cat. *J Am Vet Med Assoc.* 1999;215:501–502.

171. Kroll T, Houpt KA. A comparison of cyproheptadine and clomipramine for the treatment of urine spraying in cats. In: Overall KL, Mills DS, Heath SE, et al. eds. *Proceedings of the 3rd International Congress on Veterinary Behavioral Medicine.* Herts, UK: Universities Federation for Animal Welfare; 1995: 184–185.

172. Landsberg GM, Denenberg S, Araujo JA. Cognitive dysfunction in cats: a syndrome we used to dismiss as 'old age'. *J Feline Med Surg.* 2010;12(11):837–848.

173. Dramard V. *Pathologie du comportement du chien et du chat.* 2nd ed. Paris: Med'Com; 2007.

174. Cooper LL, Hart BL. Comparison of diazepam with progestin for effectiveness in suppression of urine spraying behavior in cats. *J Am Vet Med Assoc.* 1992;200:797–801.

175. Hart BL. Objectionable urine spraying and urine marking in cats: evaluation of progestin treatment in gonadectomized males and females. *J Am Vet Med Assoc.* 1980;177:529–533.

176. Romagnoli S. Progestins to control feline reproduction: historical abuse of high doses and potentially safe use of low doses. *J Feline Med Surg.* 2015;17(9): 743–752.

177. Mealey KL, Peck KE, et al. Systemic absorption of amitriptyline and buspirone after oral and transdermal administration to healthy cats. *J Vet Intern Med.* 2004;18:43–46.

178. Ciribassi J, Luescher A, Paloske K, et al. Comparative bioavailability of fluoxetine after transdermal and oral administration to healthy cats. *Am J Vet Res.* 2003;6: 994–998.

179. Mills DS, White JC. Long-term follow up of the effect of a pheromone therapy on feline spraying behavior. *Vet Rec.* 2000; 147(26):746–747.

180. Hunthausen W. Evaluating a feline facial pheromone analogue to control urine spraying. *Vet Med.* 2000;95: 151–156.

181. Ogata N and Takeuchi Y. Clinical trial of a feline pheromone analogue for feline urine marking. *J Vet Med Sci.* 2001;63: 157–161.

182. Mills DS, Mills CB. Evaluation of a novel method for delivering a synthetic analogue of feline facial pheromone to control urine spraying by cats. *Vet Rec.* 2001;149:197–199.

183. Griffith CA, Steigerwald ES, Buffington CA. Effects of a synthetic facial pheromone on behavior of cats. *J Am Vet Med Assoc.* 2000;217:1154–1156.

184. Gaultier E. Current research in canine and feline pheromones, *Vet Clin North Am Small Anim.* 2003;33:187.

185. Gunn-Moore DA, Cameron ME. A pilot study using synthetic feline facial pheromone for the management of feline idiopathic cystitis. *J Feline Med Surg.* 2004;6(3):133–138.

186. DePorter TL, Bledsoe DL, Beck A, et al. Evaluation of the efficacy of an appeasing pheromone diffuser product vs placebo for management of feline aggression in multi-cat households. A pilot study. *J Feline Med Surg.* 2019;21(4):293–305.

187. Meyer H, Becvarova I. Effects of a urinary food supplement with milk protein hydrolysate and L-tryptophan on

feline idiopathic cystitis – results of a case series in 10 cats. *Int J Appl Res Vet Med.* 2016;14:59–65.

188. Landsberg GM, Milgram NW, Mougeot I, et al. Therapeutic effects of an alpha-casozepine and ʟ-tryptophan supplemented diet on fear and anxiety in the cat. *J Feline Med Surg.* 2017;6:594–602.

189. Miyaji K, Kato M, Ohtani N, et al. Experimental verification of the effects on normal domestic cats by feeding prescription diet for decreasing stress. *J Appl Anim Welf Sci.* 2015;18: 355–362.

190. Halip JW, Vaillancourt JP, Luescher UA. A descriptive study of 189 cats engaging in inappropriate elimination behaviors. *Feline Pract.* 1998;26(4):18–21.

191. Marder AG, Engel JM. Long-term outcomes after treatment for feline inappropriate elimination. *J Appl Anim Welf Sci.* 2002;5:299–308.

Recommended reading and resources

AAFP and ISFM Housesoiling Guidelines - https://catvets.com/guidelines/practice-guidelines/house-soiling.

AAFP – Pet Parent Resources https://catfriendly.com/why-does-my-cat/spraying/

Carney HC, Sadek TP, Curtis TM, et al. AAFP and ISFM guidelines for diagnosis and solving house-soiling behavior in cats. *J Feline Med Surg.* 2014;16:579–598.

Dantas LMS. Vertical or horizontal? Diagnosing and treating cats who urinate outside the box. *Vet Clin North Am Small Anim.* 2018;48:403–417.

Ellis SLH, Rodan I, Carney HC, et al. AAFP and ISFM feline environmental needs guidelines. *J Feline Med Surg.* 2013; doi:10.1177/1098612X13477537.

Canine aggression

Lisa Radosta, DVM, DACVB

Introduction

Aggressive behavior is the most common behavior problem for which dogs are referred to veterinary behaviorists, representing up to 75% of all canine cases.[1-3] Veterinary practitioners report aggression as the second most common behavior complaint, just behind destructiveness, with up to 30% of pet parents reporting biting behavior.[4-6] When a dog shows aggression, it poses a risk to family members, other animals, and the public, and also puts the animal at risk of poor quality of life (e.g., relegated to living outside), euthanasia, or relinquishment. Aggressive behavior has a significant impact on the human–animal bond, leading to emotional stress for pet parent, poor quality of life for both the pet parent and the pet, increased risk of pet relinquishment and euthanasia at shelters, and pet parent-requested euthanasia.[7-10] In one UK study, over one-third of dogs were relinquished because of problematic behaviors, 14% due to aggression (7.1% to other pets and 6.4% to people).[10] Aggression which includes barking and lunging is sometimes referred to in the lay literature as reactivity.

Normal canine behavior

Aggression may be normal, adaptive, and appropriate in some contexts, and any dog can potentially bite. Aggressive behavior encompasses a wide variety of behaviors, from subtle body postures and facial expressions to threats to explosive attacks. Most pet parents do not consider their dog aggressive unless the dog has bitten, and even then only if the bite has broken skin.

Any body posture associated with threat including growling, lunging, snapping, nipping, or tense body posture should be viewed as aggressive behavior. Body language postures can be classified in several ways depending on the discipline. Ethologists may characterize them as offensive or defensive, distance increasing, or distance decreasing. Most often in veterinary medicine, they are classified as relaxed, fearful, anxious, stressed, conflicted, panicked (FASCP), and aggressive. In this text, we will most often characterize body language as relaxed or FASCP; however, distance increasing or decreasing may be used. The terms "dominance" and "submission" have specific definitions in ethology texts. Unfortunately, they have been over- and incorrectly used as a label of a personality trait in dogs, which is wholly inaccurate. Dominance describes the relationship between two individuals at one point in time, not a personality trait which can be applied to every situation.[11] Dogs do not have grand plans to take over the household, dominating each individual one by one in order to get to the top spot, an idea that is completely unsubstantiated in the literature. Instead, dogs have learned how to gain the resources needed to be happy and healthy from each individual in the household. Dogs modify their behavior to avoid conflict and retain resources, no matter where they are and with whom they are interacting. Why then is one dog aggressive and not the next? Differences in the dog's response to a person, animal, or object depends on differences in the relationship and interactions with the dog, the dog's genetic predispositions, overall wellness, and life experiences. Pet parents who are more structured and use positive reinforcement training are more likely to have relationships which do not include aggression. Because those individuals interact with the dog differently, the dog in turn asks for what he needs in different ways. This leads to differences in interactions as the dog learns the patterns of which behaviors to exhibit with which individuals in which situations.

Dominance hierarchies are evident throughout our society and animal societies. Depending on the species being studied, the most dominant animal may be the most aggressive or they be the least likely to engage in aggressive encounters. Therefore, it is a misconception to always assume that the most dominant individual is the most aggressive individual in the group. In pet dogs, often the most aggressive individual is likely to be the most uncertain dog in the group. While dominance was previously thought to be at the core of most pet parent-directed aggression, recent research suggests that many dogs that display pet parent-directed aggression are primarily fearful and often in a state of conflict (anxious and uncertain).[4,12–15]

Although it is tempting to make direct comparisons between wolves and dogs, the domestication of the dog for tens of thousands of years makes absolute comparisons inaccurate and misleading, with significant differences in cognitive ability, communication and signaling, parental and sexual behavior, cognitive ability and in both intraspecific and interspecific social behavior with humans.[16–21] Compared to hand reared wolves dogs display more human centred behaviors, and advanced abilities to respond to human behaviors and cues.[17,18] See Chapter 2 for more information on dog social structure. Hierarchies do appear to exist among domestic dogs and perhaps with family members with whom they live; however, relationships might more accurately be described in terms of resource-holding potential differences in motivation, social stress, and learned behaviors (consequences).[18,19] While pairwise relationships may be seen, a hierarchy is generally not evident.[19] However, groups of individuals do require a system of organization with some level of social asymmetry in order to resolve conflicts without aggression.

The body language of aggression

Veterinarians who diagnose and treat canine aggression cases should have a good understanding of how to interpret canine body language (see Chapter 2 and Appendix A). Aggression can be accompanied by body postures associated with fear or distance increasing (e.g., ears flattened against the head, tail tucked underneath the body, lowered body position, leaning away from the fear-eliciting stimulus, rolling over onto the back), arousal (e.g., dilated pupils, piloerection), defense (e.g., teeth bared, growling, biting, and scratching), and offensive (e.g., upright body, forward ears, tail out from body, tail curled over the back). However, body language signals can be reinforced and punished. For that reason, with repetition and learning, the body language associated with aggressive displays may appear less consistent with fear and more consistent with confidence (e.g., ears forward, upright body), and the dog may become quicker to resort to aggression rather than avoidance behavior. With the diagnostic criteria below, there is a description of body language where applicable; however, the practitioner should always keep in mind that the body language of stress is fluid and specific to the individual and often cannot be separated into distinct categories. It is a part of the picture but may not tell the entire story.

Health issues may affect a dog's ability to respond or react appropriately to a person another or dog's signals or cues. The problem may be further compounded by the differences in morphology between breeds. Facial expressions may be hidden under loose skin or distorted by alterations to facial structure in brachycephalic breeds. Eyes may be small, covered by hair and deeply inset, or large and prominent. Alterations in tail structure and ear carriage also affect important communication signals, and shortened legs or dramatic disparities in height may make reading body language signals problematic. It is also possible that sensory ability is compromised, as the size, shape, and placement of eyes, ears,

and nose are altered by breeding. In addition, with selective breeding for morphology and behavior, breeds that are less modified may have substantially retained most of repertoire of wolf signaling, while the most anatomically modified perform the fewest visual signals, which may affect the dog's social interactions and communication with other dogs.[16,20,21]

Pathology of aggression

Decreased cerebrospinal fluid 5-hydroxyindoleacetic acid concentrations have been linked to aggression in several species, including dogs.[22,23] Alterations in serum serotonin levels or turnover has been reported in some English Cocker Spaniels, English Springer Spaniels, and other breeds of aggressive dogs,[24–27] and altered prolactin levels have been identified with acute and chronic anxiety disorders.[28] Serum serotonin levels have been demonstrated to be lower in dogs immediately following displays of aggression compared to when those same dogs were calm.[29] There is evidence of a correlation between binding at the 5-HT2A serotonin receptor and aggressive behavior in dogs. In fact, a correlation was found between decreased serotonin binding at the 5-HT2A receptor prior to treatment and improvement in impulsively aggressive dogs that were treated with citalopram.[30] And in another study, dogs that exhibited aggression toward people had a higher binding index at the 5-HT2A receptor in the cortical regions of the brain when compared to dogs that did not show aggression.[31] Neurotransmitter and receptor alterations have also been postulated based on response to therapy. It is unclear if these changes cause, contribute to, or are caused by the behavior disorder.

Several studies have investigated the link between the gastrointestinal microbiome and behavioral clinical signs. One study found predominance of different bacteria in the microbiome of phobic dogs, aggressive dogs, and control dogs.[32] See chapter 13 for more information on feeding and the microbiome as it relates to behavior disorders.

Learning and aggression

Learning complicates accurate diagnosis of dogs displaying aggressive behavior because it can significantly change the body language and behaviors that are displayed. Aggressive signaling and behavior is an attempt at communication. When those signals are acknowledged with appropriate (as determined by the sender) behavior by the recipient of the signal, the aggression reduces. When it is not, the aggression increases. The progression from disengagement body language to aggressive displays can be considered a progression as if climbing a ladder. Each rung of the ladder is a different level of stress associated with certain body language signals. If a dog feels uncomfortable or stressed, they may avert their gaze, lick their lips, or blink their eyes slowly. If these signals are effective at gaining distance from the stress-eliciting situation, those body language signals are reinforced and the likelihood that the dog will continue to exhibit those signals in that situation increases. Figuratively speaking, the dog continues to sit on that rung of the ladder. However, if those signals are not effective at gaining distance from the person, animal, or stimulus, that signal is punished (i.e., the likelihood of exhibiting the lower intensity signals decreases). Imagine the rung of the ladder breaking. The only recourse the dog has is to jump to the next rung of the ladder to communicate their need to gain distance from the stressor, which appears grossly as an escalation in body language signaling. If this happens repeatedly, where lower level, more passive body language signals are punished, the dog may and often does continue to escalate until he shows aggression. Aggression is inevitably reinforced because when bitten, most people pull back, reinforcing the behavior instantly. Finally, the dog has found a way to communicate with humans! Even if the person yells at the dog 30 seconds later, it will not change that the behavior was immediately reinforced and that the behavior has a high likelihood of increasing in that situation the next time (see Figure 23.1).

Consider the dog presented for growling at the pet parent when the food bowl is removed. The dog growls at the pet parent due to a motivation to keep the food for whatever reason (e.g., genetics, previous learning, physical disease, anxiety, fear, hunger). The pet parent has removed the bowl in the past as the dog was eating. For this reason, the dog anticipates that the pet parent's approach is going to result in the consequence of the food being removed. If the pet parent takes away the bowl after the dog growls, the motivation for growling (e.g., anxiety) is still present, but the growling is extrinsically punished (the pet parent took the food, negative punishment). In this case, anxiety will increase (the pet parent's approach results in the consequence of the food being taken away) and growling will decrease over time (the growling is punished). As anxiety increases, the dog will continue to escalate the signaling to lunging or biting. If the dog bites, the pet parent will most likely recoil, even if for a split second, negatively reinforcing the bite (biting will increase). To be clear, it is unreasonable and unsafe to advise a pet parent to continue to let a dog bite to avoid negatively reinforcing that behavior; however, it is reasonable, safe, and the standard of practice to recommend that the pet parent stop picking up the bowl and seek help from a veterinarian or board-certified veterinary behaviorist.

In another example, a dog is hugged by a well-meaning pet parent. The pet parent does not notice that the dog turns its head away and licks its lips (signs of stress and disengagement). If this interaction continues, the dog will most likely progress from benign signals to more offensive ones. Finally, if and when the dog bites the pet parent, she retreats and the behavior is negatively reinforced, teaching the dog to bite instead of warn in more subtle ways. This type of dog may be presented for treatment or euthanasia with a history of unprovoked bites when for days, months, or years the dog had been attempting to signal in a nonoffensive way. For the best possible outcome, each case history should be closely examined for clues of how behaviors have been punished and reinforced to create the behavior for which the dog is being presented. See Chapter 10 for more information about learning theory.

Any stimulus can be paired with a conditioned emotional response (CER). For example, if application of topical flea and tick medication is uncomfortable, the pet may form a negative CER to the sight of the tube or the pet parent's movement to where medications are kept. This association can lead to aggression. Pets that are threatened or physically punished for aggressive displays can learn to associate pain or fear with certain stimuli, and become even more aggressive each time the situation recurs. They can also form a negative CER to certain people who perpetrate the physical punishment. Some types of aggression such as territorial aggression are reinforced by the environmental factors or stimuli outside of the pet parent's control. For example, if a dog barks at the window at a delivery person, the delivery person drops the package and leaves. The barking was reinforced (negative reinforcement) even though it was not the cause of the delivery person's departure.

Prevalence

The World Health Organization (WHO) estimates that each year, dog bites account for tens of millions of injuries.[32]

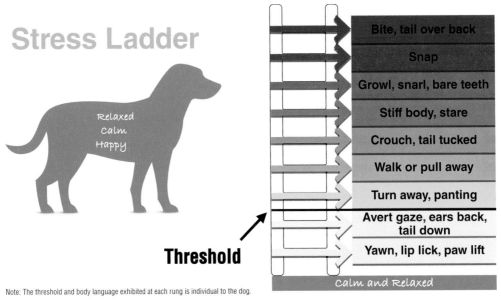

Note: The threshold and body language exhibited at each rung is individual to the dog.

Figure 23.1 The dog stress ladder. Often body language signals are exhibited prior to biting, but go unnoticed by pet parents. (*Attribution: Lisa Radosta. Modified from Shepherd, K 2009. BSAVA Manual of Canine and Feline Behaviour, 2nd edition.*)

Annually, in the United States, 1.5% of the almost 20% population (4.5 million people) are bitten by dogs, of whom 19.7% seek medical care, 0.67% need reconstructive procedures, up to 18% develop infections, and 10-20 incidents are fatal.[33,34] Dog bites are the 13th most common reason for visits to hospital emergency departments and occur approximately equally in male (53.6%) and female victims (47.4%).[35] While in some countries such as the Netherlands, the bite rate is lower (0.8%), Australia, Canada, and France have similar bite prevalence and fatality rates to the United States.[33,36] Pet parents may not report bites accurately to their doctor because they are concerned about the fate of the dog. In fact, one study found that 64% of dog bites went unreported to local health authorities.[37] For this reason, prevalence and risk factor data are skewed by the study focus and population.[38] Whether a dog bite is reported to a doctor or the local health authorities depends on the severity of the bite, the health of the victim, the willingness of the victim to fully disclose the facts surrounding the dog bite, the knowledge level of the victim as to the possible outcomes, income, and access to health care.[39]

Often, people are bitten by their own dogs or at least dogs known to them. In one area of Canada, the most severe bites took place in the family home, with children and older adults at the highest risk.[37] In another study of adult dog bite victims, two-thirds of the dogs were known to the victim, over one-third were family dogs, over half had a history of aggression, and 27% had bitten a person previously.[40] The most common context was when attempting to interact with the dog (stroking, playing, handling); however, in half the cases, the dog approached the victim.[40] In a recent Finnish study of almost 1800 dogs with aggressive behavior toward people, the likelihood of aggression was associated with the pet being the first dog adopted by the person, male, small body size, older dogs, lack of conspecific company (also reported in Dodman 2021), and fearfulness.[14] Other studies have found an association with smaller size and aggression[6,41,42] and an association of small size with increased fearfulness.[43] However, other studies have identified an association with medium size[40,44] and medium to large size.[45]

Children are at the highest risk of being bitten by dogs, with a peak incidence at 5-9 years, more commonly in boys with nearly all bites in children <10 in their own home.[34,46-48] Most children are bitten by dogs with which they are familiar, and younger children most often by the family dog in their own home.[48-50] While children are more likely to be bitten by a familiar dog, the most severe bites occur from unfamiliar dogs in public places.[36]

As would be expected, bites from larger dogs are more likely to result in hospitalization.[51] One study examined the severity of bites among dogs that were presented to veterinary behaviorists in Italy for severe aggression. In that study, dogs exhibiting aggression to other dogs inflicted significantly more severe bites and had more offensive body language than dogs that directed aggression toward people (defensive body language, inflicted less severe bites).[52]

In some populations, aggression toward unfamiliar people in public is more common than aggression toward family members, although this type of aggression may be less likely to result in a bite due to pet parent control of the dog when in public.[53] The prevalence of aggression to people depends somewhat on the population being assessed. In a survey study of pet parents in the United Kingdom, the prevalence of aggression to familiar people was 3%, to unfamiliar people in the home was 7%, and to unfamiliar people outside the home was 5%.[53]

In a retrospective study of 284 dogs referred for problem behaviors, the prevalence of fear-induced aggression was 26%.[54]

Aggression is the most common reason for pet parents to present dogs to veterinary specialists, with as many as 75% having aggression as the primary complaint[1,2,55] and up to 37% of aggressive dogs showing aggression to other dogs.[1,2,15,55,56] It should be noted that the aforementioned studies varied in their analysis of the data with some analyzing only the primary presenting complaint, while others examined if the behavior was present regardless of the presenting complaint. Possessive aggression (resource guarding) is reported as one of the most common types of aggression seen by veterinary behaviorists (16–36% of cases).[15] When data from 900 dogs that were seized by the American Society for the Prevention of Cruelty to Animals as part of criminal cruelty cases was analyzed, the prevalence of possessive aggression was only 9.2%,[57] while in a pet parent survey, approximately 50% of dogs exhibited some level of possessive aggression (resource guarding).[58] The prevalence of aggression toward unfamiliar dogs on walks has been reported to be 47% in one study[59] (see Box 23.1).

Etiology and predisposing factors

Predisposing factors and the etiology of dog aggression is varied and complex. Factors contributing to the development of aggression include genetics, epigenetics (effect of environment and external factors on the expression of genes), the dog's coping style, maternal care, neonatal handling and socialization, environmental experience, physical health, and learning. There is evidence that different areas of the brain are involved with different types of aggression. It is likely that aggression, which is associated with different motivations or functions, has different subsets of predisposing factors.

Risk factors for fatal dog bites include pet parent mismanagement (37.5%), abuse or neglect (21.1%), isolation from positive interactions with people (76.2%), absence of an able-bodied person to intervene (87%), failure to neuter (85%), and compromised ability of victims to interact properly with the dog.[60] The conclusions of a 2021 Canine Research Policy Think Tank are that dog bite fatalities are rare; there is no reliable link with breed; family dogs are rarely

---

Box 23.1 Quick facts about canine aggression

- Aggression is the most common canine behavior problem referred to behaviorists.
- It is often treatable and manageable for a positive long-term outcome.
- It is seldom curable.
- Aggression causes damage to the human–animal bond.
- It is a common behavioral reason for euthanasia.
- With aggression, there is risk of injury.
- Young children are the most common bite victims and most often are bitten by dogs that they know.
- With aggression, there may be potential liability for the pet parent and the veterinarian.

involved; children and elderly are at highest risk; that there is a higher rate of sexually unaltered males; and pet parent mismanagement abuse and neglect.[61]

Most often interdog aggression in the household involves same-sex pairs, most frequently females[62] compared to males that may be more likely to show aggression to dogs outside of the home.[63] In addition, female–female pairings resulted in more severe injuries.[63] However, in a Spanish study, males and females were represented at a comparable rate.[55] Younger dogs, dogs that are new to the household, or dogs that have been rehomed are more likely to start fights in cases of interdog aggression.[62,63]

Early exposure and socialization

Experiences during the early developmental phases of a dog's life can have extraordinary impacts on later behavior.[62,64–67] This is especially true of traumatic incidents or ones that induce a fear response. The socialization period spans between 3 and 12 weeks of age, and dogs that are properly socialized during this time are less likely to show fear and aggression. See below for prevention. Puppies that were raised prior to adoption in a kennel environment (not in a household), as is often the case with puppies shipped to pet stores, those that find themselves in shelter facilities between three and six months of age, and those that were poorly socialized to environmental stimuli are more likely to exhibit aggression toward and fear of unfamiliar people, and aggression at the veterinarian's office later in life.[65] Puppies that had negative experiences in public with dogs were more likely to show aggression toward dogs as adults. In addition, there was no correlation found between the time spent exposing the puppy to other dogs or the number of dogs met per week and a decrease in aggression.[66] This demonstrates the need for early socialization in a positive way under the tutelage of a trained professional. Socialization is not the same as exposure. In addition, dogs that are raised with positive exposure to people are less likely to develop aggression to people compared to those that were isolated from people as puppies.[67]

Acquisition

Where and at what age the dog is obtained can affect the likelihood of aggression. In one study examining aggression toward familiar people, dogs that had been rehomed were 2.6 times more likely to show aggression to family members when compared to dogs purchased from retail stores and breeders; dogs purchased from retail stores were 1.8 times more likely to show aggression when compared to dogs adopted from breeders, and dogs kept with their original breeder were 4.5 times less likely to show aggression toward familiar people.[53] In other studies, prevalence of aggression was greatest in dogs that were of mixed breeds and originating from a rescue,[4] while interdog household aggression was highest in dogs obtained from a shelter or pet stores.[62] Based on the aforementioned study, the rehoming of dogs, even when adopted from a quality breeder, may predispose them to fear, anxiety, stress, conflict, or panic. This requires more investigation before any conclusions can be made.

The age of acquisition is also important in the development of aggression, and dogs adopted at greater than 12 weeks of age were at increased risk for intraspecific household aggression.[63] A Finnish study found that puppies adopted from a breeder's domestic environment after 8 weeks (i.e. 9 to 16 weeks) had a higher prevalence of aggression and avoidance as adult dogs toward unfamiliar people both on and off the property.[64] The same study found that puppies adopted at 8 weeks of age or between 13 and 16 weeks had greater barking at other dogs compared to puppies adopted between 9 and 12 weeks.[64] These findings demonstrate the necessity of exposing puppies to the range of social stimuli outside of the breeder's environment during the socialization period.

Genetics and breed

While dogs of any breed can bite, even those widely regarded as unlikely to show aggression such as Golden Retrievers,[54,68–70] and there is no consistent evidence of a breed propensity to aggression,[71] several studies have demonstrated a higher prevalence in some breeds in relationship to breed popularity, most likely due in part to a genetic predisposition.[14,42,56] However, these studies show wide diversity due to differences in study populations and methodologies, type and target of aggression, sample size, geographic location (gene pool, housing, breed popularity at the time of the study), bite characteristics (severity, context, target), and accuracy of the breeds being reported.

While mixed-breed dogs are among the most common presented for aggression across many studies,[2,45,54,72,73] in some studies, purebreds may be most common.[14,44,48,53] In a study comparing three behavior specialty practices, English Springer Spaniels, Jack Russell Terriers (Parson Russell, Russell Terriers), and Dalmatians were overrepresented for aggression in both Canada and United States, while in Australia, the Dalmatian and Kelpie were overrepresented.[15] In another study, dogs in the utility (a diverse group of dogs bred for a specific purpose that is no longer applicable in current times) and hound groups (sight or scent hounds) were 4.4 and 2.6 times respectively more likely to show aggression to familiar people than mixed-breed dogs and gun dogs (dogs trained to hunt with people) were 2.4 times less likely to show aggression to unfamiliar people, while Cocker Spaniels and Golden Retrievers had a reduced risk.[53] Several other studies have demonstrated a reduced risk in Golden and Labrador Retrievers,[44,74] while in another study, Golden Retrievers, Rottweilers, and Bernese Mountain Dogs were the most likely purebred dogs to be presented for fear-induced aggression.[54] The prevalence of aggression in any particular breed most likely depends on the gene pool in that area at the time the study was conducted. For example, aggression has been shown to be more likely in certain lines of English Springer Spaniels (conformation-bred dogs more than field dogs), primarily in American studies,[2,6,15,44,56,75] while in European veterinary behavior specialty practices, English Cocker Spaniels (especially associated with golden coat color) were overrepresented.[55,76–78] Interestingly, for Labrador Retrievers, the field stock was more likely to show aggression than the conformation (show) stock.[44] Just as the predisposition for certain types of aggression may be present in certain gene pools, aggression can potentially be eliminated from gene pools by refraining from breeding animals that are showing signs of fear and or aggression.[79]

In another study, biting dogs tended to be female, neutered, smaller dogs that live in homes with children, show aggression over food, and are excitable and/or are fearful of children, men, and/or strangers.[41] When severe bites are examined, risk factors tend to be larger, male, purebred, and in one study, brachycephalic.[48,72,80]

Some studies have demonstrated differences in the expression of genes in aggressive dogs and nonaggressive dogs, specifically the UBE2V2 and ZNF227 genes in the amygdala, frontal cortex, hypothalamus, and parietal cortex.[81]

Stress threshold and coping style

Most types of aggression have an associated physiologic response (i.e., fight, flight, freeze, or fidget), including the mobilization of glucose, tachycardia, and tachypnea (see Chapter 7).[82] This is one of the reasons why the treatment of aggression includes techniques focused on changing the emotional state of the dog as opposed to simply attempting to change the behavior being displayed. During the stress response, there is increased memory consolidation and retrieval.[82] In other words, dogs are more likely to remember what happened and what they did to avoid the stressor when there is a physiologic stress response than they are when taught behaviors when they are calm. Changes in behavior such as aggressive responses occur once the dog has reached his individual threshold for the tolerance of stress. Genetic predispositions, environment, diet, fear, anxiety, stress, conflict, panic, systemic disease, pain, pruritus, gastrointestinal disease, hunger, and any illness causing discomfort or inflammation in the body can lower the threshold bar over which aggression is exhibited. For these reasons, aggression is best examined through a wide-angle lens, so to speak, considering overall health, environment, and behavioral history.

When a dog is under chronic stress, the threshold for aggression can decrease, causing a general increase in reactivity to stimuli. For example, if a dog has fear-induced aggression and storm phobia, the aggression may get worse during storm season due to chronic physiologic stress. In fact, in a study of 5610 responses from pet parents regarding their dog's behavior, reactivity to stimuli defined as a reaction to sudden movements or sounds in the home was associated with aggression directed at familiar and unfamiliar people.[83] Pet parents may say that the aggression is unprovoked. While this may be the case, in most cases the pet parent simply does not notice the subtle warning signs, or the warning signs may have been muted by punishment. Pet parents may describe their previously lovable dog as tense and exhibiting a glazed look before displaying aggression. This type of arousal can be associated with any type of aggression.

Gonadectomy and gender

Gonadectomy decreases gonadal steroid hormones and has been correlated with a decrease in sexually dimorphic behaviors, but the information regarding its effect on aggressive behavior in dogs is conflicting.[84–89] One study suggested marking, mounting, masturbation, and aggression toward other male dogs and territorial aggression might be prevented or reduced by castration.[88] However, a more recent study found no effect of neutering on intermale aggression, roaming, or mounting.[90] Another study suggested that neutering does not appear to decrease the likelihood of aggression in male dogs, with perhaps the exception of some cases

of territorial and intermale aggression.[91] Gonadectomy appears to reduce sexually dimorphic behaviors but appears to have little effect on those behaviors which are not sexually dimorphic. For example, if a dog is mounting as a displacement behavior, neutering is not likely to change the expression of that behavior. If a dog is mounting due to sex hormones, neutering will most likely decrease that behavior. Similarly, if marking is territorial in nature, it most likely will decrease with neutering. If it is due to house training or anxiety, it will not.

Most studies examining aggression prevalence have found males to be overrepresented,[2,4,15,54,55] specifically with aggression toward people,[14,40,48,55,60] toward pet parents,[42,55,74] toward other dogs,[55] or toward strangers,[55,92] while one study found that females bite three times more frequently than males.[41] An association with castration of male dogs has been variable. In several studies, reproductive status was found to have no significance.[41,42,53,93] Several studies have shown greater aggression in intact male dogs[48,54,56,60] as well as more severe incidents of aggression.[52] In one study, intact males were 1.68 times more likely to bite than castrated males but 0.80 times as likely to bite as intact females.[94] Several other studies have found that neutered dogs are likely to show aggression to people[4,41,95] and toward other dogs.[92] On the other hand, studies have also shown that neutered dogs may show less aggression[1] and less pet parent-directed aggression.[74] However, depending on the study population, sex and neuter status, as well as breed of many of the biting dogs, is unknown.

Some studies suggest that spayed females are more likely to display certain types of aggression when compared with intact females.[96,97] One study found that spayed females were 2.3 times less likely to display aggression to family members, 1.8 times less likely to show aggression to unfamiliar people entering the home, and 1.7 times less likely to show aggression toward unfamiliar people outside of the home when compared to neutered dogs.[53] An increase in reactivity toward humans with unfamiliar dogs and aggression toward family members has also been reported after ovariohysterectomy of bitches in several studies.[96–98] While the cause has not been determined, it may be due to a decrease in estrogen and oxytocin concentrations, both of which may have some antianxiety effects.[99] Of course, when female dogs display hormonally related signs of aggression during estrus, as a part of maternal behavior or during pseudopregnancy, these will be eliminated by spaying. In a retrospective study of 217 cases of dogs presented for interdog aggression, a little over half of the dogs were female and most were spayed. Similarly, most male dogs presented for interdog aggression within the same household were neutered.[100] Regarding possessive aggression, female dogs may be less likely to show aggression over food and chewable resources when compared to males.[57]

In a large survey study of 13,795 dog pet parents, dogs that were gonadectomized between 7 and 12 months of age were more likely to show aggression to strangers when compared to those that were gonadectomized at 18 months of age or that were intact.[101] This finding may be due to the life stage at which most dogs are spayed and neutered. Between six and eight months, many dogs enter a second fear period and between one and three years, dogs progress through social maturity. Traumatic incidents during either of these developmental stages can make a large impact on the dog's likelihood of developing a behavior disorder.

Even as we gather more information regarding how gonadectomy influences behavior, there is conflicting information and still many unanswered questions. More research is certainly needed. Veterinarians often wonder what recommendations they can make to pet parents regarding spaying and neutering and its relation to behavior. While the studies are in disagreement, the mounting evidence demonstrates that for some of our patients, the detriment of gonadectomy especially at a young age, is greater than the benefits. Decision to spay or neuter a dog should be based on that individual's risk factors for behavioral disease, unwanted pregnancies, and other concerns which will be affected by neuter status. The evidence is clear that neutering rarely affects in a positive way the most common types of aggression seen by veterinarians, although there may be rationale for neutering of dogs with established aggression, both for the potential of reducing aggression by behavior-focused breeding and neutering of dogs with potentially heritable traits.[14,48,60]

Thyroid disease

Thyroid disease has been implicated as a potential or contributing factor in the development of aggression in 1.7% of dogs.[102] Proposed mechanisms for hypothyroid-related aggression include lowered threshold for aggression due to lethargy and irritability,[103] impaired transmission of serotonin at the postsynaptic 5-HT2A receptors in the cerebral cortex,[104] and increased metabolism of serotonin in the cerebrospinal fluid.[105] Hypothyroidism has been linked anecdotally in dogs to noise and storm phobia, separation-related disorder, hyperactivity, poor focus and learning, compulsive behaviors, and aggression,[106–108] and is discussed in detail in Chapter 6. Aggression has been associated with increased thyroglobulin autoantibody (TgAA) concentrations, along with normal thyroxine (TT4) and thyroid-stimulating hormone (TSH) concentrations in dogs.[109] Hypothyroidism may potentially account for a small percentage of aggressive behaviors, occurring even in the absence of lethargy, weight gain, and other characteristic clinical signs of hypothyroidism. In a case series of four dogs that were presented for aggression to people and also had thyroid values consistent with hypothyroidism but did not exhibit signs traditionally associated with hypothyroidism, all dogs responded to treatment with supplementation, but none resolved completely. The response to treatment was variable, depending on the individual. In addition, all pet parents were given safety and avoidance instructions at the time of the appointment, which would undoubtedly affect the outcome of the cases.[110]

On the other hand, aggression is a common presentation in dogs with normal thyroid concentrations. Inappropriate or unnecessary supplementation of thyroid hormone may lead to tachycardia, irritability, aggression, nervousness, and weight loss in dogs. In addition, because thyroid hormone is functionally linked to brain dopamine and serotonergic systems, L-thyroxine supplementation, even in euthyroid patients, may affect the same systems involved in canine aggression disorders; therefore, improvement with thyroid supplementation does not confirm that the cause is thyroid

related. In a study measuring TT4, fT4, TT3, fT3, TgAA, TSH, T3AA, and T4AA in 31 aggressive and nonaggressive dogs, aggressive dogs had higher concentrations of T4AA when compared to nonaggressive dogs; however, T4AA values were still within normal range.[111] In a second study comparing TT4 and TSH in 39 aggressive and nonaggressive dogs, TT4 was higher in aggressive dogs but was not outside the normal range.[112] In a double-blinded, placebo-controlled study examining the effect of thyroid supplementation on dogs with fT4 in or below the lower 20th percentile of the normal range, TT4, TT3, or fT3 in or below the lower 30th percentile of the normal range or the presence of thyroid autoantibodies (TgAA) that directed aggression at family members, no difference was found between the supplemented and placebo groups in the level of aggression.[113] In conclusion, hypothyroid-related aggression is considered rare; however, it most likely occurs in some subset of dogs and should be ruled out in aggression cases.

Discomfort and pain

Pain is defined by the Merriam-Webster dictionary as "a localized or generalized unpleasant bodily sensation or complex of sensations that causes mild to severe physical discomfort and emotional distress and typically results from bodily disorder (such as injury or disease)" and "basic bodily sensation that is induced by a noxious stimulus, is received by naked nerve endings, is associated with actual or potential tissue damage, is characterized by physical discomfort (such as pricking, throbbing, or aching), and typically leads to evasive action." The International Association for the Study of Pain (IASP) defines pain as "an unpleasant sensory and emotional experience associated with, or resembling that associated with, actual or potential tissue damage." In addition, IASP notes that pain is always a personal experience that is influenced to varying degrees by biological, psychological, and social factors; and pain cannot be inferred solely from sensory neurons (https://www.iasp-pain.org/publications/iasp-news/iasp-announces-revised-definition-of-pain/). The most commonly reported clinical signs associated with pain in animals are behavior changes such as changes in attitude, decreased activity and ambulation, decreased appetite, fear reactions, aggression, house-training accidents, increased vocalization, hiding, restlessness, and decreased interactions with family members.[114] Any illness that causes discomfort, pain, pruritus, disability, or inflammation in the body can contribute to aggression,[115] potentially through reduced serotonin activity in the brain directly[116] or indirectly as a result of reduced mobility and exercise.[117] In dogs presented to veterinary behavior specialists, 15% of aggressive dogs were found to have a contributing medical issue,[73] while from 28-82% of cases with problem behavior were suspected to have underlying pain.[118] Dogs that were aggressive to family members were more likely to have pain than dogs with no history of aggression.[119]

Diet

Aggression has been linked to gluten sensitivity in one dog and the aggression resolved with diet change.[120] Surprisingly, underweight dogs were not more likely to display food aggression, nor was it more severe when compared to dogs that were a healthy weight.[57]

Environment and exercise

Dog parks have increased in popularity within the past decade. It is unclear at this time what impact dog parks have on dog aggression. In general, dogs at dog parks are less controlled than they would be on leash, pet parents may not be adequately supervising their dog or the children that they bring to the dog park, and incidents can occur very quickly. Even when a bite does not occur, agonistic interactions can cause fear aggression in victim dogs. With that said, in one study looking at aggression occurring at one dog park in Indianapolis, it was found that aggression was exhibited less than 0.5% of the time.[121] Certainly, dogs that are underexercised and whose needs are not being met can become frustrated, which can contribute to aggression.

Pet parent behavior and training methods

The type and amount of training that the dog receives can affect the likelihood of the development of aggression later in life. Dogs that were trained with positive punishment and/or negative reinforcement training (e.g., choke, shock, pinch collars, leash corrections, yelling, physical corrections) were 2.9 times more likely to exhibit aggression to familiar people and 2.2 times more likely to show aggression to unfamiliar people outside of the home.[53] In addition, the use of positive punishment put the pet at an increased risk of euthanasia or rehoming.[122] Despite the increased risks and overwhelming evidence that these methods contribute to aggression and fear, 72% of pet parents reported using those types of techniques.[59] This underscores the need for education of pet parents on the current scientific literature. While some may consider the use of electronic fences for containment less damaging than bark-activated or handler-controlled shock collars, in fact electric pet containment systems have been linked to severe attacks toward people and other dogs.[123] For these reasons and many more, punishment-based and negative reinforcement-based training is never recommended when training dogs. Very simply, it creates fear, stress, and aggression. Why recommend something that has been shown to contribute to a behavior disorder that can endanger the life of your patient (see Chapter 10)?

Unfortunately, dog pet parents have limited knowledge of dog communication and the risks associated with aggression. They often feel that their dog would not "cross the line" and bite someone. In one study, 82% of respondents thought it was safe for children to kiss and hug their own dogs and 45% indicated they would restrain their dog if it moved away from an unfamiliar child who wanted to pet it.[124] In that same study, mothers were most knowledgeable about the risks associated with aggression toward their children when compared with fathers and nonparents of both genders. In another survey of parents, over half felt that their 4-year-old child would be safe when left unsupervised with their dog.[125] All of these situations are common ones where bites to children occur. The disparity between the level of knowledge of pet parents and the reality of keeping kids safe contributes to the number of dog bites to children (see Chapter 4, Box 23.2 and resources in Appendix A.).

> **Box 23.2** Potential causes of, predisposing and contributing factors for aggression in dogs
>
> - Early life experience
>   - Lack of appropriate socialization before 12 (to 14) weeks
>   - Incorrect socialization
>   - Traumatic experience
>   - Illness
>   - Raised in kennel environment (commercial breeding, puppy mills, pet stores)
> - Acquisition
>   - Rehoming
>   - Purchase from pet stores
>   - Adoption at older than 12 weeks
>   - Adoption before six weeks
> - Genetics and breed
>   - No breed predispositions
>   - Inherited predisposition toward fear, anxiety, stress, conflict, panic, and aggression
> - Stress threshold and coping style
>   - Innate coping style
>   - Threshold for physiologic and emotional stress
>   - Physical disease
>   - Life experiences
> - Gonadectomy and gender
>   - Gonadectomy less than 18 months of age
>   - Female dogs more likely to instigate household aggression
>   - Male dogs more likely to instigate aggression to non household dogs
>   - Spayed female pairings within the same household
> - Thyroid disease
>   - In some cases hypothyroidism in the absence of typical clinical signs can contribute to aggression
> - Discomfort and pain
>   - Any pain or discomfort can lead to aggression
> - Diet
>   - Gluten sensitivity
>   - Protein levels
> - Environment and exercise
>   - Lack of enrichment
>   - Frustration as a result of inadequate fulfillment of pet's needs
> - Pet parent behavior and training methods
>   - Positive punishment training
>   - Negative reinforcement training
>   - Inconsistent, unstructured interactions with family members
>   - Shock collar use
>   - Electric fence use

Prevention

Because most aggression stems from fear, anxiety, stress, conflict, panic, and pain, there is overlap between the prevention of different types of aggressive behavior. A structured, predictable, and positive relationship with the pet parent, other pets in the home, and the outside environment; avoidance of punishment-based training; proper socialization; and use of positive reinforcement training can all contribute to the prevention of aggressive behavior. Puppies that show fear, anxiety, and stress are at risk of developing aggressive behavior and should be treated aggressively and immediately, including treatment at home, customized socialization programs, referral to a positive reinforcement dog training professional, or referral to a board-certified veterinary behaviorist.[126]

Socialization and early life experiences

Proper socialization between 3 and 12 weeks of age is extremely important. Socialization outside of the home should start at eight weeks of age. Puppies should meet many different types of people, animals, and objects in controlled, pleasant situations as often as possible during these months. Puppy classes should be started after the first vaccinations and deworming, and as close to eight weeks as possible for best results. Puppies that attend properly conducted puppy classes had reduced fear, reactivity, and aggression to unfamiliar people and to familiar and unfamiliar dogs, and together with pheromone collars, improved sociability and decreased fear and anxiety to new people and environments.[53,59,127,128] Puppies that attended at least two puppy classes before 12 weeks of age were 1.5 times less likely to show aggression to unfamiliar people entering the home and 1.6 times less likely to show aggression to unfamiliar people outside of the home.[53] It should be clear from the literature that there is a protective effect against aggression when puppies attend positive reinforcement puppy classes within the socialization period, which ends at 12-14 weeks. Frequent positive social interactions with non-fearful or reactive dogs can help facilitate normal social communication. Taking a puppy away from its littermates and preventing interaction with other dogs prior to six weeks of age may impede the puppy's ability to develop normal communication skills with other dogs. Veterinarians must make it a priority to recommend attendance at puppy classes as close to eight weeks of age as possible and before 12-14 weeks of age to help prevent the development of aggressive behavior. See Chapter 5 for more information on puppy classes.

Giving pet parents the information that they need in order to use positive reinforcement rather than punishment and maintain structured, predictable relationships should be started at the first puppy appointment and continued through a year of age. One study showed that when advice to new puppy pet parents was provided at the first visit by a veterinary behaviorist, there were fewer problems as adults, including aggression toward people and other dogs.[129] The puppy should be habituated to all types of handling as soon as it is adopted, provided there are no signs of fear or anxiety. Puppy socialization and basic training classes that use positive reinforcement help set the stage for consistent interactions as the dog ages. The pet parent should begin developing obedience skills in puppyhood, when learning comes easily.

Enrichment and confinement

Adequate exercise, mental stimulation, and enrichment can help prevent the development of aggressive behavior. Young dogs should not be tied out or chained outside, nor should they be confined to yards for long periods in situations where they are continuously overstimulated by passing people and dogs.

Appropriate play

Pet parents should not encourage mouthing (biting without breaking skin) in any capacity, including play. Setting boundaries early in life regarding how to play, use of the mouth during play, and which toys are appropriate can help prevent play-induced aggression later in life.

Training

Positive reinforcement training sets the stage for structured relationships which reduce conflict, fear, frustration, anxiety, and stress. Young dogs that display predatory behavior should be identified early and every attempt should be made to habituate, countercondition, or train the dog to ignore the stimuli. They should not be encouraged or permitted to engage in predatory behavior directed toward wildlife or other animals. Similar attention should be given to dogs that might be prone to chasing and herding.

Structured interactions and environment

Using a trained behavior to precede reinforcement or pleasurable interactions can help to increase structure in the pet's life. The behavior can be used to help the pet gain physiologic control (e.g. settled and focused) when aroused, enable the pet parent to ask the dog's consent for interactions with family and strangers, and give the pet and the pet parent a feeling of control over situations. For example, touch, sit, or down can be used before the dog receives anything he wants or needs (e.g., attention, play, walks, treats, food). This allows the dog to understand and communicate how to get what he wants and needs, and it allows the pet parent to feel in control of the reinforcements and resources which are doled out throughout the day. It reduces the dog's and the pet parent's anxiety. The dog can, if the pet parent is observing carefully, say "no" by not performing the behavior, which gives the pet parent insight into the dog's emotional state. For example, consider a dog that is fluent (i.e., the dog performs the behavior 9 out of 10 times consistently when asked in that situation) at hand touching (the dog touches his nose to the palm of a person's hand) when meeting new people. The dog has done this many times before with people with varying appearance and demeanor. One day, the dog is asked to hand touch with a child and the dog does not perform this behavior. This gives the pet parent insight that the dog is likely fearful, anxious, stressed, or conflicted. While it is true that the dog could be distracted or undertrained, if the dog understands the behavior, consistently performs it, and declines to do it in a particular situation, it is more likely that he is suffering from FASCP. In this case, the pet parent can withdraw the dog from the situation before the fear escalates and he shows aggressive behavior.

Gonadectomy

Gonadectomy may help to prevent intermale aggression,[87,130] territorial aggression, behavior changes during estrus, and maternal aggression (including aggression from pseudocyesis); however, it is not likely to have a positive effect on aggression outside of these specific categories (see Chapter 1 and section on "Gonadectomy and gender" above). In breeding animals, extensive socialization, handling, and reward-based training starting at an early age are the best ways to minimize the risks of maternal aggression. Intact male and female dogs that fight often begin to show this behavior at one and three years of age, respectively.

Toys and food

Pet parents should avoid sticking their hands in the dog's bowl or taking the bowl away suddenly. While many dogs are accepting of this type of intrusion, some dogs and puppies are not. Imagine how you would react if while eating a meal, your partner grabbed your plate or pulled your food right out of your mouth. What if that happened randomly? Now, imagine that you are not in a position to eat when you like. Instead, your partner (the one who keeps randomly taking away your plate) doles out food as he or she sees fit, controlling how much and when you eat. Might you feel a little anxious or even aggressive? Of course, you would, and those feelings would be understandable and justified just as they are in dogs. Because pet parents are not reliably able to read their dog's body language accurately, they are likely to miss the subtle signs of stress. As described above, through learning and consequences, dogs that are stressed about this interaction can progress to aggression, which is quickly reinforced in most cases, making it more likely in the future. Aside from the risks, this is an unnatural and unnecessary interaction. Instead, the pet parent should condition the dog to accept close contact by pairing food with their approaches to the bowl. When the puppy or newly adopted dog is eating, the pet parent should pass by at a distance that does not elicit any stress response, say the dog's name, and then toss food into the bowl. They should stay at the same distance during each session until the point where the dog steps back or moves toward the pet parent happily and calmly when he hears his name. At that point, the sessions can include passes which are closer to the dog's bowl. The same criteria should apply to each stage. The dog should be responding to the sound of his name by stepping away from the bowl or orienting in a relaxed way toward the pet parent upon hearing his name 9 out of 10 times for at least 3 sessions consecutively before moving forward. There is not a need for the pet parent to ever touch or hover over the dog while he is eating, and this is not recommended. How would a person feel if while they were eating, someone approached and hugged them or continued to touch them? In addition, each dog should learn a "leave it" cue, which means to step away from an item. This way, if the pet parent has to take the bowl away while the dog is eating (e.g., the wrong medication or food was put into the pet's bowl), they have a way to cue the dog to step back so that the bowl can be picked up. They can ask the dog to leave it, then when the dog steps back, the pet parent can reinforce with even more tasty food or treat, and then pick up the bowl. The dog has just learned that the pet parent is predictable and that when the dog is compliant, it is a win–win situation.

Pet parent behavior and training

The pet parent's behavior, while rarely the sole cause of aggressive behavior, can be a contributing factor, and thus should be addressed in its prevention. Pet parents who engage in positive reinforcement training are less likely to have dogs that are aggressive. As would be expected, pet parents who engage in punishment-based training are more likely to end up with an aggressive dog. Dogs that have been subjected to punishment and without formal training classes are more likely to show aggression and avoidance.[59,74] It is the obligation of the veterinarian to meet the standard of care and recommend only positive reinforcement trainers to new pet parents. In addition, education of pet parents in the normal communication of dogs, including subtle body language changes, can allow them to note body language signals that precede aggression, preventing its development in the first place. Proactive supervision of dogs with children and unfamiliar people is widely underutilized as a method for preventing aggression. Pet parent intervention or lack thereof in interspecies and intraspecies interactions can fuel aggression. There is no one right answer of when to intervene and when to step back except in situations where injury is likely, either the aggressor or the victim is distressed, or there is a large size disparity. The best way to help pet parents know when to intervene is to educate them on dog body language. See Appendix A for resources. Pet parents also need to be educated on how to intervene. As in all aspects of pet behavior, calm direction to the pet with reinforcement for good decisions is the best avenue.

Overall health and wellness

Although it is not possible to anticipate the effects of all stimuli, the dog that is trained to be lifted, have its nails trimmed, teeth brushed, and anal sacs expressed is more likely to tolerate handling when he is in pain or experiencing discomfort. At puppy appointments, the veterinarian should inform pet parents as to which medical diseases their dog's breed is predisposed and the type of manipulation and handling that the dog might require over time. For example, if the family has an English Bulldog puppy, they should be instructed to handle the dog's ears, facial folds, and tail fold daily while giving the dog treats. This can also be covered in a positive reinforcement puppy class. In fact, dogs that are used to gentle handling by pet parents were less stressed during veterinary examinations.[131] In addition, both puppies and juveniles that attended puppy classes had reduced touch sensitivity as well as nonsocial fear and family-dog aggression as adults.[127] At every exam, the pet should be assessed for discomfort. If the pet is diagnosed with a disorder which increases pain or discomfort, undergoes a procedure at the hospital, or is given medications which may change mood or lower the threshold for aggression, the pet parent should be informed and suggestions made to reduce the likelihood of aggression in these circumstances (see Box 23.3).

Approach to diagnosis and treatment in general practice

As with all behavior problems, the following steps should be taken whenever possible: gather history, evaluate overall health and wellness, create a differential diagnosis list, and develop a treatment plan. Veterinarians working in general practice may not have enough time in one appointment to complete all of these steps. In these cases, history taking, diagnosis, and treatment can be divided over several appointments. How the case is approached depends somewhat

- Early life experiences
  - Proper socialization between 3–12 weeks of age
  - Positive reinforcement puppy classes
- Enrichment and confinement
  - Adequate exercise, mental stimulation, and enrichment
- Appropriate play
  - Structured, consistent play which does not involve hands, feet, or wrestling
- Training
  - Positive reinforcement training
  - Prevention of predatory behavior in those predisposed
- Structured interactions and environment
  - Structured, consistent interactions with family and the environment
  - Teaching a structured, consent behavior
- Gonadectomy
  - No indication to reduce aggression in general
  - Indicated for aggression directly related to the estrus cycle, pregnancy, or pseudopregnancy
  - Indicated for any animals that are showing aggression and may be bred to reduce the likelihood of predisposition in offspring
  - Indicated for territorial aggression and intermale aggression which is not related to FASCP
  - May increase fear and aggression
- Toys and food
  - Avoid taking the food bowl away, touching the dog during eating, or when he has food toys
  - Create a positive association with approach to valuable items including food using counterconditioning techniques and positive conditioning techniques
  - Teach leave it and/or drop it cues
- Pet parent behavior and training
  - Positive reinforcement training
  - Structured, consistent interactions
  - Supervision with visitors
  - Supervision with children
- Overall health and wellness
  - Assessment for pain and discomfort at every appointment with the veterinarian
  - Immediate treatment of pain or discomfort
  - Judicious use of previsit pharmaceuticals to reduce pain and discomfort at veterinary visits
  - Use of antianxiety or pain medications in patients with ongoing home treatments

on the resources available and the education level of the veterinarian. For canine aggression cases, ideally, the veterinarian would have at the ready an educated veterinary healthcare team member for pet parent education, handouts, book, websites, and video recommendations, the name(s) of positive reinforcement training professionals in the area, board-certified veterinary behaviorist referral options for pet parents who need more help than can be provided by the primary care practitioner, and a foundational knowledge of canine behavior (see Appendix A).

Before considering how dog aggression or any type of behavior cases are seen at your practice, consider the amount of time that the veterinarian and the veterinary healthcare team has with each pet parent, the number of exam rooms, the flow of the hospital, the training of the team members, the ability of the team to perform diagnostic tests, and the

interest of the veterinary team members in behavioral medicine. Regardless of what you decide regarding workflow, always assess the overall wellness of canine patients and treat immediately FASCP and pain. See Chapters 1, 9, and 16 for more information on how to implement behavioral medicine in primary care practice.

Pain resulting from a variety of medical problems (e.g., otitis externa, arthritis, atopy, gastroenteritis, dental) can cause or contribute to aggression.[118] Physical diseases (e.g., hyperadrenocorticism, hypothyroidism, seizures, hepatoencephalopathy) can manifest with signs of aggression. Because of the possibility of an underlying medical cause or contributing disease, dogs presented for aggression should receive a physical examination and screening laboratory tests, including a complete blood count, serum chemistry, urinalysis, thyroid assessment, and fecal antigen test + Giardia. This also serves to establish a baseline of health, which is necessary before instituting pharmaceutical therapy (see Chapter 6).

The likelihood of report of aggression will vary and may be dependent on the size of the dog, pet parent age (e.g., older pet parents were less likely to report aggression) and gender of the pet parent (e.g., female pet parents were less likely to report aggression to visitors), and the family's tolerance for aggression.[53] In addition, there is an increased likelihood of aggression as dogs age,[14,42,74] which may be due to the addition of physical diseases lowering the threshold for aggression or the progression of the primary underlying behavioral disorder (e.g., FASCP).[53] It is well documented that behavioral disorders and clinical signs worsen over time if not treated. For these reasons, a questionnaire and proactive questioning of pet parents at every visit is imperative to avoid emergency and crisis situations.

Aggressive displays may be viewed directly by the clinician if the circumstance arises; however, most often the diagnosis is based on the history provided by the pet parent. A video of the behavior can be very helpful but for safety reasons, pet parents should not be encouraged to provoke aggressive behavior in order to make a recording. By the same token, clinicians should not deliberately provoke aggressive behavior. This type of activity weakens pet parent trust, worsens the behavior of the pet, and puts the clinician and support staff in harm's way. History taking for aggression cases is no different than for physical problems. For example, when a patient presents for vomiting, the pet parent describes the behavior so that the veterinarian can distinguish vomiting from regurgitation, but the veterinarian does not attempt to elicit the vomiting or regurgitation in order to witness it because that would cause undue harm to the patient. Guidelines for behavioral consultations are covered in Chapters 1 and 9. Before consulting on cases of aggression, it would be prudent to consider having a release form signed. This may not always be sufficient to protect against legal action. Liability can vary depending on the case, level of expertise, and the jurisdiction in which the case is heard. Therefore, it might be advisable to consult with an attorney to determine the type of release that most suits your practice.

The experience and behavior as a puppy, age of onset, signalment, overall health, contributing medical diseases, temperament, body language, vocalizations, inciting stimulus, situations in which the aggression is displayed, target, motivation, and progression should be considered when making a diagnosis. Repeated exposure and learning (including pet parent response and victim response) can modify the pet's behavior, so the practitioner should collect information on any change in the body language, inciting stimuli, and situations for aggression since the first aggressive displays. Aggression to strangers, unfamiliar dogs, familiar people, or family pets, and aggression caused by pain and discomfort may each have different underlying mechanisms and genetic factors.[55,79,132] In one study of 3897 dogs, most did not show aggression in multiple contexts.[53] However, it is not uncommon for dogs to present with multiple types of aggression. In these cases, the veterinarian should design the treatment plan by prioritizing and addressing the clinical signs which cause the most distress to the pet parent and the dog, and which may result in the most harm to the dog or others. Do not lose touch with these pet parents: the risks of injury, relinquishment, euthanasia, and legal liability (for the pet parent and the veterinarian) are too great. In-person or telehealth rechecks should be scheduled starting 1-2 weeks after the first appointment, at regular intervals until 2-3 months and then as needed for consistent progress. For the ESVCE statement on risk assessment, see https://esvce.org/wp-content/uploads/2021/09/risk-assessment.pdf.

Behavioral treatment may be referred to a veterinary technician with an interest in behavior or a dog training professional. Veterinarians should interview the professionals to whom they refer, verify that their methods are positive reinforcement based, watch them train various dogs, and know what techniques (e.g., clicker training) and products (e.g., no-pull harnesses) with which they are familiar. In addition, they should set up a protocol for communication each time the dog is seen by either party. Referral to a board-certified veterinary behaviorist should be considered when one of more of the following criteria are present:

1. The pet parent is considering euthanasia.
2. The case is chronic and thus far outcomes have been poor.
3. There is a threat of injury to a person.
4. There are immunocompromised, elderly, or very young family members in a household or visitors to the home who may be exposed to the dog.
5. The patient is at risk of relinquishment, self harm, exposure to positive punishment and/or negative reinforcement training or euthanasia.
6. The veterinarian has exhausted her/his comfort level regarding pharmaceutical treatments.
7. Bites are injurious.
8. The pet parent is under threat of legal action.

In addition, consider affected puppies as medical emergencies; refer them early for the best outcome.

History

Use of a short behavior questionnaire at each appointment, such as the one found in the online resources (Appendix C), can facilitate the efficient acquisition of patient history and provide the veterinarian with the opportunity to practice preventative medicine instead of reacting to behavioral crises. Ask about who is involved (targets of aggression), the body language of each dog, other pets in the household, latency to arousal (how quickly the aggression escalates), recovery time (how long it takes for the aggressor and the

victim to return to a relaxed state), severity and frequency (how often the aggression occurs over a period of time), the pet parent's stress level with this situation, whether the pet parent is afraid of the dog, and any injuries.

Many pet parents have pictures and videos on their mobile devices, which can be helpful when creating a differential diagnosis list. If the problem is stated to the client care representative at the time of scheduling, a request can be made for videos to be sent prior to the appointment. If that is not possible, viewing at the time of the appointment or after the appointment should be adequate. Videos are the gold standard; however, do not recommend that dangerous situations be triggered for the sake of a video. Videos from mild or low stress interactions and descriptions from pet parents, while not as helpful as a video, can still be adequate. History should include a description of the dog's facial expressions and body postures, targets, and a description of all situations in which the aggression occurs. Care should be taken to review the history from the initial event to the current presentation because the consequences of each interaction can alter how each dog responds. For example, the dog that at the time of presentation appears to be the aggressor toward the other dog in the household could have been the victim when they were first introduced. Illustrations can help pet parents identify their dog's postures and states of arousal, especially if they have difficulty recalling precise descriptions of the dog's behavior. Illustrations are available online which may be helpful to clinicians and pet parents (see Appendix A). Often, pet parents will have formed an opinion of the situation before presentation, which inevitably is tied to their emotions and feelings toward the dog. It is best to listen carefully, watch videos, view images, objectively collect information, and then make the decision as to how to move forward. In multidog households, where there is aggression to each other, all dogs will need to be evaluated and most likely treated, even if one is the alleged victim.

Assessment of overall health and wellness

As with every behavior case, it is essential that the veterinarian first assess the dog's physical health to determine if there are any physical problems that might have caused or contributed to the aggression, as well as to decide the effect that these problems might have on treating the aggression. Painful conditions (e.g., abscesses, arthritis, anal sacculitis, dental disease), conditions affecting the central nervous system (CNS: e.g., brain tumors, encephalitis), sensory decline, and endocrine imbalances (e.g., hyperthyroidism) can all have a direct effect on behavior (see Chapter 6). Physical conditions can act in concert with environmental, genetic, and other health factors to lower thresholds of inhibition and result in exhibition of aggression. These might include abnormal neurotransmitter/receptor activity, CNS anatomic abnormalities (genetic, congenital, acquired), neoplasia (CNS tumors), metabolic disease states (hepatic encephalopathy, endocrine disorders), infections (rabies), trauma (CNS injury), and toxins (lead, pesticides, illicit drugs), and cognitive dysfunction in senior pets. A pet's behavior may be affected during any developmental period from prenatal to adulthood but is most susceptible to pathological outcomes during the prenatal, neonatal and socialization periods (i.e., the first few months of brain development). Cognitive dysfunction (brain aging) may also be a factor in older dogs since altered social relationships are a commonly reported sign (see Chapter 8). Treat for treatable disorders as well as FASCP. Avoid waiting to treat FASCP until all medical conditions are "ruled out." Presume that there is underlying pain or discomfort until proven otherwise and treat accordingly.

Diagnosis

The most important factor in treatment is not always finding that perfect diagnosis, but instead, creating a complete list of credible differential diagnoses and identifying triggers underlying motivation, and targets of the aggression. In many cases, there may be several or conflicting motivations or differing motivations for similar situations. Most types of aggression exhibited by dogs has an underlying component of FASCP or pain. Any stimulus can cause virtually any type of aggression. The underlying motivation for the aggression is in the eye of the beholder. If, for example, a dog thinks that the vacuum is a threat, then it is. The veterinarian's job in that case is to identify what the individual views as a threat and then formulate a treatment plan. The pet parent will have formed their own opinions about the motivation of the dog, which are usually linked to their emotions together with anthropomorphic judgements about what the dog is doing. Listen to the pet parent and collect objective information before making a differential diagnosis list.

What follows is a list of diagnostic criteria for different types of aggression, or "labels" for the motivation or function of the aggression. Labels are helpful because they allow us to speak the same language. As veterinary healthcare team members, we use labeling throughout our day to communicate with each other and pet parents. We label dogs with increased serum cortisol as having hyperadrenocorticism and dogs with osteoarthritis as arthritic. We label behaviors by making diagnoses; however, this concept is accompanied by the danger of tunnel vision and omission of the fact that there is much yet to discover about the motivations and functions associated with aggression. There will be times when the practitioner may not be able to distinguish between territorial aggression and fear-induced aggression. In cases such as these, it is best to write a list of differential diagnoses which may be ruled in or out with additional time spent treating the case.

Behavioral diagnoses can be characterized as functional, motivational, or descriptive. The most common diagnoses in use at this time in North America are either descriptive or motivational. Descriptive diagnoses are as they sound, a description of what is occurring. Examples include: owner-directed aggression and petting-induced aggression. Motivational diagnoses attempt to assess the underlying emotional state or physiologic process causing the aggression. Examples include stress-or fear-induced aggression. Functional aggression diagnoses are used more infrequently at this time and might include distance-increasing aggression.

Diagnoses of disorders of any body system reflect the level of our understanding of the problems at the time that they are made. At the first appointment, the motivation may not be clear; thus the pet is given a descriptive diagnosis. After more information is gathered in follow-up or upon reexamination, a motivational diagnosis can potentially be made.

In addition, there are qualifiers which may be applied to any diagnosis. Examples include: redirected and impulsive. In the past, these might have been standalone diagnoses. However, currently they appear to be best used as qualifiers, words that modify the meaning of the aggressive diagnosis by characterizing it further. A qualifier is not always necessary, but it can delineate further the characteristics of the aggression.

There are not yet any practical or validated diagnostic tests for clinical use. However, positron emission tomography scans, measures of neurotransmitters and their metabolites, genetic testing, and electroencephalogram evaluations might hold some promise in the future. In the interim, behavioral diagnostics must focus on clinical signs and response to therapeutic trials.

Categories of diagnoses

Descriptive diagnoses
Dominance-related aggression

Dominance-related aggression is arguably the most misdiagnosed and overdiagnosed type of canine aggression. While it was previously regarded as a common disorder, it is recognized now as rare and specific to certain criteria. See above (Normal Canine Behavior and Chapter 2) for a discussion of dominance in domestic dogs. Most, if not all, aggression problems that once would have been designated as dominance-related aggression are now being diagnosed as possessive aggression (resource guarding), conflict induced (social conflict induced), stress induced, and fear induced.[13,19,41,54,55,80]

Interdog aggression

The behavior of animals with others of their species is generally more straightforward than their interspecies behavior patterns as a result of shared communication strategies. In a recent study, 11% of pet parents reported aggression toward other dogs in the home, unfamiliar dogs on walks (16% on lead and 9% off lead), and unfamiliar dogs in the home (9%).[4] Tension between dogs in the household rarely has to do with dominance, and most dogs live together with little or no structured hierarchy. The strongest evidence to explain aggression between dogs in the same household comes from three areas: FASCP (discussed above), resource-holding potential (RHP), and resource value (RV). RHP can be understood as the traits possessed by an individual which affect the ability to win a competitive contest over a limited resource, and RV is the inherent value of that particular resource to the individual dog.[133] RHP and RV may be factors in aggression between dogs in the same household, as some resources such as attention from the pet parent, food, toys, or long-lasting chews (bones) are considered by the dogs as scarce or limited. Within a household, behaviorally appropriate dogs generally work out a system for coexistence without injury, and any competition over resources is resolved through a combination of factors, including RHP, RV, which dog controls the resource at any given time (possession is 9/10 of the law), socialization, temperament of the dog, and previous consequences. Problems arise when dogs of nearly equal RHP and RV for a particular resource simultaneously inhabit the same house or one or both dogs suffer from FASCP.

With some forms of aggression and when there is a size or strength disparity between dogs, injuries or death may occur. Situations in which fights are most likely to occur are usually competitive in nature (food, toys, resting area, pet parent attention), ones in which there is high arousal or excitement (greetings, territorial barking, running through the home, play, exiting through a door into the yard), or passing through narrow doorways or tight spaces. As a matter of fact, in a retrospective study of 217 cases of dogs presented to a veterinary behavior referral practice for aggression to each other within the same household, possessive aggression (aggression related to valuable items or resources) was the most common fight trigger and comorbidity for individual dogs.[100] In that same study, consistent with other studies, the aggressor was new to the home, younger, and larger than the victim.[100]

Pet parents who interfere with normal dog interactions can cause or contribute to fighting. For example, if dog A has a bone and dog B approaches, dog A may signal to dog B by posturing and growling to stay away, and dog B may retreat. This is a normal dog interaction which has ended as intended. If the pet parent decides this is unfair, she may reprimand dog A and give dog B the bone. If this persists, dog A may become increasingly more anxious and increasingly more intense as dog B approaches, crossing the line between normal and abnormal behavior. The dog world is inherently unfair in that some degree of social asymmetry is needed to help establish stable relationships. Although there are times when pet parents should absolutely intervene (injury, abnormal signaling and/or response, size disparity, out-of-context or excessive displays), there are also times when this is contraindicated.

Approach these cases as you would any other case. Try to identify the underlying function or motivation of the aggression when possible. In some cases, the most that can be done at the initial appointment is to make a list of differential diagnoses and formulate a safety plan. The body language displayed by each dog involved in the problem will depend on the underlying motivation for function of the aggression and the learning that has occurred. For example, victim dogs, even if they have been acting appropriately (e.g., deferring, avoiding), may be more aggressive and fearful if they continue to be bitten.

Defensive aggression and defensive behavior

Defensive aggression and defensive behavior describe aggression that stems from the condition of defending, resisting, or preventing aggression, attack, or threat. It is not intended to describe a certain emotional state, as dogs that defend against an attack or fight back when attacked, for example, may have any number of emotional states and may not have FASCP. In addition, defensive behavior is not necessarily abnormal or pathologic.

Defensive aggression is displayed in situations where the dog is threatened by a stimulus which is present or has a conditioned response (not necessarily emotional or accompanied by significant arousal) to a stimulus resulting in a past undesirable consequence. Defensive aggression can be associated with any body language (confident, relaxed, or fearful) before and after the aggressive response because

dogs displaying this type of aggression are not necessarily fearful, but instead may be reacting with aggression in defense of self or a location in which they have stationed. The aggression is characterized by short duration (lasting as long as the dog needs it to in order to repel the stimulus or achieve the desired response); measured response (as much aggression or force as needed to repel the stimulus or achieve the desired response); mild to moderate arousal (e.g., pupils may be dilated), and immediate or very short recovery (dog returns to baseline immediately or after a short period of time) when the stimulus is removed. This is most likely a normal response without a fear component in behaviorally appropriate animals when there is a threat. Perhaps dogs that were previously diagnosed with dominance or status-induced aggression would now be characterized as having defensive aggression with this current terminology. For example, two dogs (Dog A and Dog B) go to the front door as the pet parent is entering. Dog A inadvertently bumps into Dog B. Dog B who has a separation-related disorder and is anxious about the pet parent's return and bites Dog A when he is bumped. Dog A fights back, biting Dog B (a defensive response). The pet parent separates the dogs. Dog A does not attempt to reinitiate the fight and does not show prolonged arousal or recovery. If this occurs repeatedly, Dog A could develop a negative conditioned response to any number of factors including the pet parent's entry and Dog B and FASCP in this situation.

Iatrogenic aggression

Iatrogenic aggression is characterized by aggression which is caused by a medication, supplement, natural product, or procedure performed by a veterinarian. Aggression as an expression of altered mood is a possible side effect of corticosteroids, any medication which alters mentation (e.g., serotonergic medications, benzodiazepines, anticonvulsants, sedatives, opioids), and natural products (e.g., silver vine, catnip pheromones), and over the counter products. Iatrogenic aggression can be the impetus for other types of aggression, such as fear-induced, which may continue to be exhibited after the inciting stimulus for the iatrogenic aggression has been removed. Dogs with iatrogenic aggression may have a long or short latency to arousal and recovery, depending on the situation, the effect of the medication or procedure, and the level of FASCP. The frequency is consistent with the presentation of the stimulus or any conditioned stimuli. When prescribing medications which can cause a change in mood, hunger, or aggression, pet parents should always be advised of the risks.

For example, a pruritic dog is prescribed prednisone. The dog experiences increased hunger and mood swings from the medication. When the pet parent goes to pick up the food bowl after it is empty, a situation which would not have elicited aggression prior, the dog lunges and growls. In each situation, regardless of whether the aggression had an iatrogenic cause originally, there is the possibility that the behavioral clinical signs will continue even after the medication has been withdrawn.

Maternal aggression

Maternal aggression refers to aggressive behavior directed toward people or other animals that approach the bitch with her puppies. All mothers have protective instincts concerning their offspring. The intensity varies between individuals, with some exhibiting only mild growling and threatening, while others may attack and injure without warning. Bitches that experience pseudocyesis (false pregnancy) may also display maternal aggression despite the lack of puppies. The well-trained and socialized bitch is most likely to allow her puppies to be handled, especially by trusted family members. The diagnosis is made when a newly whelped bitch or one with pseudocyesis barks, growls, or attempts to bite humans or other animals that approach the puppies, puppy surrogates (e.g., toys), or nest area. The prognosis is good, as there is usually spontaneous remission as the puppies mature or are weaned. There is also some risk that the behavior will persist once learned or that the problem will recur with subsequent litters.

Play-induced aggression and undesirable play behavior

Play-induced aggression, while used in the past as a primary diagnosis, may not be an accurate description of the typical presentation of aggression during play. Dogs that present for aggression during play often have normal play behavior which is undesirable or injurious due to circumstances (e.g., victim health) outside of the dog's control. They may also have been reinforced for inappropriate play behavior. If the pet parent has punished the dog for playing in a certain way, that can cause fear, anxiety, stress, and conflict with further play. If the pet parent has encouraged inappropriate play with hands and feet or wrestling on the floor, this can contribute to reinforcement and confusion on the dog's part. The function of aggression is to repel the recipient. Much of the aggression about which pet parents complain which occurs during play is not intended to repel the recipient but instead intended to perpetuate play or is a component of play. For this reason, injurious play behavior or undesirable play behavior may be more appropriate terms with which to describe this behavior.

Undesirable play behavior is typically seen in puppies and young dogs and is accompanied by playful postures and behaviors. A classic play-soliciting behavior is the *play bow*. The dog may quickly dart forward and back, barking, and thrusting its muzzle toward the target. See Chapter 2 for a description of play postures. Play attacks can be spontaneous, with bites that might be hard enough to injure. Mouthing and biting that achieve a goal of soliciting play are positively reinforced and will continue. Prolonged, deeptone growling associated with staring and stiff body postures indicates that the behavior is more serious. A large portion of canine play involves aggressive behaviors such as growling, biting, bumping, and attacking. Bites should be inhibited. If the dog is rowdy, persistent, or bites without inhibition, it becomes a problem for the family and visitors. Uncontrolled play can pose a danger to young children and adults with fragile skin or who could be knocked over. While play can be vigorous and physical, young pups will usually learn at an early age that hard bites and overexuberant play with littermates causes play to stop. The same rules must be taught when the puppy is playing with people. Puppies with insufficient training, exercise, and mental stimulation especially in breeds with high energy are the most likely to display this problem. Another scenario is the puppy that is play biting, which is a normal behavior. If pet parents use positive punishment to deter the behavior (e.g., hit, squeeze the mouth, pin to the floor), the desire to play will not be lessened, but the puppy may become increasingly anxious and conflicted about the pet parent's response. If the play biting is also sometimes successful at getting the pet parents to play, this places the pet in a situation of conflict, since the pet is still motivated to play but uncertain about how the pet parent will respond, which can progress to fear-induced or conflict-induced aggression.

When presented with human-directed aggression which resembles play, first the veterinarian must distinguish between normal play and play-induced aggression. Play behaviors include: exploration and investigation; stalking, chasing, attacking, silent ambush, pouncing, and leaping sideways; fighting; wrestling; swatting, quick recovery, self-handicapping, and vacillating between relaxed body language and spurts of energy and biting. Dogs may get overaroused during normal play and display play behavior with an impulsive component. Regardless of whether the behavior is normal or pathologic, it can still be dangerous and should be treated. Play-induced aggression occurs when the dog's bites are deep, uninhibited, out of context, or more intense than would be expected with normal play. Dogs may be overly aroused, or have a long or short latency to arousal and recovery. The body language and context are consistent with play, at least initially. There is often a component of impulsivity aggression or a history of frustration and punishment in these cases.

Motivational diagnoses

Conflict-induced (social conflict-induced) aggression

Conflict-related behaviors are seen when there are competing states of motivation and/or frustration over the inability to perform desired behaviors or achieve desired outcomes. Conflict can lead to confusion, anxiety, fear, and aggression. Dogs that exhibit conflict-induced aggression are often fearful and/or anxious dogs that are unsure how to avoid confusing or disagreeable interactions with their pet parents, in part because they lack control over outcomes. Some authors suggest that conflict-induced aggression is better deemed social conflict-induced aggression because most manifestations of aggression include some level of internal conflict, and conflict-induced aggression was originally coined to mean aggression to familiar people.[13]

Due to inconsistent pet parent signals and actions, the dog learns that aggression is the best way to stop the interaction (see Learning and Aggression, earlier in this chapter). The dog may initially exhibit signs of appeasement, anxiety, uncertainty, or fear, and then progress to aggression. If the signs (e.g., ears back, horizontal retraction of lips, lip lick, inguinal presentation) are subtle or ignored, the dog enters a state of conflict with a resulting arousal response. The state of arousal can lead to aggression, even when the threat seems to be relatively benign (e.g., pet parents attempting to pet a resting dog). For example, a fearful puppy is approached by the pet parent and told to get off the couch. The puppy has not been taught to get off the couch (the pet parent has not adequately trained the dog) and is confused. When confronted, the puppy displays submissive signaling such as ears back and tail down because he does not understand what is expected of him. The pet parent responds by pulling the dog by the collar to get it off the couch. If these interactions are repeated, the dog will progress to stronger signals such as growling and eventually biting. The dog is in conflict as to how to respond since its initial appeasing and submissive signals resulted in confrontation and punishment (considered inappropriate in the dog world), which ultimately leading to fear and conflict-induced (social conflict-induced) aggression.

Conflict-induced aggression is exhibited toward social group members when the dog is resting, during physical manipulations, and around valuable resources, often with an accompanying ambivalence, submission, or attempts at reconciliation after biting.[134] Pet parents often report that their dog looks guilty after the aggressive display. This type of aggression can be confused with possessive aggression because it may occur under similar circumstances. Possessive aggression can be exhibited toward social group members, unfamiliar people, and/or animals, and is exhibited consistently only in the presence of valued resources.

The diagnosis is made based on the situations in which the aggression is exhibited, the targets of the aggression, and the pet's overall demeanor. Conflict-induced aggression is often diagnosed with other fear and anxiety-related disorders, such as separation-related disorders or storm phobia. It is likely dogs that were previously diagnosed with dominance-related aggression would now be diagnosed with conflict-induced aggression.[19,13]

Fear-induced aggression

Fear is a common cause of behavior problems in companion animals and aggression is no exception. In a survey study in the United Kingdom of dogs that showed aggression toward people, 4% had shown signs of fear of family members and 10% had shown signs of fear of unfamiliar people.[53] In a Finnish study, highly (5 times higher) and moderately fearful dogs had a higher probability of aggressive behavior toward people than nonfearful dogs.[14] Fear-induced aggression can be displayed toward any person, animal, or object. Clinical signs include growling, snapping, biting, ears down, tail down, and low posture.[54] Dogs with fear-induced aggression may be more likely to exhibit aggression in the home toward familiar people when approached and or touched,[54] or inside and outside of the home toward familiar or unfamiliar people when they are fearful and unable to escape the stressor.[3] In the laboratory setting, fear-induced aggression can be caused by lesions in the amygdala and temporal areas of the brain.[135]

Fear-induced aggression is exhibited when a dog is exposed to someone (e.g., person, animal), something (e.g., sound, object), or a situation (e.g., veterinarian, car) that it perceives as threatening, or a stimulus which is paired with something, someone, or a situation that is or was perceived as a threat, especially if there is no opportunity to escape. Any stimulus, from cars and skateboards to unfamiliar people or dogs, can produce fear leading to an aggressive response. Body language exhibited before it is significantly altered via reinforcement and/or punishment is consistent with fear. Dogs with fear-induced aggression may have a long or short latency to arousal and recovery depending on the situation and the dog's level of FASCP. The frequency is consistent with the presentation of the stimulus or any conditioned stimuli.

Pet parent behavior can increase this type of aggression. Punishment, inconsistent responses, and removing the opportunity for the pet to escape or cope with the situation appropriately will aggravate fear-induced aggression. When faced with the fear-producing stimulus, if the pet parent does nothing to keep the dog safe (e.g., avoid the stimulus, teach the dog an alternate behavior), the dog will find a way to stay safe, which may include aggression. If the pet parent uses harsh or physical punishment, the autonomic nervous system arousal level will increase, increasing the animal's state of agitation. Warning signals may be punished, causing the dog to be more dangerous (i.e., no warning before aggression). If the pet parent acts nervous, grabs the leash tightly, or acts erratically, the dog's nervousness may be further enhanced. Fear cannot be positively reinforced, so petting the dog at this time will not make the dog more fearful and aggressive. However, unless the dog can be sufficiently calmed, it does not help the dog cope. If the dog does not understand how to cope and downregulate, the aggression will increase. In addition, petting may positively reinforce fear-related operant behaviors (e.g., growling, biting, escape, staying close to the pet parent). Genetic predisposition will play a role in determining the threshold for a fear response. Some dogs require a strong stimulus to elicit fear, while others become extremely anxious in response to mild stimuli or any auditory, visual, or perhaps even odor stimulus that is unfamiliar.

Dogs that exhibit fear-induced aggression on leash may be more aggressive when on the leash, and may display fearful or distance-increasing behaviors when off leash and allowed to approach of their own accord. This may be a result of restriction and inability to escape when on the leash. Inappropriate pet parent responses (e.g., tension on the leash, agitation, frustration, punishment) will further condition unpleasant associations when meeting new people or dogs on the leash. In one study of dogs on walks with their pet parents, threats were twice as often between dogs when on leash than off, and both males and females bit dogs of the same gender more than five times more than the opposite gender.[136]

Some dogs will approach as if they want to interact and then retreat when the person reaches for them. These dogs may be inherently fearful or insufficiently socialized and in conflict when meeting unfamiliar people or dogs. A dog may be fearful with certain people or dogs because of previous unpleasant experiences or lack of socialization to specific individuals (e.g., children, men, large dogs), or react to all unfamiliar people or dogs. History should be collected regarding dog's behavior as a puppy to determine if the dog was exuberant and friendly, uncertain, or showed avoidance of stimuli. When a person approaches, the dog may feel threatened and growl When the person turns and walks away, the aggression the dog may lunge, chase, or bite.

Dogs that exhibit fear-induced aggression are acting to keep themselves safe and remove the fear-eliciting stimuli. If a dog sits near the pet parent when afraid, it may be seeking a secure location from which it may then defend itself if the stimulus continues to approach. If the pet parent responds with cues which keep the dog safe and repel the stimuli, the dog will be more likely to exhibit those behaviors in the future. This is often misinterpreted by observers as an effort to defend the pet parent from the stimulus when in fact, the dog is fearful and retreating to the pet parent for support. It is the pet parent's responsibility to first ensure safety and to work with the dog over time to reduce fear of the stimulus.

Fear is a common cause of aggression toward children. Families often report that the dog was fine with or ambivalent toward a particular child until the child started crawling or walking. When the child starts to crawl or walk, it is much more likely to interact physically with the pet and possibly corner it. When fearful dogs cannot escape, they are more likely to react with aggression.

Frustration-induced aggression

Frustration-induced aggression is exhibited when the dog cannot achieve the desired outcome because the dog does not have the appropriate communication or coping skills, the pet parent does not recognize the signals, or the dog is physically prevented from engaging in interaction with or escape from the stimulus or situation. It can be challenging to discern if these dogs desire interaction and are over-aroused and frustrated due to lack of ability to interact in a friendly manner, or if they are fearful and anxious and are threatening the target. Dogs may have any level of arousal or a short or long latency to arousal and recovery depending on the level of frustration. Pet parents will often describe the dog as friendly except when they do not do what he wants or when he cannot get what he wants. Body language can be consistent with confidence or fear and mild to moderate arousal. Because the lives of many dogs are unpredictable and outside of their control, it is likely that this type of aggression is more common than we now recognize. Dogs diagnosed with this type of aggression may have previously been diagnosed with dominance-related aggression. Additionally, frustration-induced aggression can be difficult to distinguish from territorial aggression. Dogs who bark at passersby from behind a fence may bite the fence during the bout of barking. In cases like this, the dog may be frustrated, however the aggression might be determined to be territorial aggression which has been redirected to the fence. In another example, a dog is barking for attention from behind a baby gate. The function of the barking is to get the attention of the pet parent so that she will give the dog some of the food that she is eating. She ignores him entirely. After a couple of minutes, he bites the baby gate behind which he is confined out of frustration.

Pain-induced aggression

Dogs with pain-induced aggression act aggressively when they are pushed, pulled, handled, picked up, examined, medicated, and when feeling discomfort or pain. The diagnosis may be difficult because dogs may not show gross clinical signs of discomfort or physical disease. Pain-induced aggression should be considered if the pet has a disease or disorder which is known to cause pain or discomfort, mobility or activity has been altered, or the aggression suddenly appears in a dog with no previous aggression when being handled, approached, reached for, or moved. In a study of 12 dogs diagnosed with pain-induced aggression, hip dysplasia was the most common cause of pain. If the dog was not aggressive prior to the onset of pain, they were more likely to show an impulsive component to the aggressive behavior, show aggression when manipulated, and show defensive body postures when compared to dogs that were aggressive prior to the onset of pain.[137] Additionally, aggression was not necessarily correlated with manipulation of the painful body part potentially because the pet had established a conditioned response to manipulation based on anticipation that the interaction would cause pain. In a study comparing aggressive dogs with musculoskeletal pain and aggressive dogs without pain, pet parents described the painful and aggressive dogs as having a more negative temperament, being reluctant to move, and potentially more aggressive when the dog was lying down or approached by another dog. It is important to note that in the aforementioned study, half of the dogs in the pain group had undiagnosed pain at the time of presentation, meaning that neither the primary care veterinarian nor the pet parent was aware of the dog's discomfort prior to referral.[138]

A therapeutic response trial with pain control medication may aid in confirming the diagnosis. In addition, where pain or discomfort is a contributory factor to aggression, dogs should be closely monitored for a recurrence of aggression or associated behavior problems when analgesic therapy is reduced or withdrawn. Pain-induced aggression can be distinguished from stress-induced aggression (see below) because the action from the stimulus causes pain or discomfort, whereas stress-induced aggression is related to cumulative or chronic stress which may or may not have a pain or discomfort component and can be due entirely to emotional stress.

Even the most sociable and docile animal may exhibit aggression when it is in pain, uncomfortable, ill, or has sensory impairment (e.g., sight, hearing). If there is any presumption of pain, it should be investigated and treated. If the pet parent declines diagnostics, the pet should be treated, if safe to do so, for the presumption of pain. Both acute and chronic pain may trigger aggression. Pain and discomfort are in the eye of the beholder. Gastrointestinal discomfort associated with chronic small intestinal diarrhea or pruritus resulting from atopy may cause aggression just as much as otitis externa or osteoarthritis. Handling or the anticipation of handling when a person approaches or reaches for the dog that is painful or ill might also result in aggression, even when the dog is tolerant of those interactions otherwise. Metabolic disorders such as liver disease, pancreatitis, renal disease, endocrine disorders, CNS disorders, or sensory decline might lead to aggression due to discomfort (see Chapter 6). Sometimes the diagnosis is straightforward: the dog experiences pain and reacts aggressively. The dog might snarl, growl, or bite people if it perceives they are the cause of the pain. It is important to remedy the situation for both humane and welfare reasons for the dog as well as to prevent the problem from escalating. The dog that learns that biting accomplished its goals (i.e., stopped the painful interaction) might then use aggression when similar interactions arise in the future if it anticipates pain or has a negative association with being handled, even after the pain has resolved, as the dog may still anticipate a painful outcome as a conditioned emotional response or as learned response. Degenerative disease, trauma, and illness that lead to pain or increased irritability may be difficult to identify; therefore, a complete history plus a full physical workup are essential for all aggressive dogs. Dogs with pain-induced aggression may have a long or short latency to arousal and recovery depending on the situation and the dog's level of pain or discomfort. The frequency is consistent with the presentation of the stimulus or any conditioned stimuli.

Any handling that elicits pain or discomfort can lead to this type of aggression. The dog's reaction can become conditioned, being exhibited when the dog anticipates that it will be touched. The presence of pain may lower the threshold for the manifestation of other types of aggression, such as fear-induced aggression. The use of physical punishment or force to apply treatments such as ear medication can lead to both pain, fear and defensive aggression. Therefore, physical punishment or force should not be used, as it may lead to a conditioned fear response, which may manifest itself as aggression during similar types of handling or approach in the future. The behavior of the veterinary healthcare team can contribute to this type of aggression. For information on how to manage pets in a low-stress way in the veterinary clinic, see Chapter 16.

Possessive aggression (resource guarding)

The terminology associated with aggression around resources is somewhat controversial and currently there is disagreement among experts. When a dog is aggressive within close proximity to food or resting spaces, what is the function of that behavior? Should we label aggression around valuable items resource guarding or possessive aggression?[139] Could this behavior be caused by frustration, fear, anxiety, stress, pain, discomfort, or hunger? There is much yet to learn about why animals show aggression over resources and what items, people, or animals are considered resources.

Possessive aggression is a normal behavior which can become maladaptive. It is one of the most common types of aggression.[41,140] It may be directed at familiar and unfamiliar humans or other animals that approach the dog when it is near or in possession of something it values such as food bowls, chew toys, people, pets, or places. Novel or stolen items are especially valuable. Dogs can show any body language from fearful to confident. Dogs that exhibit this type of aggression may have a long or short latency to arousal and recovery, depending on the level of stress, but will display aggression only when valuable items are present. Dogs that may have been labeled previously with dominance-related aggression may fall under the possessive aggression category however, possessive aggression has little to do with dominance. As mentioned above, RHP, RV, and FASCP are the main drivers of this behavior.

Pet parents often negatively reinforce the pet's anxiety by taking items, chasing the pet when he has an item, and physical forcing the pet to give the item up. These dogs have not been taught to expect a reward for relinquishing an item or to relinquish items on cue. In other words, the dog is anxious about people taking his stuff and then his worst fear – that his stuff will be taken away – comes true. If the dog runs away, hides, or growls, the pet parent often chases and forcefully takes the item. Through these interactions, the dog learns fearful body postures and avoidance are not effective

in inhibiting threatening behavior. The dog then starts to growl or bite, which he quickly learns is an effective way to protect items of value. In dogs with possessive aggression, the behavior of the pet parent may be especially important. In fact, 78 dogs that showed possessive aggression in a shelter situation did not show aggression when adopted into a home,[141] demonstrating to some extent the importance of the environment on this type of aggression.

The age of onset is often prior to 16 weeks of age. Initial onset may occur in adulthood in dogs on reducing diets or medication that increases hunger (e.g., corticosteroids) or with medical conditions that increase appetite (e.g., hyperadrenocorticism). When affected puppies are identified early, the progression of the disorder can usually be stopped and the long-term outcome can be positive, at least from the standpoint of management. This can be both a normal desire to maintain valuable possessions and an anxiety-related disorder. Some dogs may bury items in the cushions of the couch and are then aggressive when someone enters the room or sits on the couch.

Predatory aggression and predatory behavior

It is a normal instinct in dogs to chase and hunt prey. However, when this behavior is directed toward people and domestic animals, it can be dangerous. Predatory behavior could include any or all of stalking, chasing, catching, biting, killing, and eating, and may be socially facilitated and more dangerous in a group. Predatory behaviors may be stimulated by anything that moves, including other animals, joggers, cyclists, playing children, or moving automobiles. Auditory stimuli, such as the cries and screams of babies or young children, may elicit a predatory response. Predation is not preceded by threats because during hunting, a warning behavior would be counterproductive. Barking and in some cases growling may occur during pursuit of prey or when the dog is frustrated. Normal predatory behavior is often mistaken for aggression. Predatory behavior is not truly "aggression" because the goal is not to increase distance between the instigator and recipient.

Predatory aggression can be elicited in laboratory animals by stimulating the lateral hypothalamus.[137] Dogs may direct predatory behavior toward other pets cohabitating in the home, especially if those animals belong to species that are normally prey (e.g., mice, rats, birds, hamsters, cats). The initial movements of this behavioral sequence are characterized by silent stalking. While predatory aggression and behavior are most likely normal, they can still be undesirable and may need treatment. If the bites are injurious or uninhibited or if the aggression causes a degradation of the quality of life of the human or animal victims, it should be treated. Dogs may have a long or short recovery and latency to arousal. Aggression is accompanied by the body language consistent with predation.

Predatory aggression may be exhibited by dogs of either sex. A moving stimulus is the usual target. The response of the dog is to chase, bite, and potentially kill prey, which is most often smaller than the dog. To some extent, chase behaviors (e.g., herding) may be genetically selected predatory behaviors that also have the potential for serious injury. The behavior may be socially facilitated, as dogs in groups may exhibit intense chase, attack, and kill behavior in situations where they may have done little or no chasing on their own.

Protective aggression

Protective aggression is defined by target, target behavior, and the presence of a pet and/or human family member and is uncommon. The behavior is directed toward unfamiliar people or animals approaching or acting in a way the pet perceives to be threatening, and may be manifested in or away from the dog's home. The defining variable is the presence of a family member. A dog with protective aggression may be friendly to unfamiliar people when the family member is not present. Pet parents often assume that their dog is protecting them at the veterinary clinic and other situations. They report that their dog is "fine" when they are not present. However, typically, the dog is inhibited when the pet parent is not there and shows fearful or disengagement body language as opposed to acting in a friendly and relaxed way. The protective dog would show body language consistent with confidence or relaxation away from the family member that he would normally protect. A common situation seen in homes with multiple pets occurs when the dog that is sitting with or near the pet parent growls as the other pet approaches. This behavior pattern could be consistent with protective aggression; however, it is more likely to be fear induced (pet parent is a secure base), pain induced, or stress induced.

Stress-induced aggression

Stress-induced aggression occurs when a dog is cumulatively (hours, days, weeks) in a state of intermittent or constant physiologic stress due to emotional or physical disease (e.g., painful, uncomfortable, metabolic) and shows aggression to a person, animal, or object which may or may not be the cause of the stress. The dog may before or after the aggressive incident show signs of fear, anxiety, and stress; however, because this type of aggression is a function of cumulative or chronic physiologic or emotional stress, there may be no clear body language precursors. Often dogs with stress-induced aggression do not show aggression consistently toward the victim or even consistently when put into the same situation or with the same stimuli. Incidents may be sporadic. This type of aggression could be described as threshold aggression or aggression as a result of trigger stacking. The dog is under cumulative stress and a single stimulus (e.g., situation, person, environment, animal) causes the dog to surpass the threshold for coping or tolerance, resulting in aggression. The difference between stress-induced and redirected aggression is that redirected aggression involves aggression to another stimulus, which is then targeted to another animal, person, or object. Dogs that express stress-induced aggression often appear to have a short latency to arousal (when in fact they are under chronic or cumulative stress); recovery can be variable and the body language can vary. For example, consider the older, arthritic dog that lives in a relatively quiet house. The adult children come to visit with their puppy that is 16 weeks old to stay for the holidays. The puppy is rambunctious and consistently tries to play with the older dog. The older dog sometimes relents and plays and at other times, would rather sleep. Little effort is made by the family to separate the dogs when the older dog is overwhelmed. This continues throughout the week. One evening when the puppy is confined to his crate, the pet parent reaches down to pet the older dog that is on the couch. He startles awake and bites her hand. In this situation, the dog is overwhelmed physiologically due to emotional and physical stress (pain). When the stressor is removed (the puppy) for an amount of time which allows him to recover, he may not show aggression to the pet parent again.

Territorial aggression

Territorial aggression is exhibited toward unfamiliar people or animals in the dog's territory and can have body language consistent with fear or confidence. The underlying cause of territorial aggression is the social tension that arises from the intrusion of a new dog or person. The behavior is generally manifested in the dog's home or yard, or perhaps the car, and is directed toward unfamiliar people or animals approaching or entering the territory. Territorial behaviors are to some extent a variant of normal behavior (i.e., intruder on territory). Problems occur when the pet has a very low threshold for arousal and is aggressive in relatively benign situations and/or the pet's response is excessive for the needs of the situation. Anxiety and fear also play a role in the development or progression of aggression since threats and aggressive displays are more likely to be exhibited toward novel, unfamiliar, or fear-eliciting stimuli. Fearful dogs will also be fearful when off property. However, if pet parents report no aggression off property, the veterinarian should question whether the dog attempts to avoid interactions with unfamiliar stimuli. If the dog is friendly off of the property and aggressive on the property, territorial aggression is more likely.

If pet parents use positive punishment in an attempt to suppress the behavior, become angry or frustrated each time the behavior is displayed, or contain the dog on an electric fence, the association with unfamiliar people and animals will become increasingly more negative. Aggression is negatively reinforced each time the stimulus (person or dog) leaves or passes by the property while the pet is displaying the territorial behavior (e.g., barking, lunging, growling). The dog barks and the stimulus retreats. Even though the barking most likely did not cause the retreat of the stimulus, the barking was reinforced nonetheless. Territorial dogs are often allowed to practice the behavior daily at doors, windows, in the yard, or on a tie-out, which adds the element of frustration. If the dog is permitted to bark at stimuli outside of the home as described above, the behavior will be more difficult to correct (see Table 23.1).

Aggression qualifiers

Impulsivity and aggression

Impulsivity can be a characteristic of almost any type of aggression. Impulsive aggression, while used historically as a stand-alone diagnosis, may be best used as a qualifier to describe an impulsive component of another type of aggression. Impulsivity has a substantial, obvious sympathetic nervous system arousal component (e.g., piloerection, dilated pupils) and is characterized by sudden action which may appear automatic and out of context and proportion to the level of the stimulus, often ramping up with

Table 23.1 Aggression diagnoses and characteristics

Diagnosis	Motivation/ function	Latency to arousal	Recovery	Target	Body language	Other characteristics
Descriptive diagnoses						
Interdog aggression	Fear, conflict, defense of resources, stress, anxiety, pain, discomfort, loss of senses/faculties/affecting ability to communicate	Varies	Varies	Other dog within the household	Varies	Most often, both dogs need to be treated for resolution
Defensive aggression	Increase distance from stimulus/target/victim	Varies	Short	Any familiar or unfamiliar person, object, or animal	Varies, not consistent with moderate to severe arousal	Can be a normal, behaviorally appropriate response
Iatrogenic aggression	Increase distance from stimulus/target/victim	Varies	Varies	Any familiar or unfamiliar person, object, or animal	Varies	Inciting cause is external (e.g., medication, supplement, procedure)
Maternal aggression	Increase distance from stimulus/target/victim	Varies	Varies	Person/animal near or handing puppies	Varies	Pregnancy or pseudocyesis
Undesirable play behavior	Decrease distance from stimulus/target/victim, continue play	Varies	Varies	Person or animal engaged in play	Consistent with play, play bow	Common in young dogs, most likely a variation of normal play
Play-induced aggression	Increase distance from stimulus/target/victim, fear, anxiety, stress	Varies	Varies	Person or animal engaged in play	Play postures, conflict, arousal, less inhibited bites	May be caused by inconsistent interactions with play partners
Conflict-induced aggression	Increase distance from stimulus/target/victim, fear, anxiety, stress	Varies	Varies	Social group members	Arousal, tense distance increasing, fearful	Dogs are often very attached to pet parent despite the aggressive responses
Fear-induced aggression	Increase distance from stimulus/target/victim, fear, anxiety, stress	Varies	Varies	Any familiar or unfamiliar person, object, or animal	Fear, anxiety, arousal, stress	Body language can look offensive as disorder progresses
Frustration-induced aggression	Increase or decrease distance from stimulus/target/victim	Varies	Varies	Any familiar or unfamiliar person, object, or animal	Fear, anxiety, arousal, stress	May be described as friendly until he does not get what he wants
Pain-induced aggression	Increase distance from stimulus/target/victim, fear, anxiety, stress, pain	Varies	Varies	Any familiar or unfamiliar person, object, or animal	Fear, anxiety, arousal, stress, pain	Always assume pain or discomfort plays a role until proven otherwise
Possessive aggression	Increase distance from stimulus/target/victim, fear, anxiety, stress	Varies	Varies	Any familiar or unfamiliar person, object, or animal	Fear, anxiety, arousal, stress	Exhibited around valuable items
Predatory aggression (behavior)	Decrease distance from stimulus/target/victim, fear, anxiety, stress, pain	Varies	Varies	Any person, animal or object which stimulates predatory response	Quiet, stalking, tense	May include a frustration component
Protective aggression	Increase distance from stimulus/target/victim, fear, anxiety, stress	Varies	When target retreats	Any familiar or unfamiliar person, animal, or object	Varies	Only occurs when the person or animal that is being protected is present
Stress-induced aggression	Increase distance from stimulus/target/victim, fear, anxiety, stress	Varies	Varies	Any familiar or unfamiliar person, animal, or object	Varies	Chronic stress is present, either physical or emotional or both
Territorial aggression	Increase distance from stimulus/target/victim, fear, anxiety, stress	Varies	When target retreats/ variable	Any unfamiliar person, animal, or object	Offensive, moderate to severe arousal, varies	Often has a fear component, leading to increased recovery time

time exposed to the stimulus, and appears to the observer to be outside of the dog's control. It often does not respond to typical distraction such as the shake of a treat bag. Dogs with impulsivity as a component of their aggressive behavior appear to have a short latency to arousal, long recovery, and body language consistent with significant arousal (e.g., widely dilated pupils, piloerection). The frequency is often intermittent and may have no identifiable stimulus. There is some evidence that self-control is a limited resource, meaning that if the animal chronically must display self-control behaviors (e.g., inadequate, frustrating environment), there will be a point at which the capacity for self-control appears to be diminished and the animal acts impulsively. As more is learned about impulsivity in dogs, the way that we characterize it will change as well.[142] See Chapter 25 for a discussion of testing related to impulsivity in dogs.

Redirected aggression or behavior

Redirected behavior or aggression occurs secondary to another type of aggression or motivation (i.e., there is an underlying aggressive motivation which is then being redirected to another target) and can occur when the dog is displaying aggression and is interrupted.[143,144] Redirected aggression occurs when a dog is exposed to a visual, auditory, or olfactory stimulus (e.g., people, other animals, objects) and redirects the aggressive response to a nearby person, object, or animal because it is physically or socially prevented from accessing the target. Classically, the aggression will occur when the victim approaches or just happens to be near the aroused dog when he is displaying aggression. Since the aggressor may be vigilantly focused on the stimulus, the victim may approach without noticing that the dog is already in an aroused state and the aroused dog may not notice the soon-to-be victim. In some situations, the victim is not nearby and the aggressor may bypass the nearest individual to target a specific victim. This is especially true if the pattern is chronic. The attacks are often acute, intense, and seem unprovoked. The latency to arousal often appears short, and the recovery and frequency will vary. If the association between reduction of stress and biting the victim becomes conditioned, which can happen presumably with any type of aggression, the aggressor may seek out the victim out and bite them as a way to reduce the physiologic stress response.

For example, a dog that is showing aggression toward another dog on leash may turn and bite the pet parent or the leash when they are restrained from approaching the other dog. The primary aggression may be territorial, protective, or fear induced (redirected). Aggression might also be redirected toward another family dog, such as when one dog exhibits territorial aggression through a window toward a stranger or dog walking across the property, and the second family dog approaches during the heightened arousal and is attacked.

Prognosis

Aggression has historically been characterized and prognosis affected by severity of injury to the victim; however, the severity of a bite or the bite level is affected by many extrinsic and intrinsic factors, including the overall health and behavior of the victim (e.g., pulling the limb away, overall health, skin thickness, bite location) and ability of the dog to do damage (e.g., length of exposure to the victim, relative size of the dog to the victim, bite strength, skull size, skull shape).[145,146] In addition, there is no literature which supports injury to victim as a predictive factor. For these reasons, injury to the victim is not an accurate predictor of the severity of the aggression, or the likelihood or severity of future aggression. Prognosis is not set for any one animal or diagnosis. The prognosis will depend to a great extent on the family's ability to live with the dog, adhere to treatment recommendations, realistic pet parent expectations for the dog and the household, and ability to keep family members and the public safe. Pet parents may be more likely to seek treatment for larger dogs where aggression is not easily avoided (e.g., aggression to family members).

As should be clear, prognosis depends on many factors, which are for the most part out of the veterinarian's control. It is impossible to predict the outcome of any particular case; however, in general, pet parents can be counseled that the best prognosis lies with cases which are predictable and avoidable. Pet parents who are able to adhere to treatment recommendations will generally have better outcomes than those who cannot. Any discussion of predictability should come with a discussion of the obvious triggers for the aggression. Many pet parents will report that their dog has unpredictable or unprovoked aggression when in most cases, thoughtful behavioral history taking reveals that it is in fact chronic, there is a learned component, and there are identifiable triggers. The decision to keep a dog that is aggressive in the family is a personal one. Pet parents need the full picture in order to make a decision as to whether or not to treat their dog. As with physical diseases, positive outcomes are easier to achieve when treatment is initiated soon after onset and predisposed individuals are targeted for prevention. It would be ideal to be able to assess the risk of injury from a particular dog without a shadow of a doubt, but that is not possible. Dogs are sentient beings and as such, their behavior cannot accurately be predicted 100% of the time. In addition, every biting dog was once a dog that had not done so, meaning that if only past behavior is used to predict future behavior, predictions will inevitably be inaccurate. Bite inhibition has been used in an attempt to assess the level of danger from a particular dog; however, bite inhibition scales have not been validated. It is not uncommon for a dog to bite with different levels of bite inhibition depending on the situation and victim.

Caution should be used when trying to predict a particular dog's level of aggression. In general, it is best to assume that the dog will bite again and cause injury. This way, bites will generally be avoided, keeping others safe. Still, the veterinarian has to be able to give the pet parents of an aggressive dog an assessment of the likelihood of a positive outcome. Six categories should be considered when determining prognosis: (1) latency to arousal (impulsivity); (2) social and physical environment; (3) complexity of the situation; (4) potential to do harm; (5) predictability; and (6) ability of family to adhere to treatment recommendations. The latency to arousal is how long it takes for the dog to show observable signs of stress. These generally precede an aggressive display and should be used for this measurement. For example, If Dog A starts to attack within 1 second of seeing someone, as opposed to Dog B that does not attack until the person is present for 10 seconds, the latency to arousal is relatively short for Dog A and longer for Dog B. Dogs with a short latency to arousal may generally be more difficult to manage and more dangerous than dogs with a longer latency to arousal.

The social and physical environments are important when considering the potential for a positive outcome. For example, if the presenting complaint is growling at children and the dog lives in a busy household with three children under five years old, the environment is a negative prognostic factor. If that same dog lived in a quiet neighborhood with a childless couple, the environment would be a positive prognostic factor. The potential to do harm includes factors such as the size of the dog, bite history, severity of previous bites, targets, and level of arousal. Dogs with a history of pursuing the victim, multiple bites per incident, or more severe bites should be considered more dangerous than dogs that have not bitten (assuming the dog has been in a situation in which it could have bitten). Dogs that have bitten multiple times in one bout, are interrupted, and then when released go back to the victim or become so aroused that they cannot easily be pulled off, should be considered more dangerous. The complexity of the problem includes the presence of concurrent behavior diagnoses, physical disease, the presence of the triggering stimuli in the environment, the pet parent's ability to implement the plan, the presence of children or the elderly in the house, and the presence of other pets. Care should be taken not to prejudge pet parents. If the veterinarian is concerned about the ability of the pet parents to implement the plan, they should be asked directly what they see as the challenges to treatment. Then those challenges can be addressed in the treatment plan. The predictability of the dog includes factors such as whether all aggression-eliciting stimuli can be identified, the presence of identifiable warning signals, and how consistently the animal responds to environmental stimuli. For example, if the pet parent cannot provide an accurate history with a list of triggers, that case will be more difficult and potentially more dangerous to treat than a case where the list is relatively complete. Dogs that display warning signals might be easier to interrupt when compared with dogs that signal in more subtle ways (see Appendix A and Chapter 2 for more information on body language). The presence of children in the home is a negative prognostic indicator for canine aggression cases.[15] Children are more unpredictable and inconsistent, and move more quickly than adults. A large, strong dog that bites children unpredictably without inhibition in a home with small children will pose an extremely high risk for a serious injury. Finally, the ability of the pet parent to adhere to treatment recommendations should be considered. This is best determined through an honest conversation with the pet parent about their goals and abilities.

No discussion of aggression would be complete without mention of euthanasia. The decision to recommend euthanasia is fraught with ethical, moral, and personal dilemmas. Since safety is the primary concern, rehoming the dog is risky. Pet parents, rescue organizations, and/or the veterinarian may be responsible for future bites after a dog is rehomed. Factors associated with pet parent decision to euthanize or rehome their aggressive dog includes heavier weight, mixed breed, aggression to familiar people over valuable items and resting places, aggression to unfamiliar people, the presence of children age 13–17 years, and a history of biting.[122] In one study, large dogs (>18.2 kg) that have a short latency to arousal (i.e., act immediately and severely to minimal or benign stimuli) and are perceived by the pet parent as unpredictable are more likely to be euthanized than smaller dogs.[147] This is most likely due to the amount of damage that results from the bites. In one study, brachycephalic dogs and dogs 30–45 kg were at the highest risk of damage for facial injury, while Akitas and Great Danes had the lowest risk and highest damage.[72]

Factors to consider when discussing euthanasia are identifying the risks and who might be harmed, the ability of the pet parent to ensure safety, and the dog's quality of life.[148] If the pet parent is considering this option, the pet should be referred to a board-certified veterinary behaviorist for evaluation. Canine aggression is often treatable, extending and improving the quality of life of the pet. Dogs should not be given a negative prognosis simply because they show aggression. If the veterinarian chooses to treat aggression cases instead of referring them to a board-certified veterinary behaviorist, phone follow-up and in-person rechecks are important for a positive outcome. Pet parents of aggressive dogs should be contacted at 2-week intervals by support staff or the veterinarian for the best outcome.[149]

For some types of aggression, the prognosis has been established historically in certain populations. Of 73 cases of fear-induced aggression which underwent treatment, 75% of the dogs improved and 7% of the dogs worsened, while 13% remained unchanged throughout treatment.[54] Regarding inter-dog aggression within the same household, factors associated with negative outcomes include same-sex pairs, bites that broke the skin, and aggression with a little provocation (on sight of the other dog).[100] In another study, 59% of dogs showing aggression to another dog in the home and 52% of dogs showing aggression to dogs outside the home improved with treatment. Once treatment was completed, 56% of dogs could be in the presence of the other household dog unsupervised without showing aggression and 76% of the dogs that exhibited aggression outside of the home could be around previous targets under leash control without aggression.[63] Negative prognostic indicators included the aggressive dog being younger than the victim dog, a person had been bitten, and fights were not able to be predicted by the pet parent.[63] In another study of interdog aggression, improvement was reported in 65% of cases when one or both dogs received medication, 22% when a head halter was used, and 26% for separation followed by gradual introduction.[62] While the response of predatory aggression to treatment has not been examined in the literature, it is generally regarded as treatable but not completely resolvable because the behavior is instinctual. The prognosis is good for play aggression with proper treatment and early intervention[150] (see Table 23.2).

Treatment essentials

Regardless of the diagnosis, the treatment approach is similar to other behavior disorders and includes the following areas:
1. Evaluation of overall wellness.
2. Avoidance of triggers.

Table 23.2 Considerations for assessing danger and risk of injury (prognosis)*

Factors	Essential points
Latency to arousal	Length of time after exposure to stimulus before stress response/aggressive display
Predictability	Identifiable situations, stimuli, and warning signals Consistency in response (latency, intensity, target, stituation)
Potential to do harm	Size and strength of animal Intensity of focus/level of arousal Number of bites per incident Degree of bite inhibition/severity of previous bites Likelihood of pursuit of the victim Target/victim health, age, likelihood of injury Size of dog compared to target/victim Behavior of victim when bitten
Social and physical environment	Ability of people in the social group to understand management and treatment Ability of people in the social group to control environment Verbal control, dependability of obedience responses Physical control (leash, harness, fenced yard) Family size, lifestyle Presence of children or elderly Experience of the family with animals
Complexity of the situation	Concurrent behavioral diagnoses Number of situations/stimuli that trigger aggression Opportunity for confrontations Number of aggression diagnoses Concurrent physical diagnoses Presence of other pets Presence of victim in home
Ability of family to adhere to treatment recommendations	Family is able to administer medications, separate from victims, treat underlying physical disorders

*Also see ESVCE risk assessment position statement (esvce.org) and Recommended Reading.

3. Modulation of fear, anxiety, stress, conflict, and panic through environmental management, medications, behavior modification, diet, and supplements as needed.
4. Management of the environment and use of training and management tools to provide adequate outlets necessary to address breed-typical needs, increase enrichment, keep the pet and the family safe, and remove reinforcement for undesirable behaviors.
5. Pathways to teach desirable behaviors with positive reinforcement.
6. Education on proper interactions with the pet, species-specific body language, and proper training.
7. Discontinuation of all positive punishment techniques.
8. Discussion of quality of life of the pet and the family.
9. Assessment of risk to others and risk to pet.

Every patient does not need all modalities; however, each case should include a risk assessment, treatment of physical disease, and reduction of FASCP.

Potentially because there is still much to learn about why dogs are aggressive or because most aggression stems from FASCP, there is much overlap between treatments, regardless of the type of aggression (see Table 23.3).

Below treatments are divided into categories of recommendations. These are general recommendations which can be made for almost every aggression case.

Safety first

Pet parents should be educated on how to recognize signs of arousal and how to handle the aroused dog. This is especially essential when situations that may trigger aroused or aggressive behavior are unknown or are not easily prevented. Pet parents can often recognize that their dog is distressed and try to comfort him, even when the dog has been aggressive toward them. Sometimes they try to move the dog away from the intended target and get bitten themselves. However, when the pet is in a high state of arousal, the ideal way to respond is to maintain physical distance from the dog or move the dog safely without touching him into a room or crate or behind a baby gate. This can be accomplished by tossing treats into the room or making a treat trail without approaching the dog or leaning toward him. Alternatively, it can be safer to simply close the door to the room where the dog is, separating him from other dogs and people, and let him decompress. Pet parents should be advised not to stand up to the dog during an aggressive display, as this will increase aggression.[151] Dogs that are aggressive, even if not toward children directly, should not be permitted to interact with children until the risk has been adequately assessed. For example, a dog that is aggressive around valuable items could easily display aggression toward a child in that situation when they might never display aggression toward that child otherwise. Children can be victims of accidental bites when two dogs in the same household are fighting or become a victim of redirected aggression as a dog is barking at the window. For these reasons, if there is any possibility of risk to a familiar or unfamiliar child, recommend separation.

In order for maximum improvement to be made, all family members should interact in the same way with the dog. Remind pet parents that society is litigious, and they can be sued for the injuries due to a dog bite or a dog that is barking and knocks a person over and injures them. For severely or chronically affected dogs, the behavior will be more difficult to resolve. Nonetheless, safe management can reasonably be achieved in most cases.

Avoid triggers

Avoidance is a reasonable strategy because it is safe, and the behavior may become weaker and dissipate if it is not elicited for a long period. For some households, it might be more practical to implement avoidance for the life of the dog. Begin by listing all aggression-eliciting triggers so that strategies can be implemented to ensure that each situation is avoided. If it is not possible to predict and prevent all situations in which aggression might arise, then it may be unsafe and impractical to proceed. Pet parent treatment adherence, in particular the willingness and ability to implement the recommendations, is critical for safety and success. A list of situations and stimuli that elicit aggressive behavior should

Table 23.3 General guidelines for treatment of aggression in dogs

Step	Comments
Safety first	Train pet parents to read canine body language to prevent and preempt before bites Separate the dog from children, elderly, or other at-risk victims even if they are not targets Warn the pet parent of liability Provide tools to manage situations such as strategies to break up dogfight and move the dog after aggressive incidents
Avoid triggers	Identify all situations that might result in aggression and instruct pet parents to avoid them Separate the dog from and avoid contact with all victims or targets at all times
Environmental and relationship management	Recommend changes to the environment to assist with segregation and avoidance of triggers (baby gates, crates, closed doors, harnesses, leashes) Educate pet parent how to properly interact with their dog, emphasizing the positive and reducing interactions which cause conflict Recommend a behavior be taught and used to increase structure within the relationship Recommend changes to the environment to make the likelihood of aggression lower
Environmental enrichment	Provide for the dog's needs regarding exercise and mental stimulation
Desensitization and counterconditioning	These exercises should only be attempted under the close supervision of an experienced behavior professional and only if deemed appropriate and necessary Progress should be slow enough that no aggression is elicited during training sessions. If aggression results, stop immediately and resume training on the next day at a level where success can be achieved, proceeding more slowly.
Surgery	Assess the likelihood of breeding and recommended gonadectomy on a case-by-case basis. Gonadectomy is unlikely to reduce aggression and may increase aggression, especially if spayed/neutered before 12 months of age and/or affected when spayed/neutered. Fear and aggressive behavior are heritable. Dogs that show these characteristics should not be bred.
Medication/supplement/ diet therapy	Selective serotonin reuptake inhibitors (e.g., fluoxetine, paroxetine, sertraline) may be helpful in decreasing arousal, impulsivity, and reactivity Medications should be prescribed with behavior modification and safety recommendations There may be a positive effect of a reduced-protein diet and concurrent tryptophan supplementation on certain types of aggression Other medications and supplements which affect the gabanergic, adrenergic, and serotonergic systems may be helpful in reducing arousal Synthetic pheromones may be helpful by decreasing anxiety
Stop physical punishment	Treatment should not include confrontation Physical punishment, choke and shock devices, and confrontational techniques such as alpha rolls or scruff shakes are contraindicated and dangerous, and result in increased aggression and avoidance
Euthanasia and rehoming	When safety cannot be ensured, euthanasia may need to be considered Except for exceptional circumstances, rehoming might not be an option because it may only move the danger to another environment
Overall health and wellness	Treat all physical disorders/diseases Assess for pain and discomfort. When in doubt, treat for presumed pain and discomfort.

be made and the pet parent should be advised to avoid them entirely. For example, if the dog is aggressive when disturbed while sleeping on the couch, the recommendation would be to keep the dog off the couch. Pet parents should be told to separate their dog from young children and anyone who cannot follow the treatment plan. Situations where conditioning desirable outcomes are impractical should be avoided for the life of the dog.

Environmental and relationship management

Management changes are intended to help the pet parent avoid bites, lower the dog's arousal while behavior modification is implemented, and improve the dog's quality of life. Management changes alone can improve the behavior and can be recommended at the first appointment. Dogs should be physically separated from all targets, including people and other dogs in the household using crates, baby gates,

and closed doors. Signs can be used on the doors so that whoever is in the house understands not to move into that room or open the baby gate. For some dogs, especially those that are aggressive toward other dogs, baby gates may need to be covered with a nontransparent cover so that they cannot see each other.

Many dogs that show aggression will need a sanctuary space in order to feel safe and keep the target of the aggression safe. Pet parents may reject the idea of a sanctuary space because they want their dog to enjoy being with their guests, they anticipate (sometimes accurately) that their dog will be stressed when alone, or they are unwilling to accept the necessary changes to their home to create a sanctuary space. The veterinary healthcare team should educate pet parents about the importance of the sanctuary space from the dog's point of view. If the dog wanted to be with the guests or child or other animals, he would not be showing aggression to them. The dog is attempting to gain space from the target of the aggression with the aggressive displays. By creating a sanctuary space, the pet parent is giving the dog what he is requesting. Unfortunately, many dogs have not been trained to accept confinement or separation from the pet parent. For these dogs, sanctuary space conditioning is necessary. More information on sanctuary spaces can be found in the section Treatment essentials: Behavior modification, Chapters 15 and 17, and in the online resources, Appendix C.

Adding structure

Changing the relationship of the dog with social group members, whether animal or human, or as it is commonly referred to, relationship building, can be an important step in reducing aggression. Veterinarians should approach this with empathy, as some parents can become insulted when they are told that their relationship with their pet may need to be modified. This can be a huge change for pet parents who are used to lavishing attention on their dogs in an unstructured and inconsistent manner. There is no reason why dogs cannot be spoiled and there is no limit to the amount of love they can and should receive. However, when interactions with the pet parent, whether reinforcing or punishing, are inconsistent, they can cause unpredictability and conflict, which increases aggression. It is not the amount of love or spoiling that needs to change but the way that the dog's needs are met as they relate to his relationship with the pet parent. The goal is to create a structured, consistent, positive relationship between the dog and the family.

Stop all physical punishment

All forms of physical punishment, such as shock, hitting, yelling, prong collars, and hanging by choke collars, should be avoided. Hitting a puppy or adult dog on the nose, squeezing the gums against the teeth, scruff shakes, alpha rollovers, bullhorns, or other forms of physical punishment should be discouraged as they are unlikely to be successful and often lead to other problems such as fear of noises, conflict-induced aggression, and fear-induced aggression.[59,152] Punishing the dog for displaying warning signals (e.g., growling, barking) may suppress those signals without treating the underlying problem and may result in the dog learning to bite without warning.

Even if punishment suppresses the behavior, it does not train what is desirable. In addition, corrections with choke collars, pinch collars, and shock collars make the problem worse over time by associating fear, anxiety, stress, and pain with the stimuli to which the animal reacts.

Positive reinforcement techniques are more effective and have less risk of inducing aggression than punishment-based and negative reinforcement-based techniques.[53,59,79,152] In a survey of 326 dog pet parents, dogs that were trained with positive reinforcement techniques were rated by their pet parents as more obedient than dogs that were trained with mixed positive-based and punishment-based training and dogs trained with solely punishment-based techniques.[153] Training with punishment was associated with more problem behaviors such as separation problems,[153,154] as well as barking, chasing and house-soiling[154] while over-excitement was reduced with reward based methods.[153] Positive punishment aversive and disciplinary training negatively impact patient welfare, have been associated with increased fear and

aggression, and both behavioral signs (e.g., tenseness, lower body posture) and physiological signs (e.g., panting, elevated cortisol) of stress.[53,59,153,155–158] Studies show that training with positive punishment and confrontation, including hitting, prong collars, hanging by choke collars, shock, physical methods such as alpha rolls, and even yelling "no" is associated with increased aggression and avoidance.[53,59,74,152,154] On the other hand, dogs trained solely with reward-based training had fewer behavior problems than dogs that had punishment as part of their training.[59,153] In addition, when positive punishment-based techniques were used in training, dogs were less likely to approach a stranger, less playful, less trainable, more fearful, and at increased risk of aggression toward family members, unfamiliar people, and in the veterinary clinic.[53,59,74,152,154,160–162] By comparison, dogs trained with positive reinforcement techniques had greater playfulness, higher training scores, performed better when taught a new task, and had fewer behavior problems including fear, aggression, and attention seeking.[79,153,158–160,162] In a study in military service dogs, positive reinforcement training was associated with higher closeness, increased attachment behavior, and more playfulness, while more fear and less closeness was associated with the greater use of punishment.[162] In a recent study examining techniques used to treat aggression and their efficacy, the use of antibark collars had a decreased probability of treatment success.[73] The scientific literature overwhelmingly supports the use of positive reinforcement techniques and refutes the use of negative reinforcement and punishment-based, aversive techniques. To recommend otherwise is to ignore the scientific literature and the standard of care in veterinary medicine. First, do no harm to your patients. Avoid these types of training techniques (see Box 23.4).

Environmental enrichment and exercise

Enrichment with positive social interactions has been shown to decrease the incidence of fear-induced aggression and the latency at which fearful dogs approached a location.[163] For dogs that have excess energy contributing to aggression at the fence line or even play aggression, increased exercise may be helpful. Long walks, play dates with other dogs, and play with toys should be provided several times daily. This is especially helpful for puppies that may not be exhibiting play aggression but may engage in unruly play that ends in bites. The environment should be enriched by providing a variety of toys. These should be kept novel by providing the puppy or dog with toys on a rotating schedule (three new toys each day). Dogs that do not become aggressive over food or toys can eat all of their meals out of food toys. This will keep the dog or puppy occupied and expend energy.

Box 23.4 Punishment and its possible effects on aggression

- Escalate aggression
- Lower the threshold for aggression
- Cause redirected aggression
- Destroy the bond between the pet parent and the pet
- Lead to fear-related aggression
- Cause conflict-related aggression
- Result in injuries
- Decrease warning signals before bites
- Increase the risk of euthanasia

Behavior modification

Behavior modification techniques are the cornerstone of treatment. When implemented correctly, they can be highly effective at reducing fearful, aggressive, and anxious behaviors. [73,164-166] The extent to which aggression is reduced by behavior modification is dependent on the abilities of the person implementing the treatment plan. For example, in one study examining aggression when visitors rang the doorbell of the family home, aggression was virtually resolved by an experienced handler; however, the pet parent was unsuccessful in implementing the procedure over time, which caused a regression.[167] In a case series of four dogs that were aggressive on the leash toward other dogs where behavior modification, including private instruction, establishment of a conditioned reinforcer, positive reinforcement training, use of a head collar, use of highly valuable food rewards, reinforcement of calm behaviors in the presence of the stimulus, and generalization training were used, aggression was resolved in three dogs and reduced to 5% of the times when exposed in one dog and maintained during follow-up.[166]

Behavior modification can be overwhelming for pet parents. An individual pet parent's decision to use one method over another or to implement a particular treatment plan can depend on many factors, such as their perceived risk, perceived ability to implement behavior modification, perceived support from family members or others in their social group who encounter the dog, guilt about their dog's behavior, perceived ability to successfully implement the program, their past experiences or lack thereof with that particular type of training method, and the perceptions of others that their dog encounters.[151] Treatment plans, whenever possible, should be tailored to the pet and the pet parent. Goals should be achievable and realistic. Pet parents need to understand the time and financial commitment involved in behavior modification and what it can yield regarding the pet's behavior. For example, in the case of interdog aggression in the same household, the pet parent's initial goal may be for the dogs to be together unsupervised. However, that goal may take 6–12 months of work on the behavioral treatment plan. The pet parent may not be able to implement a plan that intensive or may have financial restraints that do not permit that level of treatment. In those cases, the veterinarian should have a realistic conversation with the family about what can be achieved and how the plan can be changed in order to achieve alternative goals. The goal in treating aggression with behavior modification is to change the pet's negative emotional response to a positive one when presented with the stimuli that cause him to react and to replace the previous aggressive behavior with other, more acceptable, less physiologically stressful coping behaviors. Specific recommendations vary based on diagnosis; however, some aspects of behavior modification are consistent across aggression types.

Creating emotional safety and teaching foundational behaviors

Exercises which create emotional safety are those which promote desirable behaviors, allow the dog to feel safe enough not to engage in the undesirable behavior, and assist in avoiding confrontation. These are often taught before more intensive treatments such as desensitization and counter-conditioning are utilized. As with all behavior modification, the pet must be skilled in calm situations before the skills can be used in more distracting or stressful situations. For a behavior to be regarded as safe by the dog, it cannot be used by the pet parent to put the dog in overly stressful or frightening situations. For example, a dog is aggressive toward other dogs when he has walked on a leash in the neighborhood. The pet parent teaches him to sit in low-stress situations such as in the house and in the yard. Then, she takes him to a dog park and forces him to sit as other dogs run around him. The dog will learn to associate the sit behavior with frightening and stressful events, which will make him less likely to perform this behavior in the future at minimum in that situation, and potentially through the process of generalization in other situations as well.

A behavior should be trained for all animals with aggression to create consistent interactions with family members, as explained previously in Prevention: Structured interactions and environment. Historically, exercises to increase structure focused on control of resources and had various names such as learn to earn, nothing in life is free, predictable consequences, structured interactive training (SIT), and say please. In one study, 89% of pet parents indicated an improvement when a predictable rewards or nothing in life is free program was implemented.[62] As we have learned more about dog behavior, structure exercises have become more focused on proper communication and providing consistency and predictability between the family and the dog. They allow the dog to say "no" when he is too stressed to perform the behavior, giving the pet parent valuable insight into his emotional state and the likelihood of aggression. In addition, structure exercises increase impulse control, which is now recognized to be a factor in many types of aggression. They also cause the pet parent to pause before reaching for the dog or interacting with him, which will increase the likelihood that the pet parent will not be put in a situation where the dog will become aggressive. Finally, they give the dog control of its rewards by engaging in calm, desirable behaviors (what the pet parent wants the dog to learn), which can then be reinforced.

Pet parents can use touch, sit, watch (which can be standing or sitting), or down (or any other simple behavior) before the dog receives anything it desires (e.g., attention, play, walks, treats, food, going outside). This allows the dog to understand how to get what he wants and needs, and it allows the pet parent to feel in control of the reinforcements and resources which are doled out throughout the day. It reduces the dog's and the pet parent's anxiety. For example, consider a dog that is fluent (i.e., the dog performs the behavior 9 out of 10 times consistently when asked in that situation) at sit before going inside of the house (waiting at the door). One day, the pet parent asks him to sit at the door and he does not do so. This gives the pet parent insight that the dog is likely fearful, anxious, stressed, painful, over-aroused, distracted, lacking focus, or conflicted. In this case, the pet parent can direct him inside or lure him with a treat into the sit position, then assess the situation to determine the next best step.

Many pet parents think that it is sufficient to ask the dog to sit before the food bowl is put down or the leash is put on. In fact, they will often state that they have already completed this exercise because their dog sits before the food bowl is put down and also before he gets his leash put on. However, for this program to work, the behavior should be requested or offered before *any* and *all* wants are fulfilled. Within about seven days, the dog should be offering this behavior for anything of importance instead of having to be instructed to perform the behavior. Pet parents should be advised not to give attention, treats, or play, for example without requesting or the pet offering this behavior first. If it is impossible to ignore the dog, they should walk away. This exercise is simple, yet has a huge impact on the dog's life because it makes the dog's interactions with people predictable and consistent, and gives the dog control over the outcome, lowering anxiety and aggression. In some dogs, the process goes more slowly. The dog may get frustrated with inattention and the procedure may need to be modified.

In addition to a safety or structure behavior, pet parents should be encouraged to emphasize the positive. Often, they are focused most on correcting undesirable behavior. Of course, we all want the undesirable behavior to disappear. The quickest way to do that is often not to focus directly on the negative behavior and what to do after it occurs, but instead to focus on what desirable behaviors can be taught to replace the negative one. Once a behavior occurs, it may be intrinsically or extrinsically reinforced (e.g., territorial aggression), which will alter the expression of that behavior outside of the pet parent's control. Recommend that the pet parent reinforce all calm behaviors and/or a lack of aggression in situations, and pair favored rewards with the stimulus even from afar. Many dogs are told throughout the day, every day all that they do wrong and then attention is lavished on them randomly. Instead, we want to explain to the dog via reinforcement what is acceptable and desirable. Then the pet parent can prohibit the dog from engaging in undesirable behaviors and let him know when behaviors are undesirable in a humane way by withholding reinforcement, marking with a no-reward marker, or asking him to perform an alternate behavior which can then be reinforced.

Sanctuary space training is a powerful tool for creating emotional safety for the dog and keeping targets safe from bites. Sanctuary spaces can be crates, rooms, hallways, exercise pens, or any place that the dog can feel comfortable and safe. Some dogs need two spaces. One space is used for longer seclusions such as more than 5 minutes and the second space is a room close to the door where the pet parent can seclude the dog when they get a delivery. Most dogs need to be conditioned to accept sanctuary spaces, but some immediately welcome the relief from exposure to what makes them uncomfortable and aroused. Most often, dogs feel safest when they cannot see or hear the stimulus; however, some dogs feel safer with a baby gate or even in a crate where they can see or hear the stimulus. Do not recommend that the pet parent keep the dog in a crate in a room where the stimulus is present. The dog will be trapped with what frightens it. This will make the aggression more intense, worsening it over time. If the dog is not successful with sanctuary space conditioning and is clearly better when in a crate where they can see the stimulus, put the crate in the corner of the room with signage that the dog should not be approached. If the dog is barking at the stimulus, he is not calm and needs additional space from the stimulus. Some dogs are anxious when away from the pet parent, yet they must be segregated from the target of the aggression. For these dogs,

gradual conditioning to the sanctuary space when there is no exposure to the stimulus is necessary. This can be done slowly over days or weeks. The conditioning starts with something that the dog likes and will keep him occupied for at least 10 minutes, but longer is better. This is usually a food toy, but for those dogs that like to play independently, another toy might work. The sanctuary space should have ambient sound (e.g., music, white noise, brown noise), a bed, water, and anything else that the dog needs to feel comfortable. The conditioning starts with the pet parent and the dog in the room together while the dog eats out of the food toy. The pet parent should not interact with the dog. The purpose of this conditioning is to help the dog feel safe independent from the pet parent. If the pet parent is petting, touching, or talking to him, that will not teach him to stay there independently. If the dog does not have a separation-related disorder in addition to aggression, the pet parent can make short departures from the room, returning quickly at first, and then increasing the amount of time as conditioning progresses. Dogs with separation-related disorders need more systematic conditioning (see Chapter 17). When the sanctuary space is conditioned, the dog should be put into that space 10 minutes prior to the arrival of the target and then let come out 5 minutes after the target has left.

Basket muzzle training

A basket muzzle can be a useful adjunct to treatment because it improves pet parent confidence and provides an opportunity to safely assess the dog's response to stimuli. A muzzle should be used when the pet parent can monitor the dog and is working on the behavior modification plan. The dog should not wear a muzzle when alone or loose with the fear-evoking stimuli. For example, if the dog is afraid of new people, the pet parent should not muzzle the dog and then let the dog interact with no opportunity to maintain a relaxed distance. This will increase fear and the future likelihood of aggression because the dog does not have an opportunity for escape and cannot repel the stimuli. When a dog is properly trained to wear a basket muzzle, it has usefulness in the treatment of all kinds of aggression such as fear-induced aggression (e.g., on walks, at the veterinarian's office), predatory aggression, possessive aggression (e.g., reducing the likelihood of items being picked up on walks which can induce aggression), maternal aggression (e.g., to allow handling of the puppies), and pain-induced aggression (e.g., to allow administration of medications or examination). See Chapter 10, Appendix A, and online resources in Appendix C for more information on muzzle training.

Techniques to change emotional state

Counterconditioning

Counterconditioning involves pairing a positive stimulus with a negative stimulus in an effort to change the dog's emotional state. Before initiating treatment, the veterinarian should decide if counterconditioning to the stimulus or situation is necessary or safe. Consider the dog that growls at the pet parent when the pet parent rolls over in bed at night, inadvertently moving the dog. This would be a difficult stimulus to condition the dog to accept, as both the dog and the pet parent may be asleep or in a state of decreased awareness when it happens. It would be much easier to recommend that the pet parent simply change the dog's sleeping area.

Desensitization and counterconditioning

Desensitization and counterconditioning (DS/CC or CC/DS) techniques are effective treatments for aggression toward dogs and people.[63,168] DS/CC takes time and commitment and should only be done with professional supervision because the aggression can increase if the stimulus exposure is not controlled, gradually increased, and always associated with positive outcomes. Many dog training professionals and pet parents believe that they have already used this technique or that they understand the technique. Most of the time, this is not the case. True desensitization and counterconditioning is tedious work and requires a highly skilled training professional to direct the plan.

Relaxation exercises can be taught to facilitate a change in the dog's emotional state. If the dog has been taught to relax on a mat, the mat can be transported to other locations. The relaxation mat can also be used to reintroduce the dog into the situations in which the undesirable behavior occurs or as a foundation for DS/CC. See Chapter 10, Appendix A, and Appendix C for information teaching relaxation and behavior modification techniques.

Medications, supplements, and diet

Medications, supplements, and diet changes (for intolerance, allergy and neurotransmitter modulation) can be helpful adjunctive treatments. While not without their own risks, side effects are infrequent when used appropriately and can save the lives of aggressive dogs that would otherwise be euthanized. Medications are not a last resort, nor are they a cure. They are part of a complete treatment plan. Pet parents should understand that there is not a magic pill; medications will most likely cause a 50% change in the pet's behavior when they are effective; supplements and diet will cause a 25% change when they are effective; and medications, supplements, and diet will be most effective when they are used with other strategies. See Chapter 9 for more information on how to approach prescribing as part of behavioral treatment plans.

Treatment specifics

Below are tailored recommendations which can be made in addition to the ones above, which apply to specific situations or diagnoses.

Aggression toward children

Safety first

If the dog is aggressive toward children, safe management without contact is the most important approach, most likely lifelong. This is difficult for pet parents to accept because they often had an expectation of what their dog would be and what relationship he would have with their child. Regardless, of their expectation, children are vulnerable and are the most common bite victims. Dogs that are aggressive

to children cannot have any contact with or uncontrolled access to them, familiar or not.

Avoid triggers

Children can get bitten when they reach for a dog when the dog is barking or during a dogfight, in contexts of possessive aggression, and even in benign interactions such as hugging or petting. Children are at greater risk of being bitten because they are inherently unpredictable, inconsistent, smaller, and closer to the dog's eye level and mouth. For all of these reasons and additional reasons mentioned above, children often need to be separated from dogs.

If the dog is aggressive to children who visit, create a sanctuary space for the dog where the children do not have access to him. Children are curious and have been known to open doors and scale baby gates to get to dogs that are inside. The door that keeps the dog separated from the child may need to be locked. For separation from children, baby gates are often insufficient. In that case, parents may choose to use a double baby gate system with one baby gate secured in a doorway and the next one secured about 12 inches (30 cm) inside of the doorway, or use a closed door. Children should not be permitted to hang onto or stand near the gate. For the dog to feel safe, the area of confinement must be safe from the approach of children.

Crates without additional confinement are insufficient for separation because children can walk up to the crate, climb on the top of the crate, or reach inside. These types of activities are unsafe for the child and for the dog. The dog should be placed in a sanctuary space 10 minutes prior to the arrival of the children and let out after they have left the house and pulled out of the driveway (bites sometimes occur when visitors walk back into the house abruptly after initially leaving). If the children live in the house, the dog would be in the sanctuary space any time that the child is out and about in the house.

Environmental and relationship management

For older children, it may be possible to change the structure of the relationship with the exercises mentioned above. However, for small children, the risk is generally too great because their fine motor skills and impulse control are not developed enough to participate in the types of exercises needed to change the dog's emotional state. Relationship management can come through the pet parent. If the pet parent provides a safe environment for the dog where the child cannot approach and makes sure that any time that the child is within the dog's sight that the dog is reinforced for calm behavior, the relationship will most likely change to some extent. Dogs that are aggressive to children should have a sanctuary space where they will be secluded from the child.

Adding structure

As long as the situation is safe and the dog is confined or held securely on a leash, structure exercises like the ones mentioned previously might be utilized. There are many conditions where this is not safe and the dog is best maintained away from the child.

Stop all physical punishment

Positive punishment, as mentioned above, will suppress the warning signals of aggression and create a more dangerous dog. It should be avoided.

Environmental enrichment

Because dogs that are aggressive toward children in the home spend a significant amount of time away from the family, environmental enrichment is extremely important. Food and puzzle toys, walks without the child, or visits to a safe doggie day care can all be helpful to improve the pet's quality of life while confined. Confinement areas should be comfortable, with toys, water, and a bed. Dogs should be conditioned to stay there before regular use.

Behavior modification

Behavior modification to reduce fear, anxiety, stress, and resultant aggression toward children is possible; however, it is not always feasible and more often than not, is not safe to conduct. Techniques may include CC or DS/CC to the presence of the child. DS/CC is challenging to conduct with children within the same household because DS/CC must include complete control of the stimulus (intensity, frequency, duration, and distance) and slow exposure at a level which does not evoke a response. Instead, relaxation exercises can be taught and then CC can be used in the presence of the child while in protected contact (e.g., with a baby gate in between and the pet parent holding the child). Challenges with small children abound because of their lack of ability to be consistent, which makes behavior modification dangerous for the child and potentially ineffective and frightening for the dog. Behavior modification with older children may be safer in some circumstances. Most often, the behavior modification includes helping the dog to feel safe in a sanctuary space so that he can accept confinement. Instructions for sanctuary space training can be found in Chapter 17 and in the online handouts (Appendix C). In some situations, that is best achieved with a combination of medication and behavior modification. It should be noted that in many circumstances, children must also modify their behaviors so that they interact with the dog safely (see Chapter 4). It is not realistic, safe, nor ethical to allow a child to stand at, climb, or reach through a baby gate or crate into a dog's confinement area. Certainly, that would immediately make that space unsafe for the dog and create an unsafe situation for the child.

Aggression to familiar and unfamiliar adults (pain, FASCP)

Safety first

Educate the pet parents on the signs of FASCP. Help them to understand that their dog is having a hard time, not giving them a hard time. Give them resources so that they can understand how to recognize when their dog is stressed and what to do when the dog is showing aggression. Emphasize the importance of the entire family's involvement.

Avoid triggers

Avoiding exposure to the triggers (victims, stimuli) of aggression keeps the aggression from worsening, reduces risk to potential victims, and keeps the dog from continuing to be reinforced for aggression. This is an essential step which if not taken will hinder treatment. If the dog is aggressive in the yard and house, barking at unfamiliar people or passersby through windows, doors, and at the fence line, the pet parent can close drapes, move furniture in front of windows, close doors, close off parts of the home with baby gates, or cover windows with window film to keep the pet away from those areas. The dog should only have access to the yard when he is supervised. For dogs that are aggressive because they are painful or uncomfortable, avoid painful interactions as much as possible and use pain medications and antianxiety medications to reduce pain and the anxiety which often accompanies pain. At the veterinary hospital, use previsit pharmaceuticals wisely and frequently for these patients. For dogs that are aggressive to visitors, a sanctuary space should be chosen and conditioned. The sanctuary space should be in an area where the dog cannot see or hear the stimulus. For dogs that are aggressive toward family members, a list of situations in which the aggression has been displayed should be made and those situations should be avoided. If the dog is aggressive late in the evening, he should be allowed to go to bed early or put in his crate earlier in the night if he enjoys sleeping in his crate. If he is aggressive on the couch, he should not be allowed on the couch. If he is aggressive when he sits with a certain pet parent, he should not be allowed to sit there. Pet parents may be resistant to recommendations because they enjoy having their dog with them on the couch, for example; they feel that they are giving another pet in the household unfair privileges; they feel bad for the aggressive dog; or they do not feel that the aggression is severe enough to warrant the recommendation. Regardless of their perspective, the veterinary healthcare team has an obligation to protect the family and the dog. For those reasons, avoidance recommendations should be as complete as possible.

Environmental and relationship management

For the dog that is aggressive when people approach him while he is sleeping, his bed can be moved to areas where people are unlikely to pass and people can be instructed to never interact with him when he is lying on the bed. The room where he likes to sleep can also be blocked off with a baby gate so that when he is sleeping, he is confined. For dogs that are aggressive in the bed when the pet parent rolls over during the night and touches them or reaches for them, and those that are aggressive when the pet parent gets into bed, it should be recommended that the dog sleep in his own bed, preferably in the same room. Dogs that growl at their pet parents in the bed are often resistant to confinement away from the pet parents at night. In that case, an exercise pen can be set up in the bedroom and the dog's bed can be placed inside for sleeping. Alternatively, the pet parent can put a baby gate up in the bedroom. This may result in the dog whining, crying, and scratching at the gate overnight. If that is the case, instruct the pet parents to ignore the dog when possible. Most dogs stop this behavior when completely ignored between 3 and 5 days after the start of the procedure. Alternatively, medication can be used to help the dog make this transition to a different sleeping area.

For the dog that is aggressive to stimuli outside of the home while on his property, the yard should be secured. Dogs should be confined with a solid fence which is tall enough to prevent escape, does not allow anyone to reach through it, and blocks the sight of the stimuli. Pet parents should lock all gates, post signs that a dog is present, and make sure that workers and visitors stay out of the yard when the dog is outdoors. If there is any chance someone could make contact with the pet in the fenced yard, the family may need to allow the pet in the yard only on a leash.

Pet parents can use window film to block the dog's access to stimuli or confine the dog in a different part of the house. Dogs that show aggression due to underlying pain and discomfort may need modifications such as carpet runners or booties if the floors are smooth or slick. Ramps to get on furniture, and a body support devices might be used to aid the dog with mobility issues. Aggressive dogs can benefit from a sanctuary space where they can retreat to avoid frightening or stressful stimuli which induce aggression. See above and Chapters 5, 15, and 17 for more information on sanctuary space training. If the pet parent has engaged in positive punishment training, especially shock collar training, the relationship between the pet parent and the dog needs repair. Structure behaviors (see section Treatment essentials: Adding structure) should be taught immediately.

Adding structure

The pet parent should understand that consistent interactions with the pet will help the pet to feel safe and decrease aggression. Ideally, all family members would follow the same rule structure and interact in the same way. This is more challenging than it sounds, as often family members feel differently about the pet or have their own ideas about the treatment of the aggression.

Stop all physical punishment

Aggression begets aggression. If the family is physical with the aggressive dog, the dog is very likely to fight back. Aggressive dogs are stressed. Yelling, hitting, and holding dogs down just teaches them to bite. That is not the goal of treatment. The use of electric fences and shock increases aggression. In addition, they are not effective at keeping dogs inside of the yard because there is not a physical barrier, and it does not keep other animals and people out of the yard. Dogs can associate anything unpleasant (e.g., shock) in the environment with an emotional or physiologic response (elicited by shock), causing aggression to be targeted at anything in the environment.

Environmental enrichment

Dogs that show aggression may have components of impulsivity, excess energy, and frustration. Environmental enrichment as explained above and in Chapters 5 and 13 can reduce those contributing factors. In addition, dogs that are painful or older may not be able to play with toys

as they used to or may not even be able to walk on a slick floor to push a food ball. Modifications should be made for dogs that cannot engage in enrichment as they used to do. Dogs that are aggressive will invariably spend some time confined. Every effort should be made to keep sanctuary and confinement areas enriched and provide adequate exercise when not confined.

Behavior modification

Behavior modification techniques take time, energy, and the financial ability to work with a positive reinforcement dog training professional. For these reasons, some pet parents stop with management, structure, and avoidance. This is perfectly acceptable with the condition that the family is committed to those strategies for the lifetime of the pet. Foundational behaviors such as sit, settle, down, and attention to the pet parent can be taught using positive reinforcement techniques. Not only will these behaviors allow the pet parent to add structure and consistency to their relationship with the dog, but they will also lay the foundation for DS/CC.

For the dog that is aggressive toward visitors in the home, leave it, go to your bed/place, settle, sit, down, and stay can all be helpful foundational behaviors. For dogs that growl when bumped by the pet parent in bed overnight, foundational and emotional safety behaviors include go to your bed/place, off, and a structure behavior such as sit, touch, or down. For the dog that barks at stimuli (e.g., dogs, other animals, objects, people) while inside of the house, foundational behaviors such as leave it, go to your spot/place, quiet, calm, and settle can be very valuable.

Once dogs have foundational behaviors, CC or DS/CC can begin if the pet parent chooses.

Aggression on walks

Safety first

Assess if the pet parent can safely walk the dog. If there is a large size differential between the pet parent and the dog or if there is risk to injury to the pet parent or others, recommend that the pet parent limit the walks or avoid walks entirely and use the yard for elimination and exercise. Make sure that the pet parent has proper training tools (e.g., harness, head collar, leash) so that the dog can be controlled humanely. If the dog is not aggressive at day care, attendance may be a reasonable option for giving the dog the exercise that it would have received on walks.

Avoid triggers

For dogs that are aggressive on leash, the pet parent should not walk the dog near these stimuli or should walk in a fenced yard until the dog can complete the first steps of behavior modification. In addition, the pet parent should walk the dog at times when triggers are least likely to be encountered. The benefits of a long walk in this case are outweighed by the benefits of reducing the chronic stress response. For dogs that live in homes without yards and have to be taken to a more public place for elimination, indoor elimination areas might be offered. Alternatively, pet parents can be instructed to take their dog to an area very close to home for elimination and then back into the home for exercise. If the pet parent does not elect to pursue behavior modification, they should commit to avoiding the triggers to which their dog reacts on leash for the lifetime of the dog.

Environmental and relationship management

Pet parents are often very stressed about their pet's behavior on walks as not only can it be dangerous, but it also can be embarrassing. These factors may cause the pet parent to be more likely to grab the leash, tighten up on the leash, or act stressed themselves. These behaviors are not helpful to the dog. Instead, encourage the pet parent to have clear, consistent interactions with the dog that start before the walk begins. Pet parents should be instructed to make sure that they have the proper harness/head collar, leash, treat bag, and reinforcers on every walk. Discourage wholeheartedly the use of retractable leashes. It is not uncommon for pet parents to forget an essential piece of their training tools and have a negative walk with their dog, emotionally setting the dog and the pet parent back. Recommend that all gear for walks be used on every walk, no matter the length or location, and that they be easily accessible to the pet parent.

Inevitably, dogs that are aggressive on leash have had trauma (e.g., attack by another dog, exposure to frightening stimuli) either in the presence of the pet parent or at the pet parent's direction. If the dog has been conditioned or taught through the pet parent's actions to believe that the pet parent's presence on walks predicts or precedes the presentation of frightening (e.g., dogs, trucks, motorcycles, presence of or petting by people) or uncomfortable stimuli (e.g., corrections with a pinch collar or shock collar), they are more likely to show aggression in that situation. These circumstances erode the trust of the dog in the pet parent and are generally believed to contribute to the dog's aggressive responses. In order to build trust, the pet parent must be consistent, calm, and in control of their own responses. They should be careful not to put the dog in situations where he will react.

Adding structure

The dog should perform the structure cue such as sit, down, watch, or hand touch before the walk begins and then throughout the walk if he is calm enough to do so. The pet parent should strive to reinforce the absence of aggression on walks and be consistent in their interactions.

Stop all physical punishment

The pet parent should discontinue use of shock, choke, or pinch collars. Instead, direct them to humane head halters or no-pull harnesses.

Environmental enrichment

Because many dogs will be on a stress vacation (no walks) for the first two to six weeks of the treatment of aggression on leash, the enrichment in the household will need to be increased. That can be done through puzzle toys, feeding all of the dog's meals out of food toys, nosework games, indoor agility, playing in the yard, and games of fetch.

Behavior modification

Behaviors such as watch or focus (connection with the pet parent), find it (searching for treats in the grass), sit, leave it, target or touch training, here (come back to me), and let's go (turn with me and leave) can be used to give the dog other options outside of acting aggressively. Once foundation behaviors have been taught, if desired, counterconditioning can begin. More on the treatment of leash aggression can be found in Chapter 10.

Possessive aggression

Safety first

For dogs with possessive aggression, pet parents should be instructed to make a trade for a higher-value item in order to get stolen items from their pet before the behavior modification and foundation training (including drop and leave it) has been completed. Pet parents may be confused because they may think that they are rewarding the aggression when they make a trade. However, this is not the case. The aggression associated with possessive aggression is often a classically conditioned, anxiety-related behavior which will not increase with positive reinforcement. Once the dog is showing aggression, the opportunity for rational learning is gone. The pet parent should manage the crisis by trading with the dog and working on the behavior modification when the dog is not aroused or has objects that it will readily relinquish. There is a chance that the dog will learn to find or steal items and bring them to the pet parent to trade. This behavior is operantly conditioned and can easily be corrected if the pet parent so chooses with prevention, supervision, extinction, or reinforcement of alternate or other behaviors.

How the pet parent makes the trade with the dog will affect the dog's level of aggression. The item that the pet parent uses to trade should be of higher value than the item that the dog has in his possession. The pet parent should not reach over the dog or lean toward him. Instead, the high value food reward or toys should be tossed away from the dog. Some dogs will run to the food or the toy and grab it, then run quickly back to the item and bite the pet parent as the pet parent goes to pick it up. For this reason, toys should be thrown far from the valuable item, or many small treats should be scattered in a line away from the item. The pet parent should make sure that the dog is occupied and a couple of feet away before they go to pick up the item. Alternatively, they can scatter food or make a treat trail leading to a room where a door or baby gate can be closed. Once the door is closed with the dog inside the room, they can pick up the item.

Avoid triggers

Recommend that the pet parent avoid giving the pet anything that would typically cause aggressive behavior. Eliminate those items entirely. For pets for whom stealing is a part of their presentation, recommend that the pet parent close doors and pick up items that might easily be stolen. Dogs that can safely be given items when alone can enjoy their special chews and food puzzle toys in a separate space with a baby gate. If this technique is used, the pet parent should be instructed on how to move the dog out of the room without aggression. For example, the pet parent can open the door and call the dog out or let the dog come out on his own, then enter the room, closing the door or baby gate behind them, allowing them to pick up the toy safely.

Environmental and relationship management

For the dog that is aggressive when people approach valuable items, simple management changes such as securing the trash can, picking up frequently stolen items, feeding the dog in a low-traffic area, and segregating the dog out of areas where food is prepared or served should be made. When the pet parent approaches the dog and the dog has an item, the pet parent should not try to take the item away until the pet has learned foundational behaviors. If the item is unsafe, the pet parent can use the techniques outlined above. There is no need to hand-feed dogs that have possessive aggression.

Adding structure

All family members should always interact with the dog in the same way when he has an item. Either trade up for a more valuable food or item and take the item if it is safe to do so, or trade up for a more valuable food or item and give the item back to the dog. This sets up a clear contingency which starts with the pet parent's approach when the dog has an item and always ends with the dog earning reinforcement.

Stop all physical punishment

Pet parents should never attempt to take items from any dog's mouth by reaching with their hand, slapping under the chin, blowing in the nose, or prying the mouth open. These practices create situations where family members are likely to be bitten.

Behavior modification

For dogs that are aggressive around valuable items, leave it, drop it, go to your bed/place, and back are all valuable foundational emotional safety behaviors. DS/CC to the pet parent's approach to the food bowl or any other item can also be completed if necessary; however, many pet parents see a significant change in their dog's possessive aggression quickly when they change the management of the dog and change their interactions with the dog as outlined above.

Play aggression or undesirable play behavior

Safety first

Educate pet parents on the proper way to play with dogs. Wrestling and using their hands for play is never acceptable.

Avoid triggers

If a certain type of play results in aggression, ask the pet parent to avoid that entirely. Many pet parents even though the aggression is induced by a certain type of play may be resistant to avoiding that interaction because they perceive that their dog really enjoys it. While it may be true that the dog does enjoy the play in the beginning or at some point during the interaction, it is still an unsafe interaction where the dog becomes out of control. Potentially, that interaction can be resumed in the future once treatment has been initiated and has been successful. However, avoidance is best at first.

Environmental and relationship management

For dogs that show aggression during play, pet parents should encourage play with dog toys only and never play with their hands or feet. Tug games can be a good outlet for interactive play as long as they do not progress to body contact and out-of-control behavior. If a puppy or dog shows any aggression during play with tug toys, the pet parents should cease this type of play until they can train the pet to drop on cue or play without biting. Pet parents should never tease with their hands. If the puppy or dog's mouth ever contacts the pet parent's skin, even if it is unintentional, play should stop immediately. The pet parent should briskly but calmly turn and walk away. If the dog or puppy follows the pet parent, that gives the pet parent an opportunity to ask him to sit, and then resume play with games that avoid human contact (e.g., fetch, chase, train for treats). The pet parent should choose which toys are appropriate for tug and only use those toys so that the dog can understand which games can be played with which toys.

Adding structure

A structure behavior (see section Treatment essentials: Adding structure) should be taught which precedes all play. Additionally, the same behavior can be used to interrupt play. Every couple of minutes, the pet parent can ask for a sit, down, or watch, for example. When the dog complies, play can resume. Over time, the pet parent can, if desired, increase the amount of time needed for impulse control before play resumes.

Stop all physical punishment

Sometimes pet parents will get the dog excited or overaroused with inappropriate play and then punish the dog for overaroused behavior. This causes the dog to be conflicted. It is acceptable to be overaroused when playing or not? Is it acceptable when the pet parent instigates it? Is it acceptable for a certain amount of time? The pet parent is the responsible party in this scenario. Instead of waiting for the dog to make a mistake and then punishing the dog, the pet parent should orchestrate situations where the dog is likely to succeed.

Behavior modification

Dogs with play-induced aggression and undesirable play behavior often respond very well to management. However, when arousal is conditioned, behavior modification is necessary. Techniques used should focus on impulse control. Foundation behaviors such as sit, down, go to your mat, take it, drop it, and duration (time spent in the activity) can be helpful. Once trained they can be used during play.

Interdog aggression

Interdog aggression within the same household presents a unique set of challenges. This is especially true if there is one pet parent and two or more dogs in the house. Some pet parents choose not to reintroduce the dogs and instead live with the dogs separated, or rehome one of the dogs. If the pet parents choose to live with the dogs separated, that is a valid option; however, if the pet parent makes a mistake in management, there is likely to be a dogfight. Thus, the pet parent should understand that electing to use a medication and management plan only without behavior modification depends entirely on the medication's efficacy and the pet parent's ability to adhere 100% of the time to management recommendations.

The family needs to be sufficiently educated about canine social behavior and committed to behavior modification and household changes. They should understand that their dogs are not a pack, but instead roommates that might be competitive over particular resources or unable to communicate effectively. They did not choose to live together. In some cases, the dogs do get along well together in the pet parent's absence, indicating that the pet parent is a resource over which the dogs are fighting, or the pet parent's actions are in some way contributing to the problem.

Safety first

The family should be advised not to allow the dogs to fight it out. This is unsafe and rarely resolves the problem in the long term. In the event that a fight does occur, pet parents should be instructed how to break up a dogfight safely. Pet parents are often bitten and suffer worse injuries than the dogs in the process of breaking up a dogfight. Children are also at risk, as they may be emotional seeing their dogs hurting each other (see online resources in Appendix C). Although physical intervention is often required, in one study, 42% of households did not require physical intervention to break up fights.[62]

Avoid triggers

For dogs which are aggressive toward other dogs in the household, triggers should be identified and avoided. Most dogs need to be separated at all times; however, some can be allowed together when supervised. Interdog aggression in the same household often progresses over time from intermittent fights to fights on sight of the other dog. When in doubt, separate the dogs until professional help can be sought out. Separate the dogs whenever there are valuable resources such as food, toys, bones, and chewies, and potentially the pet parents' attention. If a dog shows redirected aggression to another dog in the yard when barking at passersby, do not let the dogs into the yard together. If the dog shows aggression to the other dog when they are fed together, feed them in separate rooms behind a baby gate or closed door. If the dogs fight at the door when coming inside from the yard or a walk, let them out in the yard or walk them separately. If the dogs fight at the front door when visitors come over, separate them before there are visitors expected. If they fight when the pet parent comes home, separate them when the pet parent is absent so that they are not at the door when family members come home.

Environmental and relationship management

The classical approach to treating interdog aggression within the family by choosing an individual to promote to a higher rank can be problematic. It is likely that families have already intervened in the relationship so that social behaviors occur out of context, making interpretation difficult. It is often impossible to determine which dog to support and which should learn to defer. There may be, in fact, no higher-ranking individual, or by the time that the veterinarian sees the case, the original social structure has been modified by learning and pet parent intervention. Presumably, had social structure and communication been healthy, aggression would not have an issue and problems would have quickly been resolved. In cases where older dogs are being challenged by younger dogs, the older dog may have health or mobility issues, leading to irritability or affecting its ability to communicate. An important question in any aggressive interaction is which dog, if any, is acting appropriately so that the focus of treatment can be on reinforcing what is appropriate and preventing or changing the response of the dog behaving inappropriately, or preventing the interactions that lead to aggression.

Adding structure

Sometimes it is the relationship that the dog has with other pets in the house that needs to be made more structured. When the pet parent is petting or giving treats, food, or play, one pet may invariably have to be rewarded before another. The dog who receives reinforcement first may be the behaviorally appropriate dog, the younger dog, the older dog, or the dog to whom it matters most, depending on the situation. Giving priority access to resources to a particular dog has been found to be successful in only 48% of cases. In 67% of cases, improvement was seen if the senior dog was supported.[62] If the support of one dog is ineffective, it has been suggested that after six weeks, the support program be reversed.[169] Alternatively it might be possible to consider providing resources separately so that the order in which the dogs are fed, given toys, or greeted might vary for each resource based on its relative value of each resource to each dog. Determining the "natural hierarchy," who the "alpha dog" should be, and who should get the best, the most, and first resources is fraught with problems. Poor observational skills by the family, interference with normal social signaling, and misinformation regarding dog behavior may cloud the real picture regarding the dogs' social behavior. Currently, it appears that the most effective technique is to set up a structure that will be consistently followed in each interaction of that type. In addition, consider the abilities of the pet parent and the dogs to comply with the structure when making recommendations. Most fights between dogs occur because of FASCP and pain. Some dogs will be too stressed to wait for a privilege to be doled out. Initially, those dogs may be reinforced with a treat before the other dog in situations where they are both present. That will reduce stress and lessen the likelihood of fights between the dogs. Dogs want to know what will come next; consistency and structure can help them to interact with their environment in a more peaceful way.

Stop all physical punishment

Punishment or scoldings applied after or during a dogfight between household dogs will not change the likelihood of a fight in the future, may worsen the situation, and could lead to redirected aggression to family members. Pet parents think of the fight as one behavior or incident which can be punished. However, a fight is an accumulation of many individual behaviors. Think of each individual action as a behavior which can be reinforced or punished. If a dog bites the other family dog and there is any relief from the stress that the biting dog feels or if that other dog moves away, that behavior has been reinforced. Punishment applied minutes later will not be associated with the act of biting. It will be associated with anything in the environment at the moment of punishment, which is generally the pet parent. This contributes to the dog's confusion and conflict. When a fight occurs, the damage, so to speak has been done; the fight should be broken up and the dogs separated.

Behavior modification

For dogs that are aggressive toward other household dogs, foundational behaviors include leave it, down, sit, back, and go to your bed/place. Most frequently, both the aggressor and the victim dog will need to learn these foundational behaviors for success to be achieved. Often, the victim dog has fear, anxiety, or stress surrounding the interactions with the aggressor dog. Most often, both dogs are suffering from fear, anxiety, and stress regarding their relationship.

DS/CC can be used to reintroduce dogs in the same household that are fighting with each other (one handler per dog). Initial reintroduction might begin on walks. The pets should be closely watched for appropriate social behavior and reinforced with praise and food (unless giving treats is a trigger for aggression). Each time there are any signs of arousal, cues such as leave it, watch, come, here, or let's go can be used to redirect the dog's attention. Over many walks, the dogs are walked closer and closer together until the entire walk goes smoothly, without the need for distraction or interruption. Then, when the dogs come back into the house, they go to their relaxation mats while on leash and the exercise may continue. These types of treatments should always be done with supervision and coaching from a qualified professional. Resources over which the dogs might fight should be removed. The entire time that the dogs are together, the pet parent should be watching, directing their behavior, and reinforcing desirable calm behaviors.

Maternal aggression

For bitches exhibiting maternal aggression, counterconditioning can be used with gentle, positive handling by trusted family members. If safety can be ensured, DS/CC can reduce problems for future pregnancies.

Medications

Medications, supplements, and diet changes can be used to reduce fear, anxiety, stress, conflict, panic, arousal, and aggression. These cases may require medical therapy in conjunction with management and behavior modification, both from the pet's standpoint to improve its mental health and welfare, and from a behavior modification standpoint to help achieve a satisfactory level of improvement. In other words, without medications, supplements, or diet to modulate the neurochemistry associated with the aggression, many pets will not be able to improve significantly. When using medication as part of a treatment plan for canine aggression, all recommendations should be documented and the pet parent should be informed in writing of all risks, particularly for any off-label use. To meet the standard of care, veterinarians must provide behavior modification, management, and/or safety recommendations with medication. Pet parents should also be made aware of the expected improvement after treatment with medication is instituted. For example, a reasonable expectation might be a 50% improvement with medication alone. Pet parents come to the appointment with their own preconceived ideas of what medication can do and which medication they would be willing to administer to their pet. Some pet parents prefer supplements and some prefer medications. Others have used psychotropic medication themselves and are biased toward or against certain medications based on their own responses. In a survey of dog pet parents, most were comfortable with fast-acting versus slow-acting medications. Further, they were most concerned about side effects such as sedation, potential for addiction, and negative changes in the dog's personality. In this study, pet parents considered proven efficacy, ease of administration, veterinarian recommendation, and the cost. As would be expected, those who had a personal history taking psychotropic medications were more comfortable with administering those to their pets.[170] See Chapter 9 for more information on the approach to prescribing and the most frequently asked questions and answers when prescribing psychotropic medications.

Antidepressants such as tricyclic antidepressants, selective serotonin reuptake inhibitors (e.g. fluoxetine), and selective serotonin reuptake/norepinephrine inhibitors e.g. venlafaxine are most commonly recommended as foundational (continued use) medications. Acute, situational or adjunctive medications include serotonin reuptake inhibitors/ antagonists (e.g. trazodone), alpha-2 agonists (e.g. clonidine), and gabaminergics. First-line recommendations might also include pheromone analogs, nutraceutical supplements, and behavioral probiotics. Many dogs will require medication in conjunction with environmental management (antecedent arrangement) and behavior modification (see Chapter 10) treatment plans. Any pain and underlying medical disease should be treated immediately with appropriate medications (see Chapters 11 and 12).

In a recent study of aggressive dogs presented to behavior specialists, there was no correlation found between specific medications and response to treatment.[73] This may be because of the small numbers of dogs in each medication group. In a two-phase study examining the effect of amitriptyline on aggressive behavior prospectively and retrospectively, no positive effect was seen over behavior modification alone.[171] Fluoxetine and clomipramine have both shown efficacy in the treatment of aggression in dogs.[172–174] Clonidine has been shown to reduce the intensity of aggression in dogs with fear-induced aggression when used in conjunction with fluoxetine.[175]

When deciding to institute pharmacologic therapy, the veterinarian should consider the following questions:

1. Is the environment consistent with a positive outcome?
2. What is the latency to arousal?
3. Is the animal's quality of life affected?
4. Is the animal at risk of injuring himself or others or at risk of euthanasia or relinquishment?
5. Is the behavior predictable?
6. What is the severity of the behavior?
7. What is the recovery time?
8. Would the use of a medication, supplement, or diet decrease the pet's stress and improve the likelihood of response to treatment?

Diet and supplements

Any disease or disorder which causes discomfort, pain, or inflammation has the potential to affect behavioral clinical signs. This includes food sensitivity, food allergy, inflammatory bowel disease, and intestinal parasites. Signs which may be vague such as licking, star gazing, and tail chasing have been attributed to gastrointestinal disease. In one small study, a low-protein diet with tryptophan supplementation was partially effective in the treatment of territorial aggression.[176] Gluten sensitivity has been linked to aggressive behavior in one dog. Change in diet resolved the behavior.[120] A trial with a novel antigen, vegetarian, or homemade diet could be utilized to assess if food sensitivity or food allergy is present. In one study, aggressive dogs were found to have lower omega-3 polyunsaturated fatty acids when compared to nonaggressive dogs. It is unclear if this is a predisposing factor to aggression or if it is a result of changes related to aggression; however, there may be a place for fatty acid supplementation in the treatment of aggressive dogs.[177] A recent study demonstrated that nutraceutical supplements may be efficacious in the treatment of aggression in dogs[73] (see Chapter 13).

CASE EXAMPLES

Case 1

Presentation

Simon, a 4-month-old, 10-kg intact male Rottweiler, presented for biting his pet parents during play.

History

Both of the pet parents spent long hours at work. Simon's only opportunity to exercise was when he was let out into the back yard. Against the veterinarian's recommendation, Simon had not been brought to any puppy socialization or training classes between adoption at nine weeks and presentation for the behavior change. The husband played roughly with Simon by using his hands to push Simon's head around and wrestle on the floor. Simon would respond by biting, interspersed with bouncy, relaxed behavior and play bows. When Simon did this, the pet parent would smack him lightly across the nose. In the evening, the puppy would come up to the pet parents and bark, lunge, and nip at any available body part accompanied by play bows. Attempts at verbal and physical discipline only seemed to aggravate the situation.

Workup

The physical examination and screening lab tests were within normal limits. During the appointment, Simon was friendly and interactive. He bounced around the room, biting at the legs of the veterinarian and technician. His bites were inhibited and quick. His body language was relaxed. This was similar to previous puppy visits with Simon. The difference at this visit which was noted by the veterinarian and the veterinary technician was that when they reached for Simon, he quickly jumped back and lowered his tail.

Differential diagnoses

The differential diagnoses for the behavior include species-typical play behavior, specific/situational fear (when reached for), lack of exercise and enrichment, lack of training, pain-induced aggression, play aggression, fear-induced aggression, and conflict-induced aggression. Simon was diagnosed with specific/situational fear and species-typical play behavior. In addition, contributing factors were lack of training, lack of socialization, and lack of exercise.

Treatment

The pet parents were advised of the risks of developing fear-induced aggression or conflict-induced aggression if the current interactions between the pet parents and Simon persist. In addition, they were told to avoid all interactions which induce the aggression, avoid interactions with children, enroll him immediately in a positive reinforcement training class, increase his level of exercise appropriately for his age and breed, feed him out of food toys exclusively, play with toys that are long such as tug toys so that he cannot in advertently bite their hands, add structure to their interactions, and to avoid rough play. To avoid a feeling of overwhelm, they were supplied with resources in the way of video links, book recommendations, and handout recommendations which could be found online. They were referred to a positive reinforcement training facility nearby for classes. The veterinarian advised them of the risk that this aggression could worsen over time and that they may be managing his behavior for the rest of his life. In addition, they were advised of the liability and keeping a dog that bites.

The veterinary technician followed up via phone in one week. The pet parents felt overwhelmed and had only purchased food toys and called the dog training facility to sign up for the next class. The veterinary technician helped the pet parents to understand how they could implement recommendations in a stepwise fashion. In addition, she reiterated that this was an urgent situation so that Simon did not develop aggression. Finally, she recommended that they use food toys at times when he would usually be asking for attention inappropriately.

Simon came in for a reexamination one month after his initial presentation. He immediately sat when the veterinary technician picked up a treat. The pet parents reported that they were going to class and that Simon was the smartest one in the family! He was eating out of food toys at each meal and got special treats out of his food toys at times during the night when the pet parents wanted to relax instead of playing with him. He had scheduled play sessions and the pet parents had started to utilize the day care facility nearby so that he could get adequate exercise.

The pet parents were pleased with his progress. The veterinarian emphasized that this program should be followed at least to some extent well through social maturity, ending at three years.

Case 2

Presentation

Babe was a 5-year-old, 40-kg spayed female Labrador Retriever with chronic otitis externa that was presented for growling when the pet parent tried to clean her ears.

History

Over the past year, Babe had progressively become more and more irritable, running away and growling when the pet parent tried to clean or medicate her ears. Two days before, she had bitten the pet parent who had lifted Babe's ear to instill medication.

Workup

Babe's physical examination was within normal limits with the exception of previously diagnosed otitis externa, which was under treatment. Screening lab work revealed a low TT4, fT4, and increased TSH.

Differential diagnoses

Differential diagnoses included otitis externa, hypothyroidism, pain-induced aggression, stress-induced depression, and fear-induced aggression. Babe was tentatively diagnosed with pain-induced aggression and fear-induced aggression, hypothyroidism, and chronic otitis externa.

Treatment

Babe was sedated and an ear medication instilled which would last for the remaining treatment of the otitis externa. The pet parents were instructed to avoid reaching for her in any way unless it was an emergency situation. Whenever they had to touch her around her head, even to put her collar on, they were to use smearable food in a bowl or on a plate to distract her while they touched her. Gabapentin was dispensed as a previsit pharmaceutical to be used when she had otitis flareups and had to be brought to the veterinarian. In addition, it was to be used at 10 mg/kg PO BID until the otitis had been resolved.

Thyroid supplementation was instituted, and Babe was referred to a board-certified veterinary dermatologist for evaluation. The pet parent was counseled to pay closer attention to the ears so that cleaning and treatment were begun before the problem reached a painful stage. It was recommended that the pet parents work with a positive reinforcement trainer to desensitize and countercondition Babe to having her ears handled and to teach her to accept handling at the veterinary hospital using cooperative care techniques, as this would most likely be a lifelong problem. The veterinarian advised them of the risk that this aggression could worsen over time and that they may be managing her behavior for the rest of her life. In addition, they were advised of the liability of keeping a dog that bites and that she may not ever interact with children.

The veterinary technician followed up by phone in seven days. The pet parents had declined to call the dog-training professional and reported that there had been no aggression since they had been using cream cheese to distract Babe before they reached for her head and since she was on gabapentin and thyroid supplementation. They had yet to call the dermatologist. The veterinary technician emphasized the importance of seeing the dermatologist so that any underlying problems could be addressed. In addition, she reiterated that this would likely be a lifelong problem and that behavior modification could improve the quality of life of the dog and the pet parents.

Babe presented for reexamination two weeks after the initial appointment. The otitis had resolved and the pet parents were very pleased. They were administering the thyroid supplementation as directed and had just finished the gabapentin the day before.

A week after the reexamination, Babe's pet parents called the veterinary hospital and reported to the veterinary technician that Babe's demeanor had changed and although she was not biting them, she was running from them. It was recommended that she come in for a reexamination with the veterinarian. The veterinarian found no abnormalities on physical examination and there was no evidence of otitis. Blood was drawn for a recheck TT4, which was within normal limits. At this time, the veterinarian presumed that either Babe was still painful, even though it appeared that the otitis was resolved, or she was still anxious or fearful and that regardless of which of these two was the cause, the gabapentin may need to be restarted. The pet parents were instructed to administer the gabapentin at a dose of 10 mg/kg PO BID and report back in three to five days. The pet parents called the veterinary hospital in five days and reported that Babe was back to her old self. After speaking to the veterinarian, the veterinary technician advised them to continue with the gabapentin daily.

Case 3

Presentation

Remy, a 6-month-old, 22-kg spayed female Golden Retriever, was presented for growling at family members when approached while she was chewing a rawhide, had possession of a stolen item, or was eating meals.

History

The behavior had started at two months of age when she was adopted. She was fed a commercial puppy diet twice daily in the kitchen. The family consisted of two adults and one cat. The pet parents had been taking the bowl away without warning twice each time that the dog ate a meal. If Remy growled when they approached her rawhide or bowl, the pet parents reached for her and held her by the scruff. The behavior had progressively worsened in the past two months. She had been through an obedience class starting at four months.

Workup

Her physical examination and laboratory tests were within normal limits.

Differential diagnoses

Differential diagnoses were possessive aggression, conflict-induced aggression, pain-induced aggression, stress-induced aggression, and fear-induced aggression. Remy was diagnosed with possessive aggression.

Treatment

The pet parents were instructed to stop giving her rawhides, pick up any item that could potentially be stolen, feed her in a crate out of the kitchen, and stop reaching for her when she was eating or had a rawhide. They were instructed how to safely get items from her by trading up. If they needed to get an item from her, they were to toss treats or toy away from her, making sure to use something that was higher value than the item over which she was aggressive. They were also given resources in the way of video links, handouts, and book recommendations to support the suggestions. They were given the name of a positive reinforcement dog training professional who could work with them to help condition Remy to give things back to them without aggression. They were reminded that whenever interacting with Remy, if they took something from her, she should get that item back, get something better in return, or get the item back and get something better in return. The veterinarian advised them of the risk that this aggression could worsen over time and that they may be managing her behavior for the rest of her life. In addition, they were advised of the liability of keeping a dog that bites and that she may not ever interact with kids if there are any items around over which she might become aggressive. Because it could not be predicted which items would lead to an aggressive response, it was recommended that she not be permitted to interact with children.

The veterinary technician followed up by phone in two weeks. The pet parents reported that Remy had made a complete turnaround. The pet parents had stopped giving her the most valuable items over which she had shown aggression previously; however, they were having great success with trading up for higher-value treats. The veterinary technician advised them that when possessive aggression is treated in puppies

continued

it can be highly successful. With that said, she strongly advised that they work with the positive reinforcement trainer who was recommended.

The veterinary technician followed up by phone four weeks after the initial appointment. The pet parents reported that they had been working with a positive reinforcement trainer to teach drop it and leave it. They had begun to give Remy valuable items again in a special place where they would not bother her. They let her out of the room when she was done with her chewies and food toys. They had not seen any aggression since the initial appointment.

Case 4
Presentation

Rocko, a 4-year-old, 20-kg neutered male American Bulldog, was presented for biting both of his pet parents when reached for, petted, or when they tried to remove his blanket.

History

Rocko had not been to any formal obedience training and did not respond to the pet parent's verbal cues. He lived in a house with two adult pet parents and no children. The first sign of aggression was at eight months old when the pet parents took Rocko to visit a relative with two dogs. Rocko was not well socialized and did not get along well with the other dogs. He stayed on the couch, curled in a ball for most of the visit. When the pet parent went to put his leash on, he snapped at her. The pet parents generally yelled at him or smacked him across the face with an open hand when he showed aggression. The aggression had continued to worsen over the years. Rocko was also fearful of storms and loud noises. He refused to walk outside on stormy days. In the examination room, Rocko often faced away from the pet parents, yet when the female pet parent left the room, he went to the door and whined the entire time that she was gone. When he was called to come to the pet parent, he averted his gaze and froze. He was fearful during his physical examination but was not aggressive.

Workup

The physical examination was within normal limits. Laboratory testing could not be performed due to his level of stress.

Differential diagnoses

Differential diagnoses include specific/situational fear (veterinary visits), fear-induced aggression, conflict-induced aggression, stress-induced aggression, pain-induced aggression, noise fear, and storm fear. Rocko was diagnosed with specific/situational fear (veterinary visits), conflict-induced aggression, noise fear, and storm fear.

Treatment

Trazodone was prescribed for veterinary visits. The parents were advised to give the trazodone 3 hours prior to veterinary visits. Before they used it for a veterinary visit, they were to test the dose starting at 3 mg/kg PO. They could work up the dosing range to 10 mg/kg PO 3 hours prior to veterinary appointments if needed, depending on the effect that they saw during their test doses. The veterinarian advised them of the risk that this aggression could worsen over time and that they may be managing his behavior for the rest of his life. In addition, they were advised of the liability of keeping a dog that has shown aggression and that he not be permitted to interact with children. Further, the pet parent was told to avoid pushing or pulling him, cease all punishment, institute a program of relationship building and structured interactions, and to not touch him or approach him when he was lying on his blanket. The pet parents were given resources and a recommendation for a positive reinforcement dog trainer in the area. They were given instructions on how to create a sanctuary space during storms during noise events and to avoid, if possible, all triggers for the aggression and the fear. Finally, the pet parents were educated that the source of the aggression was fear and anxiety, which was magnified by an unstructured, inconsistent relationship with the pet parent, causing conflict.

In two weeks, the veterinary technician followed up with the pet parents by phone. The pet parents had started working with the dog training professional on behaviors such as go to your spot, and conditioning to petting and structured interactions. The pet parents reported that Rocko seemed happier and more relaxed. He had not shown aggression. They understood how to read his body language and they noticed that he was stressed a lot of the time but especially on storm days.

At his reexamination appointment four weeks after the initial assessment, Rocko was visibly less stressed in the examination room. He was interactive with the pet parents and did not orient away from them as much. He was more responsive to cues as well. However, he had received 7 mg/kg of trazodone 3 hours prior to his appointment. At this time, blood was drawn for screening lab work, which was all within normal limits. The pet parents were given resources for the treatment of noise and storm phobia and instructed to use trazodone at a dose of 7 mg/kg PO 2 hours prior to storm or noise events.

In six months, Rocko continued to do well as long as the pet parents followed the treatment plan.

Case 5
Presentation

Joe, a 1.45-kg, 10-week-old male Miniature Poodle, was presented for growling and biting when held during the past two weeks.

History

The pet parent had tried holding him tightly until he calmed down (1 to 2 minutes). This occurred five to six times a week. He had no training or socialization. He was acquired from a breeder at eight weeks and lived with two retired adults and no children. The pet parents did not meet the sire or the dam. The first incident was when Joe was in the back yard and he kept running under the bushes. The pet parent continually told him "no," and pulled him out. When he ran under the bushes the third time, the pet parent grabbed him by the scruff of his neck, pulled him out, yelled "no," and carried him inside. As she was carrying him, he began to bite and growl. The pet parent held his muzzle and said "no," to which he responded with more growling, at which point she put him down.

Workup

The physical examination and screening laboratory testing was within normal limits. During the examination, Joe was quiet and spent time lying under a chair. He explored the room but was fearful when interacting with the clinician. He would approach for treats, then retreat.

Differential diagnoses

Differential diagnoses include fear-induced aggression, conflict-induced aggression, pain-induced aggression, and stress-induced aggression. Joe was diagnosed with fear-induced aggression.

Treatment

The pet parent was given the following safety recommendations: (1) stop physical punishment; (2) do not push or pull him; (3) do not let new people pet him; and (4) avoid stimuli that frighten him (e.g., picking him up). She was advised of the liability of keeping a dog that had a history of showing aggression and was warned that he was not to be allowed to interact with any children. In addition, she was to immediately enroll him in puppy kindergarten at least once a week. She was given resources in the way of books, handouts, and video links for socialization. The veterinarian outlined to her the importance of structured interactions with her dog and proper socialization, which was not the same as exposing Joe to stimuli.

Follow-up

The veterinary technician followed up in one week after the initial appointment. Joe was doing well, but they had not enrolled him in class

CASE EXAMPLES—cont'd

yet. They were having a hard time refraining from reaching for him or picking him up. He was so small and the pet parents were worried for his safety. After all, why get a small dog if you cannot pick it up? The veterinary technician recommended that they use a food lure to pick him up but even then, only in emergencies.

At Joe's next puppy visit, the pet parents reported that they had started puppy socialization classes, but that Joe was fearful in class. He was still growling at the pet parents. The pet parents were instructed to continue the treatment plan.

At the third puppy visit, the pet parent was able to handle and brush him. They were actively socializing him and he was showing less fear in those situations but was now showing aggression at the veterinarian's office. The pet parent was instructed to desensitize and countercondition him and teach him to be handled using the concepts of cooperative care with the help of the trainer that they had been using.

At his last puppy visit when he was four and half months old, he was attending puppy playtime, had started his second round of obedience classes, was more confident when he met new people, and was less fearful at the veterinarian's office.

Seven months after the initial appointment, the pet parent called the hospital and reported a bite. An appointment was made for a reexamination. At the reexamination, she reported that she tried to groom him at home and he bit her. She held him down and yelled at him. After that, he began showing more stress-related body language cues and anxiety. The pet parent was reminded that punishment was contraindicated and was reeducated on counterconditioning.

Eight months after the initial appointment, he was presented for a reexamination. At this time, the aggression and fear had stopped improving. It was not worsening, but no improvement was made. He was started on sertraline (6 mg q 24 hours) to decrease arousal and the emergence of new fears.

Twelve months after the initial appointment, the pet parent reported that the counterconditioning had reduced the aggression toward strangers, veterinarians, and the pet parent. The pet parent was advised to continue the sertraline until at least three years of age.

Three years after the initial appointment, the pet parent reported that he was friendly with people, active in agility and obedience, and was able to be examined at the veterinarian's office without incident. The pet parent asked if the sertraline could be discontinued. The veterinarian advised her that there was no way to know how much of the improvement was due to the medication and how much was due to the behavior modification and socialization. Weaning off of sertraline was a reasonable plan, but there could be a relapse. Sertraline was weaned over two weeks by reducing the dose by 50% per week. At the end of the two weeks, Joe's behavior had not worsened.

Six weeks after the last dose of sertraline, the pet parent called the hospital to report that while Joe was not aggressive since their last appointment, he was showing signs of fear at agility class and in the neighborhood. The veterinary technician enquired about changes to the environment or schedule. The pet parent reported none. The veterinarian recommended restarting sertraline at the 6 mg/kg dose once

daily. Joe continued to do well and was on sertraline until he died of heart failure at 13 years of age.

Case 6
Presentation

Rufus, a 5-year-old, 40-kg neutered male German Shepherd Dog, was presented for aggressively barking and lunging at visitors who entered the home.

History

Rufus had not bitten anyone yet. The pet parent always kept him on a leash. He did not respond to verbal cues. After the visitor entered, Rufus was moved to the basement or back yard. When the pet parent was at work, he was confined in the back yard where, he according to the neighbors, he spent most of the day lunging and barking at passersby at the fence line. The pet parents reported that he was generally friendly when he was walked in the neighborhood. When people petted him, he would lean on them and look very relaxed.

Workup

The physical examination was within normal limits. In the examination room, Rufus was friendly and confident. He did not display any aggression and was not muzzled when examined. Blood was drawn without incident and screening laboratory tests were completed. All were within normal limits.

Treatment

The pet parent was advised of the liability and risk associated with having a dog that shows aggression. Further, she was told to keep Rufus indoors when they were not home in order to keep him from repeatedly practicing the undesirable behavior. When any visitor or even a delivery person came to the house, Rufus was to be put in another room with the door closed before the visitor entered. Each time he was confined, the radio in the room was turned up and he was given treats and a favored toy. If the visitor would only be at the home briefly (e.g., delivering a package), they were to scatter treats into a nearby room, close the door after he went in, get their package or interact with the visitor, and then open the door to the room only when the visitor was gone and the door to the home was closed. He could be in the yard only on leash. They were given resources and referred to a positive reinforcement dog trainer to learn quiet, come, and leave it. The veterinary technician followed up in one month by phone. Rufus understood leave it and was able to sit and come on cue, and would go immediately to his room when company arrived at the door. They were advised to continue confinement when visitors arrived. Two months after the original appointment, the pet parents could easily call Rufus from the fence line when most stimuli went by. His reactions were much less intense. They had decided not to work with visitors in the home and instead put Rufus in his sanctuary space when visitors came over. He was relaxed there and they could more easily enjoy their visitors.

References

1. Col R, Day C, Phillips JC. An epidemiological analysis of dog behavior problems presented to an Australian behavior clinic, with associated risk factors. *J Vet Behav.* 2016;15:1–11.
2. Bamberger M, Houpt KA. Signalment factors, comorbidity, and trends in behavior diagnoses in dogs: 1644 cases (1991–2001). *J Am Vet Med Assoc.* 2006;229:1591–1601.
3. Blackshaw JK. An overview of types of aggressive behaviour in dogs and methods of treatment. *Appl Anim Behav Sci.* 1991;30:351–361.
4. Dinwoodie IR, Dwyer B, Zottola V, et al. Demographics and comorbidity of behavior problems in dogs. *J Vet Behav.* 2019;32:62–71.
5. Fatjó J, Ruiz-de-la-Torre JL, Manteca X. The epidemiology of behavioural
problems in dogs and cats: a survey of veterinary practitioners. *Anim Welf.* 2006;15:179–185.
6. Guy NC, Luescher UA, Dohoo SE, et al. Demographic and aggressive characteristics of dogs in a general veterinary caseload. *Appl Anim Behav Sci.* 2001;74:15–28.
7. Salman MD, Hutchinson J, Ruch-Gallie R, et al. Behavioral reasons for relinquishment

of dogs and cats to 12 shelters. *J Appl Animl Welf Sci.* 2000;3:93–106.

8. Caffrey N, Mounchili A, McConkey S, et al. Survey of euthanasia practices in animal shelters in Canada. *Can Vet J.* 2011;52:55.

9. Salman MD, New Jr JG, Scarlett JM, et al. Human and animal factors related to relinquishment of dogs and cats in 12 selected animal shelters in the United States. *J Appl Anim Welf Sci.* 1998;1:207–226.

10. Diesel G, Brodbelt D, Pfeiffer DU. Characteristics of relinquished dogs and their owners at 14 rehoming centers in the United Kingdom. *J Appl Anim Welf Sci.* 2010;13:15–30.

11. Mertens PA. The concept of dominance and the treatment of aggression in multidog homes: a comment on van Kerkhove's commentary. *J Appl Anim Welf Sci.* 2004;7:287–291.

12. Voith VL, Borchelt PL. Dominance aggression in dogs. *Comp Contin Educ Pract Vet.* 1986;8:36–44.

13. Luescher UA, Reisner IR. Canine aggression toward familiar people; a new look at an old problems. *Vet Clin North Am Small Anim Pract.* 2008;38:1107–1130.

14. Mikkola S, Salonen M, Puurunen J, et al. Aggressive behaviour is affected by demographic, environmental and behavioural factors in purebred dogs. *Sci Rep.* 2021;11:9433. doi:10.1038/s41598-021-88793-5.

15. Denenberg S, Landsberg G, Horwitz D, et al. A comparison of cases referred to behaviorists in three different countries. In: Mills D, Levine E, eds. *Current Issues and Research in Veterinary Behavioral Medicine*. West Lafayette, IND: Purdue University Press; 2005:56–62.

16. Bradshaw J, Rooney N. Dog social behavior and communication. In: Serpell J, ed. *The Domestic Dog. Its Evolution, Behavior and Interactions with People*. 2nd ed. Cambridge: Cambridge University Press; 2017:133–159.

17. Range F. Viranyi Z. Social cognition and emotions underlying dog behavior. In: Serpell J, ed. *The Domestic Dog. Its Evolution, Behavior and Interactions with People*. 2nd ed. Cambridge: Cambridge University Press; 2017:182–209.

18. Gácsi M, Vas J, Topál J, et al. Wolves do not join the dance: Sophisticated aggression control by adjusting to human social signals in dogs. *Appl Anim Behav Sci,*. 2013;145:109–122.

19. Bradshaw JW, Blackwell EJ, Casey RA. Dominance in domestic dogs – useful construct or bad habit? *J Vet Behav.* 2009;4:135–144.

20. Goodwin D, Bradshaw JWS, Wickens SM. Paedomorphosis affects agonistic visual signals of domestic dogs. *Anim Behav.* 1997;53:297–304.

21. Bradshaw J. *Dog Sense*. New York: Basic Books; 2011:252–276.

22. Reisner IR, Mann JJ, Stanley M, et al. Comparison of cerebrospinal fluid monoamine metabolite levels in dominant-aggressive and nonaggressive dogs. *Brain Res.* 1996;714:1–2.

23. Mehlman PT, Higley JD, Faucher I, et al. Low CSF 5-HIAA concentrations and severe aggression and impaired impulse control in nonhuman primates. *Am J Psychiatry.* 1994;151:1485–1491.

24. Amat M, Mariotti VM, Le Brech S, et al. Differences in serotonin levels between aggressive English cocker spaniels and aggressive dogs of other breeds. *J Vet Behav.* 2010;5:46.

25. Rosado B, Garcia-Belenguer S, León M. Blood concentrations of serotonin, cortisol and dehydroepiandrosterone in aggressive dogs. *Appl Anim Behav Sci.* 2010;123:124–130.

26. Çakiroglu D, Meral Y, Sancak AA, et al. The relationship between the serum concentrations of serotonin and lipids and aggression in dogs. *Vet Rec.* 2007; 161:59–61.

27. Leon M, Rosado B, Garcia-Belenguer S, et al. Assessment of serotonin in serum, plasma, and platelets of aggressive dogs. *J Vet Behav.* 2012;7:348–352.

28. Pageat P, Lafont C, Falewee C, et al. An evaluation of serum prolactin in anxious dogs and response to treatment with selegiline or fluoxetine. *Appl Anim Behav Sci.* 2007;105:342–350.

29. Andrea KT, Groszler A-S, Zarcula S, et al. The impact of dog feeding on their aggressiveness. *Vet Sci.* 2015;3:503–506. doi:10.14737/journal.aavs/2015/3.9.503.506.

30. Peremans K, Audenaert K, Hoybergs Y, et al. The effect of citalopram hydrobromide on 5-HT2A receptors in the impulsive-aggressive dog, as measured with 2l5iR91150 SPECT. *Mol Imaging.* 2005;32:708–716.

31. Peremens K, Audenaert K, Coopman F, et al. Estimates of regional cerebral blood flow and 5-HT2A receptor density in impulsive, aggressive dogs with 99mTc-ECD and 123I-5-I-R91150. *Eur J Nucl Med Mol Imaging.* 2003;30:1538–1546.

32. Mondo E, Barone M, Soverini M, et al. Gut microbiome structure and adrenocortical activity in dogs with aggressive and phobic behavioral disorders. *Heliyon.* 2020;6;e03311.

33. World Health Organization Animal Bites. Available at: https://www.who.int/news-room/fact-sheets/detail/animal-bites (accessed on 4 December 2021).

34. Gilchrist J, Sacks JJ, White D, et al. Dog bites: still a problem? *Inj Prev.* 2008;14: 296–301.

35. Loder RT. The demographics of dog bites in the United States. *Heliyon.* 2019;5(3): e01360. doi:10.1016/j.heliyon.2019. e01360.

36. Cornelissen JMR, Hopster H. Dog bites in The Netherlands: a study of victims, injuries, circumstances and aggressors to support evaluation of breed specific legislation. *Vet J.* 2010;186:292–298.

37. Caffrey N, Rock M, Schmidtz O, et al. Insights about the epidemiology of dog bites in a Canadian city using a dog aggression scale and administrative data. *Animals.* 2019;9:324. doi:10.3390/ani9060324.

38. Sacks JJ, Kresnow M, Houston B. Dog bites: how big a problem? *Inj Prev.* 1996;2:52–54.

39. Chang YF, McMahon JE, Hennon DL, et al. Dog bite incidence in the city of Pittsburgh: a capture-recapture approach. *Am J Public Health.* 1997;87:1703–1705.

40. Oxley JA, Christley R, Carri Westgarth C. Contexts and consequences of dog bite incidents. *J Vet Behav.* 2018;23:33–39.

41. Guy NC, Luescher AU, Dohoo SE, et al. Risk factors for dog bites to owners in a general veterinary caseload. *Appl Anim Behav Sci.* 2001;74:29–42.

42. Martinez AG, Pernas GS, Casalta FJD, et al. Risk factors associated with behavioral problems in dogs. *J Vet Behav.* 2011;6:225–231.

43. Puurunen J, Hakanen E, Salonen MK, et al. Inadequate socialisation, inactivity, and urban living environment are associated with social fearfulness in pet dogs. *Sci Rep.* 2020;10:3527. doi:10.1038/s41598-020-60546.

44. Duffy DL, Hsu Y, Serpell JA. Breed differences in canine aggression. *Appl Anim Behav Sci.* 2008;114:441–460.

45. Barrios CL, Bustos-López C, Pavletic C, et al. Epidemiology of dog bite incidents in Chile: factors related to the patterns of human-dog relationship. *Animals.* 2021;11(1):96. doi:10.3390/ani11010096.

46. Ozanne-Smith J, Ashby K, Stathakis VZ. Dog bite and injury prevention—analysis, critical review, and research agenda. *Inj Prev.* 2001;7:321–326.

47. Avner JUR, Baker MD. Dog bites in urban children. *Pediatrics.* 1991;88:55–57.

48. Shuler CM, DeBess EE, Lapidus JA, et al. Canine and human factors related to dog bite injuries. *J Am Vet Med Assoc.* 2008; 232(4):542–546.

49. Kaye AE, Belz JM, Kirshner RE. Pediatric dog bite injuries. A 5 year review of the experience at the Children's Hospital in Philadelphia. *Plast Reconstr Surg.* 2009; 124:551–568.

50. Reisner IR, Shofer FS, Nance ML. Behavioral assessment of child-directed aggression. *Inj Prev.* 2007;13:348–351.

51. Overall KL, Love M. Dog bites to humans – demography, epi-demiology, injury, and risk. *J Am Vet Med Assoc.* 2001;218: 1923–1934.

52. Notari L, Cannas S, Agata Di Sotto Y, et al. A retrospective analysis of dog–dog and dog–human cases of aggression in Northern Italy. *Animals.* 2020;10:1662. doi:10.3390/ani10091662.

53. Casey RA, Loftus B, Bolster C, et al. Human directed aggression in domestic dogs (Canis familiaris): occurrence in different contexts and risk factors. *Appl Anim Behav Sci.* 2014;152:52–63.

54. Galac S, Knol BW. Fear-motivated aggression in dogs: patient characteristics, diagnosis and therapy. *Anim Welf.* 1997; 6:9–15.

55. Fatjo J, Amat M, Mariotti VM, et al. Analysis of 1040 cases of canine aggression in a referral practice in Spain. *J Vet Behav.* 2007;2:158–165.

56. Borchelt PL. Aggressive behavior of dogs kept as companion animals: classification and influence of sex, reproductive status and breed. *Appl Anim Ethol.* 1983;10:45–61.

57. Miller KA, Dolan ED, Cussen VA, et al. Are underweight shelter dogs more likely to display food aggression toward humans? *Animals.* 2019;9:1035. doi:10.3390/ani9121035.

58. Jacobs JA, Coe JB, Pearl DL, Widowski TM, Niel L. Factors associated with canine resource guarding behaviour in the presence of people: a cross-sectional survey of dog owners. *Prev Vet Med.* 2018;161(December):143–153.

59. Blackwell EJ, Twells C, Seawright A, et al. The relationship between training methods and the occurrence of behaviour problems as reported by owners, in a population of domestic dogs. *J Vet Behav.* 2008;3:207–217.

60. Patronek GJ, Sacks JJ, Delise KM, et al. Co-occurrence of potentially preventable factors in 256 dog bite-related fatalities in the United States (2000–2009). *J Am Vet Med Assoc.* 2013;243:1726–1736.

61. National Canine Research Council, Dog Bite-Related Fatalities: a literature review. October 2021. https://nationalcaniresearchcouncil.com/research_library/dog-bite-related-fatalities-a-literature-review/– accessed December 18, 2021.

62. Wrubel KM, Moon-Fanelli AA, Maranda LS, et al. Interdog household aggression: 38 cases (2006–2007). *J Am Vet Med Assoc.* 2011;238:731–740.

63. Sherman CK, Reisner IR, Taliaferro L, et al. Characteristics, treatment and outcome of 99 cases of aggression between dogs. *Appl Anim Behav Sci.* 1996;47:91–108.

64. Jokinen O, Appleby D, Sandbacka-Saxen S, et al. Homing age influences the prevalence of aggressive and avoidance behavior an adult dogs. *Appl Anim Behav Sci.* 2017;195:87–92.

65. Appleby DL, Bradshaw JWS, Casey RA. Relationship between aggressive and avoidance behavior by dogs and their experience in the first six months of life. *Vet Rec.* 2002;150:434–438.

66. Wormald D, Lawrence AJ, Carter G, et al. Analysis of correlations between early social exposure and reported aggression and the dog. *J Vet Behav.* 2016;15:31–36.

67. Marion M, Beata C, Sarcey G, et al. Study of aggressiveness in livestock-guarding dogs based on rearing method. *J Vet Behav.* 2018;25:14–16.

68. Edwards RA. Aggression in golden retrievers. *Vet Rec.* 1991;27:410.

69. Heath S. Aggression in golden retrievers. *Vet Rec.* 1991;11:459.

70. van den Berg L, Schilder MBH, de Vries H. Phenotyping of aggressive behavior in golden retriever dogs with a questionnaire. *Behav Genet.* 2006;36:882–902.

71. Newman J, Christley R, Westgarth C, et al. Risk factors for dog bites. An epidemiological perspective. In: Mills D, Westgarth C, eds. *Dog Bites: A Multidisciplinary Perspective.* Sheffield, England: 5M publishing; 2017.

72. Essig GF, Sheehan C, Rikhi S, et al. Dog bite injuries to the face: is there risk with breed ownership? A systematic review with meta-analysis. *Int J Pediatr Otorhinolaryngol.* 2019;117:182–188.

73. Dinwoodie I, Zotola V, Dodman N. An investigation into the effectiveness of various professionals and behavior modification programs with or without medication for the treatment of canine aggression. *J Vet Behav.* 2021;43:46–53.

74. Hsu Y, Sun L. Factors associated with aggressive responses in pet dogs. *Appl Anim Behav Sci.* 2010;123:108–123.

75. Reisner IR, Houpt KA, Shofer FS. National survey of owner-directed aggression in English Springer Spaniels. *J Am Vet Med Assoc.* 2005;227:1594–1603.

76. Podberscek AL, Serpell JA. Environmental influences on the expression of aggressive behavior in English Cocker-Spaniels. *Appl Anim Behav Sci.* 1998;52:215–227.

77. Amat M, Manteca X, Mariott VM, et al. Aggressive behavior in the English Cocker Spaniel. *J Vet Behav.* 2009;4:111–117.

78. Perez-Guisado J, Lopez-Rodriguez R, Munoz-Serrano A. Heritability of dominant–aggressive behavior in English Cocker Spaniels. *Appl Anim Behav Sci.* 2006;100:219–227.

79. Van der Borg JAM, Graat EAM, Beerda B. Behavioral testing based breeding policy reduces the prevalence of fear and aggression related behavior and Rottweilers. *Appl Anim Behav Sci.* 2017;195:80–86.

80. Guy NC, Luescher AU, Dohoo SE, et al. A case series of biting dogs: characteristics of dogs, their behavior and their victims. *Appl Anim Behav Sci.* 2001;74:43–57.

81. Vage J, Bonsdorf TB, Arnet E, et al. Differential gene expression in brain tissues of aggressive and non-aggressive dogs. *BMC Vet Res.* 2010;6:34. http://www.biomedcentral.com/1746-6148/6/34.

82. Carlson NR. *Physiology of Behavior.* Boston: Pearson; 2016:601–603.

83. Arata S, Takeuchi Y, Inoue M, et al. Reactivity to stimuli is a temperamental factor contributing to canine aggression. *PLoS One.* 2014;9(6):e100767. doi:10.1371/journal.pone.0100767.

84. Patronek GJ, Glickman LT, Beck AM, et al. Risk factors for relinquishment of dogs to an animal shelter. *J Am Vet Med Assoc.* 1996;209:572–581.

85. Stubbs WP, Bloomberg MS, Scruggs SL, et al. Effects of prepubertal gonadectomy on physical and behavioral development in cats. *J Am Vet Med Assoc.* 1996;209:1864–1871.

86. Spain CV, Scarlett JM, Houpt KA. Long-term risks and benefits of early-age gonadectomy in cats. *J Am Vet Med Assoc.* 2004;224:372–379.

87. Hopkins SG, Schubert TA, Hart BL. Castration of adult male dogs: effects on roaming, aggression, urine marking, and mounting. *J Am Vet Med Assoc.* 1976;168:1108–1110.

88. Nielsen JC, Eckstein RA, Hart BL. Effects of castration on problem behaviors in male dogs with reference to age and duration of behavior. *J Am Vet Med Assoc.* 1997;211:180–182.

89. Hart BL, Barrett RE. Effects of castration on fighting, roaming, and urine spraying in adult male cats. *J Am Vet Med Assoc.* 1973;163:290–292.

90. Mengoli M, Cozzi A, Chiara M, et al. Survey of possible changes in undesirable behavior after neutering in male dogs. In: *Proceedings of the 2010 European Behaviour Meeting.* Belgium: ESVCE; 2010:189–193.

91. Hart BL, Eckstein RA. The role of gonadal hormones in the occurrence of objectionable behaviors in dogs and cats. *Appl Anim Behav Sci.* 1997;52:331–354.

92. Flint HE, Coe JB, Serpell JA, et al. Risk factors associated with stranger-directed aggression in domestic dogs. *Appl Anim Behav Sci.* 2017;197:45–54.

93. Bennett PC, Rohlf VI. Owner-companion dog interactions: relationships between demographic variables, potentially problematic behaviours, training engagement and shared activities. *Appl Anim Behav Sci.* 2007;102:65–84.

94. Messam LLM, Kass PH, Chomel BB, et al. The human–canine environment: a risk factor for non-play bites? *Vet J.* 2008;177:205–215.

95. Liinamo A-L, van den Berg L, Leegwater PAJ, et al. Genetic variation in aggression-related traits in Golden Retriever dogs. *Appl Anim Behav Sci.* 2007;104:95–106.

96. O'Farrell V, Peachey E. Behavioural effects of ovariohysterectomy on bitches. *J Small Anim Pract.* 1990;31:595–598.

97. Kim HH, Yeon SC, Houpt KA, et al. Effects of ovariohysterectomy on reactivity in German Shepherd Dogs. *Vet J.* 2006;172:154–159.

98. Reisner IR. Dominance-related aggression of English Springer Spaniels: a review of 53 cases. *Appl Anim Behav Sci.* 1993;37:83–84.

99. McCarthy MM, McDonald EH, Brooks PJ, et al. An anxiolytic action of oxytocin is enhanced by estrogen in the mouse. *Physiol Behav.* 1997;60:1209–1215.

100. Feltes ESM, Stull JW, Herron ME, et al. Characteristics of intrahousehold interdog aggression and dog and pair factors associated with a poor outcome. *J Am Vet Med Assoc.* 2020;256:349–361.

101. Farhoody P, Mallawaarachchi I, Tarwater PM, et al. Aggression toward familiar people, strangers, and conspecifics in gonadectomized and intact dogs. *Front Vet Sci.* 2018;5:18. doi:10.3389/fvets.2018.00018.

102. Beaver BV. Canine social behavior. In: *Canine Behavior: a Guide for Veterinarians.*

Philadelphia: W. B. Saunders; 1999; 137–199.

103. Feldman EC, Nelson RW. *Canine and Feline Endocrinology and Reproduction*. Philadelphia, PA: W.B. Saunders; 2015:70–111.

104. Henley WN, Valdic F. Hypothyroid-induced changes in autonomic control have a central serotonergic component. *Am J Physiol*. 1997;272:H894–903.

105. Henley WN, Chen S, Klettner C, et al. Hypothyroidism increases serotonin turnover and sympathetic activity in the adult rat. *Can J Physiol Pharmacol*. 1991;69:205–210.

106. Aronson LP, Dodds WJ. The effect of hypothyroid function on canine behavior. In: *Current Issues and Research in Veterinary Behavioral Medicine*. West Lafayette, IN: Purdue University Press; 2005:131–138.

107. Beaver BV, Haug LI. Canine behaviors associated with hypothyroidism. *J Am Anim Hosp Assoc*. 2003;39:431–434.

108. Fatjo J. Animal behavior case of the month. *J Am Vet Med Assoc*. 2003;223; 623–626.

109. Graham PA, Lundquist RB, Refsal KR, et al. Reported clinical signs in 8317 cases of canine hypothyroidism and 2647 cases of subclinical thyroiditis. In: *Proceedings of BSAVA*. Birmingham, UK; 2004:529.

110. Fatjo J, Stub C, Manteca X. Four cases of aggression and hypothyroidism in dogs. *Vet Rec*. 2002;151:547–548.

111. Radosta L, Shofer F, Reisner I. Comparison of thyroid analytes in aggressive and nonaggressive dogs. In: *Proceedings of the AVSAB/ACVB scientific meeting*. 2006:23–25.

112. Carter G, Scott-Moncrieff JC, Luescher AU. Serum total thyroxine and thyroid stimulating hormone concentrations in dogs with behavior problems. *J Vet Behav*. 2009;4:230–236.

113. Dodman NH, Arsonson L, Cottam N, et al. The effect of thyroid replacement in dogs with suboptimal thyroid function on owner-directed aggression: a randomized, double-blind, placebo-controlled clinical trial. *J Vet Behav*. 2013;8:225–230.

114. Monteiro BP, Lascelles BDX, Murrel J, et al. 2022 WSAVA guidelines for the recognition, assessment and treatment of pain. *J Small Anim Pract* [online]. doi:10.1111/jsap.13566.

115. Margari F, Lorusso M, Matera E, et al. Aggression, impulsivity, and suicide risk in benign chronic pain patients - a cross-sectional study. *Neuropsychiatr Dis Treat*. 2014;10:1613–1620. doi:10.2147/NDT. S66209.

116. Mellor DJ, Cook CJ, Stafford KJ. Quantifying some responses to pain as a stressor. In: Moberg GP, Mench JA, eds. *The Biology of Animal Stress. Basic Principles and Implications for Animal Welfare*. Wallingford, UK: CAB International; 2000:171–198.

117. Chaouloff F. Effects of acute physical exercise on central serotonergic systems. *Med Sci Sports Exerc*. 1997;29:58–62.

118. Mills DS, Demontigny-Bédard I, Gruen M, et al. Pain and problem behavior in cats and dogs. *Animals*. 2020;10:318.

119. Le Brech S, Amat M, Camps T, et al. Canine aggression toward family members in Spain: Clinical presentations and related factors. *J Vet Behav*. 2016;12:36–41.

120. Sunol A, Perez-Accino JP, Kelley M, et al. Successful dietary treatment of aggression and behavioral changes in a dog. *J Vet Behav*. 2020;37:56–60.

121. Shyan MR, Fortune KA, King C. "Bark Parks"—a study on interdog aggression in a limited-control environment. *Appl Anim Behav Sci*. 2003;6:25–32.

122. Siracusa C, Provoost L, Reisner IR. Dog- and owner-related risk factors for consideration of euthanasia or rehoming before a referral behavioral consultation and for euthanizing or rehoming the dog after consultation. *J Vet Behav*. 2017;22:46–56.

123. Polsky R. Can aggression in dogs be elicited through the use of electronic pet containment systems? *J Appl Anim Welf Sci*. 2000;3;345–357.

124. Reisner IR, Shofer FS. Effects of gender and parental status on knowledge and attitudes of dog owners regarding dog aggression toward children. *J Am Vet Med Assoc*. 2008;233:1412–1419.

125. Villar RG, Connick M, Barton LL, et al. Parent and pediatrician knowledge, attitudes, and practices regarding pet-associated hazards. *Arch Pediatr Adolesc Med*. 1998;152:1035–1037.

126. Godbout M, Frank D. Persistence of puppy behaviors and signs of anxiety during adulthood. *J Vet Behav*. 2011; 6:92.

127. Martinez ÁG, Martínez MF, Rosado B, et al. Association between puppy classes and adulthood behavior of the dog. *J Vet Behav*. 2019;32:36–41.

128. Denenberg S, Landsberg GM. Effect of dog-appeasing pheromones on anxiety and fear in puppies during training its effects on long term socialization. *J Am Vet Med Assoc*. 2008;233:1874–1882.

129. Gazzano A, Mariti C, Alvares S, et al. The prevention of undesirable behaviors in dogs: effectiveness of veterinary behaviorists' advice given to puppy owners. *J Vet Behav*. 2008;3:125–133.

130. Maarschalkerweerd RJ, Endenburg N, Kirpensteijn J, et al. Influence of orchiectomy on canine behavior. *Vet Rec*. 1997;140:617–619.

131. Mariti C, Pierantoni L, Sighieri C, et al. Guardians' perceptions of dogs' welfare and behaviors related to visiting the veterinary clinic. *J Appl Welf Sci*. 2017;20:24–33.

132. Zapata I, Serpell JA, Alvarez CE. Genetic mapping of fear and aggression. *Genomics*. 2016;17:572. doi:10.1186/ s12864-016-2936-3.

133. Bonnani R, Cafazzo S, Fantini C, et al. Feeding-order in an urban feral domestic cat colony: relationship to dominance rank, sex and age. *Anim Behav*. 2007;74:

1369–1379. doi:10.1016/j.anbehav. 2007.02.029.

134. Luescher AU. Veterinary Medicine Today: Animal Behavior Case of the Month. *JAVMA*. 2000;217:1143–1145.

135. Moyer KE. Kinds of aggression and their physiological basis. *Commun Behav Biol*. 1998;2:65–87.

136. Řezáč P, Viziová P, Dobešová M, et al. Factors affecting dog–dog interactions on walks with their owners. *Appl Anim Behav Sci*. 2011;134:170–176.

137. Camps T, Amat M, Mariotti VM, et al. Pain-related aggression in dogs: 12 clinical cases. *J Vet Behav*. 2012;7:99–102.

138. Barcelos AM, Mills DS, Zulch H. Clinical indicators of occult musculoskeletal pain in aggressive dogs. *Vet Rec*. 2015;176(18):465.

139. Jacobs JA, Coe JB, Widowski TM, et al. Defining and clarifying the terms canine possessive aggression and resource guarding: a study of expert opinion. *Front Vet Sci*. 2018;5:115.

140. Beaver BV. Profiles of dogs presented for aggression. *J Am Anim Hosp Assoc*. 1993;29:564–569.

141. Marder AR, Shabelansky A, Patronek G. Food-related aggression in shelter dogs: a comparison of behavior identified by a behavior evaluation in the shelter and owner reports after adoption. *Appl Anim Behav Sci*. 2013;48:150–156.

142. Miller HC, DeWall CN, Pattison K, et al. Too dog tired to avoid danger: self-control depletion in canines increases behavioral approach toward an aggressive threat. *Psychon Bull Rev*. 2012;19(3):535–540.

143. Borchelt PL, Voith VL. Aggressive behavior in dogs and cats. *Compend Contin Educ Pract Vet*. 1985;7:949–957.

144. Borchelt PL, Voith VL. Classification of canine behavior problems. *Vet Clin North Am Small Anim Pract*. 1982;12: 571–585.

145. Kim SE, Arzi B, Garcia T, et al. Bite forces and their measurement in dogs and cats. *Front Vet Sci*. 2018;5:76. doi:10.3389/ fvets.2018.00076.

146. Ellis JL, Thomason JJ, Kebreab E, et al. Calibration of estimated biting forces in domestic canids: comparison of post-mortem and in vivo measurements. *J Anat*. 2008;212:769–780.

147. Reisner IR, Erb HN, Houpt KA. Risk factors for behavior-related euthanasia amount dominant-aggressive dogs: 110 cases (1989–1992). *J Am Vet Med Assoc*. 1994;205:855–863.

148. DeMeester RH, Mills DS, De Keuster T, et al. ESVCE position statement on risk assessment. *J Vet Behav*. 2011;6:38–39.

149. Radosta-Huntley L, Shofer F, Reisner IR. Comparison of 42 cases of canine fear-related aggression with structured clinician initiated follow-up and 25 cases with unstructured client initiated follow up. *Appl Anim Behav Sci*. 2007;105:330–341.

150. Godbout M, Frank D. Excessive mouthing in puppies as a predictor of

aggressive behavior in adult dogs. *J Vet Behav.* 2011;6:93.

151. Williams EJ, Blackwell E. Managing the risk of aggressive dog behavior: investigating the influence of owner threat and efficacy perceptions. *Risk Anal.* 2019;39:2528–2542.

152. Herron M, Shofer F, Reisner I. Survey of the use and outcome of confrontational and non-confrontational training methods in client-owned dogs showing undesirable behaviors. *Appl Anim Behav Sci.* 2009;117:47–54.

153. Hiby EF, Rooney NJ, Bradshaw JWS, et al. Dog training methods; their use, effectiveness and interaction with behavior and welfare. *Anim Welf.* 2007;13:63–69.

154. Dodman NH, Brown DC, Serpell JA. Associations between owner personality and psychological status and the prevalence of canine behavior problems. *PLoS One.* 2018;13(2):e0192846. https://doi.org/10.1371/journal.pone.0192846.

155. Cooper JJ, Cracknell N, Hardiman J, et al. The welfare consequences and efficacy of training pet dogs with remote electronic training collars in comparison to reward based training. *PLoS One.* 2014;9:e102722.

156. de Castro ACV, Fuchs D, Pastur S, et al. Does training matter? Evidence for the negative impact of aversive-based methods on companion dog welfare. *PLoS One.* 2020;15(12):e0225023. doi:10.1371/journal.pone.0225023.

157. Horváth Z, Dóka A, Miklósi Á. Affiliative and disciplinary behaviour of human handlers during play with their dog affects cortisol concentrations in opposite directions. *Horm Behav.* 2008;54:107–114.

158. China L, Mills DS, Cooper JJ. Efficacy of dog Training with and without remote electronic collars vs. a focus on positive reinforcement. *Front Vet Sci.* 2020;7:508. doi:10.3389/fvets.2020.00508.

159. Blackwell EJ, Bolster C, Richards GJ, et al. The use of electronic collars for training domestic dogs: estimated prevalence, reasons and risk factors for use, and owner perceived success as compared to other training methods. *BMC Vet Res.* 2012;8:93. https://doi.org/10.1186/1746-6148-8-93.

160. Rooney NJ, Cowan S. Training methods and owner-dog interactions: links with dog behaviour and learning ability. *Appl Anim Behav Sci.* 2011;132:169–177.

161. Stellato AC, Flint HE, Dewey CE, et al. Risk-factors associated with veterinary-related fear and aggression in owned domestic dogs. *Appl Anim Behav Sci.* 2021;241:105374. doi:10.1016/j.applanim.2021.105374.

162. Follette MR, Rodriguez KE, Ogata N, et al. Military veterans and their PTSD service dogs: associations between training methods, PTSD severity, dog behavior, and the human-animal bond. *Front Vet Sci.* 2019;6:23. doi:10.3389/fvets.2019.00023.

163. Willen RM, Schiml PA, Hennessy MB. Enrichment centered on human interaction moderates fear-induced T aggression and increases positive expectancy in fearful shelter dogs. *Appl Anim Behav Sci.* 2019;217:57–62.

164. Dickinson A, Pearce JM. Inhibitory interactions between appetitive and aversive stimuli. *Psychol Bull.* 1997;84:696–711.

165. Kroll HW. Rapid treatment of dog phobia by a feeding procedure. *J Behav Ther Exp Psychiatry.* 1975;6:325–326.

166. Echterling-Savage K, DiGennaro Reed FD, Miller K, et al. Effects of caregiver-implemented aggression reduction procedure on problem behavior of dogs. *J Appl Anim Welf Sci.* 2014;1–17.

167. Echterling-Savage K. *A Comparison of Classical Counterconditioning and Differential Reinforcement of Alternative Behavior on Aggressive Behavior in Dogs* (Unpublished master's thesis). Lawrence: University of Kansas; 2010.

168. Orihel JS, Fraser D. A note on the effectiveness of behavioural rehabilitation for reducing inter-dog aggression in shelter dogs. *Appl Anim Behav Sci.* 2008;112:400–405.

169. Dodman NH, Arrington D. Animal behavior case of the month. *J Am Vet Med Assoc.* 2000;217;1468–1472.

170. Van Haaften KA, Grigg EK, Kolus C, et al. A survey of dog owners perceptions on the use of psychoactive medication and alternatives for the treatment of canine behavior problems. *J Vet Behav.* 2020;35:27–33.

171. Virga V, Houpt KA, Scarlett J. Pharmacological adjunct to behavioral modification in the management of aggressive behaviors in dogs. *J Am Anim Hosp Assoc.* 2001;37:325–330.

173. Dodman NH, Donnelly R, Shuster L, et al. Use of fluoxetine to treat dominance aggression in dogs. *J Am Vet Med Assoc.* 1996;209:1585–1587.

173. White MM, Neilson JC, Hart BL, et al. Effects of clomipramine hydrochloride on dominance-related aggression in dogs. *J Am Vet Med Assoc.* 1999;215:1288–1291.

174. Odore R, Rendini D, Badino P, et al. Behavioral therapy and fluoxetine treatment and aggressive dogs: a case study. *Animals.* 2020;10:832. doi:10.3390/ani10050832.

175. Ogata N, Dodman NH. They use a clonidine in the treatment of fear-based behavior problems in dogs: an open trial. *J Vet Behav.* 2011;6(2):130–137.

176. DeNapoli JS, Dodman NH, Shuster L, et al. Effect of dietary protein content and tryptophan supplementation on dominance aggression, territorial aggression and hyperactivity in dogs. *J Am Vet Med Assoc.* 2000;217:504–508.

177. Re S, Zanoletti M, Emanuele E. Aggressive dogs are characterized by low omega-3 polyunsaturated fatty acids status. *Vet Res Commun.* 2008;32:225–230.

Recommended reading

Duncan-Sutherland N, Lissaman AC, Shepherd M, et al. Systematic review of dog bite prevention strategies. *Inj Prev.* 2022;28:288–297.

Mills D, Westgarth C. eds. *Dog Bites. A Multidisciplinary Perspective.* Sheffield, England: 5M publishing; 2017.

Pike A. Managing canine aggression In the home. *Vet Clin North Am Small Anim Pract.* 2018;48:387–402.

CHAPTER 24

Feline aggression

Karen Sueda, DVM, DACVB and Lisa Radosta, DVM, DACVB

Introduction

Cats that are aggressive are at risk for rehoming or euthanasia, and aggression is a primary reason for behavior referrals.[1-5] Cats are smaller than dogs and it might seem that their bites would be less injurious when compared to dogs; however, cat bites pose a serious health risk, especially to those who are immunocompromised. In addition, about 50% of cat bites get infected,[6] a higher rate than dogs, and can lead to serious disease such as bartonellosis. Misunderstandings about the cat's intentions and severity of the injuries can degrade the human–animal bond and impact the welfare of the cat. Pet parents of an aggressive cat may elect to declaw them, isolate them from the rest of the family, or relegate them to living outdoors, negatively affecting the cat's quality of life. Owing to a lack of education regarding normal cat behavior, behavioral needs, and communicative signals on the part of pet parents and veterinary healthcare team members, pet cats are unrealistically expected to welcome new feline housemates, be a good neighbor when unfamiliar felines encroach on their property, and blissfully tolerate the unpredictable activities of other species, such as humans or dogs. Passive avoidance is the cat's first response, which people often perceive as rude, arrogant, or independent, and fits the traditional view that cats are not social. When those more passive attempts to communicate are not heeded, cats may resort to more overt communication which can include aggression, much like other species.

Consider the cat that has the disconcerting habit of accepting petting and attention only to respond by biting. These cats may seem to enjoy or may actually enjoy petting and interaction, initiating it by crying, rubbing or bunting (rub bing with their head) against people, or jumping into their laps. Because these are affiliative greetings, people often assume the cat would like petting or physical interaction. Some do, but some do not. The cat may desire to be near the pet parent but may not necessarily be soliciting physical handling or may only want brief physical contact.

Consider the complexities of human greetings – greetings are expressed by shaking hands, smiling, or hugging, yet solicitation and even acceptance of these human greetings do not imply acceptance of more invasive or prolonged social physical contact such as kissing, holding hands, or tickling. Humans have social boundaries and so do cats. Cats attempt to communicate those boundaries to us through body language (see below). When the body language is recognized and interpreted accurately, aggression often does not develop in the first place (see Chapter 2).

Normal feline behavior

Cats prefer not to fight. They may use a combination of visual and audible communication displays to avoid aggressive and physical confrontations. There are many reasons why the systems may fail, resulting in aggressive encounters and even serious injuries. Domestic cats evolved from solitary ancestors, the African wildcat (*Felis silvestris lybica*) and are well equipped for independent living. Many feline behaviors (hunting, eating, and resting) may be performed individually, rather than in groups. However, domestic cats may be opportunistically social when abundant resources encourage congregation or when cooperative living is most advantageous (e.g., communal rearing of kittens). In these cases, feline social structure is most commonly based on groups of related females and their offspring, with males loosely associated with a female lineage occupying central or peripheral areas.[7] With that said, there is evidence that neutered cats behave differently and may be more accepting of other cats.[8] Cats recognize colony versus noncolony members, and aggression is typically exhibited by members of a cat colony toward unfamiliar cats that are not members of the colony.[9] With persistence, some cats may be integrated into an existing colony, but this is a gradual process that usually takes many interactions over an extended period of time.[9,10]

When presented with conflict, rather than fighting, it is more common for cats to defer to or avoid a cat that already has a resource, whether a resting area, litterbox, or access to a passageway (first come, first served).[11] On the other hand, a social asymmetry helps to maintain healthy social relationships without the need for conflict. Much has been said about dominance in dogs, but what do we know about dominance in cats? Cats, similarly to dogs, appear to some extent to have a hierarchy based on resource-holding potential (how likely the cat is able to keep the resource if there is aggression) and relative resource value (how important the resource is to the cat). In this type of dominance hierarchy, the dominance is not static, but instead fluid, based on the value of the resources and the interactions between the cats around that resource. For example, in one study of feral cats, the male cats were higher ranking away from food (had preferential access to resources), while the female cats were higher ranking near food (ate first).[12] Also in this study, kittens between four and six months of age were more likely to feed first compared to either sex of adult cat, indicating that dominance is not absolute.[12] In some cases, the female cat is higher ranking even though she is of smaller body size than the male cat.[13] Similarly to dogs, the highest-ranking cat is not necessarily

the most aggressive cat.[9] The overwhelming majority of the aggression that is seen in domestic cats presented to veterinarians by pet parents is a result of fear, anxiety, stress, conflict, panic, or pain, not dominance.

Cats will utilize a repertoire of aggression and aggressive displays to communicate their needs, fears, or intentions, whether to humans or other animals. In free-roaming cats, hostility among familiar, friendly felines may be minimal and limited to passive displays, while unwelcome feline invasions may be met with intense and explosive reactivity and injury.

The body language of aggression

Aggression includes a wide variety of behaviors from somewhat subtle body postures or facial expressions to violent attacks. Some grooming interactions between cats may actually be a way of avoiding overt aggression, though agonistic behavior by the groomer may still occur following a bout of grooming.[14] Aggression can be accompanied by body postures associated with fear or distance increasing (e.g., hissing, ears flattened against the head, tail tucked to the side of the body or underneath, lowered body position, leaning away from the fear-eliciting stimulus, rolling over onto the side), arousal (e.g., dilated pupils, piloerection), defense (e.g., teeth bared, growling, swatting, biting, and scratching), and offensive (e.g., upright body, forward ears, tail out from body). However, even body language signals can be reinforced and punished, as noted above. For that reason, with repetition and learning, the body language associated with aggressive displays may appear less consistent with fear and more consistent with confidence (e.g., ears forward, upright body), and the cat may become quicker to resort to aggression rather than avoidance behavior. With the diagnostic criteria below, there is a description of body language where applicable; however, the practitioner should always keep in mind that the body language of stress is fluid and individual and often cannot be separated into distinct categories. It is a part of the picture, but may not tell the entire story (see Figures 24.1–24.4).

Learning and aggression

Aggression can be reinforced or punished as is the case with any behavior. See Chapter 10 for more information about learning theory. In the case of aggression, the progression from disengagement body language to aggressive displays might best be considered a progression of stress as if climbing a ladder. Each rung of the ladder is a different level of stress associated with certain body language signals. If a cat feels uncomfortable or stressed, they may avert their gaze, lick their lips, or blink their eyes slowly. If these signals are effective at gaining distance from the stress-eliciting situation, those body language signals are reinforced and the likelihood that the cat will continue to exhibit those signals in that situation increases. Figuratively speaking, the cat continues to perch on that rung of the ladder. However, if those signals are not effective at gaining distance from the person, animal, or stimulus, that signal

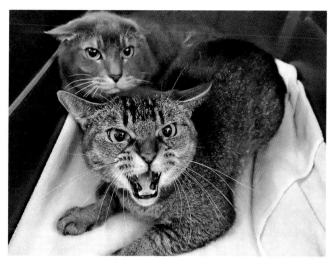

Figure 24.1 This cat is displaying body language associated with fear, including ears back, body shifted caudally, mouth open hissing. *(Attribution: Gary Landsberg, DVM, DACVB.)*

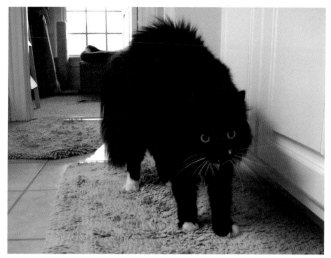

Figure 24.3 This cat has body language associated with extreme fear and arousal, including dilated pupils, arched back, piloerection, and tail down. *(Attribution: Katy Cohen.)*

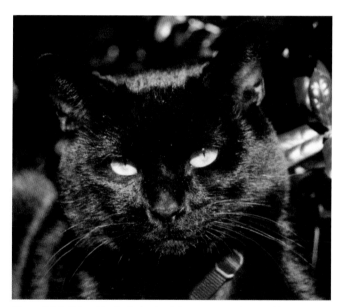

Figure 24.2 This cat is displaying body language consistent with a non-aroused state or potentially confidence including ears forward and pupils of a normal size. *(Attribution: Lisa Radosta.)*

is punished (i.e., the likelihood of exhibiting these lower intensity signals decreases). Effectively, the rung of the ladder breaks. The only recourse the cat has is to climb to the next rung of the ladder to communicate their need to gain distance from the stressor, which appears grossly as an escalation in body language signaling. If this happens repeatedly, where lower-level, more passive body language signals are punished, the cat will continue to escalate until he shows aggression. Aggression is inevitably reinforced because when bitten or scratched, most people pull back, reinforcing the behavior instantly. Finally, the cat has found a way to communicate with humans! Even if the person yells at the cat 30 seconds later, it will not change that the behavior was immediately reinforced and that the behavior

has a high likelihood of increasing in that situation the next time. Similarly, if a victim cat runs from an aggressor cat, this action may reinforce the aggression of the aggressor cat. This concept is explained further in Chapter 10. That is not to say that the solution to all intercat aggression is to help the victim gain confidence. Some types of aggression, such as impulsive, stress-induced, anxiety-induced, or redirected aggression, may not change, based on the victim's behavior (see Figure 24.5).

Any stimulus can be paired with a conditioned emotional response (CER). For example, if application of topical flea and tick medication is uncomfortable, the pet may form a negative CER to the sight of the tube or the pet parent's movement to where medications are kept. This association can lead to aggression. Pets that are threatened or physically punished for aggressive displays can learn to associate pain or fear with certain stimuli and become even more aggressive each time the situations recur. They can also form a negative CER to certain people who perpetrate the physical punishment.

Some types of aggression such as territorial aggression are reinforced by the environmental factors or stimuli outside of the pet parent's control. For example, when a cat hisses at a delivery person leaving a package at the front door, the cat's hissing was reinforced (negative reinforcement) even though it was not the cause of the delivery person's departure.

Prevalence

Aggressive pet cats can pose a significant danger to family and visitors, causing physical and emotional trauma and leading to legal action in some cases. In the United States alone, there are an estimated 400,000 cat bites and 66,000 emergency room visits each year.[15,16] The target of the aggression may be familiar or unfamiliar cats, dogs, animals, objects, or people. This may include inhabitants living in the same home, visitors, and neighboring animals or people. The prevalence of aggression in household cats ranges from 36% (people and other animals)[17] to between 49.5%[18] and 69% toward people,[19] depending on the study. Most

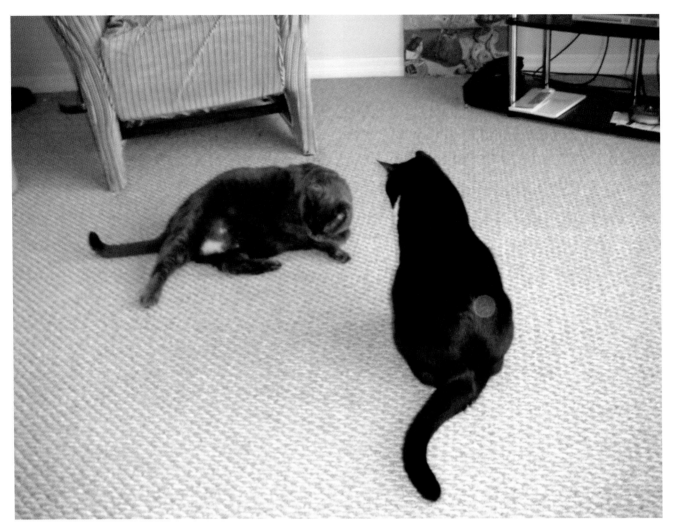

Figure 24.4 The gray cat is displaying body language consistent with disengagement and distance increasing such as grooming, averting the gaze, and exposing the abdomen. The black cat is displaying confident and threatening body language with weight shifted forward, ears forward, and tail out. *(Attribution: Lisa Radosta.)*

cases of aggression result in bites directed at family members. In one study of cats that bite, 50% of the bites are likely to be directed at family members.[4,20] Predatory play increases around eight weeks of age[21] and peaks at 18–21 weeks,[22] the same time kittens are adopted into their new home, and this behavior is often reported as one of the most common reasons for pet parent-related aggression at behavior practices.[23,24]

Interestingly, adult females were at highest risk for cat bites compared to children, who make up the largest percentage of people bitten by dogs.[19,20,25] Most wounds are scratches, but punctures and tears also occur.[19,20] Bites can occur anywhere, but are most common, when all populations of cats (i.e., stray and owned) are examined, on the hand, fingers, arms, feet, or legs, with the face and neck being uncommon unlike dogs.[19,20] Owned cats are more likely to bite family members in the face or neck, and children are more likely than adults to be bitten in these places.[19,20] These differences are most likely due to the interactions between humans and stray versus owned cats. In several studies of cat aggression toward people, female cats were more likely than male cats to exhibit aggression,[19,20] while in one study evaluating aggression in owned cats, there was

no difference between male and female cats.[18] Pet parents often report that the aggression is unprovoked; however, in one study, 92% of the cases of aggression directed at humans was determined to be provoked.[19] Aggression toward other cats is a significant problem.[23,26] In multicat households, up to 50% of cats fight upon initial introduction, with fights occurring with equal likelihood greater than and less than one week after introduction.[27] Outside of introduction, the prevalence of fighting in multicat households can be as high as 35% up to 12 months into the relationship, with fights occurring more than one time per week in 39% of the population.[27] The literature differs, with one study demonstrating that males are more likely than females to instigate aggression toward other cats and another demonstrating that females are more likely[28]; however, there does not appear to be any difference in the likelihood of the victim being male or female nor in the likelihood of resolution when gender is considered.[29]

Any cat of any breed, size, or age can exhibit undesirable aggression; however, in one study, Siamese cats most commonly exhibited aggression (42%) with European (36%), Persian (15%), mixed breed (5%), and Angora (3%) also represented.[18,19]

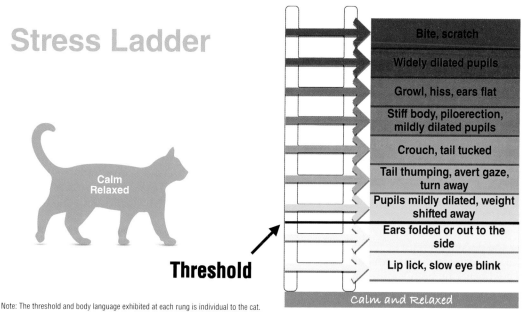

Stress Ladder

Calm
Relaxed

Threshold

Bite, scratch

Widely dilated pupils

Growl, hiss, ears flat

Stiff body, piloerection, mildly dilated pupils

Crouch, tail tucked

Tail thumping, avert gaze, turn away

Pupils mildly dilated, weight shifted away

Ears folded or out to the side

Lip lick, slow eye blink

Calm and Relaxed

Note: The threshold and body language exhibited at each rung is individual to the cat.

Figure 24.5 The cat stress ladder. Often body language signals are exhibited prior to biting, but go unnoticed by pet parents. *(Attribution: Lisa Radosta. Modified from Shepherd, K 2009. BSAVA Manual of Canine and Feline Behaviour, 2nd edition.)*

Etiology and predisposing factors

Predisposing factors and the etiology of cat aggression is varied and complex (see Box 24.1). Important factors appear to be the pet parent's behavior, early developmental experiences, traumatic experiences, and level of stress due to social and environmental factors. Factors contributing to the development of aggression include genetics, epigenetics (effect of environment and external factors on the expression of genes), the cat's coping style, maternal care, neonatal handling and socialization, environmental experience, physical health, and learning. Aggression may be normal, adaptive, and appropriate in some contexts. For example, a queen will protect her

offspring by showing aggression, even though she is typically not aggressive. This type of aggressive activity is believed to be a function of the hormonal state of the female during lactation as well as the presence of the young. Males will display ritualized threat displays (e.g., posturing, threatening, fighting) to other males, facilitated by postpubertal androgen secretion, especially at the peak of sexual and social maturity (two to four years of age) and during mating season.[30]

Experiences during early development are important for the development of all behavioral disorders, and aggression is no exception. Kittens lacking early socialization and handling are more likely to be fearful of people and thus more likely to display fear-induced and defensive aggression when approached or handled.[31–33] Paternal temperament appears to have a large effect on the temperament of the offspring, with friendly toms more likely to sire friendly kittens, even if the kittens are not exposed to the tom after birth.[33,34] The presence or absence of the queen and her behavior toward stimuli during early development of the kittens can affect the development of aggression, presumably due to the effect of observational learning and mimicry of behavior and exposure (socialization), leading to fear, anxiety, stress, conflict, panic (FASCP).[7,35] Kittens removed from the litter before 6 weeks of age are more likely to be fearful and reactive compared with kittens weaned between 6 and 12 weeks of age,[35] and those weaned before 8 weeks of age are more likely to show aggression directed at unfamiliar people than those weaned after 14 weeks.[36] Early trauma has also been linked to an increased likelihood of aggression.[18] Contrary to popular thought, several studies have found that bottle-reared kittens were not more likely to exhibit aggressive behavior compared to queen-reared kittens, although the presence of a second cat and play with wand-type toys decreased aggression to people.[28,37] When a kitten grows up without appropriate social interaction that discourages hard biting, such as a kitten that has been hand

Box 24.1 Etiology and predisposing factors affecting the development of aggression

- Intrinsic influences
  - Psychological health
  - Emotional state
- Coping style
  - Genetics
  - Learning
  - Physical health
- Extrinsic influences
  - Social environment
    - Pet parent
    - Other animals
  - Physical environment
    - In utero
    - Present
    - Past

From Mills DS, Westgarth C. *Dog Bites: A Multidisciplinary Perspective.* Sheffield, United Kingdom: 5m Books Ltd.; 2017.

reared with no contact with other cats, it may bite without inhibition into adulthood and be quite dangerous.[35,38] See Chapter 2 for more information about feline development.

At any age, cats that have aversive experiences (e.g., pain, punishment, fear inducing) associated with any stimulus (e.g., humans, other cats or animals, object, situation, sensory stimulus, sight, sound, smell) may develop an aggressive response. Some cats require a very strong stimulus to elicit fear, while others may become aggressive in response to mild stimuli, such as small movements, a noxious odor, or a novel noise.

Pain or discomfort of any sort can result in or increase aggressive behavior. Cats can be silent in their suffering whether due to the predisposition to hiding when they are ill, or the lack of understanding by pet parents and veterinarians of cat body language and species-typical behavior. For that reason, at every turn, pain and discomfort must be fully investigated and treated. When a gonadectomized cat exhibits sexual or hormonally influenced behavior, both endogenous (e.g., ovarian or testicular remnants, cryptorchidism, hormone-secreting neoplasms)[39] and exogenous (e.g., access to human estrogen or testosterone replacement creams) sources of hormones should be investigated. Hyperthyroidism may also be a cause for aggressive behavior in previously docile middle-aged or older adult cat. See Chapter 6 for more information on the physical causes of and influences on aggression.

The most common contexts in which cats show aggression are: physical interactions (e.g., petting, picking up on lap), during play, when startled, in the presence of unfamiliar animals or unfamiliar people, or when protecting food or territory (as assessed by the pet parent).[18] Pet parents who interacted with their cat by rewarding them for appropriate behaviors or ignoring undesirable behaviors instead of primarily punishing them (e.g., stern voice, verbal corrections, physical corrections) were less likely to live with cats that expressed aggression toward familiar and unfamiliar people, animals, objects, and situations, and were less likely to live with cats that expressed severe aggression.[28] Just as with other animals, structured, consistent interactions associated with positive reinforcement of desirable behaviors and lacking physical punishment reduces aggression.

Environment can play a factor, presumably due to stress and lack of enrichment, with about one-half of the households with aggressive cats reporting that their cats were not allowed outside,[18] while other studies have shown no association with outdoor access[27,40] and some have shown an increased likelihood of behavior problems including aggression.[28,41] To complicate matters, one study found that intercat aggression was more likely in situations where one cat had access to outdoors and the other did not.[27] Finally, it appears that the initial or home cat is more likely to show aggression when compared with the newly adopted cat in some households with intercat aggression.[27] Enrichment opportunities, the amount of time spent with the cat, and the absence of pet parent-directed play can affect the expression of aggression.[41] Homes with more than two cats may be at less risk for pet parent-directed aggression, presumably because the pet parent has alternative cats with which to interact and because the cat has an alternative outlet other than the pet parents; however, having additional pets in the household is likely to increase aggression toward other animals potentially due to accessibility or increased stress.[28]

Cats that, by the pet parent's assessment, did not like other animals or did not appreciate petting are more likely to show aggression.[18] In cats that show aggression to other cats, those that have previously been preferred associates and slept adjacent, nose-touched, and tail-wrapped,[42,43] may be more likely to recover from an aggressive event than cats that did not have a preferred associate relationship. The most important factor in prediction of future fighting appears to be the presence of stress or unfriendly behavior at initial introduction.[27] Cats in underenriched environments without enough physical space to maintain social distance (e.g., confined area, narrow hallways) or that do not have free, unfettered access to resources (e.g., food, water, litterboxes, preferred resting areas, human attention) will have an increased level of stress, which fuels all types of behavior problems, including aggression.

Aggression might arise between cats living in the same household where there had been little or no previous history of aggression. Increased conflicts may arise acutely or gradually when there has been a change in the social group (e.g., people or animals), environment (e.g., moving, sharing of space where cats sleep, eat, rest, or eliminate), and physical health (e.g., pain, systemic disease). As cats age and mature, their relationships may change. It is also not unusual for aggression to arise when a cat has been out of the home and then returns (e.g., from a groomer or veterinary hospital). The cat that remained in the home may be responding to some alteration in the way the cat looks, acts, or smells, which prevents familiar identification, while the returning cat may be painful and remain stressed for hours or even days, leading to conflict with other animals or people if not given sufficient time, space, and/or medication to recover.[44]

Redirected aggression is a common cause of acute-onset aggression between cats in the same household that have been living together amicably for quite some time. Occasionally, a family member will have observed the inciting event. More often this is not the case, and pet parents are often perplexed about why their pets suddenly do not get along. The injuries inflicted may be quite serious and the attacks unpredictable to the victim. In cases where there is an unexpected occurrence of intercat aggression for no apparent reason, historical evidence might suggest that one or both cats have exhibited high levels of fearful or territorial arousal, and unfamiliar cats have recently been visiting the pets' territory. In such instances, redirected aggression may be diagnosed even without knowing the inciting event.

No relationship has been found between age or source of acquisition, presence of other cats or the relationship of the cats in the household, or availability of contact with other animals or social contact with the family and the expression of aggression in general, although in one study, odds of intercat aggression were increased in cats that came to shelters as surrenders rather than strays.[18,19,27] While feline periuria behaviors such as urine marking are not classified as aggression, they are intimately involved, as both are generally motivated by FASCP.

Prevention

Selecting a friendly, well-socialized, outgoing kitten can be important, as kittens that exhibit fear and aggressiveness will likely continue to do so as adults. Kittens adopted at any age should have appropriate, low-stress socialization to as many stimuli as possible. Prevention of deficits in socialization or introduction to new people or animals by positive association will yield a better outcome and is safer than treating aggression once it has occurred (see Socialization in Chapters 2 and 5 and Learning in Chapter 10).

In one study, kittens that received addition handling, play, exposure to household sounds, and contact with people were less likely to exhibit fear responses to people at one year of age compared to the control group.[45] Veterinarians should educate pet parents about the concepts of socialization, habituation handling, and behavioral development, and how they can prevent such problems. Socialization to other cats, people, and other animals, habituation to noises, the cat carrier, and the pet parent's departure may help to prevent the FASCP which underlie most aggression. Intensity and potential for injury during play may be minimized by early socialization, provision of appropriate object and social play, positive reinforcement training, and avoiding punishment. Hand-raised kittens may be at particular risk of play-induced aggression if they do not have sufficient contact with other cats and play toys for chasing and biting during rearing.[37] Adopting two cats may be preventive (see Box 24.2).

Pet parent education regarding feline body language, husbandry, and training are also helpful, since prevention of aggression involves knowing how to recognize arousal and modifying the environment to reduce or prevent exposure to stimuli by keeping the cat from the stimuli or the stimuli from the cat. Much of the aggression displayed by cats is toward pet parents and is likely to be linked to their inability to understand and recognize stress in their cats. See Appendix A for resources. Early positive-reinforcement training to teach skills that can help manage the cats' behavior, establish a structured environment and way of interacting with others, can be helpful.

Gentle, positive handling exercises performed with kittens may help raise the adult cat's threshold for handling and petting. While the pet is being hand-fed its food or treats, the pet parent can gently handle all parts of the body. Pairing the treats immediately following the start of handling or stroking can help to develop positive associations. As days go by, the intensity and variety of handling should increase, gradually introducing brushing, touching the cat's claws with a clipper, or rubbing veterinary toothpaste on the cat's teeth. This process should be done slowly over weeks to months.

Introductions to visitors should be done at the cat's own level of comfort, rewarding it with treats or play if it approaches. Aggression can be displayed to veterinarians, to pet parents as they try to put their cat in the carrier to go to a veterinary appointment, or when the cat is painful or uncomfortable. Veterinarians should place emphasis on the use of medications, sedation, and anesthesia to minimize or alleviate pain. Gentle handling should always be used to minimize FASCP and pain at the veterinary office (see Chapters 1 and 16). Additionally, the importance of regular wellness visits to the veterinarian should be emphasized to address physical issues before they result in pain or discomfort which could lead to aggression (see Chapters 6 and 9).

When introducing a new cat, preemptive measures should be taken to allow for a slow introduction paired with pleasurable activities, ideally before the home cat establishes a home territory. Establish separate confinement areas or rooms. Initially, the resident cat can be given freedom of the entire home, while the new cat is given in its own room. Once the new cat is comfortable in its room, the situation can be reversed so that the new cat is given greater freedom while the resident cat spends time in its own room. This allows the cats to explore the area, determine escape routes, and deposit natural pheromones. The cats should be observed for FASCP during these exchanges, as the goal is calm, relaxed behaviors. Keep in mind even experienced cat parents, most likely do not understand the subtle signs of stress and need resources with which to educate themselves. Sometimes cats will react to the scent of other cats. Using scent exchange, where the scent of one cat is put on a towel which is then placed into the other cat's space, may help to acclimate cats. Food and play can be used to facilitate relaxed behaviors and condition a positive response to the other cat. The process will vary in duration and intensity and may take hours to months.[27] If done properly, it will seem as if all the steps were superfluous and unnecessary, since the cats will adjust seamlessly. In other words, if the procedure takes a while and there is no aggression but forward movement toward introduction, it is likely being done correctly. It is best to err on the side of caution, then hasten the pace if the introduction is going well rather than risk an altercation and backtrack to repair the damaged relationship. Even with proper introduction, certain individuals are genetically less social and may be more difficult to acclimate to a new member of the household.

It may be difficult to prevent outdoor cats from exhibiting territorial aggression, since this is an intrinsic behavior that is negatively reinforced through the retreat of the other cat or animal. Neutering will reduce a male cat's tendency to roam and fight with other males.[30] However, keeping the cat indoors or allowing safe outdoor access only within the pet parent's property or enclosed cattery is recommended.

Predation in cats is strongly influenced by early experience, including maternal effects and experience with prey animals.[46,47] Therefore, withholding hunting opportunities from young cats may decrease the likelihood of predation on animals with which they do not have experience. Adopting cats when they are kittens and socializing them to prey species may have a similar effect. Similarly, keeping cats indoors will reduce opportunities

Box 24.2 Factors favoring feline injurious play behavior ("play aggression")

Factor	Comments
Age of cat	The problem is more common in kittens and young cats.
Play experience as a kitten	The pet was encouraged to chase and attack hands and feet.
Number of cats in the household	The pet lives alone without other feline companions.
Type of play with pet parents	Play frequently involves rough play and teasing the pet with fingers or toes.
Amount of time spent alone	The pet is alone most of the day and spends little time with humans or other pets.

to practice predatory skills. Giving indoor cats plenty of appropriate predatory play opportunities can decrease future predatory behavior.

General environmental enrichment is paramount to the treatment of any feline behavior problem. By providing appropriate enrichment from adoption, the cat will be less likely to look for other enrichment opportunities which may lead to undesirable interactions and aggression.

Approach to diagnosis and treatment in general practice

As with all behavior problems, the following steps should be taken whenever possible: gather history, evaluate overall health and wellness, create a differential diagnosis list, and develop a treatment plan. Veterinarians working in general practice may not have enough time in one appointment to complete all of these steps. In these cases, history taking, diagnosis, and treatment can be divided over several appointments. How the case is approached depends somewhat on the resources available and the education level of the veterinarian. For feline aggression cases, ideally, the veterinarian would have at the ready an educated veterinary healthcare team member for pet parent education' handouts' book, web site, and video recommendations; the name(s) of positive reinforcement training professionals who are skilled with cats; board-certified veterinary behaviorist referral options for pet parents who need more help than can be provided by the primary care practitioner' and a foundational knowledge of feline behavior (see Appendix A).

Before considering how feline aggression or any type of behavior cases are seen at your practice, consider the amount of time that the veterinarian and the veterinary healthcare team has with each pet parent, the number of exam rooms, the flow of the hospital, the training of the team members, the ability of the team to perform diagnostic tests, and the interest of the veterinary team members in behavioral medicine. Regardless of what you decide regarding workflow, always assess the overall wellness of feline patients and treat immediately FASCP and pain if there is detriment to quality of life, the pet is at risk of euthanasia or risk to self, or the patient is in distress. See Chapter 1, 9, and 16 for more information on how to implement behavioral medicine in primary care practice.

History

Use of a short behavior questionnaire such as the one found in Appendix C, list of online resources at each appointment can facilitate the efficient acquisition of patient history and provide the veterinarian with the opportunity to practice preventative medicine instead of reacting to behavioral crises. Ask about who is involved, the body language of each cat, other pets in the household, latency to arousal (how quickly the aggression escalates), recovery time (how long it takes for the aggressor and the victim to return to a relaxed state), frequency (how often the aggression occurs over a period of time), the pet parent's stress level with this situation, if the pet parent is afraid of the cat, and any injuries.

Many pet parents have pictures and videos on their mobile devices, which can be extremely helpful when creating a differential diagnosis list. If the problem is stated to the client care representative at the time of scheduling, a request can be made for videos to be sent prior to the appointment. If that is not possible, viewing at the time of the appointment or after the appointment should be adequate. Videos are the gold standard; however, do not recommend that dangerous situations be triggered for the sake of a video. Videos from mild or low stress interactions and descriptions from pet parents, while not as helpful as a video, can still be very helpful. History should include a description of the cat's facial expressions and body postures, targets, and a description of all situations in which the aggression occurs. Care should be taken to review the history from the initial event to the current presentation because the consequences of each interaction can alter how each cat responds. For example, the cat that at the time of presentation appears to be the victim could have been the instigator originally or vice versa. Illustrations can help pet parents identify their cat's postures and states of arousal, especially if they have difficulty recalling precise descriptions of the cat's behavior. Illustrations are available online, which may be helpful to clinicians and pet parents[48] (see Appendix A). Often, pet parents will have formed an opinion of the situation before presentation which inevitably is tied to their emotions and feelings toward the cat. It is best to listen carefully, watch videos, view images, objectively collect information, and then make the decision as to how to move forward.

Most often, all cats in a multicat household should be evaluated and treated, even if one is the alleged victim. Aggression between household cats can also play a role in elimination problems. Cats may present to the veterinarian for periuria (e.g., urine marking, elimination) or perichezia (e.g., fecal marking, elimination) when in reality, the problem is related to intercat relationship difficulties.[7] Diagnosis of these conditions requires careful history taking with attention to intercat relationships.

Assessment of overall health and wellness

As with every behavior case, it is essential that the veterinarian first assess the cat's physical health to determine if there are any physical problems that might have caused or contributed to the aggression, as well as to decide the effect that these problems might have on treating the aggression. Painful conditions (e.g., abscesses, arthritis, anal sacculitis, dental disease), conditions affecting the central nervous system (CNS: e.g., brain tumors, encephalitis), sensory decline, and endocrine imbalances (e.g., hyperthyroidism) can all have a direct effect on behavior (see Chapter 6). Physical conditions can act in concert with environmental, genetic, and other health factors to lower thresholds of inhibition and result in exhibition of aggression. These might include abnormal neurotransmitter/receptor activity, CNS anatomic abnormalities (genetic, congenital, acquired), neoplasia (CNS tumors), metabolic disease states (hepatic encephalopathy, endocrine disorders), infections (rabies, feline leukemia virus, feline immunodeficiency virus), trauma (CNS injury), and toxins (lead, pesticides, illicit drugs), and cognitive dysfunction in senior pets. A pet's behavior may be affected during any developmental period from prenatal to adulthood but is most susceptible to pathological outcomes during the prenatal period and the first few months of brain development. Chronic or acute stress also plays an important role in the development of many feline health and behavioral disorders.[49,50] Cognitive dysfunction (brain aging) may also be a factor in older cats since altered social relationships are a commonly reported sign (see Chapter 8). Always conduct a thorough assessment of wellness in every involved cat, including a physical examination, screening lab work (CBC, serum chemistry, T4, U/A, proBNP, fecal float with antigen test with giardia)[51] based on age, health, and clinical signs. Treat for treatable disorders as well as FASCP. Presume that there is underlying pain or discomfort until proven otherwise and treat accordingly.

Diagnosis

Behavioral clinical signs may arise at any age, and may be of chronic or acute onset. Attempting to understand the cat's intentions, motivations, and signaling is essential for proper diagnosis and treatment. The list of potential causes of aggression is long and can seem confusing. See Box 24.3 for a complete list of diagnoses. The most important factor in treatment is not always finding that perfect diagnosis, but instead creating a complete list of credible differential diagnoses and identifying triggers for the aggression and the underlying motivation. In many cases, there may be mixed motivations or different motivations for similar-appearing situations. Most types of aggression exhibited by household cats have an underlying component of FASCP or pain. Any stimulus can cause virtually any type of aggression. The underlying motivation for the aggression is in the eye of the beholder. If, for example, a cat thinks that a pillow on the sofa is a threat, then it is. The veterinarian's job is to identify what the individual views as a threat and then formulate a treatment plan. The pet parent will have formed their own opinions about the motivation of the cat, which is usually linked to their emotions, together with anthropomorphism about what the cat is doing. Listen to the pet parent and collect objective information as well before making a differential diagnosis list.

What follows is a list of diagnostic criteria for different types of aggression or "labels" for the motivation or function of the aggression. Labels are helpful because they allow us to speak the same language. As veterinary healthcare team members, we use labeling throughout our day to communicate with each other and pet parents. We label diabetic cats as DKA (diabetic ketoacidosis) and cats with arthritis as painful. We label behaviors by making diagnoses; however, this concept is accompanied by the danger of tunnel vision and omission of the fact that there is much yet to discover about the motivations and functions associated with aggression. There is much overlap among the diagnoses below. There will be times when the practitioner may not be able to distinguish between territorial aggression and fear-induced aggression, for example. In cases such as these, it is best to write a list of differential diagnoses which may be ruled in or out, with additional time spent treating the case.

Behavioral diagnoses can be characterized as functional, motivational, or descriptive. The most common diagnoses in use at this time in North America are either descriptive or motivational. Descriptive diagnoses are as they sound, a description of what is occurring. Examples include petting-induced aggression (petting-related aggression) and intercat aggression. Motivational diagnoses attempt to assess the underlying emotional state or physiologic process causing the aggression. Examples include stress or fear-induced aggression. Functional aggression diagnoses are used more infrequently at this time and might include distance-increasing aggression.

Diagnoses of disorders of any body system reflect the level of our understanding of the problem at the time that the diagnosis is made. Just as a dog that is diagnosed with vomiting may be, after diagnostics, diagnosed with gastrointestinal lymphoma, a cat with intercat aggression may later be diagnosed with fear-induced aggression. At the first appointment, the motivation may not be clear; thus the pet is given a descriptive diagnosis. After more information is gathered in follow-up or upon reexamination, a motivational diagnosis can potentially be made.

In addition, there are qualifiers which may be applied to any diagnosis. They include redirected and impulsive. In the past, these might have been standalone diagnoses. However, currently, they appear to be best used as qualifiers, words that modify the meaning of the aggressive diagnosis by characterizing it further. A qualifier is not always necessary, but can further delineate the characteristics of the aggression.

Descriptive diagnoses

Cats that bite when petted and handled

Historically, a diagnosis of petting-induced aggression or petting-related aggression might have been used for cats that bite when handled or petted. These terms can be used as a catch-all until the motivation of the aggression can be ascertained. Any motivation can cause this behavior.

Some cats may not desire physical attention or may have a limited threshold for physical attention. This is more problematic when the pet parent's desire to interact through physical attention exceeds the tolerance of the cat. The observant pet parent may be able to tell when the bite is about to occur, as the pet usually will show typical behaviors, including fidgeting, tail twitching, tenseness, leaning away, ears flattened against the head, retraction of the lips, hissing,

---

Box 24.3 Aggression diagnoses

- Defensive aggression
- Fear-induced aggression
- Iatrogenic aggression
- Impulsive aggression
- Maternal aggression
- Play-induced aggression
- Possessive aggression
- Redirected aggression
- Stress-induced aggression
- Territorial aggression
- Predatory aggression
- Frustration-induced aggression
- Pain-induced aggresion

or even running away. These early body language cues intended to gain distance or cease the interaction may either be overlooked or misinterpreted. Pet parents who then chastise or scold the cat will often elevate the cat's stress, resulting in aggression rather than diminishing it.

Pet parents commonly ask why their cat is aggressive rather than simply avoiding, stopping, or leaving if they do not want to be petted. The reason may differ from cat to cat or even from one situation to the next. Some fearful cats may initially freeze rather than flee; when they can no longer tolerate physical contact, they become aggressive (fight). Other cats may enjoy brief amounts or petting but become annoyed with prolonged contact, similar to how a quick hug might be enjoyable, but a prolonged hug might be increasingly unpleasant or stifling. Petting or stroking on some areas of the body may be better tolerated than others. For example, gentle stroking of the facial area (temporal and perioral) is better tolerated than stroking of the caudal regions of the body,[52,53] possibly because it mimics locations where cats allogroom each other. In one study of shelter cats, following a brief handler education session, by providing cats with choice and control, paying attention to the cat's behavior and body language, and limiting touch primarily to the temporal region (base of the ears, cheeks, and under the chin), cats displayed significantly greater affiliative and positive behaviors and less aggression to humans, less conflict and a less negative emotional state.[54] In the same way, education of pet parents regarding recognizing and observing feline body language and where to pet a cat can alter the cat's response and increase the likelihood of positive interactions.

The history may reveal a cat that is initially calm and comfortable with being petted but bites after variable periods of attention. Other cats are tense and barely tolerant of any petting, but desire to rest in close proximity to family members. Tolerance for physical interaction may also vary based on the body area being petted or the circumstances during which physical contact occurs (e.g., cat versus pet parent instigated). While previously this was regarded as a separate diagnosis (i.e., petting-induced aggression), it is more likely that cats have varying motivations for aggression in this circumstance, ranging from anxiety to fear to pain. Whenever possible, the veterinarian should try to make a list of possible motivations for or functions of the behavior, regardless of the circumstance.

Aggression directed at other cats in the same household

Intercat aggression is a general term to describe aggression between two cats. Ideally, a motivational diagnosis or one that describes the function of the aggression would be made. When the diagnosis cannot be clearly found, it is best to write a list of differential diagnoses which may apply to the cats in question instead of using this catch-all term. Having a list of presumed differential diagnoses will aid the veterinarian in guiding the history taking in follow-up and will reduce the likelihood of tunnel vision in treatment. Because intercat aggression inherently involves more than one cat, a list of differential diagnoses should be made for each cat involved; the list of motivational or functional diagnoses may be different for each cat. It should not be assumed that the aggressor cat is the most confident cat when in fact the

aggressor may be the more fearful cat. That is one of the reasons why labeling the cat is not helpful, but making a list of differential diagnoses which focus on motivation or function of the behavior is more helpful. As mentioned in Chapter 2 and above, it is normal and expected for a cat to display aggression to an unfamiliar cat that enters its territory.

Defensive aggression and defensive behavior

Defensive aggression and defensive behavior describe aggression that stems from the condition of defending, resisting, or preventing aggression, attack, or threat. It is not intended to describe a certain emotional state, as cats that defend against an attack or fight back when swatted, for example, may or may not be fearful or anxious. In addition, defensive behavior is not necessarily abnormal or pathologic.

Defensive aggression is displayed in situations where the cat is threatened by a stimulus which is present or has a conditioned response (not necessarily emotional or accompanied by significant arousal) to a stimulus resulting in a past undesirable consequence. Defensive aggression can be associated with any body language (confident, relaxed, or fearful) before and after the aggressive response because cats displaying this type of aggression are not necessarily fearful but instead are reacting with aggression in defense of self or a location in which they have stationed. The aggression is characterized by short duration (lasting as long as the cat needs it to in order to repel the stimulus); measured response (as much aggression or force as needed to repel the stimulus); mild to moderate arousal (e.g., pupils may be dilated but not widely so) and immediate or very short recovery (cat returns to baseline within minutes) when the stimulus is removed. This is most likely a normal response in behaviorally appropriate animals when there is a threat without a fear component. Perhaps cats that were previously diagnosed with dominance, status-induced, or social status aggression would now be characterized as having defensive aggression with this current terminology.

Examples may include a confident cat that does not desire petting or a victim cat that is aggressive in defense of self when bitten by another cat but does not show signs of lasting fear, anxiety, or stress. For example, a friendly and confident cat is lying on the couch. Another cat with whom she gets along approaches and moves very close to lie next to her, potentially to displace her from her, comfortable resting spot. The resting cat sits up, swats the other cat in the face, and then lies back down and goes to sleep as the other cat retreats.

Iatrogenic aggression

Iatrogenic aggression is characterized by aggression which is caused by a medication, supplement, natural product, or procedure performed by a veterinarian. Aggression as an expression of altered mood is a possible side effect of corticosteroids, any medication which alters mentation (e.g., serotonergic medications, benzodiazepines, anticonvulsants, sedatives, opioids), and natural products (e.g., silver vine, catnip, pheromones) and over-the-counter products. Iatrogenic aggression can be the impetus for other types of aggression, such as fear-induced or redirected aggression, which may continue to be exhibited after the inciting stimulus for the iatrogenic aggression has been removed. Cats with iatrogenic aggression may have a long or short latency to arousal and recovery, depending on the situation, the effect of the medication or procedure, and the cat's level of FASCP. The frequency is consistent with the presentation of the stimulus or any conditioned stimuli. When prescribing medications which can cause a change in mood, hunger, or aggression, pet parents should always be advised of the risks.

Injurious play behavior

Play-induced aggression, while used in the past as a primary diagnosis, may not be an accurate description of the typical presentation of aggression during play. Cats that present for aggression during play often have normal play behavior which is undesirable or injurious due to circumstances (e.g., victim health) outside of the cat's control. They may also have been reinforced for inappropriate play behavior. If the pet parent has punished the cat for playing in a certain way, that can cause fear, anxiety, and stress. The function of aggression is to repel the recipient. Much of the aggression about which pet parents complain which occurs during play is not intended to repel the recipient but instead intended to perpetuate play. For this reason, injurious play behavior or undesirable play behavior may be more appropriate terms with which to describe this behavior.

When presented with human-directed aggression which resembles play, first, the veterinarian must distinguish between normal play and play-induced aggression. Play behaviors include: exploration and investigation; stalking, chasing, attacking, silent ambush, pouncing, and leaping sideways; fighting; wrestling; swatting; quick recovery; and vacillating between relaxed body language and spurts of energy and biting. Victims are generally familiar people or housemate animals, and the kitten may develop a preference for one target. Predatory play, which includes stalking, chasing, pouncing, grabbing, and biting, may have both appropriate (e.g., toys) and unacceptable (e.g., people) outlets. Kittens typically play hard with each other but quickly learn when they are actually causing pain. Since the bitten kitten will either stop playing or react with defensive responses, hard bites tend to become inhibited. Swatting is usually done with claws retracted. Vocalizations are rare during this type of attack, which can help differentiate it from other types of aggression (e.g., fear induced, territorial, redirected, pain-induced). In play, behavior becomes intolerable in single-cat households where the pet does not have the opportunity to engage in normal play with conspecifics.[24,55] In multicat households, problems occur when the object of play is another cat that is passive, weak, fearful, old, uninterested, or unable to respond appropriately (e.g., due to physical problems or insufficient previous socialization). This may result in the target developing fear-aggressive behavior toward the instigator. Then, the kitten that may be acting in a species-typical way can develop more serious aggression (e.g., play-induced, fear-induced). Pet parents often contribute to the problem by playing with kittens in a way that encourages attacks toward hands and feet, such as allowing kittens to bite hard at a gloved hand or moving their feet under blankets. This behavior generally begins when the pet is a kitten, peaks around 9–12 months, and then wanes as the cat grows into adulthood.

Although play directed at humans is not desirable, it is in many cases normal. Although the cat's intention is not to harm, play-related injuries can be serious, as the stalk-pounce-bite sequence of predation may not be sufficiently inhibited. In addition, humans lack the intraspecific communication and signaling responses of other cats, and human skin is not covered with a layer of fur. The behavior can be quite alarming and frightening for family members who may think they have a "mean" pet in the home. Injuries to family members may occur by attempting to handle, restrain, or punish the aroused kitten, especially if punishment leads to the development of fear-induced or defensive aggression in the cat. Regardless of the fact that the behavior is normal or pathologic, it can still be dangerous and should be treated. Play-induced aggression occurs when the cat's bites or scratches are deep, uninhibited, out of context, or more intense than would be expected with normal play. Cats may be overly aroused, or have a long or short latency to arousal and recovery. The body language is consistent with play. There is often a component of impulsive aggression or a history of frustration and punishment in these cases.

Maternal aggression

Maternal aggression refers to aggressive behavior directed toward people or other animals that approach the queen with her kittens. All mothers have protective instincts concerning their offspring. The intensity varies between individuals, with some exhibiting only mild aggression while others may attack and injure without warning. Queens that experience pseudocyesis (false pregnancy) may also display maternal aggression despite the lack of kittens. The diagnosis is made when a queen that has recently given birth or one with pseudocyesis shows aggression when someone approaches the kittens, kitten surrogates (e.g., toys), or nest area.

Motivational diagnoses
Fear-induced aggression

Fear-induced aggression is exhibited when a cat is exposed to someone (e.g., person, animal), something (e.g., sound, object), or a situation (e.g., veterinarian, car) that it perceives threatening, or a stimulus which is paired with something, someone, or a situation that is or was perceived as a threat, especially if there is no opportunity to escape. Body language before there is significant reinforcement or punishment of body language is consistent with fear. Cats with fear-induced aggression may have a long or short latency to arousal and recovery, depending on the situation and the cat's level of FASCP. The frequency is consistent with the presentation of the stimulus or any conditioned stimuli.

For example, a cat is at the veterinary clinic. The nurse reaches into the carrier to remove the cat and the cat hisses and spits. In this case, the threat is directly in front of the cat and she is fearful, so she reacts with aggression. In this situation, the presence of body language associated with fear, significant arousal, or longer than expected recovery time would help distinguish this from defensive aggression.

Finally, a cat goes to the veterinary clinic for an anesthetic dental cleaning. The cat comes home and the second cat that was left at home smells the scents (conditioned stimuli) of the veterinary clinic or sees the fearful, stressed, or painful body language of the returning cat. The second cat becomes fearful at the smell or sight of the first cat and hisses, spits, and swats when approached. This is consistent with fear-induced aggression because the stimulus causing the fear is present, the body language is consistent with fear, and there is significant arousal.

Frustration-induced aggression

Frustration-induced aggression is exhibited when the cat cannot achieve the outcome that she desires either because she does not have the appropriate communication skills, the pet parent does not recognize the signals, or the cat is physically prevented from engaging in escape or retreat from the situation. Cats may have any level of arousal or a short or long latency to arousal and recovery, depending on the level of frustration. Pet parents will often describe the cat as friendly except when they do not do what she wants or when he cannot get what she wants. Body language can be consistent with confidence or fear, and mild to moderate arousal. Owing to the unpredictability in the lives of most domestic cats, it is likely that this type of aggression is more common than we now recognize. Cats diagnosed with this type of aggression may have previously been diagnosed with status-induced or social status aggression.

For example, a friendly cat is sitting next to the pet parent as she works on her computer. The cat puts his paw gently on the pet parent's hand to solicit petting. His body language is relaxed. She stops to look at him and smiles but does not change her body posture to attend to him, and instead continues to type on the keyboard. After 10 seconds, he bites her, but does not break the skin. She pulls her hand away from him and verbally scolds him. He puts his ears back and jumps off of the desk. In this case, the cat wanted to be petted. The pet parent did not respond. The cat did not have any additional tools with which to communicate with the pet parent. When he was not petted, he bit her. When she scolded him, he had a fear response and moved away from her.

Pain-induced aggression

Pain is defined by the Merriam-Webster dictionary as "a localized or generalized unpleasant bodily sensation or complex of sensations that causes mild to severe physical discomfort and emotional distress and typically results from bodily disorder (such as injury or disease)" and "basic bodily sensation that is induced by a noxious stimulus, is received by naked nerve endings, is associated with actual or potential tissue damage, is characterized by physical discomfort (such as pricking, throbbing, or aching), and typically leads to evasive action." The International Association for the Study of Pain (IASP) defines pain as "An unpleasant sensory and emotional experience associated with, or resembling that associated with, actual or potential tissue damage." In addition, IASP notes that pain is always a personal experience that is influenced to varying degrees by biological, psychological, and social factors; and pain cannot be inferred solely from sensory neurons (https://www.iasp-pain.org/publications/iasp-news/iasp-announces-revised-definition-of-pain/). In light of these definitions, the diagnosis of pain-induced aggression can include

discomfort or pruritus caused by disorders which may not generally be regarded as overtly painful (e.g., inflammatory bowel disease, feline inhaled allergies, renal disease).

Pain-induced aggression can be distinguished from stress-induced aggression (see below) because the action from the stimulus causes pain or discomfort or is anticipated to cause pain or discomfort, whereas stress-induced aggression is related to cumulative or chronic stress which may or may not have a pain or discomfort component and can be due entirely to emotional stress.

Even the most sociable and docile animal may exhibit aggression when it is in pain, uncomfortable, or has sensory impairment (e.g., sight, hearing). Because pain monitoring is primarily a subjective assessment in cats, if there is any presumption of pain, it should be investigated and treated. If the pet parent declines diagnostics, the pet should be treated if safe to do so for the presumption of pain. Both acute and chronic pain may trigger aggression. Pain and discomfort are in the eye of the beholder. Gastrointestinal discomfort associated with constipation and pruritus resulting from atopy may cause aggression just as much as otitis externa or osteoarthritis. Handling or the anticipation of handling when a person approaches or reaches for a cat that is painful or ill might also result in aggression, even when the cat is tolerant of those interactions otherwise. Metabolic disorders such as liver disease, pancreatitis, renal disease, endocrine disorders, CNS disorders, or sensory decline might lead to aggression due to discomfort (see Chapter 6). All cats, but especially those that are presented for recent onset in aggression, should be examined for underlying physical conditions, including pain. Sometimes the diagnosis is straightforward: the cat experiences pain and reacts aggressively. The cat might hiss, snarl, and growl, or bite people if it perceives they are the cause of the pain. It is important to remedy the situation for both humane and welfare reasons for the cat as well as to prevent the problem from escalating. The cat that learns that biting accomplished its goals (i.e., stopped the painful interaction) might then use aggression when similar interactions arise in the future if it anticipates pain or has a negative association with being handled, even after the pain has resolved, as the cat may still anticipate a painful outcome. Degenerative disease, trauma, and illness that lead to pain or increased irritability may be difficult to identify; therefore, the history plus a full physical workup are essential for all aggressive cats. If pain is suspected, a trial with a pain control medication might be warranted. Cats with pain-induced aggression may have a long or short latency to arousal and recovery, depending on the situation and the cat's level of pain or discomfort. The frequency is consistent with the presentation of the stimulus or any conditioned stimuli.

For example, a cat that has osteoarthritis is lying on the couch. The large family dog approaches the couch and puts his nose on the cat, pressing on him. This causes the cat to feel discomfort. The cat bites him. In this case, the cat is painful and reacts to stop the dog from pressing on him so that he does not feel pain.

Possessive aggression

The terminology associated with aggression around resources is somewhat controversial and currently there is disagreement among some experts.[56] When a cat is aggressive within close proximity to food or resting spaces, what is the function of that behavior? Should we label aggression around valuable items resource guarding or possessive aggression? Could this behavior be caused by frustration, fear, anxiety, stress, hunger, or territorial behavior? As mentioned above and in Chapter 2, unrelated feral cats do not generally live in close proximity unless resources are plentiful. In our households, cats live in close proximity and may not only share a small feeding and watering space but also share one bowl. Resources are not limited to food and water. The pet parent is a valuable resource, as are resting and hiding spaces. Should this type of aggression be labeled based on potential motivation or function, such as fear or stress induced? There is much yet to learn about why animals show aggression over resources and what items, people, or animals are considered resources.

In this text, possessive aggression is intended to characterize a cat that is aggressive when another person or animal approaches the cat when it is near or in possession of something it values. Cats can show any body language from fearful to confident. Regardless of the body language, these cats are most likely living in a situation where the resources and/or environmental enrichment are not adequate for the population density. This is easily confused with frustration-induced aggression where the cat is eager to eat and bites the pet parent when she is not putting out the food fast enough. Cats that exhibit this type of aggression may have a long or short latency to arousal and recovery depending on the level of stress but will display aggression only when the valuable item is present. At the foundation of this behavior pattern is frustration and stress, not dominance. Cats that may have been labeled previously with status-induced or social status aggression may fall under the possessive aggression category with this classification.

Predatory aggression

Normal predatory behavior is often mistaken for aggression. Predatory behavior is not truly aggression because the goal is not to increase distance between the instigator and recipient. Cats may direct predatory behavior toward other pets cohabitating in the home, especially if those animals belong to species that are normally prey (e.g., mice, rats, birds, hamsters). Predation is a highly motivated, instinctive behavior for cats. Neurostimulation studies have mapped brain pathways evoking predatory behavior that differ from defensive aggression in the cat.[57] The initial movements of this behavioral sequence are characterized by silent stalking. The body is held close to the ground during the approach and the attack is patterned to achieve a quick kill of the prey. Predation is not preceded by vocal or postural threats in feral cats that are hunting because a warning to prey would be counterproductive. Kittens learning how to perfect their hunting skills may practice their predatory skills on any available target. Elements of predatory behavior may also appear as part of the play sequence with cats stalking, pouncing on, and biting not only toys but human feet and other pets. Parts of the predatory sequence may be exhibited during play, but in these cases the target may be nonprey animals (e.g., other cats, humans) and/or inanimate objects. While predatory aggression and behavior are most likely normal, they can

still be undesirable and may need treatment. If the bites and scratches are deep or uninhibited, or if the aggression causes a degradation of the quality of life of the human or animal victims, it should be treated. Cats may have a long or short recovery and latency to arousal. Aggression is accompanied by the body language consistent with predation.

Stress-induced aggression

Stress-induced aggression occurs when a cat is cumulatively (hours, days, weeks) in a state of intermittent or constant physiologic stress due to emotional and/or physical disease (e.g., painful, uncomfortable, metabolic) and shows aggression to a person, animal, or object which may or may not be the cause of the stress. Before or after the aggressive incident, the cat may show signs of fear, anxiety, and stress; however, because this type of aggression is a function of cumulative or chronic physiologic stress, there may be no clear body language precursors. Often, cats with stress-induced aggression do not show aggression consistently toward the victim or even consistently when put into the same situation or with the same stimuli. Incidents may be sporadic. This type of aggression could be described as threshold aggression. The cat is under cumulative stress and a single stimulus (e.g., situation, person, environment, animal) causes the cat to surpass the threshold for coping or tolerance, resulting in aggression. The difference between stress-induced and redirected aggression is that redirected aggression involves aggression to another stimulus which is then targeted to another animal, person, or object. Cats that express stress-induced aggression often appear to have a short latency to arousal (when in fact they are under chronic or cumulative stress); recovery can be variable and the body language can vary.

For example, a cat is emotionally stressed by the new baby in the house. The cat is approached by the pet parent when sleeping on the couch. The cat would usually welcome this approach and special time with the pet parent. However, the baby has been crying all evening and has just gone to bed. The pet has had to tolerate a very stressful evening, and when the pet parent goes to pet him, he bites her.

In another example, a cat with chronic rhinitis is lying on the pet parent's desk. He is not usually aggressive to the pet parent and sits with her frequently in the office. On this day, he is having particular difficulty breathing. The pet parent lifts him as she does often to put him on the cat tree in order to clear her desk, and he bites her. In this case, the cat has reached his threshold for physiologic and emotional stress and bites her potentially to try to keep her from moving him.

Territorial aggression

Territorial aggression is exhibited toward unfamiliar people or animals in the cat's territory, and can have body language consistent with fear or confidence. The underlying cause of territorial aggression is the social tension that arises from the intrusion of a new cat or person. Since cats will generally defend territory from unfamiliar cats that are not members of the colony, it might be expected that introduction of a new cat to a home with cats may initially be associated with territorial aggression toward the new cat, and that in return, the new cat might be fearfully or defensively aggressive.[9]

Territorial boundaries may vary greatly among cats, with some attempting to defend only a room in their home and others protecting a much larger area. This may be analogous to the home range of free-ranging domestic cats that contain a smaller core area where resources tend to be clumped, a larger territory that is defended, and areas outside the territory that may be shared by several individuals.[7] Thus, if one room in a home may be the cat's core area, particularly if it contains multiple resources, other rooms may be part of a territory and yet others "time-shared" without aggression as part of an overlapping home range.

Territorial aggression occurs in both females and males but can be particularly intense during the breeding season when males may protect extensive boundaries. The territorially aggressive cat may take a slow, steady approach as it stalks or it may immediately and aggressively chase the other cat. The focus on the intruder can be intense, and the cat can be very determined in pursuing and acting aggressively toward the newcomer. Though classically the victim is a cat, the target of aggression may be a person, child, or dog.

Cats exhibiting territorial aggression exhibit confident body language to actively expel perceived intruders (e.g., other cats, dogs, humans) from an area. This area may have defined boundaries, such as an entranceway to a room or house, or may be indistinct, such as the general area around one or more resources (e.g., chasing another cat out of the room that the pet parent currently occupies). For the latter, it may be difficult to differentiate between possessive aggression and territorial behavior. However, since territorial behavior often occurs because resources exist within a space, there may be considerable overlap between the two.

Diagnostic qualifiers

Impulsivity and aggression

Impulsivity can be a characteristic of almost any type of aggression. Impulsive aggression, while used historically as a standalone diagnosis, may be best used as a qualifier of other types of aggression. Impulsive aggression has a substantial, obvious sympathetic nervous system arousal component (e.g., piloerection, dilated pupils) and is characterized by sudden action which may appear automatic and out of context and proportion to the level of the stimulus, often ramping up with time exposed to the stimulus, and appears to the observer to be outside of the cat's control. It often does not respond to typical distraction such as the shake of a treat bag. Cats with impulsive aggression appear to have a short latency to arousal, long recovery, and body language consistent with significant arousal (e.g., widely dilated pupils, piloerection, ears flat back). The frequency is often intermittent and may have no identifiable stimulus. Impulsive aggression can stand alone as a diagnosis; however, it is often used as a qualifier to describe an impulsive component of another type of aggression. Other types of aggression such as fear-induced and territorial aggression can have an impulsive component or can look very similar to impulsive aggression. As more is learned about impulsivity in cats, the way that we characterize impulsivity will change as well.

For example, a pet parent is sitting calmly with a newly adopted cat nearby as they watch television. Without any new stimuli being introduced, the cat leaps up and wraps the front paws around the pet parent's arm, scratching and biting, pupils widely dilated, and tail piloerect.

Redirected

Redirected aggression occurs secondary to another type of aggression or motivation (i.e., there is an underlying aggressive motivation which is then being redirected to another target). Redirected aggression can be directed to any person, object, or animal, although in one study, when the cat could not direct the aggression toward the inciting stimulus, the pet parent was the most common target for aggression.[24] Redirected aggression occurs when a cat is highly aroused by a visual, auditory, or olfactory stimulus and redirects the aggressive response to a nearby person or animal because it is physically or socially prevented from accessing the target stimulus. Frustration can also contribute to redirected aggression. Classically, the aggression will occur when the victim (person or animal) approaches or just happens to be near the aroused cat. Since the aggressor may be vigilantly focused on the stimulus, the victim may approach without noticing that the cat is already in an aroused state and the aroused cat may not notice the soon-to-be victim. In some situations, the victim is not nearby and the aggressor may bypass the nearest individual to target a specific victim. This is especially true if the pattern is chronic. The attacks are often acute, intense, and seemingly unprovoked, with multiple deep bites and severe injuries. The aroused cat may exhibit hypervigilance, agitation, nervous pacing, piloerection, fixed gaze, tail thumping, dilated pupils, lunging, growling, yowling, and biting. The latency to arousal often appears short; the recovery and frequency will vary. If the association between reduction of stress and biting the victim becomes conditioned, which can happen with any type of aggression, the aggressor may seek the victim out and bite them, as a way to reduce the physiologic stress response.

While the most common triggers for redirected aggression are other cats, loud noises, and unknown people, any aversive sight, sound, or odor, as well as pain or other fear or stress-inducing stimuli, can elicit redirected aggression.[24] Pet parents cannot watch their cats constantly and so the triggering event and original target may not be readily apparent. If the cat displays body language consistent with fear, the behavior is likely motivated by fear.[24]

A common situation is one in which an indoor cat that is sitting by a window becomes aroused or distressed upon seeing or hearing an outdoor "intruder" cat. The cat then directs its aggression to a person, cat, dog, or object that happens to be nearby. If these episodes occur when the pet parent is away, out of the room, or sleeping, they may see or hear the results of the fight but not be aware of the feline intruder (or other stimulus) that initiated the cascade of aggression.

If an aggressive display or heightened arousal by a cat toward an unfamiliar cat outside the home is observed, the pet parent may initially attempt to disrupt the event by nudging the pet away from the window, picking the cat up to calm it, or punishing the cat. Any of these interactions may cause the cat to attack the pet parent.

The relationship between the aggressor and victim may quickly change following an episode of redirected aggression. The aggressor may continue to exhibit aggressive behavior toward the victim, even after the inciting trigger is long gone. This may be due to ongoing arousal and/or a learned association or conditioned emotional response between the victim and prior negative experience. Understandably, the victim may also be fearful of the aggressor and exhibit fear-induced aggression whenever it sees or is approached by its former attacker, even if that cat is no longer aggressive. The aggressor, in turn, may react to its housemate's change in behavior and respond aggressively in kind, perpetuating the aggression between the two.

In general, the history will suggest that the victim was nearby at the time the cat was threatened, territorially aroused, afraid, or fighting. The diagnosis involves recognizing that a specific stimulus or situation has aroused the cat and resulted in a nearby person or animal being attacked. A cat may stay in a high state of arousal long after exposure to the inciting stimulus, (hours to several days) making the initial cause difficult to identify.[58]

Prognosis

Aggression has historically been characterized and prognosis affected by severity of injury to the victim; however, the severity of a bite or the bite level is affected by many extrinsic and intrinsic factors, including the overall health and behavior of the victim (e.g., pulling the limb away, overall health, skin thickness, bite location) and ability of the cat to do damage (e.g., length of exposure to the victim, relative size of the cat to the victim, bite strength, skull size, skull shape).[59,60] In addition, there is no literature which supports injury to victim as a predictive factor. For these reasons, injury to the victim is not an accurate predictor of the severity of the aggression nor the likelihood or severity of future aggression. Prognosis is not set for any one animal or diagnosis. The prognosis will depend to much extent on the family's ability to live with the cat, adhere to treatment recommendations, and keep family members safe (see Box 24.4).

As should be clear, prognosis depends on many factors which are for the most part out of the veterinarian's control. It is impossible to predict the outcome of any particular case; however, in general, pet parents can be counseled that the best prognosis lies with cases which are predictable and avoidable. Pet parents who are able to adhere to treatment recommendations will generally have better outcomes than those who cannot. Any discussion of predictability should come with a discussion of the obvious triggers for the aggression. Many pet parents will report that their cat has unpredictable or unprovoked aggression when in most cases, thoughtful behavioral history taking may reveal that it is in fact chronic, there is a learned component, and there are identifiable triggers. The decision to keep a cat that is aggressive in the family is a personal one. Pet parents need the full picture in order to make a decision as to whether or not to treat their cat.

For some types of aggression, the prognosis has been established historically in certain populations. For example, in a retrospective study of 48 cases of intercat aggression, 62% were cured with proper treatment.[29]

Treatment

After a differential and/or final diagnoses are made and assessment of overall health (e.g., pain, discomfort, systemic

---

Box 24.4 Considerations when advising pet parents of prognosis

- Bite severity (e.g., force of bite, age of victim, victim's response, victim's health)
- Predictability of aggressive events (e.g., aggressive events occur with reliable triggers)
- Context of aggressive events
- Ability to avoid of aggressive events (e.g., the cat can be separated from the victim)
- The family's bond with the cat
- Ability of the family to adhere to treatment recommendations
- Ease with which cat takes medication
- The individual cat's ability to cope with stress and be behaviorally flexible
- The cat's genetic predispositions
- Epigenetics (e.g., environmental factors affecting genetic expression)
- Socialization, learning, training, and life experience
- Level of arousal associated with aggression
- Chronicity of problem
- Use of positive punishment
- Presence of a negative CER to stimulus
- Cat's recovery time from stressful events or aggressive bouts
- Latency to aggression when exposed to the stimulus
- Presence of immunocompromised or at-risk animals or people to whom exposure cannot be limited or avoided
- Liability to the family if the cat bites again
- Ability to identify arousing stimuli
- Frequency of stimulus exposure
- Ability of family members to recognize and avoid the aroused cat
- Innate nature of the behavior (e.g., predatory aggression)

---

disease) is under way, all behavioral treatment can begin. There are some cases of aggression which may resolve without treatment such as reintroduction of cats that had one bout of aggression after a visit by one of the cats to the veterinary hospital or iatrogenic aggression with no reinforced or punished consequences, and for which the inciting external factor has been discontinued. However, most aggression cases will at minimum need environmental management. Some will need neurochemical modulation and environmental changes. Still others will need behavioral treatment, neurochemical modulation, and environmental changes.

Treatment includes assessment of risk to others (e.g., people, other animals) and risk to self (e.g., self-injurious behaviors, euthanasia, relinquishment); treatment of comorbidities of systemic disease or pain; environmental modification; behavioral treatments; and modulation of neurochemistry (e.g., diet, supplements, medications). Every patient does not need all modalities; however, each case should include a risk assessment, treatment of physical disease, and reduction of FASCP, whether indirectly with management changes and behavior modification or whether medications, diet, and supplements would also be indicated or required.

Potentially because there is still much to learn about why cats are aggressive or because most aggression stems from FASCP, there is overlap between treatments regardless of the type of aggression. Treatments are divided into categories and particular instructions for individual types of aggression are noted where necessary (see Box 24.5).

Box 24.5 Treatment of feline aggression

Steps	Comments
Safety first	• Educate pet parents on the signs of arousal, when to approach and not approach aroused cats, risk, liability, and separation from children.
Assess overall wellness	• Conduct a thorough physical examination, screening lab work, and history. • Rule out any iatrogenic causes and physical conditions that might be contributing factors to aggression.
Identify and manage exposure to stimuli	• Identify all aggression-provoking stimuli and the thresholds (intensity or distance) at which the behavior occurs. • Avoid triggers. • Cover windows, block off rooms, and create a sanctuary space. • Stop all behaviors which trigger aggression such as touching, handling, play, or letting outdoors. • Separate from other animals or people. • Remove or repel outdoor cats.
Enrich the environment	• Enrich the environment, rotate toys, spread out resources, manage the cat's time with puzzle toys, add resting and hiding spaces.
Desensitization and counterconditioning	• Consider this treatment if the pet parent has the time and inclination to work with the cat(s) long term. Always recommend a behavior professional to assist with this procedure.
Positive reinforcement training	• Habituation to a sanctuary space or wearing a body harness and leash might need to be implemented in advance of exposure as a safety precaution. • Teach touch, go to your spot (station, place), leave it, and settle.
Drug and supplement therapy	• SSRIs, SNRIs, and TCAs may be effective at modifying the FASCP in cats. • Treat any pain or discomfort, including pruritus. • Medications such as buspirone, gabapentin, or benzodiazepines may help to reduce fear and anxiety. • Supplements such as L-theanine or alpha-casozepine can be used to reduce fear and arousal.
Pheromones	• Feliway Classic, Feliway Multicat (or Feliway Friends) and Feliway Optimum can be used to change arousal.

Also see online resources Intercat Aggression and Cat Aggression to People

Safety first

Pet parents should be educated on how to recognize signs of arousal and how to handle the aroused cat. This is especially essential when situations that may trigger aroused or aggressive behavior are unknown or are not easily prevented. Pet parents can often recognize that their cat is distressed and try to comfort the cat, even when the cat has been aggressive toward them. However, when the pet is in a high state of arousal, the ideal way to respond is to maintain physical distance from the cat to allow time for it to deescalate. This may entail leaving the cat in its current location and closing the door. The cat's view of the target may be blocked by a piece of large poster board; introducing a visual barrier may reduce arousal but should not be used to threaten the cat. If the cat must be relocated to another room for safety reasons or to avoid continued exposure to the trigger, avoid touching or approaching the cat. The cat may be called away with a lure or a reward-based command (e.g., food time, play time, mat, or carrier). If the cat must be handled, covering it with a thick blanket may be calming, reduce visual stimulation, and provide a level of physical protection from claws and teeth. Then it can be transported to another room. Settling may take several hours or several days, so the room should be prepared ahead of time with food, water, and a litterbox. It may help to keep the lighting muted or dark to facilitate calming. Avoid checking in on the cat frequently, since this may prolong arousal.

Keeping the aggressive pet in the home always includes some risk. Past behavior does not predict future behavior with accuracy, meaning that just because a cat has not bitten in a certain situation does not mean that he will not bite in that situation in the future. Also, one bite, even if severe, does not necessarily predict that the cat will ever bite again. For these reasons, counsel the pet parents on all circumstances which may result in aggression and instruct them to avoid them. Remind them that society is litigious and they can be sued for the injuries due to a cat bite.

Environmental management

Environmental management consists of creating an environment where aggression is unlikely to happen and enriching the environment to lower stress.

Stop all physical punishment

Use of positive punishment, such as squirting with water, yelling, chasing, or swatting an aggressive cat, increases its arousal and anxiety and increases the risk of injury for family members. These methods are ineffective and counterproductive in the long term and have been associated with more severe aggressive behavior.[28] Similarly repeating situations which resulted in the aggressive event to ascertain the severity of the problem typically results in the cat becoming more sensitized, rather than desensitized, to the trigger situation and quicker to escalate to a more intense aggressive response. In summary, positive punishment, which is commonly used by pet parents, is ineffective at stopping aggressive responses and increases the likelihood of aggression in the future.

Avoid triggers

Situations that may result in aggressive behavior must be avoided. In some cases, prompt separation, avoidance of stress, and allowing a recovery period may provide a simple and effortless resolution. Until the pet is successfully treated, it should be prevented from having any exposure to stimuli that trigger aggression. Repetition of unpleasant exposures for the cat is likely to worsen the fear rather than improve it – many pet parents attempt to desensitize the cat and instead, they are actually sensitizing it. Although the goal is gradual improvement through positive exposure to stimuli, prevention and avoidance are necessary for immediate management and often the most practical long-term strategies.

For cats in which stimuli outside incite aggression, limiting the opportunities to see the triggers may be useful. This may be accomplished by blocking access to windows, covering windows with window film or window coverings, making the site less pleasant (e.g., with a strip of carpet runner nubs up or double-sided tape), or confining the cat away from windows with exposure to the stimuli. Furniture and desired resting places may be rearranged to prevent a perch for vigilance and reactivity. The family may describe how much the cat "loves to look out windows," but some cats are actually on guard and reactive rather than enjoying the view. Body postures and behavior must be assessed to ascertain the true motivation, and window access may need to be denied in order to reduce the cat's state of arousal.

For cats that exhibit maternal aggression, treatment would include avoiding approach when the queen is in her nest. For cats that become highly aroused after going outdoors, they should be confined indoors. If the cat becomes aroused watching outdoor cats through windows, that opportunity should be removed by closing drapes, covering windows with window film, or blocking access to windows by closing doors to those rooms or reducing the appeal of the area such as with double-sided sticky tape on windowsills, while providing equally or more appealing locations for resting, perching, and enrichment. The pet parent could also discontinue feeding stray animals, secure trash cans to discourage scavengers, and remove bird feeders that might provide hunting opportunities for predatory cats entering the yard. Unwelcome feline visitors may be further discouraged by environmental modifications, including the use of motion-activated sprinklers, aerosol or ultrasonic deterrents, olfactory repellents (fox urine or cayenne pepper), or unpleasant surfaces such as upside-down carpet runners or rough-surfaced/shoe-cleaning welcome mats. Capture and humane removal may also be a consideration for stray animals.

For pets that are aggressive toward other pets in the home, the pets should be separated until well after arousal has subsided and when they cannot be directly supervised, which may be hours or days. Providing the victim pet with a secure location to avoid interaction with the aggressor cat, even if it is a kitten (elevated resting areas the kitten cannot reach) or seclusion in a room or crate may be helpful.

Other strategies for safe physical management include room confinement, baby gates, crates, or harnesses. Sometimes the addition of an automatic door closer can lessen the risk for an escape, thus reducing the opportunity for an aggressive event. Sometimes a cat should be boarded rather than risk exposure at an event while medication dosages are tested and the house is prepared for proper management.

For cats that exhibit pain-induced aggression, avoid handling and manipulation of a cat in pain. If the pet parent can bring the cat to the veterinary clinic for any needed treatments, that may be enough to avoid aggression until the primary disease is treated. However, this is not always practical, especially when frequent treatments are necessary to treat the cause of pain. This is one of those times where medications which reduce FASCP are necessary and humane, not only to treat the underlying source of pain or discomfort but also to treat the stress, distress, and further learning that comes with handling

and treatment. Pet parents should avoid touching their cat in places which are known to be painful.

If nonpainful petting or physical touch elicits aggression, petting should be avoided. This is very difficult for pet parents to understand and they often resist this recommendation. A peaceful compromise may be found by limiting petting (e.g., petting only on the cat's head for five strokes), then ceasing all petting and observing the cat's response. The cat is then allowed to signal consent for further physical interaction by moving closer to the pet parent, initiating contact, etc. This is commonly referred to as a consent test. If the cat moves its body closer to the pet parent's hand (consents to petting), the pet parent can pet again for five more strokes on the head, then stopping and awaiting the cat's response. If the cat does not solicit petting (move closer to the hand, bunt the pet parent), it is not desired and the pet parent may not pet him. If the cat's response to the consent test is equivocal, it is best to withhold additional physical interaction.

For cats with undesirable predatory or play behavior and play-induced or predatory aggression, play with hands and feet or any other body part should be discontinued. Cats that bite pet parents during the night as they move should be kept outside of the bedroom or put into a sanctuary space (see Chapters 5, 15, and 17). Keeping the cat's nails trimmed or temporarily covering them with claw caps may help to decrease scratch-related injury. Attempts to redirect rather than suppress the cat's predatory behavior toward more acceptable outlets will be most successful.

In order to maximize opportunities for avoidance, the locations of resources such as food, resting areas, and litterboxes should be distributed throughout the house to allow all feline household members access to them without forcing contact with another cat. This may entail providing multiple litterboxes, perches, food and water bowls, etc. in strategic locations to aid the behavior modification program.

Environmental enrichment

Environmental enrichment can mitigate stress in cats and increase the threshold for aggression. For example, aggression between cats in the same household may center around resources (possessive aggression) or access to spaces (defensive or territorial aggression). Both of these types of aggression can be improved or possibly resolved in the examples above by adding resting and perching spaces, increasing the number of and the locations of feeding and watering stations, and enrichment toys.

Cats with undesirable predatory behavior or predatory or play-induced aggression can be given motorized and remote-control toys with which to play that will distance them from the pet parent and promote independent play. The most important consideration is to provide and encourage plenty of hunting opportunities that involve acceptable chase and attack behavior. Toys that bounce, flutter, or move in a way that entices the cat to chase should be provided. The pet parent should use toys preemptively at times of night or day when the cat is likely to desire play. As cats are more likely to engage in more intense play and predation when hungry, feeding multiple small meals and placing food inside puzzle and manipulation toys may aid in reducing the problem behavior. In addition, if the cat tries to play with the pet parent inappropriately, the pet parent should immediately stop all play and move away from the cat. Allowing the cat to engage in predatory behavior directed toward toys may be an acceptable alternative. Playing with different toys that allow the cat to perform different aspects of the predatory sequence (e.g., stalking and pouncing on a feather wand; chasing, grabbing, and biting a plush toy; running after and consuming a treat tossed down a hallway) may also be helpful. Increasing mental enrichment via puzzle toys may also provide both physical and mental exercise for food-motivated cats. It may also be beneficial to add another cat to the home. However, adding an additional cat, even if the cat already in the home has play-induced aggression or inappropriate play behavior, does not guarantee a positive result.

Behavior modification

Positive reinforcement training may be used to teach cats acceptable behaviors to perform as an alternative to exhibiting aggressive responses. For example, the cat could be trained to offer an alternate behavior incompatible with the aggressive response. These might include coming to the pet parent on cue, stationing (i.e., going to a specific location) on a cat tree, relaxing on a mat, and turning away from a stimulus. Cat pet parents may not realize that cats can be taught tricks using positive reinforcement training and are often amazed at how quickly their cat learns to sit, come, or jump to an elevated perch on cue.

Training cats is not impossible and can be very rewarding. Cats are not little dogs. They learn as they do most things in life, in short spurts. In addition, because they are free fed and not exposed to different types of foods, they may be challenging to motivate. Behavioral treatments can be facilitated by feeding on a schedule and holding the sessions just prior to mealtime when the cat might be most food motivated. It is not recommended to completely delay meals or withhold food from cats in order to increase food motivation (see Chapter 13). Special food treats should be restricted to training sessions. If the cat is not particularly motivated by food, other reinforcers may be used. For instance, a toy may be used to lure a cat to a spot on the cat tree, followed by a brief session in that location. It may take a little effort and creativity to determine what motivates an individual cat.

Habituation may occur when the fear is mild and the cat is able to adjust at its own pace. Early recognition and intervention lead to the most effective outcomes. For example, a cat that hisses and jumps up on a table when a new dog is introduced to the household may eventually habituate to the presence of the dog as long as the dog is prevented from barking at, chasing, or otherwise inciting more fearful or fear-aggressive behavior from the cat over time. Full exposure to threatening stimuli that elicit a strong fear response should be avoided (e.g., flooding, response blocking).

Desensitization involves repeatedly exposing the cat to modified or attenuated representations of the fear-evoking stimuli that are below the threshold that evoke a fear response until the cat is comfortable. Desensitization and counterconditioning (DS/CC) techniques are frequently combined when treating aggression by using repeated, controlled, below-threshold exposures to stimuli that trigger the behavior while pairing with food, treats, or toys with each exposure. For DS/CC to be successful, the cat's threshold for arousal must be identified and exposure to the fear-eliciting stimuli carefully adjusted to maintain the cat below its fear-eliciting threshold. See Chapter 10 for a full discussion of behavioral treatments. There is inherent risk during these exposures and the pet parent must provide complete management of the cat to avoid aggressive responses. The situation may worsen if the cat learns that growling, scratching, and biting are effective ways to avoid fear-or stress-inducing stimuli or situations. DS/CC requires a very high skill level and knowledge of cat body language. This should only be attempted with a qualified, skilled positive reinforcement trainer or veterinary healthcare team member. Cats learn from each exposure. Behavior modification attempts that end with the cat in an aroused and agitated state are not productive (and not desensitizing), and are counterproductive. Failed attempts to perform desensitization exercises for an aggressive cat will further condition the aggression and put the cat at risk of euthanasia or relinquishment.

Many cats may be successfully treated with counterconditioning alone involving food rewards or favored play toys to encourage appropriate responses and associations with the stimulus.

Examples of desensitization and counterconditioning

Aggression related to petting

For cats that are intolerant or uncomfortable with petting and there is no underlying source of pain or discomfort, DS/CC can be attempted. Before this treatment is started, the pet parent should be educated to the concept of consent and the cat's right to say "no." In our society, we recognize the right of any human being to deny physical contact from another, even a family member. While it may be a new concept for humans, in fact for cats, much aggression would be avoided if we accepted that cats will and should be able to say "no" to physical interactions. When pet parents are educated, they often choose to refrain from petting the cat so very often or in certain places because they finally can see life from the cat's point of view.

If pet parents want to pursue DS/CC to touch or handling, the pet parent must first determine how long the cat can *always* be stroked before it becomes agitated. The body area where the cat is most tolerant of touch should be determined, as well as when the cat will most likely be in the right emotional state to engage in social interaction. These times may be limited to very specific situations. The cat's emotional state and willingness to interact should determine the pace and design of the desensitization program. Petting should then take place for a short period of time (e.g., 1 second; one stroke) and stop before the threshold for anxiety or tension is reached. A high-value food incentive or other reinforcer may be given immediately after the bout of petting. The cat should not be restrained or confined, as it is an acceptable option for the cat to elect to jump down or move away rather than become aggressive. The sessions can gradually be lengthened as the cat's arousal and tension decrease, and as the cat learns to enjoy, or at least tolerate, longer stroking sessions in anticipation of a treat or other reward. The pet parent must be instructed to always look at the cat's communication signals and to avoid absentmindedly stroking or approaching the cat between counterconditioning sessions, since this will result in arousal or tension and will counteract the conditioning sessions, causing treatment failure. If the cat solicits interactions, the pet parent may engage the cat for a brief period but not longer than the cat's baseline tolerance for petting, even if the pet seems to enjoy the interaction. As improvement is noted, the pet parent may initiate short affection sessions but must stop the affection before the cat gets aroused or aggressive. As the cat becomes more comfortable with predictable and positive physical social interactions, it may solicit attention. This is an appropriate and desirable outcome, especially if the cat was not social and solicitous previously.

Some cats may never learn to tolerate as much physical affection as their pet parent wants to give. This can be extremely distressing to some pet parents, greatly straining the human–animal bond. Positive reinforcement training, particularly clicker training, may help rebuild the bond by allowing the pet parent and cat to interact and communicate without the need for physical contact. Similarly, other forms of enrichment, such as play with wand or chase toys or provision of food-puzzle toys and catnip toys, may also give pet parents the opportunity to engage with their cats without the risk of aggression.

Aggression to cats in the same household

For cats that show aggression to other cats in the household, DS/CC can facilitate reintroduction; however, this is most successful when the cats also have been taught operantly conditioned self-control tools such as go to a place (stationing), target training, come, and settle. This is usually easiest to accomplish with clicker training (see Chapter 10).

Regardless of the method used, reintroduction should be gradual, closely supervised, and associated with positive interactions such as feeding, just as if new pets were being introduced to the home. In highly aroused cats, this reintroduction program can take from a few days to a year. Pet parents must be educated on the amount of time this will potentially take and the likelihood of relapse after the treatment is discontinued. The work of DS/CC is time consuming and tedious. In addition, there is a good likelihood of relapse if management falters or the stress level in the house gets too high. For the cats to complete the reintroduction process, one or both cats may need to be medicated to reduce FASCP because food may not be an adequate reinforcer to reduce the fear in the face of a threat such as another cat that has shown aggression or overarousal of the aggressor. Pet parents should be given the option of keeping the cats separated in the home for the life of the cats, and should be educated that this is akin to the pet parent having to live with someone that physically harmed them, sometimes repeatedly. Help the pet parent understand that this situation is very stressful for the cats. Complete separation or rehoming one of the cats are acceptable options which may improve the quality of life of one or both cats as well as the pet parents.

Cats should not be allowed to fight it out, as these fights do not settle conflicts and may make the situation worse. Cats that consistently fight should be completely separated by a closed door without sight of each other outside of training sessions. All experiences should be positive during the reintroduction process. This gives both cats an opportunity to relax (reduced arousal) without the fear of being retriggered by the presence of the other cat. Each cat may be confined for part of the day to a room or half of the house, space permitting. Basic needs including food, litterboxes, scratching posts, toys, and resting areas must be available in both locations. The cats' locations may be rotated, preferably without the cats seeing each other, to allow both cats time in different areas of the house.

Because cats communicate by leaving pheromones (skin secretions, urine) on surfaces within their living areas, permitting both cats to explore areas where the other cat has been allows for chemical communication between them without having to respond to the other's physical presence and aggressive displays. This also ensures that both cats continue to be familiar with all areas of the home and learn to access hiding places or retreat strategies. To expand on semiochemical signaling, cats may be groomed or gently toweled with a cotton cloth, including the chin, paws, and perianal regions. The cloth can then be placed in the other cat's area while giving food rewards. This may artificially mimic allomarking behavior and create a "group scent" as well as refamiliarizing both cats with the other cat's pheromones.

The door that separates the cats provides an opportune location for DS/CC; peaceful coexistence on opposite sides of the closed door may be reinforced as the first step of the behavior modification process. Both cats may be fed simultaneously or offered treats, catnip, or play on either side of the closed doors so both cats associate hearing and smelling the presence of their counterpart on the other side of the door with a positive experience. Mutual play may be encouraged through the provision of toys attached by a string threaded under the closed door; when one cat manipulates a toy, the attached toy is moved in the other cat's space.

Once the cats are comfortable hearing and smelling the other cat on the other side of a closed door, the doorway may be modified to allow varying degrees of visual desensitization or safe tactile desensitization. Pet parents can be very resourceful in making modifications, ranging from installing screen doors, plexiglass barriers, or baby gates in doorways. These may be partially covered to decrease visual contact if needed (see Figure 24.6A and B). Provision of small amounts of highly desired treats such as fresh fish, meat, shrimp, canned foods, or for some cats, whipped cream, will allow continued classical counterconditioning to the presence of the other cat, rather than just tolerance. At first, the pet parent may only allow the cats to see each other through the gate or screen door during specific, staged training periods; the solid door is closed when the pet parent is not present to manage the cats' interactions. Harness training can also be completed and used as a pathway for safe introduction once the door is opened. The family should be patient, since desensitization to the harness itself may take a couple of weeks, depending on the arousal of the cat and the ability of the pet parent. While desensitizing a cat to wear a harness is a difficult and tedious task for most pet parents, it is likely easier in comparison to desensitization to the approach of a fear-evoking stimulus. Therefore, pet parent success at the exercise with a harness may predict success in other contexts.

As the cats exhibit increased tolerance of each other's presence during pet parent-monitored interaction, the solid door

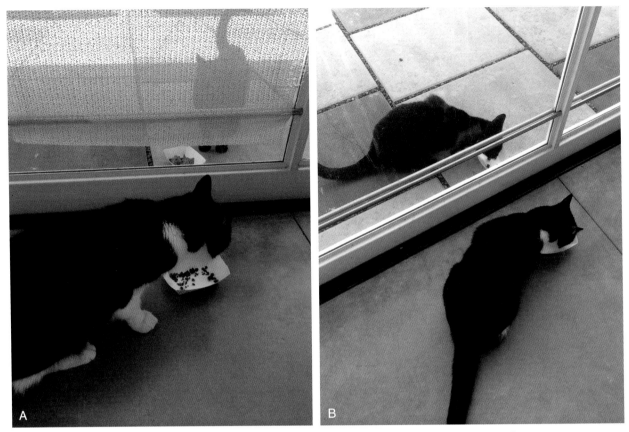

Figure 24.6 (A and B) Steps of desensitization and counterconditioning. Translucent window covering decreases visual contact (A) until both cats are comfortable enough to remain calm in each others' presence (B). *(Attribution: Karen Sueda.)*

may be left open for longer, unsupervised periods. Observation of the cats' willingness to eat, play, or sleep near the doorway indicates a positive change. If the cats are agitated and aroused by the presence of the other cat behind a door, this predicts a poorer long-term prognosis for harmonious resolution.

Over time, the goal is gradually to expose the cats to each other in very controlled situations. This can be done with the cats in carriers or controlled with a harness and leash at opposite ends of the largest room or longest hallway in the home. During the sessions, the cats are fed highly palatable food or engaged in play. During subsequent sessions, the cats are gradually brought closer together.

Once the cats are showing no tension at close proximity to each other during the sessions, the pet parent can attempt to allow them to have freedom in the same room. Initially, and until there is believed to be minimal risk for injury, this should only be allowed when the pet parent is present in the space. Training the cats to respond to few simple commands, through clicker training, for example, can greatly facilitate the reintroduction process. Both cats may be taught to go to an elevated "safe space" on cue, come when called, or look at the pet parent to end stare-downs between the cats. Cats can also be rewarded when they exhibit calm body language and behavior in the other cat's presence. When the cats are finally allowed to roam freely in the home, the home environment must be staged in order to maximize resource abundance and minimize forced interaction and physical proximity to the other cat. Multiple feeding and drinking stations, litterboxes, preferred resting areas, scratching posts,

and toys should be strategically located so the cats can avoid each other and are not trapped or surprised by the other. Along that vein, providing sufficient climbing, hiding, and perching areas (three-dimensional space) allows the victim the opportunity to prevent conflicts. Electronic cat doors (Sureflap, Cambridge, United Kingdom), which are opened only by the cat wearing the collar that activates the door, are also a means of allowing the victim cat the opportunity to access the entire home but also to retreat to a safe, secure area. Also See Online resource Appendix C - Intercat Aggression.

Aggression toward humans

For cats that are aggressive toward one family member or visitors, the pet parent should be given the option to keep the cat separated entirely from that person. Avoidance is a straightforward way to resolve the problem. If that choice is made, the focus would be on teaching the cat to accept a sanctuary space. If a cat is aggressive toward a child, it is always better to simply live separated. See Chapter 4 for more information about how to manage aggression toward children.

If the pet parent chooses not to keep the cat separated from the individual, they must accept the risk associated with injuries that may result. If the pet parent decides that introduction is appropriate or necessary, the concepts and risks are similar to the introduction of two fighting cats, above. There should be no negative exposures during the conditioning process until the cat has fully accepted the new person. The acceptance of food does not align with the acceptance of the individual.

Some pet parents begin by immediately asking a visitor to extend a hand with a food treat toward the pet's face. Reaching toward the cat may elicit a fear-aggressive response even if the intension was to offer a treat; the attractiveness of the food is initially not strong enough to overcome the close proximity of the fearful stimulus. This should be discouraged.

The first step would be to teach the cat basic skills such as go to place (station), leave it (move away), settle (sit or lie in a safe place calmly), and touch (touch a finger, pencil, or other object with the nose or paw). These behaviors establish a structure with which to interact with the person and allow the cat to choose or decline to interact in a nonaggressive way. For example, a cat may be taught to jump up on a cat tree away from the front door when visitors arrive, creating sufficient distance to keep the cat under threshold. As with harness training, it may take cats several weeks to learn these cues, and they should be taught when the cat is calm before any attempt is made to use them when a trigger is present.

When introductions with the person begin, the distance (threshold) and the intensity (person standing, sitting, speaking) which can be tolerated by the cat should have been established. The pet parent cannot cross that threshold during this process or it is counterproductive and will worsen the aggression. If visitors cause the cat to be fearful when they approach to 3 meters or closer, then sessions should be set up so that a visitor remains 4 to 5 meters from the cat while the pet parent gives a very tasty food treat or provides other reinforcement (e.g., play) if the pet shows no sign of FASCP when the person is visible. If the cat is willing to take treats or engage in a pleasurable activity during the exposure, the first step in a counterconditioning program will have been achieved. Providing extremely enticing food treats or other high-value rewards only during exposure training increases their value and ensures contingency by linking special rewards with the presence of the stimulus.

After several positive associations, the new person can be very gradually brought closer and closer. It is advisable that the visitor avoids threatening gestures or eye contact and remains quiet and calm. Additionally, the pet parent should continuously monitor the cat's body language for early signs of fear or arousal to ensure that the cat's threshold is not exceeded during the desensitization process.

Alternatively, a leash and harness may be beneficial if the cat has been previously accustomed to wearing one. This can be used to keep the cat from moving toward the victim, but not to keep the cat from escaping the situation. Remember that the cat has the right to say "no" and that any forcing of the interaction will in the long term make the situation worse. If the cat has never worn a harness, it is helpful to teach the cat to accept it by classical conditioning *before* attempting to use harness control during a conditioning exercise. Also see Appendix C and Online Resource Cat Aggression to People.

Maternal aggression

For queens that show maternal aggression, highly palatable food rewards for the queen can be offered by familiar, less threatening people at a distance which does not evoke a reactive response. If the queen can be encouraged to leave the nest or if she leaves the nest voluntarily, favored rewards (food, treats, toys) should be given. If the queen can be occupied away from the litter, the kittens can receive the handling and attention that are beneficial to their development (see Chapter 2). Depending on the severity of the mother's reactivity, it may be best to delay attempts at behavior modification until the kittens are less vulnerable since the queen's reaction will be tempered as her kittens age and are less reliant on their mother. Since kittens may learn by observation of their mother's interactions with people, it is best to avoid evoking an aggressive response.

Medications and natural products

When to use medications and natural products

Medication can be used as a part of an overall treatment plan which should always include environmental management but can also include behavioral treatments. Educate pet parents so that they understand that a medication is unlikely to cure the aggression but may decrease the intensity, frequency, or arousal associated with the aggression. Behavioral medications alter mood and emotional state. However, they do not "fix" behavior problems, meaning that without environmental management at minimum or environmental management and behavioral treatments, the medications alone will not be sufficiently effective and the behavior is likely to recur when the medications are discontinued. See Chapters 9, 11, 12, and 16 for more information on how to discuss medication with parents and how to prescribe appropriately.

Medication should be considered in the situations where exposure to fear- or stress-eliciting stimuli occurs daily, when triggering events are unpredictable or unavoidable, when arousal is high, latency to arousal is short, recovery from incidents is long, or when the cat is experiencing stress or distress interfering with its quality of life. With pharmacological support, the window of opportunity for beneficial behavior modification may be more attainable by cats and their pet parents.

In the case of intercat aggression, both cats often need to be treated with medications. Medications such as selective serotonin reuptake inhibitors (SSRIs) (e.g., fluoxetine, paroxetine, sertraline), tricyclic antidepressants (clomipramine, amitriptyline), and SNRIs (e.g., venlafaxine) are most often utilized to reduce overall arousal, fear, anxiety, and stress and reduce the possibility of new episodes, particularly if the inciting trigger cannot be avoided. Buspirone may also be effective if there is mild anxiety but may cause disinhibition and lead to increased aggression. Buspirone, a serotonin 1A partial agonist, may reduce anxiety with the added benefit of some cats becoming "more affectionate" (i.e., staying near their pet parents more, climbing and staying longer on their pet parents' laps than before)[61] and may be more appropriate for the victim cat to reduce fear and increase confidence. However, all psychotropic medications may potentially sedate or cause incoordination, changes in appetite, disinhibition, and agitation. In a study investigating buspirone treatment for urine spraying, 9 of 62 cats exhibited increased aggression toward other cats; in some cases, these cats were previously timid and fearful toward their housemates.[62] In a retrospective study of intercat aggression, the aggressor cat was treated with a TCA, buspirone, or megestrol acetate, while the victim cat was treated with diazepam.[29] No treatment was found to be more effective than another, which may indicate that treatment plans specifically tailored to the individual patients and situation have the best chance for success. Venlafaxine, a selective serotonin and norepineph-rine reuptake inhibitor (SNRI) was successfully used to treat a cat with refractory misdirected play and impulse-control aggression that initially responded to, but developed urinary retention secondary to fluoxetine.[63]

Benzodiazepines (alprazolam, lorazepam, or oxazepam) may reduce fear and anxiety, which may be an indication for treatment of a cat that is the victim of aggression by reducing the victim's fear of its previous attacker or speeding recovery of the aggressor following exposure to a fear-inducing trigger. Benzodiazepines stimulate the cat's appetite, which may be a beneficial side effect of a food-based counterconditioning program. However, it may also cause behavioral disinhibi-tion in some animals and diazepam can cause rare fulminant hepatic necrosis,[64] so care must be taken when prescribing it. The use of lorazepam, clonazepam, or oxazepam, which have

no active intermediate metabolites, might have less potential for adverse hepatic effects, although this is as yet unproven. Gabapentin is commonly used in cats to reduce anxiety and fear as well as for pain relief.

The synthetic pheromones Feliway Classic, Optimum and/ or Multicat (also marketed in some countries as Feliway Friends) might be helpful, as might anxiolytic supplements such as L-theanine and alpha-casozepine or in therapeutic diets containing these ingredients. The use of feline-appeasing pheromone (Feliway Multicat or Feliway Friends) has been shown to reduce the frequency and intensity of aggressive in-teractions between household cats with a history of aggressive behavior after three weeks compared to placebo.[65] Synthetic F3 fraction, Feliway Classic feline facial pheromone, is associ-ated with environmental marking and recommended to re-duce stress and anxiety (see Chapter 12).

CASE EXAMPLES

Case 1

Presentation

Carol was a 5-year-old, 3-kg, spayed female domestic (American) long-haired cat presented for fear and aggression toward male visitors.

History

Carol was adopted by her pet parent, Natasha, at eight weeks of age from a female friend who lived by herself and had few visitors, most of whom were women or children. In her current home, Carol was playful and con-fident when she was alone at home with Natasha, but became nervous and usually hid when a visitor entered the home, especially when the visi-tor was a man. Natasha had recently begun a relationship with a man named Bruce. She was disconcerted about the fact that Carol had not taken to her new friend. In an attempt to facilitate the relationship, she encouraged Bruce to attempt to pick Natasha up during each visit and give her a food treat. Each time that he did this, Carol would become very agitated, hiss, growl, flail her legs, and occasionally bite to get released. Instead of getting better, Carol's behavior worsened. She became more nervous around Bruce and frequently hissed at him when he visited.

Workup

Carol's physical examination and baseline lab work was within normal limits.

Differential diagnoses

Carol's differential diagnoses included fear-induced aggression, stress-induced aggression, defensive aggression, impulsive aggression, territo-rial aggression, and pain-induced aggression. Because she showed clear signs of fear, with arousal and attempts to escape in the presence of the stimulus (Bruce) without hypervigilance or attempts to pursue him ag-gressively, she was diagnosed with fear-induced aggression.

Treatment

Natasha was advised to avoid allowing Bruce to approach, reach for, or interact in any way with Carol. Instead, he was instructed to ignore her completely. A positive reinforcement trainer was recom-mended, and Natasha was given online resources and books which would help her train Carol. They were instructed to use two strate-gies outside of avoidance: teach coping or control tools and capture positive interactions. They were instructed to use a clicker teach Carol to go to a cat tree, higher than the furniture where Bruce usu-ally sat (to facilitate a feeling of safety), and lie there calmly and to touch Natasha's finger with her nose. Next, they were to capture with a click and a treat (given only by Natasha) any movement or at-tention to Bruce.

Follow-up

The veterinary technician followed up in two weeks. Natasha and Bruce had one online session with the trainer and they were amazed at Carol's trainability with tuna as a reward. They were starting to teach coping behaviors, and reported that about a week after Bruce started ignoring Carol, she had started to sit in the doorway to the living room instead of hiding when he came over. Natasha was instructed to capture this be-havior with the clicker and a treat.

The veterinary technician followed up in a month. Carol had learned to touch Natasha's finger with her nose, but they had given up on teaching her to go to the cat tree because she had continued to ven-ture closer and closer to Bruce once they had started capturing the friendly behavior with the clicker and a treat. They were pleased with how she was doing and reported that she could sit on the sofa with Bruce as long as he did not reach for her. They were given instructions at this time as to how to transition the touch cue to interactions with Bruce. Even though Carol was progressing nicely, Bruce and Natasha felt that there might be a time when he would have to handle her. When Carol was within 1 to 2 feet of Bruce, he was to use the "touch" verbal cue, extending his hand and finger. If Carol touched the finger, either Natasha or Bruce could click and Bruce could place a tasty treat near her.

Case 2

Presentation

Cap was a 9-year-old, 7-kg neutered male domestic (American) short-haired cat that was presented for aggression when petted.

History

Cap lived in a home with one male pet parent, Tony. Cap sat next to Tony frequently on the couch or bed or at the kitchen table, and he also climbed in his lap or on Tony's shoulders. Both Cap and Tony seemed to appreciate this interaction. Tony petted Cap on the head and down the back. However, within the last month if he petted Cap for longer than 1 minute or so, Cap bit him without breaking the skin and sometimes swatted with his claws out and bit at the same time. He was most ame-nable to attention in the early morning or midafternoon when Tony sat at the kitchen table for tea.

Workup

Cap's physical examination and baseline lab work was within normal limits; however, while he had no skin lesions upon questioning Tony, it was clear that Cap was pruritic. He showed skin twitching throughout the day and sometimes jumped up as if something had bitten him, then oriented toward a body part and lick, bit, and/or chewed it for up to 20 seconds. The veterinarian discussed flea allergy dermatitis, inhaled allergies, and food allergies. Tony had recently allowed Cap on the screened-in porch for enrichment.

Differential diagnoses

Cap's differential diagnoses included fear-induced aggression, pain-induced aggression, stress-induced aggression, defensive aggression, frustration-induced aggression, and impulsive aggression. Because he showed no clear signs of fear, did not try to escape, had a relatively low arousal level, was not anxious or hypervigilant, and exhibited aggression in many different situations, the differential diagnosis list was reduced to stress-induced aggression (physiologic due to pruritus and emotional) and pain-induced aggression (pruritus). In addition, a presumptive diagnosis of flea allergy dermatitis was made.

Treatment

Tony was educated on the interplay between pruritus, pain, and emotional state all affecting the threshold for aggression. In addition, it was explained that cats have a limited number of ways to communicate with us and that just because they come close does not mean that they are soliciting petting. A treatment plan was created to treat the pruritus immediately and use flea control in the long term. A Feliway Classic diffuser was plugged in near the kitchen table. Tony was instructed to only pet Cap as long as he solicited that behavior and for no longer than three strokes only on the head. He was taught how to perform a consent test and given online video resources for demonstration.

Follow-up

The veterinary technician followed up in one week. The incidents of aggression had reduced by 90%. In addition, Tony reported less startling and pruritus.

Case 3
Presentation

Wanda, a 3-year-old, 4-kg, spayed female domestic feline and Pietro, her sibling, a 3-year-old, 6-kg neutered male feline, were presented for acute onset of fighting.

History

Wanda and Pietro lived in a house with two pet parents, Stan and Jack. The pet parents reported that the cats were adopted together and had always been best friends, sleeping together and grooming each other. One day, when Jack arrived home, he found items in the sunroom knocked over, tufts of fur from Pietro on the floor, and both cats hiding in different locations in the house. Following that incident, Wanda would growl and charge at Pietro whenever they were together. Pietro currently fled the room whenever he saw Wanda. History taking revealed that previously both cats spent time together in the sunroom. The pet parents had recently started feeding an outdoor feral cat in the yard. When Wanda saw this cat, she would become agitated, growl, and pounce on the window, then run to another room to hide under the bed, while Pietro seemed unfazed by the presence of the outdoor cat.

Workup

Both Wanda and Pietro's physical examinations and baseline lab work were within normal limits.

Differential diagnoses

Wanda's differential diagnoses included fear-induced aggression, stress-induced aggression, defensive aggression, frustration-induced aggression, redirected aggression, territorial aggression (to the outside cat), and impulsive aggression. She showed signs of fear and tried to escape when she saw the cat outdoors but did not pursue him, so she was diagnosed with fear-induced aggression toward the outdoor cat. In addition, she

was diagnosed with redirected aggression and fear-induced aggression (learned through conditioning) toward Pietro. Pietro was diagnosed with fear of Wanda.

Treatment

The pet parents were instructed to stop feeding the feral cat and to use a motion-activated sprinkler to deter it from entering the yard. They were also given trap-neuter-release and local cat rescue and shelter resources for the outdoor cat. A window-darkening shade was installed to further reduce the sight of stimuli in the yard. The pet parents were given resources on sanctuary space training and environmental enrichment. Wanda and Pietro were separated when they were not able to be directly monitored. During the day when their pet parents were not at home to supervise, the rooms each cat had access to were alternated to allow each cat to explore the house equally. The cats were swapped out several times a day to explore the rest of the house for several hours. The pet parents were counseled regarding the different treatment options, including the possibility that they may need to keep the cats separated for life, teaching coping and control tools, and DS/CC. They were given resources on cat body language. They were instructed to make an online appointment with a nurse at the veterinary hospital who had training with cat behavior modification in order to teach the cats how to turn away from each other on cue, go to a mat, and relax there. Finally, they were advised to let the cats play with separate toys on either side of the glass door of the sunroom with supervision to classically condition the cats to the sight of each other as long as there was no body language displayed on the part of either cat which was consistent with FASCP.

Follow-up

The pet parents worked with the veterinary technician weekly for four weeks via an online video conferencing platform. Within that time, both cats had learned to go to their separate areas in the same room individually without the other cat in the room with fair reliability, and they played individually with motorized toys with relaxed body language on either side of the glass door. However, when they were not playing, Pietro ran to the other side of the room, away from the sight of Wanda. The veterinarian decided at this point to treat Pietro with buspirone at a dose of 0.25 mg/kg by mouth every 12 hours. The veterinary technician continued to work with the family.

Within two weeks, Pietro was more confident and would stay in the room with Wanda without a lot of coaxing. The pet parents began to let them be in the same room with supervision. If any signs of fear or arousal were demonstrated by either cat, they redirected them immediately by cueing them to go to their individual spots and reinforcing them immediately with food. They were still keeping the cats from going in the sunroom together, although they had not seen the stray cat. They were instructed that they could let the cats in the sunroom with supervision; however, they chose not to do so in case there was a relapse. Pietro continued on the buspirone for three more months and then was slowly weaned off.

Case 4
Presentation

Mobius was an 8-month-old, 2-kg intact male Siamese kitten adopted from a rescue organization at 12 weeks of age that was presented for aggression to the dog (Loki) and the people in the house.

History

Mobius was relinquished to the rescue organization at three weeks of age with one of his littermates. He was curious, active, confident, and outgoing. He bit family members' faces and hands while they were sleeping, and most attacks occurred between 5 and 8 a.m., just before they woke to feed Mobius and Loki breakfast. The household included Loki, a 10-year-old German Shepherd; Loki was also frequently attacked on his paws or tail by the kitten when he was moving around the house and wagging his tail. Mobius's claws were retracted

continued

and the bites did not break skin. When his pet parents were awake to observe him prior to the attack, he was crouched while shifting his weight on his back legs, ears forward, tail twitching. From this position, he would silently run, pounce, and bite the hands or exposed feet of his pet parents or Loki's tail. After the attack, which was always brief and noninjurious, he ran a short distance away and either played with a toy or crouched again, as if to pounce on the victim for a second time.

Workup

Mobius's physical examinations and baseline lab work were within normal limits.

Differential diagnoses

Mobius's differential diagnoses included fear-induced aggression, stress-induced aggression, defensive aggression, normal play behavior, play-induced aggression, frustration-induced aggression, redirected aggression, and impulsive aggression. He did not show any signs of fear or high arousal, did not run away or pursue the targets of the aggression, did not show any signs of anxiety, hypervigilance, or chronic stress, and had body language consistent with play. He was diagnosed with normal play behavior which was undesirable to the pet parents.

Treatment

The pet parents were educated and given resources on environmental enrichment and proper play with cats. They were also instructed to keep him out of the bedroom and use an automatic feeder, which would open up at 4:45 a.m., prior to the likelihood of the first attack.

The automatic feeder would have a small amount of food so that the pet parents would not intermittently reinforce him by getting up and feeding him at that time.

They were instructed as to how to teach him to fetch his toys and sit on cue. The family was advised to discontinue punishment strategies, use food puzzle toys for feeding throughout the day, and rotate the toys so that he had access to three new and different toys each day as well as the toys in his toybox. They were instructed how to preemptively keep him busy at the times of day where he would usually be biting Loki's tail and how to redirect him with the shake of a treat jar when they saw signs that he was going to become aggressive or bite them. Once they had his attention, they were to direct him to an appropriate toy. Loki's quality of life was addressed as well through scheduled breaks from interactions with Mobius. The pet parents described Loki as feeling most comfortable when he was sleeping on their bed. For that reason, it was recommended that at the times when Mobius was most likely to bite Loki, Loki be in the bedroom with the door closed. Finally, the pet parents were educated on how to find Mobius's preference for toys, and that it may take two or three months to find the types of toys that really stimulated him and kept his interest.

Follow-up

Mobius responded immediately to enrichment and proper play. It took about a week for him to adjust to being outside of the bedroom. His behavior was well controlled over the course of his lifetime as long as the enrichment level was kept high.

Conclusion

The causes of aggression vary and there is still much to learn about the function and motivation of aggression in cats.

With that said, feline aggression should not be intimidating. There are many treatment options and often, the prognosis can be excellent.

References

1. Rochlitz I. Feline welfare issues. In: Turner C, Bateson P, eds. *The Domestic Cat. The Biology of its Behaviour*. 2nd ed. Cambridge: University Press; 2000: 208–226.
2. Patronek GJ, Glickman LT, Beck AM, et al. Risk factors for relinquishment of cats to an animal shelter. *J Am Vet Med Assoc*. 1996;209:582–588.
3. Salman MD, New JG, Scarlett JM, et al. Human and animal factors related to relinquishment of dogs and cats in 12 selected animal shelters in the United States. *J Appl Anim Welf Sci*. 1998;3: 207–226.
4. Amat M, Ruiz de la Torre JL, Fatjo J, et al. Potential risk factors associated with feline behavior problems. *Appl Anim Behav Sci*. 2009;121:134–139.
5. Casey RA, Vandenbussche S, Bradshaw JWS, et al. Reasons for relinquishment and return of domestic cats (Felis Silvestris Catus) to rescue shelters in the UK. *Anthrozoos*. 2009;22:347–358.
6. Kizer KW. Epidemiological and clinical aspects of animal bite injuries. *JACEP*. 1979;8:134–141.
7. Turner DC. Social organization and behavioural ecology of free-ranging domestic cats. In: Turner DC, Bateson P, eds. *The Domestic Cat: The Biology of its Behaviour*. 3rd ed. Cambridge, UK: Cambridge University Press; 2014.
8. Gunther I, Finkler H, Terkel J. Demographic differences between urban feeding groups of neutered and sexually intact free-roaming cats following a trap-neuter-return procedure. *J Am Vet Med Assoc*. 2011;238: 1134–1140.
9. Crowell-Davis SL, Curtis TM, Knowles RJ. Social organization in the cat: a modern understanding. *J Feline Med Surg*. 2004;6: 19–28.
10. Wolfe R. *The Social Organization of the Free Ranging Domestic Cat (Felis catus)*. University of Georgia: PhD dissertation; 2001.
11. Beaver BV. *Feline Behavior: A Guide for Veterinarians*. 2nd ed. St. Louis: Saunders; 2003:142–143.
12. Bonnanni R, Cafazzo S, Fantini C, et al. Feeding-order in an urban feral domestic cat colony: relationship to dominance, rank, sex and age. *Anim Behav*. 2007;74: 1369–1379.
13. Natoli E, Baggio A, Pontier D. Male and female agonistic and affiliative relationships in a social group of farm cats (Felis catus L.). *Behav Process*. 2001; 53:137–143.
14. van den Bos R. The function of allogrooming in domestic cats (Felis silvestris cattus); a study in a group of cats living in confinement. *J Ethol*. 1988;16:1–13.
15. World Health Organization. *Animal Bites*. World Health Organization; 2018; Retrieved March 21, 2021. https://www. who.int/news-room/fact-sheets/detail/ animal-bites#:~:text=They%20are%20 commonly%20second%20to,hospital%20 emergency%20departments%20every% 20year.
16. Garcia VF. Animal bites and Pasteurella infections. *Pediatr Rev*. 1997;18: 127–130.
17. Grigg EK, Kogan LR, van Haaften K, et al. Cat owners' perceptions of psychoactive medications, supplements and pheromones for the treatment of feline behavior problems. *J Feline Med Surg*. 2019;21(10):902–909.

18. Ramos D, Mills DS. Human directed aggression in Brazilian domestic cats: owner reported prevalence, contexts and risk factors. *J Feline Med Surg.* 2009;1: 835–841.

19. Palacio J, Leon-Artozqui M, Pastor-Villalba E, et al. Incidence of and risk factors for cat bites: a first step in prevention and treatment of feline aggression. *J Feline Med Surg.* 2007;9:188–195.

20. Wright JC. Reported cat bites in Dallas: characteristics of the cats, the victims and the attack events. *Public Health Rep.*1990; 105:420–424.

21. Bradshaw JWS, Casey RA, Brown SL. *The Behaviour of the Domestic Cat.* 2nd ed. Oxfordshire: CABI; 2012.

22. Delgado M, Hecht J. A review of the development and functions of cat play, with future research considerations. *Appl Anim Behav Sci.* 2019;213:1–17.

23. Borchelt PL, Voith VL. Aggressive behavior in dogs and cats. *Compend Contin Educ Vet Pract.* 1985;7:950.

24. Amat M, Manteca X, Le Brech S, et al. Evaluation of inciting causes, alter-native targets, and risk factors associated with redirected aggression in cats. *J Am Vet Med Assoc.* 2008;233:586–589.

25. Patrick GR, O'Rourke KM. Dog and cat bites: epidemiologic analyses suggest different prevention strategies. *Public Health Rep.* 1998;113:252–257.

26. Bamberger M, Houpt KA. Signalment factors, comorbidity, and trends in behaviour diagnosis in cats: 736 cases 1991–2001. *J Am Vet Med Assoc.* 2006;229: 1602–1606.

27. Levine E, Perry R, Scarlett J, et al. Intercat aggression in households following the introduction of a new cat. *Appl Anim Behav Sci.* 2005;90:325–336.

28. O'Hanley KA, Pearl DL, Niel L. Risk factors for aggression in adult cats that were fostered through a shelter program as kittens. *Appl Anim Behav Sci.* 2021;236:105251.

29. Lindell EM, Erb HN, Houpt KA. Intercat aggression: a retrospective study examining types of aggression, sexes of fighting pairs, and effectiveness of treatment. *Appl Anim Behav Sci.* 1997;55: 153–162.

30. Hart BL, Cooper L. Factors related to urine spraying and fighting in prepubertally gonadectomized cats. *J Am Vet Med Assoc.* 1984;184:1255–1258.

31. Kotrschal K, Day J, McCune S. Human and cat personalities; building the bond from both sides. In: Turner DC, Bateson P, eds. *The Domestic Cat: The Biology of its Behaviour.* 3rd ed. Cambridge, UK: Cambridge University Press; 2014; 113–127.

32. Lowe SE, Bradshaw JWS. Ontogeny of individuality in the domestic cat in the home environment. *Anim Behav.* 2001;61: 231–237.

33. McCune S. The impact of paternity and early socialization on the development of cat's behaviour to people and novel objects. *Appl Anim Behav Sci.* 1995;45: 109–124.

34. Reisner IR, Houpt KA, Erb HN, Quimby FW. Friendly to humans and defensive aggression in cats: the influence of handling and paternity. *Physiol Behav.* 1994;55:1119–1124.

35. Seitz PFD. Infantile experience and adult behavior in animal subjects. Age of separation from the mother and adult behavior in the cat. *Psychosom Med.* 1959; 21:353–378.

36. Ahola MK, Vapalahti K, Lohi H. Early weaning increases aggression and stereotypic behaviour in cats. *Sci Rep.* 2017;7:1–9. doi:10.1038/s41598-017-11173-5.

37. Chon E. The effects of queen (Felis sylvestris)-rearing versus hand-rearing on feline aggression and other problematic behaviors. In: *5th International Veterinary Behavior Meeting.* Minneapolis (MN): Purdue University Press; 2005:201–202.

38. Mellen J. Effects of early rearing experience on subsequent adult sexual behavior using domestic cats (Felis catus) as a model for exotic small felids. *Zoo Biol.* 1992;11:17.

39. Sumner JP, Hulsebosch, SE, Dudley RM, et al. Sex-hormone producing adrenal tumors causing behavioral changes as the sole clinical sign in 3 cats. *Can Vet J.* 2019; 60:305–310.

40. Stelow EA, Bain MJ, Kass PH. The relationship between coat color and aggressive behaviors in the domestic cat. *J Appl Anim Welf Sci.* 2016;19:1–15.

41. Strickler BL, Shull EA. An owner survey of toys, activities, and behavior problems in indoor cats. *J Vet Behav.* 2014;9:207–214.

42. Macdonald DW, Yamaguchi N, Gillian K. Group-living in the domestic cat: its sociobiology and epidemiology. In: Turner DC, Bateson P, eds. *The Domestic Cat: The Biology of its Behaviour.* 2nd ed. Cambridge: Cambridge University Press; 2000:96–115.

43. Barry KJ, Crowell-Davis SL. Gender differences in the social behavior of the neutered indoor-only domestic cat. *Appl Anim Behav Sci.* 1999;64:193–211.

44. Volk JO, Felsted KE, Thomas JG, et al. Executive summary of the Bayer veterinary care usage study. *J Am Vet Med Assoc.* 2011;238:1275–1282.

45. Casey RA, Bradshaw JWS. The effects of additional socialisation for kittens in a rescue centre on their behaviour and suitability as a pet. *Appl Anim Behav Sci.* 2008;114:196–205.

46. Caro TM. Effects of the mother, object play, and adult experience on predation in cats. *Behav Neural Biol.* 1980;29(1):29–51.

47. Caro TM. The effects of experience on the predatory patterns of cats. *Behav Neural Biol.* 1980;29(1):1–28.

48. American Association of Feline Practitioners (AAFP). *Feline Behavior Guidelines.* Available at: https://catvets. com/public/PDFs/PracticeGuidelines/ FelineBehaviorGLS.pdf.

49. Westropp JL, Buffington CA. Feline idiopathic cystitis: current understanding of pathophysiology and management. *Vet Clin North Am Small Anim Pract.* 2004;34: 1043–1055.

50. Stella JL, Lord LK, Buffington CA. Sickness behaviors in response to unusual external events in healthy cats and cats with feline interstitial cystitis. *J Am Vet Med Assoc.* 2011;238:67–73.

51. Saleh MN. Detecting Giardia: Clinical and Molecular Identification. Dissertation submitted to the faculty of the Virginia Polytechnic Institute and State University in partial fulfillment of the requirements for the degree of Doctor of Philosophy in Biomedical and Veterinary Sciences. Accessed in 2021: https://vtechworks.lib. vt.edu/bitstream/handle/10919/89367/ Saleh_MN_D_2017.pdf?sequence=1& isAllowed=y.

52. Ellis SLH, Thompson H, Guijarro C, et al. The influence of body region, handler familiarity, and order of region handled on the domestic cat's response to being stroked. *Appl Anim Behav Sci.* 2015;173: 60–67.

53. Soennichsen S, Chamove AS. Responses of cats to petting by humans. *Anthrozoös.* 2002;15,258–265.

54. Haywood C, Ripari L, Puzzo J, et al. Providing humans with practical, best practice handling guidelines during human-cat interactions increases cats' affiliative behaviour and reduces aggression and signs of conflict. *Front Vet Sci.* 2021;8:835. doi:10.3389/fvets.2021. 714143.

55. Association of Pet Behaviour Counsellors. *Annual Review of Cases.* Available at: www. apbc.org.uk. UK: 2005.

56. Jacobs JA, Coe JB, Widowski TM, et al. Defining and clarifying the terms canine possessive aggression and resource guarding: a study of expert opinion. *Front Vet Sci.* 2018;5:115.

57. Siegel A, Roeling TA, Gregg TR, et al. Neuropharmacology of brain-stimulation-evoked aggression. *Neurosci Biobehav Rev.* 1999;23(3):359–389.

58. Sinn L. Aggression overview – cats. In: Tilley LP, Smith FWK, Sleeper MM, et al., eds. *Blackwell's 5 Minute Veterinary Consult: Canine and Feline.* 7th ed. Hoboken, New Jersey: John Wiley and Sons; 2021:56–57.

59. Kim SE, Arzi B, Garcia T, et al. Bite forces and their measurement in dogs and cats. *Front Vet Sci.* 2018. doi:10.3389/ fvets.2018.00076.

60. Ellis JL, Thomason JJ, Kebreab E, et al. Calibration of estimated biting forces in domestic canids: comparison of post-mortem and in vivo measurements. *J Anat.* 2008;212: 769–780.

61. de Souza Dantas M, Crowell-Davis SL, Miscellaneous sertonergic agents. In: *Veterinary Psychopharmacology.* 2nd ed. Hoboken, NJ: John Wiley and Sons; 2019:129–146.

62. Hart B, Eckstein RA, Powell KL, et al. Effectiveness of buspirone on urine spraying and inappropriate urination in cats. *J Am Vet Med Assoc.* 1993;203:54–258.

63. Pflaum K, Bennett S. Investigation of the use of venlafaxine for treatment of refractory misdirected play and impulse-control aggression in a cat: a case report. *J Vet Behav.* 2021;42:22–25.

64. Center SA, Elston TH, Rowland PH, et al. Fulminant hepatic failure associated with oral administration of diazepam in 11 cats. *J Am Vet Med Assoc.* 1996;209: 618–625.

65. DePorter TL, Bledsoe DL, Beck A, et al. Evaluation of the efficacy of an appeasing pheromone diffuser product vs placebo for management of feline aggression in multi-cat households: a pilot study. *J Feline Med Surg.* 2019;21:293–305.

Recommended reading

Amat M, Manteca X. Common feline problem behaviours: owner-directed aggression. *J Feline Med Surg.* 2019;21:245–255.

American College of Veterinary Behaviorists, et al. *Decoding Your Cat. The Ultimate Experts Explain Common Cat Behaviors and How to Prevent or Change Unwanted Ones.* Houghton Mifflin Harcourt; New York, New York. 2020.

Bradshaw J, Ellis S. *The Trainable Cat.* 2017.

Elzerman AL, DePorter TL, Beck A et al. Conflict and affiliative behavior frequency between cats in multi-cat households: a survey-based study. *J Fel Med and Surg.* 2020;22(8): 705-717.

Kruszka M, Graff E, Medam T, Masson S. Clinical evaluation of the effects of a single oral dose of gabapentin on fear-based aggressive behaviors in cats during veterinary examinations. *J Am Vet Med Assoc.* 2021;259(11):1285–1291.

Pike AL. Consult the expert. *Feline Aggression. Clinician's Brief,* Jan/Feb 2021:10–17. https://www.cliniciansbrief.com/article/feline-aggression-0.

Ramos D. Common feline problem behaviors: aggression in multi-cat households. *J Feline Med Surg.* 2019;21:221–233.

CHAPTER 25

The psychobiological approach to problem behavior assessment

Daniel S. Mills, BVSC, PhD, CBIOL, FRSB, FHEA, CCAB, Dip ECAWBM (BM), FRCVS, RCVS, EBVS

Chapter contents

What is a behavioral diagnosis?

When dealing with cases, clinicians make an assessment of why they think an animal is behaving in a particular way and offer treatment recommendations accordingly. This classification of the problem is important for many reasons, but the quality of the process is often overlooked and this can cause problems.

1. Imagine you and I are two people treating behavior problems. If what I consider to be a separation-related disorder is different to what you consider it to be, then we might get different outcomes using the same treatment protocols on our cases. If we do not have an agreed framework for reaching a diagnosis, we can't communicate effectively and understand each other's issues in the practice of problem behavior management. What might work for me might not work for you (or not work as well for you) because you are unknowingly giving treatment to a different profile of cases.

2. Second, when it comes to understanding the biological basis to these problems and developing new interventions, we might encounter important issues. The lack of a consistent biological basis to how we classify problem behavior might mean we come to very different conclusions. This is

more than a theoretical issue. In 2001, it was reported in the United States that intact animals were more than three times less likely to have separation-related disorders[1]; however, a few years later, a somewhat similar survey in Australia, reported that neutered animals were less likely to suffer from this problem.[2] So what is the significance of neutering as it applies to separation-related disorders based on the aforementioned studies? We simply don't know.

When it comes to consistency among clinicians in treatment recommendations, matters get even worse. In the later 1990s, we interviewed 32 veterinary behaviorists about how they recognized and managed certain behavior problems and divided them into the following geographic regions: USA, UK, France (which has a very different approach to problem behavior[3]), and the rest of Europe. In the case of separation-related disorders, agreement on the most important treatment measures ranged from 69% among the French to 44% among clinicians in the UK; but perhaps more significantly, 24 out of the 32 clinicians had at least one explicit contradiction to another clinician (e.g., one might indicate that something was important and another might explicitly say it was contraindicated). This means that what one expert was recommending as among the most important measures was what another was saying should not be done. Needless to say, this greatly hinders progress and innovation. As a result, diagnoses have often remained, subjective or vague and treatments nonspecific, with specificity being largely left to clinical judgment. Greater precision and validity in the diagnostic process can be achieved by following a systematic process grounded in a solid biological and psychological framework. This also facilitates the movement of veterinary behavioral medicine forward on a more scientific basis. It is this goal which has driven the development of a psychobiological approach to problem behavior over the last 25 years.[4]

This approach is of more than academic interest and has driven the development of a range of validated psychometric instruments, such as the Dog Impulsivity Assessment Scale (DIAS),[5] Canine Frustration Questionnaire (CFQ),[6] Positive and Negative Activation Scale (PANAS) for Dogs,[7] the Lincoln Sound Sensitivity Scale (LSSS),[8] and the Lincoln Canine Anxiety Scale (LCAS)[9] that can be used by behavior clinicians regardless of their approach to problem behavior to help gain a deeper insight into a dog's problem behavior. They are discussed in detail later in this chapter. The instruments are all freely available online at https://ipstore.lincoln.ac.uk/products/assessment-tools. However, before discussing the scales themselves, we will consider how the psychometric approach, developed at the University of Lincoln, sits relative to other approaches used in problem behavior, the most useful features of a diagnosis, and the systematic process that enables us to produce diagnoses more rigorously. We then consider the scales developed and how they can be used to help inform our judgments about the patient at any given time.

Approaches used in clinical animal behavior

Historically, there have been two dominant approaches to clinical animal behavior: one based on a model of problem behavior rooted in the scientific discipline of "behaviorism" and the other on the medical approach traditionally used in the human psychiatry. Few people exclusively follow one approach or the other, but it is useful to be aware of these different approaches as they provide insight into the priorities and biases made during problem behavior assessment and management.

The behaviorist tradition

"Behaviorism" was key to the development of the discipline of experimental psychology pioneered in the United States by psychologists such as Skinner in order to establish general laws of learning. It has a focus on observable events (rather than internal states of the brain that might control them) and so emphasizes the importance of the external environment in development, with treatment focusing on changing the behavioral signs of a problem through training. It has been instrumental in promoting a more scientific approach to training, with an increasing number of animal trainers using sound principles of reinforcement to bring about behavior change for the purposes of both cued responses (obedience exercises) and the reconditioning of problem behavior (behavioral therapy). See Chapter 10 for more information on learning theory.

In behaviorism, the emphasis on the observable means that reference is rarely made to the importance of internal processes within the central nervous system or related psychological constructs such as motivation and emotion. Accordingly, the value of considering these factors can be easily overlooked. Whether in an experimental environment or the complex multisensory environment that makes up the typical living space of most companion animals, internal processes affect behavior. The sterile, standardized experimental environments often used to study behavior do not reflect the world in which companion animals tend to live. As a result, it needs to be recognized that the work of experimental psychologists has shown us what can bring about a specific behavior but not necessarily what commonly affects behavior in the real world. As already mentioned, behaviorism has been critical to developing our understanding of general laws of learning, such as the role of positive and negative reinforcement and positive and negative punishment on shaping behavior. By their very nature, general laws apply to what typically happens (or on average) within a population, and thus individual variation is largely considered "noise" and of little importance. However, individual variability is at the heart of the science of clinical behavior. How often do we hear a pet parent say something like, "I've always treated all my pets the same, so why is this one behaving so differently?" The answer may lie in the different way this animal perceives and thinks about the physical features of its environment: its individual genetic makeup and the expression of those genes. This inevitably requires referring to internal states that cannot be objectively assessed, only inferred. Acknowledging and working with individual differences (and being able to assess them) is often important to successful problem behavior management.

With its focus on what can be described, behavior and stimuli are the foci of interest in behaviorism, but somewhat ironically, superficially similar behaviors are often considered to be controlled by similar factors, and stylistic features ignored. However, attending to such features can provide important insights into significant factors relating to the motivation and/or emotion underpinning the behavior. Consider a cat running after prey and one running away from something it doesn't like. It is only superficially the same behavior, and simply referring to both as "running" is not very helpful if you want to understand the factors affecting their occurrence, as they are under the control of very different factors. Behaviorism and classical ethology have also had a less obvious, but no less important influence on the way we think about behavior. A focus on behavior and stimuli often biases the way we think about how behavior is controlled. The relationship between a stimulus and response is often described as if there is a direct link, and while this can be true for simple reflexes and habitual responses, this often obscures important clinical considerations.

- From a neurobiological perspective, most behavior sequences are not directly stimulated by the environment but rather, released through an easing of inhibitory control. This highlights the importance of considering impulsivity and the executive control of behavior in all cases (something we return to later when we consider the assessment of behavioral tendencies later in the chapter). More impulsive animals often make poorer decisions, which can lead to problems.

- Behaviors help an individual achieve general goals (e.g., escape from a risky situation) in a certain way (e.g., by running away); however, there are many behaviors that might help an animal to escape from harm, depending on circumstances (e.g., freezing or aggressive display). Thus, animals are constantly deciding what to do as a result of the integration of vast amounts of information from both the external senses and internal systems. Shifts in the balance of these can change behavior but not necessarily the overall goal (e.g., escape). An animal most likely makes a decision about its priorities first (goals) and then the best way to achieve those goals second (behavior). This also further highlights the lack of a direct link between stimulus and response. Individual differences in predisposition (e.g., temperament traits) may play an important role in deciding the animal's strategic priority and behavioral choice, so assessment of individual predispositions (personality/temperament/character) can be very informative from a clinical perspective. Once we accept that a given behavior is simply the way in which a wider strategic objective is being addressed, then the focus of management shifts away from a focus on behavior modification toward the potential to influence higher-level cognitive and emotional influences underpinning the strategic decision-making process (e.g., the reason the animal wants to escape). This potentially allows for more efficient management recommendations with a clear functional goal.

- Since animals have a limited behavior repertoire but potentially many different goals, it is not surprising that a given behavior may have many underlying causes. If we think in terms of stimulus and response, there is a danger that we might focus primarily on the more overt associations. For example, mounting is often referred to as a sexual behavior for obvious reasons. However, it is also displayed in the contexts of play and frustration, which may be given less emphasis from a stimulus–response perspective, but should be given equal emphasis when considering the goal of the behavior an animal is exhibiting at a particular time.

Thus, although the behaviorist approach has much to commend it, it is important to appreciate both the biases it creates in our thinking and the subsequent limitations it can impose when it comes to effective clinical practice.

The medicalization of problem behavior

The medical approach to problem behavior is characterized by the definition of categories of conditions (disorders) with the goal of identifying underlying pathologies. This has emphasized the importance of assessing how different signs might relate to each other and physiological correlates. Accordingly, treatment emphasizes the need for physical interventions, such as with medications. Indeed, the valuable development of more effective medications for managing a range of problem behaviors in animals owes a lot to the influence of this perspective over the last 30 years. Although this still provides the dominant framework for psychiatric diagnosis in most of Europe and North America, there is growing concern in the human psychiatric field over the lack of progress being made using this approach (no entirely new category of medication has been discovered to treat depression since the discovering of the serotonergic agents). Like the behaviorist approach, this perspective has been critical to advancing the field, but it also has serious limitations.

Implicit within the definition of "categories" of conditions is the notion that individuals with such conditions are qualitatively different from the "normal" population (i.e., abnormal), when in reality they may simply differ by degree (e.g., have more extreme versions of adaptive traits). Much biological variation is indeed a matter of degree, and the imposition of categories on a dimensional scale results in poor diagnostic specificity. The point at which normal anxiety becomes an anxiety disorder or a fear becomes a phobia is largely arbitrary or at least without a solid biological basis. The artificial nature of categories in this context can also encourage clinicians to make multiple diagnoses when there may be a single underlying issue (e.g., the animal that is aggressive when confronted may also be more aggressive around food, but this does not mean that it has two different aggression diagnoses or motivations). This has been noted in the veterinary behavior literature as well.[10] Finally, the artificial nature of imposing categories to define a population, which vary by degree and not condition, also explains why the identification of reliable biological markers of specific behavioral problems is so rare. There is no distinctive pathology present.

Labeling conditions as disorders, also creates a bias in the way we think about managing problem behavior. If we think something is physically wrong, then there is a natural tendency to think about a physical intervention to treat or correct it. As a result, the functional benefits of the underlying state in other contexts (e.g., alternative genetic combinations, alternative environments, alternative stages of development, or in the opposite sex) may be overlooked. This limits our research focus and potentially our openness to alternative ways of managing a condition. There is also a danger of letting the diagnosis become a way of labeling the individual. Thus, if a dog is labeled as having some form of aggression disorder, then all of its aggressive behavior is seen as part of this disorder when some aspects may be considered perfectly normal in a dog not labeled in this way. For example, as a dog ages, it may become more aggressive, and this can easily be seen as a deterioration of the aggression disorder rather than the potential effects of painful arthritis.

Thus, while the medical approach has much to commend it, especially with regard to the potential value of psychopharmacological intervention, it too creates biases in our thinking that subsequently limit our potential when it comes to effective clinical practice.

The psychobiological approach

In recognition of the concerns described above, a psychobiological approach has been developed by the clinical animal behavior team at the University of Lincoln, UK. This combines an understanding of comparative psychology with evolutionary and behavioral biology within a framework which is firmly grounded in our growing understanding of the neurobiological basis to emotional behavior.[11–13] The approach takes note of the best of the two perspectives described above, while also seeking to address the limitations discussed. A consistent framework is provided for describing a problem, which must make reference to its context, motivation, and emotion. By contrast, in the general clinical behavior literature, there has often been confusing language used in relation to context, motivation, or emotion (e.g., with emotional state described as motivation for behavior, or contextual descriptions of behavior used as if they say something about the internal state of the individual), resulting in inconsistent diagnostic descriptions of behavior.[14]

- Context defines the circumstances in which the behavior arises. This should be done by reference to the observable environmental conditions surrounding the behavior. This relates to both the triggering stimuli (immediate antecedents to the behavior) and general circumstances preceding the incident (setting).
- Motivation describes the biological function/goal of the behavior, and can only be inferred in the field setting (i.e., it cannot be measured directly). However, by adapting the descriptive techniques used in Applied Behavior Analysis (ABA), it is possible to ascertain the most likely triggers (antecedents), forms (what the behavior looks like), reinforcers or inhibitors (consequences), and motivational goals of the behavior. The systematic process used makes the evidence for the final inference drawn about motivation repeatable and thus reliable, although it is appreciated that this proposal is a hypothesis that is subject to revision in light of any new evidence that becomes available at any time. Any difference in opinion in assessment should only relate to the interpretation of this evidence, not its content.
- Emotion relates to the personal significance of the event to the individual and the processes that result in an individualized response to a given situation. Like motivation, emotion cannot be measured directly in a field setting, but can be inferred using a systematic process. This also requires a careful analysis of the subject across a range of circumstances or over an extended time frame in order to elucidate information relating to four components of emotion: the potentially emotionally competent quality of the stimulus triggering the response (i.e., type of event capable of eliciting an emotional response) and how it might be personally significant to the subject, indications of arousal level, communicative signals, and the behavioral tendency that describes the sum of behaviors in the given emotionally relevant situation (see Table 25.1).[15,16]

From a pragmatic perspective, within a clinical behavior context, it is proposed that the emotional response be described in terms of a response to one of the following nine potential categories of emotionally competent stimuli:[10,15]

1. Desirables: things the animal wants at a given time which lead to seeking out opportunities to explore or acquire them.
2. Frustrations: events, objects, or individuals which limit the animal's expected control/autonomy over the environment, such as things that the animal wants but cannot access due to a barrier or are less than expected; these lead to increased, focused effort aimed at achieving the goal and removing the perceived barrier.
3. Threats: events that are perceived to be potentially harmful to the animal and therefore lead to a behavioral

Table 25.1 The four components (adapted from the component process model of emotion)[16] used to evidence an emotional response within the psychobiological approach. Evidence consistent with a fear response is described

Component	Example
Emotionally competent stimulus quality	A sudden, unexpected, loud noise is consistent with the trigger of a fear response
Arousal	Increased as evident from signs of sympathetic arousal such as pupil dilation and piloerection
Behavioral tendency	Moving away from the stimulus source, freezing, potentially barking, and other threatening behaviors toward the source; seeking of areas consistent with attempts to hide
Communicative signals	Panting, widening of the eyes, backward-pointing ears

strategy directed toward avoidance of interaction, including active and passive escape from the situation.

4. Pains: situations predicted to cause or exacerbate actual bodily damage, and which lead to withdrawal and protective responses.
5. Affiliates: individuals with whom an individual benefits from shared activity/interaction, such as members (or potential members) of a social group who provide foraging assistance or shared learning opportunities, such as social play.
6. Attachment figures and objects: those who provide safety and protection, resulting in a strong dependence on them for this, especially at times of uncertainty and insecurity.
7. Dependents: those who are perceived to be dependent on an individual animal for the provision of key resources such as safety, security, and potentially, sustenance (e.g. offspring); these will invoke a range of caring and protective behaviors around them.
8. Potential sexual partners: those perceived to provide potential breeding opportunities, leading to the expression of competitive rivalry as well as courtship and reproductive activity around them.
9. Undesirables: those who are perceived to undermine the benefits or potentially increase the net costs of the current social group; these may elicit responses associated with their active repulsion and exclusion.

Differential diagnoses are then expressed as hypotheses relating to the role of each of the above (context, motivation, and emotion), with differentials possible in any or all of them. As part of the diagnostic process, an explicit distinction is also made between different causal features: specific events that trigger (immediate antecedents) the problem behavior and circumstances which alter the predisposition on either a relatively temporary (transient moderator of response) or more permanent (moderating characteristic) basis. An example of each of these factors is given in Table 25.2 in a fictitious incident involving a pet parent who has complained about their dog biting them.

This comprehensive behavioral assessment framework, developed as part of the psychobiological approach, has the potential to bring greater structure and clarity to our thinking about the "cause" of problem behavior. In so doing, it

Table 25.2 Examples of related contextual, motivational, and emotional factors that affect the probability and/or severity of a hypothetical case of a dog that has bitten its pet parent when trying to take a ball away from it

	Immediate antecedent	Transient moderator	Moderating characteristic
Context	Removal of a ball	Dog is in its bed	The ball was the dog's favorite
Motivation	Retain possession of the ball	Dog had recently been playing with the ball	Of all its toys, the dog particularly values balls
Emotion	Frustration reaction to potential loss of a resource	Pet parent had been recently clearing up (i.e., removing a lot of the dog's toys and putting them away out of reach of the dog), reducing the autonomy of the dog to play with its toys	Poor frustration tolerance as personality trait

also brings greater focus on the way potential interventions may help and their likely impact in terms of behavioral change. The approach is also scientific in that it has a replicable method that begins with objective data (descriptions of the situation) from which logical deductions (inferences) are made. These inferences concern the internal state of the animal in terms of emotional and motivational variables and are thus hypotheses, but crucially the systematic approach and framework also provides a way to falsify these in line with the classic scientific method through the presentation of more data as it comes to light.

In summary, the aim of the psychobiological approach is to construct a functional explanation for why an animal behaves in a certain way, rather than label it as having a certain disorder; however, that does not mean that neurobiological changes have not occurred, only that they are part of normal evolved mechanisms in the vast majority of cases. The assessment considers how the current state has developed during the lifetime of the individual, both in terms of internal regulatory changes and external reinforcement, in order to construct the most parsimonious explanation of the current emotional and motivational state of the individual in the problem context and relevant factors influencing its behavior. This may involve reference to several states that reflect the real world situation. For example, the animal that is scared is also likely to seek safety, which may or may not be available, and the interaction between relevant affective systems in these circumstances needs to be carefully evaluated (see Figure 25.1).

Behavioral problems as functional states and the importance of impulsivity

Maladaptive behavior does not mean malfunctional underlying mechanism

With its focus on a functional evolutionary context for behavior, a major question that needs to be addressed is: Why does certain behavior appear so maladaptive if it does not have a pathological mechanism? In order to answer this, it is important to understand the proximate and ultimate factors governing the expression of behavior. The adaptive function of behavior has developed from evolutionary rules of thumb, which were successful within the environment that shaped the species. When these are applied in a captive environment, then adaptive processes such as shifts between internal and external reinforcement mechanisms and the streamlining of behavior which naturally occur to increase efficiency of

access to a reward with minimum effect can result in bizarre forms of behavior such as certain forms of stereotypic behavior. These may be maladaptive in the current environment, but they do not indicate that the underlying mechanisms are malfunctional.[17] Another consequence of this way of thinking is a recognition that most animals with problem behavior are not only following these rules, but trying to fit in from their own perspective. When we create the environmental circumstances for an animal to choose appropriate behavior without an overt cue, we consider the animal to be well behaved; when a problem arises with a pet parent or others, we then need to try to evaluate things from the animal's perspective and consider why the environment is not conducive to the animal being well behaved. This should draw our attention to not only how reinforcement may have shaped the original behavior, but also the reason why the initial behavioral decision was made out of all of the available options.

Impulsivity

In addition to understanding motivation and emotion, it is also important to understand the broader executive control of behavior and the factors which influence the speed with which decisions are made (i.e., the degree to which the response is influenced by cognitive input). This is often referred to as the animal's level of impulsivity and, while specific behaviors can be shaped to occur with varying degrees of delay in response to a stimulus, impulsivity refers to the animal's general tendency to react across a range of circumstances and behaviors. Thus, we might say that cats, in general, are more impulsive than dogs, but also that certain breeds of dog might typically be more impulsive than others because of the type of work they do. For example, imagine the speed with which a working Jack Russell Terrier must make decisions in order to avoid getting injured by a rat compared to the decision-making speed required by a Golden Retriever whose work is based on responding to cues from a pet parent. These differences exist not only at a breed level, but also between individuals within a breed and can be lost to some extent when we start breeding animals for their appearance rather than their work. Because there is an easing on the previous selective pressure for this trait in these circumstances, its variability may increase. As a result, there is often enormous variability in impulsivity within a given breed of dog. Whereas high levels of impulsivity can be adaptive, like any other trait, they come with a potential cost in certain environments. Individuals who are more impulsive may be prone to make poorer decisions, especially

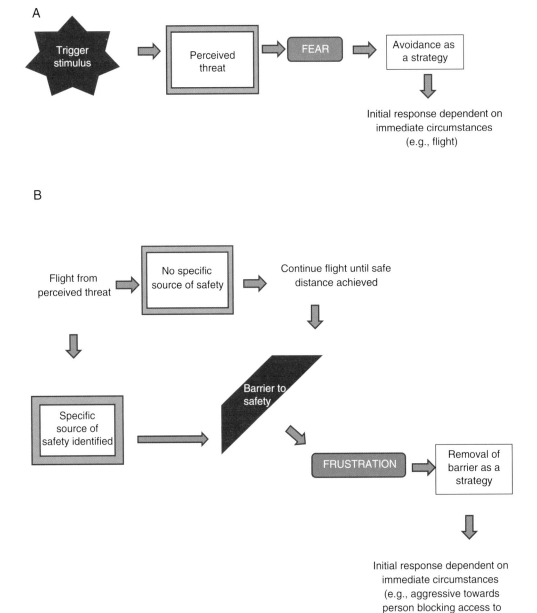

Figure 25.1 Diagrammatic representation of the functional sequence following appearance of a stimulus perceived to be a threat. Red shapes represent emotionally competent stimuli, pink boxes perceptions, orange boxes emotional reactions, white boxes strategic decisions made; note the behavior which flows from the event depends on the strategy chosen and prevailing circumstances – moderators of response which may act on any of the internal processes (represented by box shapes) are not shown. (A) The initial unimpaired response. (B) The response which might ultimately result in a bite – this arises as a result of multiple emotional changes and so could be categorized as forms of fear and/or frustration-related aggression using the classic "medical view" of problem behavior without fully explaining the role of these in the overall process; the response is not directly linked to the stimulus as implied by the classic "behaviorist view"; in the psychobiological approach, the functional response process is explained as part of the comprehensive behavior assessment (diagnosis), including the role of moderators, without labels. As a result, the potential impact of different interventions is explicitly predicted and forms part of the diagnostic validation process.

with regard to risk, since they have not fully evaluated all the available information. This is true for both humans and other animals. Understanding impulsivity can therefore be very informative when considering problem behavior and many animals are routinely screened for these traits as part of the psychobiological approach.

Impulsivity is a trait, not a condition, and can be defined as the tendency toward rapid, unplanned reactions to internal or external stimuli, potentially without functional evaluation of the consequences of this action to the individual or others.

Thus, more impulsive individuals will often make decisions on the basis of the most overt stimuli and so are potentially more likely to make decisions which might have a negative impact on others in the short term and themselves in the longer term. More impulsive individuals tend to overestimate rewards and underestimate costs compared to less impulsive individuals. This is unlikely to be a problem when the environment is safe (and there are few costs; indeed, in that circumstance evolution might favor the more impulsive individual). However, when there are greater risks, such as the risk of coming into conflict with others, this can be problematic. As a result, the individual may also be more highly aroused in general and emotionally reactive; it is also at greater risk of encountering situations that will lead to frustration. Unless the individual has appropriate skills to cope with the sort of potentially problematic situation in which it might find itself, this can lead to a wide range of problems, such as intensive vocalization (e.g., meowing in cats and whining, barking, or howling in dogs, depending on the circumstance) or aggressive displays as the animal seeks to escape from the situation.

The dog impulsivity assessment scale

Before considering how impulsivity is managed, let us consider how it is assessed. Historically, within clinical animal behavior, impulsivity has been considered in relation to aggression in the dog. The DIAS[5] was developed to allow the consistent assessment of impulsivity in dogs. It is an 18-item questionnaire which uses a 5-point Likert scale (scored 1–5) to rate the dog's behavior in general. The scale has been validated both physiologically (against urinary metabolites) and in laboratory behavior testing (with both delayed reward and spatial discounting paradigms). The former laboratory model

has been developed as a model for predicting the efficacy of fluoxetine in other species. Together these determine overall impulsivity. Using this scale, it has been found that behavior clinic cases at the University of Lincoln score ~1 standard deviation higher on average than the general dog population without problems. Accordingly, this level of difference (rather than the two standard deviations used for defining statistical abnormality) is generally used as a clinical guide to suggest that the level of the trait is an important moderating characteristic in a given case. Dogs in training classes also score more highly, but dogs at conformation dog shows tend to score lower than the general population.

The individual items making up DIAS also group to allow the identification of three facets of impulsivity (Table 25.3) which cut across behavior but may be individually important:

- Behavioral Regulation: a group of items reflecting excitability and ability to control both initiation and termination of behavior
- Response to Novelty and Aggression: items indicating active responding when faced with aversion and uncertainty
- Responsiveness: items describing a behavioral sensitivity to environmental cues

Scores on the "behavioral regulation" facet are associated with the likelihood of dogs showing signs of destructiveness

Table 25.3 Items making up DIAS, mean scores ± standard deviations (SD). Overall impulsivity questionnaire score: mean 0.52 ± 0.1. Bolded items feature in more than one facet and - items are reverse scored

Component (mean ± SD)	Constituent items
Behavioral regulation (0.47 ± 0.15)	My dog shows extreme physical signs when excited (e.g., drooling, panting, raising hackles, urination, licking lips, widening of eyes)
	When my dog gets very excited, it can lead to fixed repetitive behavior (i.e., an action that is repeated in the same way over and over again, such as tail chasing or spinning around in circles)
	I would consider my dog to be very impulsive (i.e., has sudden, strong urges to act; acts without forethought; acts without considering effects of actions)
	My dog does not think before it acts (e.g., would steal food without first looking to see if someone is watching)
	My dog can be very persistent (e.g., will continue to do something even if it knows it will get punished or told off)
	-My dog calms down very quickly after being excited
	-My dog appears to have a lot of control over how it responds
	My dog is not very patient (e.g., gets agitated waiting for its food, or waiting to go out for a walk)
	My dog seems to get excited for no reason.
	-My dog is easy to train
Aggression response to novelty (0.36 ± 0.15)	My dog doesn't like to be approached or hugged
	My dog becomes aggressive (e.g., growl, snarl, snap, bite) when excited
	My dog may become aggressive (e.g., growl, snarl, snap, bite) if frustrated with something
	My dog is not keen to go into new situations
	-My dog is very interested in new things and new places
Responsiveness (0.70 ± 0.13	My dog appears to be "sorry" after it has done something wrong
	My dog is easy to train
	My dog takes a long time to lose interest in new things
	My dog reacts very quickly
	My dog is very interested in new things and new places

and elimination problems, the "response to novelty and aggression" facet is associated with both active and passive avoidance responses; and high scores in the "responsiveness" facet are more likely to be withdrawn early, as in working police dogs. In the absence of specific behavioral intervention, it has been found that adult dog scores remain stable for more than 6–7 years.[18]

Use of DIAS in clinical practice

DIAS is not only used in the initial assessment of a case to evaluate the potential contributory role of impulsivity to a problem behavior but also to evaluate the potential value of selective serotonin reuptake inhibitors (SSRIs) (given other pharmacological and medical considerations) and to monitor case progression. As mentioned above, impulsivity is not a diagnosis, but high levels, especially, may increase the risk of problem behavior. In some cases, by using treatment measures (discussed below) to manage impulsivity, a dog may start to make better decisions without the need for more challenging behavioral interventions. Thus the instrument is not a diagnostic tool but an aid to clinical judgment, since impulsivity may be considered a moderator of behavior. The clinician must evaluate the role and potential value of addressing impulsivity in a given case. As mentioned above, we generally view scores more than one standard deviation away from the mean as potentially clinically important.

It would be wrong to think that impulsivity was the root of all problems relating to emotional arousal, but it is quite a common feature that can be moderated relatively effectively with the use of SSRIs. Accordingly, one of the main benefits to the use of DIAS is the ability to make quite reliable assessments about the potential value, or not, of instigating treatment with SSRIs, especially fluoxetine as a first-line pharmacological intervention. If scores are high overall, then in our opinion, it may be used responsibly, even in cases involving aggression, assuming the normal risks are addressed. Increased aggression when treated with an SSRI is very rare when the aggression is associated with poor decision making by the dog due to high impulsivity, assuming the animal is otherwise healthy.

We have also developed a series of impulse control exercises to help bring about more permanent changes within the individual. These exercises are similar to many that are already used in problem behavior management; however, we suggest that when used in the ways outlined, they bring about changes in behavior through altering trait level impulsivity rather than by simple generalization of learned context-specific stimulus – response associations.

As with the use of SSRIs, these exercises are used when we believe the animal may make better decisions if it were to act less impulsively. Perhaps the most widely used exercise is the "self-settle" (i.e., to calm down without specific cues being given by the pet parent) when the animal is faced with something that it wants. The critical points here are that the cause for behavioral control comes from the general environmental context and not event-specific cues (such as instructions or signals from the pet parent). Second, it is the animal's self-control and level of arousal that is the focus of the exercise and not any specific behavior; it does not matter so much what the animal does so long as it pauses, waits, and behaves in a way that we would consider well behaved. The exact circumstances chosen for a given case depend on the level of the

stimulus or situations with which the animal can cope. Although there is no scale for cats or other species, impulsivity might be important in the problems of other species; assessment in these cases is necessarily more subjective but no less important. Example situations to practice self-settle include: before going through a door, before being fed, getting out of the car, etc. The situations are also not specific to any particular one motivational or emotional state. The critical professional skill for the clinical behaviorist is to identify a range of suitable contexts that are commonly encountered every day in which the animal can practice this sort of restraint (delayed reward gratification), building on small acts of uncued behavioral restraint until a more global change is noticed in novel contexts, including the one which is the focus of the problem behavior. Indeed, by not focusing initially on the problem behavior context, pet parents are less likely to make mistakes and get frustrated at what they perceive to be their failings. It is easy to forget that pet parents are not skilled trainers, and the simpler we can make exercises, the more likely they are to succeed.

Frustration

The affective system underpinning frustration has its origin in the need for animals to respond to limits to their autonomy. From an evolutionary perspective, this perhaps began in very simple organisms with restraint, and the natural response is an invigoration of activity and in higher animals, more sophisticated processes allowing acquisition of resources from an environment where there may be many barriers. As the cognitive abilities of animals have developed through evolution, so animals have become able to not only respond in more sophisticated ways to such restrictions but also predict when these might occur, resulting in resource protection and defense strategies. From a clinical animal behavior perspective, frustration can be thought of as an emotional state which arises when an animal is thwarted from obtaining something it is motivated to gain or retaining something under its control (e.g., removing the food bowl). Frustration can also occur where previously learned expectations are not met (absent, reduced, or delayed reward, such as the absence of an expected treat) as well as those situations where there are more overt actual or potential barriers to autonomous control (e.g., restraint, intrusion into personal space, including the territory). Thus, problems such as territorial barking should be considered primarily a form of frustration response rather than an anxious/fearful response to the threat of an invader. This does not mean that circumstances involving frustration cannot also involve a degree of fear. Indeed, when there is a perceived risk of harm involved in the defense of a resource, such as when an aggressive response is involved, we would predict that most animals will show some degree of fear, and this sort of signaling ambivalence has been observed in wolf packs.[19] Such co-occurrence of affective states is common, as animals evaluate stimuli in terms of their emotionally competent potential (emotional quality) by reference to all the dimensions described above.

Many situations involving frustration are often described solely in terms of perceived threat, as if fear is the only important state. Indeed, in the English language, we commonly use terms such as "anxiety" or "worry" in a very imprecise way that can lead to confused or biased thinking. This should not be considered to be merely a theoretical issue, as it has practical implications. From a neurobiological perspective (and thus a mechanistic perspective when we consider what medications might be useful in a given situation), a distinction is made between a threat to resources (frustration) and a threat to the integrity of the self (fear). If we are worried about being mugged when we go somewhere and our primary concern is about being harmed, then fear is dominating our perspective; however, if our main focus is a concern at being robbed and losing our money or possessions, then frustration is the dominant influence. This simple example not only serves to illustrate the difference between these emotional systems but also highlights how our experience of emotional activity is the outcome of a blend of responses to a complex environment, in the same way our view of a beautiful scene is the outcome of the three primary colors (red, blue, and yellow) in space and time. This also helps to explain why psychopharmaceutical interventions may appear unreliable, as animals exist in a complex fluid emotional state arising from the continuous waxing and waning of different affective systems. This is a different perspective from that of traditional neurophysiologists who have suggested a more modular view of emotion, with discrete circuits controlling specific responses.[11] From the psychobiological perspective, affective systems are interconnected networks influencing perception, processing, decision making, and executive activity in the brain. They are not discrete structures. The outputs of affective network systems, such as behavioral systems, are controlled by the release of inhibition. Given the role of these affective networks in setting our strategic priorities at any given time (by determining the personal significance of the perceived world around us), we should not be surprised that our experience of them is typically as a blend of several emotions and rarely as a pure single state.

There has been growing appreciation of the importance of understanding fear and anxiety in companion animals, but there seems to have been much less recognition of the role of frustration. Many problem behaviors are ascribed to anxiety (in the sense of the anticipation of a physical threat to the self that is related to fear), when frustration offers a better explanation of the root cause of the problem and may help to guide more effective management. It seems many desensitization protocols may be less effective when applied to frustrating triggers, since animals process and thus scale rewards differently to aversives. A recent analysis[20] of the behavioral structure of what is commonly referred to as "separation-related disorders" indicates that the problematic responses are largely indicative of different expressions of frustration when left alone, with fear/anxiety playing only a minor role beyond the anticipation of the event. See Chapter 17 for more information on separation-related disorders. As indicated earlier and illustrated in Figure 25.1 above, in many situations, the two emotions may be combined, for example, when an animal is threatened and tries to escape, it will experience both fear in response to the threat and frustration at being unable to reach safety. The focus on fear and related anxiety in the literature can also lead us to undertake the natural tendency to seek the evidence in support of our belief, rather than to test it scientifically and consider alternative explanations; in such circumstances, the diagnostic process must be considered essentially unscientific. Accordingly, certain communicative signals, such as "lip licking" are described in support of our "diagnosis" as a sign of "anxiety" or even less convincingly, as signs of unspecified "stress" without explicitly considering them also as a potential indicator of frustration. Indeed, as mentioned above, very few if any behaviors can be understood from their form outside of context. By considering the affective systems linked to the nine types of emotionally competent stimulus described above, we have a framework for not only describing the emotional basis of behavior in a consistent way but also for testing and eliminating alternative explanations through the scientific process of hypothesis testing and falsification.

The canine frustration questionnaire

Given the above, it is not surprising that until recently, frustration responses have been poorly characterized in companion animals. To this end, the development and validation of the Canine Frustration Questionnaire, has been a major advance.[6] This was developed as a psychometric instrument, using a similar process to that used for the development of DIAS; items are scored on a 5-point Likert scale. Unlike impulsivity, which refers to the general executive control of behavior and cognition, frustration refers to a specific emotional state. The questionnaire consists of 21 items which group into five components and is described in Table 25.4.

There is clearly some overlap in content between some of the items included in the canine frustration and impulsivity questionnaires, and this is to be expected, given the tendency for higher levels of impulsivity to lead an animal into more frustrating situations. Indeed, individuals scoring highly across the dimensions will often benefit from psychopharmacological intervention with an SSRI such as fluoxetine, at least in the early stages of training while the necessary skills are established.

The structure revealed by the statistical analysis of CFQs suggests that while barrier frustration, dealing with unmet expectations, and autonomous control are all related to the overall construct of frustration in dogs, they generally partition out, suggesting that while responses within one of these components are closely related, they share less in common with the items in other components. Accordingly, within the suite of activities we have developed to manage frustration issues (coping with barriers, unmet expectations, or invasion of personal space boundaries), we carefully consider their relevance according to the component onto which they most closely map and the dog's associated score. When considering how to treat these problems, it is essential that animals are only exposed to situations with which they can cope as part of the training exercise and that tolerance is built up incrementally. Treatment programs which involve exposing the animal to the stimulus until it settles down (i.e., flooding, response blocking) should not be used, since these can be dangerous with an animal with poor frustration tolerance and risk provoking an aggressive response, either directly or as part of a redirected response. Such protocols are also of welfare and ethical concern when more humane alternatives, such as those described in the following section are available.

Table 25.4 Items making up CFQ, mean scores, and standard deviations (SD). The mean Overall Canine Frustration Questionnaire ± SD is 0.45 ± 0.12. - items (all in the frustration coping component) are reverse scored

Component (mean ± SD)	Constituent items
General frustration (0.38 ± 0.15)	My dog becomes frustrated in a large range of situations
	There are days when my dog seems to become more easily frustrated than others for no apparent reason
	My dog appears to become frustrated frequently (e.g., at least once daily)
	My dog shows increases in certain behaviors (e.g., lip licking, yawning, mounting, full body shake-off) if he/she cannot immediately access something he/she wants
	My dog engages in a repetitive behavior (e.g., tail chasing, pacing, circling) when unable to access something he/she wants
Barrier frustration/perseverance (0.55 ± 0.18)	My dog shows continued efforts (e.g., lunging, pulling toward) to approach a dog/person they wish to greet, when being restrained from doing so (e.g., when on lead)
	When on lead, my dog will persist in lunging/pulling toward something he/she would like to chase (e.g., a cat, rabbit, bird, toy)
	My dog has difficulty in responding to cues/commands (e.g., sit, lie down, stay) if there is something else he/she wants to do or access
	My dog gets upset if shut away from visitors (e.g., vocalizes or scratches/digs at the door)
Unmet expectations (0.52 ± 0.17)	My dog does not like being left out of activities with other dogs
	My dog appears agitated and unsettled when he/she wants something another dog has (e.g., a toy or food item)
	My dog becomes very excited/restless (e.g., pacing, whining, barking, jumping up) when waiting to take part in an enjoyable activity
	My dog appears unsettled when there are delays in his/her routine (e.g., if walked or fed later than usual)
Autonomous control (0.37 ± 0.13)	My dog becomes aggressive (i.e., growl, snap, or bite) if I try to remove an item he/she has (e.g., favorite toy or food)
	When my dog is not kept busy, he/she can repeatedly lick, chew, or nibble their own body parts (e.g., paws, flanks/sides)
	My dog appears annoyed/upset if given less than he/she was expecting (e.g., wants table scraps and gets a pat on the head; given less food/a lower quality of food than expecting)
	My dog will attempt to escape if I try to confine him/her (e.g., in a room, crate, or kennel)
	My dog is protective of his/her territory (house, garden, car)
Frustration coping (0.46 ± 0.16)	-My dog appears to cope well when denied access to things he/she is occasionally allowed (e.g., access to the sofa/bed or provision of table scraps)
	-I find it easy to interrupt/distract my dog from doing things he/she wants to do
	-My dog finds it easy to relax and settle when unable to access something he/she wants

Use of CFQ in clinical practice

CFQ is used as both an aid to the assessment of a case (in order to evaluate the potential contributory role of frustration to the problem), the choice of treatment interventions, and the monitoring of cases receiving treatment. A key question to consider is whether the score supports or refutes the involvement of frustration in a given aspect of behavior before considering the potential value of a particular exercise. To this end, we may make a number of predictions concerning the relationship between the behavior of dogs presenting for a given problem, their CFQ scores, and potential treatments of value.

Individuals with high scores for "General frustration" can be expected to frequently show signs of frustration in various aspects of their daily life and for these, interventions which focus on the development of frustration tolerance in general (i.e., across a range of contexts) may be required. Reducing behavioral perseverance when mildly frustrated might also be helpful. This can be achieved by using mild distractions. The key here is for the pet parent to show interest in something else of interest but not to directly offer this distraction to the dog. The dog then chooses to disengage from its current frustration response and refocus on the pet parent. In this way, inadvertent reinforcing of the frustration response is avoided. This component also contains an item related to unpredictable moodiness, and a high score on this item could indicate the involvement of pain, lowering the threshold to aversive events. A close and systematic medical evaluation is then indicated, and possibly even an analgesia trial.

If pet parent finds it difficult to distract their dog when it is trying to access something it wants, for example, when it is constrained by either the leash or some other form of containment, then it is worth paying particular attention to the score in relation to "Barrier frustration/perseverance." A high score indicates that it is not simply a question of obedience, but a more fundamental problem with this aspect of frustration. Rather than simply desensitize the dog in the context of the problem stimulus, we suggest that in situations involving the pet parent, they teach a "check-in" cue (e.g., "look at me") initially and then combine this with the pet parent taking the initiative to solve a potential problem before the dog gets too aroused, for example, opening a gate for the dog or taking the lead off (assuming it is safe to do so). These scenarios should be different from those where the problem is most obvious. As the pet parent becomes more sensitive to reading their dog when they want something, so they can begin to fade the verbal cue. The dog's behavior (glancing at the pet parent) then becomes a more reliable expression of the need for assistance and the pet parent is more able to respond appropriately. In the case of pet parent-absent problems, then teaching a prolonged settle on a mat in a variety of contexts may help to develop acceptance of later confinement.

A similar strategy of encouraging the pet to look to the pet parent (i.e., checking in) to ask for instruction or direction as to how to approach or behave during a situation, albeit using different contexts, can be used in relation to high scores for the component relating to "Unmet expectations." In this case, it is not necessary for the pet parent to necessarily provide the reward on which the dog was initially focused. Instead, we suggest ensuring the pet parent has a good relationship with their dog and rewarding the attentive behavior with some quality and enjoyable time for both. In this way, a potentially laborious exercise can also be turned into an opportunity to enjoy each other (something which has sometimes disappeared from the relationship). Increasing the delay between the "check-in," which should be performed very calmly, and the alternative activity will help to build greater tolerance, with a low risk of the problem behavior being expressed. As elsewhere, we encourage training in settings which are contextually different to those in which the problem behavior is performed but which require the same skill in order to maximize success.

Issues relating to "Autonomous control" reflect the dog's perception of itself and its various forms of personal space. Whereas humans tend to define boundaries in relation to fixed features of an environment (e.g., through the position of garden fences), many animals, including dogs, perceive the space around them much more in relation to where they are (i.e., distances from themselves which they find acceptable). This is why a territorial dog will often also appear to be protective of the car, even if it is new; it is not so much the item as the space it occupies which is important. Accordingly, managing protectiveness around these boundaries involves increasing positive associations around these barriers, especially with regard to access to resources, for example by tossing treats toward the dog and then seeing if the dog will allow a closer approach, or at least tolerate approach followed by withdrawal without becoming overaroused. The structure of this component suggests that

other exercises aimed at teaching the dog to cope with unmet expectations such as the provision of a lower-value food than expected for a given task (e.g., intermittent reward schedules, smaller treats) might also be useful in moderating this tendency.

Finally, the "frustration coping" score appears to reflect the ability of the dog to find alternative strategies once frustrated, potentially due to the rapid onset of increased arousal associated with the situation. Teaching relaxation exercises alongside more general problem-solving abilities to increase behavioral flexibility may be useful in these circumstances. Example exercises that might be considered to help teach frustration tolerance include self-control in relation to delayed rewards (as per the impulse control exercises above, but also the use of certain self-control food delivery toys such as the OurPets IQ Treat Activity Dog Rope Toy and Dog Tug Toy and the Pet Life Grip N' Play Treat Dispensing Football-Shaped Suction Cup Dog Toy). In this case, it is not that the toy delivers a delayed reward, but that a greater reward comes from more controlled behavior (this makes it different from the commonly used stuffed food toy-type activities).

As already noted, low frustration tolerance and impulsivity often co-occur. More impulsive individuals might be more likely to place themselves in more frustrating situations, not only because they make a poor assessment of the consequences of their actions (act without full evaluation), but also because of their sensitivity to rewards and/or aversives, which leads to poor decision making in a given context. Sensitivity to rewards and aversives is assessed in dogs using the PANAS[7] and is discussed in the next section. Including evaluation of these tendencies using this simple scale can bring further insight into a case and is often conducted as a matter of routine with the other scales described in this chapter. They can be self-administered and completed by the pet parent in advance of the consultation to save time and help the whole process run more efficiently.

Positive and negative activation

Positive activation describes sensitivity to salient positive qualities in the environment observable from behaviors such as investigatory behaviors and play tendencies; negative activation describes sensitivity to potentially aversive qualities demonstrated through behaviors such as aggression and withdrawal tendencies. These two tendencies are considered by some to provide the ultimate basis for emotion (core affect) since they translate into a decision by an individual to approach or withdraw from a stimulus. While they are often expressed as opposite ends of a scale, it might be more accurate to represent them as unrelated traits since aversives and rewards are processed differently by the brain and high sensitivity to one does not imply low sensitivity to the other. Individual differences in sensitivity to the emotional valence applied to external stimuli help to explain differences in behavioral style and temperament. For example, differences in positive incentive motivation have been associated with variation in dopaminergic activity or sensitivity, and individuals at the extremes of the dimension are more likely to exhibit behavior which is inappropriate and problematic in a range of circumstances.

Positive and negative activation scale

The PANAS for dogs[7] was originally developed to assess individual differences in responsiveness to rewarding and aversive experiences (Table 25.5). Positive and negative activation scores provide a measure that allows prediction of behavioral tendencies across diverse contexts involving reinforcement/punishment. This can assist in the identification of animals at risk of related problems. High negative activation scores should be associated with an increased risk of developing fears, phobias, and anxiety-related problems. However, some dogs may learn to show what appears to be a phobic response to noises as an attention-seeking device (pseudophobia)[21] and these individuals are less likely to score so highly for negative activation and in our clinical

Table 25.5 Items making up PANAS, together with overall and component mean scores with standard deviations

Negative activation (0.48 ± 0.15)	My dog is rarely frightened
	My dog is easily startled by noises and/or movements
	My dog appears nervous and/or jumpy for several minutes after it has been startled
	My dog has a specific fear or phobia
	My dog appears calm in noisy, crowded places
	My dog is frightened by noises from the television or radio
	My dog usually appears relaxed
	My dog adapts quickly to changes in its environment (e.g., being cared for by different people, moving house, or a family member leaving home)
	My dog appears afraid of the vacuum cleaner or any other familiar household appliance
	My dog appears calm in unfamiliar environments
	My dog appears unsettled by changes to its routine (e.g., if it is not fed at the usual time, if it is left alone for longer than usual)
Positive activation (0.72 ± 0.13)	
Energy and interest (0.85 ± 0.15)	My dog shows little interest in its surroundings
	My dog is full of energy
	My dog is lazy
	My dog requires a great deal of encouragement to take part in energetic activities
Persistence (0.55 ± 0.18)	My dog is very persistent in its efforts to get me to play
	My dog tries to escape from the garden
	My dog persists in being naughty despite being told off for the behavior
	My dog is very boisterous
Excitement (0.79 ± 0.17)	My dog becomes very excited when it is about to go for a walk (e.g., when it sees its lead or when it hears "walkies," etc.)
	My dog is easily excited

experience, score highly on positive activation. These individuals are also characterized by a very rapid drop in heart rate after the noise stimulus stops (this can be tested with a recording), which is inconsistent with the negative emotional arousal that would be expected for a phobic response, given the clinical signs.

The scale consists of 21 items, with 11 describing negative affect and 10 positive affect in the original version. Positive affect scores are divided into three components. Although the higher-level structure of PANAS has been found to be culturally robust, certain items may be culturally sensitive (e.g., the item referring to the dog trying to escape from the garden). Accordingly, when the scale was translated into Portuguese and used in Brazil,[22] certain items were excluded, resulting in slightly different norm references. The components of positive activation are also made up of relatively few items and so these component scores should be used with caution. Accordingly, it is important that only culturally validated versions of this (and other scales described in this chapter) are used and that international validity is not assumed.

Use of PANAS in clinical practice

As already noted, differences in emotional sensitivity can be used to assist in the diagnosis of behavioral problems and guide clinically relevant treatment considerations. An important feature of the psychobiological approach is its construction of the emotional (affective) aspect of the diagnosis at three levels: immediate antecedents (triggers), transient moderators of response (mood), and moderating characteristics (temperament). PANAS aims to provide a reliable profile for temperament in terms of positive and negative affect. This is an important clinical consideration since the underlying temperament of the individual provides insight into both the risk of relapse and also the potential need for psychopharmacological intervention. Take for example two dogs that are scared of fireworks following an aversive experience: one scores high on negative activation, whereas the other is within the normal range. The former is more likely to relapse due to a sensitive predisposition to aversive events. This individual is also more likely to be in need of psychopharmacological support not just to prevent this relapse risk but to also put the individual in a good state for behavioral modification exercises. Since the high negative activation score reflects a feature of temperament, it is unlikely that changes in this aspect of the patient's character will change very rapidly simply with behavior therapy. There is thus both a practical and moral responsibility to consider carefully the value of supportive medication. Sensitivity may also help to guide treatment recommendations in other ways, potentially predicting differential responses to set behavior-modification programs. For example, in general, dogs with fears tend to score higher for negative activation but contrary to popular belief, it is not the severity of the fear which predicts treatment outcome[23]; rather, it has been found that those individuals also scoring highly on positive activation are less likely to respond to routine behavioral modification protocols.[24]

Low positive affect is associated with depressive states in humans, which is commonly linked to chronic pain, and a similar relationship has been found between low positive activation scores and chronic pain in dogs.[25] Anecdotally, it seems that the dimension relating to persistence may be particularly sensitive to this. As with DIAS, PANAS may also be used in the assessment of the working dog. Successful working police dogs differ from both pet dogs and dogs withdrawn from service in a number of aspects of PANAS[26] and this could potentially be used in selection. Selection of suitable animals might be further improved by considering PANAS scores alongside DIAS, but this has yet to be evaluated in a longitudinal study.

Other behavior scales

There are many other behavior scales available, but few have undergone much if any validation and so need to be used with caution. Recently, some of the PANAS items have been used to develop a Highly Sensitive Dog Questionnaire in the German language. This aims to identify sensory processing sensitivity and load, which may be associated with an individual's coping ability and vulnerability to stress-related problems. The scale has undergone good validation and might provide a useful addition to the suite of instruments described here, but until the English language version is validated and clinical relationships identified, it should be used with caution in the English-speaking world. Accordingly, this instrument will not be discussed further.

The canine behavioral assessment and research questionnaire and feline behavioral assessment and research questionnaire

The Canine Behavioral Assessment and Research Questionnaire (C-BARQ)[27] and Feline Behavioral Assessment and Research Questionnaire (Fe-BARQ)[28] are popular, reliable instruments which provide a behavioral profile of an individual. The instruments group the intensity of behavior of animals in a range of contexts together to generate a score for that behavioral domain. However, these instruments are of limited value in the psychobiological approach to problem behavior management since they are not psychometric instruments of underlying traits; rather, they describe behavioral profiles. The way these instruments are designed means that they produce a score for a particular domain (e.g., stranger aggression) that is a composite of the number of contexts in which a behavior occurs with its intensity. Thus, a score of 4 in one of the domains could indicate an intense response in relation to a specific item or a very mild response across four items. This can limit their clinical and potential scientific utility[18] if this is not appreciated. Nonetheless, the individual items within these scales can be very useful for evaluating the extent of problem behavior and monitoring change.

The lincoln sound sensitivity scale

The LSSS[8] consists of 17 specific behavioral items plus an additional optional unspecified category; both the frequency and intensity of each behavioral response are considered separately (and in this way the confound described in relation to the scales described in the previous section can be avoided except when considering the total score). Excluding the item relating to an exaggerated response when startled and the unspecified behavior option, a total score of 30 has been used to define clinically significant conditions (noise phobia) for the development of an effective psychopharmacological intervention. The rationale for this cut-off is that a noise phobia is an excessive fear or anxiety of a sound, and excessive might refer to either the severity of response (i.e., at least two signs expressed in most intense form possible [score 5] every time the noise was heard [score 3]) or the number of behavioral signs shown (i.e., all 16 signs occur frequently [score 2] in the lowest intensity [score 1]). Because LSSS refers to the frequency with which specific responses occur, it is used to assess a series of events. This can be useful for monitoring certain events like a series of firework events, but if the event is intermittent or specific, then it is better to evaluate the response to a single event. The LCAS[9] was developed for this purpose.

Lincoln canine anxiety scale

The LCAS[9] is a 16-item scale that simply scores the severity (but not frequency) of behaviors associated with fear and anxiety. It has been shown to have good psychometric properties; a short version considering only the 11 items relating to running around; drooling saliva; hiding; cowering; restlessness/pacing; freezing to the spot; panting; pet parent-seeking behavior; vigilance/scanning of the environment; bolting; and shaking/trembling may be used for monitoring purposes without much reduction in its power. However, if any of the excluded items (destructiveness, aggressive behavior, barking/whining/howling, vomiting/defecating/urinating/diarrhea, or self-harm) form an important part of the pet parent complaint, then obviously, they should be specifically assessed.

Conclusion

The psychobiological approach provides a solid systematic and scientific framework for the evaluation of problem behavior. Using this approach, not only are we able to improve communication between clinicians, but also we have been able to begin developing robust psychometric instruments for the assessment of patients, both at initial presentation and following the instigation of treatment. The solid biological grounding of these instruments is providing new insights into treatment and the development of evidence-based protocols, which will ultimately be to the benefit of both our patients and their pet parents.

References

1. Flannigan G, Dodman NH. Risk factors and behaviors associated with separation anxiety in dogs. *J Am Vet Med Assoc.* 2001;219(4):460–466.

2. McGreevy PD, Masters AM. Risk factors for separation-related distress and feed-related aggression in dogs: additional findings from a survey of Australian dog owners. *Appl Anim Behav Sci.* 2008;109(2–4):320–328.

3. Pageat P. Terminology, behavioural pathology and the Pageat (French)

approach to canine behaviour disorders. In: Landsberg G, Hunthausen W, Ackerman L, eds. *Behavior Problems of the Dog and Cat.* 3rd ed. Edinburgh: Saunders Elsevier; 2013:345–366.

4. Mills DS. Conceptualising behaviour problems-separating a dog's bite from its owner's problem. In: *Proceedings of the first International Conference on Veterinary Behavioural Medicine.* Birmingham: Universities Federation for Animal Welfare; 1997:7–9.

5. Wright HF, Mills DS, Pollux PM. Development and validation of a psychometric tool for assessing impulsivity in the domestic dog (*Canis familiaris*). *Int J Compar Psychol.* 2011;24:210–225.

6. McPeake KJ, Collins LM, Zulch H, et al. The Canine Frustration Questionnaire—development of a new psychometric tool for measuring frustration in domestic dogs (*Canis familiaris*). *Front Vet Sci.* 2019;6:152.

7. Sheppard G, Mills DS. The development of a psychometric scale for the evaluation of the emotional predispositions of pet dogs. *Int J Compar Psychol.* 2002;15:201–222.

8. Mills D, Braem Dube M, Zulch H. Appendix B. *The Lincoln Sound-Sensitivity Scale. Stress and Pheromonatherapy in Small Animal Clinical Behavior.* West Sussex, UK: Wiley-Blackwell; 2013:259–263.

9. Mills DS, Mueller HW, McPeake K, et al. Development and psychometric validation of the Lincoln Canine Anxiety Scale. *Front Vet Sci.* 2020;7:171.

10. Mills DS, Ewbank R. ISAE, ethology and the veterinary profession. In: *Animals and Us: 50 Years and More of Applied Ethology.* Wageningen, Netherlands: Wageningen Academic Publishers; 2016:966–981.

11. Panksepp J. *Affective Neuroscience: The Foundations of Human and Animal Emotions.* Oxford, UK: Oxford University Press; 1998.

12. Craig AD. A new view of pain as a homeostatic emotion. *Trends Neurosci.* 2003;26(6):303–307.

13. Zeki S, Romaya JP. Neural correlates of hate. *PLoS One.* 2008;3(10):e3556.

14. Reisner IR. BSAVA manual of canine and feline behavioural medicine. In: *An Overview of Aggression.* Gloucestershire: BSAVA; 2002: 181–194.

15. Mills DS. Perspectives on assessing the emotional behavior of animals with behavior problems. *Curr Opin Behav Sci.* 2017;16:66–72.

16. Scherer KR. The dynamic architecture of emotion: evidence for the component process model. *Cogn Emot.* 2009;23(7): 1307–1351.

17. Mills DS. Medical paradigms for the study of problem behaviour: a critical review. *Appl Anim Behav Sci.* 2003;81(3): 265–277.

18. Riemer S, Mills DS, Wright H. Impulsive for life? The nature of long-term impulsivity in domestic dogs. *Anim Cogn.* 2014;17:815–819.

19. Fatjó J, Feddersen-Petersen D, de la Torre JLR, et al. Ambivalent signals during agonistic interactions in a captive wolf pack. *Appl Anim Behav Sci.* 2007;105(4): 274–283.

20. de Assis LS, Matos R, Pike TW, et al. Developing diagnostic frameworks in veterinary behavioral medicine: disambiguating separation related problems in dogs. *Front Vet Sci.* 2020;6:499.

21. Muller G. Pseudo phobias in dogs. In: Overall KL, Heath SE, Mills DS, et al., eds. *Proceedings of the Third International Congress on Veterinary Behavioural Medicine.* Potters Bar: UFAW; 2001; 114–118.

22. Savalli C, Albuquerque N, Vasconcellos AS, et al. Assessment of emotional predisposition in dogs using PANAS (Positive and Negative Activation Scale) and associated relationships in a sample of dogs from Brazil. *Sci Rep.* 2019;9(1): 1–9.

23. Mills DS, Estelles MG, Coleshaw PH, et al. Retrospective analysis of the treatment of firework fears in dogs. *Vet Rec.* 2003;153:561–562.

24. Sheppard G, Mills DS. The validation of scales designed to measure positive and negative activation in dogs. In: Seksel K, Perry G, Mills D, et al. *Fourth International Veterinary Behaviour Meeting Proceedings No: 352. Post Graduate Foundation in Veterinary Science.* Sydney: University of Sydney; 2003:37–45.

25. Reaney SJ, Zulch H, Mills D, et al. Emotional affect and the occurrence of owner reported health problems in the domestic dog. *Appl Anim Behav Sci.* 2017;196:76–83.

26. Braem M, Asher L, Furrer S, et al. Development of the "Highly Sensitive Dog" questionnaire to evaluate the personality dimension "Sensory Processing Sensitivity" in dogs. *PLoS One.* 2017;12(5):e0177616.

27. Hsu Y, Serpell JA. Development and validation of a questionnaire for measuring behavior and temperament traits in pet dogs. *J Am Vet Med Assoc.* 2003;223(9):1293–1300.

28. Duffy DL, de Moura RTD, Serpell JA. Development and evaluation of the Fe-BARQ: A new survey instrument for measuring behavior in domestic cats (Felis s. catus). *Behav Process.* 2017;141: 329–341.

Recommended reading

University of Lincoln Online Dog Behavior Calculators
https://ipstore.lincoln.ac.uk/product/online-canine-behaviour-calculators

C-BARQ
https://vetapps.vet.upenn.edu/cbarq
Fe-BARQ
https://vetapps.vet.upenn.edu/febarq/

Appendix A Behavior resources

Behavioral organizations for the veterinary team

Resource name	Website
**Academy of Veterinary Behavior Technicians	https://avbt.net
AAFP American Association of Feline Practitioners	www.catvets.com
**American College of Animal Welfare	www.acaw.org
**American College of Veterinary Behaviorists	www.dacvb.org
American Humane Society	www.americanhumane.org
American Veterinary Society of Animal Behavior	www.avsab.org
Animal Behavior Society	www.animalbehaviorsociety.org
Association for the Study of Animal Behaviour	www.asab.org
**Australian and New Zealand College of Veterinary Scientists – Behavior	www.anzcvs.org.au/chapters/veterinary+behaviour+chapter
Australian Veterinary Behaviour Interest Group	https://www.ava.com.au/about-us/ava-groups/animal-behaviourists/
British Veterinary Behaviour Association	www.bvba-org.co.uk
Certified Applied Animal Behaviorist (CAAB)	https://www.animalbehaviorsociety.org/web/applied-behavior-caab-directory.php
**European College of Animal Welfare and Behavioural Medicine	www.ecawbm.org
European Society of Veterinary Clinical Ethology	www.esvce.org
Interdisciplinary Forum for Applied Animal Behavior	www.ifaab.org
International Society for Anthrozoology	www.isaz.net
International Society for Applied Ethology	www.applied-ethology.org
International Society for Feline Medicine	www.icatcare.org
International Veterinary Academy of Pain Management	www.ivapm.org
Society of Veterinary Behavior Technicians	www.svbt.org

** designates veterinary behaviorist and technician certification organizations.

Behavioral organizations and educational courses for dog training

Resource name	Website
Academy for Dog Trainers	https://www.academyfordogtrainers.com/
American College of Applied Science, Diploma in Canine Behavior Analysis and Counseling	https://amcollege.us/diploma-in-canine-behavior-analysis-and-counseling/
Animal Behavior College	www.animalbehaviorcollege.com; animalbehaviorcollege.ca
Association of Pet Behaviour Counsellors	www.apbc.org.uk
Association of Professional Dog Trainers	www.apdt.com
Australian Association of Professional Dog Trainers	www.aapdt.org
Canadian Association of Professional Dog Trainers	www.capdt.ca
Certification Council for Professional Dog Trainers	www.ccpdt.org

Continued

Behavioral organizations and educational courses for dog training—cont'd

Resource name	Website
Fear Free Trainer Certification Program	https://fearfreepets.com/fear-free-animal-trainer-certification-program-overview/
International Association of Animal Behavior Consultants	www.iaabc.org
Pet Professional Guild	www.petprofessionalguild.com
Pet Professional Accreditation Board	https://www.credentialingboard.com/
Karen Pryor Academy (KPA)	www.karenpryoracademy.com
Victoria Stillwell Professional Dog Training	https://positively.com

Books and scientific journals

Author	Book
Ackerman L (ed)	Pet-Specific Care for the Veterinary Team. Wiley; 2021
Ackerman L (ed)	Five-Minute Veterinary Practice Management Consult. 3rd ed. Wiley; 2020
Applied Animal Behaviour Science (journal)	https://www.sciencedirect.com/journal/applied-animal-behaviour-science
Animals (journal)	https://www.mdpi.com/journal/animals
Beaver B	Canine Behavior: Insights and Answers. 2nd ed. Saunders Elsevier; 2009
Beaver B	Feline Behavior: A Guide for Veterinarians. 2nd ed. Saunders; 2003
Bradshaw JWS, Casey RA, Brown SL	The Behaviour of the Domestic Cat. 2nd ed. CABI; 2013
Crowell-Davis SL, Murray T, Dantas LMS	Veterinary Psychopharmacology. 2nd ed. Wiley; 2019
Denenberg S	Small Animal Psychiatry. CABI; 2021
DiGangi BA, Cussen VA, Reid P, et al (eds)	Animal Behavior for Shelter Veterinarians and Staff. 2nd ed. Wiley-Blackwell; 2022
Dog Behavior (journal)	https://dogbehavior.it/dogbehavior
Grandin T (ed)	Genetics and the Behavior of Domestic Animals. Academic Press; 2022
Horwitz DF	Five-Minute Veterinary Consult Clinical Companion. Canine and Feline Behavior. 2nd ed. Wiley-Blackwell; 2018
Houpt K	Domestic Animal Behavior for Veterinarians and Animal Scientists. 6th ed. Wiley-Blackwell; 2018
Horwitz DF, Mills DS	BSAVA Manual of Canine and Feline Behavioural Medicine. 2nd ed. BSAVA; 2009
Howell A, Feyrecilde M	Cooperative Veterinary Care. Wiley-Blackwell; 2018
Journal of Applied Welfare Science	https://www.tandfonline.com/toc/haaw20/current
Journal of Veterinary Behavior	www.journals.elsevier.com/journal-of-veterinary-behavior
Landsberg GM, Madari A, Zilka N (eds)	Canine and Feline Dementia. Molecular Basis, Diagnostics and Therapy. Springer International Publishing; 2017
Landsberg GM, Tynes V (eds)	Behavior: A Guide for Practitioners. Vet Clin North Am Small Anim Pract. 2014
McMillan FD (ed)	Mental Health and Well-Being in Animals, 2nd ed. CABI; 2019
Miklosi A	Dog Behavior, Evolution and Cognition. 2nd ed. Oxford University Press; 2016
Mills DS, Karagiannis C; Zulch H	Stress – Its effects on health and behavior: A guide for practitioners. In Vet Clin North Am Small Anim Pract. 2014;44:525-541
Mills DS, Westgarth C	Dog Bites: A Multidisciplinary Perspective. 5M Publishing; 2017
Mills DS, Braem-Dube M, Zulch H	Stress and Pheromonatherapy in Small Animal Clinical Behavior. Wiley-Blackwell; 2013
Overall KL	Manual of Clinical Behavioral Medicine for Dogs and Cats. Elsevier-Mosby; 2013
Pet Behaviour Science (journal)	https://www.petbehaviourscience.org/

Books and scientific journals—cont'd

Author	Book
Rodan I, Heath S (eds)	Feline Behavioral Health and Welfare. Elsevier; 2016
Scott JP, Fuller JL	Dog Behavior. The Genetic Basis. University of Chicago Press; 1965
Serpell J, Barrett P (eds)	The Domestic Dog: Its Evolution, Behavior and Interactions With People. 2nd ed. Cambridge University Press; 2017
Shaw J, Martin D	Canine and Feline Behavior for Veterinary Technicians and Nurses. 2nd ed. Wiley-Blackwell; 2023
Stelow E (ed)	Clinical Handbook of Feline Behavior Medicine. Wiley-Blackwell; 2023
Stelow L (ed)	Behavior as an Illness Indicator. In Vet Clin N Am Small Anim Clin. 2018
Tilley LP, Smith FWK, Sleeper MM, et al. (eds)	Blackwell's Five-Minute Veterinary Consult: Canine and Feline. 7th ed. John Wiley and Sons; 2021
Turner DC, Bateson P (eds)	The Domestic Cat. The Biology of its Behavior. 3rd ed. Cambridge University Press; 2013
Tynes VV, Landsberg GM	Nutritional Management of Behavior and Brain Disorders in Dogs and Cats. Vet Clin Small Anim. 2021,51.711-727
Mills DM	The Encyclopedia of Applied Animal Behaviour and Welfare. CAB International; 2010
Christine D Calder	https://cattledogpublishing.com/blog/the-low-stress-handling-movement-how-sophia-and-her-cattledog-started-it-all/

Websites and courses

Resource	Website
Animal Behavior Training Concepts	https://www.lauramonacotorelli.com/
APLB Association for Pet Loss and Bereavement	www.aplb.org
Cat Friendly Clinic/Cat Friendly Practices	https://catfriendlyclinic.org/ and https://catvets.com/cfp/cfp
Clicker Training	clickertraining.com
Cognitive Dysfunction	https://www.purinainstitute.com/advancing-brain-health
Companion Animal Psychology	www.companionanimalpsychology.com
Fear Free (Veterinary Professional Certification)	https://fearfreepets.com
Fear Free Happy Homes	www.fearfreehappyhomes.com
Fear Free Pet Professionals (Groomer, Petsitter, Boarding and DayCare Certification)	https://fearfreepets.com/fear-free-pet-professionals/
Fear Free Research	www.fearfreepets.com/fear-free-research
Fear Free Shelters	www.fearfreeshelters.com
Florida Veterinary Behavior Service	www.flvetbehavior.com
Indoor Pet Initiative	https://indoorpet.osu.edu
Low Stress Handling	www.lowstresshandling.com
Morris Animal Foundation	www.morrisanimalfoundation.org
PennVet Behavior Service	https://www.vet.upenn.edu/veterinary-hospitals/ryan-veterinary-hospital/services/behaviormedicine/patient-resources
UC Davis Behavior Service	https://www.vetmed.ucdavis.edu/hospital/small-animal/behavior-service
Tufts Cummings School of Veterinary Medicine Behavior Service	https://vet.tufts.edu/foster-hospital-small-animals/specialty-services/behavior
Pet Loss Support	https://ovc.uoguelph.ca/pettrust/petlossresources https://vet.osu.edu/vmc/companion/our-services/honoring-bond-support-pet-owners
Poisoned Cue	https://clickertraining.com/node/164
Psychology Today Decoding Your Pet	www.psychologytoday.com/ca/blog/decoding-your-pet
San Francisco SPCA	www.sfspca.org/resource-library/

Standards of care

2022 AAHA Pain Management Guidelines for Dogs and Cats	https://www.aaha.org/globalassets/02-guidelines/2022-pain-management/resources/2022-aaha-pain-management-guidelines-for-dog-and-cats_updated_060622.pdf
AVSAB Position Statements	https://avsab.org/resources/position-statements/
Canine Brief Pain Inventory (CBPI)	https://www.vet.upenn.edu/research/clinical-trials-vcic/our-services/pennchart/cbpi-tool
Canine Osteoarthritis Staging Tool (Liverpool Osteoarthritis in Dogs)	https://www.galliprantvet.com/us/en/coast-tools
Cat Stress Score	https://www.maddiesfund.org/Documents/Resource%20Library/Pet%20Behavior%20Solutions%20-%20Cat%20Stress%20Score.pdf
Chronic Pain Assessment in Cats	https://cvm.ncsu.edu/research/labs/clinical-sciences/comparative-pain-research/clinical-metrology-instruments/
Cincinnati Orthopedic Disability Index (CODI)	https://www.fourleg.com/media/Cincinnati%20Orthopedic%20Disability%20Index.pdf
Colorado State University Canine Acute Pain Scale	http://csu-cvmbs.colostate.edu/Documents/anesthesia-pain-management-pain-score-canine.pdf
Colorado State University Feline Acute Pain Scale	http://csu-cvmbs.colostate.edu/Documents/anesthesia-pain-management-pain-score-feline.pdf
Fear free Spectrum of Fear, Anxiety, and Stress	https://fearfreepets.com/fas-spectrum/
Feline Grimace Scale	https://www.felinegrimacescale.com
Feline Musculoskeletal Pain Index	https://painfreecats.org
Glasgow Canine Composite Measure Pain Scale (CMPS)	https://www.newmetrica.com/acute-pain-measurement/ https://www.newmetrica.com/wp-content/uploads/2016/09/Reid-et-al-2007.pdf
Glasgow Composite Measure Pain Scale – Feline (CMPS)	https://www.newmetrica.com/acute-pain-measurement http://www.aprvt.com/uploads/5/3/0/5/5305564/cmp_feline_eng.pdf
Helsinki Chronic Pain Index (HCPI)	https://www.fourleg.com/media/Helsinki%20Chronic%20Pain%20Index.pdf
Pet Nutrition Alliance	https://petnutritionalliance.org
UNESP-Boucatu Multidimensional Composite Pain Scale for Assessing Postoperative Pain in Cats	http://www.animalpain.com.br/assets/upload/escala-en-us.pdf
WSAVA 2022 Guidelines for Recognition, Assessment and Treatment of Pain	https://onlinelibrary.wiley.com/doi/pdf/10.1111/jsap.13566

Feline-specific reading and resources

American Association of Feline Practitioners (AAFP)	https://catvets.com/guidelines/practice-guidelines/behavior-guidelines
AAFP Pet Parent Resources	https://catvets.com/guidelines/client-brochures
AAFP Educational Videos	https://catvets.com/education/online/videos
Adventure Cats	How to Clicker train your cat
American College of Veterinary Behaviorists et al.	Decoding Your Cat: The Ultimate Experts Explain Common Cat Behaviors and Reveal How to Prevent or Change Unwanted Ones. Mariner Books; 2020
Battersea – How to interact with your cat	https://www.youtube.com/watch?v=UwqG2wLb0KQ
Bradshaw J	Cat Sense. Basic Books; 2013
Bradshaw J, Ellis S	The Trainable Cat. Hachette; 2017
Catalyst Council	www.catalystcouncil.org
Cornell Feline Health Center	www.vet.cornell.edu/FHC/
Fear Free Happy Homes – Cat Body Language 101	https://www.fearfreehappyhomes.com/video/cat-body-language-101/
Fear Free Happy Homes – Meeting the Basic Needs of Your Cat	https://www.fearfreehappyhomes.com/kit/cats-101/#video_link2
Food Puzzles for Cats	http://foodpuzzlesforcats.com

Feline-specific reading and resources—cont'd

Indoor Cat	How to Enrich Their Lives and Expand Their World, Running Press Adult; 2022
International Cat Care	https://icatcare.org/veterinary/resources/
Low Stress Handling, Fearful Aggressive Cats	https://www.cliniciansbrief.com/article/low-stress-handling-plan-fearful-aggressive-cats
Maddie's Fund – Cat Body Language	https://www.maddiesfund.org/feline-communication-how-to-speak-cat.htm
Prior K	Clicker Training for Cats. Sunshine Books; 2003
10 common Cat behavior Myths Decoded	http://www.vetstreet.com/our-pet-experts/10-common-cat-behavior-myths-decoded
Schroll S	Kitten Kindergarten. Books on Demand; 2017

Cat carrier resources

American Association of Feline Practitioners	https://catvets.com/public/PDFs/Cat%20Owners/Cat2VetDay/Turn%20your%20cat%20carrier%20into%20a%20-Home%20away%20(1).pdf
Cat Friendly	https://catfriendly.com/be-a-cat-friendly-caregiver/getting-cat-veterinarian/ https://catfriendly.com/wp-content/uploads/2022/05/AAFPCatToVetBrochure.pdf
Cat Friendly Clinic	https://catfriendly.com/wp-content/uploads/2022/05/AAFPCatToVetBrochure.pdf
Catalyst Council Cat Carrier – Friend or Foe	https://www.youtube.com/watch?v=9RGY5oSKVfo&t=33s
Making the Carrier Cat Friendly	https://www.youtube.com/watch?v=b1-1cEGN8VY
Going for a Car Ride	https://www.youtube.com/watch?v=-paBVCfeEpA

Canine-specific reading and resources

The Aggressive Dog	https://aggressivedog.com/
American College of Veterinary Behaviorists et al.	Decoding Your Dog: The Ultimate Experts Explain Common Dog Behaviors and Reveal How to Prevent or Change Unwanted Ones. Houghton Mifflin Harcourt; 2014
Anderson E	Remember Me. Loving and Caring for a Dog With Canine Cognitive Dysfunction. Bright Friends Productions; 2015
Becker M, Radosta L, Sung W, et al.	From Fearful To Fear Free: A Positive Program to Free Your Dog From Anxieties, Fears, and Phobias. Health Communications, Inc.; 2018
Becker SC	Becker SC. Living With a Deaf Dog. 2nd ed. Dogwise Publishing; 2017
Bender A, Strong E	Canine Enrichment for the Real World: Making It a Part of Your Dog's Daily Life. Dogwise Publishing; 2019
Care for Reactive Dogs	https://careforreactivedogs.com/
Crestejo K. Understanding Dog Communication	https://www.youtube.com/watch?v=8bg_gGguwzg
Donaldson J	The Culture Clash: A Revolutionary New Way of Understanding the Relationship Between Humans and Domestic Dogs. Dogwise Publishing; 2012
Dog Bite Prevention	https://doggonesafe.com/Dog_bite_prevention_for_parents/
Dog Stars – Bite Prevention for Kids	https://www.youtube.com/watch?v=MYDW2KV_TzE
Dogs & Kids Course	https://onlineschool.instinctdogtraining.com/course/kids-and-dogs
Family Dog – Stop the 77	https://www.thefamilydog.com/stop-the-77/
Hart BL, Hart LA	The Perfect Puppy: Breed Selection and Care by Veterinary Science for Behavior and Neutering Age. Academic Press; 2023
Horwitz A	Inside of a Dog. Scribner; 2009 Being a Dog. Scribner; 2013
Kaufer M	Canine Play Behavior: The Science of Dogs at Play. Dogwise Publishing; 2014
Latham E. Dogmantics	https://dogmantics.com/free-videos/

Continued

Canine-specific reading and resources—cont'd

Levine E	Doggie Dos and Don'ts, Instinct Dog Behavior & Training, 2020
Martin KM, Martin D	Puppy Start Right: Foundation Training for the Companion Dog. Sunshine Books; 2011
McConnell P, Scidmore P	The Puppy Primer. 2nd ed. McConnell Publishing Company; 2010
Miller P	Power of Positive Dog Training. 2nd ed. Howell Book House; 2008
Mills D, Zulch H, Baumber M	Life Skills for Puppies; Laying the Foundation for a Loving, Lasting Relationship. Veloce Publishing; 2020
Muzzle Training – Blue Cross for Pets	https://www.youtube.com/watch?v=6BjPpXer8lE
Muzzle up Project	www.muzzleupproject.com
Pelar C	Living With Kids and Dogs Without Losing Your Mind. 2nd ed. Dream Dog Productions; 2012
Pet Professional Guild	https://www.petprofessionalguild.com/PuppyTrainingResources
Stillwell V	The Ultimate Guide to Raising a Puppy. Random House LLC; 2019
Stillwell V	Train Your Dog Positively. Stillwell V. Random House LLC; 2019
SFSPCA Puppy Pet Parent Orientation	https://www.youtube.com/watch?v=RgQ7OmZU93g
The Blue Dog	http://thebluedog.org/en/
Tudge N	A Kids' Comprehensive Guide to Speaking Dog
Ultimate Puppy	www.ultimatepuppy.com
Van Arendonk Baugh L	Fired Up, Frantic, and Freaked Out: Training the Crazy Dog From Over the Top to Under Control. Aeclipse Press; 2013
Yin S	Perfect Puppy in 7 Days. CattleDog Publishing; 2011

Dog communication and body language resources

Battersea – Dog Body Language	https://www.battersea.org.uk/pet-advice/dog-advice/understanding-your-dog%E2%80%99s-body-language
Dog Decoder App	https://www.dogdecoder.com/
Fear Free Happy Homes – Dog Body Language 101	https://www.fearfreehappyhomes.com/video/dog-body-language-101/
iSpeakDog	http://www.ispeakdog.org/body-language-gallery.html
I speak Doggie	https://www.thefamilydog.com/i-speak-doggie/
Tuft's University Center for Shelter Dogs – Dog Communication and Body Language	https://centerforshelterdogs.tufts.edu/dog-behavior/dog-communication-and-body-language/
Zoom Room Guide to Dog Body Language	https://www.youtube.com/watch?v=00_9JPltXHI

Videos

Cat Clicker Training - Pasadena Humane	https://pasadenahumane.org/cat-clicker-training/
Domesticated Manners	www.youtube.com/domesticatedmanners
Emergency U-turn	https://www.youtube.com/watch?v=dj6FXimL8Jw
Fear Free Happy Homes – Activities and Enrichment	https://www.fearfreehappyhomes.com/video/activities-and-enrichment-101/
Fear Free Happy Homes – Training and Socialization	https://www.fearfreehappyhomes.com/video/training-and-socialization-101/
Intramuscular Sedation	https://www.youtube.com/watch?v=6EXV1_QJHP0
Mat Training – Vet Street	https:// https://www.youtube.com/watch?v=i9p8kR3n4hc
Pattern Games, with Leslie McDevitt	https://www.youtube.com/watch?v=Mtn-Bel9lHE
Preventing Behavior Problems With Classical Conditioning	https://www.sfspca.org/resource/preventing-problem-behaviors-video/
Touch Training	https://www.youtube.com/watch?v=hxuoZprlCDk
Touch Training	https://www.youtube.com/watch?v=PqD_pe67KCg

Pet parent resources

Ackerman L	Proactive Pet Parenting. Anticipating Pet Health Problems Before They Happen. Problem Free Publishing; 2020
Ackerman L, Ackerman R	Problem Free Pets: The Ultimate Guide to Pet Parenting. Dermvet; 2020
Ackerman L, Ackerman R	Almost Perfect Pets: A Proactive Guide to Selection, Health Care and Pet Parenting. McFarland & Company, Inc. Publishers; 2022
Chin L – Dog and Cat Drawings Posters	https://www.doggiedrawings.net/freeposters
Dog Nerds	www.therealdognerds.com
Family Paws Parent Education	https://www.familypaws.com
Proactive Parent Supervision	https://i.pinimg.com/originals/73/d6/be/73d6beccb258ae381688a251b9662aae.jpg
Fear Free Happy Homes – Training and Socialization	https://www.fearfreehappyhomes.com/video/training-and-socialization-101/
Maddie's Fund Training and Enrichment	https://www.maddiesfund.org/topic-animal-behavior-training-and-enrichment.htm
McGreevy PD, Boakes RA	Carrots and Sticks: Principles of Animal Behavior Training. Cambridge University Press; 2007
Patel C. Domesticated Manners	https://www.domesticatedmanners.com/resources
Pryor K	Don't Shoot the Dog. The Art of Teaching and Training. Simon and Schuster; 2019
Pryor K	Reaching the Animal Mind – Clicker Training and What It Teaches Us About All Animals. Scribner; 2009
SF SPCA Behavior and Training	https://www.sfspca.org/resource-library/
Veterinary Partner	https://veterinarypartner.vin.com/
Yin S	Perfect Puppy in 7 Days. CattleDog Publishing; 2011 https://todaysveterinarypractice.com/resources/handouts/

Guidelines for humane dog training

American Veterinary Society of Animal Behavior	https://avsab.ftlbcdn.net/wp-content/uploads/2019/01/How-to-Choose-a-Trainer-Position-Statement.pdf
Fear Free Happy Homes	https://fearfreehappyhomes.com/courses/trainer-danger-how-to-find-a-trainer-who-wont-harm-your-pet/
BC SPCA	https://spca.bc.ca/how-to-choose-a-dog-trainer/
SF SPCA	https://www.sfspca.org/behavior-training/how-to-choose-a-dog-trainer

Therapeutics

Adaptil	www.adaptil.com
Aktivait	https://www.vetplusglobal.com/products/aktivait/
Anipryl (selegiline)	https://www2.zoetisus.com/products/petcare/anipryl
Anxitane (L-theanine)	https://us.virbac.com
Composure Pro	https://www.vetriscience.com/composure-153-pro.html
Feliway	www.feliway.com
Imepitoin (Pexion)	https://www.ema.europa.eu/en/medicines/veterinary/EPAR/pexion
Mirataz (mirtazapine)	https://mirataz.com/mirataz/
Pregabalin (Bonqat)	https://www.ema.europa.eu/en/medicines/veterinary/EPAR/bonqat
Propentofylline (Vivitonin or Karsivan)	https://www.msd-animal-health-hub.co.uk/Products/Vivitonin
Reconcile (fluoxetine)	https://www.reconcile.com
Senilife	www.senilife.com
Sileo (dexmedetomidine oromucosal gel)	https://www2.zoetisus.com/products/petcare/sileo
Solliquin	www.solliquin.com
Tasipimidine (Tessie)	https://www.ema.europa.eu/en/medicines/veterinary/EPAR/tessie
Zylkene (alpha-casozepine)	www.vetoquinolusa.com/content/zylkene

Appendix B Medication dosages

Before using any of the medications or supplements, please refer to Chapters 8, 9, 11, 12, 16, and 18 for further details about indications, contraindications, and potential adverse effects. Although many of these medications have been used in veterinary medicine for either behavioral or medical indications (or both), many have not been studied and most are not labeled for veterinary use in dogs and cats. Of even greater concern is the combination of medications and the potential for enhancing therapeutic effect, which must be weighed against the possibility of adverse interactions, some of which are known and some of which are theorized. Drug combinations and the potential for beneficial and harmful interactions are also discussed in Chapter 11.

Except for medications approved for veterinary use whose pharmacokinetics have been studied (see Chapter 11) with published dose ranges, the dose is often based on case studies, anecdotal reports, extrapolations from human medicine, or clinical experience. For these reasons, it is always recommended to use products labeled for veterinary use as first-line therapy whenever possible and following the drug cascade decision tree, where required.[1] It is also important to note that there are likely breed and individual differences, variability associated with medical conditions, and the concurrent use of other medications that will require dose adjustments or discontinuation in some individuals. Therefore, pet parents should be advised of the expected therapeutic effects and side effects and to report immediately any unexpected change in health or behavior. When prescribing, always start at the low end of the dose range and increase based on the patient response and side effects after sufficient time to assess therapeutic effects. Because of the wide individual variability in effects and in intensity of fear, anxiety, stress, and panic for the situational use of medications, test dosing should be performed, wherever possible, in advance of the fear, anxiety, stress, conflict and panic (FASCP) evoking event to determine onset to peak effect, duration of effect and response and modified as required prior to the actual event.

Finally, it is the practitioner's responsibility to know the local regulations regarding off-label dispensing and compounding to have appropriate consent or release forms signed, if applicable.

All dosing is per os unless otherwise indicated. TM indicates transmucosal dosing

Class	Drug	Dosage (dog)	Dosage (cat)	Comments
Anticonvulsants				
	Carbamazepine	4–10 mg/kg 12h	2–6 mg/kg q12–24h OR 12.5-25 mg/**CAT** q12h	
	Levetiracetam	20–50 mg/kg q8h	20 mg/kg q8h	
	Phenobarbital	2–8 mg/kg q12h OR 10 mg/kg 90 minutes prior to event	1–4 mg/kg q12h	
	Potassium bromide	20–40 mg/kg daily or divided q12h	Not recommended	
Alpha-2 agonist				
	Clonidine	0.01–0.05 mg/kg q8–24h OR 90–120 minutes prior to event	0.004–0.015 mg/kg q12–24h OR 90 minutes prior to event	
	Dexmedetomidine oromucosal gel	125 µg /m^2 TM or 0.01–0.04 mg/kg TM 20–60 minutes in advance of event Can repeat after 2 hours if required (up to 5 doses per event)	One dot Sileo (0.25 mL) TM/**CAT** OR 0.01–0.04 mg/kg TM 20–60 minutes in advance of event	DOG: approved for noise aversion as Sileo
	Guanfacine	0.01–0.06 mg/kg q12h	No data	

Continued

All dosing is per os unless otherwise indicated. TM indicates transmucosal dosing—cont'd

Class	Drug	Dosage (dog)	Dosage (cat)	Comments
	Tasipimidine	10-60 µg/kg one hour in advance of onset of event or 20 µg q12h	no data	Approved in Europe as Tessie for alleviation of situational fear and anxiety triggered by noise and owner departure at 30 µg/kg
Azapirones				
	Buspirone	0.5–2 mg/kg q8–12h	0.5–1 mg/kg q12–24h OR 2.5–7.5 mg/**CAT** q12–24h OR 4 mg/kg transdermal[2]	
Benzodiazepines				
	Alprazolam	0.02–0.1 mg/kg up to q6h or 60 minutes prior to onset of stress.	0.125–0.25 mg/**CAT** q8–24h OR 60 minutes prior to onset of stress.	DOG: For some individuals, rapid onset to peak effect and short duration may require repeat dosing q4h
	Clonazepam	0.1–1 mg/kg q8–12h	0.02–0.25 mg/kg q12h–24h	
	Clorazepate	0.5–2 mg/kg q8–12h	0.2–0.5 mg/kg q12–24h OR up to 2.2 mg/kg for profoundly stressful events.	
	Diazepam	0.5–2.2 mg/kg up to q8h OR 45–90 minutes prior to event	Avoid use due to potential use of rare hepatoxicity. Other benzodiazepines may be safer.	DOG: For some individuals, rapid onset to peak effect and short duration may require repeat dosing q4h
	Flurazepam	0.1–0.5 mg/kg q12h	0.1–0.4 mg/kg q12–24h	
	Imepitoin	10–30 mg/kg BID beginning 2 days prior to event OR 2 hours prior to event	50–100 mg/**CAT** q12h or 2 hours prior to event	DOG: Pexion is approved for noise aversion at 30 mg/kg q12h beginning 2 days in advance
	Lorazepam	.02–0.1 mg/kg (up to 0.5 mg/kg) q12–24h 60 minutes prior to onset of stress	0.125–0.50 mg/**CAT** 12h to 24h OR 0.03–0.08 mg/kg q12h–24h OR 90 minutes prior to event	
	Oxazepam	0.04–1 mg/kg q12–24h	0.2–1 mg/kg q12–24h	
Beta-blockers				
	Pindolol	0.125–0.3 mg/kg q12h	0.125–0.25 mg/kg q12h	
	Propranolol	0.2–1 mg/kg q12h up to 3 mg/kg q12h or 60 minutes prior to onset of stress.	0.2–1 mg/kg q8h	
Central nervous system stimulants				
	Methylphenidate	0.5–2 mg/kg q12h	Not recommended	For dosing details, see Chapter 11
Gabaminergic				
	Gabapentin	10–30 mg/kg q8–12h OR 10–50 mg/kg 90 minutes prior to onset of stress.	10–30 mg/kg q8–12h OR 10–40 mg/kg 90–120 minutes prior to onset of stress OR 100-200 mg/**CAT** 90-120 minutes prior to onset of stress. OR 5–10 mg/kg transdermal q8h (pain)	DOG: Up to 40 mg q8h[3] CAT: Up to 30 mg/kg q8h for severe pain[4]

All dosing is per os unless otherwise indicated. TM indicates transmucosal dosing—cont'd

Class	Drug	Dosage (dog)	Dosage (cat)	Comments
	Pregabalin	2–5 mg/kg q8h OR 2–5 mg/kg 1.5–3 hours prior to onset of stress	1–2 mg/kg q12h OR 5–10 mg/kg 90 minutes prior to event	CAT: Approved In Europe as Bonqat for fear and anxiety of travel and veterinary visits
Hormones				
	Melatonin	1–9 mg/**DOG** 30–60 minutes prior to onset of stress or bedtime (for sleep) OR 0.1 mg/kg and round up to nearest 1 mg q8–24h Up to 12 mg/**DOG**	1–6 mg/**CAT** prior to bedtime (for sleep) 1–3 mg/**CAT** q8–24h	CAT: Up to 3–12 mg/**CAT** q12–24h[5]
Monoamine oxidase inhibitors (MAOI)				
	Selegiline	0.5–1 mg/kg q24h in the morning	0.25–1 mg/kg q24h in the morning	DOG: Licensed as Anipryl for cognitive dysfunction syndrome
Neuroleptics/ antipsychotics				
	Acepromazine	0.5–2.2 mg/kg up to q6h OR 1–2 hours prior to onset of stress.	0.5–2.2 mg/kg prn to q8h OR 1–2 hours prior to onset of stress.	Sedation not anxiolytic
NK-1 receptor antagonist (substance P inhibitor)				
	Maropitant	Motion sickness: 8 mg/kg 2 hours pre travel on an empty stomach or with a small amount of food q24h Prevention and treatment of emesis: 2 mg/kg q24h	1–2 mg/kg q24h	
N-methyl-D-aspartate antagonist				
	Amantadine	3–8 mg/kg q24h or divided q12h	2.2–5 mg/kg q24h up to q12h.	
	Dextromethorphan	2 mg/kg q6–12h	0.5–2 mg/kg up to q8h up to q6h	
	Memantine	0.3–1 mg/kg q24h		
Opiate agonists/ antagonIsts				
	Naltrexone	1–2.2 mg/kg q12–24h	25–50 mg/**CAT** q24h	
Serotonin 2A antagonist/ reuptake inhibitor				
	Trazodone	3–12 mg/kg q8–24h OR 3–19.5 mg/kg single dose 90–120 minutes prior to event	7.7–15.2 mg/kg single dose 90 minutes prior to event OR 25–100 mg/**CAT** single dose 90 minutes prior to event	Absorption and peak effect delayed by feeding CAT: Single doses of up to 33 mg/kg for situational use for sedation[6]
SSRIs				
	Citalopram	1–2 mg/kg q24h	0.5–1 mg/kg q24h	
	Escitalopram	1–2.5 mg/kg day divided in two to three doses	No data	

Continued

All dosing is per os unless otherwise indicated. TM indicates transmucosal dosing—cont'd

Class	Drug	Dosage (dog)	Dosage (cat)	Comments
	Fluoxetine	0.5–2 mg/kg q24h	0.5–1.5 mg/kg q24h	DOG: Up to 2–4 mg/kg q24h for hypersensitivity hyperreactivity syndrome[7] DOG: Approved as Reconcile for separation anxiety
	Fluvoxamine	1–2 mg/kg q12–24h	0.25–1 mg/kg q24h	
	Paroxetine	0.5–2 mg/kg q12–24h	0.25–1.5 mg/kg q24	
	Sertraline	0.5–4 mg/kg q12–24h	0.25–1.5 mg/kg q24h	
SNRIs				
	Venlafaxine	1–2 mg/kg q12h	2.5–5 mg/**CAT** q12–24h OR 0.5–2 mg/kg q24h	DOG: Up to 4 mg/kg q12h[8]
Tetracyclic antidepressant				
	Mirtazapine	0.5–1 mg/kg q24h	1.88 mg/**CAT** q24h 2 mg transdermal (TD)/**CAT** q24h (Mirataz)	CAT: Approved as Mirataz transdermal for veterinary use
Tricyclic antidepressants				
	Amitriptyline	1–4 mg/kg q12h	0.5–2 mg/kg q12–24h	DOG: Up to 6 mg/kg q12h[9]
	Clomipramine	1–3 mg/kg q12h	0.25–1 mg/kg q24h or 0.25–0.5 mg/kg q12h	DOG: Approved as Clomicalm for separation anxiety CAT: Approved for urine marking in Australia
	Doxepin	1–5 mg/kg q8–12h	0.5–1 mg/kg q12–24h	
	Imipramine	0.5–2 mg/kg q8–12h	0.5–1 mg/kg q12–24h	
Xanthine derivatives				
	Propentofylline	2.5–5 mg/kg q12h	5–12.5 mg/**CAT** q24h	DOG: Approved in some countries as Karsivan or Vivitonin for mental dullness in senior dogs
Supplements				
	SAMe	10–20 mg/kg q24h	100 mg/**CAT** q24h	
	Alpha-casozepine	15–30 mg/kg q24h	15–30 mg/kg q24h	
	L-theanine (suntheanine)	2.5–10 mg/kg q12h	5–10 mg/kg q12h OR 25 mg/**CAT** q12h	

q24h = sid, once per day; q12h = bid, twice per day, or every 12 hours; q8h = tid, every 8 hours or three times per day; q6h = qid, every 6 hours or four times per day; po, orally
SSRI – selective serotonin reuptake inhibitor; SNRI – serotonin/norepinephrine reuptake inhibitor; SAMe – S-adenosyl-L-methionine.

References

1. https://www.gov.uk/guidance/the-cascade-prescribing-unauthorised-medicines.
2. Chavez G, Pardo P, Ubilla MJ, et al. Effects on behavioural variables of oral versus transdermal administration in cats displaying urine marking. *J Appl Anim Res.* 2016;44:454–57.
3. Ciribassi J. The use of gabapentin to help manage anxiety in dogs. https://www.dvm360.com/view/use-gabapentin-help-manage-anxiety-dogs.
4. Mathews C, Sinclair M, Steele AM, et al. *Analgesia and Anesthesia for the Ill and Injured Dog and Cat.* Hoboken, NJ: Wiley-Blackwell; 2018:270–278.
5. Lefman SH, Prittie JE. Psychogenic stress in hospitalized veterinary patients: causation, implications, and therapies. *J Vet Emerg Crit Care.* 2019;29:107–120.
6. Orlando JM, Case BC, Thomson AE, Griffith E, Sherman BL. Use of oral trazodone for sedation in cats: a pilot study. *J Feline Med Surg.* 2015;18:476–482.
7. Bleuer-Elsner S, Muller G, Beata C, et al. Effect of fluoxetine at a dosage of 2–4 mg/kg daily in dogs exhibiting hypersensitivity-hyperactivity syndrome, a retrospective study. *J Vet Behav.* 2021;44:25–31.
8. KuKanich B. Outpatient oral analgesics in dogs and cats beyond nonsteroidal antiinflammatory drugs. An evidence based approach. *Vet Clin North Am Small Anim Pract.* 2013;43:1109–1125.
9. Crowell-Davis SL, Murray TF, Dantas LMS. *Veterinary Psychopharmacology.* 2nd ed. Hoboken, NJ: Wiley-Blackwell; 2019.

Recommended reading

Medication and supplement doses can be found in the following references and in the articles referenced throughout Chapters 11, 13, 16, and 18. Doses that have been obtained from other sources are listed:

Crowell-Davis S, Murray TF, Mattos de Souza Dantas L. *Veterinary Psychopharmacology*. 2nd ed. Hoboken, NJ: Blackwell Publishing; 2019.

Companion Animal Euthanasia Training Academy. https://caetainternational.com/oral-pre-visit-pharmaceuticals-for-euthanasia-go-big/.

Clinician's brief – www.cliniciansbrief.com.

Denenberg S, ed. *Small Animal Veterinary Psychiatry*. CABI; 2021.

Erickson A, Harbin K, MacPherson J, et al. A review of pre-appointment medications to reduce fear and anxiety in dogs and cats at veterinary visits. *Can Vet J*. 2021;62: 952–960.

North American Veterinary Anesthesia Society – https://www.mynavas.org/resources. https://www.mynavas.org/post/oral-sedatives-and-anxiolytics-for-veterinary-visits.

Papich M. *Papich Handbook of Veterinary Drugs*. 5th ed. Saunders; 2020.

Plumb's Veterinary Drugs: https://plumbs.com/.

Plumbs Veterinary Drug Handbook – Desk. 9th ed. Wiley-Blackwell; 2018.

Veterinary Anesthesia & Analgesia Support Group – https://vasg.org/.

Appendix C Resources available from book website

FORMS:
- CANINE BEHAVIOR SCREENING FORM
- FELINE BEHAVIOR SCREENING FORM
- FELINE PERIURIA FIRST APPOINTMENT QUESTIONNAIRE
- FELINE PERIURIA HOUSE SOILING DIARY
- FELINE PERIURIA LONG QUESTIONNAIRE FORM
- FELINE PERIURIA SECOND APPOINTMENT QUESTIONNAIRE
- CANINE BEHAVIOR HISTORY QUESTIONNAIRE
- FELINE BEHAVIOR HISTORY QUESTIONNAIRE

KIDS AND PETS
- DOG AND KID SAFETY 5 RULES EVERY KID SHOULD KNOW
- FAMILY PAWS THE 5 TYPES OF SUPERVISION

CATS
- CAT ENRICHMENT FOOD
- ENVIRONMENTAL ENRICHMENT AND APPROPRIATE OUTLETS FOR PLAY
- FELINE UNDESIRABLE URINATION (PERIURIA)
- MANAGEMENT OF AGGRESSION BETWEEN HOUSEHOLD CATS
- CAT AGGRESSION DIRECTED AT PEOPLE
- CAT ENRICHMENT: PREDATORY
- INTRODUCING CATS TO MULTI-CAT HOUSEHOLDS

GERIATRIC PETS
- SENIOR COGNITIVE DYSFUNCTION SCREENING QUESTIONNAIRE

FEARS AND PHOBIAS
- TREATMENT FOR PETS WITH FEAR
- NOISE AVERSION AND PHOBIA
- THE 5 Ds RELAXATION PROTOCOL
- SANCTUARY SPACE TRAINING
- SEPARATION-RELATED DISORDERS INITIAL STEPS

DOG AGGRESSION
- MANAGEMENT OF INTERDOG AGGRESSION IN THE SAME HOUSEHOLD
- MANAGEMENT OF VISITORS IN THE HOME

BEHAVIOR MODIFICATION/TRAINING
- BASKET MUZZLE CONDITIONING
- REINFORCEMENT CHOICE AND DELIVERY
- TIPS FOR EFFECTIVE TRAINING
- WORKSHEET FOR CHOOSING REINFORCEMENT
- WHY YOU SHOULD NOT USE SHOCK AS A TRAINING TOOL YOUR DOG
- JUMPING (DOG)
- DESTRUCTIVE CHEWING (DOG)
- STEALING (DOG)
- TARGET TRAINING (TOUCH) (DOGS)
- SETTING UP A SAFETY AND COMMUNICATION BEHAVIOR
- HOUSETRAINING (DOGS)

Index

Page numbers followed by "f" indicate figures, "t" indicate tables, and "b" indicate boxes.

A